P9-AFW-604

Ambulatory Surgical Nursing

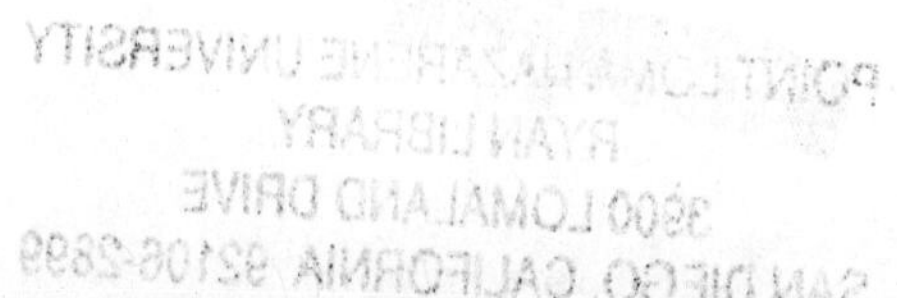

Ambulatory Surgical Nursing

Second Edition

Nancy Burden, MS, RN, CPAN, CAPA
Director of Outpatient Surgery Centers
Morton Plant Mease Health Care
Palm Harbor, Florida

Associate Editors

Donna M. DeFazio Quinn, BSN, MBA, RN, CPAN, CAPA
Henniker, New Hampshire

Denise O'Brien, BSN, RN, CPAN, CAPA
Clinical Nurse III/Educational Nurse Coordinator
Ambulatory Surgery Unit
Department of Operating Rooms/PACU
University of Michigan Health System
Ann Arbor, Michigan

Brenda S. Gregory Dawes, MSN, RN, CNOR
Editor, AORN Journal
AORN
Denver, Colorado

W.B. SAUNDERS COMPANY
A Harcourt Health Sciences Company
Philadelphia London New York St. Louis Sydney Toronto

W.B. SAUNDERS COMPANY
A Harcourt Health Sciences Company

The Curtis Center
Independence Square West
Philadelphia, Pennsylvania 19106

Library of Congress Cataloging-in-Publication Data

Burden, Nancy.
Ambulatory surgical nursing / Nancy Burden; associate editors, Donna M. DeFazio Quinn, Denise O'Brien, Brenda S. Gregory Dawes.—2nd ed.

p. cm.

Includes bibliographical references and index.

ISBN 0–7216–6847–X

1. Ambulatory surgical nursing. I. Quinn, Donna M. DeFazio. II. O'Brien, Denise, RN. III. Title.

[DNLM: 1. Perioperative Nursing. 2. Ambulatory Care Nurses' Instruction. 3. Ambulatory Surgical Procedures Nurses' Instruction. WY 161 B949a 2000]

RD110.5.B87 2000 610.73′677—dc21

DNLM/DLC 99–31873

Vice President, Nursing Editorial Director: Sally Schrefer
Editorial Manager: Thomas Eoyang
Developmental Editor: Victoria Legnini
Manuscript Editor: Marjory I. Fraser
Production Manager: Paul Harris
Illustration Specialist: Fran Moriarty
Book Designer: Steven Stave

AMBULATORY SURGICAL NURSING ISBN 0–7216–6847–X

Printed in the United States of America.

Last digit is the print number: 9 8 7 6 5 4 3 2 1

The editors and authors join together in dedicating this book to the clinical nurses who provide the day-to-day compassionate care that helps our patients endure the fears, discomforts, and uncertainties of invasive procedures and surgical interventions. And in addition . . .

Thanks and love to my family—Dave, Jeff, Nikki, and Peg—for all the years of support and encouragement as I followed the path of nursing in this wonderful specialty.

Nancy Burden

To Stephen for your love and support and to Gia and Tian who make my life complete.

Donna M. DeFazio Quinn

To Mike, Matt, and Bridget for your love, support, and perseverance while I pursue my dreams to write, to speak, and to care.

Denise O'Brien

To friends and peers who work hard to protect our patients while making patient care look easy.

Brenda S. Gregory Dawes

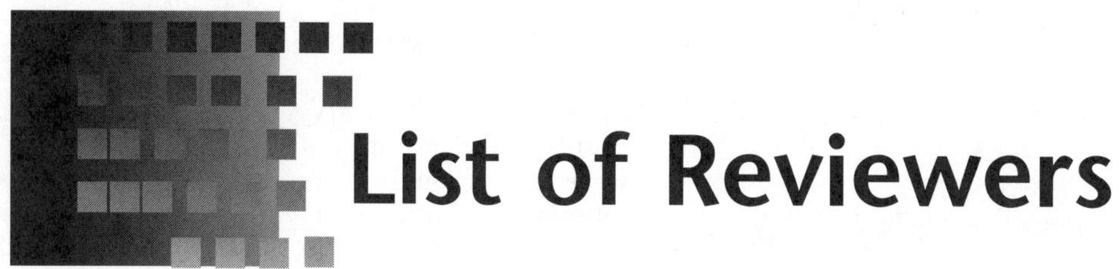

List of Reviewers

Anne Allen, RN
Patient Care Instructor
Creative Educational Options
Tulsa Technology Center
Tulsa, Oklahoma

Chuck Biddle, PhD, CRNA
Dartmouth Medical School
Hanover, New Hampshire

Patricia Brockway, BSN, RN, CPAN, CAPA
Castle Medical Center, ASF
Kailua, Hawaii

Anthony Chipas, PhD, CRNA
Anesthesia Consulting Service
Wichita, Kansas

Loree A. Collett, BSN, RN
University of Michigan Hospitals
Ann Arbor, Michigan

Jean A. Dye, BSN, RN, CPAN
St. Mary's Hospital Medical Center
Madison, Wisconsin

Karen Engledow, RN, CNOR
Trinity Mother Frances Health System
Tyler, Texas

Rose Ferrara-Love, MSN, RN, CPAN, CAPA
Pittsburgh, Pennsylvania

Joyce C. Hadley, BA, RN, CPAN
Inova Center for Clinical Education and Development
Falls Church, Virginia

Melody S. Heffline, RN, MSN, CS-ACNP, CPAN
Surgical Associates of South Carolina
West Columbia, South Carolina

Vallire D. Hooper, MSN, RN, CPAN
Medical College of Georgia
Augusta, Georgia

Deborah A. Jackson, MSN, RN, CCRN
Welborn Baptist Hospital
Evansville, Indiana

Mary E. Jenkins, BSN, CCRN, CAPA
Elliot 1-Day Surgery Center
Manchester, New Hampshire

Vicki L. Jowell, BSN, RN
East Texas Medical Center, Tyler
Tyler, Texas

Christine T. Kelley, BSN, RN, CNOR
Elliot 1-Day Surgery Center
Manchester, New Hampshire

Michael Kost, MSN, CRNA
Program Director
School of Anesthesia
Montgomery Hospital
Norristown, Pennsylvania
and
Adjunct Faculty
St. Joseph's University
Philadelphia, Pennsylvania

Lonnie G. Lane, RN
Columbia Physicians Daysurgery Center
Dallas, Texas

Sophia Mikos-Schild, EdD, RN, CNOR
Educator, Operating Room/PACU/ Outpatient and Endoscopy
Phoenix Baptist and Arrowhead Hospital
Phoenix, Arizona

Candice Murcek, RN, CPAN
Alegent Health Immanuel Medical Center
Omaha, Nebraska

Debby Niehaus, BS, RN, CPAN
Bethesda North Ambulatory Surgical Center
Cincinnati, Ohio

Judith E. Ontiveros, BSN, RN, CPAN, CAPA
St. Luke Medical Center
Pasadena, California

Mary C. (Connie) Redmond, RN, CAPA
Outpatient Surgery Department
Alegent Health Bergan Mercy Medical Center
Omaha, Nebraska

Patricia S. Stein, RN, MAOL, CNOR
Johnson and Johnson
St. Paul, Minnesota

David Tilton, BSN, RN
Post Anesthesia Care Nurse
Harrison Hospital
Bremerton, Washington

Barbara A. Urbanski, MS, RN
Department of Anesthesiology
University of Michigan
Ann Arbor, Michigan

Virginia A. Walter, BSN, MS, CGRN
Manager, Medical Procedures Unit
University of Michigan Health System
Ann Arbor, Michigan

Nancy Wheeling, RN, CGRN
Morton Plant Mease Health Care
Clearwater, Florida

Maria T. Zickuhr, MSN, RN, CPAN
Outpatient Surgery
Johns Hopkins Outpatient Center
Baltimore, Maryland

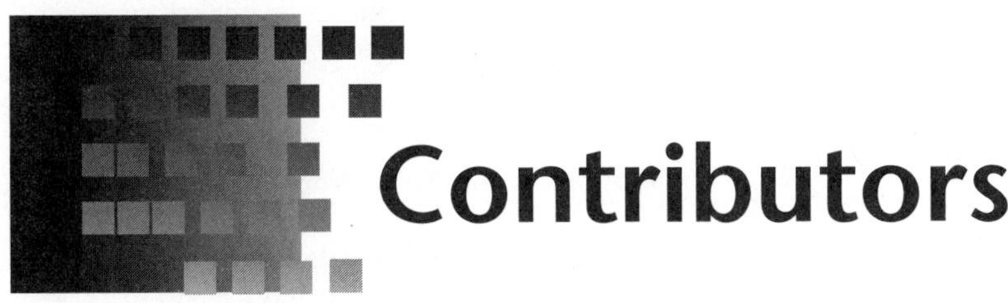

Contributors

Joan Bauer, MS, RN, CPAN
Staff Nurse, Postanesthesia Care Unit, St Mary's Hospital Medical Center, Madison, Wisconsin (Retired)
Latex Sensitivity

Joyce M. Black, RN, PhD
Assistant Professor, University of Nebraska Medical Center, Omaha, Nebraska
Plastic and Reconstructive Surgery

Patricia A. Brandon, RN
Nurse Coordinator, Anesthesia Pain Service, Ochsner Clinic, New Orleans, Louisiana
Chronic Pain Management

Nancy Burden, MS, RN, CPAN, CAPA
Director, Outpatient Surgery Centers, Morton Plant Mease Health Care, Palm Harbor, Florida
The Specialty of Ambulatory Surgery; The Environment of Care; Nursing Care of the Ambulatory Surgical Patient; Special Procedures in the Ambulatory Setting; Patients with Special Medical Needs

Pamela A. Cittan, RN, MSN, NHA, BSPA, MSA
Nurse Manager/Administrator, University of Michigan Surgery Center, Health Center Manager IV, University of Michigan Center for Specialty Care Clinics, University of Michigan Health System, Livonia, Michigan
Personnel Management Selection and Development

Donna M. DeFazio Quinn, BSN, MBA, RN, CPAN, CAPA
Henniker, New Hampshire
Business Aspects, Program Development, and Marketing; The Environment of Care

Carol DiMura, RNC, MSN
Patient Education Coordinator
Morton Plant Mease Health Care
Clearwater, Florida
Patient Education: Enhancing the Potential of the Teacher and the Learner

Deborah Dlugose, RN, CCRN, CRNA
President, Wright Professional Associates, PC, Chapel Hill, North Carolina; Staff Nurse-Anesthetist, Washington County Hospital, Hagerstown, Maryland
General Anesthesia

Rose Ferrara-Love, MSN, RN, CPAN, CAPA
Patient Services Manager, PACU/ASU, Children's Hospital of Pittsburgh, Pittsburgh, Pennsylvania
Immediate Postanesthesia Care

Denise L. Geuder, RN, MS, CNOR
Vice President, Patient Care Services, Saint Francis Hospital, Tulsa, Oklahoma
Intraoperative Care

Debra S. Goodwin, MS, BSN
ASPAN Lecturer and Nurse Manager, PACU and Preadmission Testing and Teaching, Morton Plant Mease Health Care—Countryside and Dunedin Campuses, Dunedin, Florida
Genitourinary Surgery

Brenda S. Gregory Dawes, MSN, RN, CNOR
Editor, AORN Journal, AORN, Denver, Colorado
Otorhinolaryngology and Head and Neck Surgery; Oral and Maxillofacial Surgery; Gynecologic and Obstetric Surgery; Orthopedic and Podiatric Surgery

Ginny Wacker Guido, MSN, JD
Associate Dean and Director of Graduate Studies, University of North Dakota College of Nursing, Grand Forks, North Dakota
Risk Management and Legal Issues

Delores Ireland, BSN, RN, CAPA
Clinical Nurse, Charge Nurse, POH, PACU I; William Beaumont Hospital-Troy, Troy, Michigan
Pediatric Patients and Their Families

Jay Knauer, BA
Business Systems Analyst, Purchasing Agent, and Operating Rooms Service Coordinator, University of Pittsburgh Medical Center, Pittsburgh, Pennsylvania
Materials and Equipment Management

Melissa Marshall Koehle, RN, BN, MEd
Director/Manager of Education Services, Sheikh Khalifa Medical Centre, Abu Dhabi, United Arab Emirates
Special Needs of the Older Adult

Michael Kost, CRNA, MS, MSN
Program Director, Montgomery Hospital School of Anesthesia, Adjunct Faculty, LaSalle College of Nursing, Norristown, Pennsylvania; President, Specialty Health Education, Inc., Blue Bell, Pennsylvania
Local and Regional Anesthesia

Myrna Eileen Mamaril, MS, BSN, RN, CPAN, CAPA
Nurse Manager, Preadmission Testing Center, Ambulatory Surgery Unit, Inpatient Post Anesthesia Care Unit, St. Joseph's Medical Center, Ellicott City, Maryland
Clinical Emergencies and Preparedness

Rex A. Marley, MS, CRNA, RRT
Staff Nurse Anesthetist, Northern Colorado Anesthesia Professional Consultants, Fort Collins, Colorado
Patient Discharge Issues

Gayle Miller, MS/MBA, RN, CPAN
Director of Surgical Services, St. Luke's Hospital, Jacksonville, Florida
Minimally Invasive Surgery, Laser, and Other Technologies

Beverly M. Moline, MS, RN, CNS
Acute Pain Clinical Nurse Specialist, Poudre Valley Hospital, Fort Collins, Colorado
Patient Discharge Issues

Denise O'Brien, BSN, RN, CPAN, CAPA
Clinical Nurse III/Educational Nurse Coordinator, Ambulatory Surgery Unit, Department of Operating Rooms/PACU University of Michigan Health System, Ann Arbor, Michigan
Cardiovascular Procedures; Special Procedures in the Ambulatory Setting

Jan Odom, BSN, MS, RN, CPAN, FAAN
Clinical Nurse Specialist, Forrest General Hospital, Hattiesburg, Mississippi
Conscious Sedation/Analgesia; Patients with Special Medical Needs

Sujit K. Pandit, MD, PhD
Professor of Anesthesiology, University of Michigan, Ann Arbor, Michigan
Anesthesia Management

Linda Pavlak, RN, BS, CAPA
Nurse Manager, Ambulatory Nursing Services, Morton Plant Mease Health Care, Dunedin, Florida
General Surgery

Jeanne Prin, RN
Manager, Product Evaluations, Mentor Corporation, Irving, Texas
Plastic and Reconstructive Surgery

Mary C. Redmond, BSN, RN, CAPA
Staff Nurse, Alegent Health Bergan Mercy Medical Center, Outpatient Surgery, Omaha, Nebraska
Extensions of Care: Phase III Recovery

Nancy M. Saufl, BSN, MS, RN, CPAN
ASPAN President 2000–2001 and Manager, Port Orange Day Surgery, Halifax Medical Center, Port Orange, Florida
Special Emotional, Social, and Cultural Needs

Lois Schick, BSN, MN, MBA
ASPAN Lecturer and Director, Emergency Department/Procedure Extended Recovery Unit, Exempla Saint Joseph Hospital, Denver, Colorado
Nursing Standards; Quality Improvement

Shauna Smith, RN, AD, CAPA
Compliance Coordinator, Idaho Falls Surgical Center, Idaho Falls, Idaho
Regulatory Compliance; Progressive Postanesthesia Care: Phase II Recovery

Linda Anderson Vader, RN, BS, CRNO
Head Nurse, The University of Michigan, W. K. Kellogg Eye Center, Ann Arbor, Michigan
Ophthalmic Surgery

Virginia Walter, MS, BSN, RN, CGRN
Manager, Medical Procedures Unit, University of Michigan Health System, Ann Arbor, Michigan
Special Procedures in the Ambulatory Setting

Gwen D. Williams, RN
Staff Nurse, Our Lady of Lourdes Regional Medical Center, Lafayette, Louisiana
Preoperative Preparation of the Ambulatory Surgery Patient

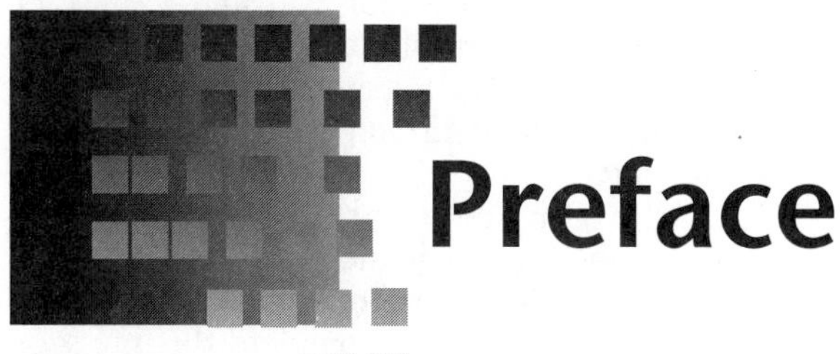

Preface

Welcome to the 2nd edition of *Ambulatory Surgical Nursing*. This edition has one distinguishing characteristic that transcends the others, and that is its broad pool of experts who contributed their knowledge and skills to both update information from the first edition and develop new avenues of learning. Contributions by my three co-editors, Donna M. DeFazio Quinn, Denise O'Brien, and Brenda S. Gregory Dawes, and the chapter authors offer readers a fresh approach to both old and new concerns that apply to our patients, from infants to seniors. For example, latex allergy, hardly a common occurrence in 1993, is a more frequent and acute problem today that we must consider as we plan our patient care. An entire chapter has, therefore, been dedicated to latex allergy in this edition.

Readers will find many Key Education Points throughout the text. This feature gives a quick overview of the most salient educational points that pertain to the chapter topic. They can be incorporated into the patient teaching plan and individualized for specific patients and situations. Another feature of this book is the expanded discussion of cultural issues that affect both patient care and teamwork within the Ambulatory Surgical Center.

Throughout the book, the reader will find Internet addresses and telephone contact information for numerous government, regulatory, association, and health-related entities. Many of these sites are geared toward professionals, but many others are resources that can be provided to patients to help them gain valuable information about self-care and decision-making. Also look for expanded information on cardiac and other special procedures as well as chapters dedicated to the concepts and content for patient education, nursing care during conscious sedation and analgesia, and pain management procedures. Chapter 9, dealing with risk management and legal issues is completely new and addresses concepts as well as patient advocacy, liability issues, and informed consent. Many actual court cases are cited as learning tools.

Managers, in particular, will find helpful information about staffing, the quality improvement process, business and financial management, and regulatory compliance. The latter chapter provides an in depth look at federal, regulatory, and accrediting compliance regarding issues such as the Americans with Disabilities Act, the Environmental Protection Agency, the National Fire Protection Association, the Food and Drug Administration, the Occupational Safety and Health Act, and many more. Illustrations of various reporting forms are provided along with key contact information and applicable standards for various agencies.

Ambulatory surgery continues to grow and develop. Since the first edition of *Ambulatory Surgical Nursing*, many changes have occurred in our practice. These changes include higher patient age and acuity, the continual evolution of procedural technology, newly developed pharmaceuticals and equipment, and more physician office-based procedures. Challenging economic trends in reimbursement, payer mix, and contractual relationships have wreaked financial havoc on facilities across the United States. In ambulatory surgical settings, these trends led not only to the drive toward even more outpatient procedures but also to greater pressure for continual and aggressive reductions of the costs of that care.

Predictions about the future supply of nurses project that in the next 15 years over half of the current nursing profession will retire and relatively few recruits will enter to take their place. In fact, fewer than 6% of nurses currently employed are younger than 30 years of age.

The search for experienced specialty nurses is often fraught with obstacles and long waits, making our roles even more critical. In this climate, the ambulatory surgical nurse continues to be looked to as a leader and innovator and as someone who has the education, common sense, and incentive to make proper professional, financial, and practice-related decisions to meet those challenges successfully. The professional nurse must be a leader in those solutions.

This reality-based backdrop to the challenges of nursing in the context of ambulatory procedures is meant to frame the importance of nurses as professionals. It is vital that nurses understand at the most basic personal level how important and essential they are, not only to the patient at whose bedside they stand but also to the bigger picture of healthcare in America and beyond. It is my earnest wish that each nurse who reads this book will find a sense of great joy and self-fulfillment in the practice of ambulatory surgical nursing and will consider becoming certified in ambulatory perianesthesia nursing.

As with any new information source, this book is only as good as the extent to which it is applied to the real world of ambulatory surgical nursing. To that end, I complete this message with my sincere gratitude for all the expert advice, reviewer input, and assistance on this project and my hope that all nurse-readers will use this information to provide focused, attentive, and professional patient care. May you all embrace the joys and challenges ahead with enthusiasm and dedication!

Nancy Burden, MS, RN, CPAN, CAPA

Contents

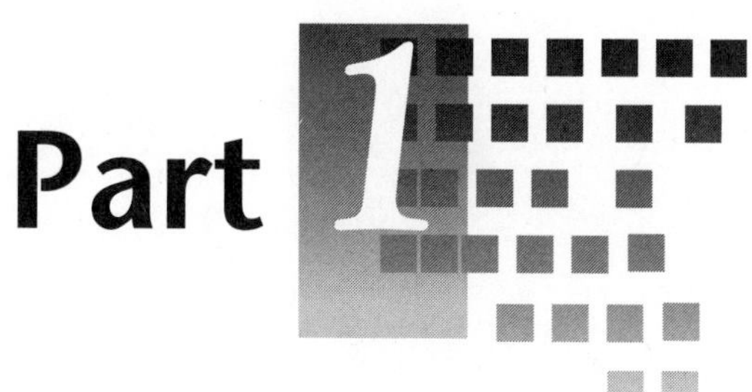

Part 1

Strategic Management

Chapter 1

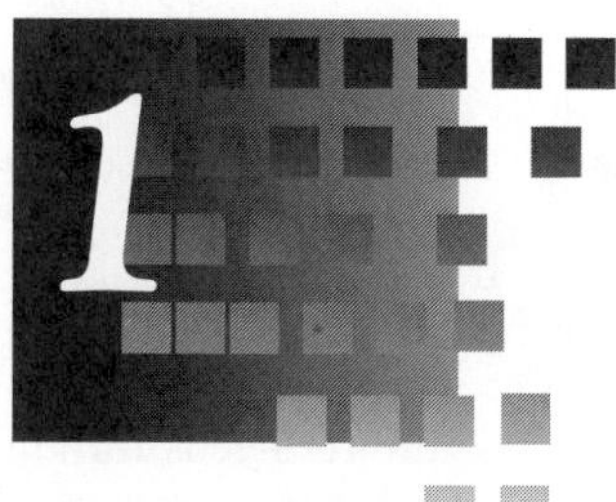

The Specialty of Ambulatory Surgery

Nancy Burden

Perioperative and perianesthesia nurses must be skilled and knowledgeable about surgery, anesthesia, and related nursing interventions. In ambulatory surgery settings, this specific knowledge, the appropriate technical skills, and a broad knowledge of the nursing process must be focused to address the needs of ambulatory surgery patients. These patients experience limited contact with healthcare providers before surgery, so it is imperative that all nursing interactions are focused and productive in assessing, educating, preparing, and caring for patients.

Patients and families are being asked to take increasingly more responsibility for aftercare in the home setting after surgical and anesthetic experiences. They are discharged soon after their procedures and are expected to deal with situations at home that involve concepts as diverse as use of aseptic technique to avoid the transmission of infection, control of orthostatic hypotension, and maintenance of neurovascular adequacy to an extremity. Most patients do not know what these concepts are or even that they are using them. Nurses, however, must know because it is the nurse who most often provides the education and support that help prepare patients to avoid or address any complications resulting from surgery and anesthesia.

Ambulatory surgical nurses must be able to predict the types of problems that might affect their patients at home. Then they must devise and execute a plan for teaching patients how to avoid such complications in terms that patients can understand. Ambulatory surgery patients have exceptional needs for education, careful assessment, and psychological encouragement. In addition, ensuring high-quality care in ambulatory surgery includes providing patient comfort and convenience, positive overall outcome, and cost-effectiveness.[1]

DEVELOPMENT OF AMBULATORY SURGERY AS A SPECIALTY

The roots of modern ambulatory surgery date back to the early 1970s, with the concept of providing surgical care for elective procedures on young, healthy patients and allowing them to return home on the same day that their procedures are performed. The program has expanded to encompass a much wider variety of procedures, patients, and structures. Complex procedures and medically compromised patients are the norm rather than the exception. Managed care companies and Medicare initiatives continue to drive this change for financial reasons. Advances in technology have improved the safety of performing more complex procedures, and effective, short-acting medications with few side effects along with improved pain management techniques have encouraged more rapid and trouble-free recovery from anesthesia.

The Beginnings

Ambulatory surgery is an ancient art, with evidence of surgery recorded in drawings dated as far back as 3500 BC. Trephining of the skull and amputations were the earliest depictions.

Documented references can also be found in ancient Babylonian, Egyptian, Eastern Indian, Greek, and Roman civilizations.[2] It was not until early Christian times that churches began to develop hospitals where patients were cared for in designated places besides their homes after surgery.

More recent times (between 1899 and 1908) saw a series of ambulatory surgeries performed with great success on 8988 children at the Glasgow Royal Hospital for Sick Children in Scotland.[3] The procedures addressed orthopedic problems, hare lip and cleft palate, spina bifida, depressed skull fractures related to birth, hernias, congenital pyloric stenosis, and others, after which none of the children required admission. Contemporary accounts describe similar results from that era.

In 1918, Dr. Ralph D. Waters at the Down-Town Anesthesia Clinic in Sioux City, Iowa, administered the first reported general anesthesia used in the western hemisphere for an ambulatory surgery patient. The medical community was apparently not ready for this innovation, and his idea was not successfully adopted in other areas. Neither were many physicians ready to accept the concept of early postoperative ambulation suggested by Dr. Emil Ries of Chicago[4] in 1899. Suggesting that patients walk and eat within hours of surgery was a radical departure from tradition and, although we now know it to be beneficial, it was not until the 1940s and 1950s that early ambulation came into widespread use.

In the 1960s, physicians began to test and stretch established traditions. Taking a cue from emergency rooms that historically have discharged patients soon after minor surgical procedures, physicians began to provide surgery without hospitalization. Economic advantages began to emerge that contributed to the trend toward outpatient surgery. Hospital beds became scarce, physicians began to undertake private surgical enterprises for profit, the public began to accept newer methods, and anesthesiologists responded with more appropriate techniques.

The Butterworth Hospital in Grand Rapids, Michigan, opened what is considered to be the country's first established ambulatory surgery program in 1961. Between 1963 and 1964, the staff performed 879 ambulatory procedures.[2] Other hospitals developed similar programs, and in 1970 the first successful freestanding ambulatory surgery facility was opened in Phoenix, Arizona. Drs. Wallace Reed and John Ford were assisted in the development and opening of this facility by a registered nurse, Sharon Schafer. This center continues to prosper and has expanded into a new facility. The freestanding facility market continues to compete with hospitals, each driving the others to develop better products and services that address community needs for ambulatory surgery.

As managed care companies, the U.S. government, and private insurers continue to decrease the amounts of payments for procedures, the most cost-effective settings will flourish. All types of facilities are striving to meet that goal. Third party payers require many surgeries to be performed in an ambulatory setting to avoid costly hospitalizations and are even requiring that certain procedures be performed in physicians' offices to further reduce costs. It is expected that competition will continue and that new concepts and services will be developed.

As the process of ambulatory surgery has evolved, nursing practice has developed ways to address varying patient needs. Specific nursing standards of practice have been developed and continue to evolve specifically for ambulatory surgery populations (see Chapter 6 for a discussion of perianesthesia standards that provide guidance for nursing care).

Various nursing processes applicable to the ambulatory surgery setting have been refined over the past decade. These include preadmission telephone calls or interviews, postdischarge telephone contacts to evaluate the effectiveness of nursing interventions, preoperative facility tours, development and application of discharge standards, and development and refinement of wellness approaches to encourage patients to participate in self-care. In many facilities, structured preadmission testing clinics have been developed to meet the assessment, educational, emotional, and physical preparatory needs of patients.

Today's Climate

Ambulatory surgery continues to change: earlier discharge occurs and more complex procedures are performed. Now, ambulatory surgery includes concepts of care other than immediate discharge of patients after initial recovery from anesthesia and minor surgery. One concept that has evolved is that of the 23-hour admission. This addresses the needs of patients who require a longer period of recuperation while still meeting acceptable criteria for ambulatory surgery, primarily to ensure third party payment.

In addition to same-day discharge, most people having major surgery now enter the hospital on the morning of surgery rather than the night before. Many of these patients are admitted and cared for before surgery in ambulatory surgery units, although some larger institutions may have separate units strictly for this category of patients, sometimes referred to as "AM admissions." Special units for these morning admission patients have many names, for instance, "To Come In Unit (TCI)," "Admission Day Surgery Program (ADP)," or "AM Admissions (AMA, AM Admit)," to name a few.

A multitude of names have been given to individual ambulatory surgery departments in hospitals and freestanding centers throughout the country, but regardless of the name attached to a department, patients on these units share many needs and problems. Sociologic, economic, and technologic influences have expanded the trend toward surgery performed on an ambulatory rather than an inpatient basis.

The high acuity and volume of critically ill patients in some hospitals result in competition for hospital beds that are becoming scarcer. Bed shortage is sometimes caused by bed closings at the hands of licensing agencies, by economic forces in the facility, and sometimes by nursing staff shortages. This situation forces less ill patients to rely on such out-of-hospital services as home care and ambulatory surgery programs.

In addition, the current financial state of the healthcare industry and pressures from the government and third party payers to contain and lower associated costs make ambulatory surgery programs economically attractive to providers and consumers. Not only does a third party payer benefit from patients being cared for in the lower cost setting of ambulatory care, but the patient can derive a benefit as well. Most people are responsible for a deductible, the amount of money that they must pay before their insurance plan pays for health benefits, regardless of the setting in which care is given. However, the co-payment amount is often defined in terms of a percentage of the total cost of care. Thus, the lower the overall charges from the healthcare institution, the less the co-payment.

The U.S. Balanced Budget Act of 1997 has affected reimbursement plans for the Medicare segment with the development of a prospective payment system, much like the hospital diagnosis-related group payment plan. Plans to implement this system in freestanding ambulatory surgery centers (ASCs) were delayed until after the year 2000 for several reasons. First, year 2000 computer compatibility needed to be ensured throughout federal systems. Also, the freestanding market, led by its professional organizations, demanded and were granted a delay in earlier implementation to allow more time for industry response and the Health Care Finance Administration's study of the proposed rule. The new payment system will be enacted along with a similar plan for hospital-based outpatient surgery reimbursement.

Technologic advances in surgery provide alternatives to more invasive major procedures, thus allowing rapid return of normal functions and earlier patient discharge. The arsenal of tools available to the surgeon has expanded significantly, and newer techniques allow surgeons to accomplish many procedures with less trauma to surrounding tissues. With the widespread use of lasers, laparoscopes, endoscopes, fiberoptic light sources, and other complex computer-assisted equipment, the numbers and the types of procedures that can be accomplished in the ambulatory arena have multiplied dramatically.[5]

Technology has affected the pharmaceutical industry as well. Specialized anesthetic approaches, availability of highly specific anesthetic agents and sedatives with short half-lives, and new analgesics and antiemetic drugs help reduce the complications of postanesthesia recovery. This, in turn, promotes early discharge and acceptable patient condition for home recuperation.

Interactive computer technology has provided both assessment and learning modalities for patients. Widespread Internet connectivity now provides patients with access to innumerable health-related sites. This medium has the potential to be the next innovation in preadmission education and postdischarge follow-up for many people. Table 1–1 provides a sample of health-related Web sites of general interest to the public and to healthcare professionals. The Internet has opened up a universe of information to the masses, including medical information that was previously not readily available to the lay public. Nurses caring for patients today must expend the energy and time to remain professionally current so that they are prepared to interpret, explain, and correct information that patients and families may learn from the Internet or various other sources.

Another advance has been the development of critical pathways (clinical pathways, care paths, care maps, clinical maps, clinical trajectories, integrated plans of care) that delineate the expected progress of a patient from beginning to end of the process related to a specific procedure or type of procedure. They plan for the provision of clinical services that have expected

Table 1–1. **Health-Related Web Sites**

WEB SITE ADDRESS	ORGANIZATION	COMMENTS
Medical/Nursing		
www.aspan.org	American Society of Perianesthesia Nurses	Standards, issues of interest re: ambulatory surgery nursing
www.fasa.org	Federated Ambulatory Surgery Association	
www.mhaus.org	Malignant Hyperthermia Association of the United States	Information on malignant hyperthermia
www.aorn.org	Association of Operation Room Nurses	Announcements, standards, conferences
www.facs.org	American College of Surgeons	
www.ama-assn.org	American Medical Association	Articles and facts for the public on a variety of topics
www.ana.org	American Nurses Association	
www.ncsbn.org	National Council of State Boards of Nursing, Inc.	State licensure information
www.nln.org	National League for Nursing	Advances quality nursing education
www.uronews.com/	Urology News	Bimonthly review of current literature in urology and related fields
www.jcaho.org	Joint Commission on Accreditation of Healthcare Organizations	Information on standards, listing of accredited organizations, and status
www.aace.com	American Association of Clinical Endocrinologists	Medical information on endocrine issues, e.g., diabetes, osteoporosis
www.aha.com	American Hospital Association	
www.asahq.com	American Society of Anesthesiologists	Link to Society for Ambulatory Anesthesia, consumer articles "Know Your Anesthesiologist," "Anesthesia and You," "Anesthesia for Ambulatory Surgery," "The Senior Citizen as a Patient," "When Your Child Needs Anesthesia"
www.aana.com	American Association of Nurse Anesthetists	
www.sgna.org	Society of Gastrointestinal Nurses and Associates	Nursing organization
www.asge.org	American Society for Gastrointestinal Endoscopists	Medical organization
www.auanet.org	American Urological Association	
www.ast.org	Association of Surgical Technologists	Association news, technology updates
www.ashrm.org	American Society for Healthcare Risk Managers	
www.aaasc.org	American Association of Ambulatory Surgery Centers	Business, political, and educational association for outpatient surgery centers
http://gasnet.med.yale.edu/apsf/	Anesthesia Patient Safety Foundation	Multidisciplinary group with main interest of safety for patients
www.apic.org	Association for Professionals in Infection Control and Epidemiology	Promotes wellness and prevents illness and infection worldwide
www.sacp-net.org	Society for Ambulatory Care Professionals	For management professionals in ambulatory settings
Publishers		
www.elsevier.nl	Elsevier Publisher	Via European section, find the international journal *Ambulatory Surgery*—contents listings
www.wbsaunders.com	W.B. Saunders Company	Medical/nursing books and journals
www.mosby.com	C.V. Mosby Company	Medical/nursing books and journals
www.lww.com	Lippincott Williams & Wilkins	Medical/nursing books and journals
www.sagepub.com	Sage Publications	Medical/nursing books and journals

Table 1–1. Health-Related Web Sites *Continued*

WEB SITE ADDRESS	ORGANIZATION	COMMENTS
www.uspharmacist.com	U.S. Pharmacist	Journal for pharmacy professional—articles of general health interest/drug updates
www.anesthesiology.org/contents.cfm	Anesthesiology	Medical journal
Organizations and General Interest		
www.mayohealth.org	Mayo Clinic Health Oasis	Self-care guides to help improve health
www.arthritis.org	The Arthritis Foundation	
www.latexallergyhelp.com	Latex Allergy Help	Information on allergy to latex with discussion section for questions and answers
http://pw2.netcom.com/~ecbdmd/elastic.html	ELASTIC	Information and emotional support to latex-allergic people
www.execpc.com/~alert/Pages/main.html	ALERT	Allergy to Latex Education and Resource Team
www.eatright.org/healthorg.html	American Diabetes Association Gateway to Nutrition	Comprehensive list of associations and organizations dedicated to proper nutrition
http://ificinfo.org/	International Food Information Council	Food safety and nutrition information. Links to antioxidants, antidotes to aging, and so on
www.ichelp.com	Interstitial Cystitis Association	Not-for-profit organization providing patient and physician education
www.medicalert.org	Medic Alert	Information on Medic Alert program
www.redcross.org	American Red Cross	Information on services, events
www.cancer.org	American Cancer Society	National data, consumer information
www.geron.org	Gerontological Society of America	Promotes the scientific study of aging
www.surgery.com	Plastic Surgery Web Site	Search engine to find surgeon by geographic location
www.netdoctor.com/	Net Doctor	Provides links to numerous health-related sites
Government		
www.healthfinder.gov	Health Finder	Consumer information about variety of healthcare issues—links to many sites
www.nih.gov	National Institutes of Health	Can enter into various institutes depending on health concern
www.nih.gov/ninr	National Institute of Nursing Research	Nursing research information with information on legislation, grants, conferences, current nursing research highlights
www.fedstats.gov/	FEDSTATS	Federal site for statistics of interest to the public from more than 70 government agencies
www.cdc.gov	Centers for Disease Control and Prevention	Information on various diseases
www.cdc.gov/nchswww/default.htm	National Center for Health Statistics	Statistical health-related information of interest to the public
www.nal.usda.gov/fnic	Food and Nutrition Information Center	Part of U.S. Department of Agriculture Research Service—interactive food pyramid, information on anorexia/bulimia, vitamins, minerals, and more
www.nci.nih.gov	National Cancer Institute	One of the National Institutes of Health

Table continued on following page

Table 1–1. **Health-Related Web Sites** *Continued*

WEB SITE ADDRESS	ORGANIZATION	COMMENTS
www.ahcpr.gov	Agency for Healthcare Policy and Research	Gateway to consumer health information, clinical practice guidelines
www.aoa.gov	Administration on Aging	Government links to vast information on aging
www.access.gpo.gov/	Government Printing Office	Access to federal publications for consumers
www.hcfa.gov	Health Care Financing Administration	Medicare and Medicaid and child health information

time frames and resources targeted to specific diagnoses or procedures. These pathways prospectively link clinical care activities and associated costs with predetermined time points and outcomes, thus allowing analysis of both clinical and economic effectiveness.

Care paths are developed by an interdisciplinary team and are based on historical data as well as on expected and desired outcomes. Care paths or maps are highly individualized to the facility or program and are dependent on collaboration among medical, nursing, and other practices as well as on patient demographics and acuity. By setting "normal" or "average" parameters expected along the patient's continuum of care, they provide a standard against which individual patients' progress can be compared and allow for interventions to improve progress and outcomes of care.

Care maps do not replace physicians' orders, but they do provide a suggested best treatment plan.[6] Given to a patient in a format the patient can understand, a care map can help the patient anticipate the timing of various stages or activities. Care maps have been developed to address progress during a hospital stay and generally are expressed in terms of day one, day two, and so on. Figure 1–1 is an example of a care map based on the shortened time frame of the ambulatory surgery process.

As new problems and challenges arise, the nursing profession must be prepared to study and respond effectively to those challenges. The continual changes in ambulatory surgery require nursing innovation. J. Allen Scoggin's classic six-step approach[7] to remaining innovative in the pharmacy profession is applicable to ambulatory surgical nursing. Nurses must keep informed of professional, community, and facility matters. Innovative nurses tend to think for themselves. They analyze problems and suggest solutions and new methods of accomplishing goals. The six steps that Scoggin suggests to become more innovative and resourceful in the pharmacy profession are presented in Table 1–2 along with potential ambulatory surgical nursing applications.

STATISTICS OF OUTPATIENT SURGERY

Surgery, with its accompanying period of recuperation, has made the transition into the outpatient arena on a grand scale. Federal statistics from the 1997 report of the National Center for Health Statistics of the Centers for Disease Control and Prevention[8] cite 1994 data collected on ambulatory surgery in hospitals and freestanding centers. Data were collected via surveys. Of the 751 hospitals and freestanding centers included in this survey, 617 were considered eligible based on the requirements of the study. Of those 617 facilities, 494 responded to the survey (80%). Further details of the survey results, methods, and limitations can be found in the cited literature, Advance Data, No. 283, March 14, 1997, available from the National Center for Health Statistics.

- Telephone: 301-436-8500
- E-mail: nchsquery.@nch10a.em.cdc.gov
- Web site: http://www.cdc.gov/nchswww/nchshome.html

During the 18.8 million ambulatory surgery visits made in the United States, approximately 28.3 million surgical and nonsurgical procedures were performed. These 18.8 million visits accounted for 49% of all surgeries, both inpatient and outpatient. Of the outpatient visits, an estimated 16 million (85%) occurred in hospitals, and 2.9 million in freestanding outpatient centers (15%).[8]

Another source of data regarding statistical issues in outpatient surgery is the SMG Marketing Group of Chicago.[9] Their June 1998 market

Table 1–2. Ways to Remain Innovative in Ambulatory Surgical Nursing

SCOGGIN'S 6 STEPS FOR PHARMACY INNOVATION	AMBULATORY SURGERY NURSING APPLICATION
Update sources of information	Maintain updated library—at work and personal Maintain current CPR, ACLS, PALS, and malignant hyperthermia protocols Keep current editions of Nursing Standards of Practice Apply results of scientific nursing research to practice Subscribe to professional journals Keep physician standing orders and preference cards current Use Internet resources Join (or start) a journal club Ask anesthesia personnel to share their journals
Sharpen observation skills	Enjoin peer nurses to challenge one another within safety of group Self-test to assess patients for predetermined criteria Role play
Attend seminars	Local, state, and national nursing seminars Facility internal programs Video and audio programs when available State and national ambulatory surgery organizations
Ask questions	Maintain a joy of learning Ask to observe new procedures Ask physicians, other nurses, CRNAs for information and insights Seek answers in literature Ask librarians for assistance
Watch for practice trends	Maintain membership in national and state nursing organizations Attend meetings to network Read professional journals and newsletters Keep abreast of national healthcare news
Look for new opportunities	Keep open mind and eyes Look toward evolution of ambulatory surgery process for ideas (e.g., home health visits before and after surgery for surgeon, anesthesia QI, family education support programs; develop Web site) Propose and/or participate in nursing research Propose new and innovative solutions for problems or challenges Develop new and improved patient education tools Seek Internet resources and opportunities Write and publish in professional journals Consider sharing knowledge as public speaker for professional or for public awareness groups

CPR, cardiopulmonary resuscitation; ACLS, advanced cardiac life support; CRNA, certified registered nurse anesthetist; QI, quality improvement; PALS, pediatric advanced life support.

Adapted from Scoggin JA: Innovation for the 90s and Beyond. Apothecary 101:9–15, 1989.

report summarized analysis from 2634 operational freestanding centers and reported an estimated 5.2 million procedures performed annually in those centers. This is a 9.1% annual growth from the previous year. Freestanding surgery centers are found in every state, ranging from two in Vermont to 417 in California. Other states with more than 100 freestanding centers include Florida (244), Georgia (126), Maryland (149), and Texas (160).

The past several years have seen a slowing of the freestanding ASC growth rate. Contributing to this slowing is the saturation of many markets as well as an economic climate that is less conducive to independently owned centers than to chain-owned centers. The SMG Marketing Group explains that further growth can be expected in states that loosen certificate-of-need controls on operating room construction.[9]

Gender plays a role in the frequency of outpatient procedures, with females having significantly more visits (10.7 million) than males (8.2 million). The rate of visits for females overall was also higher at 80.2 visits per 1000 compared with 65.0 visits per 1000 for males. With age factors taken into consideration, however, the frequency of visits varied between males and females, as noted in Figure 1–2.[8]

In regard to the disposition of ambulatory surgical patients, the vast majority (90%) returns to their customary residences after their procedures. Another 3.1% went to observation

Figure 1–1. *A*, Critical pathway applicable to ambulatory surgery.

St. Luke's Medical Center
Plan for Recovery After Same Day Surgery

	TEST CENTER	ARRIVAL TO SAME-DAY SURGERY	0 TO ½ HR AFTER SURGERY	½ TO 1 HR AFTER SURGERY	1 TO 1½ HR AFTER SURGERY	2 HR AFTER SURGERY
Activity	Phone interview or in-person interview	1. Register at desk 2. Escorted to room 3. Bedside orientation 4. Change hospital gown, robe, and slippers		Ambulate with assistance	Ambulate	Discharge per wheelchair only if necessary (RNs discretion to discharge ambulatory)
Treatments	1. Physical therapy as appropriate 2. Surgical procedure verification	1. Height, weight, pulse oximeter, vital signs 2. RN to complete preoperative checklist 3. IV to be started in SDS or HA 4. Pre-op prep if needed (e.g., Betadine scrub, Teds) 5. Surgical procedure verification	1. VS q 15 × 2 2. Surgical assessment 3. Follow MD orders	1. VS q 30 × 2 2. Surgical assessment	VS every 30 min–1 hour	Discharge vital signs Surgical assessment
Diagnostic Tests	1. Preoperative testing as ordered	If phone, CXR, ECG, Lab, physical therapy if needed				
Teaching	1. Interview by RN in Test Center or phone 2. Preoperative instruction 3. Teaching booklets as appropriate for procedure 4. Video as appropriate	1. If phone, give teaching booklets, video as appropriate. 2. Review HA or PACU visiting waiting area.		Reinforce discharge instructions	Give adult or pediatric anesthesia discharge instructions. Provide written home instructions. Provide home supplies if needed. Review instructions with significant other if present.	

Pain Management	1. Introduced to pain management after surgery 2. Distribute pain management book	1. If phone interview, give pain management book. 2. Assess for pain.	Assess for pain. Offer analgesic.	Pain assessment	Pain assessment (give Rx)	Pain assessment
Fluids	1. NPO after midnight unless otherwise instructed 2. Patient instructed by Test Center regarding medications to take if any		Nausea assessment (if nauseous, Tx immediately) Offer fluids.	Nausea assessment Assess fluid tolerance	Nausea assessment (give RX) DC IV	Minimal N/V may be present.
Discharge Planning	1. Significant other to be available 2 hours postoperative for transportation home 2. Arrangements made for adult to stay with patient 24 hours postoperatively		Send RX to pharmacy.		Patient to be seen by pharmacist regarding DC medications	Transportation home or document variance for prolonged stay.
Outcomes	Medical clearance addressed Pt/SO verbalized understanding of procedure Pt/family verbalize knowledge of activities related to surgery: Preoperative care Postoperative care Medication Preparations Testing, evaluation, and admitting complete	Patient verbalizes/ demonstrates understanding of: a. Purpose for surgery b. Surgical checks c. Postoperative activity d. Dressing/drain Patient verbalizes purpose of Holding Area and PACU. Patient identifies strategies for pain management: meds, nonpharmacologic measures, and pain scales. Patient verbalizes knowledge of importance of coughing and deep breathing. Patient verbalizes knowledge in patient path and personal responsibility. Patient verbalizes discharge plan.	Dressing and/or drain intact and evaluated Vital signs stable within preoperative parameters Responsive with stable neurologic status Pain managed Nausea managed Patient verbalizes/ demonstrates understanding of: a. Surgical assessment b. Pain assessment c. Fluid progression	Patient verbalizes/ demonstrates understanding of: a. Surgical assessment b. Discharge instructions c. Pain assessment d. Fluid progression	Patient verbalizes/ demonstrates understanding of: a. Surgical assessment b. Discharge instructions c. Pain assessment d. Fluid progression e. Activity progression f. Discharge teaching: Diet Activity Incision care Medications Follow-up with MD Community resources	Patient verbalizes/ demonstrates understanding of: a. Surgical assessment b. Discharge instructions c. Pain assessment d. Fluid progression e. Activity progression f. Discharge teaching: Diet Activity Incision care Medications Follow-up with MD Community resources

Illustration continued on following page

St. Luke's Medical Center and St. Luke's South Shore
SAME DAY SURGERY (SDS) Patient Recovery Plan

	Arrival to SDS	1/2 Hour After Surgery	1/2 to 1 Hour After Surgery	1 to 11/2 Hours After Surgery	2 Hours After Surgery
What Will My Activity Be?	• Report to the SDS Unit • You Will Be Oriented to the Unit • You May Have an IV Started • You Will Be Given Preoperative Instructions	You will be encouraged to get up to the bathroom. We will help you if needed.	You will be up and walking with help if needed	You will be up and walking.	Time to get dressed to go home!
What Can I Eat and Drink?	NOTHING TO EAT OR DRINK THE NIGHT BEFORE AND THE MORNING OF SURGERY–UNLESS YOU ARE INSTRUCTED OTHERWISE	You Will Be Given Ice Chips and Water	You May Have Any Liquids		You May Have Any Liquids Eat Light Foods at Home
How Can I Manage My Pain?	• Pain Management Booklet Will Be Reviewed • Your Nurse will teach you about the Pain Scale	• Rate Pain 0-10 • Pain Medication Will Be Given if Needed	Rate Pain 0-10	You will be given your prescriptions	Your Nurse Will Review Your Pain Management At Home
How Do I Care For Myself At Home?	Any Home Care Needs You Have Will Be Reviewed	Your Nurse Will Check Your Surgical Site	Review Discharge Instructions	Review: • Incision Care • Signs and Symptoms to Watch For • Supplies needed At Home	Instructions Reviewed
What is My Plan For Discharge?	• You will receive written instructions for home care • Your plan for transportation home will be verified	Plan for Home		Time to Contact Your Ride	Discharge Home!

05401800 (1/98)

B

Figure 1–1 *Continued. B*, Critical pathway applicable to ambulatory surgery—patient teaching copy. RN, registered nurse; NPO, nothing by mouth; Post-op, postoperative; Pre-op, preoperative; Pt, patient; SO, significant other; VS, vital signs; IV, intravenous; SDS, same-day surgery; CXR, chest x-ray; ECG, electrocardiogram; Lab, laboratory studies; PACU, postanesthesia care unit; MD, physician; Tx, treatment; RX, prescription; DC, discontinue; HA, holding area. (From Managed Care Workgroup: Diane Dombrowski, Alice Kayser, Julie Wahl. St. Luke's Medical Center, Milwaukee, WI.)

units, with 1.6% being admitted to hospitals for inpatient care. Table 1–3 provides more detailed information regarding disposition.[8]

All surgical specialties are represented in ambulatory surgery. Gastrointestinal, ophthalmic, and musculoskeletal procedures lead the list of specialties for ambulatory procedures performed, according to a comparison of the vari-

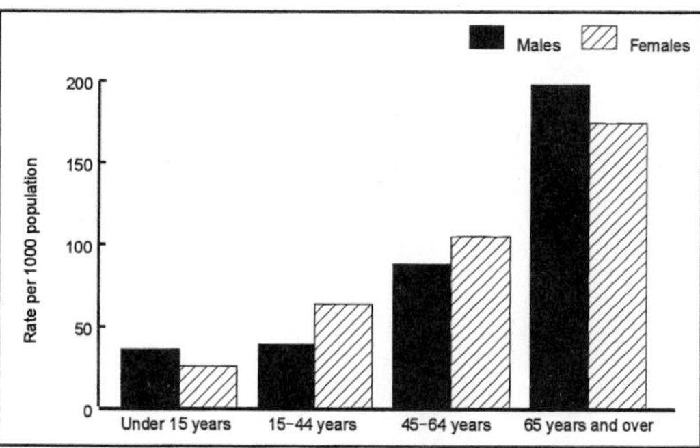

Figure 1–2. Rates of ambulatory surgery in males and females by age group, United States, 1994. (From Ambulatory Surgery in the United States, 1994. In Advance Data. US Department of Health and Human Services. Vital Statistics of the Centers for Disease Control and Prevention, National Center for Health Statistics, No. 283, March 14, 1997.)

ous specialties as reported by the National Center for Health Statistics survey of 1994 (Table 1–4).[8] In Table 1–5, data are provided from the 1998 SMG Market Group analysis of freestanding centers.[9]

The fact that a surgery is completed in an ambulatory care facility makes it no less important or serious. Safe execution of surgery requires total attention to all the details of preparation, execution, and aftercare during the perioperative period. Hospitals that offer ambulatory surgery programs must provide care that is of the same quality as that provided for hospitalized counterparts.[10]

Similarly, freestanding centers must provide a standard of medical, anesthesia, and nursing care equal to that provided in a hospital setting.

***Table 1–4.* Ambulatory Surgery by Specialty: United States—1994**

PROCEDURE	NUMBER OF PROCEDURES
All procedures	28.3 million
Nervous system	979,000
Eyes	4.6 million
Ears	870,000
Nose, mouth, and pharynx	2 million
Respiratory system	341,000
Cardiovascular system	688,000
Digestive system	6.2 million
Urinary system	1.4 million
Female genital organs	2.1 million
Musculoskeletal system	3.7 million
Integumentary system	2.8 million

Data from Advance Data. US Department of Health and Human Services. Vital Statistics of the Centers for Disease Control and Prevention, National Center for Health Statistics, No. 283, p. 7. March 14, 1997. Available at http://www.cdc.gov/nchswww/fastats/outsurg.htm September 1998.

In fact, freestanding units are sometimes obliged to show that they provide even more vigilance, patient attention, and emergency preparedness than nearby hospitals to compensate for attitudes among some portions of the public or healthcare community that a self-contained center may not be as safe as a hospital-based setting.

The past 2 decades have seen the proliferation of freestanding outpatient surgery centers in the United States. Table 1–6 illustrates that growth. The vast majority of freestanding outpatient surgery centers are either Medicare or state certified. To be eligible for Medicare reim-

***Table 1–3.* Disposition of Patients After Outpatient Surgery: United States—1994**

DISPOSITION	NUMBER IN THOUSANDS *Estimate*	NUMBER IN THOUSANDS *Standard Error*	PERCENT DISTRIBUTION *Estimate*	PERCENT DISTRIBUTION *Standard Error*
All dispositions	18,850	806	100.0	—
Routine discharge to customary residence	16,887	782	89.6	1.6
Discharge to observation status	581	78	3.1	0.4
Discharge to recovery care center	*	—	*	—
Admitted to hospital as inpatient	311	42	1.6	0.2
Surgery canceled or terminated	17	2	0.1	†
Other dispositions	141	37	0.7	0.2
Disposition not stated	678	145	3.6	0.8

—, Category not applicable.
*Figure does not meet standard of reliability or precision.
†Standard error is 0.01.
From Ambulatory Surgery in the United States, 1994. In Advance Data. US Department of Health and Human Services. Vital Statistics of the Centers for Disease Control and Prevention, National Center for Health Statistics, No. 283, p. 5, March 14, 1997.

Table 1–5. Surgeries by Specialty Performed in Freestanding Outpatient Centers: United States, 1998

SURGICAL PROCEDURE TYPE	1994	1995	1996	1997
Ophthalmology	30.8%	28.8%	27.0%	27.2%
Gastroenterology	11.9%	13.7%	17.7%	19.3%
Gynecological surgery	9.1%	8.0%	10.1%	9.7%
Orthopedics	6.1%	5.9%	8.9%	8.8%
Plastic surgery	14.8%	15.9%	8.1%	7.8%
ENT	6.1%	5.7%	7.2%	7.0%
General—other	6.2%	6.2%	7.0%	6.4%
Pain blocks	3.0%	3.0%	4.2%	4.6%
Podiatry	7.3%	8.2%	4.0%	3.7%
Urology	3.4%	3.2%	3.8%	3.6%
Dental	1.2%	1.3%	1.8%	1.7%
Neurology	0.2%	0.1%	0.2%	0.2%
Total	100%	100%	100%	100%

ENT, ear, nose, and throat.
Adapted from Freestanding Outpatient Surgery Centers Market Report, 1998 ed. Chicago: SMG Marketing Group, June 1998, p 13.

bursement, centers must meet federal standards. Medicare-certified centers totaled 2243 in 1998. Today, 41 states require state licensure.[9]

AMBULATORY SURGERY VERSUS TRADITIONAL IN-HOSPITAL SURGERY: SIMILARITIES AND DIFFERENCES

Similarities and differences can be identified in comparisons of the ambulatory setting with traditional in-hospital surgery (Table 1–7). Some relate to patients' physical and emotional needs, others, to broader facility-related issues. Obvious in both settings is the patient's basic need for surgical intervention. In both types of units, the patient is highly dependent on surgeons, anesthesia providers, and nurses. The ambulatory setting further extends that net of responsibility to families.

Patients face many of the same fears in all surgical settings, whether ambulatory or inpatient. They fear pain, the unknown, anatomic loss or alterations, possible embarrassment or loss of dignity, and financial problems. They also fear appearing ignorant when asking or answering questions. Patients may be worried about a potential change in ability to function within the family unit, an impending unfavorable diagnosis, or even the possibility of death.

Seventy-six adults undergoing ambulatory

Table 1–6. Total Number of Freestanding Outpatient Centers Operational on 12/31/97: United States, 1998

YEAR	# OF CENTERS	YEAR	# OF CENTERS
1997	2634	1983	377
1996	2425	1982	293
1995	2314	1981	250
1994	2106	1980	215
1993	1967	1979	188
1992	1807	1978	162
1991	1641	1977	132
1990	1496	1976	116
1989	1364	1975	89
1988	1213	1974	67
1987	1043	1973	47
1986	871	1972	33
1985	692	1971	23
1984	502	1970	16

From Freestanding Outpatient Surgery Centers Market Report, 1998 ed. Chicago, SMG Marketing Group, June 1998, p 2.

Table 1–7. Ambulatory Versus Inpatient Surgery

Similarities Between Ambulatory and Inpatient Surgery Programs
- Basic pathology that requires surgical intervention
- Surgical techniques/technology
- Skill and knowledge required of personnel
- Patient's need for anesthetics
- Patient fears/emotional impact
- Information/teaching needs
- Strict aseptic technique required
- Technologic support/instrumentation
- Potential for emergencies to occur
- Patient's dependence on staff during surgery and anesthesia

Differences Found in the Ambulatory Setting
- Emphasis on the concept of wellness
- Control of patient's compliance with preoperative preparations at home
- Generally healthier patients
- Alterations in anesthesia (shorter-acting agents, regional techniques)
- Use of premedicants
- Local infiltration of operative site
- Generally shorter surgical times
- Family involvement in care
- Patient and family responsibility
- Impact on home environment
- Compressed time for assessment and interventions
- Usually elective procedures

surgery for the first time were asked what concerned them the most about having their surgery on an outpatient basis. Six areas of concern were identified. Their responses focused on the following:

1. The availability of professional care following discharge
2. The need for information (this need varied considerably, with some people wanting complete information and others not wanting to know any details ahead of time)
3. Concern about the process of surgery, for instance, waiting before surgery or being discharged too soon
4. The final outcome in relation to health
5. The recovery process, including complications, pain, and integration back into home responsibilities
6. Personal vulnerability.[11]

Similarities between the two types of settings include the need for maintaining appropriate levels of asepsis in the operating suite and perioperative areas, along with the proper use of current technology and instrumentation. Appropriate quality improvement and infection control procedures must be addressed, regardless of the surgical setting. Because there is a constant potential for emergencies to occur, total preparedness of staff and equipment is essential in both freestanding and hospital settings.

Conversely, there are also differences between ambulatory and inpatient settings. Generally, a healthier patient population is found in ambulatory surgical settings than that in hospital surgical settings. Although many ambulatory units serve large numbers of elderly and systemically sick people, these patients usually present with relatively well-controlled diseases. Personnel in freestanding ASCs most often perform elective surgical procedures, but many units associated with large hospitals and medical centers frequently accommodate patients with minor emergencies in their everyday schedules.

Rapid patient turnover, shorter surgical times, reduced overall patient stays, and increased family involvement in care are all typical of an ambulatory setting. Nurses have significantly less time for preoperative and postoperative assessment, intervention, patient teaching, and evaluation. Nursing staff must be open to a practice that encourages patient and family responsibility for care. Nurses should support a medication protocol that relies on a combination of minimal sedation and aggressive pain management so that patients are able to resume self-care as quickly as possible.

Ambulatory surgery creates some unique problems for nurses. For instance, nurses often cannot monitor, much less verify, a patient's compliance with preoperative home preparations, such as bathing and complying with the NPO (nothing by mouth) status. Same-day discharge requires special discharge planning and attention to the physical set-up of the patient's home, transportation needs, home support requirements, and occasional need for unexpected hospitalization. Fear about being at home after surgery without nursing or medical supervision strongly affects some patients and should be considered in an overall nursing care plan.

An open mind and an innovative spirit are trademarks of the ambulatory surgery staff. These characteristics can result in certain advantages for an ambulatory surgery setting over traditional hospitalization. For instance, ambulatory surgery departments often provide a more home-like and inviting atmosphere, an emphasis on wellness, and a greater inclusion of family or friends in patient care and instructions.

A freestanding center is well suited to offer new ways of addressing patient needs without bureaucratic restriction. For instance, recliners may be used to replace stretchers, patients typically retain dentures and sensory aids during surgery, patients may walk to and from the operating room when appropriate, and families may wait in the immediate postoperative area. Some of these innovations are possible because of the smaller, more self-contained physical layout of the units. Others have to do with attitude changes and the freedom from hospital traditions.

Many hospital-based surgery units also offer these and other progressive services, such as facility tours before the day of surgery and radio headphones for the patient to use during surgery. Some hospital-based units find it difficult to break away from the rules requiring more traditional policies and procedures. Whenever possible, restrictive policies should be updated to support a more progressive view toward individualized patient care.

PATIENT RIGHTS AND RESPONSIBILITIES

Given the present climate of consumerism in today's healthcare industry, patients are generally better informed about what to expect, and even what to demand, from healthcare providers. High-quality care is expected. The patient is faced with the frightening experience of giving up control of both body and life for a period of time. Patients should be able to trust that the people providing care are not only medically capable but also sensitive to patients' potential fears and emotional needs. It is expected that the patient's dignity will be preserved and that any details of care will be held in confidence.

In all surgical settings, patients assume that clear, accurate instructions will be provided along with an opportunity for questions in a nonintimidating setting. That expectation has special significance for the ambulatory surgical patient who must assume a certain amount of responsibility for self-care at home very soon after surgery. Very clear discharge instructions and explanations are essential components of nursing care, as is support of the patient's sense of self-confidence, which nurses can help to nurture. In addition, ambulatory surgery patients need assurance that they will not knowingly be sent home prematurely.

Inherent in the process of providing high-quality care is a recognition that every patient cared for in an ambulatory surgery facility has both responsibilities and rights. Established policies should define and identify patients' rights and responsibilities and the facility's overall goals of care. By establishing such a philosophy, the ASC helps its staff members to focus collectively and individually on clearly defined goals that promote staff unity and purpose. There are different approaches to facility goals and to patient rights and responsibilities. Patient rights may be addressed in terms of expected outcomes or in terms of process and expectation (Table 1–8).

The goals of a program are often designed from the viewpoint of the facility staff rather than the patient. Typical goals would include providing comprehensive preoperative assessment and education, ensuring that appropriate candidates are selected, and verifying the home support for patients before giving preoperative sedation. Whatever approach is taken, the ASC should ensure that every employee is aware and supportive of its philosophy and policies. All healthcare facilities should ensure that patients' rights are communicated to patients, families, and employees. Sometimes, this is accomplished by posting the rights in public view. In other settings, a written copy is provided to each patient.

Patients also have responsibilities, such as reporting accurately on their medical histories, following the treatment protocol, and paying their bills. Ambulatory surgery demands that patients assume additional responsibilities, for example, the need to have a driver or an able adult to accompany the patient home from the surgery facility and an adult to be responsible for the patient after surgery. These are frequently abused or misapplied responsibilities that deserve serious attention. Patients who refuse to accept these or other responsibilities inherent in having surgery on an ambulatory basis may find their surgeries cancelled if other arrangements cannot be made to ensure their safe postoperative course.

NURSE'S ROLE IN AMBULATORY SURGERY

Whether patients and families actually accept the concept of same-day discharge because they are well instructed and well prepared or whether they tolerate it because they have no other alternative is not always clear. Regardless, the ambulatory surgical nurse is a primary resource for care, instruction, and support.[12] The nurse addresses a diverse and ever-changing barrage of questions and problems as the com-

***Table 1–8.* Patient Rights and Responsibilities**

As a Patient, You Have the Right to

- Considerate, respectful care at all times and under all circumstances with recognition of your personal dignity.
- Personal and informational privacy.
- Confidentiality of records and disclosures. Except when required by law, you have the right to approve or refuse the release of records.
- Information concerning your diagnosis, treatment, and prognosis, to the degree known.
- The opportunity to participate in decisions involving your healthcare.
- Competent, caring healthcare providers who act as your advocates.
- Know the identity and professional status of individuals providing service.
- Adequate education regarding self-care at home written in language you can understand.
- Make decisions about medical care, including the right to accept or refuse medical or surgical treatment and the right to initiate advance directives such as a living will or durable power of attorney. If you already have a living will or other directive or you wish to initiate one, please speak with a nurse.
- Information concerning implementation of any advance care directive.
- Impartial access to treatment regardless of race, color, sex, national origin, religion, handicap, or disability.
- Receive an itemized bill for all services.
- Report any comments concerning the quality of services provided to you during the time spent at the facility and receive fair follow-up on your comments.
- Know about any business relationships among the facility, healthcare providers, and others that might influence your care or treatment.

As a Patient, You Are Responsible for

- Providing, to the best of your knowledge, accurate and complete information about your present health status and past medical history and reporting any unexpected changes to the appropriate practitioner(s).
- Following the treatment plan recommended by the primary practitioner involved in your case.
- Providing an adult to transport you home after surgery and an adult to be responsible for you at home for the first 24 hours after surgery.
- Indicating whether you clearly understand a contemplated course of action and what is expected of you and ask questions when you need further information.
- Your actions if you refuse treatment, leave the facility against the advice of the practitioner, and/or do not follow the practitioner's instructions relating to your care.
- Ensuring that the financial obligations of your healthcare are fulfilled as expediently as possible.
- Providing information about and/or copies of any living will, power of attorney, or other directive that you desire us to know about.

plexion of ambulatory surgery changes. Ambulatory surgery patients challenge nurses to assess, plan, implement, and evaluate care on many levels. The patient's clinical, emotional, social, and educational needs must be considered concurrently.

The nurse shares the responsibility for evaluating and addressing patient needs with many members of the healthcare team. In fact, a team approach—interaction among physicians, certified registered nurse anesthetists, nurses, families, and patients—is vital to the success of the ambulatory process. Mutual trust and overlap of responsibilities exist among team members in most successful programs.

ELEMENTS OF A SUCCESSFUL PROGRAM

Many elements contribute to the ultimate success of any ambulatory surgery program. Especially important are patient and procedure selection, patient and family education, adequate home support, appropriate anesthesia technique, careful staff selection, and constant reinforcement of the wellness philosophy in a climate of caring concern. Nurses play a central role in each of these elements and are, therefore, fundamental to the program's quality and success.

Patient and Procedure Selection

Patient and procedure selection begins in the surgeon's office. The surgeon, the anesthesiologist, and sometimes other physician consultants primarily evaluate the patient's physical condition and tolerance for surgery and anesthesia. The patient's medical status must allow for adequate protection against the insult of surgery and anesthesia. Conversely, the healthcare provided must support the patient's physical condition absolutely and constantly.

Sicker and older patients are being cared for in the ambulatory setting in increasing numbers. Although these systemically sick patients face potential hazards, they may have one small advantage over some healthier people: more incentive to take care of themselves properly after returning home. Often, sick patients receive more intensive medical care after surgery because they see their own primary physicians frequently.

Contraindications to being considered for an ambulatory setting might include a poor or missing support system in the home or an educational or intelligence level that precludes the understanding of proper self-care. Emotional or mental conditions that may cause undue fear or panic for the patient (or frighten other patients in an ambulatory surgery unit) might make hospital admission advisable, especially if security or safety of patients or others is a factor. A person who has a high probability of requiring more extensive surgery than is undertaken in the ambulatory setting should be screened well before the decision is made for ambulatory care. Nurses are in an ideal position to assess and communicate many of these and other patient characteristics.

The procedure must lend itself to early patient discharge. With current economic pressures, improved technology, and constant changes in the attitudes and understanding of healthcare professionals, more and more complicated and invasive procedures are being performed on an ambulatory basis. Examples include cholecystectomy, vaginal hysterectomy, thyroidectomy, simple mastectomy, and percutaneous suction discectomy. For a particular procedure to be appropriate for an individual, however, the patient must be considered emotionally and intellectually as well as physically. Also, each surgeon's technical and supportive skills should be taken into account, as well as both the physician's and the patient's past histories of postoperative complications.

Although selection is the physician's responsibility, the ambulatory surgical nurse also has a mechanism for input on issues regarding both procedure and patient selection. The nurse often provides surgeons and anesthesiologists with information that is important to selection. An in-depth preoperative nursing interview, best accomplished before the day of surgery, provides an opportunity for both social and physical assessment.

Many patients feel hesitant to "take the doctor's time" to discuss an issue that may seem insignificant, or they may forget to mention a clinically valuable symptom or bit of history. The nurse often takes time to elicit more detail and presents patients with a demeanor that encourages discussion of what might be considered minor complaints or symptoms. The ambulatory surgical nurse who uncovers data that may have an effect on the decision to proceed with or cancel a particular surgery is responsible for communicating that information to physicians responsible for that patient.

Although all of these factors affect the selection process, third party payers, namely the U.S. government and private insurers, affect the selection process more than any other force. This requires healthcare providers to respond to the needs of many patients who may, in fact, be poor candidates for early discharge but who are placed in that situation by the reimbursement process.

Patient and Family Education

Patient and family education plays a key role in the patient's successful, uncomplicated recuperation. Without proper instruction, the family and the patient may be uninformed about the physical needs and restrictions involved both before and after a particular surgical procedure. Furthermore, they may not even realize their need for more information. They may feel uneasy asking what they consider simple or inconsequential questions, so it is the nurse's role not only to educate but also to objectively assess their learning needs. While defining preoperative and aftercare instructions and explaining the patient's and family's delegated responsibilities, the nurse must assess each learner's level of understanding and alter the teaching plan accordingly. The nurse should provide a nonjudgmental atmosphere to help patients and family feel comfortable asking any questions. Nurses should not belittle any information needs that are expressed.

The need for written instructions to accompany verbal information is paramount both before and after surgery. By supplying written directions, the nurse provides the patient with a reliable reference for later use. Before surgery, patients' anxiety levels may be competing with their attention to instructions and their ability to comprehend and retain the information being provided. After surgery, the insightful postanesthesia nurse understands that patients may seem wide awake and alert during postoperative teaching sessions, although the effects of barbiturates, sedatives, and narcotics often erase that period from patients' memories. The need to provide written instructions and to include family or support persons in the instruction process in that setting is obvious.

Ensuring an Adequate Home Support System

Reliable adult support at home should be available during the patient's surgical course, particularly for intervention in the event of complications after discharge. This support system may be a family member, friend, or a healthcare professional who is engaged by the patient for a specific period to provide care. The patient and members of the family should feel confident to handle the recuperation period at home. They must all understand that a person recuperating from anesthesia should not be left unattended after returning home on the day of surgery.

By providing personalized preoperative counseling before the day of surgery, the nurse contributes to the patient's and family's confidence, helps decrease anxiety, and helps eliminate unfounded fears and false expectations. Certainly, the adult patient has the ultimate responsibility for establishing the necessary support for home and transportation needs. However, the whole team—physician, patient, family or friends, and nurse—must work together to ensure the availability of an appropriate support system.

Preparation of the physical home environment also helps pave the way for a smooth preoperative and postoperative course. This involves having the right equipment, supplies, and medication available; providing a safe, comfortable, and clean environment; and ensuring that appropriate food and beverages are available. Sometimes the home may not be well suited to the patient's immediate postoperative needs, and modifications or an alternate plan should be instituted. Predicting and addressing these types of issues are vital to an uncomplicated recovery.

After surgery, some people may need a level of supervised medical attention in the time between hospitalization and discharge to home. Reasons for this may include an inadequate support system, a complex or lengthy surgical procedure, actual or high potential for complications, prior poor physical and emotional health, prior untoward experience with surgery, and family, physician, or patient preference.

Medical hotels, home health nursing care, overnight stays at the physician's office, 23-hour admission programs, and surgical recovery care centers are examples of systems that offer an intermediate level of care. Some facilities have established the concept of a phase III recovery area for patients who likely will be discharged within a few more hours but who require a place to rest for a slightly extended period of observation after surgery. If a person comes to an ambulatory surgery facility on the day of surgery without having established any responsible adult as a support system, surgery is often postponed if an adequate alternative cannot be established or until postoperative hospitalization can be approved.

Influencing Anesthesia Technique

Anesthesia technique is a variable that is usually beyond the nurse's direct control but is rarely beyond the nurse's influence. The nurse's documentation, suggestions, and attention to the postanesthesia patient's responses enable the anesthesia department to obtain clear information on which decisions about techniques and drugs used for ambulatory surgical procedures are based.

The trend toward less or no preoperative medication tests the nurse's professional abilities to provide reassurance and emotional support to patients and to reduce patient anxiety by use of relaxation techniques and other nursing interventions. An anesthesia and surgical team attempts to provide a postoperative course with a low incidence of pain, somnolence, nausea, and vomiting. Nursing measures in the perioperative period should complement the anesthetic approach and should be aimed at promoting readiness for discharge without complications.

Promoting a Philosophy of Wellness

During the past few decades in the United States, the concepts of disease prevention and promotion of health and fitness have emerged as major foci. The trend is for people to accept more personal responsibility for their state of health. Within this climate, the concept of ambulatory surgery has found fertile ground for growth and for increasing public acceptance. Mass-media education has provided the public with a broader awareness of health-related issues and, to some degree, sophistication regarding their expectations of the healthcare industry.

Increasing numbers of people now expect and demand to be part of the decisions that affect their health. In some cases, physician–patient relationships have taken on the flavor of partnerships. Marketing plans that promote ambulatory surgery programs are designed to increase public awareness of the benefits of the service and confidence in the process. In turn, this awareness has further added to the public's involvement in personal healthcare decisions.

Supporting a climate of wellness is certainly part of this philosophy of patient involvement and responsibility. This concept is a major element of the success of the ambulatory surgery process. In all avenues of healthcare, nurses should be attuned to patients' needs for encouragement and positive reinforcement. A person undergoing an ambulatory surgical procedure has a priority need for a positive mental outlook and for self-confidence to meet the demands of self-care at home.

Today, the healthcare profession has come to expect patients to assume more and more responsibility for their own care. In the past, the message given to patients was that "you are sick and you need us to take care of you." Now ambulatory surgery patients are asked to believe a totally different concept: that the postoperative patient is not sick and, except for a few minor limitations, often can resume normal daily activities soon after anesthesia and surgery are completed. It is quite a different message.

Communication, home-like surroundings, physical care, and attitude all have an effect on how patients perceive their condition, progress, and state of wellness. Helping patients feel confident that a procedure will not be incapacitating is sometimes a challenge, particularly with the person who has a chronically negative outlook or an overprotective family member. By constant reinforcement of wellness, not illness, the nurse helps that patient realize that a good measure of self-care is possible. Nursing skills are further displayed by the ability to encourage and foster self-care without belittling the patient's symptoms or nurturing needs.

Wellness can be promoted both by words and actions. Choosing terminology that reflects wellness promotes the goals for discharge readiness and a sense of well-being. Subtle actions, such as allowing patients who are physically able to dress themselves, tie their own shoes, make their own telephone calls for transportation, or get their own beverages all encourage a sense of normalcy.

Sometimes, convincing doting family members to allow patients to do things independently is more challenging. Just like the nurse, the family needs to be helpful, caring, and loving. Doing as much as possible for their loved one seems like a good way to express those intentions. The nurse should tactfully emphasize the family's role in wellness reinforcement as a very positive measure to encourage the patient's healthy attitude and actual recuperation.

Another concept that the nurse should understand and use to foster a sense of wellness is the powerful effect of the patient's self-concept on behavior and personality. Self-concept determines how people think of themselves, and it can influence their future behavior and that of others. Although ASC nurses cannot alter the patient's innate self-image, they can promote the patient's positive sense of self through affirmative and supportive comments and through unconditional acceptance of the patient as a valuable person.

The nurse also attempts to positively influence the patient's attitude, sense of responsibility for self-care, and response to the demands of ambulatory surgery. One way that this influence on behavior can be fostered is through a phenomenon called *self-fulfilling prophecy*, which occurs when a person's expectation of an event makes the outcome more likely to occur than would otherwise have been true.[13] For instance, a close friend told a man that the friend's arthroscopic knee surgery had been very painful. As you might imagine, the man was frightened before his own surgery and afterward complained more than usual of pain, even though his knee had been injected with bupivacaine at the end of the procedure.

Conversely, consider a child whose mother repeatedly described the anesthesiologist as a nice, happy man who would smile a lot. That child came to expect a kind person and willingly talked with him during a pleasant induction. The nurse can purposefully use the power of self-fulfilling prophecy for a positive outcome by taking the time to explain procedures well and by indicating by both verbal and nonverbal means that an ambulatory surgical process will be pleasant and uncomplicated.

Self-fulfilling prophecy is promoted when the expectations of one person govern another's actions. Consider the nurse who ends an explanation of crutch-walking technique to a man by smiling, nodding affirmatively, and saying, "You should do very well with crutch walking. Men have strong arms and shoulders, and that is a real asset for crutch walking." This nurse has set the stage for the patient to expect success from himself. To a woman, that same nurse might point out, "Women do very well with crutch walking. They tend to be cautious and take small, manageable steps, so I expect that you should do very well." The nurse has not lied to either the man or the woman but has merely found an honest reason for each to feel confident and positive.

Compare those approaches with that of the nurse who frowns and explains, "Most people take several days or more before they are able to use crutches well" or "I know crutches are hard to use, but you probably won't need them for very long." Both of these statements may be true, but the negative tone can have a subtle influence on the patient's attitude and ability to effectively use crutches. The nurse's words and body language are powerful tools in the patient's arsenal for recuperation.

SELECTION OF NURSING STAFF MEMBERS

Selection of nursing staff members is another avenue that significantly affects the quality of the ambulatory surgical process. Choosing well-prepared nurses with appropriate education, skills, and experience is essential, but with those qualities being equal among all candidates for a position, it makes sense for the manager to select the nurse who is able to quickly establish rapport with patients and others. This is especially true because time for personal interactions and making a good impression is at a premium in the ambulatory surgery setting.

A warm, outgoing, caring, animated, and happy demeanor is often what a manager seeks. The patient and family sense the attitudes of nurses as quickly as they notice nurses' skills and abilities. A positive attitude on the part of patients, which is so important to the ambulatory surgery process, is enhanced when patients meet and interact with nursing and medical staff members who genuinely care about the patient, the family, and the success of the surgery.

The manner in which nurses care for a patient's dignity, emotions, and feelings is the subject of many more compliments or complaints on postdischarge evaluations than is the patient's perception of the physical care that was received. Not only does it make ethical and moral sense to hire the nurse who shows a true concern and respect for patients and the facility, it also makes financial and business sense. Pleasant, caring nurses are the ambulatory unit's best marketing tools.

As in other busy departments, nurses in the ASC also should be able to interact pleasantly with other nurses, physicians, business and administrative personnel, and other health professionals. Well-developed time management skills are essential in ASCs, which are usually very busy departments with greatly fluctuating caseloads. Especially during times of peak volume, nurses should work well together toward a common goal of safe and efficient patient care.

To promote maximum efficiency of the department as a whole, each nurse should be willing to work in any area of need as long as that nurse is competent and has been appropriately oriented in that department. Nurses in freestanding centers have the added challenge of having no other nursing or ancillary departments to call on during emergencies. Each must have complete confidence in the dependability and the assistance of other nurses in the center.

Like most nursing settings, the ambulatory surgery unit requires nurses who are concerned with details: nurses who assess, plan, act, and reassess with vigilance. Innumerable details must be coordinated both within the facility and in the patient's home setting. Anything less than total attention to such details could lead to incomplete patient preparation before surgery, delay or cancellation of surgery, and lack of a proper support system for the postoperative period. Nurses who care about, and take action to correct, deficiencies in the patient's care plan may find themselves addressing many issues, such as missing diagnostic reports, the patient's incomplete understanding of the surgical procedure, special positioning needs for arthritic or poorly mobile patients, and special emotional support for a person suffering with depression.

Because postoperative and postanesthetic complications can have much more serious effects when they occur in the home setting, the nurse must meticulously assess, direct, and evaluate every parameter of the nursing care provided within the ASC. What the nurse does or does not notice, teach, act on, report, or intervene about greatly affects patient outcome. Caring about every aspect of the process is intrinsic to the ambulatory surgical nursing concept.

Patient and staff selection, patient education, home preparations, anesthesia care, and wellness issues are all avenues to the ultimate goal of expeditious and complication-free recovery. Nurses are instrumental in all phases of the patient's ambulatory surgical experience and should be carefully selected for the setting. When all these variables are considered, the result is a successful process that ensures patient safety, compliance, and satisfaction.

References

1. Aquavella J: Ambulatory surgery in the 1990s. J Ambul Care Manage 13:21–24, 1990.

2. Davis J: History of major ambulatory surgery. In Davis J (ed): Major Ambulatory Surgery. Baltimore: Williams & Wilkins, 1986, pp 3–31.
3. Nicoll J: The surgery of infancy. Proceedings of the 77th Annual Meeting of the British Medical Association. BMJ 2:753, 1909.
4. Ries E: Some radical changes in the after-treatment of celiotomy cases. JAMA 33:454, 1899.
5. New surgical technologies reshape hospital strategies. Hospitals 66:30–36, 40–42, 1992.
6. Adler S, Bryk E, Cesta T, et al: Collaboration: The solution to multidisciplinary care planning. Orthop Nurs 14:21–29, 1995.
7. Scoggin J: Innovation for the 90s and beyond. Apothecary 101:9–15, 1989.
8. Kozak L, Hall M, Pokras R, et al: Ambulatory surgery in the United States, 1994. In Advance Data. US Department of Health and Human Services, Centers for Disease Control and Prevention, National Center for Health Statistics, No. 283, March 14, 1997.
9. Freestanding Outpatient Surgery Centers Market Report, 1998 Edition. Chicago: SMG Marketing Group, 1998.
10. Accreditation Handbook. Chicago, IL: Joint Commission on Accreditation of Healthcare Organizations, 1998.
11. Caldwell L: Surgical outpatient concerns: What every perioperative nurse should know. AORN J, 53:761–767, 1991.
12. Burden N: The keys to success: The ambulatory approach. Breathline 7:11–12, 1987.
13. Adler R, Towne N: Looking Out/Looking In, 3rd ed. New York: Holt, Rinehart & Winston, 1981, pp 77–81.

Chapter 2

Business Aspects, Program Development, and Marketing

Donna M. DeFazio Quinn

The ambulatory surgical environment has seen many changes in the past few years. Previously, ambulatory surgery centers (ASCs) were associated with performance of simple, outpatient surgical procedures. The impact of managed care and the decrease in financial reimbursement have fostered the growth and development of the ASC. Today, numerous surgical procedures are performed in ASCs, whereas in the past, it was unheard of for some of these to be performed in an outpatient setting.

The development of recovery care centers (RCCs) in some states has allowed patients to undergo laparoscopic cholecystectomy, vaginal hysterectomy, and even total joint replacement in the ASC. The aesthetic environment and the casual setting of the ASC allow the patient to recover overnight in a more comfortable and less threatening environment than the hospital setting.

Managed care companies have forced providers to perform surgical procedures in the most cost-effective and efficient setting. ASCs can fill this need. The number of surgical procedures performed on an outpatient basis continues to grow each year. By continuing to perfect the service they deliver to patients and physicians, ASCs may soon be the norm rather than the exception for providing outpatient surgical services.

TYPES OF FACILITIES

Ambulatory surgery centers can be referred to in many ways: outpatient surgery centers, freestanding surgery centers, same-day surgery centers or units, ambulatory surgery units, one-day surgery centers, and various other titles. For the purpose of consistency, they are referred to as ASCs in this chapter.

There are many types of ASCs. They can be hospital based, freestanding, incorporated into the physician's office, associated with a health clinic, separate from the hospital but attached in some manner, and even mobile. The ASC may even have an RCC associated with it. This addition allows surgical procedures to be performed in the ASC and patients to recover overnight in the RCC.

Over the past decade, there has been a steady increase in the growth of ASCs, as the need to contain cost has become more urgent. The push from managed care companies to control costs by decreasing reimbursement to providers led healthcare managers to develop alternative means to deliver quality services at a lower cost. The 1990s saw a steady increase in the construction of new ASCs as leaders realized that methods to reduce cost would be the key to financial survival in the future.

BUSINESS STRUCTURES

The business structure of the ASC can be either not-for-profit or for-profit. Regardless of the structure that is implemented, it should ensure appropriate use of resources to deliver quality care while maintaining cost efficiency.

In the not-for-profit model, the facility may be hospital affiliated or privately owned. The ASC may be freestanding; located within a hospital, clinic, or physician's office; or even mobile. In order to be successful in the not-for-profit model, it is essential that resource consumption be carefully monitored. All too often in the hospital setting, management of resources takes a back seat. When compared with the freestanding model, the hospital-based ASC is generally not as efficient. This is in part due to the location of the facility within the hospital. Team members may have difficulty incorporating the freestanding ASC mindset into their everyday practice. Also, the fact that ASC processes must flow through the hospital system can affect efficiency. Another factor may be that hospital ASC managers may not have access to detailed financial data. If managers are not aware of actual cost as compared with reimbursement, they may be unaware that the department is losing money on certain procedures. Staff members, too, need to be aware of cost. All too often, this information is not shared with the team members who can best seek out ways to contain cost.

In the freestanding ASC environment, team members have the ability to develop processes that work well without getting caught up in the complexities of hospital processes. Here is a simple example. If an instrument tray needs to be processed, the operating room nurse or technician in the freestanding ASC decontaminates and reprocesses it. The operating room staff does not need to wait for someone from central processing to come to the operating room, take the instrument tray to central processing, decontaminate it, reprocess it, and return it to the operating room. The freestanding center is able to process the tray in a more efficient manner. On the other hand, hospital-based ASCs have more ready access to resources such as infection control and risk management specialists and high-level technology such as more innovative sterilizing equipment.

For-profit centers have expertise in providing quality service in a cost-effective manner. These centers have cultivated delivering service that meets or exceeds patients' expectations while keeping cost under control. In a for-profit model, every team member is aware of how cost affects the bottom line. Although it is difficult for some practitioners to look at the delivery of healthcare as a business, this mindset is essential to success.

Whether working in a not-for-profit or a for-profit model, team members need to ensure that they are performing their duties in a cost-efficient manner. All managers need to focus on allocation of resources to ensure that the facility receives the best "bang for their buck." With reimbursement steadily declining, the only avenue to financial success is to keep costs under control.

OWNERSHIP STRUCTURE

Hospital Owned

In the hospital environment, the ASC can be either a hospital department or a separate entity within the hospital system. Many hospitals have ASCs that function simply as a hospital department. They may be managed separately or be under the direction of the operating room, postanesthesia care unit (PACU), or surgical service director. Some ASCs also process patients who are planned admissions. In this setting, the patients are processed through the system in the same manner as outpatients, but after recovery in the PACU, they are admitted to hospital beds. The impact of managed care on cost containment has led to this process being used in many hospitals—no longer do physicians have the luxury of admitting patients to the hospital the day before surgery.

One scenario that still exists in some hospitals today is the integration of the ASC into the existing operating room and PACU environment. This allows for the hospital to use the same resources to treat both inpatients and outpatients. Advantages and disadvantages of this system are discussed later.

Another variation of a hospital-owned model is the freestanding ASC. Hospitals have realized that they are in competition with freestanding ASCs that have emerged across the country. In an effort to gain back lost market share, many hospitals have established their own freestanding ASCs.

These ASCs can have many variations, one of which is being directly attached to the hospital with a separate entrance. Another variation is to be located off campus. The hospital may choose to place the center in close proximity to the hospital, thereby making it easily accessible for surgeons who may be performing cases on both inpatients and outpatients. Another scenario is to place the center across town, in a rural setting, or in the vicinity of a competitor. By doing this, the hospital is attempting to gain market share by making it easy for patients to access the system and offering a choice to patients who otherwise would have none.

The freestanding ASC may also house many different services. The hospital may choose to put physician offices in the building. This space is then leased or purchased by physicians. This is an especially attractive option for ASCs located in a rural location. The hospital may choose to lease the office space to the physician on a full-time or part-time basis. The part-time option is good for specialty physicians who may choose to travel to the center only once or twice a month. The surgeon may choose to operate in the morning at the ASC and use the office space in the afternoon to follow up on previous patients and to see new patients.

Other possible services that may be established in an outpatient center in conjunction with the ASC include the following:

- Radiology
- Laboratory
- Endoscopy
- Pain management clinic
- Pharmacy
- Physical therapy and occupational health services
- Women's health or breast diagnostic center
- Patient education library or a community education center
- Alternative therapy center

Other services are possible, depending on the needs of the community. When development of these services is considered, it is necessary to ensure that local, state, and federal laws are followed.

Joint Ventures

The ASC structure allows participants the ability to participate in a joint venture. One likely possibility in a joint venture may be a group of physicians working with the hospital to form an ASC. The ASC is usually freestanding, although it may be attached to the hospital or placed directly within the hospital.

Establishing the structure of the joint venture can be a truly creative process. Numerous options exist. Possible structures for a joint venture include formation of partnership arrangements or establishment of a corporation. In addition, the joint venture can be established based simply on a lease or a contract arrangement.

A partnership is formed when a group of individuals come together and contribute financially (e.g., in the form of cash, property) to form a business, specifically, an ASC. The partners then share in the profits or losses associated with running the business. For tax purposes under this arrangement, the partnership files a tax return showing total profit or loss. In addition, each individual partner must show his or her distributive share of the partnership when filing individual federal income tax returns.

Establishing a corporation is another means of joint venturing. Under this structure, a group of individuals come together to form the ASC. The association conducts business and distributes profits or losses in much the same manner as the partnership. There are many different types of corporations, such as the C corporation, which is taxed as a separate entity, and the S corporation, in which the shareholders themselves are taxed. The advantage of the S corporation is that it allows the ASC to function in the corporate form, but the business income is taxed on the individual level. One difference to be aware of when establishing the business is that the S corporation has a limit of 35 shareholders, whereas the partnership has no limit.

The limited liability company is a new form of business that has been accepted in many states. The limited liability company has the characteristics of a corporation but works like a partnership in assessing profit and loss. For the purposes of federal income tax, the limited liability company is classified as a partnership.

When determining the possible structure of the ASC, it is important to consider liability and tax consequences. Also of concern are the control and governance of the joint venture, legal issues, antitrust laws, securities law, and reimbursement issues. It is important that these issues be worked out in advance in order to avoid later conflict. Experienced legal counsel should be retained to ensure proper guidance throughout the process.

Physician Owned

In addition to the previously named structures, the ASC can also be owned entirely by physicians. The established structure can take on many different configurations, such as partnership and corporation. It can also be viewed as an extension of the physician's office practice. This is especially common in the specialties of plastic surgery and ophthalmology, in which the physician performs surgery as an extension of the office practice.

Corporate Owned

A corporation may own the ASC. There are regional and national corporations across the country that own a number of ASCs. The ASC that is owned and managed by a corporation does have some advantages. The corporation may place an administrator on-site to be responsible for the day-to-day operations of the center or may have one administrator oversee a number of centers in a geographic area. In addition, a corporation can assist in designing, licensing, procuring supplies and equipment, and hiring qualified staff.

Privately Owned

Some ASCs may be privately owned. Business entrepreneurs may become involved in the ASC as an investment. In these situations, the owner is usually not involved in the day-to-day management of the center. Privately owned centers usually operate as for-profit entities.

ADVANTAGES AND DISADVANTAGES OF OWNERSHIP STRUCTURES

There are advantages and disadvantages to the different structures of ASCs and it is impossible to make a general rule about which situation is best for any given facility. Administrative leaders must evaluate their short-term and long-term goals, strategic plans, the individual facility, and the community at large to decide which scenario would work best for them. Someone experienced in the ASC arena should perform a detailed feasibility study. Until all data are carefully analyzed, it is impossible to predict which situation would be most advantageous.

Hospital-Based Ambulatory Surgery Center—Self-Contained

If the hospital-based ASC is separate from the main operating rooms but still part of the hospital, there are numerous advantages and disadvantages. The biggest advantage of being part of the hospital system is the immediate access to hospital emergency services. Should a situation develop that requires immediate emergency assistance, such assistance is readily available. In addition, if the ASC were to have equipment failure or immediately need a specific supply, the main operating room could be called on to fill this request.

Physicians also appreciate the fact that they can be in close proximity to their inpatients. In the hospital setting, they are able to make rounds, attend to emergencies, visit radiology to review films, and so on. If a patient should need an immediate consultation with a cardiologist or the primary care physician before the administration of anesthesia, the chances of this happening quickly are much better in the hospital setting than in the remote freestanding ASC.

The hospital-based ASC also offers the physician the option of performing a surgical procedure that may result in the patient's being unable to go home, in which case the patient can be easily admitted for an overnight stay. In an attempt to decrease cost, facilities are no longer admitting patients scheduled to undergo complicated surgical procedures the day before surgery. Instead, these patients are processed through the ASC unit much the same as outpatients are.

Reimbursement for services performed in the hospital setting is also not as challenging as it is in the freestanding center. The Medicare restrictions that apply to the freestanding center do not apply in the hospital-based ASC. Hospital facilities are able to perform the more complicated procedures, such as laparoscopic cholecystectomy and vaginal hysterectomy, which are not approved by Medicare to be performed in the freestanding ASC. This situation may soon change because Medicare has proposed implementation of an ambulatory payment classification (APC) system sometime in the year 2000. This plan will make Medicare reimbursement in the freestanding ASCs and the hospital-based ASCs more equitable.

Even though hospital-based centers have many advantages, they also have disadvantages. In the hospital-based ASC, duplicate services are offered. Operating rooms, equipment, and skilled personnel are employed in both the main operating room and the ambulatory center. This duplication of services requires a high capital investment. In the hospital-based ASC, efficiency may still not be as high as in a freestanding center. The overall mindset of employees is still that of a hospital setting. Managers must also abide by the hospital bureaucracy in order to get things done.

Patients do not perceive the hospital ASC to be any different than the hospital itself. Although the ASC may be providing services only to outpatients, it still operates in the hospital mode. Patients may still have difficulty finding a parking space. They may also have to walk through a maze of corridors to find the ASC.

Some hospitals are dealing with this by implementing valet parking and escort services so that patients can make their way through the system without difficulty.

The efficiencies of a freestanding center may not be seen in the hospital ASC. As previously described, the process of decontaminating and resterilizing an equipment tray may be more costly in the hospital setting because of the hospital protocols. Only when the process itself is changed to that of the freestanding ASC will the hospital ASC gain in efficiency.

Cost may be another disadvantage. In the hospital setting, the ASC is allocated overhead costs. Revenue-generating departments like the ASC are usually carrying the load for non–revenue-generating departments (e.g., administration, medical records, finance). This dollar amount can be significant enough to have a great impact on profit.

Hospital-Based Ambulatory Surgery Center—Integrated

Many of the advantages and disadvantages of hospital-based ASCs can be applied to the ASC that is integrated with the main operating room. In addition, an advantage of the integrated ASC is the decreased capital cost. There is no duplication of equipment and personnel. One distinct disadvantage in an integrated system is that there is a greater chance that the operating room schedule will be disrupted for add-on emergency cases. This can result in outpatients being delayed. Surgeons may also be dissatisfied with having their schedules disrupted. The mix of inpatient and outpatient cases does not allow the room to function as adeptly as it could in an all-outpatient setting. Staff members often have difficulty providing quick turnover times, again, because of the issues inherent in hospital operating room processes.

From a patient perspective, the integrated system may cause increased anxiety. Patients undergoing major surgical procedures are recovered in the same PACU as outpatients undergoing minor procedures. The exposure to the critical patients, as well as the potential loss of privacy in the PACU environment, may leave the outpatient dissatisfied with the entire surgical experience.

Freestanding Ambulatory Surgery Center

The freestanding ASC has many advantages. From the patient's perspective, it is not like going to a hospital—the environment is more pleasing and less threatening. This is especially beneficial if the ASC has a pediatric patient population. Freestanding ASCs can usually offer curbside parking, which is particularly helpful if the patient population is elderly.

The freestanding ASC is usually physician oriented. ASC staff members understand that physicians are the driving forces behind the business. In order to ensure their continued support, ASC leaders have developed methods to meet physicians' needs. To make the most of their time, physicians do not want to wait for the operating room to be prepared between cases. ASCs have been able to master rapid turnover time and gain physicians' approval and allegiance.

Many ASCs encourage physicians to participate in the development and planning of the ASC. Involvement can range from deciding what services to provide to determining what instrumentation and equipment to purchase. The level of involvement depends on the management of each center. This is not to say that this type of structure cannot be established in the hospital-based ASC; however, hospital bureaucracy often prevents accomplishing tasks as quickly and efficiently as they can be accomplished in the freestanding ASC.

Ambulatory surgery centers have been able to master the process of cost containment. By analyzing cost, they have been able to implement practices to decrease the cost of providing a service without having an impact on quality. In an ASC in which there is strong team involvement, staff members frequently work together to identify and implement ideas for cost containment opportunities.

The freestanding environment does not incur the high overhead cost frequently associated with the hospital setting. The ASC is not having to cover services of non–revenue-generating departments. The freestanding ASC also has the ability to shut down for the day when cases are finished. This saves on electricity, labor, and other costs.

In any highly specialized ASC in which there is a high volume of a specific specialty or procedure, staff members become very proficient at what they do. They provide the service in the most cost-efficient manner possible. In addition, because of the expertise gained through repetition, the turnover time is very quick. The staff members are well trained to anticipate and proactively respond to the surgeon's needs, be it an instrument, suture, specialized patient positioning, or other issue.

The freestanding ASC that has no ties to the hospital has the ability to accept or reject cases based on reimbursement. These centers are under no obligation to perform procedures that they know will lose money. For centers that operate in this fashion but participate with federally funded programs, such as Medicare and Medicaid, it is recommended that legal counsel be retained to ensure that the center is not inadvertently violating any laws or regulations.

An advantage to the pricing structure used in the ASC is that there is one fee for the service provided. It does not matter how many supplies are used or how long the procedure takes—the price remains the same. This can be a great marketing tool. In today's environment of patient co-payments, it is much better from the patient's perspective to pay 20% of a preset fee of $1500, for example, rather than 20% of a hospital charge that may end up being twice that amount. In the hospital setting, the cost is calculated based on charging for all supplies used to perform the procedure, the length of time the patient was in the operating room, as well as time spent in the PACU. When totaled, this cost can be significant.

The freestanding ASC is often more flexible in responding to requests for a new piece of equipment or a special supply. Consensus for (or against) purchasing can usually be obtained in a short period of time, as opposed to waiting for a predetermined annual time frame for requesting capital purchases. Also, approval from numerous levels within the organization is not necessary. By expeditiously filling the request, the ASC again gains respect from the physician.

There are disadvantages to operating a freestanding ASC. The number one disadvantage is the start-up cost and the cost of capital. If the ASC is affiliated with the hospital, the development of the freestanding ASC can be viewed as a total duplication of services. The advantage of having a freestanding ASC needs to be looked at from not only a financial perspective but also from a strategic perspective.

If the ASC is multispecialty, there may not be a sufficient volume of cases for the staff members to become proficient in performing the service. In addition, some supplies are used infrequently and remain in inventory. Expiration dates on products then become a concern.

The freestanding ASC does not have the luxury of relying on the hospital in times of need. For example, in emergency situations, the patient needs to be stabilized and then transported by ambulance to the nearest hospital. Although most freestanding ASCs focus great attention on the emergency preparedness of personnel and equipment, some patients may perceive the freestanding center to be unequipped to handle an emergency. Although emergency preparations are paramount in all ASC settings, freestanding ASC staff members have less actual opportunity than their hospital-based counterparts to implement real-life initiatives because of the types of patients and procedures found in the two settings.

The freestanding ASC may not be equipped to perform all possible ambulatory procedures. The procurement of specialized equipment for each surgical specialty is a big investment. The ASC may not make the investment until it is sure that the surgeons are committed to performing the cases in the ASC.

Additionally, the ASC may not schedule certain diagnostic surgical procedures that may result in the need to perform more extensive surgery. An example would be a diagnostic laparoscopy that is very likely to require an open incision for removal of a tumor. Although multispecialty ASCs have the basic instrumentation to respond to more aggressive operative interventions, highly specialized equipment, such as vascular and neurologic instruments, may not be available, and the staff may not be up-to-date or practiced on more complex or intricate procedures.

In addition, the ASC may not have the ability to keep the patient overnight. Because of this, procedures that tend to be performed in the ASC are often the shorter, more predictable cases that do not require increased surgical intervention. Thus, the reimbursement that could be gained from performing more complex procedures cannot be realized in most ASCs.

Physicians in the community need to be queried as to their intended support of a freestanding ASC. There may be reluctance on the part of certain surgeons to utilize the ASC, especially if it is established as a competitor to the hospital. Most hospital systems provide a public referral service to help people find and make appointments with physicians on staff; thus, a change in physician allegiance can jeopardize that referral source. The political environment is one that should be carefully investigated before the venture is pursued.

One option that may exist for both the hospital-based and the freestanding ASC is the development of an RCC. The advantage of the RCC is that it allows the facility to perform more complex surgical procedures, knowing that the patient can be admitted to the recovery facility overnight. By performing more complex procedures, facilities can recoup higher reimbursement. Local, state, and federal laws should be investigated to determine whether the RCC is allowed. In addition, individual insurance companies should be queried regarding reimbursement for services for which the patient stays overnight. Prior planning and investigating eliminate potential denial of charges by the insurance companies.

Physician's Office

The physician's office setting is usually equipped to handle minor procedures only, although some office practices include an operating room suite. This resource is common with specialty practices, such as ophthalmology and plastic surgery.

Advantages of the extended physician's office are as follows. The physicians are able to set their own schedule; thus, access to the operating room is not a problem. In addition, the office personnel are familiar with the patient, helping to decrease patient anxiety before the procedure and helping to provide for continuity of care. Depending on the specialty, start-up cost may or may not be an issue. By having the operating room as an extension of the office, the physician is able to capture increased revenue by billing for the facility fee as well as the professional fee.

Although the option of performing surgery in the office may be attractive, there are disadvantages. Staffing is a concern. Who will be responsible for preoperative and postoperative patient care and how will that affect the flow of patients coming for office visits? Will anesthesia coverage be sought or will existing staff provide adequate support for the physician for monitoring and sedation?

High on the list of disadvantages is the lack of emergency back-up. Physicians planning to perform surgery as an extension of their office need to consider how to handle emergency situations. All personnel should be trained in at least basic cardiopulmonary resuscitation, and advanced cardiac life support training is strongly recommended. Even with such training, the infrequency of using those skills makes for a setting in which office personnel may not feel comfortable or proficient in identifying or responding to a medical emergency.

Also of concern in the office setting is the issue of reimbursement. With the numerous constraints imposed by the managed care companies, authorization should be obtained before a procedure is performed to ensure that the service will be reimbursed. Additionally, it is essential that the physician's office secure contracts with the numerous payers in the marketplace. Such agreements enable the physician to perform the procedure in the office, eliminate the need for the physician to perform the procedure in the facility dictated by the insurance plan, and offer the patient a choice in where the procedure is performed.

In summary, in the decision of which type of ASC should be developed, there is no absolute right or wrong answer. Each facility must analyze the advantages and disadvantages of the different structures and decide what would work best. Leaders need to think not only of the business aspects of the center but also of the physician, community, and political environment as well. Exploration of all options and potential consequences assists leaders in making sound business decisions that result in a successful venture.

UNDERSTANDING MANAGED CARE

In the current healthcare environment, it is essential to have an understanding of managed care. In a managed care environment, access to healthcare is controlled by the insurance company (i.e., the managed care company). By controlling access to care, the managed care company can control cost, and this control in turn is passed on to consumers in the form of lower premiums.

In the past, many individuals were insured under indemnity plans. An example of an indemnity plan would be a traditional "Blue Cross" or "Aetna" policy that allowed the patient to go to any provider, and the insurance company would cover the charges. Today, we see very few individuals who are covered by indemnity insurance plans, because of their high cost.

In the 1980s, the trend moved toward putting some of the responsibility for healthcare coverage on the consumer (patient). To avoid high premiums, the consumer was asked to contribute a portion of dollars that would be applied toward their coverage. If the consumer agreed, the premiums for coverage would be lower, thus, the start of managed care plans. Although each plan differs, the typical scenario is for the patient to pay a co-payment for each office visit. In addition, the patient might also be responsible for a deductible, which is the amount of money the patient must pay out-of-pocket before the managed care company begins to pay.

Deductibles typically range from $100 to $500 per member per year.

With the institution of this new plan came the implementation of "primary caregivers" (also called primary care physicians or practitioners, or gatekeepers). Under this process, the primary care physician is the individual who directs all care for the patient. If the patient needs to see a specialist, the primary care physician must first authorize the visit. If the patient chooses to see the specialist without such authorization, the visit is not covered by the managed care company, and the patient is responsible for all charges incurred. Again, by controlling the patient's access to care, the managed care company can control the cost.

Another method of controlling cost is for the managed care company to network with providers. The managed care company sets out to negotiate with providers, such as hospitals and ASCs, that agree to provide service at a discounted rate to the individuals (members) enrolled in the managed care plan. A contract that sets forth the terms of the agreement is established between the managed care company and the provider.

Understanding managed care also involves understanding the concept of capitation. For instance, in a capitated environment, the managed care company contracts with a facility to provide all outpatient surgical services for its members. The contracted hospital or ASC provides all outpatient surgical services to the members of the plan in exchange for a set amount of money. The money received by the ASC (paid out by the managed care company) is usually expressed in units "per member per month." For example, the ASC may subcontract to provide all outpatient surgical services for all members enrolled in the plan for an amount of $1.00 per member per month. If the plan has 10,000 members, the ASC receives $10,000 per month in exchange for providing all outpatient surgical services needed for patients enrolled in the plan. The facility must decide if it wants to accept this risk, knowing that in some months, expenses for providing service may exceed $10,000 (thus, money is lost) and in some months expenses may be less (thereby profit is gained).

In the ASC, the best scenario in a capitated environment would be an operating room schedule with no patients. The ASC would collect the money, but no members would require service. The impetus in a capitated environment is to keep the members healthy. This is why in America today we have seen a push toward staying healthy. Wellness programs are offered to reduce weight, stop smoking, and reduce stress. In addition, some managed care companies and third party payers now pay for alternative health treatments, such as meditation and yoga.

A capitated environment can also include "carve outs." A carve out can be a specific category of health care that is not covered as a benefit within a contract; thus, it is carved out of the pricing structure. Usually, these are high-cost items or situations requiring special expertise, such as organ transplants and psychiatric services.

The "alphabet soup" of today's medical insurance climate makes it difficult for consumers to make an educated choice of plans and for facilities to contract to provide services simply. Some of the various medical initiatives are described in Table 2–1.

Although the focus is primarily on managed care companies, there are still patients who have private insurance. Although ASCs do not deal with nearly as many private insurance companies as they did in the past, patients still present with private coverage. The ASC may or may not have a contract with the insurance company. If no contract exists, the insurance company pays the entire charge (minus deductibles or copayments, if they exist). In an environment of shrinking reimbursement, patients presenting with private insurance are highly desirable.

The deluge of managed care has significantly affected reimbursement to ASCs. Because of the managed care companies' decreasing reimbursement and controlling access to services, both freestanding and hospital-based ASCs are in a vulnerable situation. If the ASC hopes to survive in the future, emphasis must be placed on cost containment because higher revenues from insurance companies or government health plans are unlikely.

FINANCIAL CONSIDERATIONS

The overall financial picture of health care is changing daily, and what used to be the norm a year ago is no longer true. Facilities are facing new challenges that are forcing them to be more cost effective and cost efficient. The major push of cost containment has been brought on because of reimbursement issues.

To understand reimbursement, it is essential to review how outpatient surgery is usually paid. First let us consider federal payments by Medicare. In the hospital setting, outpatient surgery charges for Medicare patients are paid by use of a complicated formula that includes the actual

Table 2–1. Managed Care Terminology

GENERAL TERMS	
Managed Care (MC) Also known as *Coordinated Care, Managed Care Plan, Alternative Delivery System*	A system of healthcare delivery in which access to service is controlled, usually by a primary care physician. Control over access attempts to ensure that services provided are necessary and that cost containment measures are employed. The term managed care can also refer to a number of healthcare arrangements including health maintenance organizations, managed indemnity plans, preferred provider organizations, and point-of-service plans. Managed care companies also establish contractual relationships directly with employers (employees become members of the managed care plan) and providers (hospitals, ambulatory surgery centers (ASCs), and so on contract directly with the managed care plan to provide service to the plan's members).
Health Maintenance Organization (HMO)	This is an organization that is responsible for managing the healthcare services of a designated population in a specific geographic location. Responsibilities include both the financial aspect as well as the delivery of care. Individuals voluntarily enroll in the organization. The enrollees pay a fixed dollar amount regardless of the services used. The emphasis of an HMO is on preventive care. Services are usually provided in facilities owned by the HMO. In a staff model program, physicians are paid a salary for treating patients, thereby eliminating the financial incentive to provide unnecessary care. Primary care physicians are used as gatekeepers to control services.
Third Party Payer	This is the party responsible for paying the patient's medical bills. It can be an insurance company, a managed care organization, a self-insured employer, or the federal government.
Provider	The provider is the person or organization that provides service to the patient. Providers include physicians, surgeons, hospitals, ambulatory surgery centers, physical therapists, and pharmacies.
Network	A network is the term used by managed care plans to delineate when a contractual arrangement exists between the managed care company and the provider of the service. When physicians, hospitals, ASCs, and so on contract with the managed care company, they are considered "in the network." Patients are expected to receive services by providers in the network. Patients who choose to receive services by providers not in the network may be responsible for all charges incurred.
Primary Care Physician (PCP) Also known as *Primary Care Practitioner, Primary Care Provider, Primary Care Network, Gatekeeper*	The PCP is responsible for coordinating the care of the plan member. The PCP can be a general practitioner, internist, family practitioner, pediatrician, obstetrician/gynecologist, nurse practitioner, or physician's assistant. Access to specialists and specialized treatment procedures is controlled by the PCP. Failure to obtain prior approval from the PCP before obtaining specialized care can result in the member's paying for the service out of pocket.
Gatekeeper Also known as *Primary Care Physician*	This is the primary care physician that is responsible for managing the care of the patient. The gatekeeper can also be referred to as the case manager or the referral source.
Preferred Provider Organization (PPO)	In this type of arrangement, the managed care plan negotiates with independent providers (e.g., physicians, hospitals) to provide services to the managed care plan members at a discounted fee. Patients maintain the right to select the provider of their choice, but financial incentives, e.g., lower co-payments or deductibles, entice the patient to use participating providers.
Physician-Hospital Organization (PHO)	Refers to an entity formed by hospitals and physicians. The entity negotiates contracts with third party payers to provide services under managed care. In a PHO arrangement, physicians usually maintain ownership of their practice but agree to accept managed care patients according to the terms of the negotiated PHO contract. The PHO may also be involved in the management of the facilities where services are provided.
Point-of-Service (POS) Plan	Under managed care, a POS plan allows members to choose where and how they would like to receive service. The member may choose to receive service from a participating provider, or the member may choose to go out of network. If the member goes out of network, benefit coverage is reduced, and the patient is responsible for a certain percentage of the charge.
Participating Provider Also known as *Preferred Provider*	A participating provider is one who has negotiated a contract with a managed care company or insurance company to provide health service to the plan members. The provider can be the physician, hospital, ASC, and so on.
Capitation	Capitation is a system in which the managed care company or third party payer prepays the provider a certain negotiated dollar amount to provide healthcare services to the plan's members. The dollar amount is usually paid on a per member per month basis. The provider receives the preset negotiated dollar amount, regardless of services provided. If the provider delivers services that cost less than the dollar amount received, it makes money. If the provider provides services that cost more than the dollar amount received, the provider loses money. The incentive in a capitated arrangement is to keep the plan members healthy so as to provide as little service as possible.

Table continued on following page

Table 2–1. Managed Care Terminology *Continued*

Carve Out	In a capitated arrangement, certain high-cost or specialty services may be carved out of the negotiated contract. An example of such services would be mental health services, cardiac surgery, or dental services. Payment for these services may be negotiated separately.
Risk	In the past, the traditional insurance carrier (indemnity plan, commercial insurance) assumed the total financial risk for the defined population it served. In a managed care system, the financial risk is redistributed to the provider in the form of financial liability for excessive and unnecessary care.
Risk Sharing	Risk sharing occurs when the financial risk for any specific disease process is distributed among the physician, the hospital, and the insurer. Risk sharing usually occurs in capitated arrangements.
Full-Risk Capitation	In a full-risk capitation arrangement, the provider agrees to accept the full financial risk of managing and providing healthcare service to the managed care plan members.
Per Member Per Month (PMPM)	This is the unit of volume used by managed care companies to measure its members. In a capitated arrangement, providers are usually paid a certain dollar amount per member per month to provide necessary service to the plan members.
Case Management	This is a system used by managed care plans and third party payers to assess, plan, refer, and follow up on patients. The goal of case management is to manage the delivery of high-cost services while ensuring delivery of quality care. Case management ensures the provision of comprehensive and continuous service so that payment and reimbursement can be coordinated for the services provided. A case manager is the professional assigned to review the patient's care and to coordinate the services needed. The case manager ensures that the services are medically necessary and are being provided in a cost-efficient manner.
Utilization Review Also known as *Utilization Management*	This is a system used by managed care plans that involves a series of techniques or processes to review and control the patient's use of medical services and the provider's use of medical resources. Some techniques used include second opinions, preadmission certification, and discharge planning. The goal is to reduce inappropriate and unnecessary care.
INSURANCE TERMS	
Commercial Insurance Also known as *Indemnity Insurance* *Fee-for-Service Insurance*	Commerical insurance refers to the traditional insurance coverage whereby the plan pays for the expense incurred, regardless of where the service is provided.
Indemnity Insurance Also known as *Fee-for-Service (FFS)* *Commercial Insurance*	When a patient has indemnity or commercial insurance, the insurance plan pays for expenses incurred, regardless of who provided the service. The patient retains the choice of seeing the provider of his or her choice. The insurance company pays either the insured individual or the provider.
Medicare	A federally funded insurance program that is part of Social Security. Medicare is specifically intended for individuals older than 65 years or disabled individuals younger than 65 years. Medicare consists of two parts. Medicare part A covers the cost of hospitalization and care after discharge from the hospital. All individuals covered by Medicare receive this benefit. Medicare part B is a supplemental insurance program that covers the cost of outpatient services, e.g., laboratory testing, outpatient surgery, and physician expenses. Individuals must pay a monthly premium to receive Medicare part B coverage. Covered services are then paid at 80% of the approved charges, leaving the 20% balance to be paid by the patient.
Medicaid	Medicaid is a federally funded insurance program that provides medical coverage to low-income individuals who meet eligibility criteria.
Workers' Compensation	Workers' compensation is generally administered by the individual state. When a worker receives an injury or illness while on duty (work-related injury), the employer is responsible for the cost of treatment. Employers are turning to managed care companies (HMOs) to treat employee injury and illnesses in order to better manage healthcare costs.
Intermediary	An intermediary may be a private company, e.g., an insurance company who is not involved in the provision of health services to the patient but acts as the intermediary to pay claims to providers and to collect premiums from patients. For example: XYZ Insurance Company of New York may be the intermediary for the payment of Medicare claims in the state of New York.
Medigap Insurance Also known as *Medicare Supplement* *Secondary Coverage*	Individuals eligible for Medicare coverage may elect to also purchase private health insurance to supplement for services that may not be covered by Medicare. For example, Medicare pays 80% of the allowable amount for a covered procedure. The patient is responsible for the remaining 20%. If the patient has private insurance, the 20% balance is paid by the private insurance.

Table 2–1. Managed Care Terminology *Continued*

Term	Definition
Secondary Insurance	Some individuals are covered by two or more insurance plans. When this occurs, there must be coordination of benefits to ensure that payment to providers is not duplicated. One insurance is established as the primary insurance, and the other(s) are secondary. Procedures are billed to the primary insurance company first. If a balance remains after payment is received from the primary insurance, it can be transferred to the secondary insurance. Frequently, documentation must be provided to the secondary insurance to ensure duplication of payment does not occur.
Co-Insurance Also known as *Out-of-Pocket Expense* *Cost Sharing* *First Dollar Coverage*	The patient (insured individual) is responsible for a certain percentage of the charges incurred. The typical co-insurance arrangement is 20/80, whereby the patient is responsible for 20% of the charges and the insurance plan for 80% of charges. Usually, in a co-insurance arrangement, there is no minimum deductible amount that the patient must pay before services are covered. Co-insurance plans generally start with first dollar coverage.
Deductible Also known as *Co-Payment*	The deductible is the amount of money the patient has to pay before the insurance plan becomes effective. Generally, the insurance plan requires the patient to meet the deductible amount each year. Some insurance plans combine deductibles with co-insurance. For example, the patient is responsible for the first $500 of expenses incurred (the deductible); the insurance plan then pays 80% of the expenses incurred and the patient is responsible for the remaining 20%.
Co-Payment Also known as *Co-Pay* *Out-of-Pocket Payments*	The insurance plan requires the patient to pay a specific dollar amount to the provider at the time of service. A typical co-payment amount is $5.00.
Charges Also known as *Fee*	The charge or fee is the dollar amount that the provider is owed for services rendered. In the ASC, the charge is the total amount due for providing surgical care to the patient. The charge owed to the ASC is usually discounted by the insurance plan. Reimbursement to the ASC can also be based on a predetermined fee schedule.
Discount Also known as *Discounted Charge* *Discounted Fee*	A discount is the amount of money the provider agrees to reduce its billed charges by. The discount can be percentage based, whereby the provider agrees to discount or reduce the billed charge by a certain percentage amount. The discount can also be based on a predetermined fee schedule. The provider and the third party payer establish and agree to the predetermined discount during contract negotiations. This discount may also be referred to as the contractual amount or the contractual allowance.
Preadmission Certification Also known as *Pre-Cert Authorization*	This is a utilization management procedure used by managed care organizations to control admission to the hospital or ASC. Preadmission certification is performed before the patient's admission (for nonemergency services) and involves obtaining approval from the managed care plan that the proposed services (surgery) will be paid for by the plan before the services (surgery) are performed.
Preauthorization Also known as *Authorization*	This is a utilization management technique used by managed care organizations. The primary care physician must authorize or give approval for services such as referral to a specialist for surgery.
Referral	A referral is the recommendation from the primary care physician that allows the patient to be treated by a physician other than the primary care physician. The referral can be to a specialist, a surgeon, and so on. The referral must be obtained in order for the services provided to be covered. Failing to obtain a referral may result in the patient having to pay for the services out of pocket.

cost of providing the service plus a blended rate based on the individual hospital's cost reports to Medicare. In the freestanding ambulatory surgery setting, payment from Medicare for services is based on a predetermined reimbursement rate for the procedure. This reimbursement is inclusive of all services and supplies that are provided by the center and includes the operating room and postanesthesia care unit fees as well as all supplies and equipment needed to perform the procedure. Reimbursement is not adjusted based on supplies used, although there are rare opportunities to receive supplemental Medicare reimbursement for specific high-cost supplies, such as certain implants and pain management pumps. In these scenarios, the invoice for the actual purchase of the device must be linked to the patient receiving it and provided to Medicare.

The pre-established charge is the same for everyone and all payers. This does not mean that the facility cannot decrease the charge by offering a discount; discount arrangements are the nature of the business. What it does mean is that the facility cannot increase the fee depending on the payer. Under no condition can the ASC charge less to any other payer than it charges Medicare.

It is no surprise that reimbursement to ASCs by third party payers will continue to steadily decline. To understand this, we need to look at how other payers reimburse the ASC. Reimbursement to the ASC can be accomplished in many ways. *Fee for service* occurs when the facility receives from the insurance company the exact amount it charges for performing the procedure. This type of payment is usually rendered when the ASC cares for a patient who has private insurance coverage. Typically, the company is not in a local network.

In the *percentage discount* scenario, the facility receives a certain percentage of its charge. The percentage discount is negotiated with the individual insurance companies. In the past, it was common for the facility and a payer to negotiate a contract for reimbursement that was amicable to all involved. These contracts usually involved the insurance company's reimbursing the facility based on a discount percentage. For example, the insurance company would pay 90% of the charges incurred to care for the patient. The facility discounted the bill 10%, thereby writing off the amount as a contractual allowance. By contracting with a payer, the facility stands to gain increased volume because patients subscribing to the insurance company are directed to the facility. This example represents what was happening in the industry in the early to mid-1990s.

More commonly, reimbursement is occurring through *fee schedules*. In this situation, a fee schedule is developed for the procedures that are normally performed at the facility. Fees may be individualized based on the different procedures performed, or they may be placed into groupings. Normally, the groupings mirror the fee schedule developed by Medicare. Each procedure is assigned to a group, and each group is paid at a predetermined rate.

Medicare uses eight different groupings to reimburse ASCs. A current procedural terminology (CPT) code is assigned to each procedure that can be performed. This is a method that provides uniform language to all healthcare workers nationwide. Each possible Medicare-approved procedure that can be performed in the ASC is assigned to one of the eight groupings, and a dollar amount is attached to each group. Medicare reimburses the facility 80% of the approved amount for a procedure based on the assigned group. The patient, or a secondary insurance if the patient has secondary coverage, is then billed for the remaining 20% of the approved amount.

For example, the CPT code 66984 is described as "extracapsular cataract removal with insertion of intraocular lens prosthesis (one-stage procedure), manual or mechanical technique (e.g., irrigation and aspiration or phacoemulsification)."[1] This CPT code is classified as a group 8. If the Medicare-approved amount for this group is $960, Medicare would reimburse the ASC 80%, or $768. The patient or secondary insurance would then be responsible for the remaining 20%, or $192. The standard ASC charge for the procedure may be $1500, but if the facility participates with Medicare, they must accept the approved amount. To further clarify, with the standard charge of $1500 being used as an example, the facility receives only $960 in total. The remaining $540 is written off to a contractual allowance, also called a *revenue deduction*. Some markets are so highly penetrated by managed care that revenue deductions amount to 58% to 60% of the ASC's charges.

By law, the facility cannot bill the Medicare patient for any amount exceeding the Medicare-approved rate, nor can it waive the patient's 20% co-payment. After the patient is billed appropriately, there may be situations in which patients do not have the financial ability to pay the 20% co-payment. At that point, existing standards and policies that are applicable to all patients, not just Medicare patients, can be applied to determine whether a charity deduction is allowed. Federal regulations must be clearly understood and followed to avoid unintentional fraudulent practices.

Not all procedures that can be performed in the ASC are approved by Medicare, and it is especially critical to understand this when accepting bookings. At the time the procedure is being scheduled, the ASC needs to determine who will be responsible for the bill. If Medicare is the primary insurance and Medicare does not approve the procedure, the ASC then needs to decide if they will accept the booking knowing that Medicare will not reimburse for the procedure and the patient will be responsible for paying the charge. By law, this information must be communicated to the patient before the procedure, preferably well in advance of the surgery day. Based on the procedure being performed, the ASC may require the patient to pay for the procedure up-front, rather than being billed after the procedure. This is especially common when cosmetic or elective procedures are being performed.

Many insurance companies have now moved toward replicating the Medicare reimbursement system. Instead of the percentage discounts off of charges offered in the past, they have changed their system of payment to providers to mirror the Medicare system. They offer to pay a percentage of the approved Medicare fee schedule. For example, the insurance company may offer to pay 1.5 times the approved Medicare rate for the procedure. If a procedure was approved by Medicare for group 1 at a rate of $320, for example, the insurance company would pay 1.5 times the rate, or $480 for the procedure.

When dealing with an insurance company that is offering this type of reimbursement contract, it is imperative to examine the agreement closely. Questions to consider include the following:

- Does the contract place all the procedures in the same groupings as Medicare or do they make their own groupings?
- What will be done about procedures that are not covered by Medicare? Are they covered in this contract, and if so, in what grouping do they fall?
- Is the insurance company willing to cover the cost of excessive supplies, such as implants and venous access devices?
- What if 1.5 times the approved amount exceeds the ASC's standard charge for the procedure? Does the ASC receive 1.5 times the amount or is the rate adjusted downward to the ASC's charge?

Placing the facility's historical volume data in a spreadsheet and running potential reimbursement scenarios assist in the negotiation of successful contracts. An added benefit is derived if cost data can also be included in the equation so that the profit or loss per case can be identified. The last thing the ASC needs to do is to sign a contract in which the facility loses money on the cases it performs. Having analyzed the data closely, the ASC administrator should be able to negotiate the reimbursement contract more wisely.

The current trend in many managed care companies is not only to shift to a "Medicare-like" reimbursement system, but some managed care companies are even offering contracts that are paying less than the Medicare-approved rate. The ASC must decide whether the competition is such that refusing the contract would be a worse alternative than accepting it. How long can ASCs survive in an environment of shrinking payments?

A new financial challenge is also at hand. ASCs must now position themselves to deal with the impact of ambulatory payment classifications. APCs are the government's way of dealing with the high cost of healthcare. The Balanced Budget Act of 1997 mandated that the Health Care Financing Administration move from a cost-based reimbursement system for hospital outpatient services to a prospective payment system. In addition, the freestanding ASCs would also follow the APC system. With this change, it is speculated that Medicare will change from the current system of eight groupings to more than 200 groupings. In short, APCs can be likened to the implementation of diagnostic related groups in the early 1980s.

To prepare for this change in reimbursement from Medicare, ASCs need to have good control of their costs. Again, facilities will no longer be able to perform procedures in which they are not reimbursed sufficiently to cover their cost. Although the implementation of APCs affects only Medicare reimbursement, ASCs should prepare for the worst. It will only be a matter of time before third party payers shift to an APC-like reimbursement system.

The biggest challenge ASCs face in the reimbursement arena is keeping track of the different contracts. ASCs need to have a system in place in which they can easily identify when they are being reimbursed correctly for procedures. With so many contracts to keep track of, it is essential that ASCs have a computerized information system to handle not only billing and accounts receivable but also all other aspects of the ASC. Information systems are available that encompass scheduling, registration, billing, accounts receivable, inventory, and general ledger. For ASCs using all components of the system, case costing is also possible. The ability to access this valuable information is extremely worthwhile. In the long run, it will assist managers in making important decisions, such as limiting nonprofitable cases and marketing highly profitable ones.

SURVIVAL IN THE FUTURE

Cost Containment in the Clinical Setting

In order to survive the future, ASCs must know their actual costs. This will be the key to success. ASCs can no longer rely on increases in reimbursement or volume, especially as we move toward a capitated environment. Therefore, the main focus should be on methods to contain and reduce cost. Even though cost containment strategies are a priority, quality should not be sacrificed.

The first step that managers need to take is to identify how much it costs to perform each specific procedure. Although it is possible to perform this calculation by hand, a computer program specifically designed for the ASC setting is best. Variable and fixed costs should be considered. Variable costs include supplies and staff salaries and benefits. Fixed costs include things that will exist whether cases are performed or not, for instance, utility bills, contractual payments for housekeeping and risk management services, leases, depreciation costs of capital equipment, and administrative overhead costs. Table 2–2 provides a template for examining the variable costs of a particular procedure. This example includes supplies and salaries associated with the procedure as well as fixed costs. Once managers know the total cost of performing each procedure, they are better prepared to negotiate realistic reimbursement rates with third party payers.

The manager should perform a number of calculations. When examining cost per case, it is also necessary to equate cost to volume. If the procedure is high cost but low volume, is it worth putting effort into reducing the cost right now? Are there other procedures that are more crucial to address? The manager should start by looking at the high-cost, high-volume procedures and focus attention on reducing the cost of these procedures.

The manager should also perform calculations that relate supply cost to surgical minutes. How much does the ASC spend on supplies for each minute of operating room time? This information can be obtained by dividing the total cost of supplies for a given period of time by the total number of operating room minutes for the same time period. For example, the ASC spent $1 million on supplies in 1998. Operating room minutes totaled 240,000. This equates to spending $4.17 on supplies for every minute the operating room has a patient in it. By plotting this information out on a month-by-month basis, managers can benchmark to determine whether the suggestions implemented for cost containment are having a positive impact on supply cost. The team may set a goal of $4.00 per minute and work diligently to reach it.

Managers must be prepared to deal with failure. Circumstances beyond anyone's control can affect whether the goal is reached. This needs to be taken into consideration and explained before a number is posted that negatively affects the goal. Explaining the cause of the variance is necessary to keep team members enthusiastic about the project. If the supply cost is increased because the ASC performed 50 more cases than projected, this is good. It also explains the reason for the variance. Conversely, if volume was significantly less than expected and costs significantly exceeded projections, a problem exists. It would be beneficial to brainstorm with staff members to identify the cause or causes.

The best approach to tackling cost containment issues is to set up a multidisciplinary team consisting of everyone involved in providing care to the patient. Team members should include registered nurses, surgical technicians, and representatives from the following departments: anesthesia, surgery, purchasing, business office, and administration. The first step is to educate everyone involved in the process:

- Explain why it is important to decrease cost.
- Use storyboards, staff meetings, graphs, and other tools to explain the effects of managed care on reimbursement.
- Present data on the cost of procedures and supplies and discuss how cutting cost is the key to survival in the future.
- After the team members have had a chance to absorb the data, brainstorm as to what exactly the focus of the group will be. Maybe it was identified that orthopedic procedures are high volume and high cost, or maybe the cost of sterile gloves has been identified as an issue. Whatever the issue, be sure that the correct team members are present.
- If physician representation from a particular specialty is needed, get a surgeon from that specialty to sit on the team.

All team members need to be apprised of the ground rules. Everyone has the right to express his or her opinion and no one is allowed to interrupt or criticize someone else's suggestion. The team should brainstorm all possible alternatives to decreasing the cost of the issue at hand. Once this is done, perform a SWOT (*s*trengths, *w*eaknesses, *o*pportunities, and *t*hreats of each suggestion) analysis for each suggestion. Although tedious and time consuming, this exercise allows thorough consideration of each suggestion.

Once strategies to decrease cost are identified, all health team members affected by the change need to be informed. A carefully considered communication plan is essential to the suc-

Table 2–2. Introduction to Case Costing

The following information is provided to assist the manager in determining the total cost of providing service for a specific procedure. Many methods can be used to determine case costing. The manager needs to identify which method of case costing works best for the facility. Information systems are also available that assist in determining the cost of performing a specific procedure.

Although time consuming and detail oriented, the method presented provides a step-by-step guideline for determining the total cost of performing a specific procedure. In order to accurately perform the calculations, detailed historical data, generally the previous fiscal years' financial records, are necessary.

The information presented represents an example of a fictitious surgery center. The activities, staffing levels, and specific financial details must be individualized for accurate information to be obtained.

STEP ONE
IDENTIFY COST PER OPERATING ROOM MINUTE

	Variable Cost per Salary and Wage Worksheet	
A.	Fiscal year (FY) 1998 clinical salary & wages	420,196
B.	Earned time, worker's compensation, and employment taxes	93,820
C.	Benefit expense	48,050
D.	Total variable workload cost per year	562,066
E.	Divided by 52 wk/yr to get weekly cost	10,809
F.	Weekly cost divided by weekly clinical hours* (see below)	520
G.	Total variable cost per hour	20.79
H.	Divided by 60 minutes = **total variable cost per minute**	**0.3465**
	Fixed Cost per Salary and Wage Worksheet	
I.	Fiscal year (FY) 1998 administrative salary & wages	164,076
J.	Earned time, worker's compensation, and employment taxes	35,762
K.	Benefit expense	33,052
L.	Total fixed workload cost per year	232,890
M.	Divided by 52 wk/yr to get weekly cost	4479
N.	Weekly cost divided by weekly administrative hours†	216
O.	Total fixed cost per hour	20.7361
P.	Divided by 60 minutes = **total fixed cost per minute**	**0.3456**

1. The following steps are used to identify the cost per operating room minute. This requires historical data, e.g., the previous fiscal year's information.
2. Identify the total cost of clinical salary & wages for the fiscal year ($420,196).
3. Identify the total cost of earned time, worker's compensation, and employment taxes paid for the fiscal year ($93,820).
4. Identify total cost of benefits for clinical staff ($48,050).
5. Total lines A, B, and C to get total variable workload cost per year ($562,066).
6. Divide by 52 (weeks in a year) to get weekly cost (line E, $10,809).
7. Calculate weekly clinical hours. Refer to chart at end of table. Identify all clinical staff and total the hours they are scheduled to work each week. Document on line F (520 hr/wk).
8. Divide weekly cost (line E, $10,809) by weekly clinical hours (line F, 520) to get total variable cost per hour ($20.79).
9. Divide total variable cost per hour ($20.79) by 60 (minutes) to get total variable cost per minute ($0.3465).
10. The total variable cost per minute ($0.3465) will be used later in calculating cost.
11. Repeat the above process using the administrative staff salary and wage information.

STEP TWO
CALCULATE FIXED COST ALLOCATIONS

	Task	*Minutes*
A.	Make preoperative phone call (interview)	10
B.	Presurgical preparation (interview patient, obtain vital signs, answer questions)	20
C.	Pick instruments and supplies for case	10
D.	Set up case in operating room	10
E.	Clean operating room between cases (2 staff members × 10 minutes)	20
F.	Make postoperative phone call	10
G.	Wash, sort, and wrap instrumentation	10
H.	Allowance for personal time, fatigue, and delay	27
I.	**Total minutes**	**117**

1. Identify tasks that are performed for each patient but are fixed in terms of the time required to perform the task.
2. Identify the total average number of minutes required to perform the task.
3. Total the number of minutes required to perform clinical tasks (117 minutes).
4. This fixed cost allocation number will be used in step nine to calculate the cost per case.

Table continued on following page

***Table 2–2.* Introduction to Case Costing** *Continued*

STEP THREE
CALCULATE FIXED OVERHEAD COST ALLOCATION

A.	Calculate annual fixed overhead cost: Includes line items such as rent expense, real estate tax, electricity, waste disposal, license and dues, subscriptions and publications, telephone, janitorial expenses, service contracts, marketing, postage, linen, audit fees, medical director fees, home office fees, travel and education, insurance, bad debt provision, and answer service fees (number can be calculated based on previous year's historical data).	553,218
B.	Divide annual fixed overhead cost by projected annual operating room minutes (total minutes can be calculated based on previous year's historical data).	861,922
C.	**Fixed overhead cost allocation (per minute)**	**0.6418**

1. Refer to department budget to identify the annual fixed cost.
2. Identify line items that are fixed—bills that must be paid regardless of the number of surgical cases performed. Refer to line A for examples.
3. After identifying all fixed items, add them to obtain a total annual fixed overhead cost ($553,218).
4. Identify the total annual operating room minutes. Historical data (previous fiscal year's actual minutes) can be used (861,922).
5. Divide total annual operating room minutes (line A, $553,218) by total annual fixed overhead cost (line B, 861,922) to obtain fixed overhead cost allocation per minute (line C, 0.6418).
6. This calculation will be used in step nine to calculate cost per case.

STEP FOUR
CALCULATE FIXED WORKLOAD STAFFING

	Staffing	***Hours***
A.	Director	1860
B.	Administrative supervisor	1860
C.	Billing clerk	1860
D.	Accounts payable clerk	1860
E.	Receptionists	2604
F.	Clinical leader	1860
G.	**Total hours**	**11,904**

1. Identify fixed staffing positions and total hours per year (52 weeks × 40 hr/wk = 2080 hr/yr; minus allowance for vacation, holidays, education, and meetings = 1860 productive hours per year). Two part-time positions account for the receptionists' 2604 hr/yr.
2. Add all hours to obtain total hours of fixed staff (line G).
3. This calculation will be used in step five to calculate fixed workload activities.

cess of the project. If team members feel that they were not informed, the chance of success will diminish.

- Who needs to know about the change?
- Does the change need to be communicated to the physicians?
- How will they find out about it?
- When will the change be implemented?
- Should some individuals be informed in person, or will a memo suffice?
- How does the change affect service?
- Is this a permanent change or just a trial?
- If the person affected has a complaint, who is it communicated to?
- When will the change be evaluated as to its success?

Taking the time to think through and answer questions like these assists in developing a communication plan that works. Including storyboards, graphs, and charts in the communication plan is also helpful.

Once the plan has been implemented, progress must be monitored. Putting up graphs depicting savings is one way to tout accomplishments. Including team members' names is also a way to recognize those individuals who participated in the project.

Regardless of the strategies for cost reduction that are implemented, it is equally important to assign accountability. If a team member takes on the issue of consolidating supplies to the use of one cost-effective brand of sterile gloves, everyone needs to know that this team member is responsible for the project. All communication should flow through the designated cham-

***Table 2–2.* Introduction to Case Costing** *Continued*

STEP FIVE
CALCULATE FIXED WORKLOAD ACTIVITIES

	Activities	*Hours*
A.	Staff meetings: 24/year × 1.5 hours × 20 staff members	720
B.	Education: 8 hours per year × 20 staff members	160
C.	Transporter services to main hospital 2 hr/day × 5 day/wk	520
D.	Purchasing: 16 hr/wk	832
E.	Data entry (preference cards, changes): 10 hr/wk	520
F.	Quality management activities: 16 hr/wk	832
G.	Restocking OR rooms/PACU with supplies 16 hr/wk	832
H.	Autoclaves Daily testing, loading, unloading (2.08 hr/wk)	108
I.	Ultrasonic cleaner/Cidex maintenance 45 min/wk (0.75 hr/wk)	39
J.	Linen: 10 min/day (0.83 hr/wk)	43
K.	Fixed workload hours per year (activities)	4606
L.	Fixed workload hours per year (staffing) from step four, line G	11,904
M.	**Fixed workload hours per year (total)**	**16,510**
N.	Fixed workload hours per day (divide by 250 work days per year)	66.04
O.	Total fixed workload hours per case (divide by average number of cases per day). To obtain average number of cases per day, divide total cases per year by 250 work days per year (3250 cases per year divided by 250 work days per year equals 13 cases per day). (66.04 hours per day divided by 13 cases per day equals 5.08 fixed workload hours per case.)	5.08
P.	**Fixed Workload Cost** = total fixed workload hours per day (5.03) times total fixed cost per hour (20.79) from step one, line G	**105.61**

1. Identify all activities that support the clinical operations. Identify average time associated with each activity. Place total yearly hours in "Hours" column.
2. Add all activities to obtain total fixed workload activities per year (K).
3. Add total fixed workload activities (K) and total fixed workload staff (step four, line G) to obtain total fixed workload hours per year (M).
4. Divide total fixed workload hours per year (M) by 250 (total work days per year) to obtain total fixed workload hours per day (N).
5. Divide total fixed workload hours per day (N) by the average number of cases per day to obtain total fixed workload hours per case (O). To obtain average cases per day, divide total yearly cases by 250 days.
6. To obtain the fixed workload cost per case, multiply the total fixed workload hours per case (line O, 5.08 hours) times the total fixed cost per hour ($20.7361) from step one, line G. This number will be used in step nine, to calculate cost per case.

STEP SIX
CALCULATE AVERAGE MINUTES PER CASE

1. Select procedure code to be evaluated, e.g., repair inguinal hernia (CPT 49505).
2. Count total number of cases performed in 1-year period, e.g., 74 cases (CPT 49505).
3. Identify total operating minutes for each case and total. Divide total by 74 to get average minutes per case, e.g., total minutes for 74 cases equals 4736 minutes.
4. Divide 4736 minutes by 74 cases to get an average of **64 operating room minutes per case.** This information will be used in step nine to calculate cost per case.
5. Identify total PACU minutes for each case (CPT 49505) and total.
6. Divide by 74 to get the average PACU minutes per case, e.g., total PACU for 74 cases equals 5550.
7. Divide 5550 by 74 cases to get the average of **75 PACU minutes per case.** This information will be used in step nine to calculate cost per case.

Table continued on following page

pion of the project. Assigning accountability helps avoid confusion in the long run.

The ability of staff members to identify potential cost savings needs to be encouraged. Managers should share financial data regarding the ASC with staff members. Only when staff members are aware of the cost can they truly realize the big picture. This does not mean that the ASC's financial books are open for viewing. Managers can customize information that will assist team members in understanding the business. For example, making a pie chart (Fig. 2–1)

Table 2–2. Introduction to Case Costing *Continued*

STEP SEVEN
CALCULATE SUPPLY COSTS

Procedure Supply Costs (CPT 49505)

1. Identify each item used for procedure (a standard preference card for CPT 49505 can be used to calculate supply cost).
2. Calculate the cost of each individual supply identified on the preference card. **NOTE:** Preference card should accurately identify the supplies being used.
3. Total all supplies to obtain procedure supply cost.

Example	*Cost*
Sodium chloride irrigation solution	$ 1.04
Tegaderm	1.31
Lap sponge	2.42
Steri-Strip	1.39
Benzoin	0.57
Surgical gown—large	2.73
Surgical gown—X-large	2.94
Suture—J285G	5.74
Prep tray	3.95
Suture—Y426H	5.21
Light handle cover	1.26
Needle counter	0.97
Lap sheet	10.00
Grounding pad	2.98
Grounding pen	2.54
Basic pack	7.97
Penrose drain	0.74
Suture J338H × 2 ($2.33)	4.66
Gloves	2.74
Gloves	2.55
Blade scalpel	0.43
Total supply cost	**$64.14** This information will be used in step nine to calculate the cost per case.

Anesthesia Supply Costs (based on historical data)

1. Identify total anesthesia supply costs for fiscal year (budget line items that can be used include oxygen expenses, anesthesia gases, anesthetic agents, and so on).
2. Divide by total cases performed during year.
   Example: total supply costs for fiscal year = $112,740.
   Total cases performed in fiscal year = 3000.
   Total anesthesia supply cost = $37.58 per case.
   This information will be used in step nine to calculate cost per case.

NOTE: Alternative method: the process utilized to identify the "procedure supply list" above can be used to calculate the anesthesia supply cost. The process requires that all anesthesia supplies used for the procedure be identified. Follow the steps as identified in the "procedure supply cost" method listed above.

STEP EIGHT
CALCULATE AVERAGE CONTRACTUAL ALLOWANCE PER CASE

1. Identify total contractual allowances for fiscal year (total amount written off due to contractual arrangements). Historical data such as the previous fiscal year's actual data can be used.

2. Divide total contractual allowances by total cases performed in fiscal year to obtain average contractual allowance per case.

Example:
Total contractual allowances for fiscal year equals $650,078.
Total cases performed equals 3000.
Average contractual allowance per case equals $216.69.
This information will be used in step nine to calculate cost per case.

Table 2–2. Introduction to Case Costing *Continued*

STEP NINE
CALCULATE COST PER CASE
REPAIR INGUINAL HERNIA (CPT 49505)

	Description	*Minutes*	*Cost*
A.	Average minutes per case (step 6, line 4)	64	
B.	Fixed cost for OR based on time (step 2, line I) (includes preoperative phone call, preoperative interview, picking instruments and supplies, set up case in OR, clean room between cases, postoperative phone call, decontamination and sterilizing of instrumentation, allowance for P, F, & D)	117	
C.	Actual OR minutes × 2 staff (circulator & scrub) (step nine, line A times 2) 64 × 2 = 128	128	
D.	Total minutes (step nine, line B + line C)	245	
E.	Fixed workload cost (step five, line P)		105.61
F.	Fixed overhead allocation (step three, line C times step nine, line D) 0.6418 × 245	245	157.24
G.	**Total fixed cost** (step nine, line E + F)		**262.85**
H.	Variable workload cost (step one, line H times step nine, line D) 0.3465 × 245	245	84.89
I.	Procedure supply costs (step seven)		64.14
J.	Anesthesia supply costs (step seven)		37.58
K.	PACU nursing cost (step six, line 7 times step one, line H) 75 × 0.3465	75	25.99
L.	Total variable cost (step nine, line H + I + J + K)		**212.6**
M.	Total cost per case (step nine, line G + L)		**475.45**
N.	Facility charge (from facility charge master)		1000
O.	Profit (step nine, line N minus line M) 1000 − 475.45		524.55
P.	Average contractual amount per case (step eight)		216.69
Q.	Profit margin (step nine, line O minus line P) 524.55 − 216.69		307.86

* **Weekly clinical hours:**
5 full-time operating room RNs × 40 hr/wk = 200 hours
3 full-time surgical technicians × 40 hr/wk = 120 hours
4 full-time PACU RNs × 40 hr/wk = 160 hours
1 full-time operating room support technician = 40 hours
Total weekly hours (200 + 120 + 160 + 40) = 520 hr/wk

† **Weekly administrative hours:**
1 full-time director = 40 hr/wk
1 full-time administrative supervisor = 40 hr/wk
1 full-time billing clerk = 40 hr/wk
1 full-time accounts payable clerk = 40 hr/wk
2 part-time receptionists = 56 hr/wk
Total weekly hours (40 + 40 + 40 + 40 + 56) = 216 hr/wk

CPT, current procedural terminology; RN, registered nurse; PACU, postanesthesia care unit; OR, operating room.

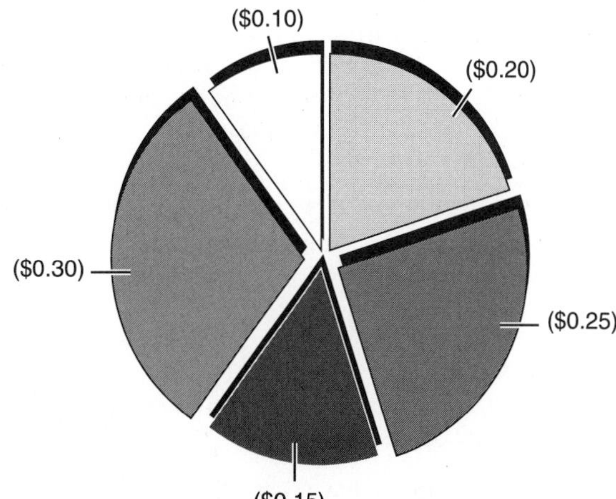

Figure 2–1. Expense allocation per $1.00 of revenues.

that shows how each dollar of revenue is spent is one way to educate staff. For every dollar spent, $.20 may go toward the lease and utilities, $.25 may go toward supplies, $.15 may go toward salaries and benefits, $.30 may go toward contractual allowances, and the remaining $.10 is profit. If the ASC's finances are broken down into easy-to-understand language and visual tools, team members will be better able to see why it is important to decrease cost.

If the freestanding ASC is in the for-profit structure, employees are very attuned to costs. For ASCs that are not-for-profit, some education may have to take place. *All* centers must have a profit margin to remain in business; the not-for-profit designation is simply indicative of where those profits go. As opposed to the for-profit center, in which profits go to shareholders and owners, the not-for-profit center typically places that money back into the center for capital purchases, staff pay increases, community service, and uncompensated (charity) care.

Making employees accountable for ensuring cost containment is one way to drive efficiency. The staff members directly involved in performing the procedures are the ones who can best identify where there is waste or excess of resources. Managers should ensure that these individuals are included in the development of any cost containment strategies. Only then can acceptance from the staff be ensured.

Inventory and Staffing Costs

One cost reduction strategy is to reduce supply inventory because having supplies sit on shelves ties up assets without producing revenue. The average operating room has anywhere from 4000 to 6000 items in stock. The manager can start by asking some simple questions:

- How frequently are supplies delivered to the ASC?
- From where are supplies being delivered, and what is the time frame required for obtaining orders?
- Could the ASC function if it implemented just-in-time ordering?
- If a certain item is needed in an emergency, can it be easily borrowed?

Once these questions have been answered, leaders can begin to make decisions affecting inventory. The first step is to move toward standardization of supplies. If there are four different suppliers for the same or similar item, consolidation should occur. Better pricing can be gained by buying an increased volume of one item through one vendor rather than four items that perform the same function from four different suppliers.

In attempts to standardize and decrease inventory, the 80-20 rule should be used to determine which items should be focused on. The 80-20 rule implies that 20% of the items on hand account for 80% of the expense. Because of this, attention must be placed on the items in the top 20%. The manager should make a list of these items and then determine whether each specific item on the list requires further attention.

- Is the purchase price reasonable?
- Is there an opportunity for potential savings?
- Is there an alternative option for procuring the item?
- If the item is used infrequently, can it be obtained from another facility when needed?
- Does the potential exist to buy one case and split it with one or more other facilities or departments?
- Is there another brand available that costs less?

Only after each item on the list is examined can an intelligent decision be made regarding the item.

When dealing with suppliers, it is crucial to have an understanding of cost. Is the facility paying freight charges? Astute managers may be able to negotiate with suppliers to eliminate freight charges, thereby saving the facility money. It is also imperative that managers work with sales representatives concerning products; managers should negotiate ethically and fairly with the different vendors to reduce the cost of their products. When pressured with competition, vendors are more likely to decrease their price in order to capture the market. Although very time consuming, comparative shopping is the only way to know whether the ASC is getting the best deal possible.

Managers should also look to alternative sources for supplies. If the ASC is part of a larger system, this can be easily accomplished. This is especially helpful for supplies that are used only once or twice a year. Creativity is the key, and any method that can be implemented to decrease cost is worth investigating.

Creative staffing patterns are another way to keep costs down. Some individuals may want to work only half days. Employing these individuals to work on an as-needed basis assists in keeping staffing levels appropriate without excess. Is it still realistic to employ a registered nurse–only staff? It may be more cost effective to employ surgical technicians. If registered nurses are performing non-nursing tasks, can these be delegated to a technical person?

Does the ASC use a formulary for medications, or can physicians request and obtain any medication they want? By limiting medications, the ASC can help to keep the cost of pharmaceuticals down. How much control does the ASC want over physician practice? Does the ASC want the anesthetics administered to be limited to only low-cost medications? What about excluding ondansetron (Zofran) because of its cost? If ASCs want to take this hard stance, they must be prepared to present hard, factual data to the physicians. In many cases, the cost of the medications does not outweigh the clinical and financial benefits. For instance, if administering ondansetron to patients with a history of nausea and vomiting would decrease the patient's length of stay in the postanesthesia care unit, then the benefit may outweigh the cost. In addition, the ASC stands to gain because the patient is extremely satisfied that he or she did not have to suffer with nausea and vomiting. Careful attention and physician input are essential when making decisions that directly affect physician practice.

In the operating room, decisions need to be made regarding resterilizing single-use items. Before the ASC chooses to resterilize a single-use item, careful consideration and legal counsel should be obtained. In addition, a letter from the manufacturer is suggested. Ethical and public relations issues are also important considerations.

Should the ASC use disposable or reusable items in the operating room? A cost analysis needs to be performed to determine what would work best for the individual facility. Disposable items are easy to use, but costly, and the cost of disposing hazardous waste needs to be considered. A reusable item may be costly initially but can be reused many times. The cost of reprocessing the item needs to be considered, as well as developing a sharpening, repair, and replacement program.

The ASC needs to identify the projected use of the item, the cost of disposable versus the cost of reusable use, and the cost of maintaining the item. Once this information is calculated, the pros and cons of each should be identified, and a serious discussion with the end-user of the item (the physician, if appropriate) should take place. It is essential that the physician's acceptance be obtained before any change is implemented. If the physicians do not agree with the intended change, the impact on the ASC could be devastating. What if the physicians decided to take all future cases elsewhere because of unhappiness with the change? Would losing volume affect the bottom line as severely as not implementing the change? Decisions should not be made in a vacuum. Involvement by all parties ensures amicable solutions and avoids conflict.

Managers should establish good working relationships with vendors. With the two parties working together, potential cost containment opportunities can be identified. It may be possible to work out an arrangement whereby the ASC buys specific supplies from a vendor and in return is able to borrow instrumentation free of charge. This is a common arrangement with vendors of orthopedic supplies.

Managers should also consider consignment arrangements for specific supplies. Vendors for intraocular lenses frequently agree to this type of arrangement. Various intraocular lenses in different sizes are stored at the ASC but remain the property of the vendor. When an intraocular lens is implanted, the information is passed on to the vendor, who then issues a bill for the lens. Consignments help the ASC keep the necessary inventory level without having to spend the dollars initially. Instead, payment occurs only after the product is used.

Additional areas that can be investigated to decrease cost are as follows:

- Increase instrument sets to avoid wasting time sterilizing instruments between cases.
- Update surgeons' preference cards frequently to avoid waste.
- Print preference cards with supply prices on them to increase staff awareness.
- Eliminate the use of cover gowns outside the operating room.
- Eliminate the use of shoe covers.
- Ensure that anesthesia gas machines are turned off at the end of the day.
- Discard dropped packages only when sterility is doubtful.
- Repair instruments instead of replacing them.
- Seek out refurbished equipment and instrumentation to decrease up-front cost of capital equipment.
- Tie cost savings into staff performance appraisals.
- Develop "operating room packs" for specialty cases.
- Medicate patients with the proper medications, for example, eliminate meperidine from the outpatient arena to decrease the incidence of nausea and vomiting.

- Encourage physicians to instill local anesthetics when appropriate (e.g., hernia repair) to decrease postoperative pain.
- Discharge patients according to specific discharge criteria, not according to time.
- Contract with a group-purchasing program to receive better discounts on supplies.

Sometimes, a significant paradigm shift can result in cost savings when there is a climate that allows and encourages the team to "think outside the box." An example is the change that some operating room teams are making related to scrubs. In some facilities, the staff members own and launder their own scrub uniforms unless the scrubs are contaminated during work. The cost savings to the facility for laundering and for replacing scrubs can be significant. The object of presenting this idea is not to debate the pros and cons of the idea itself but to illustrate that the potential ideas for cost savings can be creative and unexpected.

The ASC team, when given the opportunity, can be creative in the development of cost containment strategies. Managers should encourage and nurture staff to express their opinions without fear of retribution. Working in a team-oriented environment can enhance creative minds to explore virgin territory. The manager who encourages staff members and promotes open communication is sure to gain new insights into cost containment opportunities.

Business Office Strategies

The ASC needs to develop and implement administrative policies regarding billing. These should address issues such as self-pay patients, what to do with patients who do not pay their bills, collection of co-payments or deductibles, precertification requirements, and turnover of accounts to a collection agency.

What happens when a patient presents for surgery as a self-pay patient? Should the patient be required to pay in advance? As a general rule, insurance carriers do not cover cosmetic surgery. It is suggested that the entire amount due be paid in advance of the procedure. All too often, patients who have undergone cosmetic procedures refuse to pay for their surgery, especially if they are not happy with the results. To eliminate incurring bad debt, the ASC should require the full amount in advance.

What happens when a patient presents with no insurance and the procedure is semi-emergent? Is the patient still required to pay in advance? What if the patient has no money? Has the center established a policy not to accept patients who have no insurance?

These are difficult questions to answer, but it is essential that policies be established for such situations to help guide decision-making. The legal and ethical considerations of refusing patients also need careful analysis. Again, legal counsel should be retained to assist in establishing policies of this nature.

When does the ASC determine that an account is uncollectible? Does the ASC try for years to collect payment from patients or is there an established policy to turn delinquent accounts over to a collection agency? It is best to turn accounts over quickly. An example would be to send the patient a notice that the account is 30 days overdue. If no payment is received, a 60-days overdue notice is sent out with a warning that the account will be turned over to a collection agency if arrangements for payment are not made. When the account is 90 days overdue, a final notice is mailed referencing that if payment is not made within 10 days, the account will be turned over to a collection agency and the patient's credit report will be in jeopardy. The ASC should have established policies to work with patients to set up payment plans. This generally entails setting up realistic payment plans that the patient can meet each month. There should be clear communication that failure to follow the established payment plan will result in the account being turned over to the collection agency.

Policies also need to be established to ensure proper payment from insurance carriers. Does the patient's insurance company require that there be preauthorization or precertification before treatment? Does failure to obtain preauthorization or precertification mean that the ASC will be denied payment? If the answer is yes, who obtains the preauthorization? The patient? The primary care physician? The surgeon? Whatever process is in place, the ASC should ensure that preauthorization or precertification has occurred. The ASC may implement a policy to recheck the preauthorization number with the insurance company. Failure to recheck this information may result in the ASC's not receiving payment for the procedure performed as well as possibly being unable to bill the patient.

What about patient co-payments and deductibles? Does the ASC collect the co-payment upfront? Today, consumers feel that they already pay too much for health insurance. Having to pay a co-payment or meet a deductible seems like an excess burden on the consumer. All too often, if not collected in advance, the patient refuses to pay the co-payment or deductible. The ASC may consider instituting a policy of collecting this money in advance of the procedure.

Ensuring payment for services rendered seems like a simple task when, in fact, it is a monumental undertaking. Business office personnel need to research each patient account before the day of surgery to establish the following:

- The patient is, indeed, covered by the insurance plan named.
- A precertification or preauthorization has been obtained.
- A co-payment exists and needs to be collected.
- The patient's deductible has or has not been met (and needs to be collected).
- The patient is undergoing surgery for an injury acquired at work; therefore, there will be a worker's compensation claim.
- The patient is a Medicare subscriber, and the scheduled procedure is or is not covered under Medicare.
- The patient is in a managed care plan, and the procedure being scheduled is/is not covered under the specific insurance plan.

The business office personnel must deal with insurance companies on a daily basis. Although extremely time consuming, it is necessary to confirm payment in advance of the procedure to avoid nonpayment afterward.

After a procedure is completed, the business office coder is responsible for assigning accurate CPT codes to the record on the basis of the operative and the pathology reports. This obviates the need for rapid turnaround of these reports so that bills can be prepared and sent. Inaccurate or incomplete coding can result in incorrect or no reimbursement from the payer.

Business office personnel also need to keep close track of payments received. Payments need to be carefully analyzed to ensure that the ASC receives the proper amount of money due. The manager can start by examining the *explanation of benefits*, which is the documentation accompanying the check that the facility receives from the insurance company. Was the facility paid for all charges billed? Are some charges being denied? If so, why did the denial occur? Does the explanation of benefits state that the patient is responsible for a portion of the bill, such as the co-payment or deductible? If so, how much time should elapse before a bill is generated to the patient? What if the patient has a secondary insurance? Is the secondary insurance billed as soon as payment from the primary is received?

Insurance claims should be filed within 5 days of the procedure. A system should be established that allows review of all pending claims on a set schedule. Such review assists in trending delinquent accounts. It may be that a specific insurance carrier frequently delays payment for an extended period of time. Trending this information gives administration valuable data when it comes time for contract renewal. If payment has been an issue, an acceptable time limit for payment should be incorporated into the next contract along with enforceable penalties for late payments.

If a charge has been denied, this needs to be investigated. Why was the charge denied? If an acceptable answer is not received, the ASC should appeal the claim. Again, although time consuming, the ASC can stand to gain increased financial revenue by appealing denials.

Business office policies should address at least the following:

- Self-pay patients
  - Scheduled in advance (elective surgery)
  - Scheduled as an emergency
  - Surprise self-pay patients on the day of surgery (no advance warning)
- Insurance verification
- Confirmation of referral (if required)
- Preauthorization (if required)
- Co-payments and deductibles
  - Collection of payment up-front
- Current procedural terminology coding (CPT) procedures
- Billing
  - Time period after date of surgery before claim is filed
  - Documentation needed to complete claim (pathology report, operative report)
- Delinquent accounts
  - Establishing payment plans
  - Time period and process before turning account over to collection agency
  - Frequency of follow-up process for unpaid claims (insurance company)

The ASC should participate in electronic claim filing. Insurance carriers tend to reimburse electronic claims faster than paper claims. In addition, the cost of processing the claim is less. If issues surface regarding the length of time it takes to receive payment, an analysis should occur to determine where the problem is. Managers should determine why the average number of days it takes to receive payment on accounts is excessive. This is called the *days in accounts receivable* or *AR days*. Analysis should include:

- Is the insurance company receiving the claim promptly?
- Is the electronic claim getting where it should be?
- Is information missing on the claim?
- Are lost, missing, or late operative and pathology reports delaying the coding process?
- Is the insurance company delaying payment for some reason?
  - Waiting for documentation from the ASC (operative report)
  - Waiting for documentation from the patient
  - Investigating potential worker's compensation claim
- Did the claim go to the proper address?

Follow-up on delinquent claims needs to occur on a set schedule, be it daily, weekly, or monthly. By keeping track of the revenue due and implementing procedures to ensure prompt payment, the ASC is more likely to become financially successful.

Administrators need to establish a method to carefully monitor and trend financial data. The following data should be analyzed to identify possible trends that could affect the bottom line:

- Gross revenue (total charges before contractual allowances)
- Contractual allowances (the difference between billed charges and actual payments because of a third party contract)
- Net revenue (amount expected to be collected after contractual allowances are deducted)

In addition to the aforementioned financial data, trending of volume also needs to occur. Volume should be analyzed not only in terms of total cases performed but also in terms of types of procedures performed. Suggested analysis includes:

- Total cases performed
- Total procedures (some patients have multiple procedures performed)
- Totals by specialty (e.g., general, orthopedics, urology)

Further detailed analysis can include:

- Average number of cases per day
- Average charge per case
- Average charge per case by specialty
- Average cost per case
- Average cost per case by specialty
- Average profit per case
- Average profit per case by specialty

By further analyzing financial information, the manager is able to determine which specialty brings in the highest profit per case. In a competitive marketplace, the manager must then implement strategies to increase volume in this specialty. Trending data on a monthly basis also helps to identify potential problem areas before they become too serious. For example, has revenue declined because of a poor payer mix? Figure 2–2 illustrates the payer mix in one freestanding ASC in a Florida market that is highly penetrated by managed care companies.

There are other questions to consider. Is the ASC being denied reimbursement on certain procedures? Are preauthorizations or referrals not being properly obtained? Are payments for second and third procedures being denied as unnecessary? Are payments being posted correctly? An in-depth analysis assists the manager in identifying the underlying cause. A sudden decrease in collections for 1 month may be just a fluke, but a decrease that continues for an extended period of time must be scrutinized so that the root cause can be identified.

Contract Negotiations

An important aspect of operating a successful ASC is obtaining financially sound contracts with third party payers. The ASC should appoint one individual to be responsible for contract negotiations. This practice ensures continuity when dealing with third party payers. Some key issues to be aware of when entering into a contract are presented in Table 2–3.

Negotiation of contracts is a very complex process. As stated previously, having one individual represent the facility ensures consistency when dealing with the insurance company. Before any contract is signed, the facility should appoint a key group of individuals to review the proposal. This group should consist of at least the administrator, the finance coordinator, the medical director, the business office supervisor, and the billing supervisor. The diversity of backgrounds and the specialized interests of such a group help to identify key areas of the proposed contract that might not be the best possible negotiation for the center.

Potential problem areas should be addressed before the contract is signed. It is suggested that a careful analysis of the proposed reimbursement schedule be performed. By placing historical data into a spreadsheet along with the proposed reimbursement, the facility can calculate potential reimbursement based on past volume. Performing this exercise allows the fa-

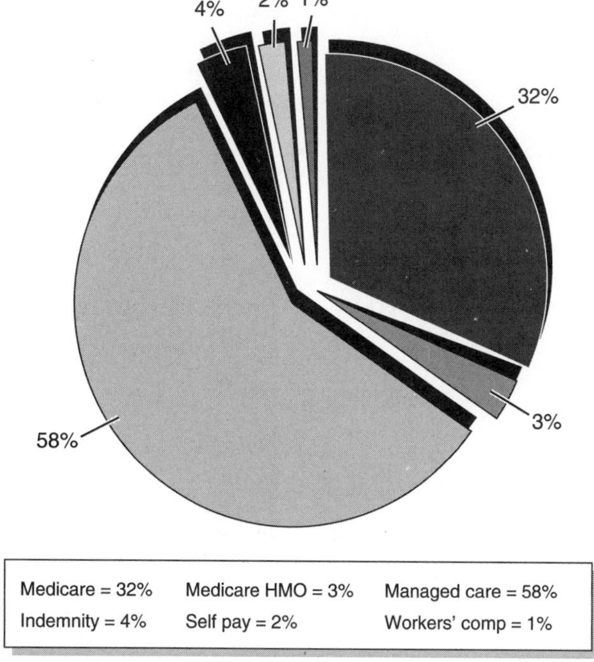

Figure 2–2. Payer mix in percentages.

cility to identify what amount of charges will be written off to contractual allowances. The contractual allowance is the amount of discount off the regular charges given to the insurance company. It is usually expressed as a percentage.

Table 2–3. Considerations For Contracting with Third Party Payers

How are claims submitted?
Do claims need to be submitted within a certain number of days after the procedure was performed?
What if the insurance company is named as secondary—does the time limit still apply?
Is there an established time limit in which the insurance company must pay claims?
What happens if claims are not paid within the established time limit?
If the contract is based on the Medicare groups, is it exactly like Medicare?
Can procedures be performed if they are not on the Medicare approved list? If so, how are they reimbursed?
What is the process if a procedure is termed "incidental"?
What is the established rate of reimbursement?
Are there precertification or referral requirements?
If charges are denied because the patient failed to obtain precertification or necessary referral, can the ambulatory surgery center bill the patient?
Are secondary and bilateral procedures covered?
Is there an established process for filing a grievance?
Is there an established process for terminating the agreement?

The data should be analyzed carefully. Can the ASC live with the proposed reimbursement? Are there certain procedures that the facility will lose money on? Is this acceptable? What happens if the money-losing procedures suddenly increase dramatically in volume? Only after comparing cost data with projected volume and expected reimbursement can an intelligent decision be made regarding the contract.

There are other issues to consider when negotiating contracts, such as the use of excessive supplies (e.g., specialized sutures, arrows, and staples used in orthopedic procedures) or the need to obtain human bone for procedures requiring bone grafting? Can the ASC bill the insurance company for these items? Will the insurance company reimburse for these? Are venous access devices or other implants reimbursable? What about the cost of using a laser or radiologic equipment during the procedure? The ASC may be able to negotiate with the insurance company to reimburse the cost of certain supplies and equipment.

As ASCs continue to be the low-cost solution to the high cost of healthcare, there will be an even greater impetus to perform more complex procedures in the outpatient setting. Managers need to ensure that the ASC remains financially viable; only through continued careful analysis of monthly data can this be accomplished.

When a negative trend appears, the cause must be quickly determined and corrective action taken.

MARKETING STRATEGIES

Marketing to Physicians

Ambulatory surgery centers need to implement innovative tactics to gain and then keep physicians using the surgery center. All personnel, including receptionists, nurses, technicians, and support personnel, need to be educated to provide exceptional customer service, not only to patients but also to physicians.

What keeps physicians happy? Whether hospital based or freestanding, the ASC that can provide doctors with available operating room time to meet their scheduling needs, quick operating room turnaround time, operating room instrumentation that is functioning properly and appropriate to meet the physician's needs, and a pleasant, cooperative perioperative team will surely gain points with the physician. But is that enough?

Marketing in a Financially Challenging Environment

In today's competitive environment, a physician's desire to use a particular facility may not be enough to keep that physician coming back. Physicians who participate in capitated plans need to ensure that they perform their surgical procedures in a cost-efficient setting. No longer can the convenience of placing an outpatient procedure between two inpatient procedures on the hospital schedule be tolerated. The high cost of performing the procedure in the inpatient setting may have a bearing on the physician's ability to continue to practice in a capitated environment. Insurance companies are scrutinizing, more closely than ever, how the physician practices and the amount of resources that are consumed to deliver services. The physician who continually consumes the highest amount of resources may be given an ultimatum to either decrease cost or face having his or her contract with that particular payer terminated.

The ASC must look at not only the charges to third party payers for their services but also ancillary services. If the ASC has contracted with other providers, such as anesthesia services and pathology services, it needs to be sure that these providers are also operating in a cost-efficient manner. If the ASC's fees are competitive but the charges of the ancillary services are high, when payers total the cost of the surgical experience, they may find that the ancillary fees have caused the total fee to be excessive. This may have an effect on where physicians are directed by managed care companies to perform surgery.

The ASC manager needs to be cognizant of the effect of outside influences and work closely with ancillary providers to negotiate contracts that keep the charges of ancillary services provided in the ASC at a cost-efficient level. The manager has negotiating power, and if services are not provided cost effectively, cancellation or nonrenewal of existing contracts with ancillary providers should be considered. When negotiating contracts, the manager should be certain that the option to cancel the contract is clearly identified. An "out" should always exist, should the conditions of the contract become unbearable to live with.

Physicians must also be assured that their patients are receiving quality care at a competitive price. Today, physicians are more aware of what patients must pay "out of pocket" to receive services. A facility that charges patients an exorbitant amount would find physicians seeking more cost-effective centers to provide service. Patients may have insurance, but they are often responsible for a co-payment. Paying 20% of $1000 is certainly a more palatable option than paying 20% of $2000. The ACS must ensure that charges are in line with, or better than, the competition.

An ASC that deals with self-pay patients may want to investigate the option of reduced fees for these patients. Instituting a discount for self-pay patients may be an attractive option for patients. If a patient is self-pay, either because he or she has no insurance or because insurance does not cover the procedure being performed, this should not preclude him or her from receiving benefits enjoyed by other patients. This can be a big marketing draw in facilities that perform procedures that are routinely self-pay, such as cosmetic surgery.

There is the rare patient who is financially able to pay for health insurance and purposely chooses not to do so but instead pays for services when needed. When this type of person presents for surgical care that is generally covered by insurance, a careful analysis of financial issues assists in determining the person's ability to pay. Then, the policy of the ASC will dictate whether prepayment or billing at a later date will occur.

Block Scheduling

What else keeps physicians practicing in certain settings? The availability of operating time is essential. The ASC needs to be sure that physicians who wish to work at the center have ample opportunity to book cases at times that work well with their schedules. A modified block schedule best accommodates physician preference, but facilities with only one or two operating rooms may have difficulty using this system. In this situation, management needs to explore options that will best meet everyone's needs. Ultimately, the center's ability to grant block time depends on the number of operating rooms, the physician mix, and the number of cases performed each day.

A modified block schedule is one in which some physicians have predetermined block time that is specifically set aside for only them to book cases. This time can be an entire day, a morning, an afternoon, or as little as 1 or 2 hours. It may be on a given day each week, every other week, or even once a month. Specialty practice physicians from the city may travel to a rural center one day a month to see patients and perform surgery. This type of setup is convenient for the patient who then does not have to travel to the city for surgery. In addition, it is a great marketing tool for the physician to gain patients by offering to travel to the rural setting. Partnerships can exist whereby the physician leases space at the surgery center to see patients on a given day.

Interspersed between assigned block time is free time, in which physicians who do not have assigned block time can schedule cases. When a block schedule or a modified block schedule is used, the manager must ensure that policies and procedures are in place to handle situations related to scheduling. For example, how many days ahead does the assigned block time get released as "free" time for anyone to book? What happens if assigned block time is not being used and a different physician wants to book that time? Do surgery center personnel contact the assigned physician to ask if the block can be released, or does the requesting physician make the contact? Is it the policy of the ASC to not get involved in these scenarios? It is suggested that assigned block time be released for open booking anywhere from 2 to 5 working days before the scheduled date. This policy allows physicians with busy practices to add on cases right up to the day of surgery.

Whatever practice is implemented, the ASC manager must be certain that the operating rooms are being utilized as efficiently as possible. If block scheduling is used, its utilization should be analyzed on a routine basis, such as monthly or quarterly. Physicians who are not using their block time can be queried as to the reason. There may be a seasonal drop, or there may have been a change in the physician's practice. Block time that is inadequately utilized may be hampering the ASC's ability to add additional cases. If physician's offices are trying to schedule cases but are unable to get prime time (first case of the day), they may be looking elsewhere for an ASC that can accommodate their needs. If blocks are underutilized, they should be released to free time in which everyone can book, or the blocks should be assigned to physicians who will adequately utilize them.

Routine reports that assign a percentage of utilization for each physician's block time assist the manager in making decisions that best serve the ASC. Utilization can also be incorporated into the ASC's quality management program. Benchmarks for utilization can be established to assist in determining when a block gets released. In this scenario, physicians know in advance what their utilization needs to be in order to keep their assigned block.

The Perioperative Team

The ASC staff members are invaluable in terms of marketing the ASC to physicians. Because of their close working relationships with physicians, they can tailor marketing efforts to the physicians' likes and dislikes. If a physician comments that he or she enjoys working with certain team members, the manager should attempt to schedule assignments so that the physician works with those team members, if possible. The disadvantages to this are that other staff members who do not have the opportunity to work with the physician may feel left out and may also feel inadequate when they are assigned to work with the physician. One solution is to rotate one or two staff members through to work with the physician so that they, too, can gain proficiency and are able to cover for vacations, call ins, and so on.

Staff members need to pay particular attention to the physician's requests. If a physician comments that a particular instrument is not functioning properly or is not sharp, the staff members need to ensure that the instrument is removed from service and repaired. A physician who comments that a particular instrument is still not working properly week after week would certainly seek a facility that shows concern for his or her needs. The same holds true for physician requests for changes to their preference cards. If a request is made to change a drape, suture, or blade size, the ASC team should have a procedure in place for enacting and communicating the change immediately. This should be automatic in most cases. Not instituting the change can result in wasted supplies and physician dissatisfaction.

A consistent process should be in place to ensure that all team members are aware of changes in physician preferences and standing orders. For example, if a physician requests to use only a certain drape for a procedure and this is a change in practice, this information needs to be communicated to all staff. One method of achieving this is to have daily morning meetings. These meetings can be held at the start of the shift and can last for no more than 5 minutes. In these meetings, staff communicate changes in physician practices, changes in supplies, back orders of supplies, or any other important issue. Documentation of the discussion is placed in a notebook, in which a separate page with all staff members' names is used each day. Staff members who are not present are responsible for reading the book and signing off once they have read it, ensuring that all important information is passed on to everyone. In situations in which meetings are difficult, just using a book may be a solution.

Communication with the physician should always be positive and professional. Physicians enjoy working in an environment that is friendly, cooperative, and easy going. Although it can be said that performing outpatient surgery is less stressful than complex inpatient procedures, the atmosphere should not be so relaxed that it is unprofessional or jeopardizes patient care. Staff must also be able to communicate with physicians in an open and honest manner. When issues arise, each staff member should do his or her best to correct the situation directly with the physician involved. Management should be supportive of team members and should coach, encourage, and empower them to seek reasonable solutions to problems without diverting complaints to higher management unless necessary.

Developing "standing orders" for physicians who routinely order the same medications or routines preoperatively is another method of increasing physician satisfaction. If preoperative instructions rarely vary, as in the eye drop regimen for cataract patients, standing orders can be developed to assist everyone. Not only does the physician not have to be called for the orders, but also the ASC staff can be assured that they know exactly what treatments to institute as soon as the patient arrives at the center. This practice prevents delays while the ASC nurse attempts to track down the physician for the order.

When implementing standing orders, the physician must review and sign the order annually. In addition, the physician is responsible for communicating any changes in the standing orders. The nurse is responsible for individualizing the standing orders based on the nursing assessment. If during the admission assessment it is discovered that the patient is allergic to the medication in the standing order, it is the nurse's responsibility to hold the standing order and contact the physician.

Another marketing draw for the center is assisting the physician by printing "postoperative discharge instructions" for patients. These surgery-specific instructions can be typed on the ASC's letterhead for added name exposure.

Physicians who work during the lunch hour should be provided with a lunch. Instituting a lunch service whereby the physician's office calls in the lunch order for the physician before a specified time each day shows that the ACS cares about the physician. This is especially true for freestanding ASCs that may not have access to cafeteria service.

The ASC manager must be knowledgeable regarding physician satisfaction with the ASC. One method of gaining insight into physician satisfaction is to develop a physician satisfaction survey (Table 2–4). Soliciting physicians' comments on an annual or semiannual basis can ensure that physician concerns are being identified. Once issues are identified, the manager must implement methods to address these issues or at least communicate why the issue is not being addressed. For example, if the survey identifies that one physician expresses dissatisfaction with the arthroscopy instrumentation, the manager might do one or more of the following:

- If the physician is identified, meet with him or her to discuss the exact issue with the instrumentation (it may be just one instrument out of the entire tray).
- If the physician has not identified himself or herself, send a follow-up letter to all the orthopedic physicians to solicit further input (identify the issue that has been raised and solicit further feedback from the group).
- Identify possible solutions to the problem (replace/repair instrument).
- Bring the issue to a higher authority (governing body, advisory board).
- Communicate outcome to all orthopedic physicians.

***Table 2–4.* Physician Satisfaction Survey**

At ABC Surgery Center, we value your input. Please take a few moments to complete this survey. Your input will assist us to better meet your needs. Thank you for your participation.

1. Are the instruments and equipment available to you at the Surgery Center sufficient to meet your needs? **Yes** ☐ **No** ☐

   Surgical Specialty:

   ____

   ____

   Comments:

   ____

   ____

2. Are you satisfied with the room turnover time at the Surgery Center? **Yes** ☐ **No** ☐

   Comments:

   ____

   ____

3. If we know in advance that your case will be delayed, are you given ample notice of the delay? **Yes** ☐ **No** ☐

   Comments:

   ____

   ____

4. Are you aware that there is a private room available to speak with patients' families pre/postoperatively? **Yes** ☐ **No** ☐

   Comments:

   ____

   ____

5. Are you satisfied with the performance of the following:

	Yes	**No**
The operating room staff?	☐	☐
The PACU nursing staff?	☐	☐
The scheduling/booking personnel?	☐	☐
Surgery Center Administration?	☐	☐

   Comments:

   ____

   ____

6. Are you satisfied with the anesthesia services provided? **Yes** ☐ **No** ☐

   Comments:

   ____

   ____

7. Are there any additional services we could provide for you? **Yes** ☐ **No** ☐

   Comments:

   ____

   ____

Please feel free to use the reverse side for additional comments & suggestions.
Name (optional)

____

The physician satisfaction survey is one method of determining whether physicians' needs are being met. Other suggestions includes:

- Visiting each physician at his or her office to discuss their satisfaction with the center
- Talking with physicians while they are at the center
- Holding an open forum with the ASC governing body to provide physicians with the opportunity to find out more about the ASC or to voice concerns
- Soliciting input from staff members working with the physicians in the operating room to identify issues raised

Ambulatory surgery center team members need to pay particular attention to detail. Performing simple, routine tasks well may seem insignificant, but such expertise actually demonstrates an organized, efficient process that benefits all members of the health care team. The surgery center team must also exhibit pride and feel that they have ownership in the ASC. One can be assured that in an ASC in which team members consistently go out of their way to please customers, their actions do not go unnoticed.

Marketing to Physician Office Personnel

A good relationship between the ASC and the physician's office staff is crucial for ensuring cooperation and understanding on both sides. If the ASC scheduling personnel have an understanding of the workings of the physician's office, they will be better able to understand the manner in which the surgical cases are being scheduled. If the physician's office personnel understand the needs of the ASC, they, too, will have a better understanding of the ASC's requirements. If the process is to be successful, scheduling personnel need to be courteous and knowledgeable regarding the booking process. It is also important that the ASC strives to make the scheduling process as time efficient as possible for the physician's office staff.

For a good working relationship to be promoted with the physician's office staff, policies and procedures should be in place to promote a positive environment. A manual prepared by the ASC that includes policies and procedures for the physician's office to follow when booking a case helps ensure a smooth process. Table 2–5 shows a table of contents for such a manual.

Table 2–5. Table of Contents of an Ambulatory Surgery Center (ASC) Manual for Physician Office Staff

Scheduling the Surgery
- Scheduling phone number
- Use of CPT codes
- Order of requested demographic information
- Cancellations

Anesthesia
- Definition of types

Brochures and Forms
- Patient brochure
- Patient bill of rights
- Preregistration questionnaire
- Preanesthesia questionnaire
- Appointment card

Preadmission Testing
- Required laboratory tests

Laboratory Preoperative Guidelines
- Fasting requirements

Important Information
- Patient appropriateness, i.e., what case can/cannot be accepted at ASC
- NPO guidelines
- Patient transportation
- Patient arrival time
- Pediatric tours

Local Anesthesia
- Definition
- Preoperative laboratory requirements
- Fasting/NPO requirements
- Arrival time
- Transportation

Financial Responsibilities
- Insurance
- Participating preferred providers—HMOs
- Self-pay policy
- Worker's compensation
- Precertification requirements

Lunch Menu

Administrative Contacts

CPT, current procedural terminology; NPO, nothing by mouth; HMO, health maintenance organization.

One marketing technique is to prepare the manual and then set up appointments with each physician's office to distribute and review the manual. Scheduling appointments during lunchtime and providing lunch for the physician's office staff are great icebreakers. The focus of the meeting should be positive and should promote open communication between the office and the ASC. Generally, having the ASC booking personnel and possibly the ASC manager attend these meetings shows genuine interest in meeting the needs of the physician's office. It is important to remember that the physician's office staff often has control over where a case gets scheduled. If the ASC makes scheduling easy and attempts to accommodate time requests, the office staff may tend to book more cases there than at a competing facility.

The ASC also needs to identify whether the physician's office staff is satisfied with the ASC. Table 2–6 provides an example of a scheduling satisfaction survey that can be used to identify areas of concern. Because it is essential that the ASC and the physician's office staff have a good working relationship, corrective action must be taken immediately regarding problem areas.

Another marketing idea is to schedule a physician office staff "get-together" at the ASC.

Table 2–6. Scheduling Satisfaction Survey

In order to best meet your needs, the Surgery Center would appreciate the person(s) who schedules surgery for your office to complete this short survey. We feel this will assist us in evaluating the service we currently provide and make us aware of necessary improvements. All responses will be kept confidential, and your identity is optional. Please return it in the postage-paid envelope provided at your earliest convenience. Thank you.

1. Do you find our scheduling system quick and efficient? **Yes** ☐ **No** ☐

   Comments:

2. Is the scheduling staff pleasant and knowledgeable? **Yes** ☐ **No** ☐

   Comments:

3. If your office does not have block time, are we able to accommodate you with the date and/or time you are requesting? **Yes** ☐ **No** ☐

   Comments:

4. Is the scheduling staff able to accommodate you with unexpected "add on" cases? **Yes** ☐ **No** ☐

   Comments:

5. Is there anything our scheduling staff can do to improve the service we are currently providing? **Yes** ☐ **No** ☐

   If yes, please explain:

Please feel free to list any additional comments and/or suggestions:

Office/Representative (optional)

This time can be used to have physician office personnel tour the center to gain a first-hand understanding of how the facility operates. Attendees are provided with ASC brochures and handouts that are normally given to patients.

At Elliot 1-Day Surgery Center in Manchester, New Hampshire, physician office staff have the experience of role playing, in which they actually see how the case gets scheduled and then follow through as if they were the patients. This allows for greater understanding of what the patient will go through. Two scenarios are presented. One scenario typifies a situation in which everything is booked correctly and the patient has a smooth experience. In the second scenario, problems are encountered: the physician's requests for special equipment are not relayed, the history and physical and laboratory work are missing, the consent is incorrect, and so forth.

This role playing shows the delays that can result when everything is not as it should be. The physician's office staff and the surgery center personnel then gather informally for refreshments while answering questions and forming relationships that will carry forward for years to come. It is much easier to deal with issues and resolve conflicts when a face can be attached to a name. The institution of a get-together such as this has done wonders in promoting positive working relations with physician offices at the New Hampshire center.

Another idea implemented by Trinity Outpatient Center in New Port Richey, Florida, is a mail-out to office schedulers of an oversized postcard with a photograph of the surgery manager and scheduler. The intended outcome is to personalize their services. An additional component of this plan is a visit to the surgeons' offices to take photographs of the office scheduler or schedulers along with the ASC scheduler, then provide a copy to the physician's office.

Marketing to Patients

Marketing the ASC to patients can be accomplished internally or externally. Internally, staff members continuously market the ASC through their interactions with patients and family members. Every conversation and interaction between a staff member and a patient should be conducted in such a manner as to promote the best image possible. Interactions should be conducted on a personal level, showing the patient that staff members care enough to ensure that all aspects of the patient's surgical experience are positive. Extending oneself to hold the patient's hand during induction of anesthesia, saying a few comforting words or offering encouragement after surgery, and providing attention to the patient's family all contribute to the patient's impression of the surgery center.

All ASC staff members should attend customer service seminars. A properly educated staff is sure to present the ASC in a positive light by being sensitive to patient and family needs. Taking the necessary time to explain postoperative instructions to the patient and the family and following up the day after surgery with a phone call all add to the image and the reality of a concerned and caring staff. Table 2–7 provides strategies for promoting a positive discharge experience.

Table 2–7. Strategies for Promoting a Positive Discharge Experience

- Explain discharge instructions in easy-to-understand terms.
- Do not make the patient feel rushed to leave the ASC.
- Encourage the physician to speak with the patient and/or family before the patient's discharge.
- Be sure anesthesia personnel see the patient and provide feedback regarding patient's care before discharge.
- Provide written instructions, preferably on ASC letterhead; include telephone numbers of ASC, physician, and nearest hospital in case of emergency.
- Call prescriptions to the pharmacy so that medications will be ready when family arrives to pick them up.
- Provide a supply of dressings, bandages, and so on, so that the patient does not have to worry about obtaining them immediately.
- Schedule the patient's follow-up appointment with the physician—it will be one less thing the patient will have to worry about; provide the date and time of follow-up appointment in writing.
- Answer questions the patient may have—encourage the patient and family to ask questions. If you are unable to provide the patient with an answer, seek out appropriate personnel who can answer questions before the patient is discharged.
- Take opportunities to provide general health information when appropriate, e.g., breast self-examination, mammograms, diet, exercise, smoking cessation, stress reduction.

ASC, ambulatory surgical center.

CONCLUSIONS

The ASC, both freestanding and hospital based, is fast becoming the center of attention as more and more business is directed to the outpatient setting. ASCs that can provide service in a cost-effective and efficient manner will certainly gain from the increase in volume. Identifying the best practices and implementing methods to ensure cost containment, delivery of quality services, and high patient satisfaction will assist the ASC in becoming the leader in delivery of outpatient services.

To ensure that the ASC maintains a positive bottom line, it is essential that the manager be skilled in financial management. A clear understanding of insurance contracts, contract negotiations, and reimbursement is imperative to survive the onslaught of managed care. With the continued decline of reimbursement, a manager experienced in cost containment techniques will be able to ensure the center's financial viability.

Development of an outpatient surgery program that meets the needs of all customers—patients, physicians, office staff, healthcare workers, and so on—takes careful planning. A staff that possesses exceptional public relations and marketing skills will assist in developing a center with a positive reputation. When customers are satisfied with the service they receive, they are certain to pass on their positive experiences.

The future of ambulatory surgery is both challenging and promising. Continued pharmacologic and technical advances are paramount to clinical innovation. Competitive pricing, astute financial management, and aggressive cost containment are essential. Added to those objectives, continual attention to a high-quality, sincere customer focus is fundamental. By concentrating on these attributes ASCs can look forward to achieving success in the years ahead.

Reference

1. CPTs for Hospital Outpatient Services, 4th ed. Chicago, American Medical Association, 1999.

Chapter 3

Regulatory Compliance

Shauna Smith

Don't look back. Something may be gaining on you.
— Satchel Paige

Many agencies regulate the day-to-day operations of the ambulatory center. These include local, state, federal, and private agencies with various and sometimes conflicting reasons for their interest. Failure to comply with the regulations or standards of these agencies may result in various forms of penalties for the facility, from monetary to punitive. To protect the overall health of the organization, administrative personnel must encourage and support in-house monitoring of all compliance issues. Some facilities have one "compliance officer" who continuously monitors regulations and standards. Other facilities have meted out the various areas of compliance to different management personnel, staff members, or departments.

For ambulatory surgery centers (ASCs) in the hospital setting, compliance with infection control, safety, environmental, and other regulatory issues is part of the overall hospital program. Adherence to hospital policies and procedures should ensure adequate compliance. Large corporate hospital organizations usually have specialists who can advise and direct each hospital member individually. Experts with specialization in risk management, employee health, engineering, environmental safety, quality improvement, third party payers, information management, as well as other resources, may be freely accessible to such organizations. Freestanding ASCs that are members of, or are managed by, such organizations may also have access to similar expertise. Small hospital and freestanding ASCs lack this support system and must rely on in-house expertise and other available resources.

Administration must be committed to protecting the organization from the complications of nonadherence to regulatory issues. Allowing adequate personnel and resources for these activities is vital to the health of the facility. Because the various regulations and standards are in a constant state of change, compliance personnel must continuously monitor new directives and adjust organizational policies and procedures. Although inspectors from the Occupational Safety and Health Administration (OSHA), the Joint Commission on Accreditation of Healthcare Organizations (JCAHO), the local fire department, or another agency will usually ask to see these policies, they may also quiz employees regarding facility procedures. Employee response is the ultimate test of facility compliance with required standards, so education of staff and physicians must be vigorous and ongoing. Each employee should be expected to understand and adhere to policies, procedures, rules, and regulations. Each job description should define this expectation, and the annual performance evaluation should reflect performance in this area.

LOCAL REGULATIONS

For new facilities, site selection is a key element. Items to be considered include zoning regulations, convenience of location, access to main streets, and type of "neighbors" in the area. City and county ordinances for building design and safety must be investigated and adhered to. Architects and contractors are familiar with codes and ordinances regarding setbacks, easements, rights of way, and building height restrictions. Other items that they can direct include fire safety measures, egress, electrical and plumbing guidelines, parking availability and plot layout, capacity of the building and individual rooms, waste management, and other structural regulations. Some locales, such as resort and vacation areas, may even regulate the overall design of the building itself to maintain a "rustic" or other type of community theme.

An understanding of local regulations also ensures that waste is managed correctly within the facility. Local landfill requirements must be considered in the planning of procedure development. A copy of the local waste and sewage ordinances may prove helpful and can usually be secured from the sanitation department.

Plot Layout

Future expansion of the facility must be considered during initial construction. Local codes usually direct that the building be located a specified distance from property lines, streets, and sidewalks. Without an understanding of these codes, expansion of the facility may be severely impaired at a future date. Planning for expansion must also allow for adequate parking as defined by local ordinances.

STATE REGULATIONS

The multiplicity of state regulations is too vast to be addressed in a single publication. Each facility must seek out and come into compliance with the numerous and varied laws and requirements of state departments that have jurisdiction over them. Generally, when state and federal regulations are similar or duplicated, the stricter regulation applies. Other state agencies that may impose regulations include laboratory, pharmacy, radiology, and health facility licensure; public health departments; medical and nursing boards; workers' compensation programs; life safety; labor and employment; Medicare/Medicaid, healthcare risk management regulations; medical records; environmental safety; and business regulations.

Americans with Disabilities Act

The Americans with Disabilities Act (ADA) ensures civil rights protection for persons with disabilities similar to that provided for individuals on the basis of race, sex, national origin, or religion. Equal opportunity is guaranteed to those with disabilities with regard to employment, public accommodations, telecommunications, state and local government services, and transportation.

Title I of the act provides requirements for nondiscrimination in employment and became effective for employers with 25 or more employees on July 26, 1992, and for employers with 15 to 24 employees on July 26, 1994. Key points of the act include:

- Who must comply with and who is protected by the act
- What the law permits and prohibits with respect to establishing qualification standards
- Assessing the qualifications and capabilities of people with disabilities to perform specific jobs
- Requiring medical examinations and other inquiries
- Making "reasonable accommodation" for disabled employees
- Nondiscrimination requirements with regard to promotion, transfer, termination, compensation, leave, fringe benefits, and contractual arrangements

If a facility has been established for some time or is part of a larger entity, compliance with these regulations should be intact and ongoing. Newly established facilities can obtain information from the Equal Employment Opportunity Commission by telephoning (800) 669-EEOC or by writing to the Equal Employment Opportunity Commission Office of Communications and Legislative Affairs, 1801 L Street, NW, Washington, DC 20507 and asking for a copy of *A Technical Assistance Manual on the Employment Provisions of the Americans with Disabilities Act*. The most recent edition of this manual was published in January 1992. The following is a list of the chapter titles in the manual:

I. Title I: an overview of legal requirements
II. Who is protected by the ADA
 A. Individual with a disability
 B. Qualified individual with a disability
III. The reasonable accommodation obligation
IV. Establishing nondiscriminatory qualification standards and selection criteria

V. Nondiscrimination in the hiring process: recruitment, applications, pre-employment inquiries, testing
VI. Medical examinations and inquiries
VII. Nondiscrimination in other employment practices
VIII. Drug and alcohol abuse
IX. Workers compensation and work-related injury
X. Enforcement provisions

The manual explains many employment provisions through the use of examples to illustrate principles of the act. It also includes a resource directory with federal and nongovernmental assistance sources.

> [U]nder Titles II and III of the ADA, public, private, and public service hospitals and other health care facilities will need to comply with the *Accessibility Guidelines for Buildings and Facilities* (ADAAG) for alterations and new construction. The *Uniform Federal Accessibility Standards* (UFAS) also provides criteria for the disabled. Also available for use in providing quality design for the disabled is the American National Standards Institute (ANSI) A117.1 *American National Standard for Accessible and Usable Buildings and Facilities.*[1]

Among other things, the standards require that new facilities and alterations to existing buildings include an accessible path of travel, and rest rooms, telephone and drinking fountains must be accessible. Detailed descriptions of hallway and door width, elevator requirements, ramp specifications, and distance to exits are provided in the guidelines.

Title III of the act addresses "public accommodations" for the disabled. The act defines public accommodations as "private entities that affect commerce." These accommodation requirements extend, therefore, to a wide range of businesses, including physician offices, pharmacies, hospitals, hotels, retail stores, parks, private schools, restaurants, theaters, and daycare centers. Private clubs and religious organizations are exempt from the ADA requirements. Items such as signage in Braille, ramps and access for wheelchairs, auxiliary aids for the vision and hearing impaired, and barrier removal are addressed.

It is the owner's responsibility to verify state and local standards for accessibility and usability, which may be more stringent than ADA, Uniform Federal Accessibility Standards, or ANSI A117.1. Local building contractors should be familiar with these requirements and should be able to assist in programs to attain compliance. Facilities considering new construction need to comply with the "new construction" regulations of the act.

With regard to patient care, application of reasonable accommodation might include such things as a paper cup dispenser next to the water fountain for patients in wheelchairs; provision of a qualified interpreter for a deaf person (a family member may not be adequate because of emotional involvement or confidentiality problems); telecommunications device for the deaf; policies that accommodate seeing eye dogs; adding raised letters or Braille to elevator buttons and office signage; rearranging furniture, vending machines, and other equipment for easier access. Policies should be evaluated within the framework of ADA guidelines to prevent unintentional violations of the act.

In the surgical suite itself, some physical disabilities may present a challenge for the staff. At one freestanding surgical center, during the preadmission interview, each patient is asked whether he or she uses hearing aids, has vision problems, and has "any special positioning needs." This allows preparation time for equipment modification, supply needs, and any changes that may need to be made in patient care.

Clinical Laboratory Improvement Act

On September 1, 1992, the Department of Health and Human Services (DHHS) published regulations implementing the 1988 Clinical Laboratory Improvement Act (CLIA). CLIA sets uniform quality standards for facilities that perform clinical tests for the purpose of diagnosis, prevention, and treatment of disease. This act provides that laboratories conducting moderately or highly complex testing must be surveyed and recertified by the Health Care Financing Administration every 2 years and must participate in proficiency testing. They must also take part in competence testing programs and comply with personnel training standards. Laboratories in clinical settings performing "simple" tests may qualify for a "certificate of waiver" from such inspections. Tests in waived category include

1. Urine dipstick
2. Fecal occult blood
3. Ovulation test–visual color comparison for human luteinizing hormone
4. Urine pregnancy test–visual color comparison test

5. Erythrocyte sedimentation rate (nonautomated)
6. Hemoglobin, copper sulfate (nonautomated)
7. Whole blood glucose, by devices cleared by the Food and Drug Administration (FDA) for home use
8. Spun hematocrit
9. Hemoglobin by HemoCue
10. Cholesterol test by Chemtrak Accumeter, Advanced Care, Cholestech LDX, or Accucheck InstantPlus
11. Microbiology: QuickVue One-Step *Helicobacter pylori*, Pyloritek Test Kit; QuickVue One-Step Strep

Examples of waived facilities include home health agencies, physician offices, long-term care facilities, health clinics, chiropractors, rehabilitation facilities, ASCs, and pharmacies.

Each facility must evaluate their laboratory circumstance and comply with federal and state regulations. Most freestanding ambulatory centers fit into the waived category, and surgical centers affiliated with a full-service hospital usually have the support of a laboratory that is already CLIA certified.

Information regarding CLIA certification can be obtained from the state agency regulating laboratory testing in each state. They also have information regarding current CLIA regulations and any current changes or updates. Generally, this agency can also assist with obtaining waived status, quality control practices, and evaluation of policies and procedures within the facility.

Environmental Protection Agency

The Environmental Protection Agency (EPA) was created in 1970 to solve urgent environmental problems and to protect public health. Polluted air and water and quickly vanishing bird and animal species made the issues obviously apparent to all Americans, and the United States Congress responded. The mission of the Environmental Protection Agency is to "protect public health and to safeguard and improve the natural environment—air, water, and land—upon which human life depends." In the medical field, Environmental Protection Agency regulations affect the disposal of waste products considered hazardous to human life. This could mean contaminated with infectious agents or chemicals.

The EPA issued final standards and guidelines on September 15, 1997 to reduce air pollution from medical waste incinerators. These are required by the Clean Air Act amendment of 1990. Historically, these rules have been much debated, litigated, and very difficult to gain any consensus on. Agreement on just the definition of medical waste has cost many man hours and taxpayer and private dollars.

The guidelines include emission limits, a compliance schedule, training of operators, monitoring and inspection, record-keeping, and site approval sections. Compliance with state regulations should be investigated thoroughly. Most facilities find that utilizing a private handler for medical waste is the most economic option.

Handling of waste contaminated with bloodborne pathogens is described in the OSHA blood-borne pathogen regulations, discussed later in this chapter.

Fire Safety

The National Fire Protection Association 101 Life Safety Code has been adopted by the Health Care Financing Administration, which is responsible for Medicare and Medicaid reimbursement. Facilities participating in Medicare and Medicaid Programs shall comply with that code.[1] The latest edition of this code became effective February 7, 1997. The document addresses life safety from fire and similar emergencies. Issues covered include construction, protection, and occupancy features. Local fire marshall offices and construction engineers usually can provide access to the code.

When new construction or remodeling is planned, building materials, wall and floor coverings, furniture, and drapery materials must all comply with fire safety regulations (see Chapter 4). Often, the specifications of these items must be submitted to the regulating agency as proof of compliance. Signage for exit routes, fire alarms, and extinguishers must also comply. Local and state as well as federal regulations and guidelines must be observed. Most professional architectural offices are well versed in these areas and direct builders accordingly. It is wise to choose builders and architects who are familiar with healthcare facilities and the regulations concerning them.

Regardless of which fire regulations govern a facility, patient safety must be the primary focus. Accrediting agencies, such as the JCAHO and the Accreditation Association for Ambulatory Health Care (AAAHC), place great weight on staff training for emergencies and disasters. Both agencies recommend quarterly fire drills for all personnel on all shifts. Fire training should include use of fire alarm systems, containment of smoke and fire, fire extinguisher use, and evacuation procedures. Involvement of staff in practice fires can reveal problems not foreseen by in-house educators. For instance, a walk-through of the evacuation of a patient on the operating table reveals many unforeseen problems. Only the operating room staff can identify these problems and plan methods to handle them. Close cooperation with in-house engineering personnel, or local fire officials for smaller facilities, can improve fire response systems and employee response to such emergencies.

Food and Drug Administration

The FDA is responsible for the safety and efficacy of all regulated marketed medical products, including drugs; biologicals; special nutritional products, such as infant formulas and dietary supplements; and medical and radiation-emitting devices. The FDA has created the MedWatch program to facilitate monitoring of these items. MedWatch is an initiative designed to educate all health professionals about the critical importance of being aware of, monitoring for, and reporting adverse events and problems and to facilitate reporting to the agency.[3]

The American Medical Association began tracking adverse drug events in the 1950s, with the FDA developing their own program a few years later. Both organizations continued this monitoring process until the early 1970s, when the American Medical Association suspended its program. Since that time, a need has been identified to track medical device problems as well as adverse drug events. In 1990, the Safe Medical Device Act was passed that expanded the FDA's authority to regulate medical devices as well. This act also provided a streamlined reporting mechanism and in 1993 was improved further with the introduction of the MedWatch program. "The purpose of the MedWatch program is to enhance the effectiveness of postmarketing surveillance of medical products as they are used in clinical practice and to rapidly identify significant health hazards associated with these products."[3] In December 1995, the FDA issued its final rule on medical device reporting, which went into effect July 31, 1996.[4]

The program has four goals:

1. To increase awareness of drug and device-induced disease
2. To clarify what should and should not be reported to the agency
3. To make reporting easier by operating a single system for health professionals to report adverse events and product problems to the agency
4. To provide regular feedback to the healthcare community about safety issues involving medical products.

The program is dependent on healthcare professionals to report product problems and adverse medication events. Knowing which medical products are reportable is important:

1. *Drugs* are primarily articles "intended for use in the diagnosis, cure, mitigation, treatment, or prevention of disease in humans, or articles (other than food) intended to affect the structure or function of the body."[5]
2. *Biological products* include any virus, therapeutic serum, toxin, antitoxin, blood, blood component or derivative, allergenic product, or analogous product applicable to the prevention, treatment, or cure of the diseases or injury to humans. Vaccines are the only biological products not included in the MedWatch program. Vaccine problems should be reported to the Vaccine Adverse Experience Reporting System.[5]
3. *Medical devices* include products with an intended use similar to a drug but that do not achieve any of their primary intended purposes by chemical action in or on the body or by being metabolized.[5] Such devices include implants of any kind, latex gloves, dialysis machines, and pacemakers.
4. *Special nutrition products* include dietary supplements, infant formulas, and medical foods.[5]

Product problems should be reported if there is a concern about the quality, performance, or safety of any medication or device. In a recent change, incidents involving operator error that result in the improper use of a medical device must also be reported. With such reports, manufacturers may identify needs for improved instructions or labeling. Problems with product quality may occur during manufacturing, shipping, or storage. They include

- Product contamination
- Defective or missing components
- Poor packaging or product mix-up
- Questionable stability
- Device malfunctions
- Labeling concerns

An adverse event is defined by the FDA[6] as "any undesirable experience associated with the use of a medical product in a patient." The event is *serious* and should be reported when the patient outcome is

- *Death*—report if the patient's death is suspected as being a direct outcome of the adverse event.
- *Life threatening*—report if the patient was at substantial risk of dying at the time of the adverse event or if it is suspected that use or continued use of the product would result in the patient's death.
- *Hospitalization (initial or prolonged)*—report if admission to the hospital or prolongation of a hospital stay results because of the adverse event.
- *Disability*—report if the adverse event resulted in a significant, persistent, or permanent change; impairment; damage or disruption in the patient's body function/structure; physical activities; or quality of life.
- *Congenital anomaly*—report if there are suspicions that exposure to a medical product before conception or during pregnancy resulted in an adverse outcome in the child.
- *Requires intervention to prevent permanent impairment or damage*—report if you suspect that the use of a medical product may result in a condition that required medical or surgical intervention to preclude permanent impairment or damage to a patient.

There are different requirements for reporting *deaths* and *serious illnesses and injuries*. All deaths must be reported to the FDA *and* to the manufacturer. Serious illnesses and injuries must be reported by the facility directly to the manufacturer (if known). If the manufacturer is unknown, then the FDA should be notified. In the case of medical devices, these reports are due as soon as possible, but not more than 10 working days after the facility becomes aware of a device problem.

A standardized form for reporting has been developed for MedWatch (Fig. 3–1). A copy of the MedWatch reporting form and the FDA form for reporting adverse vaccine events can be found in the back of every *Physician's Desk Reference*. Brief instructions and guidelines are also included with these forms, as well as important contact numbers (Table 3–1). These confidential forms should be readily available to staff members, along with training in their use, which is documented.

In case of an equipment incident, it is imperative that the device be removed from service immediately. All covers, wrappers, caps, and pieces used with the device should be saved and labeled "NOT FOR USE," and the department manager should be notified. Replacement or alternative equipment should be secured as needed. The manufacturer vendor or representative should not be allowed to examine the device if a patient injury has occurred.

***Table 3–1.* Reference Numbers for the United States Food and Drug Administration**

(800) FDA-0178	To fax report
(800) FDA-7737	To report by modem
(800) FDA-1088	To report by phone or for information
(800) 822-7967	For a Vaccine Adverse Event Reporting System form for vaccines
http://www.fda.gov/medwatch	FDA online

Each facility must respond to the FDA requirements in several ways. Procedures for compliance with the FDA requirements must be developed, and a contact person must be designated who is responsible for the program. Procedures should address the following issues:

- A review procedure to determine when an event meets the FDA criteria
- A mechanism to ensure timeliness and completeness of the reports
- Documentation and record-keeping requirements for incident information reported to the FDA and manufacturers and access to such information
- Education and training programs that focus on employee obligations to identify and report events subject to facility reporting requirements, as well as teaching use of the reporting forms

Manufacturers are required to implement tracking programs to trace medical implants. Generally, this is accomplished by requiring the healthcare facilities who purchase these devices to keep a log of each item. The manufacturer's system must be comprehensive enough to supply the FDA with the following information:

- *Device information:* lot, batch, model, serial numbers, or other identifiers; date of receipt in the facility; names of those from whom the device was received
- *Patient information:* name, address, telephone, and social security numbers; date of implantation
- *Physician information:* name, address, and telephone number

MEDWATCH

THE FDA MEDICAL PRODUCTS REPORTING PROGRAM

For VOLUNTARY reporting by health professionals of adverse events and product problems

Page ___ of ___

Form Approved: OMB No. 0910-0291 Expires: 4/30/96
See OMB statement on reverse

FDA Use Only

Triage unit sequence #

A. Patient information

1. Patient identifier — In confidence
2. Age at time of event: ___ or Date of birth:
3. Sex ☐ female ☐ male
4. Weight ___ lbs or ___ kgs

B. Adverse event or product problem

1. ☐ Adverse event and/or ☐ Product problem (e.g., defects/malfunctions)
2. Outcomes attributed to adverse event (check all that apply)
   - ☐ death ___ (mo/day/yr)
   - ☐ life-threatening
   - ☐ hospitalization – initial or prolonged
   - ☐ disability
   - ☐ congenital anomaly
   - ☐ required intervention to prevent permanent impairment/damage
   - ☐ other: ___
3. Date of event (mo/day/yr)
4. Date of this report (mo/day/yr)
5. Describe event or problem
6. Relevant tests/laboratory data, including dates
7. Other relevant history, including preexisting medical conditions (e.g., allergies, race, pregnancy, smoking and alcohol use, hepatic/renal dysfunction, etc.)

C. Suspect medication(s)

1. Name (give labeled strength & mfr/labeler, if known)
   #1
   #2
2. Dose, frequency & route used
   #1
   #2
3. Therapy dates (if unknown, give duration) from/to (or best estimate)
   #1
   #2
4. Diagnosis for use (indication)
   #1
   #2
5. Event abated after use stopped or dose reduced
   #1 ☐ yes ☐ no ☐ doesn't apply
   #2 ☐ yes ☐ no ☐ doesn't apply
6. Lot # (if known)
   #1
   #2
7. Exp. date (if known)
   #1
   #2
8. Event reappeared after reintroduction
   #1 ☐ yes ☐ no ☐ doesn't apply
   #2 ☐ yes ☐ no ☐ doesn't apply
9. NDC # (for product problems only)
   – –
10. Concomitant medical products and therapy dates (exclude treatment of event)

D. Suspect medical device

1. Brand name
2. Type of device
3. Manufacturer name & address
4. Operator of device
   - ☐ health professional
   - ☐ lay user/patient
   - ☐ other: ___
5. Expiration date (mo/day/yr)
6. model # ___
   catalog # ___
   serial # ___
   lot # ___
   other #
7. If implanted, give date (mo/day/yr)
8. If explanted, give date (mo/day/yr)
9. Device available for evaluation? (Do not send to FDA)
   ☐ yes ☐ no ☐ returned to manufacturer on ___ (mo/day/yr)
10. Concomitant medical products and therapy dates (exclude treatment of event)

E. Reporter (see confidentiality section on back)

1. Name & address — phone #
2. Health professional? ☐ yes ☐ no
3. Occupation
4. Also reported to
   - ☐ manufacturer
   - ☐ user facility
   - ☐ distributor
5. If you do NOT want your identity disclosed to the manufacturer, place an " X " in this box. ☐

FDA

Mail to: MEDWATCH
5600 Fishers Lane
Rockville, MD 20852-9787

or FAX to:
1-800-FDA-0178

FDA Form 3500 1/96)

Submission of a report does not constitute an admission that medical personnel or the product caused or contributed to the event.

Figure 3–1. A sample of the MedWatch Reporting Form FDA form 3500.

- *End-of-life information (if applicable)*: date of explantation; whether a patient death occurred; permanent disposal of device.

Manufacturers are to monitor the facilities that use their products and to notify the FDA if any healthcare organization fails to document the required information.

The FDA was given civil and criminal authority to enforce the Medical Device Reporting rule by the Safe Medical Device Act in 1991. Failure to adhere to these regulations may result in fines, imprisonment, or both, and ignorance of the regulations is not tolerated. Each facility must seek out and be in compliance with all applicable FDA regulations.

OCCUPATIONAL SAFETY AND HEALTH ADMINISTRATION

The Williams-Steiger Occupational Safety and Health Act of 1970, referred to as OSHA, was created "to assure, so far as possible, every working man or woman in the nation safe and healthful working conditions and to preserve our human resources." The intent of the act was to

- Encourage employers and employees to reduce hazards and to implement new or to improve existing safety and health programs
- Provide for research in occupational safety and health and to develop innovative ways of dealing with occupational safety and health problems
- Establish "separate but dependent responsibilities and rights" for employers and employees for the achievement of better safety and health conditions
- Maintain a reporting and record-keeping system to monitor job-related injuries and illnesses
- Establish training programs to increase the number and the competence of occupational safety and health personnel
- Develop mandatory job safety and health standards and enforce them effectively
- Provide means for the development, analysis, evaluation, and approval of state occupational safety and health programs

There are 25 states and territories with their own OSHA programs. When the federal OSHA issues new or updated standards or guidelines, the states must institute a similar program, with equal or more stringent requirements, within 180 days.

OSHA regulations for general industry have been issued in the Code of Federal Regulations (CFR), which is a codification of the general rules published in the *Federal Register* by the executive departments and agencies of the federal government. The code is divided into 50 "titles," which represent broad areas subject to federal regulation. Title 29 represents those rules pertaining to "labor." Each title is divided into volumes containing chapters, which are in turn subdivided into sections regarding specific regulatory areas. Title 29 comprises nine volumes, 1900 to 1910 (excluding 1909). Being able to identify the volumes and sections assists the reader in locating specific rules. For instance, individual regulations are usually cited in this format: "CFR 1910.111." This would refer to volume 1910, section 111.

The 29 CFR part 1910 is also called the "OSHA Standard for General Industry." Some sections of 29 CFR that are of primary interest to healthcare facilities are listed in Table 3–2. Many other issues are addressed in the CFR, and, unfortunately, OSHA does not send a list of applicable sections to each business. Each employer must seek out and comply with those standards that affect that particular business or risk penalties. Sources for OSHA information are listed in the Regulatory Agency Resource List at the end of this chapter.

Many OSHA regulations apply to ambulatory healthcare facilities. The information included in this chapter cannot possibly be all-inclusive but does summarize and highlight some of the

***Table 3–2.* Standards of Interest to Healthcare Found in Code of Federal Regulations—Title 29**

CODE OF FEDERAL REGULATIONS—TITLE 29 STANDARD TOPIC	SECTION
Access to employee exposure and medical records	1910.20
Accident signs and prevention	1910.145
Blood-borne pathogens	1910.1030
Electrical safety	1910.303-.306
Ergonomics	General Duty Clause
Ethylene oxide	1910.1047
Fire prevention	1910.38, .155- .165
Formaldehyde	1910.1048
Hazard communication	1910.1200
Ionizing radiations	1910.96
Log and summary of occupational injury and illness	1904.2
Noise exposure	1910.95
Respiratory protection	1910.134
Toxic and hazardous substances	1910.1200-.1500

most pertinent OSHA issues. Top management must be committed to provide safe and healthful working conditions and be willing to provide the necessary tools, such as personnel, budget, and support for an effective safety program. Every healthcare facility should have one person or department designated with the responsibility and the authority to fulfill necessary safety duties. For healthcare facilities, employers are responsible at least for the development of programs such as general safety and health, hazard communications, emergency action program (if 10 or more employees), fire protection program, blood-borne pathogens control program, and possibly hearing and respiratory protection programs, depending on the risk of exposure to employees. Other OSHA regulations may apply to a facility, so safety programs must be tailored individually.

General Safety and Health Program

The general safety and health program is the basic safety program that the facility establishes to comply with OSHA regulations. In it, all safety policies and procedures of the facility are defined. Management responsibility of the program within the facility should be identified, as should employee duties. Each safety program should include at least the following elements:

- Management responsibilities
- Employee participation
- Workplace analysis methods
- Identification and analysis of hazards
- Accident and record analysis
- Engineering and work practice controls
- Safety training
- Program evaluation

Posting OSHA Information

All employers are required to post information about the Occupational Safety and Health Act of 1970 as part of the employees' right to know how they are protected under the law. Under provisions of Title 29, CFR, part 1903.2(a)(1), employers must post OSHA form 2203 in a conspicuous place where notices to employees are customarily posted. The poster is sometimes called the "job safety poster" and briefly describes provisions of the Occupational Safety and Health Act (Fig. 3–2). A copy of this poster can be obtained from state or regional OSHA offices (see Regulatory Agency Resource List at the end of this chapter).

Medical and First Aid Standard

The Occupational Safety and Health Administration's Medical and First Aid Standard, 29 CFR 1910.151, is only three paragraphs long, but the third paragraph may have a significant impact on most healthcare facilities, including ambulatory centers. This paragraph, commonly referred to as "the eyewash standard," states

> (c) Where the eyes or body of any person may be exposed to injurious corrosive materials, suitable facilities for quick drenching or flushing of the eyes and body shall be provided within the work area for immediate emergency use.

Some examples of corrosives often seen in the medical environment would be glutaraldehyde, ethylene oxide, formaldehyde, chemotherapy drugs, cleaning chemicals, and developers and fixers.

This standard is a performance-based standard, and no specific guidelines are given for implementation, placement of eyewash units, or a list of chemicals that always require a full body shower or eyewash in the immediate work area. However, OSHA *does* follow the guidelines established by the ANSI Standard Z358.1 when performing on-site inspections. For eyewashes, ANSI recommends the following:

Initiation	One hand, one action to initiate, then the flow is continuous, leaving both hands free to open eyelids.
Location	Maximum 25 ft travel in 15 seconds (if solution is highly concentrated, 10 ft in 10 seconds).
Water quality	Potable with a temperature 60°F to 100°F; eyewash capable of 3 gallons/min 15 minutes; shower capable of 30 gallons/min for 15 minutes.
Maintenance	Float away covers to prevent contamination; flush units weekly for minimum of 3 minutes. Bump test eyewash daily, showers weekly, full-flow testing monthly. Document testing.
Training	Routine drills. Employees must *at least* know location and proper use of eyewash and showers.
Installation	Unit should be positioned so nozzles are 33 to 45 inches from the floor and 6 or more inches from the wall. Identify location with a highly visible sign.

Installing plumbed units in all appropriate locations can be very costly and labor intensive.

Job Safety and Health Protection

The Occupational Safety and Health Act of 1970 provides job safety and health protection for workers by promoting safe and healthful working conditions throughout the Nation. Provisions of the Act include the following:

Employers

All employers must furnish to employees' employment and a place of employment; free from recognized hazards that are causing or are likely to cause death or serious harm to employees. Employers must comply with occupational safety and health standards issued under the Act.

Employees

Employees must comply with all occupational safety and health standards, rules, regulations and orders issued under the Act that apply to their own actions and conduct on the job.

The Occupational Safety and Health Administration (OSHA) of the U.S. Department of Labor has the primary responsibility for administering the Act. OSHA issues occupational safety and health standards, and its Compliance Safety and Health Officers conduct jobsite inspections to help ensure compliance with the Act.

Inspection

The Act requires that a representative of the employer and a representative authorized by the employees be given an opportunity to accompany the OSHA inspector for the purpose of aiding the inspection.

Where there is no authorized employee representative, the OSHA Compliance Officer must consult with a reasonable number of employees concerning safety and health conditions in the workplace.

Complaint

Employees or their representatives have the right to file a complaint with the nearest OSHA office requesting an inspection if they believe unsafe or unhealthful conditions exist in their workplace. OSHA will withhold, on request, names of employees complaining.

The Act provides that employees may not be discharged or discriminated against in any way for filing safety and health complaints or for otherwise exercising their rights under the Act.

Employees who believe they have been discriminated against may file a complaint with their nearest OSHA office within 30 days of the alleged discriminatory action.

Citation

If upon inspection, OSHA believes an employer has violated the Act, a citation alleging such violations will be issued to the employer. Each citation will specify a time period within which the alleged violation must be corrected.

The OSHA citation must be prominently displayed at or near the place of alleged violation for three days, or until it is corrected, whichever is later, to warn employees of dangers that may exist there.

Proposed Penalty

The Act provides for mandatory civil penalties against employers of up to $7,000 for each serious violation and for optional penalties of up to $7,000 for each nonserious violation. Penalties of up to $7,000 per day may be proposed for failure to correct violations within the proposed time period and for each day the violation continues beyond the prescribed abatement date. Also, any employer who willfully or repeatedly violates the Act may be assessed penalties of up to $70,000 for each such violation. A minimum penalty of $5,000 may be imposed for each willful violation A violation of posting requirements can bring a penalty of up to $7,000.

There are also provisions for criminal penalties. Any willful violation resulting in the death of any employee, upon conviction, is punishable by a fine of up to $250,000 (or $500,000 if the employer is a corporation), or by imprisonment for up to six months, or both. A second conviction of an employer doubles the possible term of imprisonment. Falsifying records, reports, or applications is punishable by a fine of $10,000 or up to six months in jail or both.

Voluntary Activity

While providing penalties for violations, the Act also encourages efforts by labor and management, before an OSHA inspection, to reduce workplace hazards voluntarily and to develop and improve safety and health programs in all workplaces and industries. OSHA's Voluntary Protection Programs recognize outstanding efforts of this nature.

OSHA has published Safety and Health Program Management Guidelines to assist employers in establishing or perfecting programs to prevent or control employee exposure to workplace hazards. There are many public and private organizations that can provide information and assistance in this effort, if requested. Also, your local OSHA office can provide considerable help and advice on solving safety and health problems or can refer you to other sources for help such as training.

Consultation

Free assistance in identifying and correcting hazards and in improving safety and health management is available to employers, without citation or penalty, through OSHA-supported programs in each state. These programs are usually administered by the State Labor or Health department or a state university.

Posting Instructions

Employers in states operating OSHA-approved State Plans should obtain and post the state's equivalent poster.

Under provisions of Title 29, Code of Federal Regulations, Part 1903.2(a)(1) employers must post this notice (or facsimile) in a conspicuous place where notices to employees are customarily posted.

More Information

Additional information and copies of the Act, specific OSHA safety and health standards, and other applicable regulations may be obtained from your employer or from the nearest OSHA Regional Office in the following locations:

Atlanta, GA	(404) 347-3573
Boston, MA	(617) 565-7164
Chicago, IL	(312) 353-2220
Dallas, TX	(214) 767-4731
Denver, CO	(303) 844-3061
Kansas City, MO	(816) 426-5861
New York, NY	(212) 337-2378
Philadelphia, PA	(215) 596-1201
San Francisco, CA	(415) 744-6670
Seattle, WA	(206) 553-5930

Washington, DC
1992 (Reprinted)
OSHA 2203

Lynn Martin, Secretary of Labor

U.S. Department of Labor

Occupational Safety and Health Administration

To report suspected fire hazards, imminent danger safety and health hazards in the workplace, or other job safety and health emergencies, such as toxic waste in the workplace, call OSHA's 24-hour hotline: 1-800-321-OSHA.

The information will be made available to sensory impaired individuals upon request. Voice phone (202) 219-8615; TDD message referral phone: 1-800-326-2577.

* U.S.GPO: 1992—334-220

Figure 3–2. Occupational Safety and Health Administration Job Safety Poster, OSHA form 2203.

One acceptable solution is to install small eyewash units on existing faucets in the work areas where corrosive exposure may occur. Another option would be to install self-contained eyewash stations in areas that do not have existing plumbing. These self-contained units are available through safety equipment companies but should be evaluated for compliance with the standard before installation.

Hazard Communication Standard

Commonly called the "Right to Know Law," OSHA's Hazard Communication Standard

(HazCom), 29 CFR 1910.1200, requires that employees be protected from exposure to hazardous chemicals in the workplace. The HazCom standard covers manufacturers, distributors, and employers who use hazardous chemicals. Hazardous chemicals include any chemicals that present an actual or potential physical or health hazard. The HazCom standard does not include chemical products covered by other regulatory agencies except for the FDA, but it does cover drugs if they are hazardous and employees may be exposed to them.

This standard is based on the concept that employees have a need and a right to know which chemical hazards they are exposed to while at work, and what protective measures are available to protect them. Each employer is expected to develop a hazard communication program to aid employees in recognizing and handling hazardous chemicals on a daily basis. This program must include:

- Identification and listing of all hazardous chemicals in the facility
- A material safety data sheet system
- Container labeling and warning systems
- Personal protective equipment
- Employee information and training

Hazard Identification

The first step in developing the exposure control plan is to inventory all potentially harmful chemicals and substances in the facility. A thorough "walk-through" should be conducted, in which all cupboards, closets, and storage areas for products used by the staff are examined. Conducting the inventory itself usually results in a reduction of chemicals when dated or unused items are located and can be eliminated from stock. The product name and the manufacturer's address and phone number are noted, as well as the location or locations where the product is stored. It is a good idea to cross reference the list with that of the purchasing department to see if all products are listed. The business office area, where there are hidden hazards, like copier toner and correction fluid, should not be neglected.

Next, all items on the list are evaluated to see if any are exempt from the rule. Those items that are "a consumer product . . . where the employer can show that it is used in the workplace for the purpose intended by the chemical manufacturer . . . and the . . . duration and frequency . . . of exposure . . . is not greater than . . . that . . . experienced by consumers."[7] are exempt. For instance, bleach being used in the washer of a small laundry room in a freestanding facility would be exempt. If that same bleach is used in several areas of the facility as a disinfectant, it then falls under the HazCom regulations because this is not how the manufacturer intended it for "consumer purpose," and the duration and frequency of exposure are greater than what the average consumer would experience.

Some common hazardous chemicals in the surgical setting are formaldehyde, ethylene oxide, compressed gases, and glutaraldehyde. Procedures for proper handling, storage, and spill clean-up or emergency exposure should be well known to all employees who come into contact with these and all other hazardous chemicals found within the facility.

Hazardous Drugs

The HazCom Standard states (1910.1200 [b] (630-792-5)[vii]) that only the following drugs are exempt from the rule: "Any drug . . . when it is in solid, final form for direct administration to the patient (e.g., tablets or pills)." Literally taken, this would mean than any medication in injectable, liquid, or aerosol form would be considered as potentially hazardous. In the *OSHA Technical Manual*, section VI, Chapter 2 "Controlling Occupational Exposure to Hazardous Drugs,"[8] OSHA attempted to describe pharmaceuticals that are considered "hazardous." Whether this exempts other liquids, injectables, and aerosols is subject to interpretation.

The following questions, as posed by the American Society of Hospital Pharmacists, are suggested in the OSHA Technical Manual to assist in designating a drug as hazardous:

- Is the drug designated as therapeutic category 10:00 (antineoplastic agent) in the American Hospital Formulary Service Drug Information?
- Does the manufacturer suggest the use of special isolation techniques in its handling, administration, or disposal?
- Is the drug known to be a human mutagen, carcinogen, teratogen, or reproductive toxicant?
- Is the drug known to be acutely toxic to an organ system?

The technical manual goes on to suggest guidelines for handling antineoplastic drugs. All areas are covered, including categorization of drugs, physical effects, precautions to reduce exposure, disposal of wastes as toxic, and other handling procedures. The hazard communication program should address handling of hazardous drugs if this is part of the scope of care of the facility. Certainly, outpatient facilities have been known to administer intravenous chemotherapy, and bladder irrigation with a cytotoxic agent after a cystoscopic procedure is not unusual. More information on the OSHA antineoplastic drug guidelines is available through regional OSHA offices or on the Internet (see the Regulatory Agency Resource List at the end of this chapter for contact information).

Waste Anesthetic Gases

Waste anesthetic gases (WAGs) have been addressed in fact sheet no. OSHA 91-38, in DHHS (NIOSH) publication no. 94-100 and in NIOSH "Hazard Controls" DHHS (NIOSH) publication no. 96-107. The WAGs and vapors of concern to OSHA are nitrous oxide and the halogenated agents enflurane, halothane, methoxyflurane, trichloroethylene, and chloroform. Workers who may be exposed to these WAGs include nurses, physicians (e.g., anesthesiologists, surgeons, obstetricians, gynecologists), operating room technicians, postanesthesia recovery personnel, dentists, and veterinarians and their assistants. OSHA lists the potential effects of exposure to WAGs as liver and kidney damage, spontaneous abortions, and congenital abnormalities in children.

The American Society of Perianesthesia Nurses has issued a position statement entitled "Air Safety in the Perianesthesia Environment," which addresses not only WAGs but also respiratory pathogens and recommends "adherence to regulations and guidelines set forth by nationally recognized agencies such as NIOSH, CDC, and OSHA."[9] OSHA has recommended a WAG management program that includes a scavenging system, work practices to minimize leakage, equipment maintenance to prevent leakage, exposure monitoring, and provision for adequate room ventilation. This program is outlined in fact sheet no. OSHA 91-38. Specific guidelines for controlling nitrous oxide can be seen in DHHS (NIOSH) publication no. 94-100, which can be obtained by calling (800) 35-NIOSH. Both are available on the Internet, also.

Material Safety Data Sheets

Once the inventory is complete, the next requirement of the right to know law to be addressed is the material safety data sheet (MSDS) (Fig. 3–3). An MSDS must be in place for each item in inventory. The MSDS is a document provided by the chemical manufacturer that provides important details about the chemical. MSDSs must contain at least the following information, although no particular format is mandated:

- Chemical and common names (product identity)
- Manufacturer information: name, address, and telephone number
- Hazardous ingredients/identity information
- Physical/chemical characteristics
- Fire and explosion hazard data
- Reactivity data
- Health hazard data, including emergency and first aid procedures
- Precautions for safe handling and use
- Control measures
- Date the MSDS was printed

The manufacturer of the chemical is required to provide an MSDS to each employer the chemical is shipped to. If the chemical manufacturer becomes aware of any new information about the product, or if there are any changes in product formulation, this new information must be "added to the material safety data sheet within 3 months."[7]

It is the responsibility of each employer to maintain, in the workplace, an MSDS for each hazardous chemical used by the facility, including drugs as described in the previous section. These must be in English and must be easily accessible. In larger facilities, copies of MSDSs appropriate for each department are kept in designated areas. Employees of another employer working in the facility must also have access to the MSDSs.

Some employers keep the MSDSs in a brightly colored binder on a shelf or in a cupboard marked with large signage of some kind. Yellow and black striped binders are available from many safety supply organizations, although they are not required by the HazCom standard. Highlighting the "first aid" section of each MSDS simplifies locating this information in an emergency situation.

Personal Protective Equipment

The OSHA standards regarding personal protective equipment are outlined in 29 CFR 1910.132-140. The employer's responsibility to provide and maintain all necessary equipment to safeguard employees is included along with

Material Safety Data Sheet
May be used to comply with
OSHA's Hazard Communication Standard,
29 CFR 1910.1200. Standard must be
consulted for specific requirements.

U.S. Department of Labor
Occupational Safety and Health Administration
(Non-Mandatory Form)
Form Approved
OMB No. 1218-0072

Identity *(As Used on Label and List)*	***Note:*** *Blank spaces are not permitted. If any item is not applicable, or no information is available, the space must be marked to indicate that.*

Section I

Manufacturer's Name	Emergency Telephone Number
Address *(Number, Street, City, State, and ZIP Code)*	Telephone Number for Information
	Date Prepared
	Signature of Preparer *(optional)*

Section II — Hazardous Ingredients/Identity Information

Hazardous Components (Specific Chemical Identity: Common Name(s))	OSHA PEL	ACGIH TLV	Other Limits Recommended	% *(optional)*

Section III — Physical/Chemical Characteristics

Boiling Point		Specific Gravity (H_2O = 1)	
Vapor Pressure (mm Hg)		Melting Point	
Vapor Density (AIR = 1)		Evaporation Rate (Butyl Acetate = 1)	

Solubility in Water

Appearance and Odor

Section IV — Fire and Explosion Hazard Data

Flash Point (Method Used)	Flammable Limits	LEL	UEL

Extinguishing Media

Special Fire Fighting Procedures

Unusual Fire and Explosion Hazards

(Reproduce locally) OSHA 174, Sept. 1985

Figure 3–3. Occupational Safety and Health Administration Material Safety Data Sheet, OSHA form 174.

appropriate types of equipment and fit testing requirements. The employer must ensure safety with appropriate equipment, clothing, devices, systems, controls, and training.

The MSDS indicates what types of personal protective equipment should be worn for safety when a particular chemical is used. This information can be found in the section titled "control measures." A respirator or mask should be worn to prevent exposure to dangerous vapors, gases, or aerosols. Protective aprons, cover coats, and footwear protect the employee from liquid substances, as do protective gloves, which should be made of a substance appropriate for the chemical being used. Goggles or safety glasses, with side shields, should be worn to protect the eyes from splashes, and in some cases, a full face shield may be more appropriate.

Container Labeling

Often within a facility, chemicals are transferred into smaller containers for convenience of use. Each individual container of the product must be labeled to ensure the safety of the user. The identity of the chemical and hazard warnings regarding the physical and health hazards of the chemical must be on the new label. It must be legible, in English, and prominently displayed. The labels should also be resistant to fading or other damage from the chemical itself, should it drip or run down the container in some way. By shrinking an original label on a photocopy machine, then attaching the new label to the smaller container with wide plastic tape, all pertinent information is automatically transferred. When this technique is used, the information on the smaller labels should be readable and prominent. Another option is to use "fill-in-the-blank" adhesive labels available from suppliers of industrial safety equipment. These are available in different sizes to fit different containers and to streamline the labeling process.

When containers other than the original are used, cost of volume buying must be weighed against the purchase of smaller containers with the appropriate label already in place. The new container must be physically suitable for the product. If the product arrives in a glass container, then the smaller containers should probably also be made of glass.

In the healthcare field, there is a longstanding history of soaking instruments and other items in open trays, bottles, and canisters of disinfectant solutions. These chemicals fall under the HazCom standard, and so the containers must be labeled in some way. The standard states that ". . . signs, placards, process sheets, batch tickets, or other such labels . . . as long as the alternative method identifies the containers to which it is applicable"[7] are acceptable. A placard on the countertop next to the container and covered with clear adhesive paper is an easy option to labeling containers themselves.

"The employer is not required to label portable containers into which hazardous chemicals are transferred from labeled containers, and which are intended only for the immediate use of the employee who performs the transfer."[7] If only one employee will be using the portable container for one shift, a label is not required.

Employee Information and Training

"Employers shall provide employees with effective information and training on hazardous chemicals in their work area at the time of their initial assignment, and whenever a new physical or health hazard the employees have not previously been trained about is introduced into their work area."[7] This training should include information about the HazCom standard, the training requirements, which operations in their work area will expose employees to hazardous chemicals, and the location of the HazCom program, the inventory of hazardous chemicals in their workplace, and the MSDSs. Training of employees must include

- Methods used in the workplace to detect the presence of a hazardous chemical
- The physical and health hazards of the chemicals in the work area
- Protective measures employees can take, including work practices, emergency procedures, and protective equipment
- Use of labels and the MSDSs, and how to obtain hazard information

What OSHA Will Look For

In the course of an inspection, the OSHA compliance officer looks for evidence of compliance with the hazard communication standard. Evidence of compliance with the HazCom Standard includes

- Designation of person or persons responsible for the HazCom program, including labeling, MSDS maintenance, and staff training. This function may be performed by several persons, one for each department, or one for each task, respectively.

Table 3–3. Occupational Safety and Health Administration (OSHA) Regional Offices

Region I (CT*, MA, ME, NH, RI, VT*) JFK Federal Building, Room E34D 1st Floor Boston, MA 02203 (617) 565-9860	***Region II*** (NJ, NY*, PR*, VI*) 201 Varick Street Room 670 New York, NY 10014 (212) 337-2378
Region III (DC, DE, MD*, PA, VA*, WV) Gateway Building, Suite 2100 3535 Market Street Philadelphia, PA 19104 (215) 596-1201	***Region IV*** (AL, FL, GA, KY*, MS, NC*, SC*, TN*) 61 Forsythe St. S.W. Atlanta, GA 30303 (404) 562-2300
Region V (IL, IN*, MI*, MN*, OH, WI) 230 South Dearborn Street Room 3244 Chicago, IL 60604 (312) 353-2220	***Region VI*** (AR, LA, NM*, OK, TX) 525 Griffin Street Room 602 Dallas, TX 75202 (214) 767-4731
Region VII (IA*, KS, MO, NE) City Center Square Suite 800 Kansas City, MO 64105 (816) 426-5861	***Region VIII*** (CO, MT, ND, SD, UT*, WY*) 1999 Broadway Suite 1690 Denver, CO 80202-1600 (303) 844-1600
Region IX (American Samoa, AZ*, CA*, Guam, HI*, NV*, Pacific Trust Territories) 71 Stevenson Street Room 420 San Francisco, CA 94105 (415) 975-4310 (800) 475-4019	***Region X*** (AK*, ID, OR*, WA*) 1111 Third Avenue Suite #715 Seattle, WA 98101-3212 (206) 553-5930

* States and territories with their own OSHA programs. Connecticut and New York plans apply only to public employees. State-approved plans must be equal to or at least as effective as Federal OSHA.

- The written HazCom program itself, which includes all required elements and procedures.
- Records and documentation such as the following support the effectiveness of the program: training session records of attendance, inventory of all hazardous chemicals in the workplace, MSDS files and binders, and minutes of meetings where HazCom was discussed and outlined.

The following checklist assists personnel in determining whether they are in compliance with the Hazard Communication standard:

1. Have a copy of the rule. (see HazCom resources).
2. Read and understand the requirements.
3. Assign program responsibility.
4. Program is written.
5. Have inventory of chemicals available.
6. Ensure labeling is complete.
7. Have MSDS for each item in inventory.
8. Ensure that MSDS is available to all workers.
9. Ensure that training of all workers is on record.
10. Ensure that program is ongoing.
11. Ensure that program is evaluated and updated periodically.

HazCom Resources

In addition to the standard itself, several pamphlets are available from OSHA that help in understanding and implementing the HazCom program. These may be obtained by contacting the OSHA publications office at (202) 523-9667 or the regional OSHA Office (Table 3–3).

OSHA publication No. 3084 "Chemical Hazard Communication"

OSHA publication No. 2254 "Training guidelines from OSHA Training Institute"

Emergency Action Program

The emergency action program applies to employers with 10 or more employees and establishes the protocol to be followed in the event of an emergency. Key personnel and specific tasks are to be identified, as well as evacuation routes for employee exiting during an emergent situation. Reference to these requirements can be found in 29 CFR 1910.38. Generally, the fire evacuation plan can double as the emergency evacuation plan with just a few alterations. Many facilities have only one plan for all emergent situations.

Fire Protection Program

General fire protection issues have been addressed previously in this chapter. A more in-depth evaluation can be found in Chapter 4. OSHA requirements are specific for fire extinguisher training and testing criteria for fixed fire extinguishing equipment, among others. There is also a checklist included in the OSHA fire protection regulations that can be used to document the on-site assessments. Specific fire requirements can be found in 29 CFR 1910.155-165.

Blood-Borne Pathogens Control Program

The blood-borne pathogen standard was instituted in 1992 in an effort to protect health-care workers from pathogens transmitted through blood and other body fluids. Pathogens include hepatitis B, hepatitis C, human immunodeficiency virus, syphilis, and malaria. Those workers who, as a result of performing their daily job duties, can reasonably anticipate exposure to blood and other body fluids, are covered by this standard.

Each facility must have a copy of the entire standard available for employee reference. It is located in 29 CFR 1910.1030. Careful study of the standard reveals necessary elements of compliance. The following is a partial listing of critical points; however, each facility must demonstrate compliance with all items in the standard:

- Standard precautions
- Exposure control plan
- Engineering and work practice controls
- Personal protective equipment
- Training

Standard Precautions

Formerly known as "universal precautions," these guidelines were recently revised in a joint effort of the Centers for Disease Control and Prevention and the Hospital Infection Control Practices Advisory Committee. The new guidelines clarify confusion and standardize isolation precautions nationwide with simplified descriptions and clearer terminology. The new term *standard precautions* incorporates features of universal blood and body fluid precautions and body substance isolation precautions. Any employee performing procedures in which there is a likelihood of exposure to blood or body fluids should apply these standards, regardless of the patient's diagnosis.

Exposure Control Plan

The Occupational Safety and Health Administration requires each facility to have an exposure control plan that addresses multiple issues related to blood-borne pathogens. Table 3–4 provides a list of items to be covered in the exposure control plan. This plan must be acces-

Table 3–4. Items to be Addressed in the Exposure Control Plan

Accidents, incidents, and investigating	Handwashing
Biohazard labeling	Hepatitis B immunization
Classification of exposure categories	Housekeeping methods and records
Cleaning up spills/splashes of body fluids	Informed consent for HIV testing
Decontamination/labeling of contaminated equipment	Injury on the job
Employee health program	Laundry
Employee medical records	Masks
Employees of other employers	Needlesticks/puncture wounds/cuts
Engineering controls	OSHA 200 log
Exposure Control Coordinator duties and responsibilities	Policy review and updating
Exposure determination and categories	Postexposure follow-up
Exposure to blood or body fluids	Protective equipment
Gloves	Surveillance of risk
Goggles/eyewear/facemask	Training of employees
Gowns/aprons/labcoats	Warning labels
	Waste disposal
	Work practices

HIV, human immunodeficiency virus.

sible to all employees, and they should be familiar with it. Should an OSHA inspection occur, this plan is most likely to be scrutinized carefully and employees quizzed regarding its content.

Waste Disposal

Infectious waste (sometimes referred to as *biohazardous*, *medical*, or just *hazardous* waste) disposal, is addressed in the "Compliance Assistance Guidelines for the . . . Enforcement Procedures for Occupational Exposure to Hepatitis B Virus and Human Immunodeficiency Virus" published by OSHA in 1991. These guidelines list the following consideration for waste disposal:

- Disposal of all infectious waste shall be in accordance with applicable federal, state, and local regulations.
- All infectious waste shall be placed in closable, leakproof containers or bags that are color coded, labeled, or tagged. Biohazard symbol should be used.
- Disposable syringes, needles, scalpel blades, and other sharp items shall be placed in puncture-resistant containers for disposal.
- Puncture-resistant sharps containers shall be easily accessible to workers and located in areas where sharps are commonly used.
- Double-bagging before handling, storing, or transporting infectious waste is necessary if the outside of a bag is contaminated with blood or other potentially infectious materials.
- Laboratory specimens of body fluids shall be transported in a container that will prevent leaking and shall be disposed of in accordance with institutional policies and regulatory requirements.

Hearing and Respiratory Protection Programs

Depending on the conditions employees are exposed to involving noise levels or exposure to toxic or hazardous fumes, employers must establish written programs for hearing and respiratory protection. With regard to respiratory protection, employees must be trained in proper donning, doffing, maintenance, care, and limitation of respiratory equipment, including fit testing. In the healthcare industry, two areas that are currently under close scrutiny are cautery/laser plume and exposure to air-borne pathogens, especially tuberculosis. New information is frequently forthcoming in these critical areas and must be assessed by management continually.

Smoke from Laser/Electrical Surgical Procedures

Occupational Safety and Health Administration standard 1910.134, personal protective equipment, states: ". . . the primary objective [of respiratory protection] shall be to prevent atmospheric contamination . . . in the control of those occupational diseases caused by breathing air contaminated with harmful dusts, fogs, fumes, mists, gases, smokes, sprays or vapors."

The National Institute for Occupational Safety and Health (NIOSH) is the federal agency based in Washington, DC that is responsible for conducting research and making recommendations for preventing work-related illness and injuries for OSHA. In an October 1996 "Hazard Controls" communication, NIOSH emphasized the importance of dealing with smoke plume and offered some work practice control actions. This is a public domain document, DHHS (NIOSH) publication no. 96-128 and is available from NIOSH by calling (800) 356-4674 or on the Internet at http://ftp.cdc.gov.niosh/hc11.html.

The thermal destruction of tissue during a surgical procedure creates a smoke byproduct. Information about this laser plume has been available for many years, but recent studies demonstrate that the plume generated by electrocautery and other thermal cutting methods may be equally dangerous, or even more so.

In the NIOSH publication, several issues are addressed:

- "Research studies have confirmed that this smoke plume can contain toxic gases and vapors such as benzene, hydrogen cyanide, and formaldehyde, bioaerosols, dead and live cellular material (including blood fragments), and viruses."
- "At high concentrations the smoke causes ocular and upper respiratory tract irritation in health care personnel, and creates visual problems for the surgeon."
- "The smoke has unpleasant odors and has been shown to have mutagenic potential."

Research at NIOSH has shown there are two methods of control that effectively control the air-borne contaminants.

Ventilation

A combination of local exhaust ventilation (LEV) and general room ventilation is recommended by NIOSH:

- "General room ventilation is not by itself sufficient to capture contaminants generated at the source. The two major LEV approaches used to reduce surgical smoke levels for health care personnel are portable smoke evacuators and room suction systems. Smoke evacuators contain a suction unit (vacuum pump), filter, hose, and an inlet nozzle. The smoke evacuator should have high efficiency in airborne particle reduction and should be used in accordance with the manufacturer's recommendations . . . [with a] capture velocity of about 100 to 150 feet per minute at the inlet nozzle . . . recommended."
- "A high efficiency particulate air (HEPA) or equivalent is recommended for trapping particulate. The various filters and absorbers used in smoke evacuators require monitoring and replacement on a regular basis and are considered possible biohazards requiring proper disposal."
- "Room suction systems can pull at a much lower rate and were designed . . . to capture liquids rather than particulate or gases. If these systems are used . . . , users must install appropriate filters in the lines, insure that the line is cleared, and that filters are disposed of properly. Generally . . . smoke evacuators are more effective than room suction systems."

Work Practices

- It is most effective to keep the hose nozzle inlet within 2 inches of the surgical site, and the evacuator should remain on whenever airborne particles are being produced.
- All tubing, filters, nozzles, and related equipment should be handled as any other biohazard, disposed of properly, and completely new set-ups used for each case.
- Preventive maintenance and inspections on all systems prevent leaks and other breakdowns.

Protection of employees from this potentially harmful plume applies at least under the OSHA general duty clause, and perhaps other respiratory protection sections. As research reveals more and more dangers from smoke and plume, current literature supports taking steps to control exposure.

Ergonomics

Ergonomics is the "study of equipment design in order to reduce operator fatigue and discomfort."[10] It is sometimes called *human engineering*. In the early 1970s, the automotive industry used this engineering idea to redesign car interiors for comfort and efficiency. This science is applied in the workplace to help workers interact more efficiently, with improved comfort and safety in their work environment. Proper application of ergonomics can reduce cumulative trauma disorders, minimize on-the-job stress, and result in reductions in worker injuries.

In the early 1990s, OSHA began steps toward an ergonomic policy. In March 1995, OSHA published the "Draft Proposed Ergonomics Protection Standard," which was never adopted as official policy. This document has since been deleted, but OSHA has announced its intention to resurrect the ergonomics proposal in a four-step plan that includes enforcement, educational, and research activities. In any case, ergonomics issues will always fall under OSHA's general duty clause, and wise employers will be aware of the implications. Issues addressed in previous ergonomics standards included

- Identification of musculoskeletal disorders that occur in the workplace by using annual surveys
- Evaluation of jobs that have previously led to worker injuries
- Identification of high-risk jobs and actions to correct either the job or the working conditions of the job
- Employer adoption of procedures to respond to employee complaints and offer medical management
- Employee involvement and training in ergonomic safety issues

Cumulative Trauma Disorder

When the same task is performed on a continual basis, the repetitive motion can put excessive strain on isolated groups of muscles, tendons, and joints. Eventually, the worker feels stiffness and pain, which can lead to difficulty using the injured part of the body. This type of injury is called a cumulative trauma disorder. For example, many keyboard operators identify their job conditions as a cause of carpal tunnel syndrome. Other kinds of factors that can increase the risk of acquiring a cumulative trauma disorder include jobs requiring excessive force (lifting) or requiring the employee to be in an awkward position, work in extreme temperatures, using tools or equipment that vibrates for an extended period of time, and overall poor physical health.

Informed employers focus on prevention of cumulative trauma disorders in the workplace.

Workers and employers must work together to analyze the risk of exposure involved in each job and control the cause or change the environment around the risk. For example, a simple foot rest can reduce lower back strain for employees who spend extended time sitting at a desk. Headsets for those who must use the phone repeatedly can reduce shoulder and neck stress. Stepstools should be used when reaching for items stored overhead. Employee training is necessary on a continual basis, because human nature tends to promote unwise use and abuse of our musculoskeletal systems. This is evidenced in the constant barrage of back injuries seen in the workplace.

Information on ergonomic safety is also available through NIOSH and the American College of Occupational and Environmental Medicine (see Regulatory Agency Resource List). Reducing worker stress and injury has many positive benefits, including improved worker satisfaction and health, reduction in lost work days, fewer workers' compensation claims, and more efficient operations.

Reporting Occupational Injuries and Illnesses

The Occupational Safety and Health Administration issued the regulation regarding occupational injury and illness recording in 1971 under 29 CFR part 1904. Employers with 11 or more employees are required to keep an illness and injury record. The regulation includes criteria to determine whether an occupational injury or illness is recordable, as well as defining which records employers must give employees and OSHA access to. Understanding this regulation is easier through the use of the booklet "Recordkeeping Guidelines for Occupational Injuries and Illnesses," sometimes called the Blue Book, available from OSHA (see Regulatory Agency Resource List). The most recent edition of this was completed in 1986. There is currently a movement underway to simplify and streamline the reporting process, but nothing definitive is available at present.

The Occupational Safety and Health Administration requires that all work-related deaths and illnesses be recorded. Nonfatal injuries must also be recorded, but these are limited to those requiring medical treatment or involving loss of consciousness, restriction of work or motion, and requiring that the employee be transferred to another job. Injuries requiring only first aid treatment are not recordable.

Two forms are used for OSHA employee record keeping. The first, the OSHA no. 200, serves two purposes: (1) as the log of occupational injuries and illnesses on which the occurrence, extent, and outcome of cases are recorded during the year, and (2) as the summary of occupational injuries and illnesses used to summarize the log at the end of the year to satisfy employer posting obligations (Fig. 3–4). A portion of the OSHA 200 form must be posted for all employees to see from February 1 to March 1 of each year. This section reveals the types of injuries or illness occurring in the past year and the number of lost work days. Posting this information provides employees with information regarding possible hazards in their workplace. If OSHA conducts a "spot" inspection in February and the form is not posted, the facility is subject to stiff monetary penalties.

The second form, the supplementary record of occupational injuries and illnesses, OSHA no. 101 (Fig. 3–5), provides additional details of each of the cases that have been recorded on the log.[11]

What Is Recordable?

Understanding the difference between "medical" and "first aid" treatment is important because only those injuries requiring medical treatment are recordable. The instructions on the back of the OSHA 200 form define medical treatment as

> treatment (other than first aid) administered by a physician or by registered professional personnel under the standing orders of a physician. Medical treatment does NOT include first aid treatment (one-time treatment and subsequent observation of minor scratches, cuts, burns, splinters, and so forth, which do not ordinarily require medical care) even though provided by a physician or registered professional personnel.

The distinction between medical treatment and first aid depends on the treatment provided to the employee and the severity of the injury being treated. First aid does not include emergency treatment of serious injuries. Injuries are not minor if

- Bodily function is impaired, as normal use of senses, limbs, and so on
- Nonsuperficial damage is done to physical structure (i.e., fractures)
- Complications are involved that require follow-up medical treatment

A visit to a physician for a diagnostic procedure or examination to determine the extent of

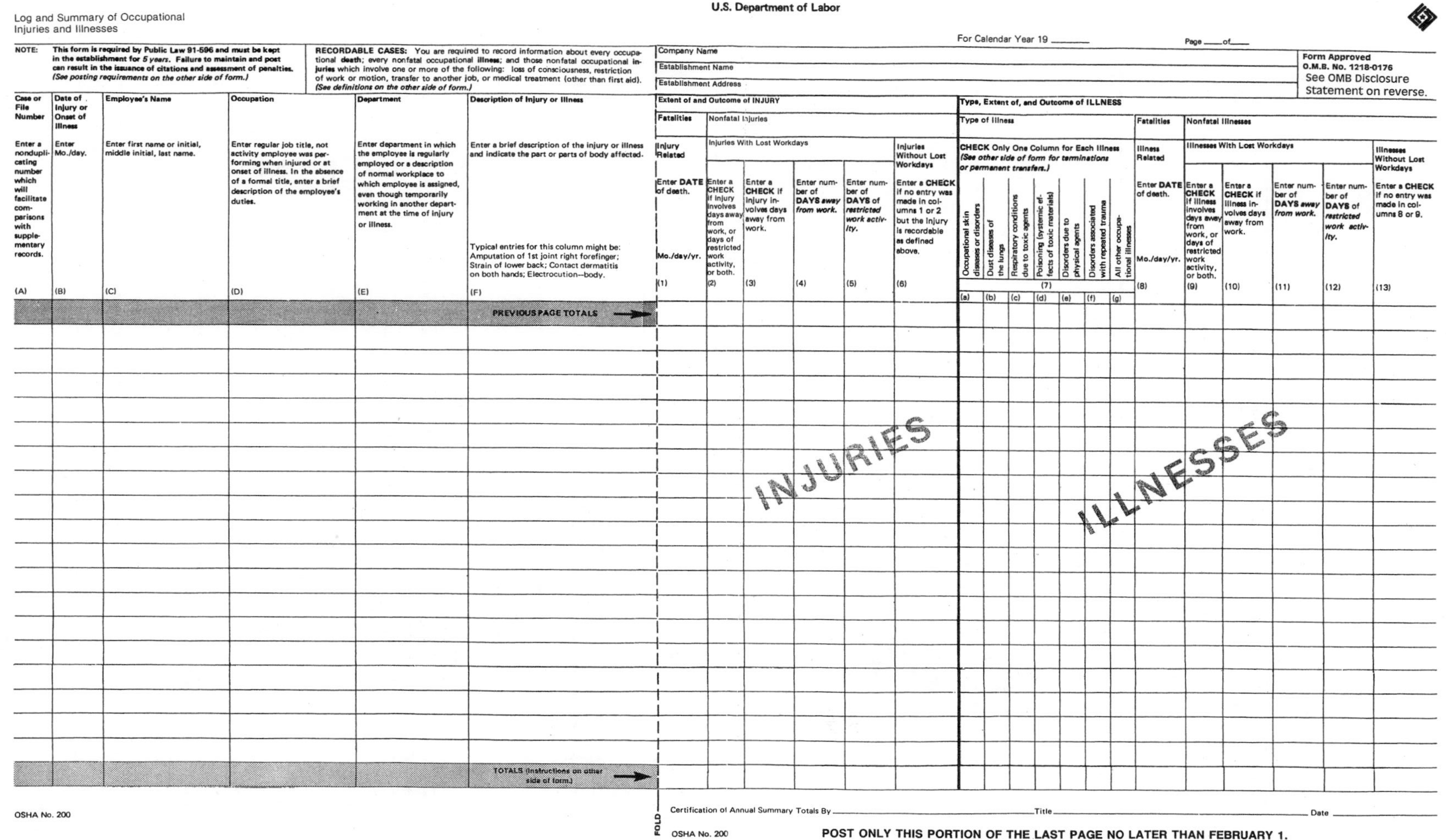

U.S. Department of Labor

Log and Summary of Occupational Injuries and Illnesses

For Calendar Year 19 ______ Page ___ of ___

Form Approved
O.M.B. No. 1218-0176
See OMB Disclosure Statement on reverse.

NOTE: **This form is required by Public Law 91-596 and must be kept in the establishment for 5 years. Failure to maintain and post can result in the issuance of citations and assessment of penalties.** *(See posting requirements on the other side of form.)*

RECORDABLE CASES: You are required to record information about every occupational **death**; every nonfatal occupational **illness**; and those nonfatal occupational **injuries** which involve one or more of the following: loss of consciousness, restriction of work or motion, transfer to another job, or medical treatment (other than first aid). *(See definitions on the other side of form.)*

Company Name
Establishment Name
Establishment Address

Case or File Number	Date of Injury or Onset of Illness	Employee's Name	Occupation	Department	Description of Injury or Illness
Enter a nonduplicating number which will facilitate comparisons with supplementary records.	Enter Mo./day.	Enter first name or initial, middle initial, last name.	Enter regular job title, not activity employee was performing when injured or at onset of illness. In the absence of a formal title, enter a brief description of the employee's duties.	Enter department in which the employee is regularly employed or a description of normal workplace to which employee is assigned, even though temporarily working in another department at the time of injury or illness.	Enter a brief description of the injury or illness and indicate the part or parts of body affected. Typical entries for this column might be: Amputation of 1st joint right forefinger; Strain of lower back; Contact dermatitis on both hands; Electrocution—body.
(A)	(B)	(C)	(D)	(E)	(F)
					PREVIOUS PAGE TOTALS →
					TOTALS (Instructions on other side of form.) →

Extent of and Outcome of INJURY

Fatalities: Injury Related	Nonfatal Injuries — Injuries With Lost Workdays				Injuries Without Lost Workdays
Enter DATE of death. Mo./day/yr.	Enter a CHECK if injury involves days away from work, or days of restricted work activity, or both.	Enter a CHECK if injury involves days away from work.	Enter number of DAYS away from work.	Enter number of DAYS of restricted work activity.	Enter a CHECK if no entry was made in columns 1 or 2 but the injury is recordable as defined above.
(1)	(2)	(3)	(4)	(5)	(6)

Type, Extent of, and Outcome of ILLNESS

Type of Illness — CHECK Only One Column for Each Illness *(See other side of form for terminations or permanent transfers.)* (7)

Occupational skin diseases or disorders	Dust diseases of the lungs	Respiratory conditions due to toxic agents	Poisoning (systemic effects of toxic materials)	Disorders due to physical agents	Disorders associated with repeated trauma	All other occupational illnesses
(a)	(b)	(c)	(d)	(e)	(f)	(g)

Fatalities: Illness Related	Nonfatal Illnesses — Illnesses With Lost Workdays				Illnesses Without Lost Workdays
Enter DATE of death. Mo./day/yr.	Enter a CHECK if illness involves days away from work, or days of restricted work activity, or both.	Enter a CHECK if illness involves days away from work.	Enter number of DAYS away from work.	Enter number of DAYS of restricted work activity.	Enter a CHECK if no entry was made in columns 8 or 9.
(8)	(9)	(10)	(11)	(12)	(13)

INJURIES

ILLNESSES

OSHA No. 200

FOLD

Certification of Annual Summary Totals By ______ Title ______ Date ______

OSHA No. 200

POST ONLY THIS PORTION OF THE LAST PAGE NO LATER THAN FEBRUARY 1.

Figure 3–4. Sample OSHA 200 form.

Bureau of Labor Statistics
Supplementary Record of
Occupational Injuries and Illnesses

U.S. Department of Labor

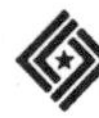

This form is required by Public Law 91-596 and must be kept in the establishment for *5 years.* Failure to maintain can result in the issuance of citations and assessment of penalties.	Case or File No.	Form Approved O.M.B. No. 1220-0029

Employer

1. Name

2. Mail address *(No. and street, city or town, State, and zip code)*

3. Location, if different from mail address

Injured or Ill Employee

4. Name *(First, middle, and last)* — Social Security No.

5. Home address *(No. and street, city or town, State, and zip code)*

6. Age — 7. Sex: *(Check one)* Male ☐ Female ☐

8. Occupation *(Enter regular job title, not the specific activity he was performing at time of injury.)*

9. Department *(Enter name of department or division in which the injured person is regularly employed, even though he may have been temporarily working in another department at the time of injury.)*

The Accident or Exposure to Occupational Illness

If accident or exposure occurred on employer's premises, give address of plant or establishment in which it occurred. Do not indicate department or division within the plant or establishment. If accident occurred outside employer's premises at an identifiable address, give that address. If it occurred on a public highway or at any other place which cannot be identified by number and street, please provide place references locating the place of injury as accurately as possible.

10. Place of accident or exposure *(No. and street, city or town, State, and zip code)*

11. Was place of accident or exposure on employer's premises? Yes ☐ No ☐

12. What was the employee doing when injured? *(Be specific. If he was using tools or equipment or handling material, name them and tell what he was doing with them.)*

13. How did the accident occur? *(Describe fully the events which resulted in the injury or occupational illness. Tell what happened and how it happened. Name any objects or substances involved and tell how they were involved. Give full details on all factors which led or contributed to the accident. Use separate sheet for additional space.)*

Occupational Injury or Occupational Illness

14. Describe the injury or illness in detail and indicate the part of body affected. *(E.g., amputation of right index finger at second joint; fracture of ribs; lead poisoning; dermatitis of left hand, etc.)*

15. Name the object or substance which directly injured the employee. *(For example, the machine or thing he struck against or which struck him; the vapor or poison he inhaled or swallowed; the chemical or radiation which irriatated his skin; or in cases of strains, hernias, etc., the thing he was lifting, pulling, etc.)*

16. Date of injury or initial diagnosis of occupational illness — 17. Did employee die? *(Check one)* Yes ☐ No ☐

Other

18. Name and address of physician

19. If hospitalized, name and address of hospital

Date of report	Prepared by	Official position

OSHA No. 101 (Feb. 1981)

Figure 3–5. Sample OSHA 101 form.

injury does not necessarily constitute medical treatment. Likewise, medical treatment may be provided to employees by someone other than a physician or registered medical professional.

The following are generally considered first aid treatment and are therefore not recordable, if the injury does not involve restriction of work or motion, loss of consciousness, or transfer to another job:

- Negative x-ray diagnosis
- Observation for evaluation of injury during a visit to medical personnel
- Superficial treatment with topical antiseptics and/or antibiotics
- Treatment of first-degree burns
- Foreign body removal from the eye if only irrigation is required
- Foreign body removal from wounds if procedure is uncomplicated, as by use of tweezers or other simple technique
- Removal of bandages by soaking, or soaking therapy on initial visit
- Application of elastic support bandages during initial visit to medical personnel
- Administration of nonprescription medications and/or administration of a singe dose of prescription medication on first medical visit for minor injury or discomfort

Exposure to blood-borne pathogens, through needlestick, puncture wound, spill, or splash, often results in a question of recordability. It is actually the result of the needlestick that determines whether it is recordable or not. The initial response is with first aid only, although it is the policy of most healthcare facilities to draw blood work on the affected employee.

Blood work in and of itself is not a medical treatment that triggers recordability.[12] If the needlestick involves loss of consciousness, restricted work assignment, transfer to another job, or a recommendation of medical treatment, it must be recorded. According to OSHA instruction CPL 2-2.44C, March 1992, "[The incident] shall be recorded if . . . [it] results in the recommendation of medical treatment beyond first aid (e.g., gamma globulin, hepatitis B immune globulin, hepatitis B vaccine, or zidovudine) regardless of dosage." Thus, if any of the aforementioned agents are given, the incident is reportable. Also, if a seroconversion occurs as a result of the incident, it is recordable.

Because loss of consciousness is usually associated with more serious injuries, when an employee loses consciousness as the result of a work-related injury, it is always recordable. "Restriction of work or motion" occurs if an employee, because of the effect of a job-related injury, is physically or mentally unable to perform any part of the normal work assignment during any part of the work day. Regardless of the type of treatment used for an injury, if the employee is required to transfer to another job, it is recordable.

Injury of Illness?

Determination of whether the case is an injury or an illness must be made by the employer. The nature of the original event or exposure is the determining factor, not the resulting condition of the employee. Injuries are caused by an instantaneous event, such as an explosion that causes a loss of hearing. If the loss of hearing were to occur as a result of exposure to high levels of noise in the workplace over a period of time, it would be considered an occupational illness. The aggravation of a previous injury almost always results from some new incident. Consequently, when they are work related, these new incidents should be recorded as new cases.

OSHA's Right to Inspect

The Occupational Safety and Health Administration's compliance and safety health officers (CSHO) have the right to inspect a facility at any time, without advance notice. This visit may be just a random event or may have been prompted by an employee complaint. The facility does have certain rights, however, so it should be prepared, as should the staff. In one facility, a "code orange" overhead page indicates that an OSHA inspector is on the premises.

Some guidelines for handling an OSHA inspection are included in Table 3–5. Perhaps the most important issue to remember is not to create an adversarial atmosphere with the CSHO. Employees should be prepared to answer questions asked by the inspector. Staff's compliance understanding can be tested with a few simple activities:

- Ask specific questions about safety issues, procedures, and facility policy.
- Spot-check compliance records.
- Evaluate understanding of safety issues during performance review.

PATIENT SELF-DETERMINATION ACT

Congress passed the Patient Self-Determination Act in 1991 as a result of the landmark

Table 3–5. How to Weather An Occupational Safety and Health Administration Inspection

1. When the compliance and safety health officer (CSHO) arrives, the officer will identify himself or herself to the receptionist. The person in charge of the safety/compliance program should be notified. Request proper identification of the officer prior to inspection.
2. You DO have the right to refuse entry to the CSHO, but exercising this right may lead to negative feelings before the compliance evaluation begins. The CSHO has the right to return with a federal marshal and a warrant to gain entry.
3. In an opening conference, the CSHO will identify the scope of the inspection, reasons your establishment was selected, and rationale for the inspection. If a complaint has been filed with OSHA, a copy will be provided to the employer. Employee representatives are to be included in the conference.
4. Answer all questions truthfully, but do not expound unless specifically asked to do so. It is best not to volunteer any information. Maintaining a *professional* attitude is important. The CSHO is an *enforcement* official and did not write the regulations.
5. During the opening conference, the CSHO may ask to see the OSHA 200 logs for the past 5 years, the written safety program, material safety data sheets and other records. He or she will also observe whether the required posters are on display.
6. Accompany the CSHO on the walk-through inspection. Document the same things the CSHO documents and if pictures are taken, take your own pictures from the same vantage point. Apparent violations will be brought to the attention of the employer and the employee representative.
7. The CSHO may wish to interview some employees privately. These interviews will be put in writing and the statements held in confidence.
8. A closing conference will be held to summarize findings and deficiencies. At this time the employer may produce documentation to support the safety program and company efforts to comply with regulations. This is the time to inform the CSHO of any unusual circumstances in the workplace. The CSHO may choose to conduct this conference via telephone at a later date. Employer and employee representatives will be informed of their rights to contest penalties and to participate in further conferences or discussions.

Missouri case of *Cruzan v Director, Division of Health* (110 S Ct 2841). The United States Supreme Court found that states have a right to require "clear and convincing" evidence of patients' wishes before allowing the removal of feeding tubes from patients in persistent vegetative states.[13] The Patient Self-Determination Act was passed with the intent to inform patients of their options and have the information available to them to exercise these options if they desire. Although the act does not create new patient rights, it does require that patients be informed of rights that already exist under individual state law.

Advance directives are documents that indicate the patient's future healthcare, should he or she become incapacitated or unable to communicate, and they provide "clear and convincing" written evidence of the desires of the patient. They give a person control over his or her medical care, ensuring that physicians and family members understand how much life-prolonging technology the patient wants employed during crisis. There are two kinds of advance directives: (1) the living will and (2) the durable power of attorney.

Living Will

The living will describes preferences for life-sustaining treatment. The provisions vary from state to state, but most describe diverse degrees of life support, from respiratory to nutritional support, do-not-resuscitate, or do-not-intubate issues. The patient identifies preferences regarding his or her own care. The living will takes effect only if the physician believes that the patient is permanently unconscious or that death is near, and that the patient is unable to verbalize his or her wishes.

The living will requires the signature of the patient and usually that of a witness or notary.

Durable Power of Attorney

The durable power of attorney designates an individual as the healthcare agent for the patient, to make healthcare decisions should the patient lose the ability to make them for himself or herself. This individual should be an adult who understands the desires of the patient regarding medical treatment in life-sustaining situations. Generally, this durable power of attorney goes into effect only if the patient is unable to make decisions. This document must be signed by the patient and, depending on state requirements, witnessed or notarized.

The specific provisions of the act require that hospitals have written policies and procedures regarding the following:

- A method of informing adult patients of their right to advance directives

- Documentation in the patient chart about whether they have designated advance directives
- Compliance with state law regarding advance directives
- Staff and public education regarding issues concerning advance directives

Hospitals cannot discriminate against individuals based on whether they have executed advance directives. At the time of admission to an inpatient facility, all adult patients must be provided with written information regarding their rights to advance directives and consent to treatment. Outpatient facilities, whether hospital based or freestanding, must have information available should the patient ask for it.

The Patient Self Determination Act applies to Medicare- and Medicaid-certified hospitals, nursing facilities, hospices, home health agencies, and prepaid health plans[14] but does not specify outpatient surgery providers. Likewise, most states do not require outpatient surgery centers to meet Patient Self-Determination Act regulations. It is best to seek the advice of whoever represents the facility in legal matters for information regarding applicable state requirements.

The patient with pre-existing advance directives may complicate the issue in the outpatient surgical setting, however. On admission, the patient should be asked whether he or she has advance directives. Some facilities include a statement about the existence of directives in the consent for admission. If the patient does have directives, a copy of them should become part of the medical record.

In the perianesthesia period, the question arises of whether the patient with advance directives is truly informed. The American Society of Perianesthesia Nurses issued a position statement entitled "The Perianesthesia Patient with a Do-Not Resuscitate Advance Directive" in April of 1996 stating in part

> A patient whose advance directive specifies no life sustaining measures may be unaware that cardiac or respiratory arrests are always potential yet usually reversible outcomes associated with anesthesia. When the patient's desires for the perianesthetic period are not specifically identified, anesthetic-related changes in physiologic function present the perianesthesia nurse with ethical conflict and confusion about appropriate interventions.

The statement goes on to suggest that preoperative patient education through the informed consent "will include discussion of the advance directive" and that the patient "must reconsider this designation and reclarify wishes about resuscitation during the perianesthetic period."[15] In the interest of the patient and the outpatient healthcare facility, a policy to suspend advance directives during the intraoperative period is often considered. When such a policy is adopted, the patient who has a do-not-resuscitate directive may not desire to waive it and should be given the opportunity to select another facility for care.

PRIVATE ACCREDITATION

There are two private agencies in the United States that ambulatory surgical centers, either freestanding or hospital based, may choose to voluntarily submit to for accreditation. JCAHO and AAAHC provide written standards regarding the environment of care, the provision of care, and the quality of care, as well as in-house reviews for compliance. Regular surveys of the organization's performance are intended to ensure the quality of care provided to each patient.

Medicare and Deemed Status

In a DHHS Health Care Financing Administration notice dated December 13, 1996, a landmark announcement was made regarding a coordination among Medicare, JCAHO, and AAAHC. The summary of this notice states

> This notice grants deemed status to two organizations, the Joint Commission on the Accreditation of Healthcare Organizations (JCAHO) and the Accreditation Association for Ambulatory Health Care (AAAHC), for their accredited ambulatory surgical centers (ASCs) that request Medicare certification. We believe that accreditation of ASCs by either organization demonstrates that all Medicare ASC conditions are met or exceeded, and thus, we grant deemed status to each organization. The provisions of this notice are effective beginning on December 19, 1996 through December 19, 2002.

Joint Commission on Accreditation of Healthcare Organizations

The mission of JCAHO is "to improve the quality of care provided to the public." The most recent revision of JCAHO standards created "performance" objectives that describe a desired outcome or goal, and each facility can be creative in methods to achieve the intent of each standard. In the past, these standards went into lengthy descriptions of committee functions, nursing processes, and other "how to" items that each facility was required to fulfill. The JCAHO has standards for and conducts surveys of

- Ambulatory care organizations
- Behavioral healthcare organizations
- Hospitals
- Home care organizations
- Laboratory services
- Long-term care organizations
- Healthcare networks

Standards for each of the aforementioned divisions of healthcare are published in individual manuals. Once the decision is made to request accreditation by the JCAHO, an application for accreditation must be submitted and the appropriate fees paid. The JCAHO sends the organization an accreditation manual and plans the date for the first survey. Surveys are generally conducted on a triennial basis. Table 3–6 provides a list of JCAHO telephone numbers.

The JCAHO has been accrediting ambulatory facilities since 1975. These standards apply to many types of facilities, including surgery centers, birthing centers, chiropractic clinics, dental centers, dialysis centers, group practices, imaging centers, and oncology centers. The ambulatory care standards are divided into two sections: (1) patient-focused functions and (2) organization functions.

Section 1: Patient-Focused Functions

Patient rights and organization ethics
Assessment of patients
Care of patients
Education of patients and family
Continuity of care

Section 2: Organization Functions

Improving organization performance
Leadership
Management of human resources
Surveillance, prevention and control of infection
Management of information
Management of the environment of care

For ambulatory centers that are part of an acute care hospital, the JCAHO hospital standards apply. These, too, are performance based and must be carefully evaluated for applicability to the unit. Questions regarding applicable standards may be directed to JCAHO.

***Table 3–6.* Joint Commission Resources and Telephone Numbers for Ambulatory Care Providers**

Common Types of Questions	
If you are new to Joint Commission accreditation and want more information.	630-792-5259 or 630-792-5732
If you have questions about how to apply for a survey, survey costs, and survey procedures.	630-792-5259 or 630-792-5732
If you have questions about preparing your application for a survey.	630-792-5509 or 630-792-5732
If you have already submitted your application for accreditation OR if you are already accredited.	630-792-5509 or 630-792-5732
If you have questions about completing your presurvey questionnaire.	630-792-5509 or 630-792-5879
If you have specific questions about survey fees.	630-792-5665
Key Resources	
Standards—If you have questions about how a particular standard applies to your ambulatory setting.	630-792-5900
Educational Programs—If you want information about, or to register for, Joint Commission educational programs.	630-792-5800
Publications—If you want information about, or to purchase, a Joint Commission publication.	630-792-5800

Table 3–7. Regulatory Agency Resource List

Accreditation Association for Ambulatory Health Care, Inc.
9933 Lawler Avenue
Skokie, IL 60077-3708
(847) 676-9610
FAX: 847-676-9628

American Association of Blood Banks (AABB)
8101 Glenbrook Road
Bethesda, MD 20814-2749
(301) 907-6977

American College of Occupational and Environmental Medicine
55 W. Seegers Road
Arlington Heights, IL 60005
(708) 228-6850

American Health Information Management Association (AHIMA)
919 N. Michigan Ave.
Suite 1400 Chicago, IL 60611
(312) 787-2672

American Hospital Association
One North Franklin
Chicago, IL 60606
(312) 422-3000

American National Standards Institute (ANSI)
11 W. 42nd St.
New York, NY 10036
(212) 642-4900

American Society of Anesthesiologists
520 N. Northwest Highway
Park Ridge, IL 60068-2573
(847) 825-5586
E-mail: mail@ASAhq.org
Internet: http://www.asahq.org.

American Society of Perianesthesia Nurses (ASPAN)
6900 Grove Road
Thorofare, NJ 08086
(609) 845-5557
FAX: 609-848-1881
Internet: aspan@slackinc.com

Association for the Advancement of Medical Instrumentation (AAMI)
3330 Washington Blvd. Suite 400
Arlington, VA 22201-4598
(703) 525-4890

Association of Operating Room Nurses (AORN)
2170 S. Parker Road #300
Denver, CO 80231-5711
(800) 755-2676
Internet: http://www.aorn.org/

Centers for Disease Control and Prevention
Office of Public Affairs
P.O. Box 13827
Research Triangle Park, NC 27704
(404) 332-4555
FAX Information Service (404) 332-4565
Internet: http://www.cdc.gov/

Environmental Protection Agency (EPA)
401 M Street, SW
Washington, DC 20460
(800) 858-7377
Internet: www.epa.gov
RCRA (EPA) HotLine (800) 424-9346

Federal Register
Superintendent of Documents
P.O. Box 371954
Pittsburgh, PA 15250-7954
(202) 512-1800

Food & Drug Administration (FDA)
9200 Corporate Blvd.
Rockville, MD 20850
(301) 443-6310

Guidelines for Design and Construction of Hospital and Health Care Facilities
American Institute of Architects
Academy of Architecture for Health
1735 New York Avenue, N.W.
Washington, DC 20006
To order: 800-365-2724

Joint Commission on Accreditation of Healthcare Organizations (JCAHO)
One Renaissance Boulevard
Oakbrook Terrace, IL 60181
(630) 792-5000
FAX: 630-792-5005
(see Table 3–6)

National Library of Medicine
8600 Rockville Pike
Bethesda, MD 20894
(800) 496-6095

National Fire Protection Association (NFPA)
1 Batterymarch Park
Quincy, MA 02269-9101
(617) 770-3000
Internet: www.nfpa.org

National Institute for Occupational Safety and Health (NIOSH)
U.S. Department of Health and Human Services
4676 Columbia Parkway
Cincinnati, OH 45226
(800) 35-NIOSH
Internet: www.cdc.gov/niosh/homepage.html

National Safety Council
1121 Spring Lake Drive
Itasca, IL 60143-3201
(312) 527-4800

OSHA FAX on Demand
($1.50/min):
(900) 555-3400
OSHA Information Line:
202-219-8151

OSHA on the Internet:
http://www.osha.gov

OSHA Publications Office
200 Constitution Ave., N.W.
Room N3101
Washington, DC 20210
(202) 219-4667

OSHA Standards:
Commerce Clearing House Inc.
4025 W. Peterson Ave.
Chicago, IL 60646-6085
(800) TELL-CCH

Superintendent of Documents (GPO):
(202) 512-1800

OSHA Training Institute
US Department of Labor
1555 Times Drive
Des Plaines, IL 60018
(847) 297-4913

Regional OSHA Offices
(see Table 3–3)

Accreditation Association for Ambulatory Health Care

The AAAHC was created in 1979 with the goal "to organize and operate a peer-based assessment, education, and accreditation program for ambulatory health care organizations as a means of assisting them to provide the highest achievable level of care for recipients in the most efficient and economically sound manner."[16] Their standards in the *Accreditation Handbook for Ambulatory Health Care* have been revised eight times since the original manual, with the most current edition being dated 1999. Reference information for Medicare and National Fire Protection Association are included in the most current manual for ease in compliance with multiple agencies.

The AAAHC functions in a way that is similar to the JCAHO. Application must be made for accreditation, at which time a fee is determined based on the number of surveyors and the number of days required to complete an onsite survey. Surveys are conducted on a triennial basis, and the AAAHC may deny accreditation if the organization is not in substantial compliance with their standards. These standards cover the following topics:

- Rights of patients
- Governance
- Administration
- Quality of care provided
- Quality management and improvement
- Clinical records
- Professional improvement
- Facilities and environment

Adjunct standards follow divided by specialty of the facility, e.g., surgical, dental, emergency, and radiology.

Contact information for the AAAHC can be found in the Regulatory Agency Resource List (Table 3–7).

In the current atmosphere of managed care and strong influences of health insurers and third party payers, many facilities find that accreditation provides credibility for them. Additionally, as the public takes a greater and greater interest in their own healthcare, accreditation provides assurance of a quality level of care.

References

1. Guidelines for Design and Construction of Hospital and Health Care Facilities, 1996–1997 ed., Washington, DC: The American Institute of Architects Academy of Architecture for Health and the US Department of Health and Human Services, 1996.
2. Doucet L: EPA prescribes "painless" rules for med waste incinerators. Health Facilities Manage 9:12, 1996.
3. What is MedWatch? FDA MedWatch Online. Available at http://www.fda.gov/medwatch. June 1997.
4. Harris A, Ziel S: Reporting requirements under the safe medical device act. AORN J 64: 460–462, 1996.
5. Medical Products Regulated by the FDA. FDA MedWatch Online. Available at http://www.fda.gov/medwatch. June 1997.
6. What is a Serious Adverse Event? FDA MedWatch Online. Available at http://www.fda.gov/MedWatch. June 1997.
7. Department of Labor, Occupational Safety and Health Administration, 29 CFR 1910.1200; Hazard Communication Standard, February 1994.
8. Office of Science & Technology Assessment. OSHA Technical Manual. TED 1-0. 15A Washington, DC: Occupational Safety and Health Administration, January 20, 1999.
9. American Society of Perianesthesia Nurses. ASPAN Position Statement on Air Safety in the Perianesthesia Environment. Thorofare, NJ: Published by Author, April 1996.
10. Webster's II New Riverside University Dictionary. Boston, MA: Riverside Publishing, Houghton Mifflin Company, 1984.
11. Recordkeeping Guidelines for Occupational Injuries and Illnesses. US Department of Labor, Bureau of Labor Statistics, September 1986.
12. Bernhart WM: Experts: OSHA 200 Logs. Facility Care 2:5, 1997.
13. Murphy E: Advance directives and the patient self-determination act. AORN J 55:270–271, 1992.
14. Surgery centers confused by obligations under PSDA. Same Day Surg 17:2, 1993.
15. American Society of Perianesthesia Nurses. ASPAN Position Statement. A Position statement on the Perianesthesia Patient with a Do-Not-Resuscitate Advance Directive. Thorofare, NJ: Published by Author, April 1996.
16. Accreditation Association for Ambulatory Health Care: Accreditation Handbook for Ambulatory Health Care. Skokie, IL: Published by Author, 1996–97.

Chapter 4

The Environment of Care

Nancy Burden and Donna M. DeFazio Quinn

Safe, efficient patient care is supported by an appropriate physical structure. Patients, family members, and visitors are significantly affected emotionally as well as physically by the environment and the decor, so efforts should ensure that the impression of the physical structure is a positive one and that it enhances, rather than detracts from, the patient's ultimate perception of the care received. Although there is diversity in design, structure, and utilization in various practice settings, the general concepts of traffic flow, patient needs, and equipment usage are homogeneous and apply to all ambulatory surgery programs.

From the planning and building stages to the actual use of the center, the architectural and interior design of an ambulatory surgery center (ASC) should reflect concern for the comfort, privacy, and safety of patients, visitors, staff, and physicians. It should foster a calm and pleasant atmosphere to help reduce anxiety and promote confidence. Patients and physicians are more likely to provide the center with repeat business when they have felt welcome and comfortable in the facility.

Nurses and other professionals should be involved in the earliest planning stages of development or renovation of any ASC because their clinical experience can provide significant insight for the initial design. Each specialty and procedure intended for the center should be evaluated so that their specific needs are planned into the initial design.[1]

The development team for any new building or renovation should comprise administrative, business, maintenance, clinical, and physician members along with the design and construction experts. Every step of each clinical process should be detailed, such as patient flow, family waiting needs, information flow, equipment storage, waste handling and storage, and sterile processing. Visualizing these multifunctional processes in the early blueprints will help the team identify and redesign problem areas.

It is important for each member of the team to provide as much input as possible during the design phase, mentioning every idea, no matter how insignificant it may seem. From these many ideas will come a final design that works well for the patients and staff. Embarrassment or timidity should not prevent team members from speaking up, because any professional health-care architect will welcome all ideas from the user group.

Making changes during the construction phase is much more expensive than accommodating ideas in the planning stage. It is also important for the staff to seek expert guidance from the architect, whose role is to be knowledgeable about all local, state, and federal building and safety requirements.

Creativity is particularly important when renovating an existing building or area. The team should avoid allowing new ideas to be restricted by the current structure, flow, and design so that fresh and imaginative ideas can originate. The leaders of any preconstruction design committee should set a tone of open, two-way communication to allow all members of the team to feel comfortable in group discussions.

From the simplest to the most sophisticated designs, ASCs provide the setting for a select patient population: short-stay patients who require a combination of acute care for a portion of their stay and a home-like, family-oriented setting before and after that acute care period.

Ideally, these two environments are in physically separate areas. Combining admission and discharge functions in a critical care unit such as a postanesthesia care unit (PACU) is generally counter to the promotion of wellness and patient independence, which is the hallmark of ambulatory surgery programs.

Most facilities show a preference for providing separate areas for admission and discharge of patients, but the use of the main PACU for the care and discharge of late or overflow ambulatory surgery patients may still be necessary. Because the PACU environment is often chaotic, nurses sometimes address this issue by separating the two populations in different areas of the existing PACU.

The intent of this chapter is not to provide an inclusive discussion of the physical layout and equipment needs of the PACU and operating room (OR). Rather, discussion concentrates on the preoperative and postoperative care areas and visitor areas. References to the OR and PACU are made when appropriate to specific issues.

CODES AND REGULATIONS

All federal, state, and local building codes that address the safety and effectiveness of the facility must be addressed. National nursing organizations, such as the Association of Operating Room Nurses (AORN) and the American Society of Perianesthesia Nurses (ASPAN) recommend voluntary adherence to particular physical specifications. Conversely, many regulatory agencies demand compliance with their respective standards. Some of these include the United States Department of Health and Human Services, individual state licensing bodies, and accrediting organizations (e.g., the Joint Commission on Accreditation of Healthcare Organizations (JCAHO), the Accreditation Association for Ambulatory Health Care, and other specialty specific agencies.

The Joint Commission on Accreditation of Healthcare Organizations standards relating to the environment address both the structure and the management of related processes. Joint Commission standards related to the environment of care address many areas. Some include the design and maintenance of the physical plant; management issues related to safety, security, life safety, utility systems, and emergency preparedness; orientation of staff members so that proper implementation of safety and security plans are effective; and adequate and safe space for specialized services.[2] The commission stresses orientation and ongoing education and practice for employees, physicians, and volunteers within each facility to ensure that safety and security issues are addressed.

Building codes for health facilities mandate specific construction materials, fire walls and exits, size and locations of doorways and windows, wall surface finishes, illuminated exit signs, and other requirements. Sophisticated regulations exist for ORs, including air exchange and directional airflow systems, elimination systems for anesthetic waste gases, isolation of electrical circuits, an electrical back-up generator, temperature and humidity controls, and separation of sterile, clean, and soiled utility and storage areas. Patient care areas outside of the OR must comply with many standards as well, for instance, room size; mechanical, electrical, lighting, and plumbing systems; nurse and emergency call systems; patient safety features, such as handrails and dual-access doors for patient bathrooms; and access for the physically challenged that complies with the Americans with Disabilities Act.

Probably among the most stringent of all codes are those pertaining to fire prevention. The Department of Health and Human Services requires adherence to specifications and safety practices. The National Fire Protection Agency (NFPA) has no intrinsic legal authority, but its regulations are considered mandatory by most regulatory and accrediting agencies, so NFPA requirements come to the ASC secondarily from those regulatory bodies. Ambulatory surgery facilities are addressed in Chapters 12 and 13 of the *NFPA 101 Life Safety Code*.[3] A discussion of some of the requirements of this code is included in Chapter 3. A copy of the book, an NFPA catalogue, or other materials can be ordered from NFPA (NFPA, Fire Analysis and Research Division, NFPA, One Batterymarch Park, Quincy, MA 02269-9101; telephone: [800] 344-3555). For general information, the telephone number for the NFPA is (617) 770-3000, and the fax number is (617) 770-0700. The Internet address is http.// www.nfpa.org.

LOCATION

When selecting a building site for a freestanding ASC, planners consider geographic proximity to a full-service facility for expedient emergency transfers of patients, public visibility, and traffic flow. Access roads and driveways should be well lighted, and signs should clearly direct the public and emergency vehicles to the facility. If nearby street signs are missing or unclear, an effort should be made to have appropriate ones installed.

Within the hospital setting, several locations are frequently used for the addition of an ambulatory surgery unit. A self-contained ASC that includes dedicated ORs and PACU may be constructed adjacent to or near the hospital. However, building costs are considerably reduced when major mechanical systems and support department services can be shared, so the more economical choice to renovate existing internal space is often favored.

Consideration must go beyond the economics of the site selection, however, to include issues of patient access, mixing versus segregation of inpatient and outpatient populations, access to hospital entrances, and convenience for physicians and patients. A separate hospital entrance for the ASC department is ideal. It should be well lighted, free from obstacles, and protected from the weather, with appropriate security devices in place. The internal route to the ambulatory surgery department must be well identified, with clearly visible signs at frequent intervals along the route between the hospital entrance and the ASC.

For patient convenience, consolidating all aspects of the ambulatory surgery program in one area is preferred to requiring the patient to travel from one floor to another for admission, diagnostics, and actual surgical care. A self-contained unit also allows the ambulatory surgery department to maintain more control over the whole process and to better share staff members from one department to another during peaks and lulls in patient flow. A secondary gain with this type of staffing pattern is the added comfort patients may feel when seeing the same nurse in different locations during their operative experiences. The cost of duplicating support services within the ASC must be considered and balanced against the positive impact of providing convenience and maintaining internal control.

An example of one facility's implementation can be found at Morton Plant Hospital in Clearwater, Florida. This facility has designed their preadmission testing and assessment area in a highly accessible and visible location adjacent to the hospital's main lobby. The department includes nursing, anesthesia, and diagnostic services. For patient convenience, a radiologic suite capable of performing chest examinations was added to avoid the need to send patients through the large facility's winding hallways.

Adequate, clearly marked parking should be available near the entrance. Most ASCs offer free parking on the day of surgery and for any preadmission visits. Valet parking is another amenity provided by some metropolitan hospitals. Not only is the service a marketing tactic that fosters goodwill and customer satisfaction, it also has a positive impact on the OR schedule when patients are not delayed as a result of parking problems. In an attempt to attract business, some programs supply patients with the convenience of free bus or van transportation to and from the center.

STRUCTURAL DESIGN AND DECOR

Choices made for both outside structure and interior design are typically constrained by budget issues. The challenge is to provide the desired image and tone while holding costs to a predetermined level. Budgetary issues make it imperative that multiple options are explored for each step of the planning. Can less costly desks be found that are acceptable to allow more money to be spent on flooring or reception area furniture? Will a better grade of ceiling material or window coverings ultimately reduce operational costs for electricity? These and many other questions should continue throughout the decision-making process.

The initial design should allow for future expansion. Patient census may increase significantly, or there may be the opportunity to add new equipment. Placing the groundwork for projected future needs at the time of the initial construction usually costs less than adding them to an existing structure. Examples of such needs are ceiling tracks, electrical wiring, medical gas lines, and plumbing for specialized equipment that is likely to be added later.

The interior decor reflects the image that the facility wishes to convey. In a hospital unit, that image may be an extension of the hospital as a whole. Most often, it is an approach that provides ambulatory surgery patients with a pleasant, low-stress environment without the traditional institutional flavor of many hospitals. It is important to strike a balance between a warm and home-like setting and the feeling of safety and stability, so that patients feel secure in the clinical and professional services delivered. People walking through the door will likely form opinions about whether they feel welcome and whether their anxieties are minimized or exacerbated in the facility on the basis of their initial reactions to the surroundings.[4]

Furnishings should provide comfort, durability, and ergonomic support. Acoustical considerations include building materials as well as walls, barriers, and distances between various services and work stations. Appropriate lighting and temperature controls should enhance comfort levels. Depending on the clientele and the administrative stance of the ASC, the environment may be sophisticated, sedate, casual, or child oriented. Color choices range from soft, relaxing tones to primary colors, again depending on the customers being served.

An example of designing a facility with the customer in mind is a women's center in Staten Island, New York, that identified the elements of design most important to women to be music, soft lighting, natural materials, floral carpets, unusual tile designs, and bright, colorful bathrooms. This center used rounded corners on cabinetry and furniture for a soft, feminine look. It placed mirrors in helpful locations and ensured privacy in areas where women would need to undress.[4] Consider the differences in design when planning for a center specializing in men's health, children's surgery, or a geriatric population.

Traffic should flow logically from one area to another without overlap or backtracking, from the front entrance to the discharge area where patients and families are reunited. Separate doors should be provided for patient entrance and exit to the facility and for staff and physician use. Generally speaking, patients should not be required to enter or remain in an area of high-acuity care longer than necessary for their conditions. For example, those receiving uncomplicated local or upper-extremity regional anesthesia usually bypass the PACU, and patients undergoing pain clinic or other special procedures may not enter the ORs.

Patients in the ASC are best served by separate admission and discharge areas for many reasons. Segregation of preoperative patients from those who have already undergone surgery is aesthetically and psychologically important. Some units use the two areas interchangeably, and others do so only when there is an overflow of patients in one or the other area. This separation prevents the mixing of patients who cannot have food or fluids before surgery with postoperative patients who are allowed nourishment. Not only can preoperative patients be tempted or upset by seeing others eat and drink or affected with nausea secondary to the odors or sight of food, but a staff member could unwittingly provide a beverage or food in error. Also, the emotional strain of seeing postoperative patients who may be experiencing some type of distress can prove unsettling to those who are still awaiting their procedures.

Discharging a patient through the main reception room or lobby can be an embarrassing event that does not support the patient's right to privacy or uphold his or her dignity. Such an arrangement also contributes to congestion in a busy lobby and removes nursing personnel from the patient care areas for each discharge. Also, the sight of a postoperative patient who is bandaged, vomiting, or in pain is unpleasant for visitors and for patients being admitted and can ultimately lead to loss of return business. Figure 4–1 provides a schematic drawing oftypical traffic flow for patient admission, care, and discharge.

In a hospital setting, there should be little or no mixing of outpatients with inpatients, who tend to be sicker, with acute care needs. Hospital-based outpatient programs that share the main OR often address this issue by designing units where patient traffic patterns and designated entrances and exits to the OR suite encourage separation of the two patient populations. Separation of patient populations is advisable for patient satisfaction, emotional response, and infection control.

Floor Plan

The floor plan should support the control of infection and cross-contamination. There must be restricted traffic flow through sterile areas, with provisions made for alternate routes to reduce or avoid staff and visitor travel in these areas. Sterile supplies should be stored adjacent to the restricted area, and a separate receiving area should be available near the delivery entrance for acceptance and unboxing of goods from the outside.

Soiled and clean linen should be stored separately, and appropriate provisions must be made for the short-term storage of contaminated waste until its periodic removal. Waste removal policies should conform to state mandates and to federal requirements of the Environmental Protection Agency and the Occupational Safety and Health Administration. An adequate number of sinks must be available for handwashing in patient care areas, and separate bathroom facilities should be provided for patients, staff, and visitors. All staff and physicians should have an entrance to locker room facilities, which allows them to change into scrub suits and other protective gear and enter the operative areas without retracing steps.

Structural provisions must be made for the

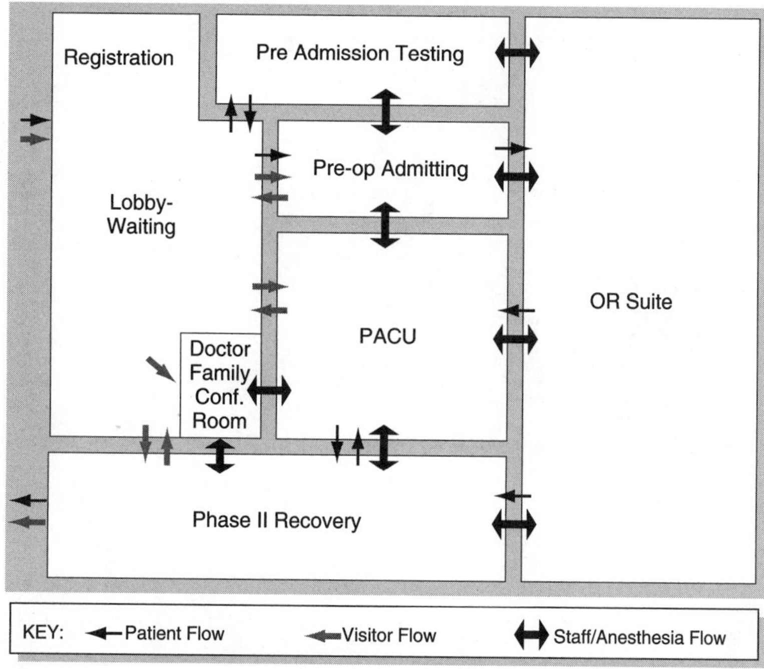

Figure 4–1. Schematic of traffic flow for patient care.

physical isolation of patients with infectious or contagious diseases and for patients with decreased immunity to disease who require a reverse isolation technique for their own protection. Even if the center's patient appropriateness policy precludes the known admission of an infectious patient, the JCAHO requires that ASCs identify a specific location for the isolation of anyone found to be infectious after admission to the unit.[2]

Lobby and Reception Area

The reception area provides the first impression. There should be no confusion about the location of a reception desk, which should be situated within sight of the entrance door or have signs to clearly indicate the route. It should immediately give the person who enters a sense of safety, cleanliness, warmth, comfort, and professionalism. The area should be free of clutter. A short rise in the counter between the customer and the receptionist can help camouflage necessary paperwork and tools and act as a visual barrier to prevent access to sensitive patient information. Conversely, tall barriers or walls with small glass windows and bells to summon assistance are impersonal and create an immediate feeling of isolation and distance. Often, visitors, family members, or vendors may see only this area, so they make a judgment about the entire facility based solely on the reception area.

Along with the physical amenities should come a smiling, pleasant, and knowledgeable person to help direct people and answer questions. The receptionist has the important role of providing a positive first impression. Often, the manner in which that person handles a situation, such as a lengthy waiting period or an angry visitor, makes a significant difference in turning the person's attitude into a more positive one. The receptionist should be attentive to the waiting periods for various customers and intercede appropriately.

The lobby is often the area where families or friends wait during a surgical procedure. It should be a comfortable and relaxed setting. Carpeting softens the noise level and adds a warm dimension. Plants, wall decorations, paintings, and sculptures are often included to promote a home-like decor. Furnishings should be plentiful to accommodate the expected number of people at any given time. Comfortable sofas and chairs, well-positioned reading lights, nearby restrooms, and telephones should be available. Many centers provide both pay telephones and courtesy telephones that can be used for local calls without charge. All areas should be accessible to handicapped and wheelchair-bound people.

Figure 4–2 illustrates the lobby at Morton

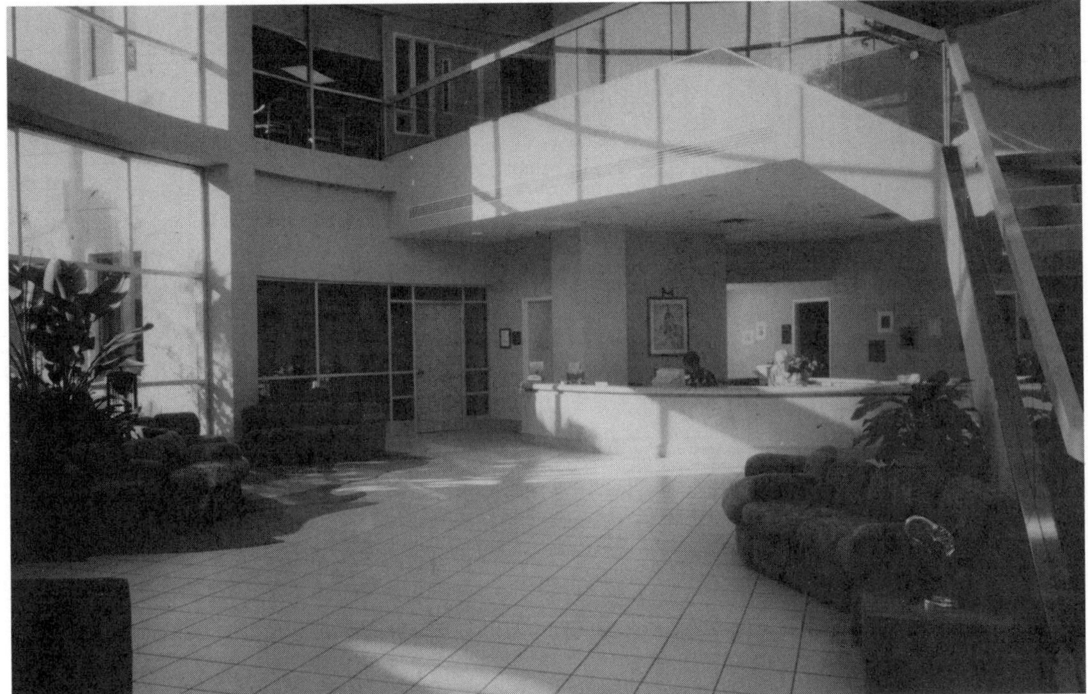

Figure 4–2. Lobby of Trinity Outpatient Center. Morton Plant Mease Health Care, New Port Richey, FL.

Plant Mease Trinity Outpatient Center in west central Florida. It is designed to reflect the natural setting of the massive oak trees and wetlands surrounding it, from its two-story windows to the privacy windows etched with cranes and oak trees that separate the patient registration area from the lobby. Not shown in the photograph are the large watercolor paintings of classic Florida scenes over the staircase.

Diversionary items can help ease the stress of the waiting period. A television or piped-in music system, general-interest reading materials of recent publication, newspapers, vending machines, complimentary nourishments, and coffee are all appreciated. If a drinking fountain is provided, it should be accompanied by a sign that limits use by preoperative, fasting patients. Some centers provide playing cards, board games, children's books and toys, and other recreational games in the waiting areas. Recent additions in some facilities are Internet access terminals.

Another idea is to provide recipe cards imprinted with the surgery center's name. These allow waiting visitors to copy recipes from magazines in the lobby. Not only is this a diversionary method to help people pass the time, it is also a way to prevent destruction and loss of magazines.

The innovative patient access services department of Morton Plant Mease East Lake Outpatient Center has developed a "survival kit" for waiting families. According to Kandy Swanson, manager of patient access services at the center, the kit contains a nutritional snack, a "stress card," a healthy search-a-word puzzle, a pencil, cartoons, motivational thoughts, a laminated first aid guide for the home refrigerator, and procedure-specific information about what to expect during the family member's recuperation at home. The cost of this kit, including the personalized white paper bag, is under $1.[5]

Many ASCs provide a separate, enclosed play area for families with children to enjoy where noise and play do not disturb other people. These special areas are often furnished with scaled-down furniture, special toys that are easy to clean, and youthful decor. Equipment and supplies that allow parents to care for infants are much appreciated, for instance, baby care centers in the restrooms. There should be special attention to the disinfection of toys and child-care surfaces to reduce the chance of spreading infections from one child to another.

The issue of providing a smoking area is one that must follow the facility's policy. More and more health facilities and campuses are now smoke-free. Although this may be a hardship for some waiting visitors, the overall service provided to both nonsmokers and smokers is two-fold: (1) the environment provided is healthier and more pleasant, and (2) the facility projects a statement that promotes healthy living. In smoke-free buildings, an outdoor area for smokers may be provided unless the entire campus is smoke free. Signs should be conspicuously posted to inform people of smoking regulations.

Business and Administrative Area

The administrative area in a freestanding center usually houses offices for clerical, case scheduling, registration, and billing services; the administrative director; the nurse manager; medical records; and sometimes, the anesthesia business office or the medical director's office. A separate conference room near the lobby provides for private conversations between a physician and a family or patient, for a billing specialist to discuss financial concerns, for vendor presentations, and for other private needs, such as visits with clergy and family discussions. An area with audiovisual capabilities should be available for staff educational programs somewhere within the center, in either the administrative or the clinical areas. The hospital-based center often shares business and administrative office space within other areas of the hospital. Thus, its internal business area may be simply a reception area.

Important components for the health and emotional well-being of the business staff include appropriate lighting and temperature control, windows that provide natural light and a view of the outdoors, and furnishings that promote comfort and good body mechanics. Noise reduction measures in a busy clerical setting can involve physical isolation of particularly noisy equipment, insulating enclosures for printers, acoustical ceiling tiles, carpeting, and fabric-covered furniture. Partial walls may help with noise control by their sound-absorbing quality. For registrars and schedulers who are frequently on the telephone, hands-free headsets may provide positive physical advantages.

Sufficient numbers of files and storage cabinets for office supplies are necessary. A telephone answering system should be in place to direct callers to alternate sources of assistance during hours when the facility is closed. During working hours, it is preferable that a human voice answer all calls. If staffing in relation to the volume of incoming calls does not allow that, it is important that any recorded message prompts be concise and allow the user familiar with the system the choice of quickly inputting the code to bypass the message. The least number of recorded options is the most customer friendly approach.

Computerized management information systems (MISs) are available to address such multiple needs as billing, scheduling, inventory, payroll, quality improvement, utilization, and cost per case data. Confidentiality of data is essential, so passwords and security levels must be implemented. Policies should be in place that specifically address access and security. The measures that will be taken for breeches of security should be clearly spelled out for all staff members.

MIS also can be an acronym for "medical information system," in which the primary use of the computer system may be for nurses' notes, physicians' orders, laboratory test ordering, and other clinically focused functions. This type of system, when available, may allow physicians to enter as well as to access information from their offices. It can provide immediate access to laboratory and other diagnostic tests as soon as they are completed—a feature that is especially beneficial for nurses preparing patients for surgery. Other possible features of such a system are: (1) generating individualized, patient-discharge instructions preprinted with the patient's name, physician's name, and other pertinent information; (2) integrating inventory and case scheduling; and (3) providing information about supply cost versus pricing of procedures. Nursing personnel can use terminals in clinical areas for documenting nursing care, auditing, quality improvement follow-up, and inventory needs.

There are also programs that generate patient bills for surgeons and anesthesiologists in conjunction with the information already within the system. Most physicians contract for such services anyway, so the easy accessibility can be a marketing tool for the ASC. Some physicians do not feel comfortable if that information is in the hands of the facility administration; however, the ability to provide patients with a single bill for all services, including professional medical fees, is a strong marketing tool.

Consultation and Diagnostic Areas

Ambulatory surgery centers that offer diagnostic services within the center usually locate these areas close to the lobby or entrance for ease of access. Direct access between diagnostic and other clinical areas that bypasses the lobby is also a benefit in case a patient faints or has an unexpected reaction during testing. Two-way communication, which may be a call system with speaker or a telephone and paging system, must be available in diagnostic areas to summon help.

Consultation rooms for preadmission interviews by anesthesia and nursing personnel should include a table and at least three chairs to provide seating for the interviewer, the patient, and a family member. Space should accommodate wheelchairs. Lighting must be appropriate for paperwork, and storage for supplies should be provided for immediate documentation and educational needs. The interview area should provide privacy for physical assessments and a quiet atmosphere where dialogue can be heard easily by the participants but not by others in adjacent areas. This type of setting allows the patient and the interviewer to focus their attention on each other without distraction. Pages should be audible in the area, but piped-in music is usually distracting. The interviewer should not sit in front of a brightly lit window, because this may interfere with the patient's ability to see and concentrate. This area may house audiovisual equipment used in the education process.

A laboratory for obtaining patient specimens must be immaculate with a sink for handwashing. It should be arranged so that patients do not see specimens from others. A chair designed with a surface to support the patient's arm while blood is being drawn is ideal. Appropriate supplies must be available, along with spirits of ammonia ampules and a place for patients to recline should they feel faint. A stretcher for use during electrocardiograms is often in the same room.

Patients who are required to undress for tests should have a private area with a secure place for belongings. If radiology services are provided within the ASC, appropriate safety measures to ensure protection of all people in the area must be in place. For example, lead aprons must be provided for staff members and to shield areas of the patient's body that are not being filmed.

Admitting (Preoperative) Unit

Some centers provide private rooms for each patient and use the same location for the admission and discharge phases of the patient's stay. Although affording the most privacy and comfort, such a system may be impractical because of limited space. Private rooms also preclude visual observation from a central location.

When an open floor plan is used, constant observation is possible. Staff efficiency may be enhanced, but patient privacy can suffer. At the least, patients should be separated by curtains. Partial walls that can provide visual and some audio separation between patients but allow visual contact with the nursing station are more appropriate. When unit separations do not provide audio privacy, the patient should be asked if the location is satisfactory for answering personal questions before any interviews commence. A more private area is required for confidentiality purposes. This type of setting is best addressed with distinct separation of preoperative and postoperative areas, a design often found in freestanding centers. A bathroom should be within the area or in close proximity.

Provision must be made for storage of personal belongings. Lockers may be used. One design suggests the use of lockers that provide for dual-sided access, with one side in the admitting area and the other side in the postoperative area. Another system that works well is the use of closed containers or plastic bags carried with the patient from one area to the next as long as security can be ensured.

Differences in anesthesia practice affect the types of furnishings and equipment necessary for the admission area. Many centers have recliners for their preoperative patients and encourage them to walk to the OR. This type of atmosphere fosters the concept of wellness and may be less intimidating than others. It does not, however, accommodate the patient who will be given preoperative sedation or regional blocks. For those patients, beds or stretchers remain the appropriate mode for admitting and transferring them to the OR.

When intravenous access is established or when sedating drugs or regional anesthetics are administered in the admitting area, oxygen delivery and suction equipment must be immediately available, along with monitoring devices and emergency equipment and drugs. Each patient should have access to a nurse call device and patient safety features, such as handrails. In addition, clean, dry, and uncluttered floors; well-lighted hallways; rounded corners on cabinets and furniture; and wide-based step stools should be available.

The decor of the admitting area should be relaxing. Calming colors, quiet surroundings with restricted traffic, and soft music help patients to relax. Many newly constructed facilities install wall-mounted consoles to provide hidden storage for supplies near beds or chairs. These eliminate nursing steps while maintaining an uncluttered, nonclinical look.

Operating Room

If any area of the ASC can be identified as most frightening for a patient, it has to be the OR. There is an unavoidable, intrinsic clinical atmosphere in ORs because of their technical and aseptic requirements. Depending on the philosophy of care in the facility and the specific needs of each patient, the ambulatory surgery patient may not receive sedating drugs to decrease the anxiety associated with the actual transfer to the OR. The attitudes and actions of staff members can turn the OR into a less frightening and friendlier environment for all patients. Staff attitude is the key to reducing the emotional trauma and fear that can be associated with an intraoperative experience.

The basic requirements of the OR environment remain the same for all types of surgical settings. Both freestanding and hospital-based units should follow AORN recommended practices. The OR must have equipment and access to emergency supplies, such as malignant hyperthermia and latex allergy carts, a crash cart with emergency medications and a defibrillator, an emergency power generator and lighting fixtures, and a back-up oxygen supply. Within or adjacent to the OR suite, anesthesia supplies and drugs are often located in a designated area that includes a double-locked cabinet for storage of restricted drugs. A two-way communication system is also necessary within each OR.

Other considerations in the OR environment must address storage, cleaning, sterilizing, clerical, infection control, patient privacy, and communication needs. Safety issues are of primary concern in the OR, where there is high risk for patient and staff injury from specialized equipment. Electrical devices must be inspected routinely, and educational programs to instruct staff members on their proper use should be ongoing.

Protective devices for preventing patient injury include such equipment as grounding devices, restraining straps, pillows and padding for positioning, fail-safe mechanisms on anesthesia administering equipment, and back-up oxygen, suction, and electrical sources. The principles of asepsis must be maintained to provide a safe environment, regardless of the patient population.

Outside windows in both the OR and the PACU are being considered in building and renovation projects. Windows can provide an emotional boost to the spirits of staff and patients when visual contact with the outdoors can be maintained throughout the day. Still, social and clinical issues must be addressed. Privacy should be ensured through the use of tinted or one-way glass or by the positioning of windows in an area where people walking by the facility cannot see in the OR. Patients cared for in a windowed room should be advised of the method used to ensure their privacy so that they do not worry unnecessarily that they will be viewed from outside the building. Adequate methods of cleaning the window must be instituted and consideration given to the fact that the diffuse outdoor light might create glare and interfere with effectiveness or intensity of a surgical spotlight. Blinds used to provide privacy and to darken the rooms for specific cases should be encased between two permanent layers of glass so that they do not attract or harbor dust.

Privacy must also be considered in regard to the windows and doors that open into corridors. Windows should be covered, and the operating table should be positioned in a manner that enhances patient privacy, particularly for the more sensitive procedures, such as gynecologic and plastic surgical cases.

Postanesthesia Care Unit

The PACU, often called phase I recovery, has intrinsic requirements for design, equipment, and supplies, regardless of whether they accommodate strictly ambulatory surgery patients or a mixed population of both hospitalized and ambulatory patients. Adequate space must be available to allow nursing care from either side of the patient's stretcher. Every patient station should be supplied with oxygen, suction, and monitoring devices, such as cardiac monitors, oximeters, and noninvasive blood pressure monitors. Other essential PACU equipment includes a ventilator, an emergency cart with defibrillator and medications, and an emergency call system. In addition, there must be easy access to the malignant hyperthermia cart and the anesthesia department. An ice machine and a blanket warmer or other means of patient warming are especially helpful to provide optimal patient comfort.

Design of a PACU should promote safe and efficient nursing practice. Patient care supplies should be readily accessible so that nurses are not required to leave the area frequently to obtain necessary materials. One or more work desks within sight of patients are essential, and observation is further enhanced by a visually open room design. Often, the main medication storage area for the OR suite is stationed within the PACU as well.

A few differences may exist in PACUs that are dedicated strictly to the care of ambulatory surgery patients. For one, an ASC may favor a more liberal "open door" policy for visitors in PACU, so the proximity of the waiting room and an entrance that connects the two are especially desirable. A specialized ambulatory PACU is likely to be used for chronic pain management procedures, preoperative administration of regional blockade, and other nonsurgical procedures. Room size and design should favor separation of various patient populations.

Historically, the general rule of thumb for number of recovery beds has been 1.5 to two beds for each OR or two to three beds in facilities with a high volume of short, uncomplicated cases. This concept should be challenged in any new construction or renovation based on the actual history of the facility in question. Rather than overbuild or underbuild an expensive unit, data relating to the facility's prior usage and projections related to the physicians and staff who will be using the new construction must be taken into account.[6]

Outpatients who remain in a hospital-based PACU for an extended time or those who are discharged directly from the PACU to home should be physically separated from more critical patients whenever possible. Ambulatory surgery patients should have access to an easy chair at the bedside, a bathroom, privacy for changing clothes, and enough space available for a family member or other adult to sit with the patient. Arrangements for beverages and snacks should be provided as well. Such amenities are not physically possible in some PACUs, but when possible, such things can help to enhance the patient's return to independence and help neutralize the otherwise clinical atmosphere of a PACU.

Ease of transfer to a second-phase recovery unit is enhanced if the two areas are adjoining. Virtually all freestanding centers are constructed in that manner or with combined phase I and phase II recovery areas. Hospital-based ASCs are often in more distant locations, some even located on different floors from the PACU. The transporting route should be designed to avoid public areas of the hospital.

A freestanding center has another issue to address. When the patient requires ambulance transfer to a hospital, there should be outside access to the PACU for the transport team. Ideally, this entrance should not be in view of other areas of the surgical facility, especially the views of preoperative patients or waiting family members. Prior contact with community ambulance personnel should apprise them of the appropriate door for emergency access.

Phase II Recovery (Discharge, Sit-Up) Areas

Ideally, a second-phase recovery area provides the patient with a more casual, home-like atmosphere. Its purposes are to provide continued nursing care and observation; to provide a setting for education and instructions; to allow reunion with family or friends, if that has not previously occurred; and to encourage self-care, ambulation, and a return to a level of function as close to the preoperative state as the procedure will allow. To these ends, the environment must address varied physical, social, and emotional needs.

Just as preoperative areas differ in design, various interior floor plans are found in phase II recovery units. Private rooms may be provided. This type of setting is especially useful for patients who are expected to remain for several hours after surgery or for those who require an extended period of recumbency or privacy, for instance, after facial or abdominal surgeries. An open design is less private but is usually adequate for most patients by this stage of recovery. In fact, socialization with other patients and families is often considered pleasant by many patients. In open areas where patients and families are in view of others, provisions should be made for necessary privacy related to care. Partial walls, curtains, or movable screens may be used.

Because patients arrive in this area in various stages of recovery based on the types and duration of the anesthesia and surgery performed, some may need to remain on stretchers or beds. Most patients are able to ambulate to recliners, which encourages movement and a sense of return to normalcy. Recliners provide the ability to lower the patient's head in response to a drop in blood pressure, nausea, or faintness. The discharge area should be large enough to accommodate one or more family members or friends for each patient, thus supporting what many consider to be an essential component in a successful ambulatory course. In facilities with a significant pediatric practice, a separate area for children is usually preferred to avoid proximity to adult patients.

When a nourishment center is close by, family members and patients can take care of some of their own needs, again encouraging a return to normal preoperative independence. A television may be a helpful diversion or too distracting, depending on the setting, and may contribute to delayed discharge if patients or visitors become interested in a particular program. Television may be used for teaching videos for more alert patients or for family members. Cabinetry or furniture that allows for storage of patient care items out of public view promotes a nonclinical atmosphere. A bathroom should be nearby for patient use.

The internal floor plan should take into consideration the special attitudes and policies of the ambulatory surgery program. Access linking the phase II recovery unit and a waiting area is important so that family members are readily available to the patient after surgery. A phase II unit should be positioned for efficient patient discharge to the outside. A separate exit door is favored to provide the most convenience and privacy for patients. The exit should be blocked from the view of passing motorists and pedestrians.

Because many centers prefer that patients walk to their automobiles to promote independence and to allow for a final assessment of their abilities, the route should be as short as possible. Some programs require wheelchair discharge, either because of the philosophy of care or due to the physical layout of the building. In either case, a wheelchair ramp should be available, as should provision for protection from the weather. A portico or canopy at the exit door is ideal. If such a cover is not in place, umbrellas should be provided. Protective floor mats are important inside doorways to help prevent accidental falls on rain- or snow-soaked flooring or carpets.

SUPPORT SERVICES

Supplies and Equipment

Storage for equipment and supplies must be available and efficiently positioned. Shipments from outside sources should be unboxed in a receiving room separate from sterile supplies to decrease the potential of presenting outside contaminants and vermin to the restricted areas of the surgery center. An efficient inventory system allows for rapid location and retrieval of specific items by staff members.

Equipment should be stored adjacent to or near the areas in which it will be used. Adequate, protected space must be assigned for delicate instrumentation and equipment to prevent accidental damage. All electronic medical equipment should be inspected and certified for use by a knowledgeable and experienced person before its use and periodically thereafter, according to any applicable safety and inspection codes.

Employees who are expected to use technical equipment must be trained in its proper use, storage, and maintenance. They should demonstrate competency through periodic skills checks. A user's manual must be available for all equipment, and a simplified list of basic instructions attached to technical equipment is helpful for quick reference.

Housekeeping and Linen

Cleaning supplies and equipment must be stored out of the sight of patients and visitors. Because most ambulatory surgery units have down times in the evening and night, general housekeeping chores are usually accommodated at those times. Dangerous chemicals and insecticides should not be used near patients or personnel. Cleaning solutions and chemicals must be stored safely with adequate ventilation, and care must be taken to identify and label caustic or poisonous items. In the OR suite, there must be provision for supplies and personnel for cleaning ORs between cases. Mop sinks must be separate from other uses.

Separation of soiled and clean linen must be maintained. Storage for scrub clothing should be within the confines of the changing rooms. Linen delivery carts are kept outside of restricted areas to avoid contamination from outside the building. Separation of patient and staff linen is advisable, and all linen should be stored in covered areas.

Mechanical and Electrical

Operation of the physical plant is dependent on effective electricity, telephone, water, and sewage services. In a hospital setting, the plant manager or any number of employees from the maintenance department are available and responsible for the proper function of all such services. In a freestanding center, only one person may be assigned to, and knowledgeable in, the mechanical working of the building. Because the constant attendance of this person cannot be guaranteed, other members of the staff, including nurses, should have a basic understanding, along with written instructions for essential functions. These might include a general understanding of electrical breaker switches, water shut-off valves in bathrooms, back-up oxygen sources, piped-in gas shut-off valves, the emergency generator, the security system, and air conditioner and humidifier controls.

Telephone numbers for various emergency service technicians should be prominently displayed. Table 4–1 is an example of the contact information for essential utilities failure. It is essential that all staff understand what to do should the telephones fail because communication is essential for the safety of patients and staff alike. A plan such as a messenger system among departments may be enacted for internal needs. For external communication, a cellular telephone may be available within the center, or a single-line telephone, separate from the main telephone system, may provide a back-up process.

***Table 4–1.* Essential Utilities Failure Plan**

UTILITY SYSTEM	FAILURE	ACTION	PHONE NO.
Electricity	Loss of **power** to normal power outlets	Plug all critical patient support devices into red outlets. **NO new procedures or surgery will be initiated if we are on generator power.** Check refrigerators for medications that may be altered if not kept at specific temperature. Check refrigerators for food spoilage.	
Electricity	Loss of **power** to all outlets	Manually support all critical patient devices. Use any equipment that runs on batteries in the meantime, e.g., patient monitors. Batteries are stored in refrigerator in back store room. Use flashlights. Check refrigerators for medications that may be altered if not kept at specific temperature. Check refrigerators for food spoilage.	
Water	Loss of **water** pressure	Reduce use to minimum; toilets may run constantly. **Call your maintenance department.** Have sterile water available when water must be used for instruments or scopes.	
Water	Loss of all **water**	Do not attempt to use water; turn off all faucets. **Call your maintenance department.**	
Oxygen	Loss of **oxygen** from wall outlets	Provide tank oxygen to dependent patients. We have portable oxygen tanks available, located in:	
Vacuum	Loss of **vacuum** from wall outlets	Use portable suction devices to support patients.	
Medical air	Loss of **medical air** pressure	Manually support patients on medical air devices. Ventilator works off of air but can run without an air supply as well.	
Air conditioning	Loss of **air conditioning**	Use fans temporarily. **Call your maintenance department.** Ensure surgery rooms are within acceptable range of temperature and humidity. Inspect integrity of sterile supplies and sterile packaging. Reschedule patients if loss of air conditioning continues.	
Heating	Loss of **heat**	**Call your maintenance department.** Use extra blankets as necessary. If loss of heat continues, check with manager for instructions to proceed with daily schedule.	
Communications	**Telephones** not working	Follow communication failure plan. Use cellular phones if available. Designate a messenger runner to relay information.	
Communications	Loss of **data system**	Use manual data processes—schedule using book.	
Elevators	**Elevators** not working	Use stairs. **Call your maintenance department** or **fire department.**	
Elevators	Stuck in elevators	Use emergency phone to call operator. Stay calm. Do not try to get out of car.	

STAFF SUPPORT SERVICES

Along with providing a safe and pleasant environment for patients and visitors, staff members and physicians should be comfortable and safe in their working environment. Decor and furnishings, color choices, and other amenities combine to create the overall work atmosphere.

Physicians who use the facility appreciate conveniences, such as ample parking near an entrance that is separate from the patients' entrance. A quiet area for dictating physicians' notes, telephoning, and completing paperwork is essential and is often found near the physicians' locker room or adjacent to the patient discharge area. Easy access to prior medical records is important to the busy surgeon and is a great boon in effecting completion of charts. Some centers provide hand-held dictating devices that accompany each patient's medical record throughout the building. The physician need only slip a completed mini-cassette into a plastic bag attached to the patient's medical record.

A lounge area for relaxation and meals is necessary. A single lounge is often shared by physicians, nurses, and other staff members to encourage interaction and promote a friendly climate. A lounge should provide a place to laugh and let down the more restrained demeanor necessary when in direct patient contact. Thus, the area should be positioned a distance from the clinical areas of the center. Comfortable furniture, kitchen facilities, a bathroom, and a telephone should be provided.

Another need of the staff is a quiet area for educational sessions, independent study, and completion of special assignments. A reference library for materials pertinent to ambulatory surgery and anesthesia should be maintained and updated in an ongoing manner. This may be addressed by an on-site unit, an agreement with a neighboring facility, through a lending reference library system, or on-line through the Internet.

SAFETY CONSIDERATIONS FOR PATIENTS, VISITORS, AND EMPLOYEES

Provision of a safe environment is a primary consideration in every healthcare setting. The physical conditions of the facility, the policies in place, the attitude of staff members, and the practice habits of all employees and physicians all play a part in the provision of a safe environment. Also essential is administrative support that reflects the importance of compliance with safety standards.

Safety precautions protect patients, visitors, staff, and physicians. It is unlikely that every accident is preventable, but with planning and concern for details, the ambulatory surgery environment can be one in which unexpected events and accidents are infrequent. Periodic surveys of the environment assist in monitoring safety practices. Table 4–2 is an example of one such survey that is performed by a different employee each time (monthly or quarterly) so that all become aware of essential safety issues. A second environmental survey, again performed by varying individuals, focuses more on processes than structure of the environment. Table 4–3 illustrates this survey tool, which much be completed by actual observation of the behavior and practices of various employees during the care of the patient. Its major focus is reducing environmental risks related to processes.

After the issues of building and environmental safety are addressed, the staff must turn its attention to internal policies and practice habits. Attentive, safe nursing care is the patient's major defense against injury. Patients who come to an ASC have a right to believe that they will be protected from harm during periods of personal vulnerability. Table 4–4 lists reasonable patient expectations regarding safety that should be addressed by the ambulatory surgery staff.

Family members and other visitors to the ASC must be provided with a safe environment as well. Dry, nonskid floors in waiting areas and uncluttered, well-lighted hallways are essential. Toys with small parts should not be stored where small toddlers and infants have access to them. Visitors should not be expected to help with the transport of patients through the center, because they may not be knowledgeable of the proper use of stretchers and wheelchairs or of proper body mechanics.

Hazardous wastes or needles should be disposed of properly and should not be left where they could injure a visitor or staff member. Sharps containers should be placed above child heights and should be anchored in racks so that they cannot tip over. Safety closures are available that prevent spillage should tipping occur.

It is important to follow up on any reported or observed injury to ensure that the person has adequately recovered, to maintain rapport with the injured person, and to identify problem areas so that adjustments can be made to reduce similar injuries in the future. Objective

Text continued on page 103

Table 4–2. Environmental/Safety/Infection Survey Tool

Reviewed by: ______________________ Date: ____________ Area Reviewed: ____________

Personal Protective Equipment (PPE) ***Availability of PPE in necessary areas.***	***Yes***	***No***	***N/A***	***Comments***
1. Utility gloves are available for housekeeping, maintenance, and other personnel whose duties may require such protection.				
2. Exam gloves, available in treatment/OR areas. Both sterile and nonsterile.				
3. Location of goggles/protective eyewear is posted and available as posted.				
4. Cover gowns (water impervious) are available when soiling of clothing is likely.				
5. Face masks (water impervious) are available at scrub sinks, patient care areas.				
6. Soap and towel dispensers are located at each sink, are full, and are in good working order.				
7. Eye splash equipment is available.				
Staff Compliance with PPE—Use PPE properly when in contact with blood and body fluids. ***OSHA and infection control policies practiced***	***Yes***	***No***	***N/A***	
8. Gloves, gowns, and masks used and disposed of properly.				
9. Eye protection/shields used when indicated.				
10. Hands washed after removing PPE.				
Proper Handling of Biohazardous Material ***Proving a hazard-free area.***	***Yes***	***No***	***N/A***	
11. Sharps containers are available, secured, and replaced when full.				
12. Sharps are disposed of properly.				
13. Biohazardous and white trash is sorted and stored in a secured area for pickup.				
14. Biohazardous containers are clearly identified with proper logo and are available in patient care areas.				
15. Red bags are appropriate leakproof ply and labeled with facility name.				
16. Infectious waste logs are current. (Includes receipts, invoices signed by agent.)				
17. Soiled linen is stored in appropriate laundry bags and removed at end of day.				
18. Soiled equipment is covered/decontaminated.				
19. Vector control program is in place.				
Proper Storage of Supplies	***Yes***	***No***	***N/A***	
20. No cardboard boxes are stored within the sterile zone.				
21. Supplies are stored above the floor and free of moisture and free from clutter.				
22. Clean linen stored in covered cabinets/carts.				
23. Food and drugs are stored separately.				
Sterilization Control of Equipment and Instruments ***Processes are being carried out consistently to ensure proper sterilization.***	***Yes***	***No***	***N/A***	
24. Sterilization logs are current and complete, including chemical, cold, steam, and flash.				
25. Sterilizers are cleaned as scheduled.				

Table 4–2. Environmental/Safety/Infection Survey Tool *Continued*

26. Biologic indicators are used as indicated and results documented.				
27. Chemical indicators used in each tray.				
28. Instrument trays and sterilization pouches are wrapped and sealed properly.				
29. Sterile supplies/trays are inspected for integrity before use.				
30. Equipment, instrumentation is cleaned and in good working order.				
Employee Infection Control Compliance All employees are oriented to:	***Yes***	***No***	***N/A***	***Comments***
31. Exposure control, infectious waste, HIV/HBV, housekeeping practices, location of PPE, infection policies and procedures, employee health program.				
32. Handwashing performed between patients.				
33. Employee health records are current, stored separately from personnel files, and secured.				
Quality Assurance in Infection Control	***Yes***	***No***	***N/A***	
34. Monthly infection control surveys are performed to determine postoperative infections.				
35. Postoperative infection research is performed to investigate possible source of infection.				
36. Infection control issues are discussed at quality improvement and/or risk management meetings.				
Safety Inspection	***Yes***	***No***	***N/A***	
37. Are fire extinguishers of proper size and type readily available?				
38. Are there fire alarm boxes and emergency call systems?				
39. Are staff alerted to and responsive to peer and patient negligence in fire safety?				
40. Are supplies stored on open shelves 18 inches from the ceiling?				
41. Are standpipes, fire extinguishers, and hoses examined monthly?				
42. Are personnel instructed in fire safety and the use of extinguishers and communication system?				
43. Is the "No Smoking" prohibition being enforced?				
44. Are electrical cords and plugs designed for use without use of adapter plugs?				
45. Is there adequate test and inspection program for electrical devices and wiring?				
46. Is the use of extension cords prohibited?				
47. Is equipment turned off or unplugged when repairs are being conducted?				
48. Is defective or inoperative equipment removed from use?				
49. Are all electrical distribution and shut-off boxes clearly marked with unobstructed access?				
50. Are oxygen and other gas tanks or bottles properly stored and secured?				
51. Is lighting intensity at all workstations at proper level with no glare?				
52. Do employees use proper body mechanics?				
53. Are safety practices stressed as part of employee orientation and training?				

Table continued on following page

Table 4–2. Environmental/Safety/Infection Survey Tool *Continued*

COMMENTS: ____

Total # of criteria 53   Criteria Not Met ______   Total Score ______
N/A Criteria ______

OR, operating room; OSHA, Occupational Safety and Health Administration; HIV, human immunodeficiency virus; HBV, hepatitis B virus; QA, quality assurance.

Courtesy of Morton Plant Mease Health Care, Dunedin, FL.

Table 4–3. Quality Assurance Review Risk Management Checklist

PREDETERMINED CRITERIA	Yes	No	N/A	Comments
General *Environment* 1. Free of dust and dirt				
2. Chairs clean				
3. Vacuum and O_2 at each station or readily available				
4. Humidifiers dated for proper changing interval				
5. BP cuffs and manometer clean and working				
6. Emergency equipment available and in good repair (O_2 cannula, airway, and tongue blade)				
7. No exposed wires on monitors and other equipment				
8. No spills on floor				
9. Prescription pads in secure area				
Patient Care 10. Surgical counseling documented and complete				
11. Physician flow follows patient flow				
12. Preoperative testing and preps scheduled and reviewed with patients				
13. Side rails up all times and beds in low position				
Lobby and Reception *Environment* 14. Free of dust and dirt				
15. Emergency equipment available/good repair				
16. All staff aware of location of emergency equipment				
17. No object or packages that could cause accidents left unattended				
18. No wet areas or slippery surfaces				
Confidentiality 19. Patients registered in a cordial manner				
20. Assistance offered to complete registration information				
21. Patient privacy maintained.				
22. No medical records or x-ray films left unattended				
23. Patient names and procedures not posted in view of public				
24. Schedules not posted in view of public				
25. Medical charts secured and locked				
26. Insurance and financial counseling available and completed—includes payment plans				

Table 4–3. Quality Assurance Review Risk Management Checklist *Continued*

PREDETERMINED CRITERIA	Yes	No	N/A	Comments
Anesthesia 27. Anesthesiologist accompanies patient to the OR				
28. Anesthesiologist speaks to patient before transfer to OR room				
29. Anesthesiologists directly available at all times during patient care				
Operating Room *Preparation of OR and Team Transportation of Patient to the OR*				
30. Floors clean				
31. Fixtures free of dust				
32. Supplies ready and in order; cupboard adequately stocked				
33. Routine equipment ready and checked for proper functioning: suction, autoclave, overhead lights, spotlight, microscope				
34. Emergency equipment and procedures known				
35. Special equipment ready: table, monitors, microscopes				
36. Instrument tables set up according to standard procedure				
37. Room temperature within proper ranges				
38. Anesthetic gases scavenge system working				
Transportation of Patient to OR 39. Proper identification of patient conducted				
40. Appropriate, safe mode used according to patient need				
Surgical Checklist Noted, Assessed, and Acted on Accordingly 41. Patient belongings secured				
42. Jewelry removed or secured to patients' finger				
43. Underwear removed according to procedure				
Initial Patient Interaction by Nurse in Operating Room				
44. Patient identified and called by name.				
45. ID band checked with chart and OR schedule				
46. Nurse identifies self, indicates his or her presence, and states his or her role				
47. Ability to verbalize determined				
48. Patient's right to privacy respected (e.g., door closed, no exposure)				
49. Explanation to the patient of actions taken by nurse				
Operating Room Team Clad Properly 50. Masks: nose and mouth covered, with no gaps at sides				
51. Caps: hair completely covered, with no wisps hanging out				
52. Clean shoes or shoe coverings worn				
Patient Care in Anesthesia and Surgery 53. The circulating nurse stands quietly by patient during induction				
54. Observes and reassures patient				
55. Prepares local injections and identifies drugs to person administering injection and records same properly				
56. Assists person administering anesthesia				
Position of Patient 57. Safe transfer (two people) to table with safety strap in place				
58. Correct body alignment with no obstruction to circulation or respiration				
Patient Preparation 59. Grounding pad properly placed and secured				
60. Exposure of surgical site adequate				
61. Prep adequate				
62. Proper draping procedure followed				

Table continued on following page

Table 4–3. Quality Assurance Review Risk Management Checklist *Continued*

PREDETERMINED CRITERIA	Yes	No	N/A	Comments
Maintenance of Environment				
63. Packs opened correctly				
64. Proper movement of personnel in room				
65. Team members perform stated duties and proper procedures				
66. Doors kept closed				
67. Traffic controlled to minimum				
68. Safety maintained regarding liquid contact or wires in OR				
Scrub Nurse's General Knowledge of Basic Steps in Procedure				
69. Surgeon's preference cards accessible and current				
70. Anticipates and asks appropriate questions				
71. Uses supplies judiciously				
72. Organizes surgical instruments efficiently				
73. Has knowledge of proper equipment use				
74. Time and motion are used economically				
Tenor of Room				
75. Effective/professional conversation				
76. Noise level at minimum				
End of Procedure				
77. Removal of drapes appropriate				
78. Exposure avoided to protect patient privacy				
79. Circulator and anesthesia with patient for transportation				
Specimens				
80. Handled appropriately by technician				
81. Labeled correctly with patient, number, and specimen				
82. Recorded in specimen log book appropriately				
Maintenance and Re-Establishment of Aseptic Environment				
83. Gowns and gloves are removed in room				
84. Instruments, linen, and wastes disposed of properly				
85. Appropriate cleaning procedures conducted between patients				
Postoperative Care and Evaluation				
86. Patient information report given to PACU nurse.				

Total No. of Criteria 86 Criteria Not Met ________ Total Score ________
N/A Criteria ________

Completed By: ____________________ Date: ________

BP, blood pressure; ID, identification; PACU, postanesthesia care unit; OR, operating room.
Courtesy of Morton Plant Mease Health Care, Dunedin, FL.

Table 4–4. Patient Expectations for a Safe Environment

1. The competence of all health providers is ensured.
   - All professional healthcare providers are currently licensed.
   - All nonprofessional healthcare providers are appropriately trained and supervised.
   - Providers are currently certified in basic cardiac life support (BLS/CPR) and, in the PACU, in ACLS or its equivalent.
   - Providers are knowledgeable of specific perianesthesia healthcare needs.
   - Providers continually update and demonstrate necessary competencies.
   - Emergency drills are practiced by all providers periodically.
   - All employees are knowledgeable of the policies and practices of the facility.
2. The patient is appropriately attended.
   - Patients have a method for summoning assistance within reach at all times.
   - Heavily sedated or anesthetized patients and children are attended at all times.
   - Patients at high risk for falls are identified, and interventions are employed.

Table 4–4. Patient Expectations for a Safe Environment *Continued*

- An anesthesia provider or other physician who is appropriately qualified in resuscitative techniques is present or immediately available until all patients operated on each day have been evaluated and discharged.

3. Safety practices are in place to protect the patient during times of dependence.
   - An identification bracelet is provided and visually checked before administration of medications or start of a procedure.
   - The name of the patient's primary physician is documented on the medical record for reference in case of an emergency situation.
   - Safety devices are used, e.g., nonskid slippers or flooring, side rails and safety straps, locks on stretchers and wheelchairs.
   - Providers protect the patient from pressure and injury through knowledge of proper body mechanics, positioning, and padding of pressure points.
   - The patient is asked for verbal identification and the type and site of surgery before transfer into the OR.
   - Sharp objects and unprotected needles are not placed in contact with or near the patient at any time.
   - Sponges, needles, and instruments are accounted for before closing of body cavities.
   - Radiopaque sponges are used whenever a body cavity is entered.
   - The patient is appropriately protected from radiation, electrical, and laser injuries.
   - Intubated patients in the PACU will have endotracheal cuffs inflated until the time of extubation unless specific contraindications exist.
   - Patients with artificial airways in place are constantly attended and are positioned to prevent aspiration.
   - Suction is immediately available for unconscious patients.
   - Two licensed providers, one of whom is a registered nurse, are present at all times when a postoperative patient is in the building or department.
   - Two providers are available to help with the initial ambulation of patients who are at high risk for falling—the very elderly or physically weak, postspinal or postepidural patients, those unable or not allowed to bear weight on one leg, and those with a history of fainting or difficulty in ambulating.
   - Discharge of the patient who has received anesthesia or sedation is allowed only when that patient is accompanied by a responsible adult.
4. Appropriate and safe equipment is available.
   - All technical and electronic equipment is tested for safety by the clinical engineer or equivalent before initial use and in an ongoing manner.
   - Unsafe or questionable equipment is taken out of service and labeled immediately.
   - Monitoring devices are calibrated and serviced periodically as designated by the manufacturer.
   - Directions for use are readily available for all equipment.
   - Emergency equipment is checked periodically for function and staff familiarity.
   - Stretchers and wheelchairs are periodically inspected.
   - There is emergency access to replacement equipment in the event of a failure.
   - Portable emergency equipment allows for safe transport to another unit or facility.
   - An internal and external communication system is available throughout the facility.
5. Medications are stored and administered safely.
   - An adequate stock of medications is maintained.
   - Security of medication from tampering, theft, and unauthorized use is ensured.
   - All medications remain in their original wrapping. If they are transferred to another container, they are conspicuously labeled by the pharmacist who transfers them.
   - Expiration dates, color, and clarity are checked before use.
   - Outdated medications are removed from the storage area of medications in use.
   - Emergency drugs are checked for expiration dates at least monthly and are replaced immediately if used or outdated.
   - Storage of medication is temperature and humidity controlled as indicated for individual drugs.
   - Oral, injectable, and topical drugs are stored separately.
   - Allergies are identified and consistently documented in a prominent and consistent location on all patient records. This may include having the patient wear a bracelet noting any allergies.
   - Nurses follow safe standards of practice by identifying the drug, dose, route, time, and patient's name and allergies before administering any medication.
   - All patients are observed for untoward or allergic effects of medications administered.
6. The principles of asepsis are maintained.
   - All providers are knowledgeable of and practice proper techniques to prevent the spread of disease and germs.
   - Strict aseptic technique is followed in the OR and for invasive procedures such as catheter insertion or irrigation, venipunctures, dressing changes, and injections.
   - All personnel are truthful and ethical about any break in sterile technique. They immediately report such an occurrence and take necessary steps to correct or address any resulting problems and to avoid future occurrences.
   - Sterility of supplies is ascertained through ongoing monitoring of autoclave function, checking of expiration dates, rotating of stock, and monitoring of individual techniques of packaging for sterilization.
   - Providers with highly contagious diseases will not be involved in the care of surgical patients.
7. Decisions about healthcare are made thoughtfully and with regard to the individual.
   - A physician knowledgeable of the patient directs the patient's care, including the discharge.
   - All pertinent data and diagnostic test results are available and are assessed before administration of anesthesia or the onset of the procedure.

PACU, postanesthesia care unit; BLS, basic life support; CPR, cardiopulmonary resuscitation; ACLS, advanced cardiac life support; OR, operating room.

Table 4–5. Staff Expectations for a Safe Environment

1. Personal security is addressed.
   - Alarm systems, security devices, and locks are maintained as appropriate to the risks inherent to the geographic location of the ASC.
   - Entrances and parking lots are well lighted.
   - A security guard is provided in high-risk areas.
   - One person is not left alone in the facility.
   - Narcotics, needles, syringes, and prescription pads are appropriately locked or kept out of sight when not in use.
2. Policies and practices are in place to prevent the spread of disease.
   - Universal precautions approved by the CDC (Centers for Disease Control and Prevention) are practiced.
   - The facility provides sufficient protective clothing, gloves, goggles, storage containers for wastes, antiseptics, and sinks for handwashing.
   - Needles are discarded without recapping or breaking.
   - Personnel and patients with highly communicable diseases (measles, chickenpox, influenza) are not allowed in the facility.
   - Aseptic technique is maintained.
3. Policies and practices are in place to prevent exposure to, or injury from, radiation, laser equipment, electrical, and other equipment.
   - Defibrillators are stored in the "disarmed" mode.
   - Appropriate gear (goggles, lead aprons) is available for protection against injury from potentially dangerous equipment.
   - Warning signs are posted conspicuously when laser equipment or radiation is in use.
   - Radiology technicians announce their intentions before taking an exposure to allow staff members to put on protective apparel or to leave the immediate area.
   - Adequate instruction regarding equipment usage is provided for all staff members.
   - Equipment is safety checked before its use and periodically thereafter.
   - Equipment that is faulty or suspected to be faulty is removed from service immediately and is labeled for repair immediately.
4. Individual health practices are encouraged.
   - The facility provides or requires a periodic physical examination of all employees. This includes appropriate diagnostic testing.
   - The facility supports and provides immunization against hepatitis B for high-risk personnel.
   - The facility requires appropriate skin testing for tuberculosis.
   - Vacation and personal leave time is supported administratively for the emotional and physical well-being of employees.
   - Appropriate stress reduction practices are encouraged.
5. Ongoing educational programs and information sessions are provided to instruct personnel on safety habits.
   - Information is available regarding body mechanics, use of electrical equipment, storage and disposal of toxic wastes, and so on.
   - Information is available in the native language of employees who are unable to understand English.
   - Periodic fire and disaster drills are held to increase employees' awareness of personal responsibilities and ways to protect themselves and patients from danger during an emergency.
6. Storage of chemicals and toxic or dangerous materials protects personnel.
   - Unit-specific material safety data sheets for all toxic materials stored in the building or department are available and are easily accessible to all employees.
   - Adequate ventilation and sturdy storage shelves are provided.
   - No smoking is allowed near volatile materials or other combustibles.
   - Policies for handling dangerous materials are available and are communicated to all employees.
7. Employees in high-risk areas are protected from anesthesia waste gases.
   - A scavenging system is in place for retrieval and elimination of anesthetic waste gases from the OR.
   - Anesthesia equipment is maintained and inspected for leaks and cracks. Damaged equipment is discarded or repaired.
   - Ventilating systems are cleaned regularly.
   - Anesthetic gases are not turned on before actual induction of the anesthesia.
   - Female employees of childbearing age receive appropriate medical care and counseling.
   - Employees in high-risk areas receive annual physical examinations; these may include liver and kidney function tests if deemed appropriate by the employee's physician.
8. A policy is in place regarding employee incidents, injury, or exposure to a biologic hazard.
   - Access to emergency care is available should an employee be injured.
   - A mechanism is in place for reporting any incident involving staff safety.
   - Follow-up of injuries or incidents includes a plan to prevent similar future occurrences.

ASC, ambulatory surgery center; OR, operating room.

documentation of the injury should be completed according to facility standards.

It is the responsibility of the institution to provide a safe environment for its employees and other professionals and contract workers who work in it. On the other hand, it is the responsibility of those people to conduct themselves in a manner that exhibits knowledge of safety policies and a regard for personal protection. Table 4–5 lists some of the expectations that should be maintained for and by employees and other healthcare providers for their own protection.

The Occupational Safety and Health Administration (OSHA) requires employers to inform their workers about the potential dangers of chemical and toxic hazards and to provide training to help employees avoid harm on the job. This mandate identifies a worker's right to know about the dangers to which he or she may or will be exposed. One component of this requirement is the employer's compilation of material safety data sheets (MSDSs) for all chemicals and toxic agents used in the facility.

The MSDS manual should be individualized to the facility as illustrated in Table 4–6, the

Table 4–6. **Material Safety Data Sheet Informational Sheets—Index**

General Items

Acetic acid
Acetone
Alcohol, ethyl (70%)
Alcohol, ethyl (denatured)
Alcohol, isopropyl
Ammonium chloride (dimethyl)
Autoclave tape
Benzalkonium chloride
Benzoin
Betadine (povidone iodine)
Buffer solution 7.01
Bugger solution 1.09
Carbon dioxide
Chloroxylenol 4% hand scrub
Chlorhexidine gluconate—Foam Care 2%
Chlorhexidine gluconate—Foam Care 4%
Chlorhexidine gluconate—Hibiclens 4%
CLOtest
Cocaine hydrochloride
Collodion
Comfort Care roll-on deodorant
Dantrium (dantrolene sodium)
Duraprep (iodophor/ETOH)
Ethrane (enflurane)
Fix-Rite cytology fixative
Forane (isoflurane)
Formaldehyde
Formalin
Halothane
HemoCue calibrator hemoglobin
HemoCue glucose cuvettes
HemoCue hemoglobin cuvettes
Isoflurane
K-Y lubricating jelly
Lead
Lidocaine viscous 2%
Lugol's solution
Mercury (Maloney & Hurst esophageal dilators)
Mineral oil (sterile)
Monsel's solution
Mucolex
Nitrogen
Nitrous oxide
Oxygen
Pentothal
Petrolatum gauze
Phenol
pHisoHex
Povidone iodine
Pyloritek hydration reagent
Saccomanno fluid
Silver nitrate sticks
Soda ash (soda canisters)
Sodium chloride
Sterno—canned heat
Subsulfate solution—Ferris
Sulfuric acid
Suprane (desflurane)
Surgicel—absorbable hemostat
Tannic acid
Trichloroacetic acid
Ultane (sevoflurane)
Urine dipstick control (human urine)
Whisk (adhesive removers)
Xeroform petroleum gauze
Zephiran (benzalkonium chloride)

Insecticides, Herbicides, and Plant Products

Baygon 2%
Bait Blocks
Drione
Dursban
Engage
Fican W
Gentrol
Maxforce
Orthene
PT 565 Plus XLO

Outdoor products:
20-20-20 soluble fertilizer
Atrazine 4L herbicide
Dursban + with fertilizer
Malathion
Ortho Orthene
Roundup

Table continued on following page

Table 4–6. Material Safety Data Sheet Informational Sheets—Index *Continued*

Antimicrobial and Cleaning Agents	
Accent Plus—antibacterial amino lotion/skin care	Medline enzymatic detergent
Bleach—Hilex	Nutra pH instrument milk
Bleach—Clorox	Orthozime (bacteriostatic enzyme cleaner)
Cavicide	Peracetic acid (STERIS-20 sterilant concentrate)
Cidex	Ruhof Biocide (detergent disinfectant spray)
Klenzyme	Scott liquid soap
Lap Cholyzime bacteriostatic cleaner	Spectra Care (hand cleaner)
Instrument Cleaning Agents	
ACTS (autoclave cleaning treatment system)	m317 power instrument lubricant (3M)
AMSCO Enzycare 2 detergent	Metricide 28
AMSCO Liquid Jet-2 detergent	Surgi Stain (removes rust and corrosion)
Calgon Manu-Klenz (Instru-Klenz)	Vespore (glutaraldehyde)
Contrad 70 (Ultan Sonic Detergent)	Xomed—Treace Micro Craft drill system cleaning solution
Lubricating Oil—Wolf	
Physical Agents	
Noise	Ionizing radiation
Heat	VDT computer terminals
Office Supplies	
D-Q23 developer	T-Q23 toner
Toner and developer	Smoke detector tester
Lasers	
CO_2 laser	Nd:YAG laser
KTP/YAG laser	
Environmental Services Products	
Butchers Speedtrack floor polish	Lysol phenolic disinfectant
Comet Creme	Lysol hard water stain cleaner
Contempo Stat carpet sanitizer	Neutrodor spray
Lysol disinfectant	Pledge aerosol furniture polish lemon
Lysol IC foaming disinfectant	Resolve Procare carpet spot cleaner
Lysol IC quaternary glass cleaner	Shimmer metal surface cleaner
Living Plants and Greenery (All Are Nonpoisonous)	
Bird of paradise (White)	Pothos
Bromeliads	Raphis palm
Cham palm	Silver Queen
Licus Ali	Spath (Peace Lily)

VDT, visual display terminal; KTP, potassium titanyl phosphate; YAG, yttrium-aluminum-garnet; Nd; neodymium.

index from one freestanding ASC's MSDS manual. It is important to survey the entire facility to identify all substances for which MSDSs are needed. Forgotten products may be found under sinks, in locker rooms, and in desks. Common household products that are sold retail in the sizes stocked in the facility and are being used for their intended commercial purposes need not be listed. Examples include dishwashing soaps, fragrance sprays, hair sprays, deodorants, and erasure liquids. It is the responsibility of the employer to identify these products and implement policies that preclude bringing unapproved products into the work environment.

These data sheets provide information about the potentially harmful ingredients or dangers of chemicals and other toxic products in the workplace. They must be available for reference by all employees. Manufacturers are required, by law, to supply material safety data sheets on all their products. Sheets can be obtained by calling the company. MSDSs should be kept only for those products within the department or center; thus, the manual must be individualized. All chemical products should be stored in their original containers or approved containers and must always be labeled. Data on some generic chemicals may need to be secured by the employer from other sources, for instance, a pharmacist.

All employees should be required to read and document that they have read the safety data sheets on hire periodically, for instance, annually. In addition, education on the proper method of containing or cleaning up spills and protecting oneself must be provided at least annually. Table 4–7 can be adapted to provide employees with a quick reference to the location of spill control supplies. A further discussion and a sample material safety data sheet can be found in Chapter 3.

It is helpful to have someone who is not familiar with the ASC survey the environment for potential risks. The hospital-based ASC may ask that the director of safety and security assign someone to this task, or the center may have an employee from the business department survey the clinical locations while a clinical person reciprocates within the business areas. One helpful idea is to ask this person to use the "eyes of a child" approach and look for dangers at low levels, for instance, sharps containers or live plants that are accessible to a toddler. As unlikely as it may seem, small children could chew on leaves of plants in waiting areas. "Do you know the names and poisonous status of plants in your center?" This was a direct question from a JCAHO surveyor to one receptionist.

An ambulatory surgery facility possesses all the inherent dangers of any surgical setting. It is made into a safer environment by the healthcare providers who are responsible for patients' care and by support personnel who tend to environmental needs. Forward thinking, along with thoughtful observation of the environment, helps nurses to identify potential problem areas and make changes to prevent accidents before they occur.

***Table 4–7.* Biohazardous and Chemical Spill Control Equipment**

SPILL KITS CONTAIN

Personal protective equipment (gown, mask with eye shield, gloves, head and foot covers), absorbent material, bleach, biohazardous red bags and sharps containers, "Caution spill" signs

EYE CARE KITS CONTAIN

Ophthalmic—Blephamide drops, Garamycin drops, Dacriose eye wash, tetracaine 0.5% drops, 1000 mL 0.9% saline IV bag w/flush solution, eye pads, tape, small ice pack

Enter the location of PPE in various departments

DEPARTMENT			
Spill kits			
Absorbent rolls			
Eye wash station			
Full body shower			
Eye care kit			
Chemical filtration mask			
Mercury spill kit			
MSDS manual			

MSDS, material safety data sheet; IV, intravenous.

INFECTION CONTROL ISSUES IN THE AMBULATORY SURGERY CENTER

In general, infection control issues in the ASC mirror the issues common to the inpatient hospital setting. The differences that exist can be attributed to how certain practices are implemented. The mere fact that a patient is undergoing an invasive procedure in the perioperative area sets the stage for potential infection. The ASC environment needs to be surveyed to assess, identify, address, and implement actions to reduce and eliminate potential infections in the perioperative patient. The focus of this section is not to review basic infection control principles and practices, but instead to review how infection control practices interface in the ASC setting.

The ASC should have a detailed infection control program in place. According to the JCAHO, the program should be designed to guard against infection by preventing it, breaking the chain of transmission, and improving the ability of individuals to avoid infectious agents, such as those that cause vaccine-preventable diseases.[2]

Infection Control Program

The ASC should develop an infection control program specific to the population served. If the facility treats patients in all age groups from infants to elderly, the program should address concerns for all individuals in this population. For example, facilities treating pediatric patients would screen for potential exposure to communicable diseases, whereas facilities treating immigrants would screen for possible exposure to tuberculosis. The ASC must develop processes that work in tandem with physician offices to ensure that proper screening occurs before the patient enters the facility.

According to the JCAHO, specific aspects of the infection control program include:[1]

- Surveillance
- Identification
- Prevention
- Control of infections
- Reporting

The infection control program needs to identify how surveillance activities are accomplished in the ASC. The purpose of surveillance is to collect data about infections in order to detect any changes in infection trends. Leaders need to identify what they want to focus on, what data will be collected, who will collect the data, and who will examine the data.

Once the data are collected, they are assessed to determine whether there are negative outcomes or trends. If an infection is identified, an investigation needs to occur to determine whether the infection was acquired in the ASC or in the community. To do this, predetermined criteria are applied. If it is determined that the infection was acquired in the ASC, further investigation is needed to determine any common factors that could have led to the transmission of the infection. Potential sources include equipment, staff members, ORs, surgeons, and anesthesia personnel. A thorough and complete investigation should occur to rule out or confirm common factors.

The infection control program should include a process for developing and implementing policies and procedures relative to infection control practices. Table 4–8 includes a sample of infection control policies and procedures that should be available in the ASC setting. Policies and procedures are essential to ensure that all staff members are performing procedures uniformly. The ultimate goal of having a policy and procedure manual is to reduce or prevent the transmission of infection.

The ASC must also identify how it will control the transmission of an infectious disease once it has occurred. For example, an employee who tests positive for streptococcus is required not to report to work until cleared by the employee health nurse.

The ASC must also develop a policy that outlines the process for reporting any diseases or infections that are reportable as required by law and regulation. The local health department can assist in identifying the reportable diseases. Normally, the primary physician is responsible for reporting to the authorities, but the ASC should follow up to ensure that the physician has seen the report and is reporting the disease.

***Table 4–8.* Sample Index of Infection Control Policy and Procedure Manual**

Exposure control plan
Infection control plan
Handwashing
Aseptic technique in the operating room
Gowning and gloving
Removing soiled gloves, gown, and mask
Accidental exposure to blood and body fluids
Disposal of contaminated sharps
Hepatitis B vaccine
Personnel attire
Handling soiled linen
Procedure for autoclave testing
Response to sterilizer malfunction
Flash sterilization
Disinfection of supplies, instrument, and equipment used in the operating room
Reporting infectious diseases or conditions
Routine disinfection of toys and juvenile furniture
Sterile processing of equipment
Medical waste
Personal protective equipment
Identification of communicable diseases

Identification of Postoperative Infections

In the ASC, there should be a process in place for identifying surgical site infections. One method of surveillance is consistent follow-up with each physician to identify whether any patient who underwent surgery in the ASC had an identified postoperative infection. The ASC can generate a list of each physician's patients and ask for follow-up information. For example, the ASC can generate a list of patients who underwent orthopedic procedures the previous month, or it can survey all physicians and include all patients. A letter can be sent to each physician indicating the patient's name, date of surgery, and so on. A checklist such as that in Table 4–9 accompanies the letter to the physician. The physician is asked to check off the appropriate information and return the form to the ASC.

Another method of following up on patients after surgery is to contact each patient. One method of accomplishing this is to have a preprinted letter asking for follow-up information concerning the patient's surgery. A letter can be sent to each patient asking whether they experienced any postoperative infections. This

Table 4–9. Sample Letter to Physician Regarding Postoperative Infections

AMBULATORY SURGERY CENTER
INFECTION CONTROL SURVEY

SURGEON:	Dr. S. Smith
PATIENT:	John Doe
SURGERY DATE:	01/04/99
PROCEDURE:	Left knee arthroscopy

1. Did the patient experience any postoperative complications? Y N

   If yes, please explain. ______________

   ____
2. Did the patient have any postoperative infection? Y N

   If yes, please complete questions 3 through 8.
3. When did the symptoms first occur? ______

   ____
4. What symptoms did the patient experience?

   ____

   ____
5. Was drainage purulent? Y N
6. Was a culture performed? Y N
   Was an I & D performed? Y N

   If yes, indicate site: ______________
7. What organism was cultured? ______________
8. How was the infection treated? ______________

   ____

I & D, incision and drainage.

letter can be combined with a patient satisfaction tool, thereby allowing the ASC to gather information for not only postoperative infection information but also patient satisfaction with the ASC. The drawback to this type of follow-up is that the response rate may be low.

An alternative method is to call the patient anywhere from 2 weeks to 1 month after surgery. The telephone interview can be used to gain insightful information regarding the patient's postoperative recovery. Although time intensive, the follow-up phone call can provide valuable information as to how the patient's recovery progressed, when they returned to work, and any complications they may be experiencing. Sample questions that the nurse might ask the patient include the following:

1. Are you experiencing any signs or symptoms of an infection?
2. Do you have an elevated temperature?
3. Is your surgical site clean and dry?
4. Is your surgical site reddened, swollen, or warm to touch?
5. Is there any drainage from your incision?
6. If yes, what color is the drainage?
7. Is the drainage foul smelling?
8. Have you contacted your physician?
9. If yes, did the physician prescribe an antibiotic?
10. If yes, are you taking your antibiotic as ordered?

Any patient who identifies a potential infection should be directed to contact the physician's office. The ASC nurse should also contact the physician's office to report the conversation. All nursing actions should be documented in the patient's medical record.

The infection control follow-up phone call is not meant to replace the postoperative follow-up phone call that usually occurs the day after surgery. One way to obtain better compliance when following up by telephone is to ask when and where the patient can be reached 2 to 3 weeks later. Is the patient receptive to being contacted at work? To gain higher compliance, a method of placing phone calls in the evening may need to be instituted.

Employee Health Issues

The ASC needs to ensure that a program exists to identify employee health issues. Table 4–10 identifies possible policies and procedures that should be in place. A mechanism for instituting the specific policies also needs to be identified. The ASC can employ their own em-

Table 4–10. Sample Employee Health Policies and Procedures

1. Pre-employment health screening requirements
2. Annual health screening requirements
3. Annual tuberculosis testing
4. Personal illness or injury
5. Work-related illness or injury
6. Staff incident report form
7. Medical leave of absence
8. Return to work clearance
9. Occupational exposure to blood-borne pathogens
10. Guidelines for treating possible hepatitis B exposure
11. Guidelines for treating possible human immunodeficiency virus exposure
12. Measles, mumps, and rubella immunity
13. Hepatitis B vaccine
14. Employees with infectious diseases
15. Work exposure to communicable diseases
16. Latex allergy

ployee health nurse, or they can contract with a nearby hospital or clinic to provide this service.

The purpose of an employee health program is to screen and monitor the health of employees, both at the time of hiring and on an ongoing basis. The program should provide for immunizations, monitoring for infections, and follow-up care for occupational exposures to communicable diseases. The function of the employee health nurse should be to screen new employees; assess, treat, and track work-related illness and injury; provide immunizations; monitor infections; and work with all department managers on health- and safety-related issues.

Infection Control in the Operating Room

In the OR, prevention and control of infection is paramount. Asepsis is the foundation of controlling infections in the operative setting. Perioperative nurses are instilled with the basis for aseptic technique during their orientation to the operative setting. The reader is referred to the numerous sources of information available for detailed practices of infection control in the operative setting. One such source is the AORN *Standards, Recommended Practices and Guidelines* published by AORN.[10]

Issues that the ASC needs to address in their infection control program include

- Autoclave policies and procedures
- Equipment decontamination
- Flash sterilization
- Surgical attire
- Environmental cleaning
- Hand scrubs
- Traffic control

Establishing policies and procedures that are in accordance with accepted standards of practice ensures that the ASC is committed to reducing the risk of exposure to infections.

The ASC must have a comprehensive, effective infection control program in place. The program should contain methods to identify, prevent, control, and report infections. A multidisciplinary team should meet on a regular basis to address issues identified, develop policies and procedures, discuss identified infections, and develop methods to reduce potential exposure to infections in the ASC.

THE FUTURE IS NOW

Nothing is so constant as change. That old saying is particularly applicable to the healthcare profession. Mobile lithotripsy units and magnetic resonance imaging units have become relatively common. Now, surgery can be added to the list of mobile services.

An innovation in surgical care is the advent of the mobile surgery unit developed by the Mobile Medical International Corporation of St. Johnsbury, Vermont. Virtually all of the structural and clinical features previously discussed in this chapter have been integrated into the world's first fully mobile surgical and recovery suite. The ambiance is clearly clinical, with-

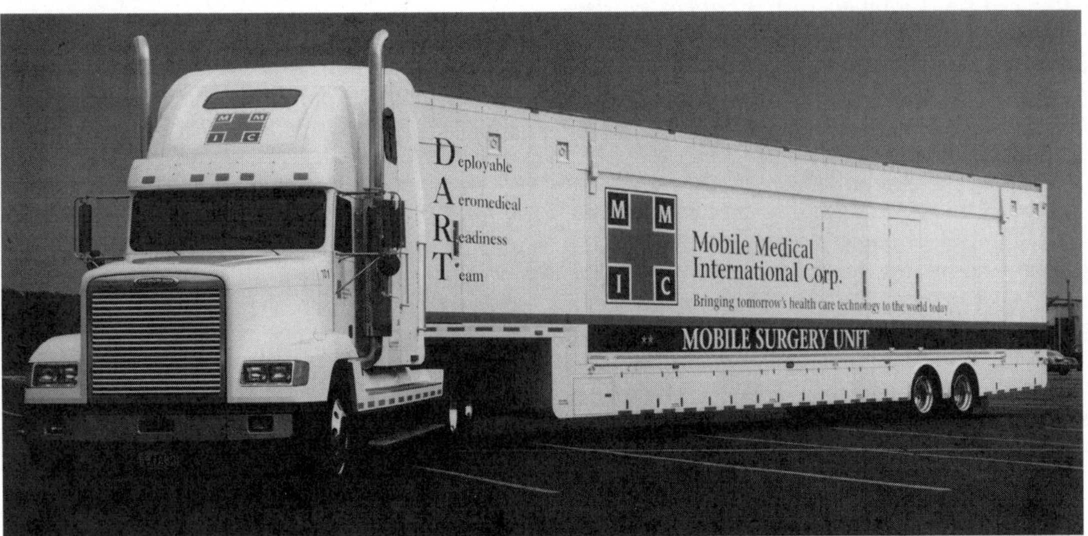

Figure 4–3. Mobile surgical unit. (Reprinted with permission of Mobile Medical International Corporation, St. Johnsbury, VT.)

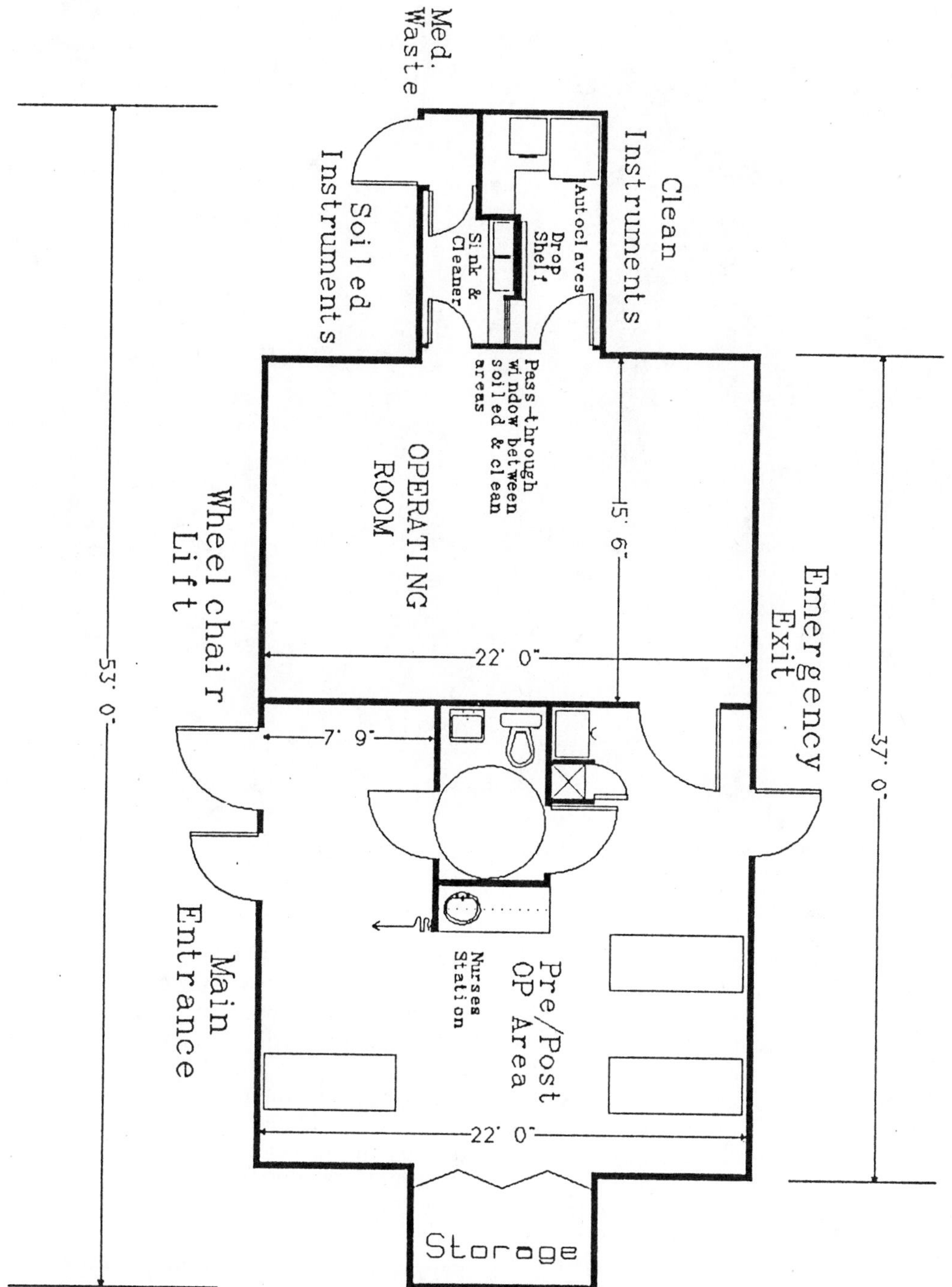

Figure 4–4. Floor plan of mobile surgical unit. (Reprinted with permission of Mobile Medical International Corporation, St. Johnsbury, VT.)

out a focus on the environmental "niceties" for the patient and family, but the amazingly compact unit is impressive. Figure 4–3 illustrates the unit as it appears during transportation. Figures 4–4 to 4–6 illustrate the floor plan and the interior operating and admission/recovery areas, with the unit fully expanded on each side of the vehicle to allow more floor space for operational use.

President and chief executive officer Rick Cochran[7] explained that although the unit is fully deployable to combat areas by military

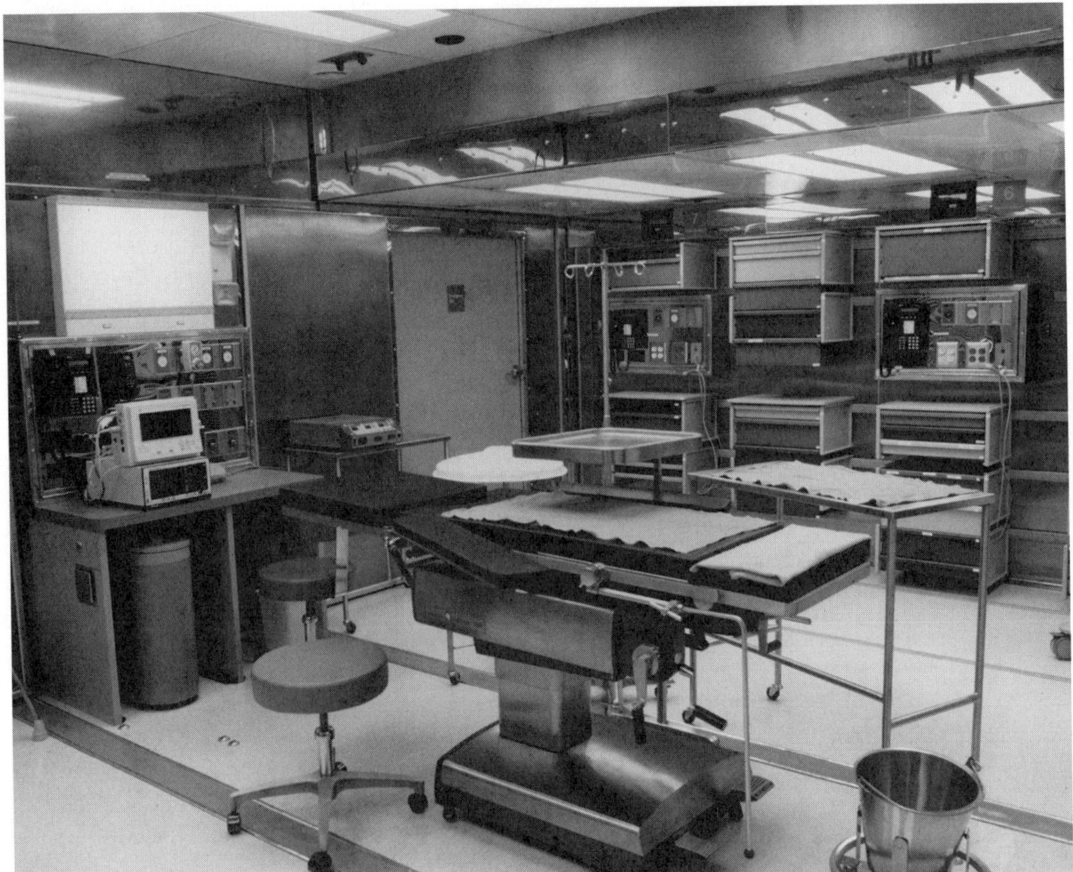

Figure 4–5. Operating room in mobile surgical unit. (Reprinted with permission of Mobile Medical International Corporation, St. Johnsbury, VT.)

cargo plane, its commercial uses are also broad. These range from providing care to underserved, wilderness, and international relief areas, to prisons and disaster zones, and to hospitals that are renovating interior surgical suites.

Clinical trials found surgeons from across the United States using this mobile unit for cases as divergent as hernia repair, cataract removal, and aortic resections. Stability, efficiency, and effectiveness were tested with favorable outcomes, particularly with regard to turnover times; separation of soiled, clean, and sterile areas; and ease of cleaning. The recovery area serves three patients at a time and includes blanket warmer, crash cart, portable cabinetry, full patient monitoring, computerized work stations, and telecommunications at each bed. Each telephone is capable of land, satellite, and cellular broadcast.

The design allows for maximum conservation of supplies in this self-contained unit. Redundant systems for power, communications, water, and vacuum allow for operation of the unit, even if portions should fail as a result of external forces. The diesel generator can operate around the clock for 8 days. This unit is designed to comply with Medicare standards. Although most of us are not providing care to our ambulatory surgical patients in such a unit, its very existence should make every nurse cognizant of the need to maintain objectivity and open, creative minds in the ever-changing environment of healthcare.

ENVIRONMENTAL EMERGENCIES

Look around the ambulatory surgery unit. The possibility of an environmental disaster in such a seemingly safe setting seems extremely remote. In rare instances when a fire, explosion, or another disaster occurs, the situation can turn into a medical emergency quickly if personnel or patients are injured or in jeopardy. Regardless of the extraordinarily small chance of such an occurrence, every ASC, whether freestanding or hospital based, must have a doc-

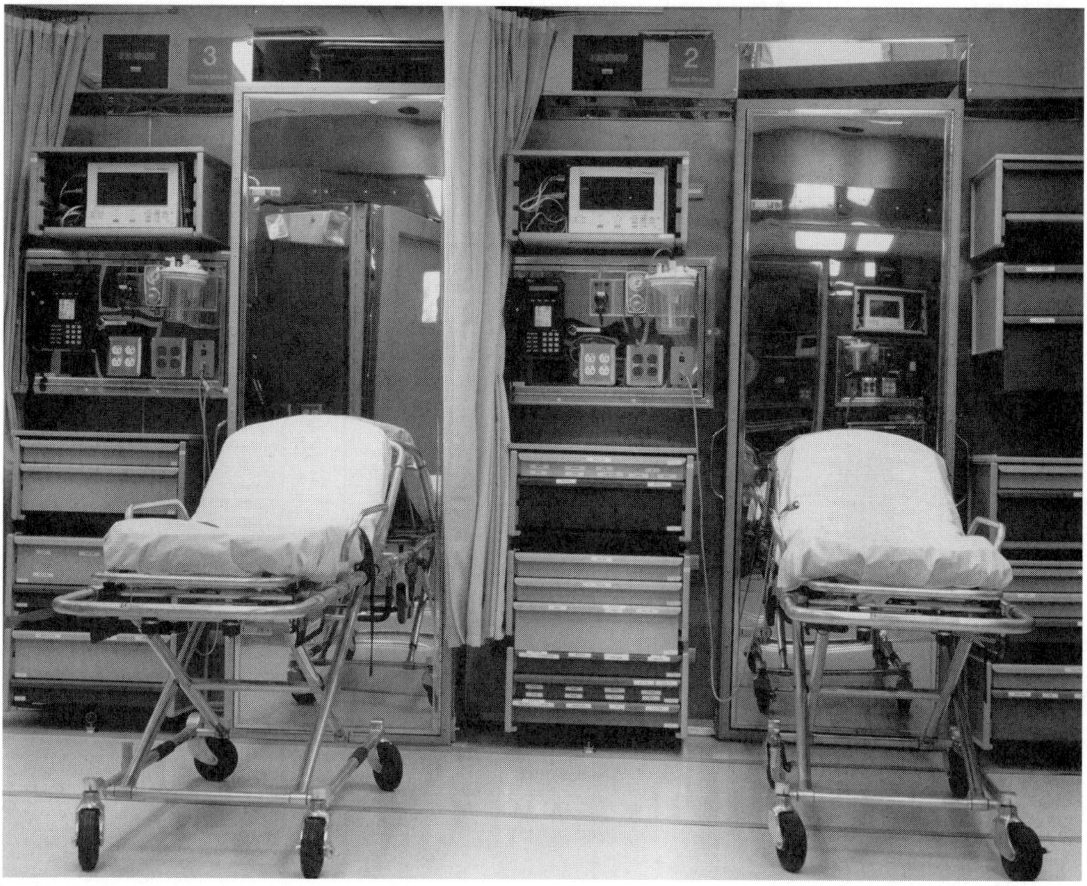

Figure 4–6. Pre- and postoperative care unit in mobile surgical unit. (Reprinted with permission of Mobile Medical International Corporation, St. Johnsbury, VT.)

umented and rehearsed plan for responding to unexpected disasters. This plan should be reviewed and updated annually by a cross-section of administration, staff, and disaster authorities. It should be easy to understand, widely disseminated, easy to implement, flexible, comprehensive, and coordinated with other plans within the facility and community.[8]

The relationship of the unit to the community disaster plan should be clearly defined. For instance, would the center's ORs and personnel be available to provide treatment of victims of a widespread community disaster? The freestanding center should provide information and discuss such matters with civil authorities to ensure that the community understands that the unit is not staffed 24 hours a day. Other questions to ponder include whether a telephone tree can and should be implemented among staff members of the ASC to apprise them of the need for their assistance in local hospitals or other departments.

People come to a health facility expecting a safe environment. Rarely is a patient consciously considering the possibility of an environmental disaster, but the staff members responsible for the patient's care must be in constant readiness for both internal and external disasters. Internal problems can include fire, explosion, bomb threat, gas leak, and confrontation by a dangerous or threatening person. External disasters may be natural, for instance, tornado, lightning strike, hurricane, earthquake, snowstorm, and flood. Man-made problems can include toxic chemical spills, gas leaks, and electrical or telephone blackouts. In facilities with a geographic predisposition to environmental emergencies, institutional programs should be in place that deal with specific preparedness plans. For instance, a surgery unit in the midwest should frequently rehearse tornado drills, and a unit along a natural fault line must have clearly defined earthquake protocols in place.

Prevention and preparedness are essential elements in any internal disaster plan. Prevention includes practices that help to eliminate unsafe

***Table 4–11.* Drills, Codes, and Surveys Checklist: Enter team members' names in first column and add dates as they complete various drills and surveys.**

	FIRE DRILLS	FULL EVACUATION	MOCK CODE DRILL	RISK MANAGEMENT SURVEY	SAFETY/ INFECTION SURVEY	COMMENTS
Year: Team Members:						

situations in the environment, for example, smoking regulations, proper storage of chemicals and housekeeping supplies, laser safety precautions, and periodic inspection of electronic equipment and of fire prevention and detection systems. Preparedness lies in communicating and practicing established policies and practices for immediate and appropriate action in the event of an emergency. General rules of preparedness include posting of fire, police, and ambulance telephone numbers near all telephones; establishing a relationship with outside emergency response resources; having more than one person in the center at all times; providing written instructions for use of emergency equipment and ancillary support equipment; educating more than one person about the building's mechanical and emergency systems; and educating all personnel about their individual roles during emergencies.

Ongoing staff education teaches necessary response skills and helps to promote an attitude of personal responsibility among staff members. Internal evacuation routes should be established and communicated to all staff members. Only a few people may be immediately available to respond to an emergency, especially in a freestanding unit, so roles and responsibilities must be predetermined and practiced. Managers should ensure that all employees have been given the opportunity to take part in practice drills and environmental surveys so that they feel comfortable with the safety practices of the facility. The grid illustrated in Table 4–11 can help to identify who has and who has not participated in drills, so that future drills can be planned at times to include those who have not already practiced.

For a practice emergency drill to be of real value, it is essential that staff discuss the effectiveness of response and address both triumphs and deficiencies. An evacuation drill review sheet, as illustrated in Table 4–12, can be used to document the emergency response. Typical problems can include failure of an alarm box, failure of fire doors to close, inability to hear an alarm in all areas, and equipment blocking fire exits. Staff-related errors might include failure to close doors or windows or to turn off gas valves, failure to check all areas for people remaining in the department before evacuation, failure to bring a fire extinguisher to the evacuation route, and evacuation attempts in the wrong direction.

Should an actual disaster occur, a predetermined spokesperson should be available to make statements to the press and to provide appropriate information to the public. Other employees should not address outsiders, particularly the news media. The designated person must have a previously developed plan that is designed to provide a well-coordinated command post and to avoid as much negative publicity as possible. Given free access to the facts, outsiders are not as inclined to believe or spread information that is not true. Immediate response also impresses the public that the facility's personnel have acted appropriately in response to the disaster.

Another consideration is that of diverting further patients from coming to the hospital or freestanding center. A clerical person may be assigned to telephone patients and physicians to cancel any imminent arrivals. This action can help to avoid the formation of an even larger crowd outside the facility.

FIRE THREAT

Fire and explosion are always possibilities in any surgical and anesthetic environment. Electrical sparks or short circuits from electrocautery units, laser machines, defibrillators, and other sophisticated electronic equipment can ignite sheets, clothing, and hair and can injure personnel and patients with electrical shock. Other predisposing factors include storage of volatile liquids and gases, frequent use of oxygen, increased use of disposable paper products, presence of complex electrical wiring as a feature of the structural requirements, and concurrent use of numerous pieces of equipment in the same area. Even a seemingly benign piece of equipment, such as a toaster and coffee maker, can be at fault, so periodic inspection for frayed or broken wires is imperative. Personnel must take responsibility for turning off electrical sources before closing the department for the day.

Prevention

No amount of prevention can be considered too much when fire safety is the issue. Ambulatory surgery patients are extraordinarily vulnerable to their environment during periods of anesthesia, recovery, and immobility, so it is the responsibility of the staff to protect them. Staff meetings should address ways to prevent fires. Also, periodic questioning of individuals can help keep information fresh in their minds. Table 4–13 illustrates such a questionnaire that is used by a staff member in the role of safety officer.

Inherently dangerous situations that exist in the ASC setting can be decreased by the following actions:

Table 4–12. **Fire/Disaster Evacuation Drill**

SUMMARY	S	U	N/A	COMMENTS
Actual Alarm or Rehearsed (circle one) Date: ______ 1. Fire department response time				
2. Overhead page accuracy/clarity				
3. Response time				
i. Reception				
a. Main reception desk				
b. Business office personnel				
c. Administration				
ii. Clinical units				
a. Admitting desk				
b. PACU team				
c. OR staff				
d. Endoscopy staff				
e. Gas valves				
f. Stairwells/extinguishers				
g. Doors/telephones				
4. Facility engineering response				
a. Power supply				
b. Generators				
c. Sprinklers				
d. Mechanical				
e. Electrical				
f. Fire doors				
Total No. of Criteria: 20 Criteria Not Met ______ Criteria N/A ______ Completed by: ______ Total Score ______				

OR, operating room; PACU, postanesthesia care unit; S, satisfactory; U, unsatisfactory.
Courtesy of Morton Plant Mease Health Care, Dunedin, FL.

- Building inspections by the local or state fire protection agency at least annually
- Flame-retardant fabrics for patient clothing and for window and cubicle curtains
- Appropriate smoking restrictions with signs placed in highly visible areas
- Safety inspection and approval of all new equipment before use and periodically
- Ongoing educational sessions regarding electrical equipment and fire safety practices
- No extension cords or portable space heaters or fans in use
- Removal of equipment with damaged, frayed, or questionable cords or plugs
- Storage of equipment in disarmed mode (i.e., defibrillators returned to zero joules, electrocautery units turned to "off" position)
- Leaving electrical equipment turned off or unplugged when the building/department is not occupied
- Structural design according to fire codes (i.e., fire doors at stairwells, automatically closing fire doors)
- Appropriate automatic sprinkler systems (required in many states)
- Keeping fire doors closed, not propped open
- Appropriate enclosures for storage of gases and volatile liquids

Table 4–13. Fire/Disaster Questionnaire: Spontaneous Review of Team Member Awareness

Date: ________ Reviewer: ________________ Person Reviewed: ________________

QUESTION	OK	NEEDS REVIEW	COMMENTS
1. Where are all fire and disaster plans kept? How often must each team member review the plans?			
2. What is our fire plan?			
3. Where is the closest fire pull station?			
4. Where is the closest fire extinguisher or hose?			
5. What does the acronym PASS stand for?			
6. What is your specific job during a fire?			
7. How do you notify the operator about a fire or other emergency?			
8. Where do you find the location of fire walls?			
9. What is the code to page for fire?			
10. What is the code to page for an evacuation?			
11. Who initiates a full building evacuation?			
12. What is the code for bomb threat?			
13. What do you do to communicate when telephones are not working?			
14. How is all clear sounded?			
15. What is the code for a medical emergency?			

Comments and Follow-Up:

Name of Team Member: ________________ Dept: ________
Total No. of Criteria: 15 Not Met: ________ N/A Criteria: ________

Courtesy of Morton Plant Mease Health Care, Dunedin, FL.

- Appropriate storage of cleaning solutions and cloths and mops
- Immediate investigation of unfamiliar odors or smoke

Preparedness

Equipment, supplies, and personnel must be in a constant state of readiness for a fire emergency. Many requirements that must be followed are specific to state regulatory agencies. The following are a few general examples.

1. Fire extinguishers and alarms should be in highly visible, accessible, and labeled locations near escape routes and known to all staff members.
2. Extinguishers should be periodically tested to ensure their adequacy.
3. A fire blanket should be accessible to smother any flames.
4. Smoke alarms and sprinkler systems should provide early warning and response for unobserved fires.
5. Halls and doorways should be free of obstructions.
6. Illuminated exit doors should be present that are identified with lighted exit signs to help locate them in the event of a power failure.
7. The emergency power generator should be periodically inspected and tested. Fuel must be immediately available on site.
8. Exit doors should be easy to open without the use of a key.
9. Simplified floor plans that illustrate evacua-

tion routes and fire walls should be posted in various areas of the surgery center.
10. Locations of oxygen shut-off valves and circuit breakers should be posted.
11. More than one person should know how to operate the emergency power supply, alarm systems, gas sources, and other emergency systems. Written instructions should be posted in a highly visible area.

An auxiliary generator provides electrical power independent of the external electrical supply to the building. It should provide lighting in the event of a power failure or an internal disaster that incapacitates the usual supply. An emergency generator generally provides service for the exit lights; patient and emergency call system; fire alarm system, including the fire doors; public address system; some hall lights; specific emergency electrical plugs (usually indicated by a red color cover plate); electrically locked exit doors; and all refrigerators and freezers. The exact services restored by the emergency generator in each institution should be communicated to the staff.

No matter how well the environment seems to be protected from fire, personnel must be prepared to respond. All employees, including float personnel, must have access to a written procedure that includes an evacuation plan. Managers must ensure that staff members who rarely or occasionally work on the unit, as well as physicians and any contract service workers, are provided with basic information about emergency response. Besides the locations of extinguishers, exits, gas shut-off valves, and fire alarms, all personnel must know how to use the internal telephone and paging systems.

A training session should be provided at least annually, often by the local fire protection agency. Hands-on use of fire extinguishers allows employees to feel more confident about their abilities to use the equipment. Unannounced fire drills should be conducted at least quarterly and planned at various times of the day. Unexpected placement of a red "fire pillow" is an effective method to test employees' responses. Any staff member who comes on the pillow is expected to treat it like a real fire. Response to a fire should include the following actions:

- Immediately call for help (sound the fire alarm, telephone the switchboard, or report to unit manager as directed by unit policy).
- Remove patients and personnel who are in immediate danger.
- Close any sources of oxygen or other gases to the area (Note: check with anesthesia provider before shutting off main valves).
- Close all doors to prevent the spread of fire.
- Pull electrical plugs in the vicinity of the fire if possible.
- Only then, attempt to fight the fire if you feel capable and comfortable doing so.

An acronym that can help remind staff of the proper sequence of response is RACE—*r*escue patients, sound the *a*larm, *c*onfine the fire, and *e*xtinguish it or *e*vacuate.

Three elements are essential to support a fire—combustible material (fuel), heat, and oxygen. Removing one of these elements extinguishes the fire. If a flame is contained in a wastebasket, covering the basket prevents oxygen from reaching the materials. Similarly, a fire extinguisher smothers the fire by removing its source of oxygen. Extinguishers labeled A, B, C, and D are intended for different types of fires. Usually, the healthcare setting is supplied with ABC extinguishers, which are multiuse types. All personnel should be able to identify the types of fires their extinguishers are designed to fight before the need arises.

Basic safety rules apply to the use of fire extinguishers.

Use a fire extinguisher to smother flames:

1. If the fire is contained in one area
2. If you have the proper type of extinguisher
3. If the fire department has been called
4. When all patients and personnel are out of danger
5. If you can fight the fire with your back to a safe escape route
6. If you feel confident in the use of the extinguisher

If one or more of these criteria are not met, all personnel should immediately leave the area, close the door, and wait for the fire department. Elevators should not be used.

When using a fire extinguisher, one should remain low to the ground and avoid breathing fumes from the fire or the extinguisher. The National Fire Prevention Association suggests the acronym "PASS" to help people remember the proper use of most extinguishers—*p*ull the pin, *a*im the nozzle, *s*queeze the handle, and *s*weep from side to side at the base of the fire.

BOMB THREATS

Discussing the danger from a bomb explosion may seem absurd, yet there are situations that compel ASC staff to be prepared, situations in which an individual person or group might act out violently against a surgery center for real or imagined reasons. However unlikely it may seem, political or social activists, angry family members, former patients, and mentally ill persons are all potential offenders.

Personnel in an ASC must be aware of the potential effects of information they give to telephone callers. It is unwise to provide callers with any information that could be considered controversial. Individual ASC managers must be conscious of local issues that might predispose callers to anger or violent outbursts and should discuss proper telephone protocol with appropriate employees. Personnel also must be alert for unfamiliar people in the center or in restricted areas where the public is not usually allowed.

A written plan should be available for staff members instructing them on how to respond to a threatening telephone call. It should describe their individual responsibilities during an actual bomb search. The United States Department of the Treasury, Bureau of Alcohol, Tobacco, and Firearms has developed a booklet entitled "BOMB, Threats and Search Techniques," which is available from the Superintendent of Documents, US Government Printing Office, Washington, DC 20402. This booklet suggests that certain telephone numbers be identified and available for emergency use well in advance of any threatening situation. These include police, sheriff, and fire departments; ambulance; telephone; security department; Bureau of Alcohol, Tobacco, and Firearms; FBI; Army Explosives; and the Civilian Defense Unit numbers.

Information should be available to staff on how to handle a threatening telephone call. Although switchboard operators are the most likely recipients of a call, a nurse or other staff member may be involved. Authorities suggest the following protocol when a bomb threat is received.

1. Remain calm and carefully assess all information presented by the caller.
2. Ask the caller when the bomb will detonate and where it is located.
3. Keep the caller on the telephone as long as possible and inform another staff member in writing about the call.
4. Inform the caller that the building is occupied and that detonation of a bomb could result in injury or death to many innocent people.
5. Listen closely to the voice, background noise, and so on.
6. Look at the telephone to see whether the call has originated internally or externally.
7. Report the call to the manager and to the authorities immediately after the caller hangs up.

If possible, another staff member should listen in and report the call while the recipient of the call remains on the line. A worksheet should be available to document information during or immediately after a threatening call. In listening to the caller, the staff person should consider the following descriptive characteristics that are suggested by the Los Angeles City Fire Department:[9]

- *Voice*: Is it loud, high or low pitched, soft, deep, pleasant, scratchy, raspy, or intoxicated? Is it a man or a woman, or is it difficult to tell?
- *Speech*: Is it fast, slow, distant, disoriented, or nasal? Does the caller stutter or mispronounce words?
- *Language*: Is it good, foul, poor, uneducated, sophisticated, or technical?
- *Accent*: Is there none? Is the accent local, foreign, regional, or racial?
- *Manner*: Does the caller sound calm, coherent, deliberate, righteous, rational, angry, irrational, incoherent, or emotional? Does he or she have a nervous laugh?
- *Background noise*: Do you hear any noises? Are there sounds of traffic, machines (office or factory), trains or airplanes, animals or birds, children or park noises, music, or other voices? Is the background totally quiet?

Before the arrival of the responding civil agency, the highest ranking manager present may make the decision about whether to evacuate the building and conduct an immediate bomb search. That person directs the staff on the basis of facility protocol and his or her judgment at the time. Once the fire, police, or bomb experts arrive, they take charge in appropriately directing personnel. The decision to evacuate is one that should be made very carefully. Panic is contagious, and the ensuing activity dramatically increases the potential for personal injury or property damage. Some surgery centers have a standard policy to evacuate in response to any threatening call, whereas others consider it best to search first and evacuate only if a suspicious object is found.

The coordination of a bomb search is best addressed by a professionally trained team, but sometimes, the element of time requires more rapid action. If staff members are directed to search for a bomb, they should have been provided with basic information about proper search techniques. They should clearly understand that they are not to touch any suspicious object they may find. Any search should be undertaken with as little fanfare as possible, without alerting or upsetting visitors or patients.

PERSONAL THREATS

Although the chance of being personally threatened by a patient, family member, or outsider is remote, each staff member must be prepared to summon appropriate help if such a situation occurs. Criminal, emotional, addictive, or psychiatric behavior may motivate a person to threaten the physical well-being of a patient, visitor, or staff member. The fact that narcotics and barbiturates are in plentiful supply in a surgical facility predisposes the staff to some degree of danger from a person searching for drugs. Many people also realize that cash is on hand in any business setting.

Preventing a situation of physical threat begins with attention to the security system of the facility. The amount and type of security required is dependent on the actual or potential threat that the center's geographic location poses. Locks, alarms, lighted entries, security guards, and personal practices for entering and leaving the building are all features that help to provide a safe environment. One person should not be left alone in the building in the early or late hours of operation.

All personnel should watch for and report the presence of strangers who appear threatening or who are found in secured areas that are usually open only to staff members. An intruder who appears menacing should not be approached by a solitary employee. There are occasional, innocent intrusions into restricted areas by visitors or family members who are confused or lost. A staff member is often called on to quickly decide and respond appropriately if a stranger is a threat or is merely lost.

Other methods of preventing crimes stem from common sense. Staff members should keep money and purses out of sight. A safe or locked drawer that is out of public view should be provided. Basic rules for drug safety should be followed. Nurses should keep narcotic keys and prescription pads out of sight. Drug storage cabinets should be out of public view, and the door to the area should remain closed. Prescription pads should be locked up each night and when not in use during the day. Keeping a low profile regarding the availability of such drugs is a wise practice. If a staff member is threatened with violent behavior, resistance should not be directed at the intruder. No amount of money or drugs is worth personal injury or death.

Staff members should know the most efficient way to summon help to any particular area. A large facility is usually staffed with security guards who are equipped to handle such an emergency. In a freestanding center, however, there may be only employees with no formal security training or abilities, so they must rely on outside help. Telephone numbers for the police should be available at all telephones.

A threatening person in an acute psychiatric state can be very difficult to handle. Staff members must remain calm and should not further anger or upset the person in question, because such action could precipitate more violence and potential injuries. Outside help that is trained to handle such a person should be summoned. If possible, any bystanders in the immediate area of the threat should be quietly evacuated.

EXTERNAL DISASTERS

Some external disasters provide warnings that allow time for evacuation or other preparations, for instance, hurricanes, snowstorms, and flooding. Others strike without warning: natural disasters like lightning, earthquakes, and tornadoes, and man-made problems, such as toxic chemical spills and electrical blackouts. Whatever the external problem may be, the surgery facility must be prepared with an appropriate internal response. Cancellation of the day's surgery schedule and closing of the facility are appropriate when time allows, but should a sudden occurrence leave the occupied center in danger, internal plans to provide a safe shelter must be available. The confines of this chapter preclude provision of such broad-range plans appropriate for specific centers, but individual units should develop their own plans that include communication with outside authorities, internal power sources, provision of food and water, and safe evacuation.

Freestanding surgery centers should be aware that local or county authorities have a record of facilities that are licensed as being equipped with ORs. These facilities are often included in the county's overall disaster preparedness plans for use during external disasters. A center that is not staffed or open 24 hours a day or on weekends should ensure that its name is removed from the list of facilities that are prepared to accept and treat such unexpected casualties.

OWNERSHIP

Patients, family members, and visitors assume that they are safe in a healthcare institution, no matter what type it is. The structure, mechanics, and maintenance of the facility should honor that trust. In unexpected emergency situations, the nursing staff's primary role is to ensure the safety of patients, themselves, and other personnel. Strict adherence to all safety regulations is essential, without exception. Periodic practice drills and instruction classes should be conducted, and an attitude of interest and concern should be cultivated among all staff members.

The design and fabrication of a beautiful and functional environment is only as effective as the people who maintain it. Every team member has a unique role in making the environment not only safe but also attractive and welcoming. The following ways of asserting a positive concern about the facility should be considered:

1. Own your space—it is part of you.
   - Remember, neatness counts—and helps you work more efficiently.
   - Personalize your work area; remember, you spend one third of your day there.
   - Watch for and correct safety concerns; for example, use only approved chemicals.
   - Separate food and medications and date each when opened.
2. Consider the customer's point of view.
   - You are the most important part of the environment.
   - Smiles, genuine concern, and neat appearance count.
   - No food or beverages should be in clinical areas or where patients can see them.
   - Avoid loud noises and private conversations near patients.
   - Provide privacy for your patients and honor confidential information.
   - Childproof your area to keep little customers safe.
3. Be responsible for conserving resources.
   - Use supplies wisely.
   - Label supply locations and maintain appropriate stock par levels.
   - Do not hoard supplies and linens.
   - Log out and turn off all computers at the end of the day.
   - Turn electricity off when a room or piece of equipment is not being used.
   - Set room temperatures for comfort and do not continually change settings.
4. Know your facility, for you, your team, and your customers' safety and to provide excellent customer service.
   - Learn and remember the security systems and locking mechanisms in your facility.
   - Know how to summon help for any type of emergency.
   - Ask if you are unsure of how to use a piece of equipment.
   - Take responsibility to learn about all the departments and processes in your facility so that you can answer your customers' questions.
   - Be prepared to give accurate directions to customers for both outside and inside the facility.

Pride of ownership is reflected in the way that team members take care of their own work spaces in these four important areas. Staff members should ask themselves: Are you the one who walks past a discarded paper a dozen times a day without picking it up? Or, are you the person who always goes one step beyond your job description to ensure that every corner of the work environment looks like you would want your home to look? The difference between adequacy and excellence of service is reflected in the manner in which all team members understand and use all the resources at hand. The environment is a combination of both mortar and mindset.

References

1. Staff: Minimally Invasive Surgical Nursing 9:54–56, 1995.
2. Joint Commission 1998 Comprehensive Accreditation Manual for Ambulatory Care. Chicago: Joint Commission on Accreditation of Healthcare Organizations, 1998.
3. NFPA 101 Life Safety Code, 1997 ed. Quincy, MA: National Fire Protection Association, 1997.
4. Malaga S, Huckvale Arann S: Creating a peaceful, comfortable, and functional health care setting for women. Surg Services Manage 2:12–15, 1996.
5. Swanson K: Personal communication, July 1998.
6. Snyder D, Pasternak R: Facility design and procedural safety. In White P (ed): Ambulatory Anesthesia and Surgery. Philadelphia: WB Saunders, 1997, pp 61–76.
7. Cochran R: Personal communication, February 1998.
8. Counts C, Prowant B: Disaster preparedness: Is your unit really ready? ANNA J 21:155–161, 1994.
9. Stace WC: Personal communication, September 19, 1991.
10. Association of Operating Room Nurses: Standards and recommended practices. Denver: AORN, 1997.

Chapter 5

Materials and Equipment Management

Jay Knauer

COST CONTAINMENT

The first ambulatory surgery center (ASC) opened in the United States in 1970. Today more than 2400 ambulatory surgery centers exist, and 2200 procedures are approved for payment by Medicare. Of all surgery performed today, more than 50% is done on an outpatient basis. The phenomenal growth of ambulatory surgery programs is likely to continue.[1] With all this recent growth and a forecast indicating that more growth should be expected, why is there such immense pressure for ambulatory centers to contain their costs?

Experts in the ambulatory care–consulting field have identified many factors that contribute to the current cost-cutting environment, but they all seem to point to one major factor. The revenue and reimbursement paradigms have shifted significantly. Consider the following facts. Outpatient reimbursements have decreased by 25% during the last 3 years. This is compounded by Medicare rate increases, which have been frozen for the last 2 years.[2] As a result of the decrease in the reimbursement structure, surgery centers must control their costs in order to keep pace with the decline in income.

As cost containment discussions dominate healthcare conference rooms, progressive health systems have adopted new paradigms in just about every facet of operation. One of those areas is the arena of materials management. In this chapter relating to materials management, we discuss strategies that parallel these new paradigms.

GROUP BUYING

An increasing number of medical practices and healthcare facilities belong to some kind of group purchasing organization. This group purchasing concept can substantially lower supply costs through what is essentially power buying. Affiliations with healthcare purchasing groups or associations with healthcare institutions that are already connected with major buying groups can give a freestanding ASC purchasing power that it would otherwise never have.

A group purchasing organization is responsible for providing marketing and support services and for negotiating volume discount contracts with medical suppliers and manufacturers on behalf of the members. Participating members consist of hospitals, clinics, medical group practices, nursing homes, managed care organizations, long-term care facilities, pharmacies, ASCs, and others. These member facilities pay a participatory fee to activate the benefits. One group purchasing organization claims incredible discounts of up to 70% for its group members on any clinical and office supplies, equipment, office and exam room furniture, pagers, computers, cell phones, whole office set-ups, whole hospital set-ups, and so forth.[3]

The choice of which group purchasing organization to form an affiliation with depends on the distinctive goals and mission of the healthcare facility and on those of the buying group. If an ASC's management team is concerned primarily about cost savings on purchases, perhaps an organization like the one mentioned earlier should be considered. If financial constraints are a concern, the ideal group purchasing organization might conceivably be one that advertises a greater interest in its members than in its own income, offers moderate average savings (e.g., 15% to 20%), or offers low membership dues.[4] The ASC interested in developing an innovation or new project may look for groups advertising expertise in implementation of shared services.[5] For further inquiry, a directory exists that may enhance the decision-making process entitled the *Directory of Healthcare Group Purchasing Organizations 1998*. This book provides important information on more than 550 group purchasing organizations.

In addition to direct cost savings, there are buying groups that offer other benefits, such as self-education opportunities. Included among topics of interest are products and services research and even facility design and planning.[6]

The growth of the group buying trend has been impressive over the last decade. In fact, it is safe to say that this concept has reached critical mass. Group purchasing contracts are probably the best cost containment strategy for direct cost reduction. If cost containment is the goal, participation in group purchasing is strongly advocated.

JUST-IN-TIME INVENTORY MANAGEMENT

The conventional wisdom concerning ambulatory center construction planning in these days of great change in terms of reimbursement is to build smaller structures as a cost-saving measure. This trend has caused ASC administrators to consider improving space efficiency in every facet of a center's operation. One of those areas is the space management of materials and supplies. The just-in-time inventory method is an innovative tool for achieving better application of the smaller work area and is also an excellent method of managing supply costs.

The just-in-time inventory is so-called because it refers to a technique of supply distribution that gives the end-user the perception that supplies arrive just in time for use. Essentially, the original intention of this approach was designed for exactly that purpose. The aim is to reduce the amount of each supply stored at every distribution point from the warehouse shelf to the end-user's shelves. The logical outcomes of the just-in-time inventory provide the main reasons for its popularity in modern healthcare's cost containment–driven environment. The advantages of a just-in-time ordering system are as follows:

1. Decreased space requirement
2. Less money tied up in inventory

By reducing the amount of space required for supply storage, the facility is better able to deal with space management struggles more effectively. Also, management teams considering new ASC construction can reduce initial overhead costs by building smaller, less expensive buildings. When there is less inventory on the shelf, there is a reduction in the amount of stationary money tied up in inventory. Inventory sitting on the shelf is equated to money that could be better spent elsewhere.

One of the challenging aspects of the just-in-time inventory is that the flow of materials cannot be interrupted without creating a negative effect on the client's operation. With a decrease in supplies physically sitting on the shelf, timely replenishment has become more important than ever before. Because there is less margin for error in the just-in-time inventory model, Materials Management departments have had to increase their efficiency or else accept blame for a supply system that does not work.

Manufacturer backorders are particularly problematic to Materials Management departments. Some supply vendors have studied the current healthcare trends and have enough insight to realize that manufacturer backorders, which are inevitable, present a more significant challenge to all healthcare entities using the just-in-time approach than at any previous time. These companies will have already prepared for backorder situations by researching the market for adequate substitutes. Of course, not all supply houses are as progressive. Given these conditions, it is beneficial to have someone (preferably an on-site materials manager or nurse product specialist) who is familiar with the supply market and knows the users' preferences. This person should be well equipped to make alternate supplies suggestions and arrange for expedient deliveries.

The alternative to backorders is to have a system in place whereby supplies can be borrowed. It becomes essential to maintain good relationships with other facilities in the area—even with competitors. When a crisis situation develops, it is comforting to know that you can procure necessary supplies quickly.

Other logical ramifications of the just-in-time approach involve the increased responsibilities borne by the ASC staff related to ordering procedures. These include:

1. An increase in the number of times that an item must be reordered
2. More careful attention during the reordering process
3. Less margin for error in reordering
4. Establishing emergency delivery procedures with the distribution source

The reality is that many factors can cause the need for emergency delivery procedures, such as reordering mistakes, manufacturer backorders, incompetent customer or sales representatives, delivery errors, and computer system failures. Emergency arrangements, especially with the distribution source, are critical to the success of the just-in-time inventory. The facility should be aware that ordering supplies on an emergency basis increases the cost of freight charges. Paying express delivery charges can increase the cost of an item significantly. If the original delivery error can be traced to the distributor, the ASC should negotiate shifting responsibility for excess delivery charges to the distributor.

Despite these concerns and challenges, the benefits of keeping inventory as small as possible far exceed the drawbacks. The evidence is seen in the growing popularity of the just-in-time concept, not only in the healthcare field but also in retail distribution and many other areas in which inventory costs have been targeted for re-engineering.

ROTATION OF STOCK

This rather basic idea is crucial to waste reduction in an ASC, thus increasing its cost efficiency. It should be everyone's responsibility when replacing stock to position older stock more accessibly than the newer goods. The idea of consuming older stock before newer stock is to reduce the chance of supplies aging to the point at which they are unusable and must be discarded. For example, scrub sponges dry up; adhesive tape becomes brittle; and certain sterile items and medications become outdated.

The cost can be high, particularly if sterile implants or other expensive supplies are permitted to become worthless. Industries that rely on profitability for survival provide a good example in this area by assigning employees on a daily basis to monitor items with a dated shelf life. Some supplies and implants can be resterilized without compromising their effectiveness. However, there are still costs involved, such as autoclave operation and employee time that could be avoided by simply rotating stock. If resterilization of a supply is a consideration, it is advisable for the ASC to obtain written recommendations from the manufacturer regarding sterilization guidelines.

SUPPLY STANDARDIZATION

Perhaps one of the most painful, yet necessary, steps in cost containment is standardization of supplies. It is not a pleasant task to tear a surgeon away from his or her favorite brand of knife, but, in today's environment, if standardization to another brand results in significant savings, it must be done. Remember that outpatient reimbursements have decreased 25% over the last 3 years, and Medicare is developing ways to decrease reimbursements. Of course, the key is to maintain quality while reducing costs. This is where the products specialist or inventory support technician in the ASC is vital. Standardization can be achieved through a program of product evaluations that should be coordinated by the products specialist and a materials/purchasing agent, if available. Ideally, the materials/purchasing agent coordinates with the vendor, while the products specialist works with physicians. As with any change, if physicians are involved in the change process from the beginning, this can help to secure their support for new products.

CUSTOM STERILE PACKS

How often is a pack of some sterile supply opened during a procedure and the majority of the contents wasted because only one or two items were needed? Depending on the answer, there may be a waste problem in need of a solution. A good way to reduce supply waste is to use customized packs. A custom or specialty pack is a combination of supplies that are totally customized to the particular needs of a clinical service or facility. The logic behind the concept of customized packs is simple. Clinical management is usually on the lookout for ways to cut costs. Curbing supply waste results in less frequent supply replenishment, which translates into cost savings.

The creation of a customized pack may be more complicated. Because this concept is especially useful for preparatory supplies that remain constant for every procedure, identify a clinical service or group of clinical services that typically use similar prep supplies. Choose the supplies that should be included in the specialty pack. The goal is to establish a customized pack that would meet the needs of all physicians in a specialty group. For example, establishing a customized pack for ophthalmologists who perform cataract extraction would include drapes, suture, knife blades, needles, gowns, and other supplies specific to that procedure. All ophthalmologists would use this customized pack. It is essential that the end-user has input in the process to guarantee user satisfaction with the pack. This is important because future modifications to the pack may be expensive owing to its customization.

The final step in customizing a specialty pack is to assign quantities to each of the items in the pack. By referring to charge sheets from actual surgeries, the usage information needed to secure adequate quantities can be obtained. One benefit of customizing packs is that it causes standardization.

In addition to standardization, cost savings can also be linked to case preparation. When pulling supplies for a procedure, the staff member only needs to pull one pack, rather than numerous supplies. This reduces the amount of time taken for preparations and decreases potential problems or physician dissatisfaction with the inadvertent omission of a necessary supply.

CONSIGNMENTS

A consignment is an arrangement that is negotiated with a vendor to house items owned by the vendor on-site in the facility at no charge to the customer until items are actually used. A payment invoice or purchase order and consignment replacement is then arranged with the vendor. Items with consignment potential include intraocular lenses, toe and finger implants, humeral implants, penile prostheses, pulse generators, and breast implants. Consigning rather than outright purchasing of implantable devices or other costly consumables can result in the following benefits.

1. Consignment programs can effect substantial reduction in the amount of money involved in inventory sitting idly on the shelf.
2. Because the vendor retains ownership of the consignment item on a customer's shelf, vendor representatives will provide another watchful eye on items with shelf life limits. Legal ramifications prevent turning the entire responsibility to outside salespeople.
3. Supplies are in stock when needed.
4. Potentially costly delivery charges may be avoided.
5. Better pricing may be achieved by creating competition while negotiating the consignment.

Better pricing on products can be achieved by creating competition when negotiating a consignment. The ASC should bid out consignment items to several vendors and ask for the vendor's best pricing while informing the vendor that the same opportunity will be offered to other vendors. Aggressive sales representatives will do their best to ensure that their products reach your ASC shelves. If the first round of bids reveals that the vendor whom you hoped to deal with has made a higher bid than you had hoped for, offer the vendor an opportunity to rebid. Most negotiations take time. Successful negotiations require that a person be dedicated to the process and granted the authority and time it takes to act on the issues at hand.

If the ASC is affiliated with a Purchasing/Materials Management department, enlist their help because they probably have already established business relationships with the vendors used to purchase these items. Many purchasing departments service multiple healthcare facilities and may be able to influence negotiations more effectively than a stand-alone ASC. Because the primary goal of consignments is cost reduction, bidding out should create a competitive atmosphere that will accomplish the primary goal.

The bidding process can be initiated in the ASC by evaluating various vendor product lines. An ASC should assign a product specialist for this task. Market education can be achieved by networking with other facilities, tapping into purchasing resources, or surfing the Internet. As inquiries begin, salespeople will, no doubt, start to make their own inquiries. It is important to communicate the intent to pursue a consignment program with them. Not all vendors offer consignment programs, and even those who do must be convinced that the increased responsibility and service that they will assume will be advantageous to them. From the vendor's standpoint, if a facility agrees to use their product in exchange for the benefits listed earlier, and the facility neglects the product, the vendor may pull the consignment out of the facility. It may also mean that the physician must adapt to a different brand if the best deal is not achieved with the one that is presently used.

Again, involve the physicians from the start. In the current competitive environment, physician support plays an important role. Having physicians network with the vendors shows not only the ASC's real interest in the product but also carries weight when negotiating the price. When a physician's preference is on the line, the vendor may work harder to reduce the cost.

RENTAL FEES

When specialized equipment is available only through a vendor, and it cannot be obtained from neighboring facilities, the vendor will customarily charge a rental fee. The fee could be substantial, but it can sometimes be avoided. Many healthcare organizations that are committed to cost containment strategies have engaged in negotiations with vendors who impose rental fees. They have found that some vendors are willing to negotiate discounts—even up to 100%—on rental fees if the surgery center agrees to use other product lines, especially consumable product lines.

If an ASC presently uses a vendor's other product lines, it holds a potential bargaining chip. Depending on the products involved, companies are usually willing to sacrifice a one-time income producer (e.g., a rental fee) rather than risk losing the on-going revenue characteristic of consumables. Knowledge of the market is particularly advantageous in this area, which is why having a product specialist is so strongly advocated. If the product specialist is aware of what is available in the medical supply marketplace, that knowledge may translate into cost savings during the ensuing negotiations with a vendor representative.

A good way to gain a vendor's attention is to casually mention any possible benefits that their competitor's products may have. Another very effective negotiating tool is to be prepared to switch a currently used product to their competitors. Negotiating this way may be difficult for some staff because trained salespeople can sound very nice and helpful while "playing hard ball." Having a purchasing agent's negotiating experience available is an advantage. It should be noted that negotiations can be tough while still remaining ethical and professional.

INSTRUMENT AND EQUIPMENT REPAIRS

Proper care, maintenance, and repair of surgical instruments is an important part of containing costs. Various companies repair surgical instrumentation—both instrument manufacturers and independent repair companies. Repairing instead of replacing instruments can contribute significantly to the cost efficiency of the customer institution. The advantages of employing an independent instrument repair vendor are as follows:

- Rapid turnaround time
- Pick up and delivery service
- On-site repair service
- Cost containment

Other than the cost issues, independent instrument repair vendors can provide excellent services. Some of these independent repair vendors send a representative to the center to pick up broken instruments (usually on a specified day that is convenient for the ASC), repair them at their own facility(ies), and hand-deliver them to the center on the next scheduled pickup day. Some repair vendors require clients to use a delivery service or the postal service as the means of distribution.

The most convenient option for instrument reparation is the same-day repair concept. These vendors have developed the concept of a repair shop on wheels wherein at a predetermined time, a truck replete with tools, grinders, polishing agents, and so forth arrives on-site to perform repairs. The entire process (including labeling nonrepairable instruments and invoicing) is accomplished in 1 day. Some of the aforementioned repair services offer immediate replacement for nonrepairable instruments. Either way the common thread is speed. Generally speaking, reputable independent repair services turn over instrument repairs faster and cheaper than do instrument manufacturer repair departments.

This process can be time consuming, thus the surgery center staff must be willing to investigate various options. It may take some experimentation with many different independent repair services to determine which type of service makes the most sense for a particular center because of the number of different independent repair services available on the market.

The surgery center also needs to consider how the center will continue to function without the instrumentation or equipment. Are back-up instruments or equipment available? Does the repair service supply a loaner? Is there a fee attached to the loaner? All this information needs to be considered. If a piece of equipment malfunctions, what is the alternative? Is there a back-up on site or can a loaner be acquired immediately so as not to cancel cases? All the options must be weighed in this case. It may cost more to have a contract with the vendor, but canceling surgery owing to inoperable equipment is generally most costly in terms of real money as well as patient and physician convenience and satisfaction.

Many equipment contracts are set up with preventive maintenance agreements. By entering into these agreements, a facility can ensure that equipment is properly cared for and serviced. When a center pays from $70,000 to $100,000 for a piece of specialized equipment (e.g., a laser, microscope, or phacoemulsifier), it is in the best interest of the facility to ensure that the machine is well cared for. A special consideration is that some vendors specify that having work done on equipment by anyone other than that company may void the warranty on the equipment. The management team, sometimes with input from physician users, must weigh the options for equipment maintenance to decide the best course for each piece of major equipment.

INFORMATION SERVICES

Surgery centers that have access to an Information Services (IS) department should take advantage of the systems solutions that it can offer. Some of the areas where information systems can provide improvements are in cost reporting, scheduling, schedule reports, patient tracking, patient billing, revenue reports, inventory systems, charge processing, specialized reports, physicians' notes, quality assurance, and clinical notes.

A good IS department employs either information systems professionals with the programming expertise to develop customized software programs or personnel who are knowledgeable in the vendor software market and can help select and apply software or customize its application to the needs of the center. If these departmental resources are not available, there are alternative ways to seek out information about systems applications. Person-to-person networking with other ASCs is one method. Through simply tapping the knowledge base of colleagues, one can gain significant contacts with software vendor representatives. Another way is to attend seminars that cover subjects related to informatics and inventory management systems.

When choosing a software vendor, an ASC should look for more than just a company that offers software applications. Owing to the continued migration in healthcare to computer-related solutions, developing a quality relationship with a software vendor will pay dividends in the future.

Many companies sponsor seminars that can help ASC staff overcome some of the challenges inherent in computer education, from very basic computer literacy to in-depth software training. They also offer specific user help in the areas of software enhancements and development, troubleshooting techniques, implementation support, Windows conversion assistance, basic Windows user tips and navigation techniques, supply management, as well as software industry developments such as the Year 2000 compliance issue.

Other information systems tools exist that provide an even greater level of service. One system incorporates quick and accurate procedure costing and inventory management tools with an outside vendor product information database and actual per case supply data specific to the user institution. This system offers benefits that:

1. Enable an institution to capitalize on standardization opportunities
2. Provide clinically accepted product alternatives
3. Systematically reduce supply demand
4. Tangibly assess the impact of process and product changes through benchmark calculations

When investing in systems modernization, it is important to bear in mind that information systems should create greater cost efficiency for the center. When discussing systems solutions with an IS department or an outside vendor, that goal should guide decision-making. Look for direct savings as well as for the secondary gains to be found through the enhanced data management and reporting capabilities that the system can provide.

DOCTOR'S PREFERENCE CARDS

Another beneficial information systems' solution is the electronic physician's preference card. Many institutions currently use some type of tool for capturing doctors' preference information. This information is used chiefly to help nursing staff prepare for a surgical procedure. A typical doctor's preference card includes medical/surgical supplies, equipment, instruments, procedure charge information, and other procedure- or physician-related comments for every procedure that the physician performs. This information is beneficial in any format, but many

ASCs use typed or hand-written sheets of paper covered with many scribbled notes and changes.

Compared with the electronic doctor's preference card, this system is very inefficient. Furthermore, the electronic doctors' preference cards that have the capability of interfacing with inventory systems provide more than just a case prep guide.

One of the additional benefits of implementing an electronic preference card module is that it provides another excellent tool for standardizing supplies. Under the paper system, using preference cards to standardize supplies is extremely time-consuming and arduous. By utilizing the electronic card, the same work can be done in a fraction of the time through the use of the procedure or physician card-grouping mechanism.

The same mechanism can quickly facilitate cost comparison studies among surgeons who perform like procedures if the preference card module can interface with the inventory system. With the paper system, this task could take weeks.

If a doctor's office is granted access to their doctor's preference card number, and will provide it to the scheduler during the scheduling of a case, there may be a reduction in the time that it takes to enter the schedule data.

Under the paper system, if a request is made to modify all of the preference cards, or if a surgeon requests changes to all of his or her cards, each individual card must be pulled from the filing cabinet and changed. The electronic card will allow a time-starved staff member to make one-time global modifications to all of the cards. Similarly, changes can be copied to all of a physician's cards in seconds simply by querying the physician's cards by physician name.

Other benefits include:

- The ability to document supply consumption during a case
- The convenience of clear and legible pick lists
- The elimination of paper preference card storage, unless it is kept as a back-up in the event of a system crash
- The ability to use preference cards as a patient charging mechanism, if card data are interfaced with the charging system
- A reduction in lost charges

During the development of the doctor's preference cards, master files must be built for each component within the preference card. For example, each piece of equipment in the surgery center will be entered into a database called a master file. The same procedure must occur for instruments, inventory, and so forth. This exercise enables better coordination of resources and provides other benefits similar to those described in the next section. In fact, if master files are properly maintained and updated, the physical counting of the items within a master file that would normally occur during a physical inventory would not have to be done.

The trend across the healthcare field is to get rid of paper systems whenever possible. If software investment is not feasible, or, if the aforementioned advantages are deemed unnecessary, a spreadsheet, word processor, or database application program can be used to eliminate the paper preference card system.

PHYSICAL INVENTORY

One way to evaluate the effectiveness of cost containment strategies is to take physical inventories. This involves physically counting every supply and piece of equipment owned by a facility at a specific time. The next step is the accounting procedure in which each item is priced to determine the amount of money tied up in inventory. The last step is the evaluation. During this step, the totals from the current year are compared with those from previous physical inventories, and evaluations are made concerning product usage, purchasing practices, space management, and employee issues. This is a valuable exercise, because the data obtained from physical inventories can illuminate many unseen concerns and clear the pathway to resolution of others.

The key to a successful physical inventory project is the physical count. The count intervals must remain constant. Most facilities perform a physical inventory once a year usually during the least busy time of the year or at the end of the fiscal year. In this case, tradition rules. A variance of 1 or 2 days won't skew the results irreparably, but if the inventory is taken every July 12, for example, make it a tradition.

To avoid more work and confusion, complete the count in a day. The idea is to not use any inventory items once the counting has begun. This will ensure the integrity of the total count. If supplies are used after counting has started, they should be included in the tally as if they were on the shelf. Keeping track of these used supplies takes more time and more work, thus stretching the count over a few days increases the work. The count must be accurate. If it is inaccurate, the data will be skewed and so will the evaluations drawn from it. Double and triple check the data if necessary.

There are two schools of thought concerning pricing of supply items from the physical inventory. Some organizations apply an average weighted cost to determine the price of an item. Others use simply the current cost. Whichever one is used, continue with it for the entire inventory process. The inconsistencies resulting in the data from a change in pricing methods will create useless information.

The pricing of the supplies has been simplified in recent years because of computer-related innovations. Information systems personnel can help in this area. One way is to create dump files from the Purchasing/Materials Management item catalog. If IS resources are not available, a software spreadsheet can be used to compile data for analysis and for comparison with future physical inventories.

COST-PER-CASE ANALYSIS

Every ASC must develop its own strategies for dealing with the realities of the modern healthcare environment. A good way to stay competitive is to remain competitively priced. Analysis and control of the cost per case may make the difference between staying competitive and forfeiting business to competitors.

Cost-per-case encompasses almost all of the costs associated with performing a procedure and providing related patient care. There is a formula for determining cost per case that must be determined by each surgery center. What follows are components of a typical cost-per-case formula:

1. Supply charge—all the supplies used for a specific type of case
2. Core charge—all the basic, routine supplies that are applicable to every patient
3. Anesthesia charge—all anesthesia supplies, drugs, medical gases
4. Clerical charge—all forms, paper supplies, office supplies
5. Labor charge—nursing and ancillary staff
6. Ancillary charge—electrical power, water service, ancillary services
7. Preoperative, phase I and II unit charge—intravenous line set, linen, equipment repair, central supply, instrument processing

The aforementioned list is intended to serve as a guide for the determination of a basic cost-per-case formula. Each ASC will have additions and subtractions to and from this list and its own variables.

Determining cost-per-case is important before charges are set for procedures. It definitely helps to have purchasing and information systems departments available to provide cost information and reports. Every clinical service does not necessarily require that a flat fee be designed strictly for that service. Grouping similar clinical services together, thus creating one cost-per-case rate for the group of services, can be a useful measure. Once cost-per-case is established, billing is simplified greatly—and even the time saved on billing patients can be included in the flat fee.

CONCLUSION

Cost containment is a way of life in the healthcare field and, is a constant, rather than a passing, phase. Some healthcare centers have fought the paradigm shift and have died or are dying a slow death. For the ASC that performs proactively, the present challenges will prove to be a training ground for the future.

References

1. Federated Ambulatory Surgery Association: History and growth of the ambulatory surgery center. Industry. Available at: http://www.fasa.org. 1998.
2. Zasa RJ: Trends in the development of ambulatory care centers. Available at http://www.asdconsulting.com. Article 10, 1998.
3. Advocates Purchasing Services, Inc.: Information page. Available at http://www.advocatesmedical.com. October, 1998.
4. SSH, Inc.: About Shared Services Healthcare, Inc. Available at http://www.sharedservices.org. September, 1998.
5. The Vantage Health Group: Shared Services Development. Available at http://www.vhcn.com. September, 1998.
6. Neoforma: The healthcare business community. Available at http://www.neoforma.com. October, 1998.

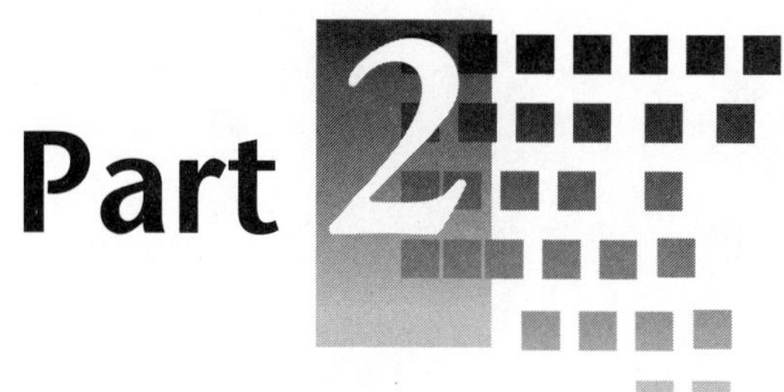

Professional and Management Issues

Chapter 6

Nursing Standards

Lois Schick

Nursing standards define specific criteria that can be used to determine whether quality care has been provided and to clarify nursing responsibilities, reducing the nurse's exposure to risk and liability. Standards provide direction to organizations, people, and patients to obtain optimal results.[1] A standard is defined as a level of performance (in staff) or a set of conditions (in the unit or the patient) that are determined to be acceptable by some authority. Standards have been defined as "authoritative statements by which the nursing profession describes the responsibilities for which its practitioners are accountable."[2] The Joint Commission on Accreditation of Healthcare Organizations (JCAHO) identifies standards as a statement that defines the performance expectations, structures, or processes that must be substantially in place in an organization to enhance the quality of care.[3] Nurses must formulate standards that are concrete and understandable to other nurses, other healthcare professionals, accrediting agencies, and consumers.

Standards provide direction, define accountability, identify outcomes, provide a framework for evaluation of practice, and define a competent level of nursing practice. Standards are written in measurable terms[2] and must be explicit and meaningful to the nurse who must implement them. The quality of nursing care defined by the standard will be evaluated. Because nursing staff have varied experiences and different educational backgrounds, meaningful standards can provide the framework of reference to ensure that all nursing staff members are providing a high quality of nursing care. Three identified sources of standards include professional nursing associations, institution-specific agencies, and regulatory agencies.[4] Nurses are held accountable by law to standards regardless of membership in any organization.

Two methods of establishing nursing standards are validation and consensus. Validated standards are formulated on the basis of well-conducted research and excellence in nursing practice. Consensus is formulated on the basis of patterns of clinical practice of nurses within a particular unit or healthcare agency. The consensual standards reflect unit policies and procedures and medical idiosyncrasies specific to the institution. If standards are already validated, one should never use consensual standards in their place, nor should consensual standards ever be in conflict with validated standards.

The existence and use of standards help to ensure quality patient care and to further develop quality assurance, particularly the quality improvement program. Quality improvement is defined through standards and leads to an outcome. Auditing according to the prescribed standards does provide specific data on the quality of nursing care and goal attainment. Developing standards and staff achieving the standards yields more consistent competent documentation of care given. Continued research is essential to ensure that new practices are in line with established standards. Nursing must assume responsibility for the development of the standards by which the services that are provided are evaluated.

CATEGORIES OF STANDARDS

There are three categories of standards according to what they are designed to accomplish: (1) structure (content) criteria; (2) process criteria, and (3) outcome criteria.[5–7]

Structure Standards

Structure criteria are designed to identify the administrative processes that need to be in existence and the structure that is required for an activity to take place. Conditions and mechanisms needed to provide quality patient care should be in place. Structure criteria constitute the institution's "thing-oriented" or policy format and embody the substance of nursing care that is shared with others. Structure standards include data to be recorded; data to be reported to others; nursing decisions; teaching needs; and standards for interactions with patients and inter/intradisciplinary planning conferences. Issues range from physical and environmental ones to philosophical and administrative problems. Structure standards incorporate all aspects of patient care delivery that are not associated with process criteria.[5]

Process Standards

Process criteria have numerous formats. They are action oriented and are designed to reflect the actual activities that take place to ensure that the standard is met. Process criteria define the quality of the implementation of nursing care. They specify series of actions or behaviors needed by the nurse to carry out patient care as well as what constitutes that care. The different formats may include job descriptions, which are written statements generally outlining duties and responsibilities of a specific-level worker; performance standards, which are statements that define the level of practice required to maintain the desired quality of nursing care; procedures, which are step-by-step outlines of how to perform a psychomotor skill that is technically and theoretically based; protocols, which define what is to be implemented in specific terms for a broad category of patient care problems; and guidelines, which outline how a nursing tool is used.

Standards should not be confused with guidelines. Guidelines establish standards for documentation and expectations for assessment and care that are to be carried out. Guidelines are more narrow in scope and describe specific recommendations for the care of a particular clinical condition or diagnosis. Guidelines are developed systematically and are based on scientific evidence and expert opinion.[1, 2, 5–7]

Outcome Standards

Outcomes are the end result and are designed to measure the results of an activity. These criteria form the basis of a quality improvement program. If the outcome is negative, structure and process criteria should be reviewed to determine whether the problem lies in either of those areas.[5]

Standards of care constitute a plan of care developed for a group of patients about whom generalizations and predictions can be made, because patients share certain common problems and characteristics. Two approaches to standards of care are standard care plans and standard care statements. Standard care plans are preprinted written column-format care plans for common groups of patients, whereas standard care statements are preprinted written statements of care that outline nursing actions for groups of patients who are commonly admitted to an area. Frequently what occurs is that the most common admitting diagnoses are identified, and approximately four to six significant nursing care problems are defined. Goals and actions are then written to address these problems. The goals must be relevant to nursing and patient interventions.

When viewing standards, one can view the Standards of Clinical Nursing Practice, which include Standards of Care and Standards of Professional Performance (Table 6–1). Specialty

***Table 6–1.* Standards of Clinical Nursing Practice**

STANDARDS OF CARE *(Based on the nursing process)*	STANDARDS OF PROFESSIONAL PERFORMANCE *(Reflect common activities of professional nursing role)*
Assessment	Quality improvement
Diagnosis	Performance appraisal
Outcome identification	Education
Planning	Collegiality
Implementation	Ethics
Evaluation	Collaboration
	Research
	Resource utilization

Reprinted with permission from American Nurses Association: Standards of Clinical Nursing Practice, 2nd ed, © 1998 American Nurses Publishing, American Nurses Foundation/American Nurses Association, Washington, DC.

standards may demand a higher level of expectation than that of the American Nurses Association (ANA) standards, but this level must never be less than the ANA standards level.[6] Standards of Care define the nursing process, which includes assessment, diagnosis, outcome identification, planning, implementation, and evaluation. Standards of Care are patient focused and outcome oriented. Standards of Professional Practice define a competent level of professional behavior and, therefore, are practitioner focused and process oriented and describe a competent level of professional nursing care and performance common to all nurses working in clinical practice. Describing behaviors expected in the professional role demonstrates nurses' ongoing commitment to professionalization of the specialty.[4]

SCOPE OF PERIANESTHESIA PRACTICE

While looking at specific standards the nurse must consider the scope of practice in perianesthesia nursing. Characteristics identified within the perianesthesia specialty area are defined in the ANA framework of core, dimensions, boundaries and intersections (Table 6–2).[5, 6]

The core of perianesthesia standards addresses the environment, consumer, type, and essence of perianesthesia and postanesthesia practice. Throughout the years, the environment has expanded to include preadmission, day of surgery/procedure ambulatory care settings, postanesthesia care unit (PACU), extended recovery facilities, pain management facilities, and special procedures area such as cardiology, radiology, gastroenterology, oncology, physician and dental offices, and labor and delivery suites. The core identifies the essence of preassessment and postoperative/procedure care.[5]

Dimensions of perianesthesia standards are multidimensional and comprise the responsibilities, functions, roles, and skills that involve a specific body of knowledge and are manifested through perianesthesia nursing processes and behaviors. The behaviors inherent in perianesthesia practice include the application of a specialized body of knowledge and skills, accountability and responsibility, communication, autonomy, and collaborative relationships with others. The American Society of Perianesthesia Nurses (ASPAN) has identified in the standards those areas characteristic of perianesthesia practice, which involves the preanesthesia phases of preadmission and day of surgery/procedure, postanesthesia phase I, postanesthesia phase II, and postanesthesia phase III.[5]

Boundaries are identified as both external and internal. External boundaries include legislative and regulatory factors, societal demands, economic climate, and healthcare delivery needs. Legislative and regulatory factors are federal and state health codes, JCAHO guidelines and mandated reporting requirements. State nurse practice acts provide the basis for interpretation of safe nursing practice. Internal boundaries are those that fall within the practice of professional nursing within the institution and include the ANA guidelines for practice such as the social policy statement or the code for nurses, risk management, quality improvement monitoring techniques, and the hospital's mission, strategic objectives, and policies and procedures.[5]

Intersections include interacting with multiple professional organizations for the common purpose of improving healthcare through education, administration, consultation, collaboration in practice, research, and policy making. ASPAN intersects with multiple professional groups to address common concerns and issues. See Table 6–3 for some of ASPAN's intersecting professional organizations. Although several of

***Table 6–2.* Scope of Perianesthesia Nursing Practice**

Core	Boundaries
Dimensions	Intersections

From ASPAN: Standards of Perianesthesia Nursing Practice 1998. Thorofare, NJ: ASPAN, 1998.

***Table 6–3.* Professional Organizations**

American Board of Perianesthesia Nurses (ABPANC)
American Nurses Association (ANA)
National League for Nursing (NLN)
American Association of Critical Care Nurses (AACN)
American Association of Nurse Anesthetists (AANA)
Association of Operating Room Nurses (AORN)
American Society of Anesthesiologists (ASA)
American College of Surgeons (ACS)
National Federation Specialty Nursing Organizations (NFSNO)

From ASPAN: Standards of Perianesthesia Nursing Practice 1998. Thorofare, NJ: ASPAN, 1998.

Table 6–4. **ASPAN Standards of Perianesthesia Nursing Practice**

Standard I	Patient rights and ethics
Standard II	Environment
Standard III	Personnel management
Standard IV	Continuous quality improvement
Standard V	Research
Standard VI	Multidisciplinary collaboration
Standard VII	Assessment
Standard VIII	Planning and implementation
Standard IX	Evaluation
Standard X	Advanced cardiac life support
Standard XI	Pain management

From ASPAN: Standards of Perianesthesia Nursing Practice 1998. Thorofare, NJ: ASPAN, 1998.

these specialty organizations develop specific standards that can be applied to the ambulatory surgery patient, the focus of this chapter is on ASPAN's standards, because the content applies to the pre- and postprocedural care of all or most patients in the ambulatory surgical unit (ASU).

ASPAN STANDARDS OF PRACTICE

The 1998 ASPAN Standards of Perianesthesia Nursing Practice include five separate parts. The first part identifies the scope of practice (see Table 6–2); the second part looks at the 11 specific standards of perianesthesia nursing practice written in the format of structure criteria, process criteria, and outcome criteria (Table 6–4); the third part looks at resources that augment or enhance the standards (Table 6–5); the fourth part addresses competency-based practice; and the fifth part addresses ASPAN position statements, such as what position the organization takes on a specific topic (Table 6–6).[5, 8]

ASPAN's 1998 Standards address patient classification/recommended staffing guidelines, initial/ongoing/discharge assessment, recommended equipment requirements, and emergency drugs and equipment for the perianesthe-

Table 6–5. **Resources for Enhancement of Perianesthesia Nursing Practice Standards**

Resource 1:	A Patient's Bill of Rights
Resource 2:	American Nurses Association Code for Nurses
Resource 3:	Patient Classification/Recommended Staffing Guidelines
Resource 4:	Data Required for Initial, Ongoing and Discharge Assessment PreAdmission Day of Surgery/Procedure Initial Assessment: Phase I Ongoing Assessment: Phase I Discharge Assessment: Phase I Initial Assessment: Phase II Ongoing Assessment: Phase II Discharge Assessment: Phase II Initial/Ongoing/Discharge Assessment: Phase III
Resource 5:	Recommended Equipment for Preanesthesia Phase, PACU Phase I, Phase II, and Phase III
Resource 6:	ACLS/PALS and Equivalent
Resource 7:	Emergency Drugs and Equipment
Resource 8:	American Society of Anesthesiologists (ASA) Standards Statement on Routine Preoperative Laboratory and Diagnostic Screening
Resource 9:	Latex Allergy
Resource 10:	AHCPR Guidelines on Pain: Nursing Interventions
Resource 11:	Critical Elements for the Competent Perianesthesia Registered Nurse (RN) and Licensed Practical Nurse (LPN)
Resource 12:	Competent Support Staff
Resource 13:	Use of Support Personnel in the Postanesthesia Care Units and Ambulatory Care Units. Joint Statement of ASPAN and ASA, October 1990
Resource 14:	The Role of the Registered Nurse in the Management of Analgesia by Catheter
Resource 14a:	AWHONN Position Statement: Role of the Registered Nurse (RN) in the Management of the Patient Receiving Analgesia by Catheter Techniques (Epidural, Intrathecal, Intrapleural, or Peripheral Nerve Catheters)
Resource 15:	The Role of the Registered Nurse in the Management of Patients Receiving IV Conscious Sedation for Short-term Therapeutic, Diagnostic, or Surgical Procedures

From ASPAN: Standards of Perianesthesia Nursing Practice 1998. Thorofare, NJ: ASPAN, 1998.

sia phase. Phase I is the period of time when the nursing roles focus on providing immediate postoperative care during the patient's transition from a totally anesthetized state to one requiring less acute interventions. Phase II is the period of time when the postoperative nursing roles focus on preparing the patient for self or family care or for care in a phase III or extended care environment. Phase III is the period of time when the postoperative nursing roles focus on providing the ongoing care for a patient requiring extended observation/intervention after transfer/discharge from phase I or II. Interventions are directed toward preparing the patient for self or family care.[5, 8] Table 6–7 presents an example of how one hospital implemented ASPAN Patient Classification/Recommended Staffing Guidelines.

With the continual change in perianesthesia nursing practice, ASPAN has committed to revising the standards as needed in even years and monitoring and reviewing them in the odd years. ASPAN standards reflect the values and priorities of the perianesthesia profession. Standards address legal implications, because the nurse enters into a relationship as a healthcare provider to act in the patient's best interest and provide sound, safe care, thus ensuring quality patient care. Standards represent what is believed to be an optimal level of practice. The public has the expectation that high-quality care will be provided; therefore, nursing has the professional responsibility to meet the public's expectation by applying and continuously updating the standards of clinical practice.

Table 6–6. ASPAN Position Statements

A Position Statement on Entry into Nursing Practice
A Position Statement on Air Safety in the Perianesthesia Environment
A Position Statement on the Perianesthesia Patient with a Do-Not-Resuscitate Advance Directive
A Position Statement on Perianesthesia Advanced Practice Nursing
A Position Statement on Minimum Staffing in Phase I PACU
A Position Statement on Registered Nurse Utilization of Unlicensed Assistive Personnel
A Position Statement on ICU Overflow Patients

From ASPAN: Standards of Perianesthesia Nursing Practice 1998. Thorofare, NJ: ASPAN, 1998.

Copies of the 1988 ASPAN Standards of Perianesthesia Nursing Practice are available for purchase by contacting:
American Society of Perianesthesia Nurses
6900 Grove Road
Thorofare, NJ 08086
Phone: 609-845-5557
Fax: 609-848-1881

Table 6–7. Example of Standard Implementation Using ASPAN Patient Classification/ Recommended Staffing Guidelines

Hospital A has a call team that covers the PACU on nights and weekends. A single nurse is assigned call and may be the only RN in phase I. To meet ASPAN standards, the hospital provides assistance to this nurse when a patient is physically present in the unit. This second RN must be immediately available when a call for assistance is made. This second nurse could be another RN, an LPN, an OR nurse, the Nursing Supervisor, an Emergency Department nurse, or an ICU nurse. The standards read: "Two licensed nurses, one of whom is an RN competent in phase I postanesthesia nursing, are present whenever a patient is recovering in phase I."[5] Staffing in the PACU is based on patient acuity, the census, and the physical facility.

Phase II is the period of time when the nursing roles focus on preparing the patient for self or family care or for care in a phase III or extended care environment. During this phase, the standard states that two competent personnel, one of whom is an RN who is competent in perianesthesia nursing, be present whenever a patient is recovering in phase II. An RN must be present at all times in phase II.

Each nurse should know the scope of practice in the individual state regarding what the RN role should be and what the UAP role should be. It has been recommended that the PACU nurse play a role in the education and training of those UAPs who are interested in working in a PACU setting.

ASPAN, The American Society of Perianesthesia Nurses; PACU, postanesthesia care unit; RN, registered nurse; UAP, unlicensed assistive personnel.

References

1. Kirk R, Hoesing H: The Nurses' Guide to Common Sense Quality Management. West Dundee, IL: S-N Publications, 1991.
2. NFSNO Biotechnology Nursing Core Curriculum. Pitman, NJ: Anthony Jannetti, 1995.
3. Joint Commission 1998 Hospital Accreditation Standards. Oakbrook Terrace, IL: JCAHO, 1998.
4. Rowland H, Rowland B: Nursing Administration Manual. Gaithersburg, MD: ASPEN Publishers, 1987.
5. ASPAN: Standards of Perianesthesia Nursing Practice 1998. Thorofare, NJ: ASPAN, 1998.
6. American Nurses Association: Standards of Clinical Nursing Practice. Kansas City, MO: ANA, 1991.
7. Association of Operating Room Nurses: 1998 AORN Standards, Recommended Practices, and Guidelines. Denver, CO: AORN, 1998.
8. Mammaril M: How to Maintain ASPAN Standards. 17th ASPAN National Conference in Philadelphia, PA, April 22, 1998.

Chapter 7

Personnel Management Selection and Development

Pamela A. Cittan

Those having torches will pass them to others!
Let yours burn brightly

— Plato

Managers of ambulatory surgery centers (ASCs), both freestanding and hospital based, are challenged daily within today's healthcare environment of constant turbulence. I hope to provide managers, not so much with solutions for problems that arise, but with ideas and information that will help them to see not only a fixed point on the healthcare horizon, but also the horizon itself (healthcare environment). In order to be a successful manager today, it is important to be communicative, consistent, creative, conscientious, curious, and challenged by the constant change.

MANAGEMENT OF THE ASC STAFF

Change Facilitator

Today's ASC managers are required not only to manage in the traditionally defined elements of planning, organizing, implementing, and controlling within their designated environment but also to be leaders and facilitators of change within those basic concepts. "Good leaders are generally respected for their knowledge, skills and methods of dealing with people and are considered to have a high level of social conscience."[1]

As managers in an ASC, it is important to first accept that change is here and will be a constant issue for the healthcare environment. Second, success will come to those who learn to work within the change productively. This does not mean that change is always pleasant or easy, but as Napoleon Hill wrote: "Every adversity carries with it the seed of an equivalent or greater benefit."[2] As successful managers, we must look for and embrace opportunities. If change has become a familiar climate in which you work, regard this as a good sign. An organization that is not aligning itself for the future (change being an indicator) will probably not have a future.[2]

Regardless of the actions and dispositions of others in the organization, an effective ASC manager should make choices according to his or her own values, purposes, and vision supporting the "big picture" and within the framework of the management role.[3]

A few suggestions for helping a manager handle change and approach it in a positive manner are:

1. Accept that change is here and work on resilience.

2. Accept that unless you can handle your own reactions to change in a productive, positive manner, you will be unable to help your staff.
3. Remember that you have a lot of company and share the same concerns with your peers within and outside of your organization.
4. Be creative and re-engineer your own job.
5. Remember that *worry* never *changed* anything, but it does increase stress and use up energy.
6. Take care of yourself so that you can take care of your staff, because you are the facilitator.

Last of all, remember that the manager is paid to handle the challenge or change. This fact remains even if the challenge constantly changes![2]

Communication Process

When employees no longer believe that their manager listens to them, they start to look for someone else who will.[3] Communication in an ASC is especially important today and can directly affect the overall performance and morale of the unit if not successfully practiced by the manager. This includes verbal and nonverbal communication. One common barrier to communication is the lack of listening skills. When disseminating information, it is important to try to understand the perceptions of the staff. Critical to giving information is validating how the information is heard. When a manager truly listens and validates how information is understood, the staff will engage with the manager in a more successful communication process.

Usual weekly or monthly staff meetings still have a place, but these should be supplemented with small informal groups and one-on-one encounters. In this manner, information can be disseminated quickly and gives the employee a sense of control. All persons in the ASC team look to their manager as the credible source of information. If the manager is able to meet these expectations, changes will be less difficult because the team will know what (to the best of the manager's knowledge) is occurring and what is expected of them. Team members can then make decisions based on the latest information.

Stress Management

It is important for ASC managers to become skilled at stress management techniques. Adjusting to the various changes that constantly flow through healthcare facilities today is a drain on psychological energy. "Even if the changes don't require more physical effort, there is always more emotional labor involved."[4] If stress becomes constant with no stress management plan in action, burnout can result. A stress management plan consists of both keeping a positively focused attitude and having a plan for physical exercise to release tension.

A few stress management tips that can help alleviate emotional and physical stress are:

1. Deep breathe.
2. Exercise, such as stretching, walking, and swimming.
3. Put things in perspective and don't take yourself too seriously.
4. Take a 5-minute "mental" break from work at an appropriate moment.
5. Have a good laugh; get yourself a book of jokes or humorous anecdotal stories; laugh at yourself; go to see a funny movie.
6. Hugs a day—hug your spouse, children, pets, and yourself.
7. Nature—look out your window; do some gardening; listen to the birds sing.
8. Vacation—plan a few days away; take a day off and pamper yourself.
9. Sleep—get a few extra hours of rest.
10. Diet—eat a well-balanced diet.

Finally, don't engage in or listen to negative conversations or gossip. Mental energy can be drained by rumor mills. "Worry is misuse of the imagination,"[2] thus invest that mental energy into positive thinking and behavior and doing your job well.

PERSONNEL SELECTION

The Process

The best way to ensure a quality ambulatory surgery department staff is by hiring the appropriate staff members. The selection process for new or vacant positions on your team is both an art and a science. By using a positive, orderly, and well-informed approach, the process becomes one that will help you choose those individuals who are suited both by skill and demeanor for your team.

When team members work in harmony, they have a greater ability to provide their clients (patients, families, and physicians) with the type of patient satisfaction that has become a healthcare standard for the industry today. A well matched team also promotes job satisfaction and team pride.[5] The manner in which care is provided as well as the care itself is important.

Many managed care companies regularly seek feedback in regard to services rendered, and if the response is less than anticipated, they may choose not to continue the contract.[6] Well cared for and satisfied patients not only provide good surgery results; loyal patients and their families also promote job security.

Although there are many different approaches to the hiring process, using both a qualitative (behavior based) interview process and quantitative skills (performance based) component, as well as credentialing verification when indicated, is an excellent method that provides both the candidate and interviewers with the information needed to make a good decision. Because new staff members must integrate into the care team, having team members participate in the interviewing and selection process can be vital to help select successful candidates. The inclusion of multiple interviewers helps to ensure a broader overview from both the candidate's and manager's perspectives.

Without question, the entire hiring and interviewing process must be completed in total compliance with the applicable state and federal guidelines that affect the organization (Table 7–1). It also takes into consideration collective bargaining agreements when applicable. The quantitative components are those that can be taken from the job description and are, for the most part, skill related. Incidentally, updated job descriptions should be on file for each position in your ASC team.

The qualitative characteristics are those behavior traits that will have a greater tendency to affect or achieve unit goals (Table 7–2). Generally in an ambulatory surgery setting, a positive, warm, and caring individual is the ideal personality type. These traits are critical to establish rapport quickly with the patient and responsible adult companion during the short length of contact in the facility. A sanguine personality generally seems to assimilate into the core team quickly and to take ownership of the work environment (seeing work not only as a "job" but as a creative expression of his or her professional skills).

Both hospital based and freestanding ASCs must be committed to having teams that render exceptional service within their existing organizational cultures.[5] For the candidates who do meet the minimum skills criteria, an interview sheet should be designed for the behaviorally based interview portion. To begin, the interviewers should select from three to five behaviorally based questions that should be asked consistently of each candidate. Have separate sheets for each candidate to be interviewed. When conducting an interview, it is important to ask open-ended questions such as "What do you feel that you could bring to this Ambulatory Surgery Center team?" as opposed to "Do you feel you could contribute to our Ambulatory Surgery Team?" The open ended questions give the candidate the ability to be an active part of the interview process. It also gives the interviewer more free flow of information about the candidate. The second type of question could illicit a possible "Yes, I am sure I could" response.

***Table 7–1.* Legal Considerations**

Civil Rights Act of 1964 (Title VII)*	Forbids discrimination regarding race, color, national origin, religion, sex, and pregnancy
Civil Rights Act of 1991*	Forbids discrimination against employees who are minorities or women
Age Discrimination in Employment Act (ADEA)* (effective 1967)	Forbids age discrimination in employment against individuals who are 40 years of age or older
Americans with Disabilities Act (ADA)* (effective 1990)	Forbids discrimination against employees on the basis of a disability, which is defined as a physical or mental impairment that significantly limits one or more major life activities
Rehabilitation Act of 1973 (Section 503)†	Forbids discrimination against defined handicapped employees and applicants. A handicap is a physical or mental impairment that significantly limits one or more major life activities.
Vietnam Era Veteran's Readjustment Assistance Act of 1974 (VEVRA)†	Forbids discrimination against disabled veterans and veterans of the Vietnam era

*These primary laws and regulations with their basic provisions relate to the employment selection process.
†Employers who participate in various government contracts and subcontracts (Medicare, Medicaid) may be subject to these laws.

***Table 7–2.* Examples of Behavior-Based Qualities (Qualitative Characteristics)**

CLIENT FOCUSED CARE

Clients

1. Internal—Physicians, other department members
2. External—Patients and patients' family and friends

Words/actions that convey this behavior

1. Helps, assists, asks for client (internal and external) input
2. Works with, collaborates with, partners
3. Committee, evaluate

COMMUNICATION

Necessary skills

1. Listening
2. Speaking
3. Writing
4. Body language

Words/actions that convey this behavior

1. Asks questions during interview at appropriate times
2. Does not interrupt to interject ideas or ask questions
3. Restates information to communicator to clarify statement
4. Uses body language appropriately and positively (smiles, nods head affirmatively, makes eye contact)
5. Provides sample of clear concise written communication

TEAM CONCEPT

Group skills

1. Likes to perform as part of a group
2. Accepts group identity as well as individual autonomy when appropriate

Words/actions that convey this behavior

1. Tries to understand another's idea or position
2. Is flexible
3. Values group achievement as well as individual achievement
4. Finds working as team enjoyable
5. Works and plans for common goal
6. Recognizes and respects that change is constant

After explaining and obtaining the candidate's permission to take notes during the interview, write the candidate's answers to these questions on the prepared sheet, being alert to responses that reflect the key words, phrases, or ideas that you are seeking that also reflect the surgery center's values and mission. It may be less intimidating for the candidates if note writing is left until after the interview. In that case, notes should be completed before another interview to avoid confusion.

Licenses and certification should be verified during the interview phase. Ask the candidate to provide the original, and make copies that should be clearly marked "copy" to prevent misuse. If the center has a human resources department, this department should verify these documents, otherwise verification is the responsibility of administration. The interview and screening process of candidates primarily serves the purpose of choosing the best possible candidate for your facility or unit, and it should also (if the interview is appropriately conducted) help to develop the manager, other interviewers, and the candidate.

After interviewing all of the candidates, an analysis of their answers may help in the selection process. By using a number scale of 1 to 6 (assuming there are six candidates), read the first question and give a 6 to the best response, a 5 to the next best response and so forth. After doing this with each question, total the scores of each of the candidates. The candidate with the highest score may or may not be the best person for the position. Open discussion among the interviewers will provide other insights about the candidates that may not have been captured in the notes written. After considering both scores and discussion, a choice can then be made for the best candidate.

The manager should come away with a greater depth experience of the process itself, and each candidate should come away with information to help in future career choices. A candidate should leave the interview with the feeling that the experience was a valuable one, that the time was well spent, and that he or she is affirmed as an individual and professional.

Without fail, all candidates should receive a personal contact in a timely manner. For the candidates who were not successful in obtaining the position, it is important to help them remember the fact that because they were not chosen does not mean that they are not qualified, only that another candidate better meets the needs of the unit at this time.

Staffing Mix and the Role of Unlicensed Assistive Personnel

The ASC team has various staffing mix types defined by such differences as freestanding or hospital based, service specific, or multiservice. The staff mix should be determined by the patient needs involved. One common feature of all ASCs remains the same; that is, to render quality care in a cost-effective environment in a manner in which patients, families, physicians and third party payors are well satisfied. The team consists of those individuals working together for a common goal. Teams can take various configurations, such as a staff that consists of registered nurses (RNs) or a mixture of licensed and nonlicensed personnel.

All-RN Staff

An all-RN staff provides the greatest flexibility, because these professionals can ostensibly work in any given area. RNs can teach, provide health counseling, and perform all activities that require specialized nursing knowledge, skill, or judgment.[7] Theoretically, with appropriate cross-training, any RN should be able to staff the preoperative unit, the operating room (circulator and scrub), and all phases of postanesthesia care. Realistically, most RNs can cross-train to one area, but it is the exceptional nurse who can work in all three areas interchangeably. "There has been a long held belief that care administered by an RN has a positive effect on patient outcomes. Unfortunately, it has been difficult to document the effects."[8] An all-RN staff becomes a budgetary as well as a care-centered consideration, particularly in today's climate of decreased reimbursement and cost containment.

Unlicensed Assistive Personnel

Fiscal imperatives encourage the use of unlicensed assistive personnel (UAP) when appropriate. The use of UAPs has increased across the United States. As early as 1992, data were released indicating that more than 90% of acute care hospitals were using UAPs in various areas and in different ways.[9] Today the question arises with regard to how the use of UAPs affects the quality of care, team morale, and overall effectiveness in an ASC.

It is essential that only selective duties be delegated to assistive personnel and that unlicensed workers are not used as substitutes for professional nurses, but as assistants to whom the nurse delegates appropriate activities. For example, duties that should remain with the nurse include assessment, care planning, teaching, health counseling, and other activities that require specialized nursing knowledge, skill, or judgment.[7]

Whether the use of UAPs is the correct approach for a particular ASC must be a decision made for each facility. Some institutions have made a conscientious decision to keep an all-RN staff in certain specialty areas such as the postanesthesia care unit, endoscopy, and ambulatory care areas.[7] Other organizations with similar data and that also value the role of the RN have made decisions to hire UAPs to assist the nurse with carefully chosen tasks in order to free time up for nurse-specific tasks.[10] When changing from an all-RN staff or integrating a greater number of UAPs into the perioperative areas within a facility, there are steps that will help facilitate the transition.

Before determining which areas and tasks will be delegated to the UAP, it is essential to have job descriptions in place. Job descriptions will clearly delineate for both the RN and UAP what is expected of each of them, decrease role ambiguity for the UAP, and assist the RN to delegate appropriate tasks. Role clarity issues can be a major road block to team harmony if one team member does not understand the role responsibilities of the other.[11] It is important for ASCs to have well trained UAPs who have basic skills and have worked in a clinical setting for a period of time.

It is also equally important for them to have good interpersonal skills that will help them in establishing rapport with the core team and patients. To meet the ASC patient's needs, unit-specific skills must be developed.[10] Working with an assigned staff RN preceptor for a designated period of time also allows for a comprehensive orientation. RNs who work with UAPs must be partners in their training and clinical evaluations.[11] A computerized or manual database that is accessible by all nursing staff identifying the UAP's training and level of expertise is helpful, particularly when the UAP is floated among departments.

Concern, feedback, and affirmation by the professional nurses for the UAPs contribute to the overall well-being of the team and allow the UAP to contribute helpful information that affects patient care results within an effective integrated and self-motivated team.

Assertive steps should be taken by the ASC manager to assist the RNs in developing skills that can enable them to work effectively with UAPs. Delegation is an essential RN skill for helping UAPs to work as effective members of the team.

During the past several years, primary and total patient care was the main focus in an RN's education and practice within health care institutions. The team that cared for the patient consisted of peers. Delegation is a skill that needs to be reviewed or taught to the staff RNs.[9] Setting aside blocks of time to review conflict resolution, collaboration, and delegation of assignments is time well spent.

It would be beneficial to the staff to arrange a half-day review session through nursing education for RNs or an all-day session to provide a basic understanding of delegation skills to assist them in learning to cope with the changing role in their work area. It will also give support both from peers and educators by providing a vehicle where questions and concerns can be addressed in a structured forum. Staff meetings also provide an avenue for discussion.

Team Building

Teams can be defined as a group of people who willingly and productively work toward common goals and objectives, satisfy the client's needs, and meet the goals of the unit and organizations. A team member has an interdependent set of personal and professional skills. Teams help to eliminate barriers and enable better decision-making by utilizing each individual's various experiences, strengths, and talents in a combined manner. A team effort is exhilarating. Team synergy is achieved when mutual support exists among team members. Collective effort empowers and sustains the team through difficulties.[12]

The manager should be like a magnet—pulling every person in the unit (into the team)—drawing all the people together, while taking pains to see that each individual feels accepted and has a place on the team. "A weak sense of belonging makes any of us feel like a bench warmer rather than a real player."[13]

Team relationships develop through sharing interactions with other team players, having structured responsibilities, and collaborating with team members and those who are outside of the team. Real team players will be productive and flexible and will have a sense of commitment as well as a positive outlook. Good morale in the workplace promotes group cooperation and cohesiveness. ASC managers who provide opportunities for positive reinforcement for individuals in a consistent manner will be able to keep committed employees as part of the team. "Research shows that all staffs (teams) want to be recognized and to feel important and worthwhile."[14]

Team members should also be provided with opportunities for leadership development. One mechanism for accomplishing this is by allowing the team to develop and use on a regular basis a core covenant as illustrated in Table 7–3. A core covenant is an agreement among the team about what is expected and valued by the team. Upon completion, each member will sign in agreement to its content. Leadership development not only gives a sense of ownership to the team but, more important, provides a sense of satisfaction and shared leadership.

After implementation, a core covenant evaluation sheet can be given to team members to use for providing feedback to others (Table 7–4). In this process of peer review, each team member is able to affect the team as a whole by helping to decide what is valued by the team in the core covenant. By completing an evaluation for every other team member, each member is able to help to develop peers on the team.

Public recognition and appreciation of the team's successful accomplishments and the manager's pride in its accomplishments is important. One way in which this can be achieved is by verbally acknowledging the team accomplishments at staff meetings. Honoring the team can be achieved by recognizing its members on special days and celebrating events as a group. A team that works and shares life's experiences cannot help but be cohesive and committed.

In today's healthcare environment with downsizing, work redesign, and almost constant change, morale sometimes seems less than optimum. In these times of uncertainty it may be unrealistic to expect high morale; however, a sense of commitment and purpose can still be a team focus. The first person to show this sense of commitment should be the manager. "Commitment can't survive when the leader doesn't seem to care. So be obvious."[13] A sense of purpose is a contagious thing. Individuals want to find meaning in their work. One way to allow this to happen in the ASC is to permit them to have some effect and control on circumstances that are within their sphere of influence.

Let your staff know that they are valued and needed as a very necessary part of the team, especially after a downsizing effort. Team members who feel valued for the work that they provide and for the input that they are able to share will feel a sense of empowerment and ownership in the team. Teamwork can make each player a "winner" in the care of patients, ourselves, and our profession.[15] It is good to remember that the whole (team) is only as good as the sum of its parts (team members), and no matter how unstable the environment seems, a cohesive team cannot only weather the storm but can also control the climate within the team parameter.

STAFF DEVELOPMENT

Major Components of Staff Development

Staff development is an area of importance to the employee as an individual and adds dimension to the team as a whole. Learning, updating,

***Table 7–3.* Core Covenant Pledges**

1. Assume the best before assuming the worst. Check for accuracy of information before acting on it.
2. Attempt to resolve issues and conflict directly with the person or people involved. Involve other parties only when direct attempts have failed and assistance is required in solving the problem.
3. Vent frustration in a constructive, nondestructive way and conclude with solutions and action steps.
4. Treat every team member as a human who deserves respect and positive regard. Recognize an individual's worth and value to the team. Respect the diversity of all team members.
5. Treat team members as they would like to be treated themselves. Do not make demands of team members; ask for what is needed politely and express appreciation for the support received.
6. Do not engage in gossip and negative dialogue about team members or the team. Discourage such dialogue whenever possible.
7. Communicate openly; listen actively; clarify understanding; summarize understanding; and conclude with action steps.
8. Indicate that you are true to your own thoughts and feelings, as well as those of the team, by showing that consensus is the goal, but that decisions should not be reached in haste or at the expense of team members' input and comfort.
9. On a periodic basis, act as team captain/leader and facilitate selected team activities.
10. Expect that you may be challenged on your thoughts and ideas. Do not take it personally. Seek to understand that feedback (both positive and negative) is critical to team's success.
11. Understand that all meetings will start and end on time and that meetings should have an agenda with a specific purpose.
12. Understand that team discussions and decisions will proceed in the absence of team members unless specific team members are affected by the discussion or decision and are absent.
13. Refer to the facility dress code and when in doubt always dress up, not down. Acknowledge that every activity/project is important and that every team member's participation and involvement is crucial toward each successful endeavor.
14. Try to return all phone messages, voice mail messages, and e-mail messages within 4 hours and by the end of each workday. Recognize that communication systems must be used responsibly in order to meet the clients' needs.
15. Show that trust, accountability, and team member or team support are crucial to daily work functions and the successes that are experienced.

I pledge that the above goals are important to me and achieving them will add quality and efficacy to my work. I realize that achieving these goals will not be easy, but I am making this commitment toward team success. I also expect and welcome being approached by teammates regarding monthly assessment feedback.

____________________ ____________________ ____________________
____________________ ____________________ ____________________
____________________ ____________________ ____________________
____________________ ____________________ ____________________

From David J. R. Wayman, M.S., Manager of Corporate Fitness Centers Operations, The University of Michigan Health System, 1996.

and sharing new information and skills is a process that will not only keep the staff current but also boost morale and keep staff enthusiastic about their work and professional development.

Staff development can be separated into orientation of new staff members and development of the current staff as well as ongoing competency testing.

Orientation Program

An orientation program should be based on Joint Commission of American Hospital Organizations (JCAHO) standards and should include purpose, objectives, content lists, strategies, and evaluation methods.[16] The program should focus on integrating the new staff member's skills and knowledge base into the patient flow process. Just as important is the awareness by the manager that opportunities should be provided that help to facilitate a sense of belonging in the work group (ASC team) as well as ownership of the unit.

Some organizations require a new employee to first attend a human resource's orientation that will define the mission statement, explain benefits, allow time for filling out the necessary tax forms, and provide information required by Occupational Safety and Health Administration (OSHA) and accrediting bodies. The nursing/technical skills lab will allow a clinical employee to review patient care skills and issues relating specifically to patient care. Finally, the on-site orientation introduces the new employee to the unit policies and procedures; quality improvement programs; fire, safety and evacuation

Table 7–4. **Core Covenant Assessment and Action Plan**

ASSESSMENT KEY: 0 = Doesn't do
1 = Does sometimes
2 = Does continually
3 = Not observed

__________ 1. Assumes the best before assuming the worst. Checks for accuracy of information before acting on it.

__________ 2. Attempts to resolve issues and conflict directly with the person or people involved. Involves other parties only when direct attempts have failed and assistance is required in solving.

__________ 3. Vents frustrations in a constructive, nondestructive way, concludes with solutions and action steps.

__________ 4. Treats every team member as a human and shows respect, and positive regard. Recognizes individual worth and value to the team. Respects the diversity of all team members.

__________ 5. Treats team members as they themselves would like to be treated. Doesn't make demands of team members; asks for what is needed politely and expresses appreciation for the support received.

__________ 6. Does not engage in gossip and negative dialogue about team members or the team and discourages such dialogue whenever possible.

__________ 7. Communicates openly. Listens actively. Clarifies understanding. Concludes with action steps.

__________ 8. Demonstrates that team members are true to their own thoughts and feelings as well as the team's by showing that consensus is the goal, but voicing that it should not be reached in haste or at the expense of the team members' input and comfort.

__________ 9. On a periodic basis, acts as team captain/leader and properly facilitates selected team activities.

__________ 10. Demonstrates an understanding that they may be challenged on their thoughts and ideas; that feedback—both positive and negative—is critical to team success and doesn't take personally.

__________ 11. Starts and ends all meetings on time and when appropriate prepares a meeting agenda that also states its specific purpose.

__________ 12. Demonstrates an understanding that team discussions and decisions will proceed in the absence of team members unless specific team members are impacted by the discussion/decision and are absent.

__________ 13. Follows the dress code and when in doubt always dresses up, not down.

__________ 14. Behaves in a manner that demonstrates every activity/project is important and that every team member's participation and involvement is crucial toward each successful endeavor.

__________ 15. Returns all phone messages, voice mail messages, and e-mail messages within 4 hours or by the end of each workday. Demonstrates that communication systems employed must be used responsibly in order to meet our clients' needs.

__________ 16. Shows that trust, accountability, and team member/team support are crucial to daily work functions and the successes that are experienced.

Please place additional comments on the back of this form in order to give feedback that doesn't fall into any of the above categories. Thanks!

This assessment is to be filled out
for ______________________________
to receive feedback
from ______________________________

Please return this form using an envelope to individual named above and place in his or her mailbox. Thank you.

From David J. R. Wayman, M.S., Manager of Corporate Fitness Centers Operations, The University of Michigan Health System, 1996.

Reprinted with permission.

plans; as well as incident sheets, and other documentation that is needed in order to function in a safe and regulatory compliant environment.

The new employee should also be required to review the Patient's Bill of Rights, standard precautions, HIV reporting, material safety issues, medical information systems and reporting, and the confidentiality policy. A form listing what programs were introduced and reviewed and also the date and the employee's signature should be kept in the employee's personnel file (Table 7–5). If a computerized system is in use, it should be placed in the staff education database. A unit specific tour should be provided for orientation to the physical plant, including the emergency fire exits and equipment, medical gas shutoff, personal protection

Table 7–5. Orientation/Staff Development Record

Employee Name ______________________ Unit Name ______________________

Employee I.D.______________________ Unit Code ______________________

MANDATORY INSERVICES	Date	Signature
BCLS		
Electrical Safety		
Fire Safety and Evacuation		
Infection Control		
Incident Sheets		
Patient's Bill of Rights		

ORIENTATION PRESENTATIONS	Date	Signature
Medical Device Reporting		
Standard Precautions		
HIV Reporting		
Material Safety Data Sheet		
Medical Information Systems		
Patient Confidentiality		
Quality Improvement		

GENERAL UNIT PRESENTATIONS	Date Completed	Participation Type*	Signature
General Orientation ASC			
Clinical Area Orientation			

EO*—Employee orienting
AO—Assisting with orientation

STAFF MEETINGS

Date Attended	Date Attended

CONTINUING EDUCATION PROGRAM

Title	Speaker	Date(s)	Contact Hours (CEUs)

equipment, storage areas, shipping and receiving docks, and other essential issues.

Assigning the new staff member to a unit liaison or orientation leader is an excellent opportunity to assist the new team member into feeling that he or she is part of the team. The liaison can become the new person's resource for answering questions, directing him or her to the correct persons in the organization when and if circumstances warrant it, and providing introductions. When new team members feel that they *belong* and there is a place for them on the core team, they will be able to proceed in acquiring a feeling of ownership in the work team in the ASC. This process serves to facilitate unit productivity, promote job satisfaction for the employee, and enhance team morale.

One way to provide the core team with an opportunity to assist in the orientation process is to have a few of the experienced employees volunteer to participate in making a videotape in which they share their experiences working on the unit, how they perform their jobs, and what they think that they uniquely contribute to the ASC team. Cohesiveness comes when members of the team work toward a common goal. In this case, that goal is strengthening the team by sharing in the responsibility of orienting the new team member.

Development of Current Staff

Staff development is a concept that a good manager should adopt in the same manner as a gardener waters the flower beds. A manager, similar to a gardener, should be sensitive to the fact that each flower requires a certain amount of water, and some team members will respond to opportunities for education and development in different manners. This may be for various reasons, such as a demanding home life, emotional or social crises, sickness in the family, or an interest in engaging in many social activities outside of work. Some consider educational offerings such as mandatory inservices, regular staff meetings, staff development opportunities, and the minimum educational units required for licensure renewal to be sufficient for their needs. Others, because of a desire for leadership opportunities, career advancement, thirst for knowledge, or love of technology, will aggressively pursue these and other opportunities such as advance degrees and certifications.

As long as overall minimum skill levels, patient care requirements, licensure, and accrediting body requirements are met, the ASC manager should respect and show the same degree of approval for all staff members. The ASC manager must remember that the good of the team is reflected in the self-esteem and satisfaction of each individual team member.

The ASC manager should share information on opportunities for attending inservice conferences. Posting notices on a centrally located bulletin board or in a designated area gives team members easy access to the materials.

Each ASC team member must know and comply with at least the minimum annual required inservices for the facility. Encouragement should be given to those who seek to do more, but the ASC manager should openly show approval and acceptance of the individual choices of the team members, whatever they may be within the unit and organizational parameters.

Cross-Training

The ability of a qualified employee to work in several areas of the ASC is invaluable. Cross-training should be considered as a routine part of the unit staff development and education. Before a cross-training program is implemented for an employee, it is important that the employee should demonstrate a proficiency in all skills in the primary work unit. A preceptor should be assigned to the staff member who is cross-training.

In cases where there are no formally designated individuals to act as liaisons or leaders, a staff member who has good clinical skills, sound judgment, good decision-making skills, is familiar with the process of functioning in that particular area of the ASC, has strong communication skills and a desire to help people orient to the area can be well suited to assist in this capacity. Keen observation and good communication between the learner and the preceptor helping with the unit orientation can help determine if the staff member who is cross-training is responding successfully to the cross-training process.[15]

Staff members who have been working in a unit for a minimum of 6 months and have shown proficiency in the area can be cross-trained to another area in the unit. Ideally in the ASC, the nurses should be able to rotate through all phases of care. Generally speaking, there seems to be a strong affinity to cross-training individuals from the preoperative area to all phases of the recovery process.

Staff members should be encouraged and acknowledged when completing their cross-training in another area. It is important to document which skills and information were satisfactorily reviewed and performed, the date when the training was completed and the signatures of both the staff person who was cross-trained and the lead person who assisted in the process. The signed copy should be placed in the individual's personnel file and entered into the Staff Education database.

Barriers to Cross-Training

Sometimes, the barriers to cross-training are more with the staff working in an area than with the person cross-training to the area. Individuals may feel territorial with regard to their unit, and having someone cross-training is considered to be an infringement upon their space. During these times of downsizing, it may also be viewed as a threat to their positions and job security. Therefore, it is important for the ASC manager to freely explain and obtain group consensus for facility cross-training before any implementation. This discussion should address issues of staff fears of work reduction and emphasize the greater viability and flexibility of the overall staff.

Certification

Certification as defined by the National Specialty Nursing Certifying Organizations (NSNCO) is the process by which a nongovernmental agency validates, based on predetermined standards, an individual nurse's qualifications and knowledge for practice in a defined functional or clinical area.[16]

RN licensure, granted by each state, provides the legal authorization for an individual to practice professional nursing, whereas private voluntary certification such as that sponsored by The American Board of Perianesthesia Nursing Certification (ABPANC) reflects achievement of a standard beyond licensure for specialty nurse practices. The ABPANC offers two certification programs: Certified Post Anesthesia Nurse (CPAN) or Certified Ambulatory Perianesthesia Nurse (CAPA). Both programs are nationally recognized in scope, and the examinations are administered by Professional Examination Services (PES). These examinations are given at sites around the United States twice a year.

For those RNs working in an ASC site, the CAPA certification program is an excellent choice. Table 7–6 lists criteria related to both CPAN and CAPA certifications.

For all ASC RNs who are interested in validating the knowledge and experiences required to care for perianesthesia patients, the CAPA certification is an excellent opportunity to do so. This certification also reflects professional commitment and provides a competitive edge into the job market. More information can be obtained by writing to the following address: ABPANC, 475 Riverside Drive, 7th floor, New York, New York 10115-0089 or by calling 1-800-6ABPANC.

Those ASC RNs who practice in the operating room may obtain information on certification from The National Certification Board: Perioperative Nursing. This organization offers two certificates: Certified Nurse Operating Room (CNOR) and Certified Registered Nurse First Assistance (CRNFA). Information on this certification process can be obtained by calling 1-888-257-CNOR or 1-303-369-9566.

Table 7–6. CAPA and CPAN Certification

The **CPAN** certification program is appropriate for nurses caring for patients who:

- Have received general or regional anesthesia, or IV conscious sedation, are in the immediate postanesthesia phase, and require constant observation and assessment
- Are unstable or are at significant risk for physiologic instability or life-threatening complication
- Require sophisticated, technologic interventions—for example, hemodynamic monitoring, ventilators, administration of blood products, a wide variety of IV medications
- May be ASA three or four patients

The **CAPA** certification program is appropriate for nurses caring for patients who:

- Have received general or regional anesthesia, or IV conscious sedation
- May be in the immediate postanesthesia phase and require constant observation and assessment
- Have recovered from the immediate postanesthesia period and require frequent monitoring
- Have completed a preoperative assessment interview and perioperative teaching with the ambulatory nurse
- Are at minimal risk for life-threatening complications
- Have fewer invasive procedures performed
- Have a low risk of hemodynamic alteration
- Will be discharged home or to an extended care facility
- Require discharge teaching by the perianesthesia nurse

From American Board of Perianesthesia Nursing Certification: Discover The Nursing Certification Programs That Give You the Competitive Edge. New York: ABPANC, 1997. Reprinted with permission.

ASA, American Society of Anesthesiologists; IV, intravenous; CAPA, certified ambulatory perianesthesia nurse; CPAN, certified postanesthesia nurse.

Performance Appraisal

Performance appraisals are an important and necessary part of an ASC manager's responsibilities. A manager should always keep in mind that the purpose of the review process is to assist the employee in better performance of job responsibilities. An annual evaluation is equally a function of operations, as well as of staff development. Performance appraisals should be a participative and dynamic process in which there is a flow of communication between the employee and the manager. It is important to not allow the process to become a static one-way flow from the manager to the employee.

The process should not be viewed by employees as a punitive measure. If deficits have been identified in an employee's performance, it is necessary for the manager to address and help the employee to correct them as soon as possible and not wait until the evaluation time. This does not mean that consistently less-than-satisfactory performance should not be addressed during a review. Being perceived as fair in the evaluation process is as important for the manager as for the employee. Giving examples of unsatisfactory performance allows the employee to acknowledge that certain standards of performance are recognized and expected outcomes of their job function. The employee at this time can assist the manager to formulate a plan that will help him or her work toward performance improvement within a mutually agreeable time period. It may also allow the employee to decide if a change in career path is desired or appropriate.

It is important during the evaluation process to keep to a few general topics, for instance the following five general topics: (1) the employee's skill proficiency, (2) team/peer interaction, (3) employee concept of what has been accomplished since the last review, (4) goals to be set and met within the next year, and (5) discussion of how the employee views his or her position within the team structure.

Standardized evaluation forms are helpful in several ways. First, an established format can help in meeting the requirements of regulatory agencies. Also, an objective tool assists the manager in being consistent from one team member to another. One effective and interactive method of evaluation is to give the employee a blank copy of the appraisal form to complete and bring to the appraisal session. The manager and employee can then review both forms and discuss differences. Generally speaking, many individuals rate themselves lower than their supervisor rates them and are pleasantly surprised to see how they are valued as employees. If the contrary does occur, this is a good opening to discuss why there is a difference.

SUMMARY

The challenges in management in an ASC are compounded by change. The basics of providing good patient care and having a cohesive, productive team that provides the support for patients' families and physicians have been (and continue to be) a touchstone. Changes in reimbursement, downsizing, re-engineering, increased information via cyberspace, and advances in technology will continue, but a nurse manager who is a good leader will harness the energy of change and allow it to illuminate the way for team creativity and productivity.

References

1. Peters T: Thriving on Chaos. New York: Alfred A. Knopf, 1988.
2. Pound R, Prichett P: The Employee Handbook for Organization Change. Dallas: Prichett & Associates, 1990.
3. Keeling E, Linnen B: Managing communication in times of rapid change. Semin Nurse Man 5:18, 1997.
4. Pound R, Prichett P: The Stress of Organizational Change. Dallas: Prichett & Associates, 1995.
5. Cittan P: Level of Nurse's Job Satisfaction in a Multihospital Osteopathic Corporation: A Research Project. Livonia, MI: Madonna University, 1994, p 15.
6. Dykstra P: Same-day surgery experts look into their crystal balls. Same Day Surgery 21:43, 1997.
7. Brazino J: Reinventing nurse extenders: The emergence of UAP. Nurs Spectrum (Florida) 7:6, 1997.
8. Koch F: Staffing outcomes: Skill mix changes. Semin Periop Nurs 5:32–35, 1996.
9. Salmond S: Models of care using unlicensed assistive personnel. Orthop Nurs 14:47–56, 1995.
10. DelTogno-Armanorsco, Harter S, Jones J, et al: Health Care Work Redesign. Thousand Oaks, CA: Sage Publications, 1995, pp 98–125,
11. Barter M, McLaughlin F, Thomas S: Registered nurse role changes and satisfaction with unlicensed assistive personnel. J Nurs Admin 27:29–38, 1997.
12. Prichett P: Firing Up Commitment During Organizational Change. Dallas: Prichett & Associates, 1994.
13. Davidhizar R, Shearer R: Boosting morale in the workplace. Today's OR Nurse 16:626, 1994.
14. Noyes B: Hiring to build a better team. Semin Nurse Man 3:11, 1995.
15. Heizenroth P: Key components of perioperative orientation. AORN J 63:183–190, 1996.
16. American Board of Perianesthesia Nursing Certification: Discover the Nursing Certification Programs That Give You the Competitive Edge. New York: American Board of Perianesthesia Nursing, 1997.

Chapter 8

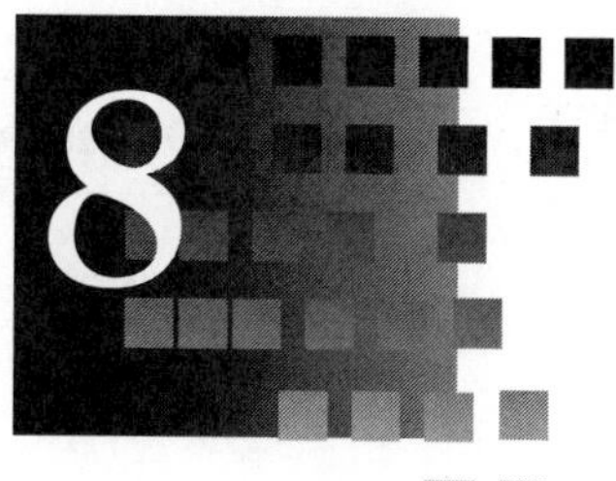

Quality Improvement

Lois Schick

DEFINITIONS OF QUALITY

The word *quality* has different meanings, depending on the context in which it is used. When applied to goods in the marketplace, "quality" can mean "deluxe" or "expensive." The American Society for Quality Control defines quality as "the totality of features and characteristics of a product or service that bear on its ability to satisfy stated or implied needs."[1] Some user-based definitions propose that quality lies in the eyes of the beholder. Manufacturing-based customers define quality as conforming to specifications by "making it right the first time," whereas product-based customers view quality as a precise and measurable variable—to many customers, higher quality means better performance, nicer features, and improvement, sometimes at higher costs.[1] The classic definition of quality in healthcare has been "conformance to current standards and achievement of expected outcomes."[2] Standards are set by health regulatory agencies, such as the Joint Commission on the Accreditation of Healthcare Organizations (JCAHO), Accreditation Association for Ambulatory Health Care, state boards of health, and professional organizations. Quality has been defined in healthcare as meeting or exceeding the customer's needs. Customers in healthcare are not just the patient but everyone associated with the industry.

Today, healthcare facilities require a broader definition of quality. Healthcare facilities have been exposed to many of the same pressures that industry faces—escalating costs, increased competition, increased quality concerns, and accountability to the public.[3] In fact, experts in the quality process have adapted many of the tools and philosophies developed by industries and have described a completely different approach to quality issues in healthcare. The term *quality assurance* refers to a program and activities intended to guarantee or ensure quality of patient care; however, the term *quality assurance* has been replaced by the term *quality improvement* (QI) or *continuous quality improvement* (CQI). CQI is the process that uses clinical and technical skills to produce a service. The focus is on whole systems, not just on performance of individual practitioners.

Total quality management (TQM) is a holistic, organization-wide approach to maintaining and improving quality. TQM requires a highly participative style of management and crosses both departmental and disciplinary lines. TQM focuses on results, not on activities. Three key differences between quality improvement and TQM are that TQM focuses on everyone as customers in a process; places emphasis on improving the process for everyone, not just the few people who have been affected; and demands continuous improvement rather than static thresholds for quality indicators (Table 8–1).

Four aspects of healthcare are evaluated in the CQI program. These four are the structure within which the care is given, the process of giving that care, the outcome of that care, and the cost of the care. *Structure* refers to the setting in which the care is given and the resources that are available. *Process* refers to the actual activities carried out by the healthcare provider. Collection of data can be by observation, self-report of the caregiver, and audits of data documented. *Outcome* refers to the results and the observable behavior.[2] *Cost* refers to resources, revenues, and profits. The standard of finance can serve as guidelines for determining specific indications and is monitored by the financial information system. The financial standards are linked to patient care outcome. The American Society of Perianesthesia Nurses' standards[4] (see Chapter 6) have identified three of the four elements. CQI advances the method for ensuring quality beyond the confines of nursing.[5] TQM requires CQI, with an end goal of perfection sought, employee empowerment and involvement in every step, and benchmarking, which involves selecting a demonstrated standard that represents the best performance for activities in similar organizations. Benchmarking is a critical tool for standards development because it searches for the best practices that lead to superior performance and is a continuous measurement against the best. Benchmarking can be used to validate the fact that a worker or facility is already performing in an efficient manner.[6]

QI is everyone's ongoing job. It affirms that quality can always be improved and that providing quality actually saves time and money, resulting in tangible rewards. QI looks at process and outcome; it is multidisciplinary and is evaluated in terms of customer satisfaction. It focuses on patient care, quality of service, and prevention of problems. QI grants that perfection cannot be guaranteed but that a continuous process designed to be internally driven by the motivation and involvement of many team members can lead to continual improvement.[7] QI is directed toward the process of care delivery and encourages all employees to improve their services within that process. It asks the question "How can improvement occur?"

Table 8–1. Differences Between Continuous Quality Improvement and Quality Assurance

CONTINUOUS QUALITY IMPROVEMENT	QUALITY ASSURANCE
Outcome	Process
Teams	Individual
Facilitation	Direction
Continuous	Intermittent
Proactive	Reactive
Information	Intuitive facts
Learning opportunity	Corrective action
Customer defined	Provider defined
Excellence	Minimal standard
Growth	Consolidation

Table 8–2. Dimensions of Performance

DOING RIGHT THINGS	DOING RIGHT THINGS WELL
Efficacy	Availability
Appropriateness	Timeliness
	Effectiveness
	Continuity
	Safety
	Efficiency
	Respect and caring

From Joint Commission on Accreditation of Healthcare Organizations. © 1998 Hospital Accreditation Standards. Oakbrook Terrace, IL: Joint Commission on Accreditation of Healthcare Organizations, 1998, p 122. Reprinted with permission.

The identified major components of quality in the healthcare setting include the *dimensions of performance*. These dimensions of performance address *doing the right thing*, which involves examining the efficacy of procedures in relation to the patient's condition and appropriateness of procedures and tests to meet patients' needs. Another component is *doing the right thing well*, in which the availability of services, the timeliness of provided services, the effectiveness of care provided to achieve the desired outcomes, and the continuity of services are

Table 8–3. 10-Step Quality Process of the Joint Commission on Accreditation of Healthcare Organizations

1. Assign responsibility for monitoring and evaluation activities.
2. Delineate the scope of care provided by the organization.
3. Identify the most important aspects of care provided by the organization.
4. Identify indicators (and appropriate clinical criteria) for monitoring the important aspects of care.
5. Establish thresholds for the indicators to trigger evaluation of the care.
6. Monitor the important aspects of care by collecting and organizing data for each indicator.
7. Evaluate care when thresholds are reached to identify opportunities to improve care or problems.
8. Take actions to improve care or correct identified problems.
9. Assess the effectiveness of the actions and document the improvement in care.
10. Communicate the results of the monitoring and evaluation process to relevant individuals, departments, or services and to the organization-wide quality assurance program.

From Joint Commission on Accreditation of Healthcare Organizations. © 1998 Hospital Accreditation Standards. Oakbrook Terrace, IL: Joint Commission on Accreditation of Healthcare Organizations, 1998. Reprinted with permission.

***Table 8–4.* Continuous Quality Improvement Plan Using the FOCUS-PDCA Model**

FOCUS-PDCA	EXAMPLES OF FOCUS-PDCA PROCESS USED FOR INFECTION CONTROL
Find a process to improve	Surgical site infection rate increasing
Organize a team that knows the process	Infection control nurse Physicians Nurses (directors, managers, staff) Information services Pathologist Chair of Infection Control Committee Pharmacist
Clarify current knowledge of the process	Classification of infections according to class Data collection regarding wound class and risk class
Understand causes of process variation	Differentiate between infection wound class and risk class Differentiate between practices of HMO and private physicians
Select the process improvement	Look at antibiotic usage in operating rooms Identify proposed solutions
Plan improvement, data collection	Provide education to physician, pharmacy, nursing staff Make definitions of wound class versus risk class known to all Identify methods to improve antibiotic administration
Do improvement, data collection, data analysis	Collect data on appropriate antibiotic administration Review data for improvement of administration times
Check data for process improvement and customer outcome	Analyze lessons learned from collected data
Act to hold gain, to reconsider, to continue improvement	Hold the gain Continue the improvement process

HMO, health maintenance organization.

Data from Joint Commission on Accreditation of Healthcare Organizations: JCAHO Ambulatory Health Care Standards Manual. Oakbrook Terrace, IL: Published by Author, 1997; Gaucher E, Coffey R: Total Quality in Health Care. San Francisco: Jossey-Bass Publishers, 1993; McLaughlin C, Kaluzny A: Continuous Quality Improvement in Healthcare. Gaithersburg, MD: Aspen, 1994.

examined. Additional aspects incorporated into doing the right thing well include patient safety, efficiency with which services are provided, respect, and caring, which involves the patient in his or her own care decisions. The dimensions of performance (Table 8–2) can be tracked over time to measure how well the organization is doing, where improvements are needed, and what impact improvement activities have had.[8]

Quality improvement programs may be structured in many ways. The JCAHO 10-step process[9] (Table 8–3) can be applied, but numerous models exist with mechanisms and tools that help guide the team to develop a comprehensive and effective QI program. Some sample models identified are the Hospital Corporation of America's FOCUS-PDCA (Plan-Do-Check-Act),[9, 10, 11] the Organization Dynamics FADE approach,[10] the Joiner Associates five-stage plan,[10] the Juran Institute's three-part approach to quality,[10] Plan-Do-Study-Act,[12, 13] and the University of Michigan Medical Center seven-step ROADMAP model. These models all have similar characteristics (see Tables 8–4 to 8–9).[10]

***Table 8–5.* FADE Model**

Focus: Verify/define the problem and write it down.
Analyze: Decide what needs to be known, collect data, and determine factors which lead to baseline data.
Develop: Generate potential solutions, select solutions, and develop implementation plan.
Execute: Gain commitment and execute the plan. Monitor the impact.

From Labovitz GH: Implementing TQM. Reprinted with permission, Organizational Dynamics, Inc. Billerica, MA, pp 12–13, 1992.

PLANNING THE QUALITY IMPROVEMENT PROGRAM

Each ambulatory surgery center (ASC) should identify which TQM process best suits its environment and then should tailor that program for implementation. The similarities of the different models are that they focus on the customer, use a scientific problem-solving ap-

Table 8–6. Joiner Associates Five-Stage Plan

Understand the process—describe the process; identify the customer needs; and develop a standard process.
Eliminate the errors.
Remove slack—streamline the process and remove those steps that do not add value.
Reduce variation—bring both the measurement systems and process into statistical control.
Plan for continuous improvement—conduct the Plan-Do-Check-Act process.

From Schotes PR et al: The Team Handbook, p 5–5. Portions of these materials are copyrighted by Oriel, Inc. and are used here with permission.

proach, identify the root causes of problems for improvement, perform pilot testing, and include staff members in the process. The differences among the models include the scope of the model, which in some focuses on problem solving and in others expands the TQM principles, and the treatment of variation, meaning that some models do not explicitly list the steps even though all models reduce variation. This is because TQM is based on the scientific process, uses data rather than hunches, employs systematic methods, is planned, and is organized for problem solving and the decision to act.

The techniques and charts used to display the data that are collected can be used for different purposes in various stages of the problem-solving process. Some of the tools that can be used for problem solving and problem analysis as depicted in diagrams and include flowcharts, cause-and-effect diagrams, histograms, trending graphs, scatter diagrams, and control charts.[14–17]

Table 8–7. Juran Institute: Three-Part Approach to Quality

Juran Institute Three-Part Approach to Quality

Quality planning: Determine who the customers are and what their needs are.
Quality control: Evaluation of performance to identify discrepancies between actual performance and goals.
Quality improvement: Establishment of infrastructure and project team to carry out process improvement.

Plan-Do-Study-Act (Nolan, 1994)

Plan: Questions and predictions; plan to carry out the cycle (who, what, where, when).
Do: Carry out the plan; collect the data; begin analysis of the data.
Study: Complete the analysis of the data; compare data to predictions; summarize what was learned.
Act: What changes are to be made; next cycle?

Courtesy of the Juran Institute, Inc., Wilton, CT. Plan-Do-Study Act (Thomas Nolan, 1994).

Table 8–8. University of Michigan Seven-Step QI Process—ROADMAP

Recognize the process: identify customers and major work processes.
Organize the data: collect and stratify data to identify specific problems.
Analyze root causes: what are contributing factors (causes) to the process flow (effect)?
Determine options: select options that will decrease or eliminate identified root causes.
Measure the change: measure results and success of proposed options.
Apply to workplace: standardize and maintain successful options.
Plan for the future: generalize improvements to other areas—celebrate achievement.

From the University of Michigan, Ann Arbor, Michigan.

The process of QI follows a pattern based on problem solving that can be retrospective, concurrent, or prospective and may focus on structure, process, outcome, or all three.

Brainstorming

Generating as many ideas, concerns, problems, or options in as short a time as possible is called brainstorming. Accepted guidelines for brainstorming include never criticizing others' ideas, considering every idea, and writing all ideas on a flipchart or bulletin board so that all participants can see. All ideas are written as given, and the recorder does not interpret; in addition, everyone agrees on the question being brainstormed. Brainstorming should be performed as quickly as possible—within 15 to 20 minutes. The leader must ensure against long discussions regarding an idea presented during the brainstorming session.

Flowchart

A flowchart shows pictorial steps of a process. Flowcharts use symbols to represent the process performed (Fig. 8–1). After the problem is discussed, a list of tasks involved in the process is created. The draft is then organized into a flowchart by drawing arrows to link each activity. Flowcharts can be used to discover actual or potential problems and to compare current processes to an "ideal" process. Different shapes are used in a flowchart to document the sequence of activity and to depict the beginning and the end of a process step, a point of deci-

***Table 8–9.* Seven-Step Meeting Process**

A meeting is a process that produces results. In order to improve the results of a meeting, one must begin by defining and improving the meeting process.

STEP 1: Clarify the objective: ensure that everyone understands and agrees on what is to be accomplished in the meeting.

STEP 2: Review roles: team confirms who will be taking on the specific roles—team members, leader, recorder, timekeeper, and facilitator.

STEP 3: Review the agenda: each item includes the methods to be used for that item (brainstorming, cause and effect diagram, tree diagram, etc.) as well as the amount of time to be devoted to each item.

STEP 4: Work through the agenda items: there may be one or several agenda items for a particular meeting. Work through them using the methods and the time frame decided upon in step 3.

STEP 5: Review the meeting record: review information recorded on flip charts/chalkboard to refresh attendee memories about what has occurred and what has been decided. Check for any corrections or additions to the meting record and decide what information should be kept in the team permanent record.

STEP 6: Plan next steps and next meeting agenda: the team takes the opportunity to think about and agree on the work that needs to be done next in order to advance the project. The team plans the next meeting. In this way, the team clearly identifies the work to be done and ensures that all members will have the opportunity to prepare for the next meeting.

STEP 7: Evaluate the meeting: respond to "What went well that we should continue doing? How could we improve the next meeting?"

From Godfrey M: Quality thinking in healthcare: The magical mystery tour. Presentation at Ambulatory Surgery Conference sponsored by Contemporary Forums, Boston, Massachusetts, September 15, 1995.

sion, and the direction of the flow. Figure 8–2 illustrates a simple flowchart depicting patient wait time.

Cause-and-Effect Diagram

A cause-and-effect diagram represents the relationship between some "effect" and all the possible "causes" influencing it. This is a graphic tool used to arrange possible causes of the observed effect or problem. This diagram is also called a fishbone or Ishikawa diagram (Fig. 8–3). The major effect is written at the right, and the reasons or causes listed are drawn as spines along the backbone. Team members identify all possible causes of the identified problem (effect) by brainstorming. The causes are then grouped into categories. The major causes can be categorized. Some examples of major categories include methods, manpower, machinery, material, policies, procedures, people, plant, information, and facilities. The benefits of cause-and-effect diagrams depend on breaking the problem down into the smallest components.

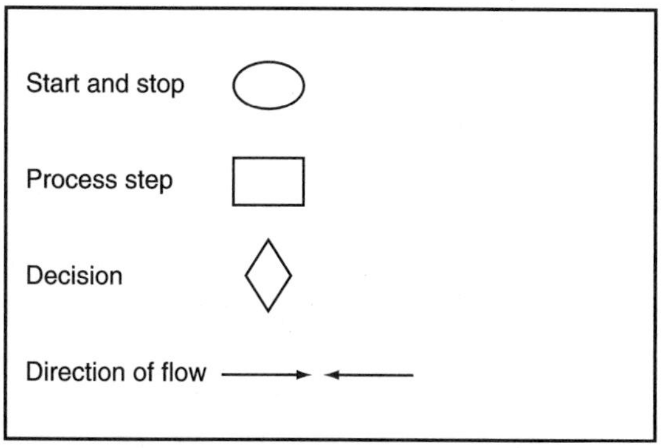

Figure 8–1. Symbols used on a flow chart. (From Katz J, Green G: Managing Quality, 2nd ed. St. Louis, CV Mosby, 1997, pp 188–189.)

Check Sheet

Data based on sample observations made in order to begin to detect patterns are displayed on a check sheet, as shown in Figure 8–4. This is a logical point to start in most problem-solving cycles because the question "How often are certain events happening?" is asked. ASCs receive multiple telephone calls, which can be disruptive to the care provider, especially if the secretary is away from the desk. One institution identified where the calls were coming from by documenting whom the calls were from with a check list.

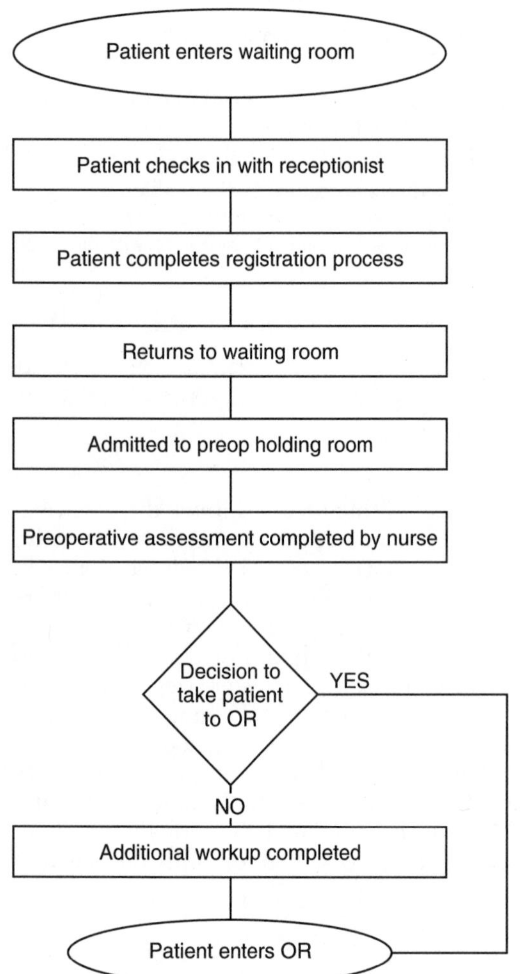

Figure 8–2. A flow chart depicting patient wait times.

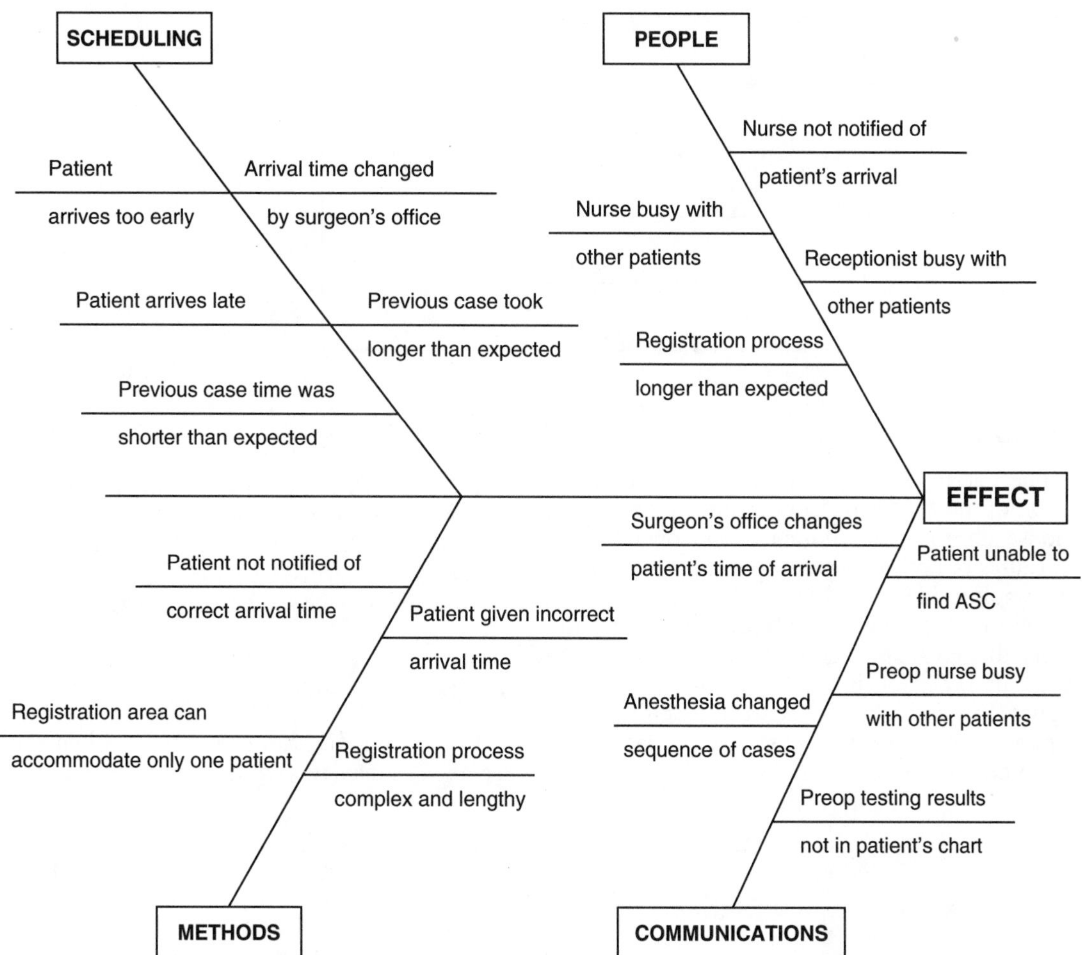

Figure 8–3. Cause and effect diagram representing patient wait times.

<table>
<tr><th></th><th>Physician's Office</th><th>Patient/Family</th><th>Staff Personnel</th><th>Other Units</th><th></th></tr>
<tr><td>7 AM</td><td>|||</td><td>|</td><td>||</td><td>||||</td><td></td></tr>
<tr><td>8 AM</td><td>|</td><td>|</td><td>|||</td><td>|</td><td></td></tr>
<tr><td>9 AM</td><td>||||</td><td></td><td>|</td><td>|||</td><td></td></tr>
<tr><td>10 AM</td><td>||</td><td>||</td><td>|</td><td>|</td><td></td></tr>
<tr><td>11 AM</td><td>||</td><td></td><td>||</td><td></td><td></td></tr>
<tr><td>12 PM</td><td>||||</td><td>|</td><td></td><td>|||</td><td></td></tr>
<tr><td>1 PM</td><td>|</td><td></td><td></td><td>|</td><td></td></tr>
<tr><td>2 PM</td><td>|</td><td></td><td></td><td></td><td></td></tr>
<tr><td>3 PM</td><td></td><td></td><td></td><td>||</td><td></td></tr>
</table>

Figure 8–4. A check sheet representing telephone calls to an ASC.

Pareto Chart

The Pareto chart displays the relative importance of problems or conditions in order to choose starting points for problem solving. Basic causes of problems are displayed in a vertical bar graph to identify which problems should be solved in what order. Simply stated, the Pareto chart displays the frequency of occurrences listed in order of importance and frequency. Figure 8–5 is a Pareto chart illustrating the departments having the most and the least occurrences of needlesticks.

Run Chart

Run charts need to display simplest possible trends of observation points over a specified time period. Run charts visually represent data and monitor a process to see whether the long-range average is changing (Fig. 8–6).

Scatter Diagram

The scatter diagram can be used when there is a need to display what happens to one variable

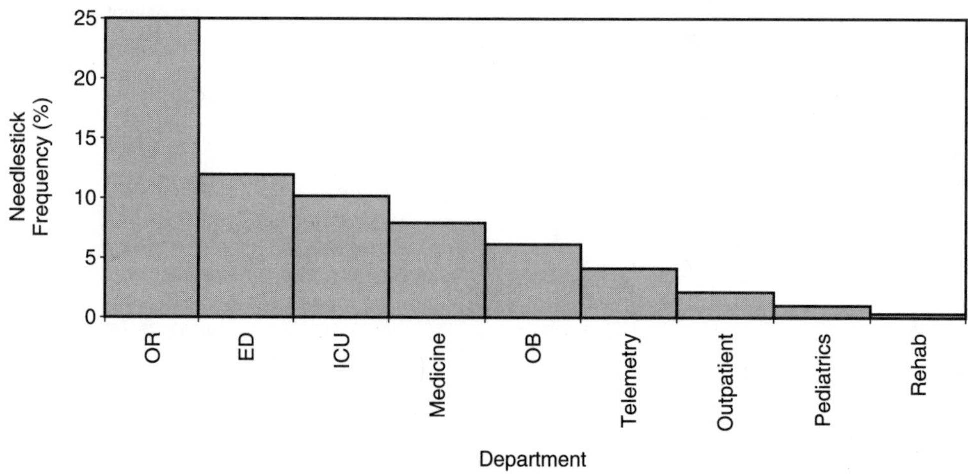

Figure 8–5. A Pareto chart illustrating needlesticks for the year 1997.

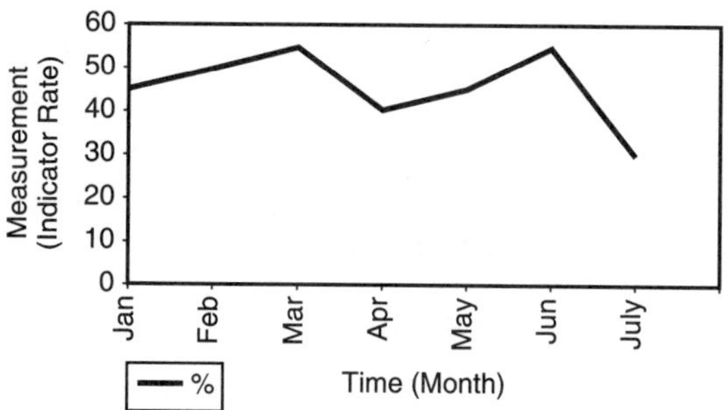

Figure 8–6. A run chart is used to illustrate data over a period of time.

when another changes in order to test whether variables are related. This method enables study of possible relationships between variables and testing for cause-and-effect relationships. It does not prove that one variable causes the other but shows that there is a relationship between the two variables. The more the cluster of plotted points resembles a straight line, the stronger the relationship between the variables. Figure 8–7 represents the relationship between patient satisfaction and preoperative wait time.

Force-Field Analysis

Force-field analysis identifies forces that oppose or support options selected. A force-field analysis helps the group identify exactly what will be involved in changing a situation. It also allows the group to discuss realistic options for creating solutions. Once an issue is identified, the group determines the ideal solution. Brainstorming is used to identify the positive, or driving, forces and the negative, or restraining, forces. The results are then prioritized, and an action plan is implemented. Figure 8–8 illustrates a force-field analysis relating to preoperative patient wait times.

Histogram

Histograms display the frequencies of numbers and present patterns that are difficult to view in a table format. Histograms reveal the amount of variation that any process has within it. Histograms display a distribution in a bar graph format (Fig. 8–9).

Numerous tools can be used in the performance improvement process. Some tools assist with planning, whereas others are useful for data collection, data analysis, or root cause analysis. The focus of the performance improvement tools is to look at the process, not the individuals, involved. It eliminates finger pointing and instead focuses on actions to correct the root cause. Whether used alone or in combination with other tools, the purpose of the performance improvement tools is to support and enhance the improvement process.

QUALITY IMPROVEMENT PROGRAM—OVERVIEW

The goal of QI is to achieve optimal patient outcomes while keeping costs to a minimum. One of the main reasons QI programs are a part of healthcare institutions' functions is that

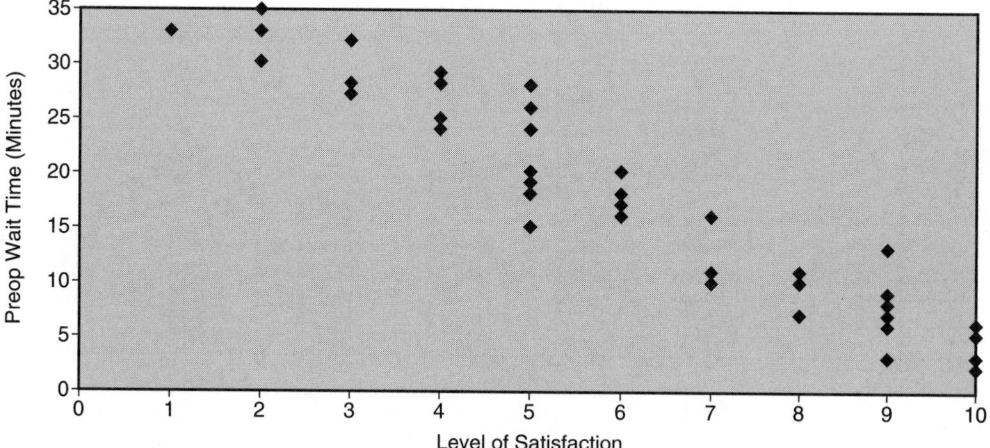

Figure 8–7. A scatter diagram representing the relationship between patient satisfaction and preoperative wait time; the longer the wait time, the lower is the level of satisfaction; the shorter the wait time, the higher is the level of satisfaction.

Problem: Patients complain that preoperative wait time is too lengthy

Ideal state: Preoperative wait time is less than 30 minutes

PROPOSED SOLUTION	**SUPPORT OPTION**	**DO NOT SUPPORT OPTION**
(OPTION) - To decrease preoperative wait time	(POSITIVE) - Driving Forces	(NEGATIVE) - Restraining Forces
	→→→→→→→→→→→→→→→→	←←←←←←←←←←←←←←←←
	Patients who wait for less than 30 minutes preoperatively will have increased satisfaction.	The receptionist is busy admitting other patients and is unable to admit the patient in a timely manner.
	Patient flow will be on schedule.	The preoperative holding nurse is busy with other patients.
	Physicians will start cases on time as scheduled.	The physician is late.
	The preoperative holding nurse will process patients when they arrive.	Anesthesia is busy with other patients.
		The patient arrives late.
		The patient did not complete the preoperative admission paperwork.
		The patient has questions regarding consent forms.

Figure 8–8. A force-field analysis is used to identify the forces that will lead to increased patient satisfaction (driving forces) and those forces that are impeding (restraining forces) the organization from accomplishing its goal.

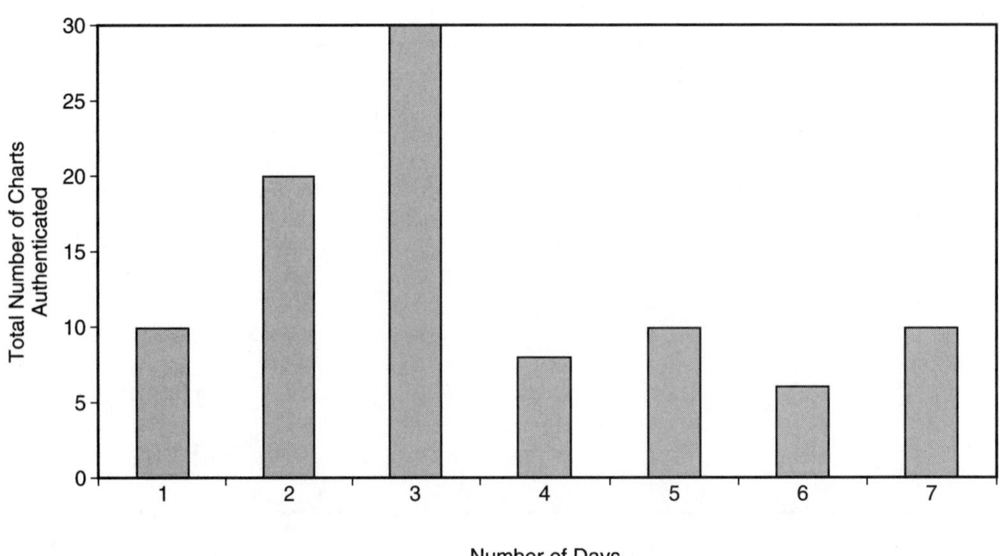

Figure 8–9. A histogram illustrating the number of days that it takes to authenticate the dictated operative report.

they can be used to identify areas in which cost savings can occur without adversely affecting the processes and outcomes of care. A definition of clinical quality care must include the patient as a customer. This is particularly true of ASCs because they are in an extremely competitive market. Emphasizing the goals of the patient is fairly unique in healthcare. Thus, a facility might satisfy the standards of all regulatory agencies without providing good quality care unless it also meets the patients' goals. Although the focus of this chapter is on patient care, it must be remembered that physicians, physicians' office staff, vendors, ancillary departments, and numerous other departments interface with the ASC on a daily basis. It is important that the QI process not exclude these ancillary providers because they are also considered valued customers.

The term *continuous quality improvement* implies a cyclical process in which ongoing efforts are made to improve the quality of patient care. The local definition of quality varies not only from facility to facility but also over time in any given institution. Continuous change in the definition of quality demands continuous efforts to satisfy this definition. All members of the ASC are involved in the effort. QI cannot be relegated to a single person or a committee. Every employee must feel a part of the program, and each must feel that suggestions are respected and considered by management. Furthermore, a serious commitment by top-level management must be very visible in the QI program.

The four basic elements of CQI are (1) teamwork, (2) patient perspective, (3) work processes, and (4) resources.[3] Teamwork is accomplished through the use of a multidisciplinary team. Membership often includes physicians, nurses, and representatives from departments such as laboratory, radiology, dietary, pharmacy, and social services. The patient's perspective is considered through the use of patient satisfaction surveys and outcomes measurement. Work processes include baseline measures and measures after change has been instituted. Data collection procedures and evaluation of the data are used to address the work processes. The final element is the adequacy of resources. Administration must be supportive of the entire process.

The facility must meet the needs and expectations of customers; however, meeting needs is not enough. Patients and other customers must have a clear understanding of the center's policies and procedures so that their expectations will coincide with what actually happens when they arrive. Customers are defined as anyone who is affected by the product or the process. This includes patients, surgeons, anesthesia providers, third-party payers, patients' families, and the sales force. Internal customers are frequently overlooked in the QI programs, but these customers may affect the overall function of the facility. At any given time, a department is both a supplier to and a customer of other people and departments. For instance, the perioperative nurse is a supplier of nursing care to the patient and a customer of the people in the business office who bill cases and those in central supply who wrap sterile instruments. Various segments of any organization interact with others on a provider-customer basis, and each of these relationships may be examined in the QI program.

Compliance with standards for licensing and accreditation does not appear in the aforementioned definition of quality. Meeting these standards may be regarded as a requirement for doing business and should be included in the QI program, but meeting external standards must not be considered as a satisfactory QI program by itself. Meeting the needs and expectations of patients satisfies most external standards. For instance, patients do expect facilities to have emergency carts, emergency power, and other appropriate equipment, as required by licensing agencies. However, the emphasis should be on the patient and other customers.

Occasionally, the needs of various customers conflict, and it is necessary to make a choice. Then, it may be helpful to distinguish between the "vital few" and the "useful many."[12] In most businesses, a few customers account for most sales. The needs of this vital few should obviously receive the greatest attention. Other choices depend on the corporate image or the philosophy of the organization.

It is said that businesses compete in one of three areas: (1) quality (Hallmark's "when you care enough to send the very best"), (2) cost (Meineke's "nobody beats our prices"), and (3) service (Burger King's "have it your way"). The patient typically wants the service performed well (quality outcome), the third-party payer wants it performed cheaply (cost), and surgeons want it performed at their convenience (service). The choice between these sometimes competing desires depends on the emphasis and the orientation of the particular facility and the market niche it seeks to occupy.

A facility's risk management program also carries out studies, reviews, and evaluations similar to, or as an adjunct to, those incorporated in the QI program. It is the responsibility of each facility to have a formal risk management program that considers aspects of the physical plant or the clinical program that expose patients, visitors, or employees to potential hazards. Risk management and QI activities frequently overlap, but the motivation for the activity is different (see Chapter 9).

An audit is a retrospective technique for measuring the degree of compliance with some set standard. There are three general types of audits:

1. The *structure audit* examines paperwork and machinery.
2. The *process audit* asks whether patients are treated the way the paperwork said they would be treated.
3. The *outcome audit* seeks to determine whether everything went as expected.

Monitors, also called *generic screens* or *clinical indicators*, are aspects of patient care that are examined routinely (e.g., infection rate, hospital admissions, length of postanesthesia care unit stay). *Incidents* are events that should not happen and need to be examined carefully when they do, for instance, cardiac arrest, death, and other grave events.

Quality in healthcare requires a commitment from management and involvement of everyone in the facility. Every written QI plan should be revised annually, and the results obtained from various studies should be used to revise the plan. A portion or all of the QI plan may also be incorporated into an orientation program to ensure that quality patient care techniques and practices are taught to new employees. QI information related to physicians should be used in the re-credentialing process. All of the aforementioned requirements recommend the participation of all departments at the ASC.

EXTERNAL REQUIREMENTS AND STANDARDS

Once quality has been defined, external requirements and standards that affect a facility's program should be examined. Standards define quality and are those practices that are accepted by a given profession. Guidelines and standards are set up by regulatory agencies, such as the JCAHO, the Accreditation Association for Ambulatory Health Care, the American Society of Anesthesiologists, the Association of Operating Room Nurses, the American Society of Perianesthesia Nurses, and state and federal government agencies. Some of these agencies deal with a specific area of the ASC, and others are concerned with all departments.

All external agencies stress an ongoing QI program. Data should be continuously collected and assessed to identify problems or potential problems in all areas of patient care. These requirements can be met by careful documentation of QI minutes, studies, revised policies and procedures, and ongoing data collection.

The JCAHO requires that "there is an ongoing QI program designed to objectively and systematically monitor and evaluate the quality and appropriateness of patient care, pursue opportunities to improve patient care, and resolve identified problems."[7] The JCAHO calls for the establishment of a written, organization-wide plan implemented by a designated group or person.

The Accreditation Association for Ambulatory Health Care requires an ongoing QI program to address "clinical, administrative, and cost-of-care issues, as well as actual or potential problems affecting patient outcomes (results of care). Exclusive concentration on administrative or cost-of-care issues does not fulfill this requirement."[17] QI activities include the following characteristics:

1. Identify problems or concerns in care of patients.
2. Evaluate frequency, severity, and source of suspected problems or concerns.
3. Resolve identified concerns and problems.
4. Re-evaluate—after studies are completed there is a restudy process to ensure that corrective measures instituted have achieved the desired results.
5. Report QI activities to the proper personnel, chief executive officer, and governing body.
6. Take suggestions and directives from the governing body to the staff for review and implementation.

These six steps are known as "closing the loop." All studies and actions must be well documented.[17]

Readers should refer to their individual state health codes for state-specific requirements for ASCs. The basic requirements vary from state to state.

For the ASC that wishes to participate in the Medicare program, the federal government also sets guidelines for QI which require participation of medical staff, ensuring medical necessity and appropriateness of the care provided. This includes the process of medical peer review.

Accreditation and government standards and requirements address the ASC as a whole. Each of the specific clinical and clerical departments also has individual department requirements for providing and monitoring quality of services. Many requirements are set nationally as described in professional organizations.

The American Society of Perianesthesia Nurses standard IV of the 1998 ASPAN Standards of Perianesthesia Nursing Practice is devoted to CQI.[4] Through a combination of associated and interdependent structure, process, and outcome criteria, these standards require that "perianesthesia nursing practice is monitored and evaluated on an ongoing basis. Identified problems are resolved in order to assure the quality and appropriateness of patient care."[4]

The Association of Operating Room Nurses standard for quality improvement for perioperative nursing states: "There shall be a quality improvement program for operating room services."[18] An operating room's QI program identifies a real or potential problem, assesses data, forms a plan of action, and recommends changes. Findings are then compared with standards of established practice. Restudy after a reasonable period allows the staff to evaluate the effectiveness of implemented changes. The criteria that the Association of Operating Room Nurses has established for a QI program include continued competence of personnel, safety and cost-effectiveness of goods and services, maintenance of a therapeutic environment, and confidentiality of information.

The American Society of Anesthesiologists has set up performance standards for basic intraoperative monitoring and postanesthesia care, including continuous evaluation of the patient's oxygenation, ventilation, circulation, and temperature. Professional judgment, within the scope of training and experience, is allowed in the evaluation of these characteristics.[4]

A successful ambulatory surgery program combines external requirements with experience-based information to develop standards for itself. This ensures that the quality of care remains high even after inspectors from various regulatory agencies have departed. Well-written bylaws, policies, procedures, and orientation and credentialing programs are essential. However, it is the actual implementation of these standards and the subsequent evaluation of their appropriateness that determine whether an ambulatory surgery facility has an adequate, progressive, and effective QI program. The QI program may address issues such as whether the credentialing process, policies, and procedures; the practice of safe anesthesia; the chart documentation; and the established business office protocols are established and are being followed.

ORIENTATION PROGRAMS

ASCs, both hospital based and freestanding, have a different focus than that of inpatient facilities and require an orientation period that reflects that difference. Nurses, physicians, and business office staff are shown in a systematic fashion their responsibilities and expected interactions with various departments. Interaction among those departments makes the facility function effectively. As a minimum orientation, each new member of the staff should have a physical plant tour, an explanation of appropriate paperwork, a review of the literature offered to patients, and ample opportunities to ask questions.

While reading policy and procedure manuals during orientation, new employees should be encouraged to point out areas in which current practice does not conform to the manuals. If practice is correct, the manual is in need of a revision or a new policy to reflect the change. If practice is incorrect, it serves as a learning tool for the new employee as well as the rest of the staff. Ultimately the goal is to improve quality. Providing adequate orientation and displaying openness to suggestions and comments are important aspects of that goal.

The internal requirements and standards set by ASC staff determine the quality of care they strive to deliver. Periodic record reviews should be performed by both the physician and the nursing staff. Medical records of cases in which significant complications have occurred require physician peer review. QI projects begin with assignment of responsibility and identification of an area of study. Once the scope of care is defined, the problem is further analyzed in terms of its important aspects, generally accepted standards of care, indicators that the standards have been met, and criteria for deciding whether they were sufficiently met. An important standard is the makeup of the multidisciplinary QI committee and its agenda. The interval that the QI committee decides on (e.g., monthly, bimonthly) is not as important as the actual compliance to the policy that is set.

Involvement of staff from each department on the QI committee enhances the functioning of the ASC. A multidisciplinary approach encourages all staff to feel involved in planning and implementing quality care at the facility. The meeting agenda, like the example in Table 8–9, should follow a set format and should allow for participation from all departments of the ASC. The QI team consists of members, a timekeeper, a recorder, a leader, and a facilitator/advisor. The duties can be shared from meeting to meeting, except those of the facilitator/advisor. The facilitator/advisor is someone who has developed special expertise in the QI process and serves as a consultant to the team. This person focuses on the meeting process and assists the team in improving the process being addressed and to improve the skill and competence of the team. All other participants are active team members, even though they may have additional roles.

GENERIC QUALITY SCREENS

Topics for generic screening are dynamic and facility specific. Each facility establishes what their problems are and the causes of the problem. For example, when cancellations are discussed, it is important to determine whether the procedure was canceled the day before the proposed surgical date or the day of the case. Identifying whether the case was canceled after the patient completed the admission process (clerical, nursing, and anesthesia departments) directs the study that may result from this problem. It also helps identify potential actions that can be taken to eliminate the problem. For example, if cancellations are occurring on the day of surgery and are the result of problems identified during the anesthesia interview, the extent of the preoperative review of the patient history performed on days prior to surgery should be examined. Perhaps the information collected by the nurse interviewing the patient before surgery is inadequate. The physicians or their office staff booking the procedures may not be aware of the extent of information that they should routinely provide at the time of booking. Obtaining more information at the time of booking should not be considered more work for the booking physician; it should be presented as a means by which there will be fewer cancellations on the operative day and therefore a more efficient use of time on the day of surgery.

Another area that requires examination is unplanned admission to an acute care facility immediately after surgery. The first parameter for consideration is the definition of "unplanned" and "immediately." When examining the charts of these patients, investigators look for common elements, such as the surgeon, the procedure, the anesthetic technique, the starting time in the operating room, and the patient selection factors, such as age, American Society of Anesthesiologists classification, preoperative status, and home environment. QI planners should develop a study that considers these parameters and includes additional review committees as necessary (e.g., utilization review, peer review, tissue review). Examples of generic screens or indicators include

- Number of charts delinquent (>30 days)
- Number of patients arriving in the operating room with inappropriate apparel or jewelry
- Number of patients requiring antiemetics
- Number of patients without transportation after surgery is completed
- Number of surgery cancellations
- Number of times the wrong side or site is booked
- Number of times consent requires changes on day of procedure
- Number of times team members cannot answer fire protocol survey questions

There is, in the course of doing business, a need for the facility to establish an acceptable level of quality care. The definition of that level is based on a comparison of standards within the community, the influence of outside agencies, and the opinions of recognized professionals in the field of ambulatory surgery. Once criteria have been established that define acceptable levels of quality, the need to measure achievement of those levels will follow. The monitors that the facility uses rely in part on statistical analysis. Without such analysis, it would be difficult to assess the extent of a problem and the impact or the scope of that problem.

CONCEPT OF BENCHMARKING

Quality Improvement Studies

There is no firm rule regarding the development of a format for QI studies. The study itself requires that the following specifics be included: (1) problem identification, (2) extent of problem defined, (3) actions taken, (4) result of the actions on the problem, and (5) follow-up. Most studies provide the facility with valuable information. The value of the study is in the quality of the information, not in the quantity of cases reviewed.

The sample of patients' charts, for example, may reflect a time period, such as 1 week or 1 month. Short-term studies need not encompass thousands of cases to be valid. Investigators should judge the extent of the problem realistically before plunging into retrospective studies on 6 months of patient visits. Some of the best data are obtained from a small population, especially if the appropriate information is available. A sample size of at least 30 patients or 5% of the total population in question (whichever is larger) is suggested for a routine review. If a query review is to be performed (a study in which the investigator asks questions to resolve a doubt), a sample size of 60 patients or 10% of the population of interest (whichever is larger) is recommended. If an intensive review is to be performed, the sample number is 90 patients or 15% of the population of interest (whichever is larger). If a sentinel event is being investigated (when the event sends a signal or sounds a warning that requires imminent attention), review of 100% of the cases is recommended.[8] It is important to share particularly relevant information by publication or group presentations, but every study need not be a major research effort.

With either retrospective or concurrent studies, it is important to confine the retrieval of data to the problem at hand. In other words, one must not take on more than can be handled. Computers provide easier analysis of the data. The organization's billing department must retrieve certain data to bill the insurance carriers for patient services. There may be an opportunity to piggyback on this system additional information for the generic screens developed by the committee. Technology can enhance CQI so that automation will become an essential tool for measuring performance. "Doing things better is what Continuous Quality Improvement is all about."[19]

The example QI study included in Table 8–10 is complete, understandable, and effective. It was followed by a repeat study to evaluate the long-term effects of the action taken and has therefore "closed the loop." To prove effectiveness of a study, the actions must be re-examined. Some suggested topics for study are included in Table 8–11.

Table 8–10. **Quality Improvement Narrative Analysis**

DATE: October–March

PROBLEM IDENTIFICATION: Informed consent forms were incomplete on patient admission to the ASC. Either they were not signed by the patient or they were not signed by the physician. It is the responsibility of the admitting nurse as well as the circulating nurse to be sure that these signatures are procured from the patient and the surgeon.

RESULTS: A study was devised to monitor the problem for 2 weeks. The weeks of September 26 and October 3 were used. Eighty-three patient consent forms were reviewed for completeness. At the end of 2 weeks, 25 consent forms were found to be complete, and 58 were either not initiated or not complete, requiring the nursing staff to intervene before the start of the operative procedure (30% complete/70% incomplete).

ACTION: A letter was sent to the surgeons reminding them that an informed consent and its documentation are their responsibility. A copy of the QI study accompanied this letter. A follow-up study will be performed to monitor policy compliance and the results of the reminder.

FOLLOW-UP: Four random days were chosen for restudy, February 27 and 28 and March 2 and 3. Fifty-seven patient informed consents were represented. Eighty-five percent of these consents were complete with both patient and physician signatures before patients entered the OR. Seven percent needed the physician's signature only, and 8% still required the patient's and the physician's signatures before the procedure started. The results of this restudy indicated that physicians have responded to the letter and staff reminders. The remaining noncomplying physicians will be spoken to about the policy and their responsibility regarding informed consents. Anesthesiologists and circulating nurses still remain responsible for checking the consent form before a patient enters the OR.

Restudy to be performed in 3 months.

ASC, ambulatory surgery center; OR, operating room; QI, quality improvement.

INVOLVEMENT IN A QUALITY IMPROVEMENT PROGRAM

There may come a point when members of the QI committee believe that they have looked at everything. This signifies the need for wider involvement in QI activities. QI must be an ongoing, organization-wide effort to ensure that the facility is a competent, caring, efficient, progressive site for healthcare delivery. Participation by physicians, nurses, clerical staff, directors, supervisors, ancillary staff, and administration is essential to a successful program.

The purpose of a QI program is beyond meeting the criteria for accreditation. It is more involved than pushing papers and finding busy work for staff. QI should be the basis of doing things right and doing the right things for caregivers throughout the facility. The delivery of quality care and the assurance that the care delivered today will improve in years to come must be part of the mindset of every employee.

Table 8–11. Common Continuous Quality Improvement Indicators Used in the Ambulatory Healthcare Setting

Patient satisfaction
Preoperative delays and incidents
Preoperative cancellations
Postoperative follow-up
Readmission to hospital following discharge
Occurrences in PACU and phase II
Turnover times
Discharge delay
Unexpected admissions from the ambulatory surgery unit
Infection control
Incident (variance) reports
Equipment repairs/failures
Physician surveys
Environmental safety

PACU, postanesthesia care unit.

It is an attitude that will be adopted when everyone realizes that the organization believes in what it does and works hard to maintain and improve the standards that have been set.

References

1. Heizer J, Render B: Production & Operations Management. Englewood Cliffs, NJ: Prentice-Hall, 1996.
2. Tappen R: Nursing Leadership and Management, 3rd ed. Philadelphia: FA Davis, 1995.
3. Lopresti J, Whetstone WR: Total quality management: Doing right things right. Nurs Manage 24:34–36, 1993.
4. American Society of Perianesthesia Nurses: ASPAN Standards of Perianesthesia Nursing Practice 1998. Thorofare, NJ: American Society of Perianesthesia Nurses, 1998.
5. Buss H: Continuous quality improvement: Adaptation of the 10-step model with postanesthesia care unit application. J Postanesth Nurs 8:238–248, 1996.
6. Curran C: An interview with Linda Slezak. Nurs Econ 14:141–144, 1996.
7. Joint Commission on Accreditation of Healthcare Organizations: Viewers Guide: Improving Organizational Performance: Joint Commission Standards and Survey Process. Oakbrook Terrace, IL: Published by Author, 1998.
8. Katz J, Green E: Managing Quality, 2nd ed. St. Louis: Mosby–Year Book, 1997.
9. Joint Commission on Accreditation of Healthcare Organizations: JCAHO Ambulatory Health Care Standards Manual. Oakbrook Terrace, IL: Published by Author, 1997.
10. Gaucher E, Coffey R: Total Quality in Health Care. San Francisco: Jossey-Bass Publishers, 1993.
11. McLaughlin C, Kaluzny A: Continuous Quality Improvement in Healthcare. Gaithersburg, MD: Aspen, 1994.
12. Hinkle A: What You Need to Know About Total Quality Management Techniques: Refresher Courses in Anesthesiology. Philadelphia: Lippincott-Raven, 1996.
13. Godfrey M: Quality thinking in healthcare: The magical mystery tour. Presentation at Ambulatory Surgery Conference sponsored by Contemporary Forums. Boston, MA, September 15, 1995.
14. Brassard M (ed): The Memory Jogger. Methuen, MA: GOAL/QPC, 1988.
15. Joint Commission on Accreditation of Healthcare Organizations: Using Quality Improvement Tools in a Health Care Setting. Oakbrook Terrace, IL: Published by Author, 1993.
16. Levin D: Assessing and improving quality in the post anesthesia care unit. Nurs Clin North Am 28:581–596, 1993.
17. Accreditation Association for Ambulatory Health Care: 1994/1995 Accreditation Handbook for Ambulatory Health Care. Skokie, IL: Published by Author, 1993.
18. Association of Operating Room Nurses: 1998 Standards and Recommended Practices. Denver, CO: Published by Author, 1998.
19. Simpson R: How technology enhances total quality improvement. Nurs Manage 25:40–41, 1994.

Chapter 9

Risk Management and Legal Issues

Ginny Wacker Guido

This chapter reviews the concept of risk management from the perspective of the nurse working in an ambulatory surgical practice area, with emphasis on nurses' roles in all aspects of ambulatory surgery. The chapter presents a variety of legal concepts to assist nurses in understanding the legal responsibility in this area of practice. The chapter concludes with a discussion of the benefits of professional liability insurance for all nurses in management or in staff positions.

RISK MANAGEMENT CONCEPTS

Risk management is a process that identifies, analyzes, and treats potential hazards within a specific setting. The object of risk management is to identify potential hazards and to eliminate them before anyone is harmed. Often confused with quality management with its emphasis on individual patient care problems, risk management relies on data from prior patient care errors. Risk management personnel analyze and evaluate the data, then design methods to prevent or minimize losses in the future. The functions of risk management are: to (1) define situations that place the entity at some financial risk; (2) determine the frequency of situations that have occurred; (3) intervene and investigate identified events; and (4) identify potential risks that exist and opportunities to improve patient care.

All nurses, whether in key management positions or staff positions, participate in an organization's risk management program. The administration of the ambulatory surgical center (ASC) develops a philosophy that encourages safe, competent patient care. The administration also provides an atmosphere that encourages the prompt identification and control of risks within the ambulatory surgical center.

Administrative personnel achieve these goals in various ways. One of the first priorities is to identify which types of surgical procedures will be performed in the ASC. A freestanding center must determine which services can be performed safely without the immediate availability of a full-service hospital. Second, the administration will have in place the procedure to be followed when patients experiencing unanticipated complications have to be transferred to institutions offering a full range of services, including intensive care, or require a broader range of surgical procedures.

Administrative personnel are responsible for ensuring that all persons who work at the ASC are licensed and qualified to perform within their job description. This is normally accomplished through the facility's credentialing committee and the annual review and evaluation of licensed personnel. Administrative personnel are also accountable for the supervision and education of those who work in the facility. Regular educational programs are offered regarding the safe and effective use of new and regularly used equipment, with mandatory attendance that is documented. Educational programs are also offered concerning competent nursing care and effective patient teaching.

The courts have in recent years carved out a duty to orient, educate, and evaluate nurse managers and administrators. This duty incorporates the daily evaluation of nurses performing in a competent manner and also orientation of new personnel. In larger centers, continuing education may be provided by specialized staff; in smaller centers, continuing education normally becomes the responsibility of administrative staff. The key to meeting these expectations is reasonableness. Nursing administrations meet this risk management expectation by thoroughly investigating all allegations of incompetent or questionable nursing care, by recommending alternatives for correcting the situation, and by including follow-up evaluations in nurses' records, which show that the nurses are competent to care for patients within the ASC.

A case that enforces this responsibility is *St. Paul Medical Center v Cecil.*[1] In that case, a term obstetric patient presented to the hospital. The woman stated that her "water had broken." The nurse assessed the patient and also did a vaginal examination. An hour later, the patient was reassessed, this time by a medical resident, who determined that the membranes had ruptured and that meconium was present. During the third hour after admission, the resident attached an internal fetal monitor. The printout showed severe fetal hypoxia and bradycardia, and more meconium was observed. The resident told the nurse to alert the attending physician of the need for an immediate cesarean section, but there was still an hour delay before a severely brain injured infant was delivered.

An issue that arose in the defense of the nurse defendant concerned evaluations that had been written about the nurse's performance 3 months before this incident arose. At that time, the nurse had been rated as an unsatisfactory employee who sometimes fell asleep while on duty, had difficulty in using electronic fetal monitors, and was reluctant to seek advice or consult with the supervisory nurse when problems arose concerning labor and delivery issues. No subsequent evaluation could be found to support that any of these problems had been addressed or that any had been resolved. The court found both the hospital and the nurse liable to the patient.

Lessons to be learned from this case include the importance of following through on incompetent staff members, either by reassigning them to less critical areas of the facility, by retraining the nurse so that safe performance of nursing skills could occur, or by discharging the nurse. A second lesson is the need for reevaluation and ensurance that current evaluations show the improved competency of the nurse in question.

A second case that illustrates the need to orient and document such orientation and competency to perform required tasks is *Healthtrust v Cantrell.*[2] In this case, the issue concerned the adequate training of operating room personnel prior to performing required tasks. To protect itself from liability, the court concluded, a surgical facility should document, before the fact, that personnel have been properly trained for the specific tasks that they will be asked to perform and that they are familiar with the specific procedures to which they will be assigned.

Surveillance of the environment and equipment used for patient care is the responsibility of administrative personnel. There should be a documented procedure for the timely inspection of patient care equipment as well as educational programs ensuring that nursing staff know the correct use of all equipment and remain competent in this area. Nurses are expected to conform with the manufacturer's recommendations as well as the facility's policy and procedure when using patient care equipment.[3] Nurses are also expected to give quality, competent nursing care despite equipment failures and faulty equipment. Liability can result from using unsafe or defective equipment, and at least one court has held that nurses have a duty to make a reasonable inspection and are to refrain from using equipment that is defective or not working properly.[4]

Staff nurses in ASCs actively participate in risk management programs in various ways. They participate through their attendance and attention at continuing education programs, adherence to facility policy and procedure manuals, prompt reporting of identified risks and potential hazards in the environment and also of patient care equipment, and in continually ensuring the competency of their patient care.

STANDARDS OF CARE

Many legal issues in the ASC may be averted through ensuring that standards of care are continually met. Standards of care are the level or degree of quality considered to be adequate by a profession. Standards of care are the skills and learning commonly possessed by members of a profession and describe the minimum requirements that define an acceptable level of care.

Standards of care are established in several

ways. To establish an acceptable standard of care, courts look to the individual's job description, level of expertise, and education as well as applicable facility policy and procedure manuals. Courts also consider standards as set by the state nurse practice act, speciality nursing organizations, previous court cases, and current literature. Nurses are accountable for these standards in practice settings, because deviations from standards of care form the basis for most lawsuits.

To ensure that standards of care are being met in the ASC, it is recommended that a periodic review of selected charts be performed by staff nurses. Areas of the charts that should be fully assessed include patient assessment data, preoperative checklists, interoperative nursing notes, sponge and instrument counts, postoperative nursing notes, and patient teaching records. The nurse reviewing the chart should be able to reconstruct an accurate and adequate picture of the patient, care received, and discharge information. Areas of inadequacy or lack of documentation note areas where standards of care may be lacking and give direction for focus of future educational offerings for nurses within the ASC.

BASIS FOR LIABILITY

Everyone dreads the possibility that a malpractice suit may be filed, and defensive nursing does exist. Malpractice, or professional negligence, is the failure to follow a reasonable standard of professional care, which failure results in or causes injury to a patient. To understand how to prevent such unprofessional negligence, one must first recognize what elements are crucial to a successful malpractice suit. Essentially, there are six elements that the patient must show at court in order to be successful in a malpractice suit. Table 9–1 gives an overview of these six elements.

Table 9–1. **Elements of Malpractice**

ELEMENT	EXAMPLES OF NURSING ACTIONS
1. Duty owed to the patient	Failing to report a change in the patient's status
Existence of the duty	Failing to provide for the patient's safety
Nature of the duty	Improper administration of medication
2. Breach of duty owed the patient	Improper use of patient care equipment
3. Foreseeability	Inadequate monitoring of the postoperative patient
4. Causation	
Cause-in-fact	Allowing a patient to be burned
Proximate-cause	Inaccurate sponge count
5. Injury	Failing to provide patient education and discharge information
6. Damages	
General	Failing to question an inappropriate medical order
Special	
Emotional	Failing to report another healthcare provider's incompetence
Punitive/exemplary	

The first element is that a duty is owed to the patient. This can be broken down to determine to what extent that duty is expected. Some legal experts label this second aspect of duty owed to the patient as the nature of the duty owed. The first part of the element means that the patient has the expectation that persons caring for him or her will act in a reasonable and professional manner. Usually, this element is easily shown by the employer-employee relationship. The patient has the right to rely on the fact that the nursing staff has a clear-cut duty to act in the patient's best interest.

The second aspect of duty owed is the standard of care that must be delivered. The standard of duty owed is that of the reasonably prudent nurse under similar circumstances as determined by expert testimony, published standards, and common sense. The court will determine what a reasonable prudent nurse with similar education and experience would do under similar circumstances and then apply that standard to this case.

The second element of malpractice is the breach of duty owed to the patient. This element involves the demonstration of a deviation from the standard of care owed and that something was done that should not have been done or that nothing was done when something should have been done. Remember that in malpractice, the omission of required care is just as important as the performance of care in a careless or harmful manner. This element is usually explained in trial courts by calling on expert nursing or medical witnesses and allowing these experts to explain how the standard was not met by the defendant nurse or facility.

The third element is that of foreseeability. This means that certain events may be reasonably expected to cause a specific result. For example, if no sponge count is taken during a surgical procedure, it is reasonable to expect that a sponge could be overlooked and retained in a patient's body cavity. The challenge is to show that one could reasonably expect a certain result, based on the facts and technology at the time of the occurrence, rather than on what could be said, based on retrospective thinking and newer technologies and facts.

Some of the more common cases concerning foreseeability include those involving medication errors and patient falls. The question of when and how to provide patient restraints and other protection also falls within this element of malpractice.[5] Patients have prevailed on the issue of malpractice when the postoperative patient was escorted to the bathroom and left there unattended or when a patient was escorted to take a shower and left in the shower unattended shortly after the patient, an elderly woman, had received an injection of trimethobenzamide (Tigan). Nurses have also been sued for a patient falling when the nurse allowed a preoperative patient, after receiving his preoperative sedation, to ambulate unescorted to the bathroom.

Interestingly, in a review of claims reported by operating room nurses between the years 1994 and 1996, most claims involved retained foreign articles, burns to patients during surgery, improper positioning of patients during surgery, operations on a wrong body part or extremity, and medication errors.[6] In all of these cases, no technology was involved and no advanced nursing skills were needed. All cases concerned commonly occurring injuries that happen to patients. The lesson to be learned is to use common sense and foresight in all cases of patient care and to adhere to standards of care.

The fourth element is causation, which means that the injury must be directly related to the breach of duty owed to the patient. Causation is frequently divided into cause-in-fact cases and proximate-cause cases. The cause-in-fact cases denote that if there had been no breach of duty, then the injury would not have happened. Most medication injury cases come under this classification. For example, in *Nicole Adams v Children's Mercy Hospital*,[7] a child was given three times the amount of a saline solution indicated during skin graft surgery and suffered permanent brain injury as a result of the infusion.

Proximate cause attempts to determine how far the liability of the nurses and facility extend for consequences following a negligent activity. Thus, proximate cause is a natural extension of foresight. The question asked is "Could one foresee the extent to which consequences will follow a negligent action?" For example, in *Crosby v Sultz*,[8] the court held that a physician was not liable for a patient's driving habits and found that the physician had no duty to protect third parties from injuries occurring in unforeseen accidents. In that case, a diabetic patient temporarily lost consciousness and harmed Mrs. Crosby and her children. The injured parties were unable to show that diabetes made it impossible for the patient to drive safely and, therefore, could not show that the physician's failure to prevent his patient from driving was a proximal cause of the harm done.

Cases involving the failure to monitor or assess the patient involve this area of causation. Legal cases surrounding failure to monitor encompass all types of nursing procedures and all areas of practice. In the postanesthesia care unit (PACU), monitoring is one of the most important responsibilities of nurses. Thus, failure to monitor in this setting does enhance the nurse's potential liability. An example of a case showing failure to monitor is *Eyoma v Falso*.[9] In Eyoma, the patient was admitted to the PACU after gallbladder surgery. Upon admission to the unit, the anesthesiologist requested that the admitting nurse monitor the patient frequently, because the patient had just received sufentanil, a potent respiratory depressant. The admitting nurse immediately asked a second nurse to monitor the patient and failed to inform the second nurse about the injection of sufentanil. The admitting nurse then left the PACU. When she returned, the patient was alone and his respirations were less than 8. The anesthesiologist returned soon after the admitting nurse and was informed by the admitting nurse that the patient "was fine." However, when the anesthesiologist checked the patient for himself, he found that the patient was in a full respiratory arrest. The court concluded that the sole negligence and cause of the respiratory arrest was the admitting nurse's failure to monitor the patient.

Courts often add communication with the duty to monitor. Nurses have a duty to both communicate what is happening as well as to listen to the patient's communications. In *Parker v Bullock County Hospital Authority*,[10] the patient fell while taking a shower. The patient had had surgery, and she told the nurse that she was feeling light-headed and dizzy. The nurse left the patient unattended to take her shower and ignored the patient's statement.

Injury or harm is the fifth element in a malpractice action. The patient must demonstrate some type of physical, financial, or emotional injury that is the result of the breach of duty owed to the patient. As a rule, emotional injury is only allowed if it accompanies some type of physical injury. The exception to the rule is when parents actually witness an injury done to their children. In these cases, courts have frequently allowed damages for purely emotional injuries.

The last element involves damages, which means that the patient must have suffered financially from the breach of duty owed to the patient. The purpose of damages is compensatory, and the law attempts to restore the injured party to his or her original position as much as is financially possible. Thus, the goal of damages is not to punish but to assist injured patients. Damages may be general (those inherent to the injury itself), special (all losses and expenses incurred as a result of the injury, including future losses), emotional, and punitive or exemplary (awarded only if malicious, willful, or wanton misconduct is involved). For punitive damages to result, the injured patient must show that the healthcare provider acted with total disregard for the patient's safety. With punitive damages, the court attempts to deter similar conduct in the future. An example of a case in which punitive damages occurred was *Manning v Twin Falls Clinic and Hospital.*[11]

In the case of Manning, nurses made the decision to move a patient from one room to another room on the unit without the use of supplemental oxygen. The patient's condition was terminal and he was not expected to live for more than 24 hours. The family begged that supplemental oxygen be given during the move. The nurses declined and the patient, who had a valid no-code order in his chart, arrested about 15 feet from his original room and was pronounced dead by the attending physician. The court held that punitive damages were appropriate in this case, because the nurses' action constituted an extreme deviation from standards of care.

In the ASC as well as within perioperative areas of larger facilities, the doctrine of res ipsa loquitur is frequently used in malpractice cases. Essentially, this doctrine allows a negligent action without requiring that all six elements of malpractice be proved. Res ipsa loquitur, meaning "the thing speaks for itself," is a rule of evidence that emerges when plaintiffs are injured in such a way that they cannot prove how the injury occurred or who was responsible for the occurrence. Injuries that occur during surgery, to comatose or heavily sedated patients or to infants, may be plead using this rule of evidence. Essential to the injured patient's case is that the nature of the incident and the circumstances surrounding the incident lead reasonably to the belief that, in the absence of negligence, the injury would not have occurred.

Courts still rely on a precedent case for the elements that the injured party must show to prevail on a res ipsa loquitur case. Although the case is now approximately 50 years old, the elements have not changed and they include the following.

1. The accident or injury must be the kind that does not usually occur in the absence of a person's negligence.
2. The accident or injury must be caused by the agency or instrumentality within exclusive control of the facility and its employees.
3. The accident or injury must not have been caused by the voluntary action or contribution on the part of the injured party.[12]

Once these three elements are shown, the hospital and staff must disprove them. Res ipsa loquitur has evolved as the courts view the defendant facility and staff as being in a better position to actually explain what happened, because the defendants had the exclusive control during the time when the incident occurred.

This doctrine is normally applied in a variety of cases. Examples of successful res ipsa loquitur cases include those in which a foreign body is retained in a patient's body cavity, when infection occurs owing to unsterile or improperly sterilized instruments, when neuromuscular injury occurs owing to improper positioning of an unconscious patient, when a patient receives burns during surgery, and during surgical procedures that were performed on a wrong limb or part of the body.

A recent case in Louisiana that nurses should carefully note is that of *Shahine v Louisiana State University Medical Center.*[13] In this case, a patient sued the surgeon and facility because of persistent numbness in her right hand, which she first noted after surgery for a total hip replacement. Her suit alleged that the numbness was the result of an ulnar nerve injury, which occurred because of improper positioning or from the surgeon pressing against her arm or hand during surgery.

The court found in favor of the facility and surgeons, based on the circulating nurse's notes that documented in precise detail how the patient had been positioned, stabilized, and padded before surgery and specifically her documentation of the steps taken to extend the patient's arms out of harm's way as well as the padding of the patient's arms and hands to prevent positioning or pressure-related injuries. Expert medical witnesses, who all read the nurse's notes, concluded and testified that the notes established affirmatively that the proper standard of care had been met for positioning and stabilizing the patient's body and arms and for cushioning her right arm and hand during the surgical procedure.

The court held that the nurse's note was proof that no negligence had occurred and thus that the doctrine of res ipsa loquitur did not apply to these facts. Note how critical to the case was the fact that the nurse's notes contained a factual statement of exactly how the patient was positioned and padded and that the nurse refrained from unsubstantiated judgment assertions such as stating that the patient was positioned properly or in a manner designed to avoid injury.

An additional area of potential liability for nurses concerns the legal concept of intentional torts. Intentional torts are civil wrongs committed against a person or a person's property with full knowledge to commit the act. Although the law recognizes a variety of intentional torts, there are three intentional torts that nurses should recognize and avoid.

Assault is any action that places another person in apprehension of being touched in a manner that is offensive, insulting, or physically injurious without the person's consent or authority. Note that no actual touching of the person is necessary and that the person must be fully capable of the potential touching. Assault is, therefore, not seen with unconscious patients or sleeping patients, because there is no knowledge of the potential touching.

An interesting perioperative case in this area is *Baca v Valez*.[14] In this case, an operating room nurse sued for assault and battery when an orthopedic surgeon struck her on the back with a bone chisel. In finding that no assault had occurred, the court concluded that because the nurse was struck on her back, "no act, threat or menacing conduct that causes another person to reasonably believe that he is in danger of receiving an immediate battery."[15]

Words alone are not enough for an assault to occur, although words may accompany an overt act. For example, the nurse moves toward a patient with a syringe in one hand while telling the patient to "lie still or this will really hurt!" Necessary to the assault is that the patient was placed in apprehension and that the nurse had the ability to carry through with the injection as well as the fact that the patient had not given consent.

Assault is rarely seen without the accompanying tort of battery. A battery involves the harmful or unwarranted contact with the patient and is based on the person's right to be free from unconsented invasion or touching. Battery is the most frequent intentional tort seen in the practice of nursing and medicine. Battery in perioperative settings usually entails procedures to which the patient did not consent. An example of such a case is that of *Perna v Pirozzi*.[16] In this case, the patient gave consent for a surgical procedure to be performed by his personal surgeon. Two other surgeons, however, performed the procedure. Even though the patient sustained no injuries that could be attributed to the surgery, he sued for battery and contended that he would not have had the surgery if he had known that his personal surgeon was not going to perform the procedure. The court held that this was a battery, and the patient was awarded damages.

An interesting line of cases for which nurses may incur both civil and criminal liability includes the sexual molestation of sedated, unconscious, or highly vulnerable patients. Though more frequently seen in psychiatric facilities, nurses have also been held liable for sexually molesting sedated patients in hospitals and clinics as well as for assaulting patients in drug and rehabilitation facilities. Although most of these cases have been brought against the healthcare provider by the victim of the abuse, some of the cases have been brought against healthcare providers by licensing boards.[17, 18]

To protect both the ASC and the individual nurse, there should be a policy in place for reporting any suspicion or knowledge of such activity within the ASC. Administrative and risk management staff may address the issue internally or notify external licensing boards as needed.

Battery can be prevented when nurses remember that competent patients have the right to refuse specific aspects of therapy. Patients retain the ultimate accountability and responsibility for their actions and cannot then bring a successful malpractice suit against the nurse or healthcare facility. For example, the postoperative patient cannot refuse to take prophylactic antibiotics or do necessary wound care and then bring a successful lawsuit for postoperative infection.

The third type of intentional tort is what the law terms false imprisonment. This is the unjustifiable detention of a person without legal warrant to confine the patient or person. Nurses frequently encounter this tort with patients who wish to leave against medical advice. The nurse's responsibility in this area includes ensuring that the patient understands the potential consequences of leaving prematurely and that the patient has assumed all accountability for his or her actions. If possible, ask the patient to sign a discharge against medical advice form, but do not retain him or her if the patient refuses to sign the form. Likewise, detaining the patient until a supervisor or the attending physician can see the patient should be avoided. To protect the nurse, carefully document all information given to the patient, potential complications that may occur because of early termination of care, and potential risks against which the patient should protect himself or herself.

Nurses should use language that does not constitute a threat to the patient, with the knowledge that postoperative infections and pneumonia are always a very possible outcome if the patient does not comply with follow-up care. Telling a patient that one's insurance carrier will not reimburse any part of the ASC's or physicians's costs if the patient leaves against medical advice is not a threat, but rather a truism. Third party reimbursers do not pay for any part of the treatment when the patient fails to follow medical prescription.

There are some circumstances that allow the detention of a patient against his or her will. Like all intentional torts, the key to false imprisonment is the patient's knowledge and consent. Nurses as well as the facility face potential liability for allowing patients who are still under sedation to exert their ability to leave or drive from the facility. Patients who are not fully aware of the potential risks or in a mental state to appreciate potential risks may be detained until they fully understand the situation. Hospitals and clinics have a common law duty to detain persons who are confused or disoriented as well as those who are mentally ill and a direct danger either to themselves or others. Common law also recognizes a limited right to detain persons until the entire procedure to which they have consented is completed. Under this aspect, courts have allowed patients in the transition from anesthesia to full comprehension to be detained until the effects of the anesthesia can be safely overcome. Essential to showing this limited right is documentation, both by nurses and medical or anesthesia staff.

The facility has a duty to ensure the patient's safety, even the patient who insists that he or she is leaving against medical advice. Thus, if the person cannot drive himself or herself home and there is no family available to safely transport the patient home, nurses and the ambulatory surgical staff are justified in detaining the patient until transportation can be arranged. A similar argument exists for the patient who has no one at home to assist in the early postoperative hours. Patients may, in limited circumstances, be detained until competent care can be ensured outside the facility. Again, the key to a successful application of such detainment is appropriate documentation in the patient's record.

A final area under basis for liability is what the law recognizes as quasi-intentional torts. Invasion of privacy and defamation are the two main areas under this concept. The patient has a right to have protection against unreasonable or unwarranted interference with his or her solitude. The right to privacy concerns one's peace of mind in that a person is allowed to be left alone without unwarranted publicity. Within the medical context, the law recognizes the patient's right against:

1. Appropriation or use of the patient's name or picture for the defendant's sole benefit
2. Intrusion on the patient's seclusion or affairs
3. Publication by the defendant that places the patient in a false light
4. Public disclosure of private facts about the patient by hospital staff or medical personnel

Information about the patient is confidential and may not be disclosed without authorization. Authorization may be given either by patient waiver or by a valid reporting statute. Usually, the patient is asked directly about taking pictures during an operation, particularly before and after pictures for plastic surgery and some skin deformities. There is no need to request permission for pictures if they are to remain solely as part of the medical record; this is often done today with burn patients, because pictures provide a better method of monitoring the patient's progress. Additionally, pictures that in no way identify a particular individual (e.g., endoscopy pictures) can be made without prior permission, although the better course of action is to obtain permission in advance, especially in cases where it is known that pictures are to be made. If a picture or personal information is to be used in a medical journal or disseminated to others, then prior written permission must be obtained.

Reporting statutes are usually state mandates that certain types of diseases or injuries be reported through the department of health. Examples of such reporting statutes include good faith suspicions of abuse (particularly in children and elders), communicable diseases, and gunshot injuries. The Centers for Disease Control and Prevention (CDC) mandate reporting by case only newly diagnosed human immunodeficiency virus (HIV) or acquired immunodeficiency syndrome (AIDS). The primary purpose of reporting statutes is to ensure the health of persons within the community. If reporting under a valid reporting statute, give only the information that is required, because additional information could result in a lawsuit for invasion of the patient's privacy.

Nurses may also become involved in invasion of privacy lawsuits for the release of patient information to persons who are not entitled to such information. To prevent the unintentional release of such information, nurses should refer callers to the patient's family or ask in advance to whom patient information may be given. For insurance and third party payers, information is usually obtained through the medical records department, and patients are required to sign in advance release forms for this type of information.

Defamation involves wrongful injury to an individual's reputation (i.e., his or her good name, respect, or esteem) through either oral or written communications to persons other than the person defamed concerning a living person's reputation. Nurses are advised to avoid any type of subjective language when charting and to avoid derogatory comments about patients or their family members.

Objective charting, especially when reinforced with appropriate examples, is not seen as defamatory to patients or family members. For example, charting "family member could not restate discharge information accurately after first or second set of instructions were given to the family member" or "patient was unable after second demonstration to use the proper technique in changing dressing" is not defamatory. Crucial to this type of charting is the follow-up that is then done with regard to the person to whom the discharge information is given when the designated family member is unable to comprehend its significance or the person who was taught to do the dressing changes when the patient was unable to perform the task.

INFORMED CONSENT

Generally the healthcare provider's right to treat a patient, barring true emergency conditions or unanticipated happenings, is based on a contractual relationship that arises through the mutual consent of parties to the relationship. Consent is the voluntary authorization by the patient or the patient's legal representative to do something to the patient. Consent is based on the mutual consent of all parties involved, and the key to true and valid consent is patient comprehension.

Consent becomes an important issue from a legal perspective in that the patient may sue for a battery (unconsented touching) if he or she does not consent to the procedure or treatment and the healthcare provider goes ahead with the procedure or treatment. This means that the patient may bring a lawsuit and be awarded damages, even if the patient was helped by the procedure or treatment. The more current trend, though, is to argue consent under a negligence or malpractice cause of action.

Consent is an issue in its own realm. Consent does not always become a factor in a malpractice suit, although it may be a concurrent issue in a malpractice suit. Consent concerns the healthcare provider's right to treat a given individual, not the manner in which the treatment was delivered. Thus, one can deliver safe and competent care and still be sued for lack of consent.

The right to consent and the right to refuse consent are based on a long-recognized, common law right of persons to be free from harmful or offensive touching of their bodies. In a landmark case during the early part of this century, the court declared the reason for consent, and that case is still quoted today when referring to the consent doctrine. "Every human being of adult years has a right to determine what shall be done with his own body, and a surgeon who performs an operation without his patient's consent commits an assault for which he is liable in damages."[19]

Thus two concepts are involved: (1) the prevention of a battery, and (2) the person's right to control what is done to his or her body. Because of these rights, the healthcare provider has a duty to obtain consent before the patient's treatment begins. Consent, therefore, is not contingent upon a request for information or clarification by the patient but must be actively sought by the healthcare practitioner.

Consent, technically, is an easy yes or no. "Yes, I will allow the surgery" or "No, I want to try medications first, then maybe I will allow the surgery." The patient may not understand or may understand only vaguely what it is he or she is allowing.

The law concerning consent in healthcare situations is based on informed consent. This doctrine of informed consent has developed from negligence law as the courts began to realize that, although consent may have been given, not enough information was imparted to form the foundation of an informed decision. Informed consent mandates to the physician or independent healthcare practitioner the separate legal duty to disclose necessary facts in language that the patient can reasonably understand so that the patient can make an informed choice. There should also be a description of the available alternatives to the proposed treatment and the risks and dangers involved in each alternative. Failure to disclose the necessary facts in understandable terms does not negate the consent, but it does place potential liability upon the practitioner for negligence. In other words, without any consent given, the practitioner may be sued for battery (an intentional tort). Without informed consent, the practitioner opens himself or herself to a potential lawsuit for negligence.

Some courts have extended the right to informed consent to what might be called informed refusal. The practitioner may be liable for failure to inform the patient of the risks of not consenting to a therapy or diagnostic screening test. *Truman v Thomas*[20] was one of the first cases to recognize this important corollary to informed consent. In that case, the court awarded damages against a physician for failure to inform the patient of the potential risks of not consenting to a recommended Papanicolaou (Pap) smear.

To be informed, the patient must receive, in terms that he or she can understand and comprehend, the following information: (1) A brief, but complete explanation of the treatment or procedure to be preformed; (2) The name and qualifications of the person to perform the procedure and, if others will assist, the names and qualifications of those assistants; (3) An explanation of any serious harm that may occur during the procedure, including death if that is a realistic outcome (pain and uncomfortable side effects, both during and after the procedure, should also be discussed); (4) An explanation of alternative therapies to the procedure or treatment, including the risk of doing nothing at all; (5) An explanation that the patient can refuse the therapy or procedure without having alternative care or support discontinued; and (6) The fact that he or she can still refuse, even after the procedure or therapy has begun. For example, all of the suggested radiation treatments need not be completed.

Consent may be obtained in various ways. Perhaps the easiest method of obtaining informed consent is when the consent is expressed. Expressed consent is consent given by direct words, written or oral. For example, after the nurse informs the patient that he or she is going to start an intravenous infusion, the patient says, “Okay, but could you put the needle in my left hand, as I am right handed?” In this latter example, if there is a reason not to use the left hand, as in the case in which the left antecubital vein is needed for the surgical procedure, then the nurse should explain why the left hand is inappropriate and the right hand must be used. As a rule, expressed consent is the type most often sought and received by healthcare providers, particularly nurses.

Implied consent is consent that may be inferred by the patient’s conduct or that which may legally be presumed in emergency situations. Many patients hold out their arm and roll up their sleeve when the nurse approaches with a stethoscope and blood pressure cuff. This is an example of implied consent, because the reasonable person would infer by the patient’s action that he or she is consenting to the procedure. Implied consent is frequently obtained by healthcare practitioners for minor procedures and routine care.

Implied consent may be presumed to exist in true emergency situations. For such consent, the patient must not be able to make his or her wishes known, and a delay in providing care would result in the loss of life or limb. An important element in allowing emergency consent is that the healthcare provider has no reason to know or believe that consent would not be given were the patient able to deny consent, and one cannot rely on implied consent if the patient had already denied consent. For example, the healthcare provider may not wait until the patient loses consciousness to order treatment that the patient had previously refused, such as a blood transfusion for a known Jehovah’s Witness patient. Implied consent is frequently relied on during surgery when an untoward event occurs and an immediate decision must be made to prevent further injury to the patient.

Consent may be given orally or in writing. Unless state law mandates written consent, the law views oral and written consent as equally valid. As a precaution, healthcare providers should recognize that oral consent is much more difficult to prove if consent or lack of consent becomes a legal issue. As a convenience and to prevent such court issues, most healthcare institutions require written consent.

The courts recognize four exceptions to the need for informed consent in circumstances in which consent is still required. These exceptions are: (1) emergency situations; (2) therapeutic privilege; (3) patient waiver; and (4) prior patient knowledge. From a practitioner's standpoint, consent is still needed to prevent charges of a battery, but the informed consent requirements are eased.

Emergencies give rise to implied consent. Some courts have recognized that if there is time to give information, a limited disclosure may be valid. If no time exists or the patient is incapable of understanding by virtue of the physical disability, then no information need be given.

Therapeutic privilege, which has its origins in the common law defense of necessity, allows primary healthcare providers to withhold information and any disclosures that they consider would be detrimental to the patient's health. The detrimental nature of the information must be more than fear that the information would lead to the patient's refusal. It must be a recognized and documented increased anxiety in the patient. Physicians and independent healthcare practitioners, when using this exception, must be able to show that full disclosure of material facts would be likely to: (1) hinder or complicate necessary treatment; (2) cause severe psychological harm; or (3) be so upsetting as to render a rational decision by the patient impossible.[21]

Therapeutic privilege is not favored by the courts and comes into play only when the patient is severely and emotionally disturbed and the current medical status presents an imminent danger to the patient's life. Some courts have held that a relative must concur with the patient decision to consent and that the relative must be given full disclosure, whereas other courts have held that no relative need give concurrent consent. Once the risk to the patient has abated, the physician or independent practitioner must fully disclose the previously withheld information to the patient. Understandably, therapeutic privilege is rarely relied on in ASCs.

The patient may also waive the right to full disclosure and still consent to the procedure. The caveat in this case is that the healthcare provider cannot suggest such waiver. The waiver, in order to be valid, must be initiated by the patient.

Prior patient knowledge involves the patient to whom the risks and benefits were fully explained the first time that the patient consented to the procedure. Liability does not exist for nondisclosure of risks that are public or common knowledge or that the patient had previously experienced. Many medical and nursing personnel fall under this category when giving consent for themselves as the patient.

The physician or independent practitioner has the responsibility for obtaining informed consent.[22] Individual hospitals have no responsibility for obtaining informed consent unless: (1) the physician or independent practitioner is an employee or agent of the hospital, or (2) the hospital knew or should have known of the lack of informed consent and took no action. Court cases and individual state statutes have repeatedly upheld this last principle.

Nurses who are not independent practitioners may become involved in the process of obtaining informed consent in one of several ways. When one realizes that consent must be obtained for all procedures and treatments, not just medical procedures, one realizes the vast impact of this doctrine. This does not mean that nurses obtain written consent each time that they give an injection or turn a patient. Most nursing interventions rely on oral expressed consent or implied consent that may be readily inferred through the patient's actions.

What the doctrine of informed consent means is that nurses must continually communicate with a patient, explaining procedures and obtaining the patient's permission. What it also means is that the patient's refusal to allow a certain procedure must be respected. The healthcare provider should know the state laws on allowing the patient to refuse life-sustaining treatment. Even if the patient validly refuses life-sustaining treatment, the nurse could face charges for honoring or failing to honor this request. Each state has its own laws and applications of the laws. If the patient is unable to communicate, permission may be derived from the patient's admission to the hospital or obtained from the patient's legal representative.

Brazell[23] notes that the important challenge for nurses is to verify the patient's understanding of the information that has been provided before surgery. Simple ways to ensure the patient's understanding is to have the patient repeat in his or her own words what will happen during surgery and why surgery is necessary. Interpreters may be needed if English is not the patient's primary or first language.

Under the Americans with Disabilities Act of 1991, hospitals and healthcare facilities are required to provide interpreters for patients with sensory disabilities. A recent case that upheld a hearing-impaired patient's right to sue when she was denied access to an American Sign Language interpreter illustrates this fact.[24] In that case, a patient incurred two separate admissions to a suburban hospital within a 2-week time span. The court applauded the hospital for securing a sign language interpreter for the patient and her husband (both hearing impaired) but found the hospital at fault for not securing the interpreter immediately when the patient was admitted. The court also found the hospital at fault for not coordinating the interpreter's presence with the patient's physicians' visits, so that the patient and her husband could communicate with the doctors.

If interpreters are used, the nurse should first discover if the facility has an interpreter on staff and use that person for questions and verification of understanding. A family member who speaks both English and the patient's language may also be used, but is not preferred. There is no way to verify that the interpreter is actually translating what the nurse is saying or that the patient's responses are translated correctly for the nurse. Also, some patients are reluctant to give full medical information through a family interpreter, because the patient may not want the family members to know the full extent of the illness or surgery or are embarrassed to answer questions asked by family members. Interpreters employed by the facility will have a better understanding of medical terminology and the importance of relaying all information that the patient supplies.

When an interpreter is used, nurses should document what information was obtained or facts that were given, who served as interpreter, and how the nurse verified that comprehension took place. Nurses may ask simple questions and require that the patient answer the questions, or they may ask the patient to tell the nurse, in his or her own words, what to expect and why they are having surgery. Although virtually no cases have been filed in this area to date, causes of action based on noncomprehension and the failure to follow instructions due to nonunderstanding may be on the horizon.

A second way to enhance understanding is to allow time between the actual giving of information and when the patient must make a decision. Such time intervals allow patients to consider what has been suggested, to put into words their questions and concerns, and then make the final decision and sign the informed consent forms.

A very real concern for the nurse is in obtaining consent for the nursing aspects of medical procedures in which the primary procedure is performed by another practitioner. An example of such a concern is with postoperative care. Should the patient be taught about postoperative care before surgery, or should the nurse wait until after the surgery has been performed? Who is responsible for teaching postoperative care—the primary practitioner or the nursing staff? The answers from a legal perspective are far from clear. Possibly the best way to handle this dilemma is to wait until after the patient has consented to the surgical procedure for the nurse to give postoperative care information. This approach prevents interference with the physician-patient relationship and avoids potential conflicting explanations. Another approach is to have postoperative teaching materials and films developed to orient the patient to the entire procedure. This approach may be augmented by having a nurse available for questions or clarifications as needed. Many ASCs have now implemented this latter approach.

A third area of concern for the nurse is in obtaining informed consent for medical procedures provided completely by another practitioner. This obvious area of concern was perhaps the first one identified by most nurses. For years, nurses have been the healthcare providers obtaining the patient's consent for surgical or medical therapies performed by physicians. Some hospitals continue to permit nurses to obtain the patient's signature on the consent form. Other hospitals, in order to avoid this potential liability, prohibit nurses from obtaining signatures on consent forms.

It is important that nurses understand that physicians may legally delegate the responsibility of obtaining the patient's informed consent to the nurse. The physician delegates this task at his or her own peril, for most medical practice acts decree that the physician or independent practitioner is the responsible party for obtaining informed consent. Thus, any deficiencies in the informed consent that are obtained by the nurse may be imputed back to the responsible physician.

The nurse so delegated to obtain the patient's signature acts in the role of the physician or independent practitioner and must ensure that all material information is given to the patient in language that he or she can understand.[25] Therefore, the nurse may incur potential liability along with the delegating physician for the patient's informed consent.[26] Any additional information that the patient requests should be supplied by the physician, and the nurse is well advised to contact the physician immediately rather than attempt to talk a reluctant patient into the proposed procedure.

Because the nurse may be potentially liable for the failure to obtain informed consent when delegated to do so by the primary medical practitioner, many hospitals and healthcare centers now mandate that nurses may only witness the signature of patients. This means that nurses may accompany the surgeon and sign as a witness to the patient's signature only after the physician has first explained the procedure to the patient and met all requirements for informed consent. Witnessing the signature attests to the fact that the nurse saw the patient sign the form, there was no duress, and questions were answered by the primary practitioner.

An alternative form of witnessing the signature is to have all the necessary information given by the primary medical practitioner and a form signed when the patient actually presents to the ASC. Many centers contend that this is not obtaining informed consent, but merely witnessing the signature because the physician has already informed the patient about the surgery, complications, risks, and expected outcomes. Courts are divided on the issue of who actually obtained the consent in such cases. A better solution from a legal perspective is to ensure that informed consent forms are available in the physician's office and that the signed form is sent by the office to the ASC. Provision of the signed form to the ASC ensures that the primary practitioner is the one who has obtained the signature and that all necessary teaching has been done.

The nurse has an important role if the patient subsequently wishes to revoke his or her prior consent or if it becomes obvious that the patient's already signed, informed consent form does not meet the standards of informed consent. Most nurses have been faced with the problem of what to do when it becomes all too clear that the patient does not understand the procedure to be performed or believes that there are no major risks or adverse consequences inherent to the procedure. Remember that the nurse and the hospital may incur liability if there is reason to know that the standards of informed consent have not been met. In such a case, the nurse should contact his or her immediate supervisor and the responsible physician. Both entities need to be informed of the patient's change of mind or lack of comprehension.

Essentially two types of consent forms are presently in use. The blanket consent form that one is required to sign prior to admission is sufficient for care that is routine and customary. Routine and customary care may also be implied from the patient's voluntary admission into the hospital, so that this initial blanket consent form is only needed for insurance coverage and assignment of benefits.

Specific consent forms provide information, such as the name and description of the procedure to be performed, to be specifically named. Usually, the form also includes a section stating that: (1) the person who signed the form was told about the medical condition, risks, alternatives, and benefits of the proposed procedure; and (2) any and all questions have been answered. With this type of form the physician and hospital could show that no battery occurred because consent was given. However, the plaintiff may still be able to convince a court that informed consent was not given.

A second type of specific consent form attempts to prevent this latter possibility. This second specific type of form is a detailed consent form that lists the procedure, consequences, risks, and alternatives. Many states are now mandating this type of form through statutory medical disclosure panels.

Most of the latter forms have the following elements: (1) signature of the competent patient or a legal representative; (2) name and full description of the proposed procedure; (3) description of risks and alternatives of the proposed procedure, including nontreatment; (4) description of probable consequences of the proposed procedure; and (5) signatures of one or two witnesses according to state law. Interestingly, at least one court has held that this type of informed consent form also mandates that the physician must use the surgical technique that was promised to the patient and to which the patient consented.[27] In that case, the physician was found liable for not using mesh during a hernia repair when the consent form specified that mesh would be used.

The nurse with such detailed forms should remember three things. First, witnesses are not required to make the consent valid. Witnesses merely attest to the competency of the patient signing the form and to the genuineness of the signature, not that the patient had all the information needed to make an informed choice.[28] Although the nurse need not be the witness for the consent form to make it valid, if he or she does observe the signature and chart that such information was given at the time of the signing of the consent form, he or she would make an excellent witness in a pursuing medical malpractice case.

Second, consent may be withdrawn at any time. There is nothing in the written form that precludes the patient's right to withdraw his or her consent at will. Third, consent forms, although strong evidence of informed consent, are not conclusive in and of themselves. Several challenges have surfaced, including: (1) technical language that precluded the reasonable patient from understanding what he or she actually signed; (2) signature that was not voluntary but was coerced or forced; and (3) incompetency of the signer due to impairment by medications previously received.

Consent forms are considered to be valid until withdrawn by the patient or until the patient's condition or authorized treatments change significantly. Some hospitals use a 30-day guideline, but most hospitals prefer to have no set guidelines.

Equally important that the patient be given all material facts needed upon which to base an informed choice is that the correct person(s) consent to the procedure or therapy. Informed consent becomes a moot point if the wrong signature is obtained.

The basic rule is that if the patient is an adult according to state law, only that adult can give or refuse consent. Most states recognize 18 as the age at which one becomes an adult, although some actions might serve to classify the person as an adult before the legal age (e.g., in the case of marriage). The adult giving or refusing consent must be competent to either sign or refuse to sign the necessary consent forms. Competency at law means that: (1) the court has not declared the person to be incompetent; and (2) the person is generally able to understand the consequences of his or her actions. There is a strong legal presumption of continuing competency.

The actual determination of legal competency is not necessarily the function of the psychiatric medical staff. It is usually made based on the assessment of the person by a physician or other member of the healthcare profession. This assessment is often performed when the informed consent is requested. Consultation with other healthcare professionals is always a possibility and should be performed if there is: (1) underlying mental retardation; (2) an obvious mental disorder; or (3) a disease that affects the patient's mental functioning.

Courts generally have held that there is a strong presumption of continued competency. Such cases involved persons whose minds sometimes wandered, who were disoriented at times, and, in one case, an individual who was confined to a mental institution. Each time the court sought evidence to show that the person was capable of understanding the alternatives to the procedure as proposed and could fully appreciate the consequences of allowing or refusing consent to the procedure.[29]

Similar issues arise with the patient who desires to leave against medical advise (AMA) while in the postoperative phase of care. If it can be determined that he or she understands the full ramifications of that decision, then his or her signature would be valid on the AMA form. Nurses are advised to carefully document objective patient information when confronted by such a situation. If the patient has received sedatives, narcotics, or anesthesia, then the documentation should be clear as to the length of interval that has passed since the administration of the drug or drugs, and objective statements that the patient has made showing competency and understanding. If there is a doubt about the patient's ability to comprehend or to make sound judgments, then the documentation should show why the patient was not competent and what was done to protect the patient from harm or injury.

There are two exceptions to the legal adult's right to give or to refuse informed consent. The hospital must seek and abide by the decision of: (1) a court-appointed guardian; and (2) a person with a valid, written power of attorney. Such persons will present themselves to the hospital administration if they have previously been appointed and if the adult patient is incapable of giving or refusing consent.

Some persons are never adjudicated as incompetent by a court of law, and in selected states the family is asked to make decisions for the incompetent patient. For example, an automobile accident may render the patient incapable of making decisions and giving consent, and the physician will frequently ask the family about medical matters for the unconscious patient. The order of selection is usually: (1) spouse; (2) adult children or grandchildren; (3) parents; (4) grandparents; (5) adult brothers and sisters; and (6) adult nieces and nephews.

The practitioner is cautioned to validate state laws and judicial decisions, because family consent may not be valid consent in a few states. Lack of valid consent may become a court battle, especially if the practitioner acts upon family consent and there was disagreement among family members as to the course of action to take.

Most states recognize the child younger than 18 years of age to be a minor. Parental or guardian consent is necessary for medical therapies unless: (1) the emergency doctrine applies; (2) the child is an emancipated or mature minor; (3) there is a court order to proceed with the therapy; or (4) the law recognizes the minor as having the ability to consent to the therapy. Some states also allow in loco parentis or the ability of a person or the state to stand in the place of the parents. Look to statutory law to see who may consent in the absence of a parent. If there is a family consent doctrine, it will be a grandparent, adult brother or sister, or adult aunt or uncle. A newer trend is to allow minor parents to consent for their children's medical and dental treatments.

As with adults, the law applies the doctrine of implied consent with medical emergencies, unless there is reason to believe that the parents would refuse such therapy. An example could be the child of Jehovah's Witness parents. Medical personnel would have reason to believe that the parents might not consent to the giving of blood. The best course for the medical staff to follow if there is doubt about whether consent would be forthcoming is to seek a court order for the therapy unless there is a true emergency or life-threatening condition.

If the child's parents are married to each other or have joint custody, usually either parent can sign the consent form or make treatment decisions. If divorce results in a sole custody arrangement or in total abrogation of parental rights, then generally the parent with custody is considered the party to give or deny consent. Step-parents are allowed to give informed consent if the child has been legally adopted by that step-parent.

Emancipated minors are persons under the legal age who are no longer under their parent's control and regulation and who are managing their own financial affairs. Some states require the parent to completely surrender the right of care and custody of the child to prevent runaways from coming under this classification. Such emancipated minors may validly consent for their own medical therapies. Examples of emancipated minors are married persons, underage parents, or those in the armed service of their country. Some states allow college students, living away from their parents, to fall in this category.

Mature minors may also consent to some medical care. This is a relatiely new concept that is gaining legal recognition. The mature minor is one, between the ages of 14 and 17, who is able to understand the nature and consequences of the proposed therapy, and who is making his or her own decisions on a daily basis and is independent. The medical practitioner is encouraged to seek parental consent along with the consent of the mature minor in most circumstances. Such a practice aids in limiting potential liability and encourages family involvement.

Obtaining valid informed consent when the minor declares himself or herself to be emancipated or sufficiently mature to consent in his or her own stead can be problematic. The best course of action when there is a question of valid consent is to temporarily postpone any elective procedure or treatment until it is determined if the minor can consent for himself or herself within state law. If a true emergency presents, then the practitioner may proceed under an emergency consent doctrine. The practitioner should carefully document in the medical record existence of valid informed consent or the need for emergency care.

The law also recognizes the right of the minor to consent for some selected therapies without informing parents of the treatment. The reason for these exceptions is to encourage the minor to seek needed treatment. Informing the parents of the treatment might prevent the minor from receiving the necessary therapy. Cases for which the minor may give valid consent include: (1) the diagnosis and treatment of infectious, contagious, or communicable diseases; (2) the diagnosis and treatment of drug dependency, drug addiction, or any condition directly related to drug usage; (3) the need for birth control devices; and (4) treatment during a pregnancy so long as the care concerns the pregnancy. A caveat in this area is the issue of abortion. Some states allow the minor to sign for abortions arguing that abortions concern the pregnancy, and other states have held that abortions are outside the concerns of pregnancy. Nurses are encouraged to seek clarification from legal counsel within their given state.

PATIENT SELF-DETERMINATION

Patient self-determination involves the right of an individual to decide what will, or will not, happen to his or her body. Usually the right of self-determination is addressed in issues surrounding death and dying, but self-determination concerns all aspects of consent and its refusal.

The durable power of attorney for healthcare (DPAHC) or the medical durable power of attorney (MDPA) allows the competent patient to appoint a surrogate or proxy to make healthcare decisions for him or her in the event that the person is incompetent to do so. Power of attorney is a common law concept that allows one person (an agent) to speak for another (the principal) and is a concept of the agency relationship. At common law, the power of attorney terminated upon the death or incapacity of the principal. To prevent this occurrence when the patient most wanted the power of attorney to be effective, legislatures adopted the Uniform Durable Power of Attorney Act. This act sanctions the right of an individual to grant a durable power of attorney—one that would be valid even if the principal was incapacitated and legally incompetent.

Under most of the Durable Power of Attorney for Health Care Statutes, an individual may designate an agent to make medical decisions for him or her when the individual is unable to make such decisions. The power includes the right to ask questions, select and remove physicians from the patient's care, assess risks and complications, and the right to select treatments and procedures from a variety of therapeutic options. The power also includes the right to refuse care or life-sustaining procedures. Healthcare providers are protected from liability if they, in good faith, act on the agent's decisions.

Agents further have the authority to enforce the patient's treatment plans by filing lawsuits or legal actions against healthcare providers or family members. Agents have the right to forego treatment, change treatment plans, or consent to additional treatment. In short, they have the full authority to act as the principal would have acted. Thus, the durable power of attorney for healthcare is the best form of substituted judgment available for an otherwise incompetent patient.

In November 1991, the Patient Self-Determination Act of 1990 was enacted into law as part of the Omnibus Budget Reconciliation Act of 1990. This act was in direct response to the Nancy Cruzan case in Missouri, and it mandates that patients in "hospitals, skilled nursing facilities, home health agencies, and hospice programs" that serve Medicare and Medicaid patients must be queried about the existence of advanced directives and that such advanced directives must be made available to them if they so wish. ASCs have grappled with their role in meeting the intent of PSDA in their outpatient settings. See Chapter 3 for further discussion on regulatory compliance relating to this issue.

The act merely lets people know about existing rights and does not create any new rights for patients. The act does not change state law. The act may have served as an incentive for more states to pass DPAHC statutes, but it does not mandate such passage. The act does not require that patients execute advanced directives. It merely provides for patient education about such directives and provides assistance for those patients who wish to execute such directives. The legislation specifically states that providers may not discriminate against a patient in any way based on the absence or presence of an advanced directive.

Furthermore, the act does not legislate communication or conversation. Yet one of the purposes of the act is to encourage communication and conversation about existing directives, at a time when the patient is competent to understand and to execute advanced directives.

Some healthcare organizations have initiated do-not-resuscitate directives that patients may execute upon admission to healthcare institutions. Per the patient's request, the physician will then follow hospital policy in attaching such orders to the patient record. Most institutions require that there is documentation that the patient's decision was made after consultation with the physician regarding the patient's diagnosis and prognosis. The order should then be re-evaluated according to institution policy.

Patients who do not wish to be resuscitated may present for surgery in ASCs. If these patients were admitted to other hospitals, they would have valid do-not-resuscitate orders written. Reasons for which the patient may have surgical procedures is to prevent further pain and suffering or to improve the quality of the patient's remaining life. Medical staff and nurses are urged to seek clarification about the patient's do-not-resuscitate status before undergoing the surgical procedure, understanding that there is a significant difference between a cardiopulmonary arrest that occurs spontaneously and one that results from induction of anesthesia and invasive procedures.[30] Generally, patients will allow stabilization and aggressive treatment for the latter but do not desire full resuscitative procedures initiated for conditions not related to the administration of anesthetic agents. Clarification preoperatively is the key to understanding and giving appropriate care in such circumstances.

NURSES AS PATIENT ADVOCATES

As the nursing profession develops, it has become apparent that nurses owe a higher duty to patients than merely tending to their comfort and following a physician's orders. Professional nurses serve in the role of patient advocate. They develop and implement nursing diagnoses and exercise good judgement as they monitor the care given to patients by physicians as well as by their peers. This independent role of the nurse as a patient advocate has long been recognized by the courts, and court decisions continue to emphasize this vital function of nursing.

The professional nurse has a duty to report medical care or medical orders that jeopardize the care of patients. One of the first cases to illustrate this point was *Catron v The Poor Sisters of St. Frances.*[31] In this case, a patient was admitted for an unintentional drug overdosage. While in the hospital, the patient was intubated via a nasotracheal tube for several days before the tube was removed. He then had a tracheostomy to prevent respiratory failure. The patient brought this cause of action due to inability to speak in a normal voice after removal of the endotracheal tube and tracheostomy.

The hospital defended the case by asserting that it was medical judgment when to remove an endotracheal tube and how long one could remain in place without causing the patient harm. The court, in finding against the hospital and nursing staff, held that although a hospital is not usually liable for nurses following physicians' orders, an exception exists when the nurses know that the practice does not follow usual procedure. The nurses had an affirmative duty to report this deviation to their supervisors.

A more current case is that of *Dixon v Freuman.*[32] In this case, the physician ordered the removal of a Foley catheter and the nurses removed the catheter per hospital policy. When the patient brought suit that the catheter should not have been removed, the court held that in the absence of proof that the order to remove the catheter was "clearly contraindicated by normal practice," the nurses and hospital could not be held liable for the subsequent fistula.

Thus, nurses have a duty not only to question incomplete and illegible orders but also to question orders that deviate from the usual standards of practice and to inform hospital administration, via nursing supervisors and mid-management nurses, of such deviations. Fiesta suggests that this affirmative duty involves not only questions of competence or inappropriate medical decisions but also the reporting of "bizarre and disruptive behavior or conduct which may be a symptom of impairment."[33]

The duty to serve as a patient advocate may also require nurses to directly disobey the physician's orders. In *Cruzbinsky v Doctor's Hospital,*[34] a circulating nurse was ordered by the physician to leave the operating room before the patient had been sent to the PACU. While the nurse initially questioned the order, she finally left at the doctor's insistence. After her departure, the patient arrested, suffering significant permanent damage. The patient then brought suit against the hospital and nurse for abandonment.

The court held that the nurse had a duty to remain with the patient, following the hospital policy and procedure manual, even if the physician was insistent and "yelling at her." The court further concluded that this abandonment was so obvious that no expert witness was needed for the jury to conclude that abandonment had occurred.

Premature patient discharge is another area in which nurses have a duty to be the patient's advocate. Court cases such as *Wickline v California*[35] and *Wilson v Blue Cross of Southern California*[36] speak to the harm that can befall patients if discharged from acute care settings before they are sufficiently improved or stabilized. In the first case, the patient lost her leg due to infection, and in the second case a psychiatric patient committed suicide after his early discharge. While these two cases were directed at physicians and utilization reviewers, there seems little doubt that the courts would also extend such holdings to nurses who failed to serve as a patient advocate, speaking directly to the involved physicians and to nursing supervisors, when patients are discharged inappropriately. In the case of *Koeniquer v Eckrich,*[37] that was the court's holding. Nurses do have a duty to question physician's discharge orders or to delay the discharge if they believe that the discharge violates acceptable standards of care.

The issue of early discharge also addresses the crucial need for early and ongoing discharge planning and education of patients. In a home healthcare case, *Ready v Personal Care Health Services,*[38] a child was discharged from home healthcare services, developed pneumonia, and died. The parents brought suit, in part, for the failure of the nurses to adequately address potential complications and to educate the parents about the possibility of such life-threatening conditions. Table 9–2 gives a variety of educational tips that may assist in preventing potential liability in this area.

Nurses, especially those in ASCs and other outpatient clinic settings, have a duty to ensure that the responsible adult to whom the patient is discharged is not intoxicated or otherwise incapacitated. If nurses suspect the latter is true, using a good faith standard based upon presenting appearance, conduct, and communications of the responsible party, they have a duty to retain the patient until a friend or family

***Table 9–2.* Key Points in Education**

1. Patients should receive the majority of the needed education regarding both the surgical procedure and discharge information during the preoperative visit. Discharge information and education will also be done after the surgical procedure. Having heard the information at least twice and having the opportunity to ask questions at least twice will assist the patient and family to remember vital instructions. At least one study has concluded that patients do best when they receive needed information well before the day of surgery.[41]
2. Incorporate a variety of teaching methodologies into the educational sessions. This will assist in ensuring that all types of learners (visual, audio, hands-on) have ample opportunity to learn in the style that best suits them. Suggested methodologies include discussion, role play, question and answer, demonstration/return demonstration, and group interaction.
3. Incorporate a variety of teaching media into the educational session. Again, this is to assist individual learning styles. Videotapes, posters, booklets/pamphlets, and samples of actual equipment may be used. Essential instructions should be provided in both verbal and written format.
4. For special learners, such as those for whom English is not their primary language or for deaf patients or family members, the use of a facility approved interpreter or sign language facilitator is essential for learning sessions. The facility approved facilitator will understand medical terminology, ensure that all information is given to the patient, and correctly translate the patient's questions and answers so that the nurse can evaluate learning and understanding.
5. Incorporate adult learning principles as possible. Let the patient guide the teaching session based on his or her needs for education, how to order the content, and how much can be absorbed in a given session.
6. Use the information/discharge instruction forms to organize teaching and ensure that the patient and family understand the information contained on the form before discharge. Fill in the exact names, purposes, and times for scheduled medications so that the patient has a ready reference sheet at home. Document in the patient's chart all instruction forms that the patient was given prior to discharge or at discharge.
7. Document all teaching that is done. Include in the documentation how the nurse ensured that the patient understood the information as given or was able to perform necessary tasks, such as dressing changes at home. Appropriate answers to the nurse's questions or return demonstrations can be used to evaluate that learning has occurred.

member meeting the definition of responsible party is available to take the patient home. To protect the nurse, clear documentation in objective (not subjective) terms must be included in the patient's record.

Nurses have a duty to protect patients, to question orders that are inappropriate or likely to cause harm to the patient, and to provide adequate, early discharge education. In one study concerning the inability to interpret a physician's orders due to illegibility and incompleteness, it was found that 4% of the orders were totally illegible, another 16% were legible with great difficulty and time consumption, and 23% of medication orders lacked at least one essential component of the order, with route of administration being the most common omission.[40]

If directly speaking with the attending physician does not result in the desired outcome, then nurses have a duty to inform their supervisors and mid-management personnel so that other means of providing safe and competent healthcare may be obtained. Communication is vital, and interventions taken on behalf of patients should be promptly and adequately charted in the patient's record.

DOCUMENTATION

Patient Records

Perhaps the surest method of preventing potential malpractice suits is correct and proper documentation in the patient's record. The focus of documentation should be that the record is complete and adequate to demonstrate to third party readers that patient care met the prevailing standards of care.

Some areas to consider when documenting patient care include the following:

1. Make an entry for every observation, because the lack of documentation will allow the inference that no observation was conducted or noticed.
2. If the observation leads to the conclusion that medical personnel should be notified of a change in the patient's condition, then document everything that was done to ensure follow-up care. If a physician does not answer a page or decides not to order a new intervention, chart that there was no answer to the page or that no new orders were given at present. If the nurse truly cannot contact medical personnel, he or she should page the nursing supervisor and note that the supervisor was contacted.
3. Always make an entry, even if it is a late entry. Entries that are made timely are more likely to be a truer picture of what really happened, because time dulls the memory and nurses may be unable to recall exactly what was done and when it was done. If information is omitted, late entries

are acceptable and far superior to no entry. Chart the entry as soon as possible, and ensure that it is legible. If out of time sequence, note that a late entry is being made.

4. Never chart before providing care, taking vital signs, or administering medications, because there is no assurance that the care or medications will be accepted by the patient or that it will be given as the nurse intended to give the care. Likewise, vital signs recorded in advance of the time indicated on the chart may have changed drastically. More than one nurse who "charted ahead" that the patient had acceptable vital signs found himself or herself trying to explain why the patient had a blood pressure of 120/70 and was being resuscitated.
5. Use language that describes objectively and clearly. Remember that the person reading the charting should be able to reconstruct an accurate picture of the patient solely from the written communication. To prevent a possible issue of defamation, state the patient's behavior and responses objectively. Use language that is definite when charting about patients. For example, "in good condition" does not adequately describe the patient's status. "Patient awake, oriented, vital signs stable" does give an accurate description of the patient's current status.
6. Be realistic and factual in charting, particularly if the patient is noncompliant, verbally abusive, or physically violent. Recording what the patient actually states and how he or she acts may prevent a future lawsuit. Attorneys are understandably reluctant to pursue a malpractice suit when the patient prevented prescribed and necessary care by his or her behavior or stated repeatedly during teaching about postoperative medication that he or she had no intention of taking the ordered medications or performing the required dressing changes.
7. Nurses should chart only what they actually saw or did, not what other nurses said or reported. Because patient records may be used in various ways and for several purposes, the nurse who charts for another may not be able to recall particular information about the patient's care or special needs. If necessary, as in a code situation, then charting what others have done or what medications are given is essential.
8. Ensure that the chart is corrected by following facility policy and procedure to correct charts. Incorrect entries should be crossed out with a single line, leaving the original entry legible. Nurses should note why the entry was incorrect if necessary to ensure that subsequent readers of the chart will understand. If no information regarding why the entry was incorrect is necessary, then nurses can draw a single line through the entry and make a correct entry next to the lined-out entry. Often a misspelling or a wrong limb comprises the lined-out entry, such as when one changes the intravenous (IV) line from the left forearm to the right forearm.
9. Use standardized flowsheets or a checklist to ensure that charting is complete without having to write everything in longhand. A simple checklist approach is legal and sufficient for subsequent lawsuits that may develop. Leave no blank spaces in the checklist, lest it be inferred that the nurse failed to assess or complete necessary aspects of care.
10. Use only abbreviations approved by the facility to ensure that all who read the chart understand what is being communicated.
11. Identify the nurse who made the entry by signing with proper name and status.
12. Charting should include nursing diagnoses or observations, including potential complications that could occur in the postoperative setting. Also include in the record any care that pertains to prevention of such complications.
13. Include in the documentation patient care equipment that is utilized and procedures that are undertaken to ensure patient safety, such as side rails in place, call bells within easy reach of the patient, and so forth.

All documentation should be legible and neat, including one's signature and credentials. Printing is acceptable if the writer's handwriting is illegible. Neatness is essential because many attorneys for injured patients have drawn the conclusion that nurses who are sloppy in their charting are also sloppy and unprofessional in their nursing care. Although this last statement is not necessarily true, juries have been willing to find against nurses merely because of sloppy and illegible charting.

Incident (Variance) Reports

A second form of documentation is an unusual occurrence report, sometimes called an incident report or a variance report. These reports are created and designed to be part of the risk management process by allowing written documentation of issues that concern patient care in the aggregate. Documentation that is pertinent to the follow-up care after patient incidents or injuries, documentation that is needed to ensure the smooth functioning of all departments of the ASC, and documentation that is required to report occurrences not directly concerning patients may be found on incident reports.

Nurses are cautioned to remember that the purpose of incident reports is confidential and that no reference to the report should be included in the patient care record. Indication that a report exists may allow the report to be discovered by both parties to a lawsuit through incorporation by reference. The ideal incident report is a checkoff list, with a limited area for a brief written description of the occurrence and its follow-up by risk management personnel. An example is given in Figure 9–1.

Note that sufficient information is given to follow-up on the report, that the report is a single copy addressed to a specific person or department, and that no photocopies have been made of the report. Nurses complete the form using objective language of what occurred and patient care follow-up, as indicated. Language that would imply guilt or causation by individuals is excluded, and only observable facts are given. Patients' accounts are incorporated into the form by quoting exactly what is said by them. If more than one person observed the occurrence, then the report is signed by both nurses or staff members. Any actions taken to discover the extent of the patient injury, such as x-rays after a patient fall, are included.

Although every effort is made to prevent the incident report or unusual occurrence report from being discovered at trial, the nurse may still be asked if such a report was made. Because the Joint Commission for Accreditation of Healthcare Organizations (JCAHO) mandates such reports, most attorneys now know to ask about existing incident reports. The report then becomes discoverable to both sides of the complaint. For that reason, nurses should use objective, clear language throughout the report.

PROFESSIONAL LIABILITY INSURANCE

No discussion on risk management would be complete without a discussion on professional liability insurance. Such insurance transfers the risk of financial loss from the nurse to the insurance carrier. While nurses are included in general policies carried by individual ASCs or hospitals, there are cases in which the nurse could not benefit from this coverage. For example, if an issue arises with the state board of nursing and the nurse needs representation at a board hearing, the facility's policy does not provide for such coverage. Likewise, the nurse may no longer be in active employment at the facility and may not be covered under its policy. Thus, individual coverage is recommended.

An insurance policy (sometimes called an insuring agreement) is a formal contract between the insurance carrier and an individual or corporation. For a stated premium (fee per year), the insurance policy will provide the insured party or policy holder with a specific dollar amount of protection when certain injuries are caused by the person(s) insured by the policy. The conditions of the coverage and the extent of coverage are detailed in the policy itself.

Regardless of the policy chosen, there are some common elements of all professional liability policies. The policies provide payment for a lawyer to represent the insured nurse in the event of a claim or lawsuit. Most insurance carriers insist that the nurse use a lawyer whom the insurance company has on retainer, because this ensures both the nurse and the insurance carrier that the selected lawyer will be versed in medical malpractice issues. All policies specify the limits of legal liability. Insurance carriers will pay settlements or jury awards but will not cover the cost of any moral obligations that the nurse might feel he or she owes the injured party.

There are essentially two ways of classifying types of insurance policies. The first way is as occurrence-based insurance coverage. Occurrence-based policies cover the nurse for any injuries arising out of incidents that occurred during the time when the policy was in effect. This holds true even if the subsequent lawsuit is filed after the policy has expired and the policy was not renewed by the policy holder.

The second means of classifying insurance policies is as claims-made insurance coverage. Claims-made policies provide coverage only if an injury occurs and the claim is reported to the insurance company during the active policy period or during an uninterrupted extension of that policy period. An uninterrupted extension or "tail" allows the claims-made policy to be enforced for a specific period of time following the policy period.

The occurrence-based policy is preferable for most nurses, because lawsuits may not be filed immediately, particularly in cases involving

Special Instructions:
- Confidential - Do Not Duplicate
- Do not place or note in the medical record
- Send original to Risk Manager designee w/in 48hrs
- Do not release to any external agencies

Occurrence / Incident Report

Date & Time Report Filed:____________________

Department: ______________________ Phone: _______

Incident Date:____________ & Time:______ A.M. / P.M. Date Incident Identified:____________

A. Person Affected by The Occurrence

☐ Patient ☐ Visitor ☐ Physician ☐ Facility /Property ☐ Other

Name (Last, First, MI)	Date of Birth:	Gender: M F	Phone:
Address:	City/State/Zip:		
Patient Medical Record Number:	Referring Physician (if applicable):	Notified? Y N	
Diagnosis:			

B. Type of Incident / Occurrence (Circle all that apply)

Medications
200 Other
201 Wrong dose
202 Wrong patient
203 Reaction
205 Wrong time
206 Count/key
207 Omission
208 Wrong drug/IV solution
209 IV flow rate
210 Injection site
211 Transcription
212 Route
213 Procedure
214 Not mixed
216 Not ordered
217 Not infused
218 Allergy
219 Mishandled Controlled Substance

Other
100 Fall
400 Other
401 Self inflicted injury
402 Suicide attempt
403 Verbal dissatisfaction
404 Left AMA
405 Injured other pt/employee
407 Left Without Treatment/being seen
408 Burn (non-procedure related)
410 Property missing/damaged
411 Bruise/skin tear noted
412 Accident
413 Angry pt./family
415 Sprain/strain/fracture
416 Upset at long wait
417 Act Team
418 Pt. uncooperative
419 Sexual behavior
420 Injured while playing
421 Fainting / Seizure

Procedure
301 Refused
303 Preparation
305 Misdiagnosis
306 Omission
307 Injured during
308 Lost specimen
309 Untoward Reaction
310 Incorrect count/no count
311 IV infiltrate/reseal
314 Ate/medicated before exam
317 Wrong test/procedure/x-ray
320 Not drawn/redrawn
321 Unnecessary
324 Equipment
325 Oxygen ran out
328 Bruise/red area
334 Chipped tooth
335 Duplication
337 Needle stick
342 Injection site
345 Break in sterile procedure
346 Unable to complete procedure
375 Other

Complications
500 Other
501 Return to procedure
502 Bleeding
503 Unplanned admission
504 Code blue/Cardiac Arrest
505 Cardiac event
506 Neuro event
507 Respiratory event
508 Infection
509 Death
510 Prolonged Post-op course

Non-clinical Procedure
300 Other
302 No ID band
304 Wrong patient
312 Repeat films missing
313 Needles left out
315 Not entered/wrong
322 Stamped wrong/mislabeled
323 Delay/late
329 Wrong time
330 Wrong doctor
331 Charting
332 Not notified
338 Request not received
339 Page not answered
341 MD not notified
343 Unable to interpret
344 Confidentiality
350 Incorrect procedure scheduled
351 Improper consents
352 Inconsistent H&P

C. Equipment Involved in The Occurrence (If applicable) - Secure equipment and all disposables and wrappers involved. *Do not send for repairs or allow vendor to examine/repair. Contact Risk Manager.*

Equipment ______________________ Vendor __________________ Manufacturer's ID ________________

Figure 9–1. Example of an occurrence/incident report.

D. Objective Statement of Facts Surrounding the Occurrence. (Do not draw conclusions or state opinion.)

____

____

____

____

____

Witness (s) 1. ____________________ 2. ____________________

Report Completed By:	Report Date:

E. Outcome of Incident "☐" Check all that apply:

- ☐ No apparent injury
- ☐ Loss of limb/digit
- ☐ Vascular phlebitis
- ☐ Dental impairment
- ☐ Cardiac/Resp arrest
- ☐ Contusion/laceration
- ☐ Neurologic impairment
- ☐ Psychologic impairment
- ☐ Drug reaction
- ☐ Injury to/loss of organ
- ☐ Death
- ☐ Hematoma
- ☐ Blindness
- ☐ Infection
- ☐ Concussion
- ☐ Hemorrhage
- ☐ Foreign Body
- ☐ Asphyxiation
- ☐ Sprain/Strain/Fracture
- ☐ Wound Dehiscence

F. Treatment Required *☐ None ☐ Invasive procedure ☐ Non-invasive procedure ☐ Hospital Care (ER or Admit)*

(Please explain)____________________

G. Occurrence Follow-Up Determine what action should or can be done to prevent this occurrence:

____

____

____

Team Leader/Manager Signature:	Date Reviewed:

INCIDENT REPORTS TO RISK MANAGER WITHIN 48 HOURS OF IDENTIFICATION

H. FOR USE BY RISK MANAGER:	
RM Designee Signature: Date Reviewed:	Risk Manager's Signature: Date Reviewed:

		Code # & MPI code	Reported	
GRAVE	A			Posted: ________
MAJOR	B			Card: ________
MINOR	C			Claim #: ________
NO ADVERSE	D			

Figure 9–1 *Continued*

children and neonates. Claims-made coverage is adequate if the policy is continuously renewed and kept active or if a "tail" is purchased for extended coverage. If there is doubt regarding needed coverage, the insurance agent should be consulted.

There are several sections in a policy contract. The first part of the policy is known as the declarations. Included under this section are the policy holder's name, address, covered professional occupation (e.g., general staff nurse, advanced family nurse practitioner, or emergency center staff nurse), and the covered time period. This section also lists the company's limits of liability coverage and state requirements for information that may modify the policy.

The insurance policy should have a section marked "Limits of Liability." This section usually has language about two separate dollar figures. For example, it could read $500,000 for each claim and $1,000,000 for the aggregate, or $1,000,000 for each claim and $3,000,000 for the aggregate. These dollar figures indicate what the insurance company will pay during a given policy period. The company will pay up to the lower limits for any one claim or lawsuit and up to the upper limits of the policy during the entire policy period.

Deductibles include any amounts that the insurance carrier deducts from the total amount available to pay for the plaintiff's damages. Some policies deduct the amount paid for the nurse's legal defense from the total limits of liability.

Exclusions are items that are not covered in the insurance policy. In professional liability policies, such exclusions frequently describe circumstances or activities that will prevent coverage of the insured party. Exclusions also include the absence of appropriate licensure or certification. These exclusions may be covered in the policy under the general title Reservation of Rights, so entitled because the company reserves the right to deny coverage once the facts are known. When and if it is determined that a restricted activity has been involved, then the insured nurse must reimburse the insurance company for incurred expenses of legal defense. Other insurance companies insist that the insured nurse pay all expenses out of pocket until it is shown that an excluded activity has not been involved.

Some of the more common examples of excluded activities involve inappropriate behavior including: (1) criminal actions; (2) incidents occurring while the insured was under the influence of either drugs or alcohol; (3) physical assault, sexual abuse, molestation, habitual neglect, licentious and immoral behavior toward patients whether intentional, negligent, inadvertent, or committed with the belief that the other party was consenting; and (4) actions that result in punitive damages to the plaintiff. More recent additions to the aforementioned list include exclusion for the transmission of AIDS/HIV from the healthcare provider to a patient and exclusions for expanded roles in nursing. This last exclusion is sometimes worded as exclusions for liability incurred in the position of proprietor, superintendent, or executive officer of a clinic, laboratory, or business enterprise. Exclusions also include any claims or suits resulting from the practice of a profession that does not appear on the certificate's declarations. Nurses should alert their insurance company when there is a change in professional status to ensure that the nurse is fully covered during the policy period.

Terms in the coverage section indicate when the insured is actually covered and for what activities. Policies that have fairly broad coverage sections include language similar to the following: ". . . professional services by the individual insured, or by any persons for whose acts or omissions such insured is legally responsible . . ." will be covered in this policy. Such verbiage indicates that the insured person is covered both for his or her own actions and for actions performed by nurses under his or her direct and indirect supervision. This coverage is vital for nurses who hold supervisory positions, such as nursing supervisors, charge nurses, and nursing faculty.

Defense costs are included in most policies. These include all reasonable and necessary costs occurred in the investigation, defense, and negotiation of any covered claim or suit. Most companies pay these in addition to the limits of liability. Additionally, if the nurse is required to appear before the state board of nursing or a governmental regulatory agency, the company will pay attorney fees and other costs resulting from investigation or defense of the proceeding, up to $1000 per policy period. This latter amount is in addition to the coverage limits.

The section on covered injuries outlines the types of injuries and provisions that the insurance company will honor. Insurance companies usually include personal (bodily) injury, mental anguish, property damage, personal injury to a patient such as invasion of privacy, libel, and slander, and economic damages as covered injuries. The lawsuit must specifically note that the suit is for monetary damages. In other words, the insurance company will cover the cost of litigation and awards if monetary damages are involved. The insurance company will not cover the cost of litigation if the action sought is a specific performance as in the case of a lawsuit brought to prevent a nurse practitioner from performing medical acts. *Sermchief v Gonzales* is a good example of such a specific performance lawsuit.[41]

The Sermchief case was brought by a group of medical doctors who contended that nurse practitioners, working in rural areas of Missouri, were exceeding the scope of the nurse practice act in both recommending and prescribing birth control medications and devices to their patients. The doctors alleged that the nurse practitioners were thus practicing medicine without a license and, rather than monetary damages, they sought to prevent nurse practitioners from performing such services in the future. The Supreme Court of Missouri, after reviewing both the nurse practice act and the intent of the legislature when the wording of the nurse practice act was passed, ruled in favor of the nurse practitioners and stated that these nurses were well within the scope of acceptable nursing practice.

A Supplementary Payments section includes provisions for additional payments to the insured party. Some policies may supplement lost earnings or reasonable expenses incurred by the insured as well as the cost of appeal bonds and costs of litigation charged against the insured. These latter provisions may also be termed defense costs.

Conditions or Coverage Conditions outline the insured nurse's duties to the insurance carrier in the event that a claim or lawsuit is filed, provisions for cancellation of the policy, prohibition of assignment of the policy, and subrogation of rights. Many insurance policies will only cover the policyholder if he or she gives written notice to the insurance carrier immediately upon the filing of a claim or lawsuit and forwards to the insurance carrier every demand, notice, summons, or other process received.

Also included in this section are the nurse's right to select counsel and the right to request a settlement. Most policies allow the insurance carrier to settle without the policyholder's consent and deny the policy holder the right to retain counsel apart from the insurance company. As explained under general provisions, most insurance companies prefer to retain attorneys known to have expertise in medical matters, rather than allow the insured the right to obtain an attorney who is unknown to them.

Should a nurse have individual professional liability coverage or should the nurse rely upon the employer's insurance policy in the event of a malpractice action? Many nurses have been assured by hospital administrative staff and by competent lawyers that one can depend upon the hospital's insurance policy to cover the nurse in the event of a subsequent legal action. However, the actual truth is that those nurses who relied upon hospital policies most often were not adequately protected monetarily nor were they adequately represented by legal counsel in the lawsuit.

There are several reasons for the aforementioned statements. First, many institutional liability insurance policies have limited coverage and only cover employees while they are performing work as hospital employees. Second, the hospital's policy is designed to meet the needs of the large institution, and hospital attorneys may not be able to protect the individual nurse's best interests. For example, the hospital may elect to settle out of court rather than pursue a particular case, even though the nurse's best interests can only be served through a court hearing. Also, should the hospital wish to bring an indemnity claim against the nurse for the incident that triggered the lawsuit, the hospital policy will not cover the nurse nor will it pay for his or her representation. Indemnity claims are those brought by the employer for monetary contributions from the nurse or nurses whose actions or failure to act caused the original patient injury.

Finally, most hospital insurance policies do not have supplementary payments for the nurse-defendant. This means that if the nurse incurs additional expenses while investigating the claim or loses days of work defending the claim, then he or she must cover the expenses out of pocket.

Employer-based coverage, though, is a good starting point for the prudent nurse. The nurse should ask to either see and read the hospital policy or ask about specific provisions in the employer-sponsored coverage and then acquire his or her own individual coverage to augment the employer's policy. The nurse should also take into consideration the following factors: (1) the type of nursing that he or she normally does (staff versus charge versus supervision); (2) the monetary amount of the average awards in his or her particular geographic area; (3) the unit or type of nursing in which he or she normally works, and (4) the propensity for lawsuits against nurses in that same geographic area. The hospital attorney can provide the nurse with information regarding trends in malpractice in his or her locality. Then the nurse should find a policy that provides the necessary coverage. The nurse can extend coverage as his or her job status changes or as he or she expands practice roles.

There is, on the other hand, no good reason for nurses to be caught in a lawsuit without professional liability insurance. A favorite argument of many in-hospital attorneys is to remind nurses that they are more lawsuit prone if they have an individual insurance policy. In today's society the nurse is, in essence, the conduit either to the hospital's potential liability or to the physician's potential liability through the doctrine of respondeat superior or through a dual servant role. In fact, in some state tort reform acts, the amount of economic liability against individual defendants may be limited. Thus, nurses may find themselves named in more, not fewer, lawsuits as attorneys seek means to find additional sources of revenue for injured clients.

It is immaterial to the patient bringing the lawsuit whether or not the nurse has insurance. When the injured party originally files the lawsuit, he or she has no idea of whether or not the nurse is insured. But it should matter greatly to the nurse, because the cost of defense could very well financially destroy an individual nurse. In most states the judgment remains open until satisfied or dropped. That means that a nurse may be paying on a prior judgment for several years after the judgment, or in states that allow garnishment of wages for adjudicated debts, that one's wages may be garnished for several years after the initial judgment.

SUMMARY

This chapter has highlighted the concept of risk management with selected legal concepts. Nurses are encouraged to be an active part of the ongoing risk management program within the ambulatory surgical center, remembering that adherence to sound legal practice may be the best way of ensuring continuing, competent care for all patients.

References

1. *St. Paul Medical Center v Cecil,* 842 SW 2nd 809 (Texas, 1992).
2. *Healthtrust v Cantrell,* 689 So 2nd 822 (Alabama, 1997).
3. *Stark v Children's Orthopedic Hospital and Medical Center,* Case no. 87-2-12416-9. Medical Malpractice Verdicts, Settlements, and Experts 9(10):28, 1990.
4. *Beltran v Downey Community Hospital.* Medical Malpractice Verdicts, Settlements, and Experts 8(5):30, 1992.
5. Guido GW: Legal Issues in Nursing, 2nd ed. Stamford, CT: Appleton & Lange, 1997.
6. Murphy EK: Types of legal claims brought against perioperative nurses. AORN 65(5):972–973, 1997.
7. *Nicole Adams v Children's Mercy Hospital,* Case no 73867. 1992.
8. *Crosby v Sultz,* 592 A2nd 1337 (Pennsylvania Superior Court, 1991).
9. *Eyoma v Falso,* 589 A2d 653 (New Jersey, 1991).
10. *Parker v Bullock County Hospital Authority,* Case no. A90A0-762. Medical Malpractice Verdicts, Settlements, and Experts 6(10):28, 1990.
11. *Manning v Twin Falls Clinic and Hospital,* 830 P2d 1185 (Idaho, 1992).
12. *Ybarra v Spangard,* 154 P2d 687 (California, 1944).
13. *Shahine v Louisiana State University Medical Center,* 680 So2d 1252 (La. App., 1996).
14. *Baca v Valez,* 833 P2d 1194 (App. New Mexico, 1992).
15. *Baca v Velez,* 833 P2d 1194 (App. New Mexico, 1992), at 1197.
16. *Perna v Pirozzi,* 457 A2d 431 (New Jersey, 1983).
17. *Heinecke v Department of Commerce, Division of Occupational and Professional Licensure,* 810 P2d 459 (Utah App., 1991).
18. *Johnson v Amethyst Corporation,* 463 SE, 2d 397 (N.C. App., 1995).
19. *Schloendorff v Society of New York Hospitals,* 211 NY 125, 105 NE 92 (1914).
20. *Truman v Thomas,* 27 Cal.3d 285, 611 P2d 902 (1980).
21. Rozovsky FA: Consent to Treatment: A Practical Guide, 2nd ed. Boston: Little, Brown, 1990.
22. *Petriello v Kalman,* et al, 576 A2d 474 (Connecticut, 1990).
23. Brazell NE: The significance and application of informed consent. AORN J 65(2):377–386, 1997.
24. *Negron v Snoqualmie Valley Hospital,* 936 P2d 55 (Wash App., 1997).
25. *Grabowski v Quigley,* 684 A2d 610 (Pa. Super., 1996).
26. *Hoffson v Orentreisch,* 543 NY2d 242 (New York, 1989).
27. *Lugenbuhl v Dowling,* 676 So2d 602 (La. App., 1996).
28. Switzer KH: Informed consent for inserting a CVC. AJN 95(6):66–67, 1995.
29. In re Milton, 29 Ohio App.3d 20, 505 NE 2d 255 (Ohio, 1987).
30. Golanowski M: Do not resuscitate: Informed consent in the operating room and postanesthesia care unit. Post Anesthesia Nurs 10(2):9–11, 1995.
31. *Catron v The Poor Sisters of Saint Francis,* 435 NE2d 305 (Indiana, 1982).
32. *Dixon v Freuman,* 573 NYS2d (New York, 1991).
33. Fiesta J: Failing to act like a professional. Nurs Man 24(8):15–17, 1994.
34. *Cruzbinsky v Doctor's Hospital,* 188 Cal. Rept. 685 (Cal. App., 1982).
35. *Wickline v State of California,* 192 Cal. App. 3d 1630, 239 Cal. Rept. 810 (1986).
36. *Wilson v Blue Cross of Southern California,* 222 Cal. App. 3d 660, 271 Cal. Rept. 876 (1992).
37. *Koeniquer v Eckrich,* 422 NW 2d 600 (South Dakota, 1988).

38. *Ready v Personal Health Care Services*, Case no. 842472 (California, 1991).
39. Caldwell LM: The influence of preference for information on preoperative stress and coping in surgical outpatients. Appl Nurs Res 4(11):177–183, 1991.
40. Winslow EH, Nestor VA, Davidoff SK, et al: Penmanship related to error risk. Heart Lung 26(2):158–163, 1997.
41. *Sermchief v Gonzales*, 600 SW 2d 683 (Missouri, en banc 1983).

Chapter 10

Latex Sensitivity

Joan Bauer

WHAT IS LATEX?

Latex is natural rubber. *Dorland's Dictionary*[1] defines latex as "a viscid, milky juice secreted by some seed plants." More than 200 plant species produce latex, including poinsettia and milkweed, but the latex for manufacturing purposes is derived from the milky sap of the *Hevea brasiliensis* plant.[2–5] The sap from the plant is treated with a stabilizer, such as ammonia, so that it does not coagulate. Accelerators, activators, antioxidants, and chemicals such as sulfur are added to increase flexibility and strength.[6, 7]

Hardening agents are added to produce vulcanized rubber such as that used for automobile tires, hockey pucks, and various pieces of medical equipment, but liquid latex is used to manufacture gloves and other rubber products that require flexibility. The liquid latex is sent to factories where it is centrifuged to remove some of the proteins, and this liquid is then stored in large vats for up to 6 months for curing. The time taken for centrifuging differs with various manufacturers, and the length of time determines how many proteins are removed—the longer the time, the more proteins are removed. This is important because proteins are thought to cause an allergic response, although accelerators and activators may also cause allergy.

During the glove manufacturing process, molded hand-shaped forms are dipped into liquid latex and then partially dried.[4, 8] After drying, the latex-coated forms are bathed in hot water to remove more of the proteins; the length of time of the washing determines the amount of proteins removed. The washed, latex-coated forms are dried in large ovens; donning powder may be added at this stage because products made from natural rubber latex may stick to each other when handled. Talc is generally used as a surface treatment because it gives a very smooth feel, but medical gloves are powdered with a bioabsorbable starch such as cornstarch powder. Slater[9] states that allergies can occur from latex protein in gloves. A report from a 1987 study by Fisher[10] stated that cornstarch powder itself contains no detectable protein, yet it has been associated with allergic reactions.

As the dried gloves are removed from the molded forms, they are turned inside out, causing the outside of the gloves to become the inside once the gloves are removed from the drying forms. The gloves are immediately packaged and sterilized by γ-radiation or gas sterilization using ethylene oxide; they are not autoclaved, because autoclaving affects the protein content and the integrity of the gloves. Because the gloves have been turned inside out when they are removed from the forms, much of the remaining protein is on the outside and can cause problems for healthcare workers and patients.

Latex consists of rubber hydrocarbons, water, lipids, proteins, and carbohydrates, but only the proteins in the latex appear to be the primary cause of an allergic response.[3, 5, 6, 11, 12] It is thought that the manufacturing process may fail to remove all of the soluble proteins that could cause an allergy. With the advent of universal precautions in the 1990s, there was a sudden increased demand for gloves. To meet the increased demand, the manufacturers may have speeded up the manufacturing process by shortening the time taken to wash away allergy-causing proteins.[2, 3]

ALLERGIC RESPONSE

What Is an Allergic Response?

An allergic reaction is any harmful immunologic reaction that causes tissue injury.[13] It is a reaction in which the body reacts with an exaggerated immune response to a foreign substance. It is caused by the release of vasoactive substances such as histamine, kinins, and prostaglandins from tissue mast cells and circulating basophils.[3]

Types of Allergic Responses

Hypersensitivity reactions are categorized into four types: Type I is the most severe. It is an immediate, local, or systemic reaction that is mediated by immunoglobulin gamma E (IgE) antibodies and can cause anaphylaxis. This is aggravated by the type and amount of allergen, the portal of entry of the allergen, and the duration of exposure. Type II is a cytotoxic reaction, meaning that a toxin or antibody exerts its action on a specific target organ (e.g., nephrotoxicity). Type III is immune complex; and type IV is a cell-mediated delayed response. Type IV reactions, or local skin reactions with redness, itching, swelling, and rash, occur mainly in healthcare workers.[5, 9, 14–18] Type IV response is aggravated by accelerators, surfactants, antioxidants, and glove powder. Hypersensitivity reactions to latex are classified as immediate hypersensitivity (anaphylactic symptoms) and delayed hypersensitivity (allergic contact dermatitis). A severe life-threatening allergic reaction is defined as anaphylactic or anaphylactoid, depending on the mechanism that causes the release of these mediators.[5, 14–15] The clinical presentations are identical.

True anaphylaxis (type I) is mediated by IgE.[3] This means that an allergic antibody is made in response to something in the environment that attaches to the mast cells and causes them to release histamine. Clinical manifestations include systemic anaphylaxis and atopic allergy such as hives, eczema, wheezing, conjunctivitis, contact urticaria, and angioedema. An anaphylactoid or pseudoallergic response is nonimmunologic.

There are three clinical stages of sensitivity. Contact dermatitis is characterized by local redness and edema. Contact urticaria syndrome exhibits rhinitis, nasal pruritus, wheezing, or blisters. Systemic reactions are characterized by hives, edema, conjunctivitis, asthma, and anaphylaxis.

Risk Factors for an Allergic Response to Latex

Persons with a history of asthma or atopy that includes multiple allergies to foods, drugs, or environmental factors are at increased risk for allergic reactions. Food allergies of special note for those potentially allergic to latex are allergies to tropical fruits such as bananas, pineapple, avocado, and water chestnuts, and, to a lesser degree, kiwi, apricots, grapes, cherries, and peaches.[2, 3, 19–27] Others who are at risk are persons with frequent exposure to latex, such as healthcare workers who wear rubber gloves, rubber industry workers, and restaurant workers who wear gloves.[6, 14, 16, 28–34] Reactions in healthcare workers are usually type IV reactions. Multiple or frequent exposures to a substance can increase the chance of a reaction as can the interval between exposures.[2, 3, 16]

The highest risk of type I reactions occurs in children with myelodysplasia and myelomeningocele or those with urogenital abnormalities.[3, 5] These patients undergo multiple operative procedures during which mucous membranes come in contact with latex gloves, or these children require frequent catheterizations during which latex catheters and gloves come into contact with mucous membranes, so that they are at a higher risk for developing latex sensitivity.[13, 35–39] Patients with spina bifida are often exposed to latex during surgical interventions during the first week of life, thus increasing their risk. Additionally, these patients require frequent bowel disimpactions with rubber gloves, which increases exposure to latex.

Clinical Manifestations of an Allergic Response to Latex

During an allergic response, skin changes such as erythema, rash, flushing, urticaria, itching, and edema may occur. Symptoms of dizziness and malaise, hypertension, tachycardia, cardiac dysrhythmias, neurologic changes, and confusion may be present. Respiratory symptoms may occur, including dyspnea, coughing, sneezing, wheezing, stridor, bronchospasm, angioedema, and laryngeal edema. The person may also have nausea, vomiting, diarrhea, abdominal pain, and even clotting defects.[3, 16, 17] Initially, these responses may go undetected, particularly if the person is undergoing anesthesia.

Routes of latex antigen exposure can be cutaneous, mucosal (contact and inhalational), and parenteral (intramuscular or intravenous). Irritation reactions may appear as dry, crusty, hard bumps that occur gradually over days and may be caused by antiseptics, scrubbing solutions, or frequent handwashing.[18, 32, 40–50] Chemical allergy may manifest as dry, crusty bumps with fewer lesions or horizontal cracks and may be caused by accelerators or other chemicals used during the glove manufacturing process.[12] Local skin reactions may appear as redness, itching, swelling, rash, and scaling, which occur several days after contact (type IV reactions).

Protein allergy (type I reaction) may manifest within minutes to hours as moist, pink, raised hives blanched in the center. These hives may spread from the hands to all over the body.[19] There may be swelling of the eyelids, lips, face, and respiratory tract; hypotension; or anaphylaxis. It is unclear whether persons with mild responses can become more sensitive if they are exposed repeatedly to latex, but some studies have shown a pattern of increased sensitivity that results in anaphylaxis.[45, 51]

Symptoms involving the mouth and oral mucous membranes, which may occur after eating tropical fruits, are similar to the skin reactions but are most likely to lead to systemic reactions.[45] The larynx and throat may be involved, and laryngeal edema may occur during such reactions. Type I reactions to protein are the most dangerous. These reactions occur immediately and include responses such as generalized flushing, nausea and vomiting, urticaria, watery eyes, sneezing, wheezing, stridor, and bronchospasm and can progress to hypotension, tachycardia, dysrhythmias, shock, cardiorespiratory arrest, and death.[3–5, 19, 46, 49, 52, 53]

Reactions may appear intraoperatively, and identification of the responsible agent can be difficult.[46–49, 53–54] One thing that seems to distinguish a latex-induced reaction is the delayed response after the start of the surgical procedure. In one study by Gold and colleagues,[39] the earliest time of onset was 50 minutes after the induction of anesthesia. Intraoperative reactions may be manifested by changes in vital signs, peak inspiratory pressures, oxygen saturations, and changes in end-tidal CO_2.[18] During surgery, these symptoms can be mistaken for reactions from other causes such as anesthetic drugs and other medications given during the operative procedure.[41] For this reason, a thorough health history including investigation into possible latex sensitivity should be conducted before administering an anesthetic agent.

Treatment of an Allergic Response to Latex

For those with a localized response, the best treatment is prevention of further exposure to latex. In the event of a generalized response, it is essential to stabilize the patient and stop the exposure to the latex, maintain the airway, administer 100% oxygen, and discontinue the anesthetic agents if the patient is already undergoing anesthesia.[2, 3, 5, 21, 55] Intravascular volume expanders are given because hypovolemia occurs rapidly owing to the loss of intravascular fluid into the tissue spaces. Epinephrine (5 to 10 μg/kg) given intravenously reduces bronchospasm and hypersensitivity reaction; subcutaneous or intramuscular routes may be used in less severe reactions. Doses of epinephrine may need to be repeated or increased. An infusion of epinephrine is indicated for refractory hypotension. According to Holzman,[18] "Doses of epinephrine recommended for resuscitation during cardiac arrest are not the same as those required for the treatment of anaphylaxis and may lead to severe supraventricular tachycardia requiring resuscitation." Secondary treatment consists of the administration of antihistamines, catecholamines, aminophylline, and corticosteroids.[2, 3, 18, 21, 48]

Incidence of Latex Allergy

Latex gloves are readily available and inexpensive.[2] Healthcare workers who wear latex gloves are at increased risk for developing hypersensitivity to latex. A study by Turjanmaa[30] found that 7.4% of doctors and 5.6% of nurses were allergic to latex. In 1992, Gonzalez[41] reported that 3% of hospital nurses and doctors are sensitive to latex. Kelly[2] reported that of 250 million people in the United States, 3 million are sensitive to latex. According to Kelly, "Being in the hospital is like standing in a ragweed field of latex" because of all the products containing latex used in hospitals. Persons who are sensitive to latex may also be allergic to formaldehyde or to ethylene oxide that may be used for sterilizing products used in the operating room.[3, 14, 42]

Allergic reactions to latex have been reported from the use of condoms, balloons, anesthesia equipment, tourniquets, barium enema tips, finger cots, and other products in the community such as rubber toys, swim caps, bath mats, sports equipment, and clothing. (See Table 10–1 for a partial listing of hospital products that may contain latex and Table 10–2 for a partial listing of products in the community that may contain latex.) It is interesting to note that "latex paints are water soluble and acrylic based and contain no latex."[5]

Table 10–1. Items in the Perioperative Environment That May Contain Latex

Endotracheal tubes	Paper operating room attire with adhesive
Nasal airways	Occlusive dressings
Anesthesia masks	Gloves/finger cots
Mask straps	Nasogastric tubes
Anesthesia hoses/tubing	Drains/chest tubes/ostomy tubes
Anesthesia machine bellows	Ostomy appliances/straps
Manual resuscitation bags and masks	Renal dialysis equipment
Monitoring electrodes	Intra-aortic balloons
Bladder catheters	Clamp covers
Rubber catheters in prep trays	Intravenous tubing injection ports
Gloves in prepackaged packs	Back check valves
Bulb syringes in prepackaged packs	Volume chamber ports
Sampling port in catheter bags	Heparin lock ports
Leg straps	Syringes
Adhesive tape/elastic tape	Tourniquets
Band-Aids	Moisture pads
Elastic bandages	Sanitary belts
Ace wraps (brown)	Rubber bands
Paper drapes with adhesive	Bite blocks
Patient identification bands	Enema kits
Blood pressure cuff/tubing	Epidural trays
Stethoscopes	Antigravity splint devices
Wheelchair tires	Oximetry adhesive finger wrap probes
Wheelchair arm pads	Antigravity splint devices
Crutch handles	Splints with foam rubber lining
Pulmonary catheters	

Data from Kelly,[2] Setlock,[3] Markey,[17] Holzman,[18] Barton,[19] Young and Associates,[49] and Brown.[56]
The above is a partial listing and is not intended to cite all possible products that may contain latex.

Table 10–2. Products in the Community That May Contain Latex

Balls	Hot water bottles
Balloons	Handlebar grips on bicycles and tricycles, other sports equipment
Beach balls	Handlebar grips on stationary cycles, rowing machines, and other exercise equipment
Bathing caps	Rain gear
Beach thongs	Rubber boots
Swim/snorkeling gear	Foam pillows/pads
Shower caps	Air mattresses/water flotation mattresses/waterbed mattresses
Bath mats	Wheelchair tires
Bath tub/shower decals	Wheelchair arm pads
Kitchen gloves	Crutch handles
Sink drain plugs	Rubber seat rings
Rubber bands	Elastic or elastic thread in clothing
Bulb syringes/eye droppers	Pantyhose
Art supplies/adhesives	Shoes
Chewing gum	Condoms
Baby bottle nipples/pacifiers	Diaphragms
Teething rings	Erasers
Rubber pants and pads	Waterproofing paints
Disposable diapers	Antifreezes
Crib mattress pads/liners	Repellents
Toys	Fungicides
Makeup (foam tip applicators)	
Some soaps/shampoos	
Handles on tools, racquets, golf clubs	

Data from Kelly,[2] Setlock,[3] Markey,[17] Holzman,[18] Barton,[19] Young and associates,[49] and Brown.[56]
The above is only a partial listing and is not intended to cite all possible products that may contain latex.

Prevalence of Latex Allergy

Nutter first reported latex allergy in 1979.[28] It was confirmed by skin-prick testing by Turjanmaa in 1984.[29] During the 1980s and early 1990s, there were multiple reports of urticaria in healthcare workers[30–34]; anaphylaxis from reactions to barium enema tips[48, 49]; occupational asthma in healthcare workers[17] and in rubber industry workers; epidemic clusters in spina bifida patients in Milwaukee, Wisconsin[2]; and reports of latex allergic responses in Canada.[44] The cluster cases reported in Milwaukee were later attributed to an intravenous volume chamber system that contained a rubber floating valve.[2]

There may be many reasons why the problem of latex allergy has become more prevalent in recent years. One explanation may be that the problem was not recognized as latex allergy in the past or that increased awareness has led to increased reporting. As mentioned earlier, the use of universal precautions led to the increased use of gloves and, therefore, increased exposure to latex. Additionally, the increased demand for gloves may have led to speeding up of the manufacturing process, causing more of the proteins that produce an allergic reaction to be left in the latex.

Testing for Latex Allergy

Markey[17] reported that no commercially licensed or standardized latex allergen *skin* tests are available commercially, and Kelly[14] reported that there is no latex *skin* test extract approved by the Food and Drug Administration (FDA) for testing. Methods have been developed to test for latex allergy, but all of the tests include the potential for a full systemic reaction.[52] A skin test may be used in which a drop of latex extract is diluted in saline, placed on the skin, and scratched with a needle. If the person is allergic, a wheal will develop within 10 minutes. A test called the use test involves placing the wetted finger of an individual into one finger of a glove; if two to three wheals appear on the contact area after 15 minutes, the test is considered to have a positive result. The intradermal test is similar to the skin prick test, but the test solution is more dilute and is injected intradermally. Sensitive persons show localized erythema after about 10 minutes.

The radioallergosorbent (RAST) test is a laboratory test. Serum is separated from a blood sample and mixed with the latex concentrate, and the specimen is examined to identify the amount of binding between the IgE antibodies and the latex antigen.[2, 3] However, this test is more expensive, not widely available, and unreliable in 53% of cases.[53]

The FDA has cleared for marketing the first test to measure latex antibodies in *blood*. The test, ALASTAT, is a latex-specific IgE allergen test available in a kit made by Diagnostic Products Corporation of Los Angeles. The test is to be used on people who are suspected of having had an allergic reaction to latex. It is not recommended for screening purposes.

Transmission of the Latex Antigen

The latex antigen can be transmitted through direct skin contact (cutaneous), direct mucosal contact, parenteral exposure, or inhaled ambient particles in the air.[3, 17, 19, 21, 34, 50] Intraoperative anaphylaxis from latex hypersensitivity has been reported frequently in the literature.[20, 49, 53, 57–61] Thus, latex allergy can be a problem for personnel and for patients in the operating room, because latex is a common component of surgical and anesthesia equipment.[2, 3, 62, 63] Avoidance is the only method that has been shown to prevent latex-induced anaphylaxis.[2]

PREVENTION OF LATEX EXPOSURE

Administrative Policies

It is important to develop administrative policies and procedures for the care of latex-sensitive healthcare workers and patients.[2, 3, 17, 19, 49, 58, 59, 63] These should be developed collaboratively by an interdisciplinary task force with representatives from every department working toward making the institution safe from latex and decreasing exposure for patients and healthcare workers.[2, 3, 17–19, 50, 59–61] (See Table 10–3 for a sample policy.)

Because latex dust is present in the hospital, a latex-sensitive patient should be placed in a private room, preferably one that is isolated from the rest of the hospital's ventilation system. In ambulatory surgery centers (ASCs) and freestanding ambulatory surgery centers (FASC), the patient should be placed in a room away from other patients in order to avoid exposure to latex products. Initially, known latex-sensitive patients were brought into the hospital and their procedures were performed in the main operating room; however, more of these patients are being treated in ASCs and freestanding facilities. The decision as to whether a

Table 10–3. Management of Latex-Allergic Patients

PURPOSE: To identify the methods necessary to provide a safe environment for the nursing care of the latex-allergic/sensitive patient, to avoid anaphylactic reactions related to latex sensitization, and to ensure a positive patient outcome.

POLICY: All patients will be questioned during the preadmission/preprocedure interview about any previous reaction to latex products to identify those at risk. A history of topical reaction to latex may indicate that the patient is at high risk for a perioperative allergic reaction.

Latex-free alternative products will be identified and available for care of the latex-sensitive person. Any known latex-allergic patient will be cared for in a latex-free environment.

PROCEDURE:

Identify high-risk populations:

Healthcare professionals (or others with occupational contact with latex)
People with spinal cord injuries, spina bifida, myelodysplasia, and chronic illness
People with history of multiple reconstructive surgeries
People with urologic deformities or conditions requiring multiple catheterizations
Those with history of intraoperative anaphylactic reactions
Possible: People with atopic dermatitis, eczema, or fruit allergies

Identify people with allergic histories:

Preadmission or preprocedure assessment will include questioning about prior allergic reactions. The response is documented on the patient's record, and any positive history is also communicated immediately to the surgeon, anesthesia personnel, and perioperative nursing team. Tables 10–1 and 10–2 provide insight as to some of the products that may contain latex in the home, community, or healthcare setting.

A latex-free cart is kept in the operating room corridor and contains supplies and equipment that are known to be latex free. For any potentially allergic patient, the following patient care protocols will be instituted.

1. Post latex allergy signs on the door to the patient's room and at the foot of the patient's stretcher.
2. Place a latex allergy sticker on front of the medical record and a latex allergy identity bracelet on the patient.
3. Provide sterile nonlatex gloves in all sizes.
4. Use a nonrubber tourniquet for venipunctures.
5. Tape intravenous injection ports to avoid an inadvertent puncture when administering medications. Place inline stopcocks for use when administering intravenous medications.
6. Avoid use of volume control chambers that contain rubber injection ports or floating valves.
7. Remove rubber stoppers from multidose medication vials, and withdraw medication directly from vials. Use all-plastic syringes.
8. Use medications from glass ampules that can be snapped open. Do not use medication from prefilled glass syringes, because a rubber stopper is punctured to initiate the injection.
9. Avoid rubber anesthesia equipment.
10. Rinse ethylene oxide–sterilized endotracheal tubes in saline before use; rinse nonlatex suction catheters if they have been sterilized in ethylene oxide.
11. Wrap the patient's arm with gauze or cotton before applying a tourniquet cuff or blood pressure cuff; wrap tubing so that it does not touch the patient's skin.
12. Wrap cords for the pulse oximeter and temperature monitoring equipment.
13. Use silicone instead of latex or red rubber bladder catheters or suction catheters.
14. Avoid use of red rubber bulb syringes for irrigation/suction.
15. Avoid use of Penrose drains or other rubber drains.
16. Use clear or silk tape; do not use paper tape or adhesive.
17. Use white cotton Ace wrapping, not a brown Ace wrapping.
18. Use gauze dressing with clear tape or a transparent dressing.
19. Schedule latex-allergic patients as first case in the day, before other cases during which latex products are opened, thus contaminating air with latex particles.
20. Ensure that patient allergies are communicated fully to all team members.

Data from Barton E: Latex-allergy: Recognition and management of a modern problem. Nurse Practitioner 18(11):54–58, 1993; Brown J: Latex allergy requires attention in orthopaedic nursing. Orthop Nurs 13(1):7–11, 1994; and Markey J: Latex allergy implications for healthcare personnel and infusion therapy patients. J Intravenous Nurs 17(1):35–39, 1994.

Adapted from and reprinted with the permission of Morton Plant Mease Health Services, Palm Harbor, Florida.

known latex-allergic person is an appropriate candidate for the FASC setting should be made by a multidisciplinary group with consideration given to emergency resources. Nevertheless, patients with unknown latex sensitivity may present in the ambulatory center; thus, personnel must be knowledgeable about latex allergy and equipped to handle an allergic reaction if it occurs.

A latex allergy bracelet should be placed on the patient on admission, and a latex allergy sticker should be displayed prominently at the front of the chart or medical record. Patient information on latex allergy should be placed in the pharmacy database, and drugs dispensed for latex-allergic patients should be labeled with a latex allergy sticker.

Nonlatex products should be used when caring for these patients. Representatives from the materials supply department, using information from product manufacturers, can assist with developing a list of nonlatex products that are safe for use. These lists need to be updated continually because manufacturers' products change, suppliers change, or supplies on backorder are substituted with supplies from a different vendor.

Prevention of Latex Exposure for Healthcare Workers

Healthcare workers wear gloves on a daily basis to protect themselves from blood and body fluids and, in the operating room, to maintain sterile conditions during surgical procedures.[64] Latex gloves have been used because they are tear resistant and strong. They have good elastic properties and only minimally inhibit the sense of touch, and they also provide a good protective barrier.[4, 8, 58]

According to Russell,[8] latex provides nine times the barrier protection of synthetic substances such as vinyl. Barton[19] cites a 1989 FDA report that says that the barrier that prevents filtration of blood-borne pathogens can be compromised within 60 seconds if a person is exposed to products containing mineral oil or petroleum. Healthcare workers need to be informed of the reduction in protection of nonlatex gloves from blood-borne pathogens. The use of powder-free gloves can prevent ambient particles containing the antigen from floating in the air.[2, 3]

Korniewicz[65] presents criteria for selecting quality latex gloves in addition to the quality-control measures of the manufacturer. Important glove characteristics include barrier integrity, cost, personal comfort and fit, sensitivity, basic research about the brand, and evidence of clinical tests related to the brand. For the latex-sensitive healthcare worker, however, vinyl or other nonlatex gloves are readily available and should be provided.

Sensitized healthcare workers should not be exposed on a daily basis. Kelly[2] recommends that sensitized healthcare workers stop personal use of latex; wear a medical alert identification bracelet, medal, or tag; and submit to testing and respiratory symptom monitoring. Employers should make reasonable accommodations for these individuals. Institutions should change to powder-free gloves or nonlatex gloves to decrease exposure. The employer must provide the employee the opportunity and experience to work within Occupational Safety and Health Administration (OSHA) standards.

Prevention of Latex Exposure for Patients

Preoperative Assessment

A detailed patient history is the best way to identify high-risk patients.[2, 3, 19, 49] Patients or parents of children should be questioned about history of asthma or allergies to food or drugs. If food allergy is mentioned, question patients or parents further about specific allergies to tropical fruits or oral symptoms after eating fruits, because oral symptoms are usually the first indication that a person is allergic. One should obtain information about dermatitis or eczema and about any localized or respiratory response to rubber products, such as pacifiers or balloons or any specific symptoms (e.g., local erythema, itching, hives, swelling, sneezing, runny nose, itching and tearing eyes, coughing, wheezing, or chest tightness) after previous contact with rubber products. A specific question to ask is one about problems with swelling of the lips after a visit to the dentist. Adult patients should be questioned about any local swelling and itching after the use of condoms or diaphragms.

If any of these symptoms are found in the history, findings should be communicated to other perioperative providers and documented in the chart, including details such as the patient's signs and symptoms of reaction, the treatment and medications received, and the procedure performed. It is important to determine if any immunodiagnostic tests were performed. The patient may require a referral to an allergist for follow-up testing. It is imperative to be vigilant when caring for these patients, but one must be prudent and not falsely "label" a patient. This could cause the potential for problems with health insurance coverage or obtaining specific employment in the future.

Prophylactic Premedication Regimes

Kelly[21] states that "the utility of premedication is unclear." It can be effective for prevention of radiocontrast dye reactions, but "use of medications has not been recognized to block IgE-mediated reactions." Premedication may lessen the severity of intraoperative reactions but not the frequency. However, premedication with antihistamines is recommended by some.[37, 58] Merguerian and associates[54] recommend that a regimen of antihistamine, diphenhydramine, cimetidine, and prednisone be started 24 hours before the scheduled surgery. Slater reported that "Premedication with corticosteroids, H_1 agonists, ephedrine and, in some series, H_2 agonists, has been used to prevent or ameliorate anaphylactoid reactions to radiocontrast media" and recommended in 1990 that this regimen be used before major surgical procedures in patients allergic to rubber.[9] Since then, Slater has reported that he is "aware of several cases in which anaphylaxis has occurred in rubber-sensitive individuals in spite of medical prophylaxis."[5, 54, 57, 66] According to Kelly,[2] although premedication may lessen the severity of a reaction, it may also allow a longer length of exposure to the anitgen, and this can lead to increased sensitization and an increased response later. Therefore, it remains important to avoid antigen exposure.

Potential Allergens in the Perioperative Phase

Many products in the operating room can potentially cause an allergic response.[2, 3, 17–20, 49–51] Nonlatex products such as muscle relaxants, hypnotics, and opiates may cause an allergic reaction, although this is rare. More commonly, antibiotics, blood products, and volume expanders can cause an allergic response, as can implantable devices such as vascular grafts. Latex-containing products such as anesthesia equipment, monitoring equipment, and intravenous equipment are widely used during surgical procedures and can cause reactions in hypersensitive patients. Patients can also be exposed to latex products in preoperative and postoperative areas, in the laboratory, and also in the radiology department.

Perioperative Patient Management

Intraoperative Patient Management

There are many suggested techniques to prevent latex exposure in the perioperative environment.[2, 3, 17, 19, 49, 62, 63] Patients with known latex allergy should be noted on the operative schedule. These patients should not go to a preoperative holding area where they could be exposed to latex products. When the patient arrives at the operating room, a latex allergy sign should be placed on the patient's stretcher, bed, or crib, as well as a sign on the door of the operating room where the procedure is to be performed so that persons will not bring latex supplies into the room. Guidelines for latex allergy precautions should be displayed prominently in the operating room.

It is advisable to assign these patients as the first case of the day to prevent exposure to ambient particles in the air from latex gloves used during preceding cases. There was a case report by Kelly[2] in which a woman experienced an anaphylactic reaction as soon as she was wheeled into the operating room before even being moved to the operating table. Multiple packages of gloves had been opened during the previous procedure in that room, and she inhaled ambient latex particles that were still present in the air.

Some institutions maintain one dedicated operating room stocked entirely with nonlatex products for use with these patients. If this is not feasible, every attempt should be made to clean the operating room thoroughly and allow extra time after the previous case before bringing a latex-sensitive patient into the room. According to Kelly,[2] it takes about 1 hour for the ventilating system to clear ambient latex particles from the air. A cart can be maintained in the operating room that contains all nonlatex supplies for use during the operative procedure (Table 10–4). It is advisable that patients with known latex allergy have anesthesia personnel present even during a local procedure so that aggressive treatment can be initiated immediately if an allergic response occurs.

If endotracheal tubes have been sterilized with ethylene oxide, it is advisable to rinse them with saline before use, even though this may be controversial regarding effectiveness. Ensure that no rubber touches the patient. Depending on the type of pulse oximetry in use, wrap the patient's finger in plastic wrap. Wrap the arm with gauze before placing the blood pressure cuff and wrap the tubing with gauze so that it doesn't touch the patient's skin. Protect the patient's skin from monitoring lead wires. Cover cautery tips with gauze or a stockinette. Tape the patient's eyes and endotracheal tube with nonlatex tape. Wrap black rubber anesthesia hoses to prevent them from touching the patient, or use nonrubber disposable equipment. Use clear vinyl rather than a black rubber bag and mask for an unintubated patient.

Table 10–4. Suggested Contents of Nonlatex Products Cart in the OR

List of latex precautions guidelines
List of signs and symptoms of an allergic response
Guidelines for treatment of an allergic response
Latex precaution signs to post on door to operating room
Latex allergy patient bracelets
Latex allergy chart labels
Latex allergy medication labels
Various sizes of nonlatex sterile gloves
Various sizes of single-hand vinyl gloves
Various sizes of nonlatex tape
Various sizes of pediatric and adult airways
Adult and pediatric nonrubber manual resuscitation bags/masks
Unsterile straight hemostat and metal can opener to remove rubber ports and stoppers
Male Luer Lok caps (sterile)
Glass syringes
Disposable sterile stopcocks
Disposable stethoscopes
Unsterile Webril or cotton wrap
Stockinette
Isolation gowns without latex
Sterile nonlatex operating room drapes
Intravenous tubing sets and extension sets
Nonlatex urinary catheters
Patient gowns in adult and pediatric sizes
Nonlatex suction catheters
Nonlatex temperature monitoring devices
Nonlatex warming blankets

The above is a suggested list; other nonlatex items may be used.

Because the latex protein is water soluble, contact with intravenous fluid could actually wash the antigen into the patient's circulation; therefore, flush the intravenous tubing thoroughly before initiating the infusion. Putting a needle through a rubber port can cause minute rubber particles to fall into the solution. Use intravenous tubing without rubber ports, or cover the rubber ports with tape to prevent inadvertent injection. Use three-way stopcocks placed in line for medication administration. An intravenous filter does not prevent latex from entering the infusion line, because the latex proteins are small enough to pass through a filter.[21] If a volume administration chamber is used, remove the rubber medication administration port and place a male dead-end device. Some manufacturers now make latex-free tubing which is preferable to the other processes described.

Do not withdraw from or inject drugs through any rubber stoppers. Administer drugs drawn up directly from a glass ampule. If multidose vials must be used, remove the rubber stopper before drawing out the contents. A straight clamp and a metal can opener work well to remove the metal ring around the top of the vial and to pull out the stopper. Prefilled glass syringes containing narcotics or other medications should not be used, because a rubber stopper is punctured to initiate the system. Nonglass syringes also contain rubber plungers, thus the medication should not be allowed to sit for any length of time in the syringe. Draw up the drug, and administer it immediately. Supply narcotics in glass ampules from which the tops can be snapped off and the medication withdrawn.

Postoperative Patient Management

Unless there is an isolation room stocked with nonlatex products within the postanesthesia care area, latex-allergic patients should be recovered in the operating room where the procedure was performed to prevent exposure to latex particles in the air in another room where latex products are being used for other patients. Before entering the operating room to care for the patient during recovery, postanesthesia care unit (PACU) personnel must change into fresh scrubs and cover jackets and remove identifications pins and watches that may have bands containing latex. They should wash their hands thoroughly before entering the room to remove all latex and glove powder from their hands. Some institutions maintain a separate isolation room within the PACU and stock it with all nonlatex products. Other institutions that do not have a separate nonlatex PACU maintain a latex precautions box of postanesthesia supplies to take to the operating room for use during the recovery phase (Table 10–5).

According to standards set forth by the American Society of Perianesthesia Nurses, two licensed nurses should recover the patient in the operating room.[67] This could be two postanesthesia nurses or one postanesthesia nurse and an operating room nurse. Often, the patient is still receiving oxygen via the anesthesia machine, and the oxygen saturations and vital signs are being monitored with the operating room equipment, thus it is imperative that postanesthesia personnel learn to use the equipment prior to the time of need. Suction equipment used in the operating room may differ from that used in the PACU, and the nurses recovering the patient must be able to use the equipment rapidly and efficiently. The postanesthesia nurses must observe the same intravenous and medication administration techniques and latex precautions as those used during the surgery.

Table 10–5. Suggested Contents of PACU Box to Take to the Operating Room for Recovery

LATEX-FREE
Adult and pediatric size oxygen cannulas and oxygen masks
Oxygen tubing
Styrofoam cup for pediatric oxygen administration
Suction equipment and tonsil tip suction apparatus
Various sizes of oral airways
Disposable medication syringes
Disposable tuberculin syringes for pediatric medication administration
Diapers
Nonlatex pacifiers and nipples; glucose water
Blood-drawing equipment and Vacutainer needles
Disposable stethoscope
Nonlatex thermometer
Adult and pediatric patient gowns
PACU record/charge slips
Red and black pens as appropriate

PACU, postanesthetic care unit.

DOCUMENTATION

One should document on the medical record (operating room record and postanesthesia record) that latex precautions were maintained throughout the patient's care. It is best to avoid using the term "latex free" in charting, because that is difficult to guarantee and to prove. Kelly[2] recommends the term "latex safe," because it is almost impossible to make an operating room totally free of rubber. Rubber cords for anesthesia machines and for other equipment lie on the floor; however, these do not come into direct contact with the patient.

DISCHARGE INSTRUCTIONS

Patients, parents, or an accompanying responsible adult should be given oral and written information explaining latex allergy, including signs, symptoms, and risk.[68] Patients should be instructed to wear a medical alert bracelet or an identification tag on a necklace indicating their latex allergy and warned about problematic foods, especially tropical fruits.[3] Patients should be taught about rubber products to avoid at home and in the community (see Table 10–2), such as rubber toys or adhesive glues at school or daycare. Adhesive carpet glues should not be a problem once carpeting has been installed and the glue is dry; however, during the actual glue application process, it is advisable that the latex-sensitive individual avoid the area until the glue has dried and the room has been well ventilated.

Kelly[2] recommends that patients be given a supply of sterile nonlatex gloves to take home with them to have available if needed. They must be taught to inform future healthcare providers of their condition and to notify staff at the dentist's or doctor's offices so that they can supply a latex-safe environment. Patients should carry nonlatex gloves with them to appointments and keep a supply of these gloves in the car.

Teach patients with known latex allergy how to protect themselves from future latex exposure and allergic reactions. Upon physician's order instruct them fully in the use of autoinjectible epinephrine and the use of bronchodilators, and caution them to have these readily available at home, at work, at school, and in the car. Patients should be prepared and be alert to the potential of latex exposure when going to hotels, restaurants, gymnasiums, and the like. If the patient is a child, tell parents to inform school officials of the child's condition, signs, symptoms, and treatment should a reaction occur. Parents should also inform grandparents, daycare providers, and baby sitters.

Patients having had orthopedic procedures must take special precautions with rubber crutch handles, wheelchair arm pads, and rubber wheel rims.[56] It is also interesting to note that products labeled hypoallergenic do not necessarily protect from latex exposure; therefore, it is important to read all labels carefully.

Instruct adult patients about condoms and diaphragms that contain rubber. Unfortunately, "latex condoms are the only proven barrier to the sexual transmission of human immunodeficiency virus and other sexually transmitted diseases."[5] An article by Fisher[10] suggested double sheathing with rubber and lambskin condoms, with the rubber condom on the outside for the rubber-allergic man and on the inside for the rubber-allergic woman. Slater believes that this method may be "unwise until objectively tested" because of the high degree of sensitivity in rubber-sensitive patients.[5] Patients should be counseled to weigh the risk of an allergic response from rubber and the risk of a sexually transmitted disease.

REPORTING

Reports of anaphylaxis associated with a latex product should be reported directly to the FDA through the Medical Device Problem Reporting System.[2, 7, 17] This is a mandatory reporting system for cases where death or serious injury may have been caused by a medical device or

***Table 10–6.* Phone Numbers to Call to Report Allergic Reactions to Latex**

United States Food and Drug Administration (FDA-Med Watch):	Telephone 1-800-FDA-1088
Centers for Disease Control and Prevention (CDC)	Telephone 1-800-311-3435 or 1-404-639-2888
For information: Latex Allergy News 176 Roosevelt Ave. Torrington, CT 06790	Telephone 1-860-482-6869

equipment. The FDA and its branch, the Practitioner Reporting Program (PRO), list more than 1000 reports documenting latex sensitivity reactions.[6] The top three product-related complaints reported involved barium enema tips, latex examination gloves, and surgeons' gloves (see Table 10–6 for contact information).

EDUCATION

Healthcare workers must be cognizant of latex allergy and alert for its manifestations. (See Table 10–7 for Key Educational Points.) Education and training should be provided to all healthcare workers. Personnel should be provided with education about reactions and treatment and instructions on how to prevent latex exposure for themselves and for allergic patients. It may be necessary for healthcare workers who are sensitive to latex to relocate to other work areas if they cannot avoid latex exposure on the job.

Those working in employee health departments are responsible for disseminating information about latex allergy to employees. Healthcare workers' participation in educational sessions should be documented, and a record should be maintained. According to Thompson,[40] "We are likely to see more occupational disorders surface, and thus, it is important that a means of effectively dealing with such problems be developed to protect both patients and healthcare workers." Kelly states that "as latex allergy in workers becomes more common, an evaluation for occupational exposure contributing to the sensitization of the patient is necessary."[21] Patients or healthcare workers with respiratory symptoms may not be able to continue working in the same environment. Thompson[40] recommends that healthcare workers who are sensitized be moved to areas where they are not exposed to latex. Occupational health workers and worker's compensation analysts must be thoroughly educated in order to best serve these persons.

Healthcare administrators and employee health personnel must view latex allergy as an occupational disorder that, if left untreated, can rob them of valuable experienced staff and may result in worker's compensation disability claims, lower productivity, and absenteeism. Kelly notes that many individuals have needed to seek legal counsel on these matters, and he suggests that the patient's allergist must be willing to support the patient through these struggles.[2, 21] Latex-allergic healthcare workers have developed support groups to provide emotional and educational reinforcement. Likewise, similar support groups have developed for patients with spina bifida.

The Internet now provides a wealth of information for healthcare workers and the public regarding latex allergy (Table 10–8). As with all information gleaned from the Internet, the user should ascertain the reliability of the source.

FUTURE RESEARCH

Kelly[2] indicates that future research should center on developing a standard, safe skin test

***Table 10–7.* Key Educational Points**

1. Latex is natural rubber and can be found in many products in the healthcare environment and in the community.
2. Persons with latex allergy may be asthmatic or exhibit allergies to multiple substances. Oral symptoms after eating fruit should be carefully investigated, because many persons who are allergic to fruit are also allergic to latex. It is imperative to take a thorough patient health history.
3. Every attempt should be made to keep the allergic patient's healthcare environment free of latex gloves and other equipment that may contain latex.
4. Develop administrative policies and procedures for management of patients and healthcare workers who are allergic to latex.
5. Provide patient discharge instructions/teaching packets on latex precautions and the treatment for an allergic reaction.
6. Provide educational inservices for healthcare workers regarding the management of latex-allergic patients and employees.
7. Provide nonlatex gloves for latex-allergic employees; provide alternative employment for those unable to work in an environment where latex products are routinely used.

Table 10–8. Internet Sites for Latex Allergy Information

http://allergy.mcg.edu/physicians/ltxhome.html 85 West Algonquin Road, Suite 550 Arlington Heights, IL 60005	Latex home page of American College of Allergy, Asthma and Immunology (ACAAI)	Clinical information
http://www.aaaai.org/ 1-800-822-2762	American Academy of Allergy, Asthma and Immunology	Clinical information
http://www.execpc.com/~alert/index.html Toll-Free: 1-888-97ALERT (972-5378) FAX: (414) 677-2808	American Latex Allergy Association (A.L.E.R.T., Inc.)	Many links to other sites, Crash Cart list, names and telephone numbers of many suppliers of non-latex products, OSHA updates
http://www.cdc.gov/niosh/homepage.html	Centers for Disease Control and Prevention, National Institute for Occupational Safety and Health (CDC–NIOSH)	Latex issues related to employment
http://www.fda.gov/	Food and Drug Administration (FDA)	Federal alerts and reporting mechanisms
http://www.cpsc.gov/	US Government Consumer Product Safety Committee	Reporting mechanisms
http://www.anesth.com/lair/lair.htm	Anesthesia Department, Case Western Reserve	Clinical information and links to other databases

reagent. He recommends further research on hypoallergenic gloves and also research into the role of food allergens and latex allergy. He suggests investigation into coating of gloves and development of creams that can be used as topical skin barriers under gloves to prevent skin contact with latex.

SUMMARY

Latex allergy remains a growing threat for healthcare professionals and sensitized patients. Medical schools and nursing schools need to include information on latex protein allergy as part of the curriculum. Healthcare administrators and employee health personnel must be ever cognizant of new developments and communicate changes and protocols to their personnel in order to protect patients and healthcare workers. Employees with known latex protein allergy must make every effort to protect themselves from latex exposure. Healthcare workers must take the time to screen their patients by conducting a thorough patient history and then must take every precaution to protect sensitized patients from latex exposure. Educational information about latex protein allergy must be provided for patients, healthcare workers, and the community. Emphasis should be on prevention of exposure to latex, because avoidance to exposure is the only certain way to prevent a latex allergy reaction.

References

1. Dorland's Illustrated Medical Dictionary, 28th ed. Philadelphia: WB Saunders, 1994, p 903.
2. Kelly KJ: Latex allergy (Oral presentation). Madison, WI: St. Mary's Hospital Medical Center, 1994.
3. Setlock M: Allergy and anesthesia (Oral presentation). Brookfield, WI: WISPAN 5th Annual Fall Seminar, September 1993.
4. Source to Surgery (videotape) Ansell Medical, a Pacific Dunlop company. Madison, WI: St. Mary's Hospital Medical Center, 1994.
5. Slater JE: Allergic reaction to natural rubber. Ann Allergy 68:203–211, 1992.
6. Subramaniam A: The chemistry of natural rubber latex. Immonol Allergy Clin North Am 15:1–43, 1995.
7. Truscott W: The industry perspective on latex. Immunol Allergy Clin North Am 15:89–121, 1995.
8. Russell C: Ansell Medical: Oral presentation on latex glove production. Madison, WI: St. Mary's Hospital Medical Center, 1994.
9. Slater JE, Mostello LA, Shaer C, et al: Type I hypersensitivity to rubber. Ann Allergy 65:411–414, 1990.
10. Fisher AA: Contact urticaria and anaphylactoid reaction due to cornstarch surgical glove powder. Contact Dermatitis 16:224, 1987.
11. Kurup VP, Murali S: Latex antigens. Immunol Allergy Clin North Am 15:45–59, 1995.
12. Yuninger J: Variances in antigenicity of latex products. Immunol Allergy Clin North Am 14:70, 1995.
13. Dorland's Illustrated Medical Dictionary, 28th ed. Philadelphia: WB Saunders, 1994, p 47.

14. Kelly KJ, Kurup VP, Reijula KE: The diagnosis of natural rubber latex allergy. J Allergy Clin Immunol 93:813–816, 1993.
15. Leynadier F, Pacquet C, Dry J: Anaphylaxis to latex during surgery. Anesthesia 44:547–550, 1989.
16. Fritsch DE, Frederick-Pilat DM: Exposing latex allergies. Nursing 93:46–48, 1993.
17. Markey J: Latex allergy: Implications for healthcare personnel and infusion therapy patients. J Intravenous Nurs 17:35–39, 1994.
18. Holzman R: Latex allergy: An emerging operating room problem. Anesth Analg 76:635–641, 1993.
19. Barton EC: Latex allergy: Recognition and management of a modern problem. Nurse Pract 19:54–58, 1992.
20. Swartz J, Braude BM, Gilmour RF, et al: Intraoperative anaphylaxis to latex. Can J Anaesth 37:589–592, 1990.
21. Kelly KJ: Management of the latex allergic patient. Immunol Allergy Clin North Am 15:139–174, 1995.
22. Ceuppens J, Van Durme P, Dooms-Goosens A: Latex allergy in patients with allergy to fruit. Lancet 339(8791):493, 1992.
23. Lavaud F, Cossart C, Reiter V, et al: Latex allergy in patients with allergy to fruit. Lancet 339:493, 1992.
24. Rodriguez M, Vega F, Garcia MT, et al: Hypersensitivity to latex, chestnut and banana. Ann Allergy 70:31–34, 1993.
25. Fernandez de Corres L, Moneo I, Mjnoz D, et al: Sensitization from chestnuts and bananas. Ann Allergy 70:31–34, 1993.
26. Anibarro B, Garcia-Ara M, Pascual C: Associated sensitization to latex and chestnut. Allergy 48:130, 1993.
27. Crist G, Belsils D: Contact urticaria for latex in patient with immediate hypersensitivity to banana, avocado and peach. Contact Dermatitis 28:247, 1993.
28. Nutter AF: Contact urticaria to rubber. Br J Dermatol 101:597–598, 1979.
29. Turjanmaa K, Reunala T, Tuimala R, et al: Severe IgE mediated allergy to surgical gloves (Abstract 35). Allergy (Suppl 2), 1984.
30. Turjanmaa K: Incidence of immediate allergy to latex gloves in hospital personnel. Contact Dermatitis 17:270–275, 1987.
31. Turjanmaa K, Rasanen L, Lehto M, et al: Basophil histamine release and lymphocyte proliferation tests in latex contact urticaria. Allergy 44:181–185, 1989.
32. Gerber AC, Jong W. Zbinden S, et al: Severe intraoperative anaphylaxis to surgical gloves: Latex allergy, an unfamiliar condition. Anesthesiology 72:800–802, 1989.
33. Spaner D, Delovich J, Tralo S, et al: Hypersensitivity to natural latex. Clin Immunol 83:1135–1137, 1989.
34. Baur X, Jager D: Airborne antigens from latex gloves. Lancet 335(8694):912, 1990.
35. Slater JE, Mostello LA: Routine testing for latex allergy in patients with spina bifida is not recommended (Letter). Anesthesiology 74:391, 1991.
36. Ethmans J: Current concepts review: Allergy to latex in patients who have myelodysplasia. J Bone Joint Surg 1102–1109, 1991.
37. Lager R, Meeropol E: Children at risk: Latex allergy and spina bifida. J Pediatr Nurs 7:371–379, 1992.
38. Meeropol E, Kelleher R, Bell S, et al: Allergic raction to rubber in patients with myelodysplasia (Letter). N Engl J Med 323:1072, 1990.
39. Gold M, Swartz J, Braude B, et al: Intraoperative anaphylaxis: An association with latex sensitivity. J Allergy Clin Immunol 87(3):662–666, 1991.
40. Thompson R: Educational challenges of latex protein allergy. Immunol Allergy Clin North Am 5:159–174, 1995.
41. Gonzalez E: Latex hypersensitivity: A new and unexpected problem. Hosp Pract 27(2):137–151, 1992.
42. Moneret-Vautrin DA, Laxensaire MC, Bavaux F: Allergic shock to latex and ethylene oxide during surgery for spina bifida. Anesthesiology 73:556–558, 1990.
43. Moscicki RA, Socklin ST, Corsello BF, et al: Anaphylaxis during induction of general anesthesia: Subsequent evaluation and management. J Allergy Clin Immunol 86(3 Pt 1):325–332, 1990.
44. Kelly KJ: Complications of latex allergy: A pediatric allergist's perspective. Dialogues Pediatr Urol 15:3–4, 1992.
45. Sussman GI, Tarlo S, Dolovich J: Natural latex hypersensitivity reactions (Abstract 521). J Allergy Clin Immunol p 270, 1991.
46. Setlock MA: Complications of latex allergy: A pediatric anesthesiologist's perspective. Dialogues Pediatr Urol 15:4–6, 1992.
47. Ownby DR, Tomianovich MD, Sammons N, et al: Anaphylaxis associated with latex allergy during barium enema examinations. AJR Am J Roentgenol 156(5):903–908, 1991.
48. Gelfand D: Barium enemas, latex balloons, and anaphylactic reactions (Commentary). AJR Am J Roentgenol 156:1–2, 1991.
49. Young M, Meyers M, Mc Cullock L, et al: Latex allergy: A guide for perioperative nurses. AORN J 56:488–508, 1992.
50. Baur X, Ammon J, Chen Z, et al: Health risk in hospitals through airborne allergens for patients presensitized to latex. Lancet 342:1148, 1993.
51. Jaeger D, Lkeinhans D, Czuppon AB, et al: Latex-specific proteins causing immediate-type cutaneous, nasal, bronchial and systemic reactions. J Allergy Clin Immunol 89:759, 1992.
52. Turjanmaa K, Makinen-Kiljenen S, Reunala R, et al: Natural rubber latex allergy. Immunol Allergy Clin North Am 15:71–88, 1995.
53. Nguyen DH, Burns, NW, Shapiro GG: Intraoperative cardiovascular collapse secondary to latex allegy. J Urol 146:571–574, 1991.
54. Merguerian PA, Klein, RB, Graven MA, et al: Intraoperative anaphylactic reaction due to latex hypersensitivity. Urology 38:303, 1991.
55. Jackson D: Latex allergy and anaphylaxis: What to do? IV Therapy Nurs Vol 19, 1995.
56. Brown JP: Latex allergy requires attention in orthopaedic nursing. Orthop Nurs 13:7–11, 1994.
57. Kwittken PL, Becker J, Oyefara B, et al: Latex hypersensitivity reactions despite prophylaxis. Allergy Proc 13:123–127, 1992.
58. Shapiro E (Guest ed): Complications of latex allergy. Dialogues Pediatr Urol 15:6–7, 1995.
59. Meyers P: Complications of latex allergy: A pediatric urology nurse's perspective. Dialogues Pediatr Urol 15:8, 1995.
60. Socklin SM, Young MC: Perioperative prophylaxis of latex anaphylaxis (Abstract 520). J Allergy Clin Immunol pp 87–269, 1991.
61. Roy C, Barton C: Intraoperative latex anaphylaxis compounded by atracurium sensitivity: A case report. AANA J 59:399–404, 1991.
62. Charpin D, Lagier F, Lhermet J, et al: Prevalence of latex allergy in nurses working in operating rooms (Abstract 520). J Allergy Clin Immunol 87 (part 2), 1991.
63. Sharma R, Buckley CE: Latex hypersensitivity in healthcare workers (Abstract 522). J Allergy Clin Immunol p 270, 1991.

64. Suwalski KL: Complications of latex allergy: An operating room nurse's perspective. Dialogues Pediatr Urol 15:123–137, 1992.
65. Korniewicz D: Barrier protection of latex. Immunol Allergy Clin North Am 15:123–137, 1995.
66. Setlock MA, Cotter TP, Rosner D: Latex allergy: Failure of prophylaxis to prevent severe reaction. Anesth Analg 76:640, 1993.
67. American Society of Post Anesthesia Nurses: Standards of Perianesthesia Nursing Practice. Thorofare, NJ: American Society of Post Anesthesia Nurses, 1995, p 11.
68. American Society of Post Anesthesia Nurses: Standards of Perianesthesia Nursing Practice. Thorofare, NJ: American Society of Post Anesthesia Nurses, 1995, p 59.

Chapter 11

Clinical Emergencies and Preparedness

Myrna Eileen Mamaril

Ambulatory surgery centers (ASCs) promote wellness and a simplistic style of surgical care. However, the composition of the human body mandates uncertainty regarding the response to surgery and anesthesia. The ambulatory surgery patient's recovery process is a dynamic response that is continuously changing owing to each individual's variable reactions. Early recognition of potentially life-threatening conditions coupled with astute nursing assessments and interventions plays an integral part in not only the prevention but also the effective management of urgent or emergency situations. Consequently, unplanned events, such as aspiration, anaphylaxis, pulmonary edema, peripheral ischemia, pulmonary embolism, and myriad other potentially life-threatening events—even cardiopulmonary arrest—may occur in these perianesthesia care settings.

The very nature of surgery and anesthesia requires astute nursing vigilance as well as aggressive nursing interventions for every patient. While these patients are under the ASC's care, the surgeon invades body tissues and cavities, and the anesthesiologist administers anesthetic drugs and gases that cause unconsciousness and paralyze muscles, effectively eradicating spontaneous respirations. The cognitive essence of the experienced ambulatory surgery nurse's practice is the ability to differentiate predictable versus unpredictable responses, synthesize the patient's inherent risk factors, critically analyze the ongoing pathophysiologic disease processes, and astutely make decisions in the emergency management of the patient.

Proper equipment and supplies, as well as informed patients and personnel, are vital to ensuring a safe ASC environment. The current trend of accepting higher patient acuity and more complicated surgical procedures, coupled with the greater number of high-risk patients (very young neonates to fragile geriatric patients), increases the incidence of complications.

Even with a generally healthier clientele, a variety of other factors combine to create complacency among staff: the elective nature of most surgeries, the frequent use of local or regional anesthetics, short operative times, an environment of wellness, and the rarity of actual emergencies. But misplaced confidence in thinking that life-threatening emergencies "just don't happen at our ASC" may lead to unpreparedness and unfavorable outcomes for ASC patients. In addition, ASCs need to be prepared for visitors or caregivers who experience distress or unplanned emergencies. Figure 11–1 illustrates helpful documentation for use when such an event occurs. Finally, ASCs must have policies that address clinical medical and nursing competencies as well as essential protocols that aggressively manage clinical emergencies.

HOSPITAL-BASED VERSUS FREESTANDING CENTERS

The type of setting—hospital-based or freestanding—is not the primary determinant of safety. Rather, it is the fiscal and clinical dedication and attention of the administrative, medi-

OUTPATIENT CENTER
Visitor Distress Record

Date & Time ____________

Name:______________________ ________________ Person accompanying patient______________________
last first

Patient's Primary Physician(if known)____________________ Allergies:______________________

Complaints /Symptoms:____

Name of Responders: 1.__________________ 2.____________________ 3.__________________

VITAL SIGNS **SKIN**

Time:	Time:	Time:	________Pink, Warm & Dry ________ Cool/ Clammy/Pale
BP	BP	BP	Other:
P	P	P	
R____ ☐ Easy ☐ Labored	R____ ☐ Easy ☐Labored	R____ ☐ Easy ☐ Labored	

Patient's physician notified______ Physician's Name:____________________ @______________am /pm

Comments/Discharge Instructions____

____

911 notified: ☐ No ☐ Yes Time of notification________am / pm Time of arrival________ am / pm

DISPOSITION: Person transported to:____________________by:________________@_____am /pm

Signature(s) of person providing care:____________________ ____________________

*** complete next portion only if treatment is initiated***

Medical treatment administered **Physician giving orders: Dr.** ____________________

Respiratory Status:

Arrest	☐ yes	☐ no	O2 @ ___l/m
Oral airway	☐ yes	☐ no	
Ambu Bag	☐ yes	☐ no	
Endotracheal Tube	☐ yes	☐ no	Tube #________

Cardiac Status:

Arrest	☐ yes	☐ no	
CPR	☐ yes	☐ no	Time:_______
Pupils Constricted:	constricted	dilated	fixed
EKG Rythmn :__________________			

IV needle established @______**site**______________

Medications:

__________________time________________

__________________time________________

__________________time________________

Other:

Outcome: ______________________

Patient transported to______________________

by:____________________@______________

Physician remarks:

Figure 11–1. Example of an outpatient center visitor distress record. Reprinted with permission of Morton Plant Mease Trinity Outpatient Center, New Port Richey, FL.

cal, and nursing staffs. Although some critics have voiced concerns that freestanding facilities are not as safe as hospital-based units, this is not the case. The excellent safety record of freestanding centers compared with that of hospital-based centers is recognized and accepted by American consumers.[1]

A freestanding facility must, however, address certain safety issues specific to its setting. Certainly, a hospital-based unit has the advantage of ancillary departments for support, including an emergency response code team, but ASCs can contract for similar resources. A smaller pool of nurses and anesthesia personnel is available, so people from other departments, such as administration, the business office, housekeeping, and maintenance, should be educated and expected to provide support in emergencies. This type of assistance frees the professional staff for essential clinical duties.

A freestanding center must have the resources to meet inherent emergency needs, such as transportation of patients to hospital facilities; portable equipment for transfer needs; back-up equipment in the event of a malfunction; and protocols for securing and transporting necessary supplies, blood products, and laboratory specimens. Outside sources of emergency support for the freestanding center include paramedical emergency personnel, specialized physicians such as cardiologists and vascular surgeons, a consulting pharmacist, and even taxi drivers to transport specimens or needed drugs or equipment. A pre-existing relationship with an ambulance service or a critical care transport service that understands the ASC's business and emergency needs is a great asset.

Although hospital-based ambulatory units have the advantage of immediate support from other hospital departments, there can be challenges in providing emergency responses in hospitals as well. A unit's location within the hospital may delay the response of other departments, or its internal physical layout may be cumbersome and lack privacy or effective space for a patient in need of emergency attention. The possibility of a concurrent emergency in another department may delay the arrival of the code team, making it essential that the primary nursing staff be able to act appropriately until assistance is available.

PREVENTION—THE BEST CURE

Preparing for emergencies is essential. Preventing them is better. Thorough preoperative assessment of all patients is a critical step in the ambulatory surgical process, particularly for predicting and intervening to prevent complications. Completing a thorough nursing history and physical examination and reviewing the results of an appropriate diagnostic workup help the nurse plan interventions aimed at identifying potential problems and avoiding complications during the patient's surgical experience. Consequently, the preoperative nurse should judiciously probe, question, and use appropriate explanations in the process of obtaining a complete history that includes information the patient may "forget" or consider "inconsequential."

Because the patient is an integral part of emergency prevention, the patient has important responsibilities in giving reliable information to the nurse. First, the patient must give healthcare providers a thorough and accurate history, which includes allergies, pre-existing diseases, previous anesthesia experiences, and medication usage (prescription and nonprescription drugs, tobacco, alcohol, and illicit substances). Patients must comply with the preoperative nothing by mouth (NPO) and medication protocols as instructed by the physician and should bring appropriate medications to the surgery center as directed. These include, for instance, nitroglycerin, insulin, and respiratory inhalers.[2] The nurse assesses the patient's understanding of these responsibilities before surgery and ascertains the level of compliance on the day of surgery.

Many other nursing interventions are simple steps that can help prevent emergency situations. For instance, the nurse should:

- Carefully note drug allergies and sensitivities and document them in a consistent and highly visible location on the medical record.
- Avoid medication errors and overdoses: read labels three times before administering the drug, always label syringes and intravenous (IV) containers, and identify the patient both by name bracelet and verbally.
- Use safety devices appropriately—side rails, safety straps, canes, walkers, wheel locks on stretchers, and the like.
- Ensure that diagnostic test values have been medically assessed before surgery.
- Provide specific directions for NPO restrictions and ascertain compliance.
- Monitor blood glucose levels of insulin-dependent diabetics, and reinforce instructions regarding insulin and diet.
- Appropriately attend and monitor anesthetized and sedated patients.

- Be alert to minor variances from normal (laboratory values, vital signs, physical complaints), and investigate before they become major problems.
- Allow adequate time for comprehensive preoperative assessments and postoperative assessments before discharge; do not rush the patient.
- Provide patient call bells and answer them promptly.
- Attend sedated or postoperative patients at all times (phase I throughout phase II), especially in the bathroom.

Healthcare providers cannot predict or prevent every emergency, even when they devote close attention to preventive measures, so preparing the personnel and the facility for the unexpected is essential. Appropriate policies and procedures must be in place; the physical plant, supplies, and equipment should be in readiness; and staff members must be properly educated in emergency preparedness protocols. Every nurse in an ambulatory center must be responsible for maintaining personal readiness.

POLICIES AND PROTOCOLS

Responsibility for the policies in any healthcare setting ultimately lies with the administrative team. There must be administrators and managers who enthusiastically support the emergency preparedness of the ASC by:

1. Communicating an expectation that all staff members will be competent for clinical emergencies
2. Providing a comprehensive orientation program for new employees
3. Providing time and financial support for ongoing education
4. Endorsing policies that contribute to the overall quality of patient care by helping to avoid and to prepare for potential emergencies
5. Supporting the interaction and joint responsibilities of all persons involved in the patient's care—nurses, certified registered nurse anesthetists (CRNAs), anesthesiologists, physicians, technicians, office staff, and others

Personnel policies should address the need to provide competent nurses in all departments of the surgery unit. For instance, consider:

1. Qualifications (education, previous experience) that an applicant should possess to respond safely and effectively in an emergency
2. Orientation program guidelines and standards for periodic demonstration of clinical skills
3. Minimum requirements, such as successful completion of basic life support/cardiopulmonary resuscitation (BLS/CPR) and advanced cardiac life support (ACLS) courses or the equivalent
4. Availability of adequate nursing and medical personnel when any patient is in the facility
5. Ongoing educational and staff development programs that update and refresh knowledge of emergency interventions

Clinical Issues

Anesthesia and nursing department leaders should endorse a policy that requires comprehensive preanesthesia assessment and appropriate diagnostic workup. Inadequate assessment and instruction increase the potential for complications and possible emergency situations. Consider the patient in shock who took a routine dose of insulin before coming to the center because she was not given, did not understand, or did not remember the preoperative instructions. Think about an electrocardiogram (ECG) that was done before surgery but not interpreted by a physician until after the procedure; the patient had experienced a silent myocardial infarction (MI) two nights before his surgery and suffered a reinfarction in the postanesthetic care unit (PACU).

Policies for response to a variety of specific emergency situations should be available and periodically reviewed by all nursing personnel. These might include cardiac arrest or malignant hyperthermia protocols, insertion of a central venous line or arterial line, chest tube insertion, mechanical ventilation, administration of aerosol treatments, and tracheotomy. Other clinical policies that affect the emergency preparedness of an ambulatory facility include IV access on all patients before their procedures, diagnostic requirements, admission and discharge criteria, and nursing response times to the patient call system.

Equipment

Policies should establish a schedule of inspection and preventive maintenance for all essential equipment: defibrillator; ventilator; oximeters; anesthesia, suction, and oxygen machines; and alternative oxygen sources. Regular, documented checks of emergency equipment should be performed by the nurses who are expected to use it in emergency situations. This responsibility should be rotated among staff members so that everyone becomes and remains familiar with the equipment.

Outside Resources

Pre-established relationships also should be in place with the pharmacist, blood bank, laboratory or radiology services for emergency work, medical specialists, and ambulance service. Policies and procedures for using outside resources should be established and communicated to all personnel. In many freestanding facilities, these supports are located outside of the physical building. Ambulance personnel should be familiar with both the geographic location and the interior layout of the building, including the door to use for emergency transfer situations. Inviting local paramedics to tour the facility provides them with firsthand knowledge of the system and building layout. The same is true for firefighters or police in the event of nonmedical emergencies. Periodic emergency drills should include actual contacts with these outside sources to ensure that changes within their organizations do not affect their ability to respond to emergency requests from the ASC. Hospital-based centers should orient other support departments (e.g., respiratory therapy, emergency code team, laboratory) to the types of patients who are being cared for in the ambulatory unit and the potential emergencies that can occur. Protocols for interdepartmental responsibilities should be established.

Communication

Each person in the ambulatory surgery unit has responsibilities for communicating information during emergency situations. The internal call bell system and the telephone are both essential elements for communicating between departments and personnel. Two-way communication in all patient care areas allows any person calling for help to know if the call has been heard. Emergency telephone numbers must be available and clearly visible at all appropriate stations. Preset speed dialing is an asset and should be used if the telephone system has the capability. Although the telephone number of a taxi service seems a trivial need, in a freestanding center, the necessity for the immediate transport of an arterial blood gas specimen, blood products, or dantrolene sodium justifies having that number readily available. Office or other support personnel should be available to make such calls and should be prepared and rehearsed in their individual responsibilities in the emergency communication system.

Immediate telephone access should be in place for the anesthesiologist, surgeons on staff, one or more cardiologists, a vascular and a thoracic surgeon, and each patient's primary physician. A notation of the patient's primary (family) physician's name and telephone number should be in a pre-established place on each chart. Also, the telephone number of the patient's family member or responsible adult should be documented before any procedure in case an emergency contact is necessary.

The internal call bell system is another vital link in the communication network. The call system should be audible both in the clinical areas and in other parts of the ASC: offices, lounges, and storage areas. A policy should be in place that requires periodic testing of all stations of the call system to ensure that it is functional. An attitude and practice of immediate response to call bells by staff members must be encouraged and required.

PERSONNEL

Emergency preparedness is a shared responsibility. From the receptionist to the nurse to the anesthesiologist, each person is a vital link in the effectiveness of an emergency plan.

Nurses are the constant attendants to the patient throughout the surgical experience. Especially in the pre- and postoperative areas, it is generally the nurse who is first to observe symptoms indicating impending disaster. The nurse's skills of observation and ability to react appropriately and quickly to those symptoms are the patient's first line of defense.

Preparedness of the nursing team begins with selection of properly educated and experienced nurses to work in the unit. A comprehensive orientation program that includes appropriate assignment to and supervision by a preceptor and successful completion of a competency skills checklist helps to ensure that each new nurse understands and supports the philosophy, policies, equipment, and physical components of the ASC.

Because of the relative rarity of emergency situations, the ASC nurse must rely on study and practice techniques to keep skills and knowledge current. Personal responsibility to read, review, and practice emergency skills and protocols requires self-motivation. Ongoing professional education both within the unit and through outside sources helps the nurse maintain and upgrade knowledge, which should be shared with other members of the staff as well.

Policies should require nurses to periodically demonstrate perianesthesia competencies. Annual certification in BLS or CPR should be required for all nurses and others involved in direct patient care. National standards now recommend ACLS or its equivalent for all phase I postanesthesia nurses.[3] Periodic, structured reviews of emergency drugs (indications, dosages, contraindications, and preparations) and protocols should be planned. A notebook or card system indicating drug dosages and administration information is helpful for quick reference. Table 11–1 provides guidelines for administration of a number of emergency drugs.

A nurse who assumes responsibility for personal readiness will review emergency protocols at intervals, practice with equipment (e.g., ventilator, defibrillator, cardiac external pacing, emergency drug cart, laryngoscope) at least monthly, be familiar with drug dosages and the location of medications and supplies, attend appropriate classes, read current nursing literature, and ascertain the function and availability of proper equipment in the work area each day. Is the oxygen humidifier functional? Is suction working, and is a suction catheter attached and ready to use in every PACU patient location? Does the laryngoscope have a working battery and bulb and available back-ups? Is the emergency cart quickly available to the phase II or discharge areas? Table 11–2 proposes some personal nursing skills and knowledge that might be used as a checklist for self-assessment.

The responsibility for checking the emergency cart should be rotated so that each nurse is familiar with its location and the function of all supplies and medications. If one or two nurses are consistently responsible for the completeness of the cart and they are not available during a crisis, the nurses involved in that crisis may not be adequately prepared for the urgent needs of the situation.

Rehearsals of staged emergencies allow nursing personnel to identify weaknesses and strengths. Hands-on drills better identify time requirements for response and are more effective than discussion of projected emergency needs. These rehearsals should include a variety of locations and potential emergencies, such as malignant hyperthermic crisis, adult and pediatric cardiopulmonary arrest, anaphylaxis, and massive hemorrhage with cardiovascular collapse. One nurse might set up a drill and then observe and document the response of the staff. Documenting the performance of mock code participants is helpful, and time should be allotted for discussion and evaluation after the drill. It is essential to act on the results of the observer's comments and the ideas generated during group discussion for improving future responses.

Collaboration among all departments in the ASC should be a major goal in any emergency preparedness program. Nurses should help educate office and technical support staff members about the "whys" of certain emergency protocols so that they are able to respond with better understanding. For instance, the immediate need for a plentiful supply of ice during a hyperthermic crisis may seem a rather trivial request to an orderly without some insight into the severity of fever and what it means to the patient's prognosis. The receptionist can be a vital link in communications if he or she understands the need to keep telephone lines open to summon specific help quickly at the emergency team's request.

Interaction between nursing departments also contributes to an effective response to emergencies. The postanesthesia staff is often most familiar with emergency medication protocols and, when possible, should respond to an intraoperative emergency. In contrast, location of emergency surgical supplies is best addressed by the operating room nurse, who is familiar with the storage area and can quickly gather necessary items. Such situations illustrate the interdependent needs of perioperative nurses in all areas of care.

A nurse who is cross-trained in all departments has the advantage of a broader knowledge base and familiarity with the equipment and supplies throughout the facility. However, there is an advantage to having nurses specialize in one area, because they may possess more knowledge of specific information and practices within their specialties. Regardless of the personnel policies in place, all nurses must be prepared to respond to emergencies in all areas of the ASC.

Medical staff members have responsibilities for preparedness as well. The anesthesia provider is responsible for each patient until the major effects of anesthesia have passed. The surgeon should be available until the patient's initial recovery is complete or should notify the nursing staff of the physician who will be covering the practice. In a freestanding center, physicians are usually required to have admitting privileges at a nearby hospital in case an emergency admission is required for one of their patients. Thoracic and vascular surgeons as well as medical specialists (cardiologist, internist) should be available for emergency crisis intervention. ACLS courses should be required for all anesthesia care providers. This provides a national standardized approach to managing cardiac arrests. Offering CPR refresher courses for staff physicians is a wise investment that communicates the facility's commitment to emergency preparedness and provides a service to the physicians as well. Finally, annual or periodic competencies should be successfully completed and documented on each staff member's permanent record. If a deficiency is noted, a plan for improvement over a specific period should be documented, and the date for successful completion of the competency should be added.

EQUIPMENT, SUPPLIES, AND PHYSICAL PLANT

The potential for clinical complications exists in all locations of any surgery center, but particularly where patients are given medications or anesthesia, including local and regional blocks. Each bedside unit in the pre- and postoperative areas should be supplied with airways, tongue blades, nasal cannulas, face masks, and nonrebreather masks. Oxygen and suction must be immediately available with tubings and catheters attached. Bedsides should have monitoring equipment as identified in the facility's policies. Within each patient care area there should be:

- IV fluids and devices for securing IV access
- Emergency resuscitation equipment
- Pulse oximeter
- Cardiac monitor/defibrillator
- Emergency medications
- Portable oxygen for use in transport and as back-up in the event of failure of a piped-in source
- Adapters on every oxygen flow meter for attaching oxygen tubing from resuscitation equipment

An emergency cart should include medications and supplies to respond to a variety of situations. The American Society of Perianesthesia Nurses' Standards of Perianesthesia Nursing Practice 1998 provides a detailed list of suggested equipment and crash cart contents (Table 11–3). A method should be in place to ensure that all medications in emergency carts are within their expiration dates.

A locking device that must be broken to remove any item from the crash cart helps identify tampering. Once the lock is broken, the cart is considered incomplete until checked, restocked, and relocked. Spare locks should be kept in a secure location. In a hospital setting, the pharmacist is usually responsible for restocking. In a freestanding facility, a nurse generally holds that responsibility.

Other emergency supplies and equipment such as a ventilator, oxygen tanks, and Doppler devices should be checked at least monthly to ensure proper function and to provide the nurse with hands-on familiarity with the equipment. Daily testing of laryngoscopes and defibrillators while on battery power is recommended to ensure that the battery remains both charged and chargeable. It is also suggested that a printed strip be run from portable monitor/defibrillators to exercise their batteries. Manufacturer recommendations for specific testing protocols should be followed. Testing calibrated equipment such as glucose or hemoglobin meters with standardized solutions ascertains both the accuracy of the equipment and the competency of the practitioner.

Supplies and medications for a malignant hyperthermic (MH) crisis may be included on the emergency cart or may be placed on a separate cart. Because ice and refrigerated IV and irrigating solutions are required, a centralized location for cold storage is desirable. One freestanding center responded to that need by positioning a small (19 × 19 inch) refrigerator on top of the MH cart. It can be unplugged and taken with the cart when needed, just like a defibrillator is kept on a crash cart.

It is also recommended that a full 36-vial supply of dantrolene solution be kept within the surgical suite to deal with MH crisis.[4] Because a patient's prognosis is specifically linked to the speed of treatment, if 36 vials are not stocked, comprehensive preparations to obtain a full complement of dantrolene must be in place. In a freestanding center where there is no resident pharmacist on duty, it may be more complicated to obtain dantrolene quickly. On the MH supply cart, there should be a card listing the telephone numbers of a taxi service and nearby hospital pharmacies (including the names of the chief pharmacists) and directions for the caller to say, "We have an emergency need for dantrolene." With such explicit instructions, the card can easily be passed to a clerical or technical person to make the calls in an emergency.

Text continued on page 216

Table 11–1. Guidelines for Administration of Emergency Medications to Adults

DRUG	ROUTE	INITIAL (I)/SUBSEQUENT (S) DOSE	COMMENTS
Adenosine (Adenocard)	IVP	(I) 6 mg rapid IVP over 1–3 sec; if no response within 1–2 min, go to (S) 12 mg IVP over 1–3 sec; may repeat once	Depresses AV node and sinus node activity; terminates PSVT involving re-entry pathway; half-life is <5 sec; patient may experience short episode of asystole; patients taking theophylline may require higher doses
Atropine sulfate	IVP	(I) Bradycardia: 0.5–1 mg q 15 min (I) Asystole: 1 mg q 3–5 min Maximum dose 0.04 mg/kg Minimum dose 0.5 mg	1st line: reverses cholinergic-mediated ↓ HR, ↓ SVR, ↓ B/P; useful in treating symptomatic bradycardia; may be useful in treating AV block/asystole; may be harmful in patients with 2nd- or 3rd-degree heart block; use with caution in MI, ↑ HR, ↑ myocardial O_2 2nd-line drug in asystole
	ET	2–2.5 times peripheral IV dose	
Bretylium tosylate (Bretylol)	IV	PVCs and stable VT: (I) 5–10 mg/kg in 50 ml D5W over 8–10 min (I) Cardiac arrest (VF): 5 mg/kg (S) 10 mg/kg IVP repeat q 5 min Maximum dose: 30–35 mg/kg	2nd line: antiarrhythmic after lidocaine for ventricular dysrhythmias (PVCs, VT, VF); hypotension common side effect
	IV inf	(S) 2 g/500 ml NS/RL per AHA	
Dexamethasone (Decadron)	IVP	(I) 4–10 mg	Used in anaphylaxis/ ↑ airway edema
Diltiazem hydrochloride (Cardizem)	IV	(I) 0.25 mg/kg given IV over 2 min	1st line: for atrial fibrillation/flutter with fast ventricular response; transient ↓ in arterial pressure due to peripheral vasodilatation
	IV inf	(S) Maintenance infusion at a rate of 5–15 mg/hr titrated to HR	
Dopamine hydrochloride (Intropin)	IV inf	(I) 800 mg/500 ml D5W produces concentration of 1600 μg/ml (I) infusion of 2.5–5 μg/kg then titrate to desired effect	1st line: for hypotension; monitor U/O and B/P; do not mix with alkaline solution; do not discontinue abruptly—taper gradually; infiltration causes sloughing of tissue
Epinephrine (Adrenalin) (1 : 10,000 solution 1 mg/10 ml)	IVP	(I) 1 mg (1 : 10,000) q 3–5 min Option to ↑ dose (S) Escalate 1 mg, 3 mg, 5 mg IV q 3–5 min; Intermediate: 2–5 mg q 3–5 min High: 1 mg/kg IVP q 3–5 min	1st line: α- and β-adrenergic receptor stimulator; should be used frequently and in unlimited amounts in cardiac arrest; do not mix with alkaline solutions; use with extreme caution in patients with a pulse
	ET	2–2.5 times peripheral IV dose	
Flumazenil (Romazicon)	IV (slow)	(I) 0.2 mg IV over 15 sec (S) 0.2 mg may be repeated at 60-sec intervals to maximum dose of 1 mg	Reversal agent for partial/complete sedative effects of benzodiazapines; in event of resedation, repeat dose of 0.2 mg at 20-min interval as needed; flumazenil may cause seizures
Isoproterenol (Isuprel)	IV inf	(I) 2–10 μg/min IV infusion; Dilute 1 mg/250 ml RL per AHA (4 μg/ml); (I) 2 μg/min IV infusion Use volumetric infusion pump	2nd line: infusion; pure β-adrenergic agonist avoided in patients with ischemic heart disease; exaggerates tachyarrhythmias; harmful at high doses
Lidocaine (Xylocaine) (100 mg/10 ml)	IVP	(I) 1–1.5 mg/kg (S) 0.5–1.5 mg/kg Maximum dose 3 mg/kg	1st line: antiarrhythmic for ventricular ectopy and VF; in VF (after defibrillation and epinephrine) (I) 1.5 mg/kg
	IV inf	IVP always followed by maintenance infusion to maintain blood level 2 g in 500 ml D5W or NSS at 2–4 mg/min	Prophylactic use in MI not recommended; observe for signs of toxicity (dizziness, ↓ LOC, headache); ↓ dose in low cardiac output, patients >70 yr, hepatic dysfunction

Table 11–1. Guidelines for Administration of Emergency Medications to Adults *Continued*

DRUG	ROUTE	INITIAL (I)/SUBSEQUENT (S) DOSE	COMMENTS
Magnesium sulfate	IV IV inf	(I) Refractory VF: 1–2 g in 100 ml RL/NS over 2 min (I) Hypomagnesemia: 1–2 g in 50–100 ml over 5–60 min 0.5–1 g/hr—follow up to 24 hr	↓ Mg^{2+} can precipitate refractory VF and hinder replacement of intracellular K^+; rate and infusion should be determined by clinical situation or degree of hypomagnesemia
Midazolam (Versed) (1 mg/ml)	IV	(I) 0.5–1 mg over 1 min (S) 1–1.5 mg individualized to patient clinical response; evaluate 2 or more minutes	Before drug administration, ensure immediate availability of O_2, resuscitation equipment, and competent skilled personnel in advanced life support; administer in IV port closest to IV site; midazolam may cause high incidence of partial or complete impaired recall for next several hours
Naloxone (Narcan) (0.4 mg/ml)	IV (slow)	(I) 0.4 mg IV titrated to effect (S) 0.2–0.4 mg (IM/SC/ET)	Reverses narcotic effects; as drug is metabolized, renarcotization may occur
Norepinephrine bitartrate (Levophed) (4 mg/4 ml)	IV inf	1–12 μg/min IV infusion; (I) 0.5–1 μg/min (S) 2–12 μg/min	2nd line: severe hypotension; use extreme caution with ↑ dose may cause renal failure
Physostigmine salicylate (Antilirium) (2 mg/2 ml)	IV (slow)	(I) 0.5–2 mg (IV slowly); no more than 1 mg/min	Rapid administration may cause bradycardia and excessive salivation leading to respiratory difficulty and possible convulsions; may cause nausea/vomiting if given too fast
Procainamide hydrochloride (Pronestyl)	IV IV inf	(I) 20 mg/min VF 30 mg/min may be given Maximum dose 17 mg/kg 2 g in 500 ml at 1–4 mg/min	2nd line: ventricular arrhythmias; indicated when lidocaine has failed or is contraindicated; end points of administration: hypotension, QRS widened by 50%; ↓ maintenance infusion dose for patients with renal failure
Sodium bicarbonate	IV	(I) 1 mEq/kg (S) half initial dose q 10 min if ABG unavailable	Bicarbonate therapy should be considered in cardiac arrest only after more definitive treatments: defibrillation, CPR, intubation, ventilation, plus at least one dose of epinephrine; may be beneficial in pre-existing metabolic acidosis, hyperkalemia, tricyclic or phenobarbital overdose
Sodium nitroprusside (Nitropress or Nipride) (50-mg vial)	IV inf	(I) 0.1 μg/kg/min (S) 0.5–8 μg/kg/min	Arterial line needed for continuous monitoring; wrap in foil to prevent deterioration; use infusion pump

ABG, arterial blood gas; AHA, American Heart Association; B/P, blood pressure; CPR, cardiopulmonary resuscitation; D5W, 5% dextrose in water; ET, endotracheal; HR, heart rate; IM, intramuscular; IV, intravenous; IVP, intravenous push; LOC, level of consciousness; MI, myocardial infarction; NS/RL, normal saline/Ringer's lactate; NSS, normal saline solution; PVC, premature ventricular contraction; PSVT, paroxysmal supraventricular tachycardia; RL/NS, Ringer's lactate/normal saline; SC, subcutaneous; SVR, supraventricular rate/systemic vascular resistance; U/O, urine output; VF, ventricular fibrillation; VT, ventricular tachycardia.

Data from Adult Advanced Cardiac Life Support. JAMA 268:2199, 2227, 1992.

Table 11–2. Skills Assessment Checklist

Can you do the following?
- Adult, child, and infant cardiopulmonary resuscitation
- Maintain a patent airway
- Properly insert nasal and oral airways
- Use a bag-valve-mask without assistance
- Explain appropriate treatment for laryngospasm
- Operate ventilator
- Couple laryngoscope blade and handle
- Replace bulb or battery of laryngoscope
- Locate and operate portable suction and oxygen
- Open a new portable tank of oxygen
- Calculate approximate PaO_2 from SaO_2
- Cannulate a peripheral intravenous line
- Operate infusion pump or calculate doses from minidrip
- List 10 covert symptoms of bleeding
- Identify symptoms of acute myocardial infarction, pulmonary edema, and pulmonary embolism
- Identify major arrhythmias and treatment protocols
- Operate monitor/defibrillator
- Change the paper in cardiac monitors
- Correctly attach pediatric paddles to the defibrillator
- Calculate defibrillation power (joules) per kg weight
- Assist with or operate external pacemaker
- Distinguish between toxic and allergic reactions
- Accurately reconstitute dantrolene and other emergency drugs
- Locate emergency drug dosage and reconstitution data
- Convert pounds to kilograms
- Calculate emergency drug dosages based on mg per kg
- Locate an alternative source of ice and cold solutions
- Locate all potentially necessary emergency telephone numbers
- Procure blood for emergency transfusion
- Initiate an emergency transfer to another facility or nursing unit
- Locate and operate fire alarms, fire extinguishers, and medical gas shut-off

Could you set up necessary supplies and assist with the following?
- Chest tube insertion with underwater sealed drainage
- Cutdown
- Central venous access catheter placement
- Emergency intubation
- Tracheotomy
- Cricothyrotomy
- Vaginal packing
- Resuture of wound
- Arterial blood gas sampling
- Malignant hyperthermia crisis

From Figley E, Burden N: Preparing for the unexpected in the ambulatory surgery unit. J Post Anesth Nurs 6:118, 1991.

Table 11–3. Recommended Equipment for Preanesthesia and Postanesthetic Care Unit (PACU) Phases I–III

PREANESTHESIA PHASE

I. Preadmission
   A. Equipment for the preadmission area includes but is not limited to:
      1. Means to measure height and weight for pediatric to adult patients
      2. Blood pressure monitor
      3. Pulse oximeter
      4. Access to laboratory, electrocardiogram (ECG), x-ray, and other diagnostic equipment as needed
      5. Access to a fax machine
      6. Means to call for help in emergency situations
      7. Access to latex-free supplies
      8. Means to ensure patient privacy
   B. Stock supplies should include:
      1. Facial tissue
      2. Gloves
      3. Syringes and needles
      4. Emesis basins
      5. Alcohol wipes
      6. Tongue blades
      7. Personal protective equipment
      8. Tourniquets
      9. Cotton balls
      10. Tape
      11. Latex-free supplies

***Table 11–3.* Recommended Equipment for Preanesthesia and Postanesthetic Care Unit (PACU) Phases I–III** *Continued*

PREANESTHESIA PHASE *Continued*

II. Day of surgery/procedure preparation area
  A. Every patient bedside unit should have the following:
    1. Means to deliver oxygen
    2. Means to provide constant and intermittent suction
    3. Means of monitoring blood pressure
    4. Adjustable lighting
    5. Capacity to ensure patient privacy
  B. The following equipment should be present in the day of surgery/procedure preparation area:
    1. Means of monitoring patient temperature
    2. Means of monitoring patient blood glucose
    3. Means of measuring height and weight
    4. ECG monitor
    5. Pulse oximeter
    6. Bag-valve-mask (age specific)
  C. A method of calling for assistance in emergency situations
  D. An emergency cart
  E. A defibrillator with adult and pediatric paddles and cardiac pacing capability
  F. Stock medications that should be available include the following:
    1. Antibiotics
    2. Antiemetics
    3. Analgesics
    4. Anxiolytics
    5. Alkalizing agents
    6. Reversal agents
    7. Steroidal agents
  G. Intravenous supplies
  H. Stock supplies should include:
    1. Facial tissues
    2. Gloves
    3. Bedpans and urinals
    4. Syringes and needles
    5. Emesis basins
    6. Patient linens
    7. Alcohol wipes
    8. Tongue blades
    9. Denture cups
    10. Personal protective equipment (universal precautions)
  I. A means to safely transport patients to the operating room or procedure unit; portable oxygen, suction, cardiac monitoring equipment, and pulse oximetry must be available for those patients requiring such equipment during transport
  J. Access to latex-free supplies and equipment

PHASE I PACU

I. Each patient bedside should be equipped with the following:
  A. Various types and sizes of artificial airways
  B. Various means of oxygen delivery
  C. Constant and intermittent suction
  D. Means to monitor blood pressure
  E. Adjustable lighting
  F. Capacity to ensure patient privacy
  G. ECG monitor
  H. Pulse oximeter
  I. Bag-valve-mask
II. Equipment should be available to assess:
  A. Hemodynamic status
  B. Blood glucose
  C. Arterial blood gases
  D. End-tidal CO_2
III. A means to monitor patient temperature should be available. A method to warm patients with low temperatures should also be available. Supplies to handle a malignant hyperthermia crisis must also be available. These supplies include:
  A. Means to deliver 100% oxygen
  B. Datrolene
  C. Mannitol
  D. Bicarbonate
  E. Antidysrhythmic agents
  F. Cool IV fluids and irrigants
  G. External cooling methods
IV. At least one ventilator must be accessible to the PACU at all times. A sufficient number of ventilators should be available to care for any postanesthesia patient who requires one. Bag-valve-masks of appropriate sizes for patient population must be in the PACU and easily accessible at all times.
V. A method of calling for assistance in emergency situations must be provided.
VI. An emergency cart should be in the PACU at all times and contain the following:
  A. Supplies necessary for insertion of arterial lines, central venous lines, and pulmonary artery catheters
  B. Intravenous (IV) pole
  C. Emergency drugs and equipment
VII. A defibrillator with adult and pediatric paddles and cardiac pacing capability must be readily available.
VIII. Stock medications should include the following:
  A. Antibiotics
  B. Medications for control of blood pressure and heart rate and respiratory drugs
  C. Antiemetics
  D. Anesthesia reversal agents
  E. Analgesics, opioid and nonopioid
  F. Muscle relaxants
  G. Steroids
  H. Sedatives
  I. Nonsteroidal anti-inflammatory drugs (NSAIDs)
IX. Intravenous supplies should include:
  A. Various types of solutions
  B. Various types of IV catheters
  C. Various types of IV tubing
  D. IV dressing supplies per hospital protocol
  E. At least one IV infusion control device
X. Patient protective devices should be available to use per hospital policy.
XI. Stock supplies should include:
  A. Dressings
  B. Facial tissues
  C. Gloves
  D. Bedpans and urinals
  E. Syringes and needles
  F. Emesis basins
  G. Patient linens
  H. Alcohol swabs
  I. Ice bags
  J. Tongue blades
  K. Irrigation trays
  L. Foley insertion supplies
  M. Personal protective equipment

Table continued on following page

Table 11–3. Recommended Equipment for Preanesthesia and Postanesthetic Care Unit (PACU) Phases I–III *Continued*

PHASE I PACU *Continued*

XII. Access to latex-free supplies and equipment must be provided.

XIII. A means to safely transport patients from phase I PACU is necessary; portable oxygen, suction, cardiac monitoring equipment, and pulse oximetry must be available for those patients requiring such equipment during transport.

PHASE II PACU

I. Each patient care unit should be equipped with the following:
   A. Means to deliver oxygen
   B. Constant and intermittent suction
   C. Means to monitor blood pressure
   D. Adjustable lighting
   E. Capacity to ensure patient privacy
   F. Means of monitoring patient temperature

II. An ECG monitor and pulse oximeter must be readily available for use in phase II PACU.

III. A bag-valve-mask, adult and pediatric, must be easily accessible at all times.

IV. A means to monitor patient temperature must be available. Supplies to handle a malignant hyperthermia crisis must be easily accessible. These supplies should include:
   A. Means to deliver 100% oxygen
   B. Dantrolene
   C. Mannitol
   D. Bicarbonate
   E. Antidysrhythmic agents
   F. Cool IV fluids and irrigants
   G. External cooling methods

V. A method of calling for assistance in emergency situations must be provided.

VI. An emergency cart must be in the phase II PACU at all times.

VII. A defibrillator with adult and pediatric paddles must be readily available.

VIII. Stock medications should include the following:
   A. Antibiotics
   B. Antiemetics
   C. Anesthesia reversal agents
   D. Analgesics, opioids and nonopioids

IX. Intravenous supplies include:
   A. Various types of solutions
   B. Various types of IV catheters
   C. Various types of IV tubing
   D. IV dressing supplies per hospital protocol

X. Stock supplies should include:
   A. Dressings
   B. Facial tissues
   C. Gloves
   D. Bedpans and urinals
   E. Syringes and needles
   F. Emesis basins
   G. Patient linens
   H. Alcohol swabs/wipes
   I. Ice bags
   J. Tongue blades
   K. Foley insertion supplies
   L. Personal protective equipment
   M. Access to latex-free supplies and equipment

XI. A means to safely transport patients from phase II PACU is necessary; portable oxygen, suction, cardiac monitoring equipment, and pulse oximetry must be available for those patients requiring such equipment during transport.

PHASE III PACU

Supplies and equipment for phase III are determined by the facility based on the patient population and the level of care to be provided.

From American Society of Perianesthesia Nurses: Standards of Perianesthesia Nursing Practice. Thorofare, NJ: ASPAN, 1998.

During a nationwide survey, Dr. H. A. Tillmann Hein of Baylor University in Dallas, Texas, estimated that 7% of American hospitals and 22% of ASCs did not stock any dantrolene. Further, only 55% of hospitals and 28% of freestanding ASCs had immediate access to a full 36 vials; these were the only facilities he deemed prepared to handle an MH crisis.[5] He further estimated that from 47 to 274 deaths occur in the United States each year as a direct result of the unavailability of dantrolene.[6]

Emergency equipment is diverse and ranges from simple to sophisticated. It is imperative that staff members accept responsibility for replacing any item that is used, damaged, or incomplete. If a staff member cannot personally replace an item, a mechanism for communicating the need to the proper resource person should be in place. Most important, the responsible staff member should follow up to ascertain that this item has actually been replaced.

By preparing as much as possible ahead of time, the crisis response time can be improved. For instance, drug labels to affix to IV solution bottles can be written and taped to the boxes or vials of unprepared drugs. Requisitions for laboratory and other diagnostic tests can be partially filled in, awaiting only the specifics of the patient in question. Remaining areas on the requisitions that need to be completed can be identified with a colored highlighting pen for ease of execution in times of emergency. The telephone number of the laboratory or blood bank can be affixed to the equipment necessary for obtaining the specimen.

It is each nurse's responsibility to treat equipment with respect at all times and to use it in accordance with the manufacturer's directions so that it remains in ideal working condition. Monitor alarms should be enabled while equipment is in use. Misuse or improper storage of equipment could result in the need for costly repairs or replacement or, more important, in patient injury. If there is confusion about the proper use of any piece of equipment, the manufacturer's representative should be asked to demonstrate or provide clarification.

Preventive maintenance for sophisticated biomedical and electronic devices generally is provided by the hospital's technical support department or by an outside contractor on a routine schedule. Maintenance of less technical equipment and provision of adequate supplies are usually the responsibility of the nursing staff. Nurses should be assigned specific responsibilities and tasks to ensure that the system works without misunderstanding.

CASE STUDY

Jennifer M., an 8-year-old girl, was admitted to the PACU after a tonsillectomy under general anesthesia. The operating room (OR) nurse reported that JM bit down on the endotracheal tube while the anesthesiologist was extubating the patient. The patient was transported into the PACU unresponsive; her temperature was 36.4°C; her pulse was 92; her respirations were 24/min and somewhat labored; and her oxygen saturation was 84%. Next, an oxygen mist mask at 40% was applied, and she was placed on a cardiac monitor; her skin and lip mucosa were pink. Three minutes after admission to the PACU, the nurse noted that JM was beginning to respond by coughing pink, frothy sputum; her respiratory rate had increased to 32/ min; and her SaO_2 had dropped to 80% even with attempts to increase the oxygen concentration to 100%. JM's skin and lip mucosa color had changed from pink to dusky. Her respiratory effort had increased so that she was using her accessory muscles to breathe.

The second PACU nurse immediately brought a bag-valve-mask with a reservoir, connected it to the oxygen flow meter at 15 L of oxygen, and began to ventilate JM unsuccessfully. No resistance was felt during ventilation, copious amounts of pink, frothy sputum filled the mask, and JM's oxygen saturation continued to fall to 70%. The first PACU nurse arrived with the emergency code cart and began to assist the second nurse by suctioning the patient to clear the airway. The anesthesiologist arrived and took over the ventilatory attempts, which remained ineffective. Both noticed an unusual amount of nonresistance from the bag. The SaO_2 was now 69%, and the patient had become cyanotic. An oral airway from the bedside stand was inserted immediately and a second bag quickly obtained from the emergency cart. Resuscitation was then successful, with the patient's oxygenation status immediately improving to SaO_2 86%, and JM's color began returning to normal. Then the anesthesiologist proceeded to reintubate JM without difficulty, and she was placed on a ventilator with assisted breathing with positive end-expiratory pressure (PEEP) (tidal volume [TV] 500, FIO_2 50%, assist control [A/C] 10, and 5 PEEP). A Foley catheter was inserted, and furosemide 5 mg IV injection was given. Within several minutes the patient began to respond, opened her eyes, and was breathing easier. Two hours later, JM was able to be extubated. Her vital signs were temperature 36.9°C, pulse 100, respiratory rate 18 to 22/ min, SaO2 94% to 98%. The rest of her postanesthesia course was uneventful, with no sequelae from the incident.

After the emergency, the nurses examined the initial resuscitation bag-valve-mask and found that the leaf valve was installed backward, which had rendered the bag ineffective. Periodic checks should have uncovered the problem. Fortunately, a second bag had been readily available. The staff discussed ways to avoid similar incidents and decided that beyond checking for the presence of the equipment, all resuscitation bags in the unit would be given a routine "hands-on" check for defects. It was discussed that squeezing the resuscitation bag should produce some resistance against the hand. If there is no resistance and no air is felt, the valve is either absent or malfunctioning. The staff also discussed that the patient's response to effective ventilation would be the chest rising and falling. Finally, the staff decided that everyone would participate in emergency preparedness and that there would be a rotating responsibility added to the assignment for checking the emergency cart and medications.

The emergency preparations of any unit are only as good as the dedication of its staff members. In an ambulatory surgery setting, patients are generally healthier than most and undergo elective and minor procedures with the expectation that their daily lifestyles will barely be interrupted. However, many more serious procedures are being done in ambulatory settings today than in the past. Currently, third party payers or insurers are regulating more complicated surgical procedures to be done in an outpatient setting. "Elective and minor" procedures can become unexpectedly complicated—even life-threatening. A fatality in that setting is a devastating and intolerable occurrence. The close observation and continual preparedness of nurses may be the single most important factor in preventing a patient's death or disability.

POTENTIAL EMERGENCIES

Anesthesia, surgery, the patient's pre-existing health status, and the administration of medications combine to predispose ambulatory surgery patients to complications. Cardiopulmonary sequelae and hemorrhage are the foremost concerns because they may occur secondary to depressant anesthetic agents and surgical intervention, but any number of different crises are possible. The following discussion is not exhaustive, but it attempts to provide ambulatory surgical nurses with the basics of predisposition, prevention, symptoms, and treatments for a variety of potential emergency situations.

Airway Obstruction

Predisposing Factors. Airway obstruction is a common problem in patients who have been given anesthesia, muscle relaxants, narcotics, hypnotics, and sedative drugs. Mechanical airway obstruction in the postanesthetic period is usually due to relaxation of the soft tissues of the upper airway, often the tongue. Excessive secretions, blood, foreign bodies, and kinked or blocked endotracheal tubes can create obstruction as well.

Prevention. Proper positioning of the patient's head and neck using a jaw thrust–chin lift maneuver, together with suctioning of the mouth and upper airway, is the primary deterrent to obstruction. Lateral, head-down positioning is recommended for an unconscious patient unless contraindicated by the surgery. Blankets, pillows, or incorrectly placed oral or nasal airways must not be allowed to obstruct an unconscious patient's mouth or nose.

Symptoms. Airway obstruction may be partial or complete. Partially obstructed respirations are noisy, often with stridor or snoring sounds. There may be any degree of the following signs: decreased tidal volume, retraction of the chest, use of accessory neck and intercostal muscles, abdominal breathing movements, decreased oxygen saturation, and cyanosis. Complete obstruction results in silent, exaggerated attempts at inspiration. If not corrected, cyanosis, progressing to respiratory and cardiac arrest and death, follows.

Until obvious symptoms appear, complete airway obstruction can be difficult to diagnose without auscultation of the lungs. This fact makes chest auscultation an imperative part of the assessment of unconscious or sedated patients, both on initial assessment and after attempting to arouse or reposition them. When lung sounds are difficult to hear, another helpful assessment is auscultation over the trachea to check for clear and easy airflow.

Treatment. When soft tissue obstruction prevents proper ventilation, repositioning of the head and neck and insertion of an oral or nasal airway, if necessary, are usually effective in correcting the problem. A nasal airway tends to be better tolerated by a partially awake patient. Occasionally the patient's tongue must be physically extended by the nurse. Suctioning may be necessary if secretions, blood, or foreign objects are blocking the airway. Oxygen therapy should be administered until respiratory inadequacy has been corrected.

Laryngospasm

Laryngospasm is a form of airway obstruction that can be a transient, self-limited problem or can progress to total obstruction that results in respiratory arrest. It is a condition that should be immediately identified by an attentive postanesthesia nurse. Early recognition and intervention are usually successful in reversing the condition in its initial stages.

Predisposing Factors. Stimulation of the vocal cords due to mechanical irritation by an endotracheal tube, laryngoscope blade, or secretions may cause partial or complete laryngospasm, which is most likely to occur as a complication of general anesthesia, particularly during periods of light anesthesia and emergence. Blood or mucus from the upper respiratory tract may be the causative agent, or a foreign object may be implicated. Furthermore, an irritable airway may be due to an incomplete neuromuscular blockade causing a highly reactive airway. In children, improper hand placement on the anterior neck when supporting an airway may also be a contributing factor.

Prevention. To avoid irritation of the cords during light planes of anesthesia when reflexes are hyperactive, patients are extubated either while they are deeply anesthetized or after they are awake and their protective airway reflexes have returned. Humidified oxygen is helpful in soothing an irritated airway. Gentle suctioning and positioning can help prevent secretions from pooling near the glottis and vocal cords. Oral airways can irritate the posterior pharynx and should be removed when reflexes return and the patient can maintain his or her own airway. No oral fluids should be given until protective airway reflexes have returned.

Controversy exists about the efficacy of IV lidocaine as a preventive measure for laryngospasm.[7] When given preoperatively on induction or intraoperatively, it is administered about 1 minute before extubation. It should be given slowly to avoid causing respiratory depression and bradycardia.[8]

A lightly anesthetized patient who is not displaying any signs of respiratory distress or inadequacy usually does better when awakened slowly, without the aggressive intervention of outside stimulation. Once the patient is awake, purposeful coughing helps clear secretions from the upper airway. In children, proper hand placement on the bony structure of the chin or lower mandible is prudent to avoid manipulating the immature musculature of the anterior neck.

Symptoms. The hallmark symptoms of laryngospasm are dyspnea and inspiratory crowing; however, total closure of the vocal cords results in complete airway obstruction and no noise. Other symptoms of laryngospasm are diminished breath sounds, little or no evidence of airflow at the nose or mouth, and reduced oxygen saturation levels. Observation of the patient's chest is an unreliable assessment in this situation because the patient may be making vigorous but ineffective attempts at ventilating, with exaggerated abdominal and chest movements. Awake patients who experience laryngospasm are usually extremely frightened or panicky. The pulse oximeter may read a relatively "acceptable" oxygen saturation in the early stages of hypoxia while the patient is actually retaining carbon dioxide. One should always remember that cyanosis is a late sign of hypoxia. Therefore, the nurse should not rely on the color of the skin and mucous membranes alone.

Treatment. The initial response is second nature to a postanesthesia nurse. Mechanical airway maintenance (head extension, jaw thrust–chin lift) and oxygen administration should be initiated immediately. A calm demeanor is an essential nursing action, particularly if the patient is awake. Often a soothing voice, gentle airway maintenance, and humidified oxygen are effective in breaking the spasm. An awake patient who is able to follow the nurse's directions can be asked to take a slow, deep breath and cough. This action can be effective in removing offending debris or secretions from the vocal cords.

No time should be wasted if respiratory distress continues or progresses. Oxygen under positive pressure by bag-valve-mask along with gentle suctioning of the pharynx and concurrent notification of the anesthesiologist are the steps to take. If spasm does not stop, administration of IV succinylcholine to paralyze the vocal cords and assisted ventilation may be necessary, with or without reintubation. An awake patient is generally given a short-acting IV hypnotic immediately before receiving the muscle relaxant. Atropine may be added to the regimen to decrease secretions in the upper airway.

Oxygen is continued until the patient's respirations are adequate and other vital signs have returned to normal. The patient's airway may continue to be irritated, so the possibility of another episode of laryngospasm cannot be ruled out. Allowing the patient to rest undisturbed, but fully observed, for a period of time is advisable. Reassurance of the family and patient is important to decrease anxiety and fear.

Bronchospasm

Bronchospasm is another problem that can result in diminished ventilation. This narrowing of the lower airways is due to increased tone in the circular smooth muscles in the bronchi or bronchioles. Hyperirritability of the tissues is a result of partial β-receptor blockade; a concurrent release of histamine causes increased mucus production and swelling of the respiratory mucosa.[9] Bronchospasm is a reversible event, contrasting with the irreversible bronchospastic changes and tissue destruction seen in a patient with emphysema.

Predisposing Factors. This reflex constriction of the bronchioles is more common in patients with pre-existing bronchospastic disease, such as asthma. Other predisposing factors include cigarette smoking, emphysema, irritation of the airways with blood or other secretions, respiratory tract infections, pulmonary overload due to IV fluids or cardiac failure, and allergic reactions.[10] Environmental factors—cold or dry air, perfumes and odors, and environmental or drug allergens—and emotional distress can precipitate occurrences in a predisposed person.

Prevention. Careful preoperative identification of predisposed people allows prophylactic measures to be used. Pretreatment with bronchodilating drugs and anesthetic choices that favor bronchodilation can help avoid problems in these patients. For instance, volatile agents are preferred over narcotics. Curare and morphine are also avoided in predisposed people.[11]

Preparing the patient before the day of surgery is important and may be undertaken by the anesthesiologist or by the patient's primary physician or pulmonologist. A patient who smokes should be directed to abstain from smoking before surgery. The bronchoconstrictive effects of one cigarette can last from 12 hours to 3 days. Predisposed people may be placed on an antibiotic and corticosteroid regimen as well.

Avoiding interventions that cause irritation of the tracheobronchial tree follows the principles outlined in the previous discussion of laryngospasm. Additionally, reducing anxiety and stress is a prophylactic measure in known asthmatic or bronchospastic patients. These patients should continue their usual medications up to the time of surgery and are usually instructed to bring any inhalant medications with them on the day of surgery.

Symptoms. High-pitched wheezing and coarse rales due to mucus buildup can be heard on auscultation. Additionally, the nurse may note skin color changes, flaring nostrils, increased respiratory rate, cough, and restlessness. Dyspnea, tightness in the chest, and apprehension are subjective symptoms often described by awake patients.

Treatment. If positioning to improve ventilation, providing a calm environment, having the patient cough deeply, suctioning, and administering oxygen do not alleviate symptoms, more definitive therapy is indicated. Both parenteral and inhaled bronchodilating drugs can be used. Parenteral medications include subcutaneous epinephrine or terbutaline and IV theophylline, but inhalation therapy with a β-agonist is the primary treatment. Either a hand-held aerosol or a machine-driven inhaler can deliver these bronchodilating drugs, but the usual route is a hand-held spray if the patient is able to cooperate. Awake patients are often able to cooperate by inhaling their own medications brought from home.

A number of β-receptor agonists are effective. Albuterol (Ventolin, Proventil) is the most frequently prescribed and is given in a dose of 2.5 to 5 mg diluted with approximately 3 ml of sterile normal saline. This dose can be given every 2 to 4 hours. Tachycardia of greater than 140 beats/min rarely occurs but is reason to discontinue therapy with this drug. Other inhalants are also used. Metaproterenol (Alupent, Metaprel) has a slow onset but a long duration of action. Isoproterenol (Isuprel) has a rapid onset but is not as frequently used because of its propensity to cause tachyarrhythmias and premature ventricular contractions (PVCs). Other agents include isoetharine (Bronkosol, Bronkometer) and terbutaline (Brethaire). Atropine is another inhalation drug used to reduce secretions and reverse mucus buildup. It may be added to the bronchodilating medication. A dose of 0.25 mg/kg in the aerosol is conservative and can be repeated every 4 to 6 hours.[11]

Aspiration

Aspiration secondary to vomiting or regurgitation can occur in patients under general anesthesia or sedation. It can occur at any time but is most likely during induction of and emergence from anesthesia. Aspiration can result in partial or complete mechanical obstruction of the tracheobronchial tree with ensuing hypoxemia or in chemical damage to pulmonary tissue.[2]

Both the volume and the acidity of material aspirated are important indicators of the severity of outcome. Aspiration of a small amount of material may cause laryngospasm, bronchospasm, pulmonary edema, and hypoxia.[12] As little as 25 ml of gastric material can cause widespread lung damage. Blood, the most common type of material aspirated, is relatively benign unless a large volume is involved.[13] The acidity of aspirated gastric secretions is the most important factor to be considered. Material with a pH of 2.5 or less causes intense bronchospasm and destruction of tracheal mucosa. Aggressive treatment must be instituted immediately, because there is often progression to aspiration pneumonitis, pulmonary edema, and eventually adult respiratory distress syndrome (ARDS) and death.[14]

Predisposing Factors. Obesity, hiatal hernia, pregnancy, peptic ulcer, extreme nervousness, old age, diminished pharyngeal reflexes, diabetes, insufflation of the abdomen during laparoscopic procedures, and a full stomach increase the risk of aspiration. Recent alcohol ingestion slows digestion, contributing to a full stomach. Narcotic administration or partial airway obstruction during anesthesia, Trendelenburg's positioning, or the presence of an artificial airway when the patient is under a light level of anesthesia can predispose as well.[15]

An ambulatory surgery patient is particularly at risk if the NPO restriction has not been followed before admission. The results of two studies demonstrating the outpatient's risk for aspiration have prompted many anesthesiologists to administer prophylactic medications, including antacids, preoperatively. Ong and colleagues demonstrated that ambulatory surgery patients come to surgery with larger volumes of acidic gastric contents than those noted in inpatients,[16] and the study by Manchikanti and Marrero demonstrated that 60% of ambulatory anesthesia patients had a gastric pH of 2.5 or less and gastric content volumes of 25 ml or more.[17]

Prevention. Adherence to NPO status is the most essential preventive measure. After surgery, unconscious or heavily sedated patients must be constantly monitored and should remain in a side-lying, head-down position to promote gravity drainage of secretions. Extubation by the PACU nurse should occur only after protective airway reflexes return. Until the gag and swallow reflexes return, gentle oral suctioning may be needed. Artificial airways should be removed promptly when the patient begins to respond to prevent gagging.

Patients who have had topical anesthesia of the trachea or pharynx should demonstrate a return of all protective airway reflexes before taking oral liquids. Even then, water should be given first while the nurse observes the patient's ability to swallow.

A combination of any of the following pharmacologic interventions may be used for prophylaxis. The effectiveness of some is controversial, and anesthesiologists make decisions about the use of these medications on an individual basis.

Anticholinergics such as atropine and glycopyrrolate (Robinul) may be given to decrease salivary, pharyngeal, tracheal, and bronchial secretions. Glycopyrrolate reduces the volume and free acidity of gastric secretions. Because current anesthetic agents provoke fewer secretions than those used in the past, anticholinergics are not considered routine for the premedication of ambulatory surgical patients by some authorities.[18] In fact, because they reduce lower esophageal sphincter tone, some clinicians feel that they may actually predispose to regurgitation.[19]

Nonparticulate antacids such as sodium citrate (Bicitra) neutralize gastric secretions. Because this medication is rapidly absorbed orally, it can be administered preoperatively after admission. The pungent taste can be reduced if administered cold. Cimetidine (Tagamet), a histamine H_2-receptor antagonist, is used to decrease acidity and volume and is also given preoperatively either as an oral liquid or parenterally. Another premedication, metoclopramide (Reglan), fosters gastric emptying, although it does not reduce gastric acidity. Antiemetics often are given before or during anesthesia to patients with a significant history of anesthesia-related nausea or motion sickness; antiemetics reduce the potential for vomiting, and thus aspiration, in the immediate perioperative period.

Symptoms. Aspiration of small amounts of material can occur "silently"—without manifesting discernible symptoms or serious consequences. With larger amounts of aspirate, initial symptoms typically include bronchospasm, wheezing, rales, and expiratory rhonchi. Progression to tachycardia, dyspnea, hypoxemia, pulmonary edema, hypotension, and cyanosis can occur rapidly. Immediate cardiorespiratory arrest is also a possibility if the volume of aspirate is significant.

Treatment. Treatment depends on the severity of symptoms. Immediate intervention includes suctioning as appropriate, oxygen administration, and positioning to prevent further aspiration. If obstruction of the trachea has occurred owing to particulate aspiration, the airway must be cleared immediately. If an artificial airway is required, caution must be observed to avoid pushing a solid aspirant further down with the airway.

Dexamethasone or another corticosteroid may be given IV to a patient in whom aspiration is considered a possibility even if symptoms do not confirm a definitive diagnosis. A patient with substantial aspiration often requires intubation and ventilation with PEEP, antibiotics, theophylline (aminophylline), and steroid therapy. Sometimes an aggressive cardiopulmonary resuscitative course is necessary. Arterial blood gases and a chest radiograph help confirm the diagnosis. Hospitalization is indicated in significant cases.

Pulmonary Edema

Pulmonary edema occurs when fluid accumulates in the interstitial spaces or alveoli of the lungs. Onset is usually insidious and may be typified by early signs such as wheezing, cough, exercise intolerance, orthopnea, and restlessness. It is not until the process is advanced that the classic signs and symptoms of rales, frothy sputum, and hypoxemia are observed.[14] Although pulmonary edema is not a frequent complication in ambulatory surgery units, when it occurs, intervention must be immediate, for it is a true emergency.

Predisposing Factors. Aged and debilitated patients suffering from cardiopulmonary disease, particularly those with left ventricular failure, are at special risk for pulmonary edema. IV fluid overload is the most common environmental cause, but other factors include administration of narcotic antagonists, aspiration,[20] narcotic overdose, anesthesia, and pulmonary embolism.[21] In addition, if the patient does not understand the importance of continuing to take cardiotonic medications the morning of surgery, the omission of these drugs before surgery may place the patient in a state of congestive heart failure. Also, allergic reaction to medications and a number of factors unrelated to ambulatory surgery (e.g., burns, ARDS, head trauma) may result in pulmonary edema.[22] Laryngospasm-induced pulmonary edema is also a threat to the healthy outpatient population and is discussed separately.

Prevention. Thorough preanesthesia assessment of predisposed patients should help identify those at particular risk. After admission, careful attention must be given to IV fluid replacement, with the rate of infusion and total amount of solution monitored and given according to physician's orders. All medications should be administered prudently and according to manufacturers' directions. In all patients, lung sounds should be auscultated throughout the perioperative period.

Symptoms. Classic symptoms and signs include dyspnea and orthopnea; cough with pink or white sputum progressively becoming frothy and copious; anxiety and panic due to a sense of suffocation; borderline to low SaO_2 refractory to 100% oxygen administration; cyanosis and perspiration with clammy, cold skin; wheezing and audible rales; distention of neck veins; and tachycardia with weak, thready pulse.[23] Blood pressure rises, and sometimes chest pain secondary to stretching of the alveoli is present. Angina may occur because of decreased cardiac output.[24]

Treatment. Treatment for cardiogenic pulmonary edema should be initiated to improve left ventricular function, correct fluid overload, and decrease pulmonary blood flow. Anxious patients benefit significantly from the nurse's calm manner. Oxygen is given in high concentrations, and intermittent positive-pressure breathing (IPPB) may be required using PEEP. Patients should be placed in a sitting position to facilitate breathing. Although the use of rotating tourniquets has largely been replaced by newly developed medications, placing legs in a dependent position (over the edge of the stretcher, if possible) causes pooling of blood and helps decrease venous return. Patients should be supported with pillows because they are usually unable to move well or hold up their arms and legs because of the effort required to breathe. Continuous cardiac monitoring is essential.

IV morphine is often given to reduce anxiety and decrease respiratory effort. It also causes vasodilatation, thus further reducing venous return. Diuretics such as furosemide (Lasix) or ethacrynic acid (Edecrin) are given to reduce preload, and a Foley catheter is inserted to provide accurate assessment of the fluid status.

The nurse should observe for hypotension secondary to treatment. Hypotension accompanied by tachycardia and decreased urinary output indicates that the patient is not tolerating the diuresis and that hypovolemia may result. Treatment for cardiogenic pulmonary edema may include (1) a rapid-acting digitalis derivative given to increase cardiac output and enhance contractility, (2) administration of vasodilators (nitroprusside, sublingual or IV nitroglycerin) and diuretics (furosemide) to decrease preload and afterload of the heart, and (3) administration of other drugs such as dobutamine.[22]

Noncardiogenic Pulmonary Edema

Another type of pulmonary edema, noncardiogenic pulmonary edema (NCPE), is characterized by an increase in the permeability of the alveolar-capillary membrane and is also referred to as adult respiratory distress syndrome (ARDS). The term NCPE is usually reserved for a less severe form of the disorder that is limited to the interstitium. NCPE following relief of airway obstruction (laryngospasm at the end of extubation) may be due to a marked increase in the negative interstitial hydrostatic pressures.

Negative-pressure pulmonary edema (NPPE) is a rare occurrence that originates from complications following airway obstruction and attempts to breathe against a closed glottis. Oswalt and colleagues first identified the association in 1977 after three patients in a study developed acute pulmonary edema after re-establishment of obstructed airways.[25] NPPE (as well as hypertension, ventricular arrhythmias, and cardiac arrest) also can follow the administration of naloxone, an opioid antagonist occasionally used as a reversal agent at the end of anesthesia.[26–28]

Predisposing Factors. Healthy young adults and children may be affected after benign procedures. The patient often has a perioperative history of airway obstruction. The occurrence of laryngospasm, epiglottitis, and croup should alert the nurse to the potential for development of NPPE.[29]

Prevention. Because occurrence is rare and unpredictable, actual prevention is difficult. The anesthesia provider's reporting of any airway problems, such as the possibility of a "silent" or actual laryngospasm, is essential and should be passed on to all subsequent caregivers so that they can anticipate any pathophysiologic sequelae that may occur. Any interventions aimed at avoiding laryngospasm should be considered preventive for NPPE. Close observation for early symptoms should follow any episode of airway obstruction or administration of naloxone. Avoiding early discharge of an ambulatory surgical patient who has experienced significant laryngospasm is prudent.

Symptoms. The patient may present with a variety of signs and symptoms, ranging from only cough and tachypnea to all the typical symptoms of pulmonary edema, with the accompanying restlessness; respiratory distress; tachycardia and tachypnea; pink, frothy sputum; rales or rhonchi; presence of infiltrates on chest films; and decreased SaO_2, even with oxygen administration. In contrast to the elevations seen with cardiogenic pulmonary edema, pulmonary artery pressures remain normal.[30]

Treatment. Severity of symptoms dictates treatment. Oxygen therapy may be all that is needed, and its effectiveness can be ascertained by pulse oximetry rather than invasive means. Should a short period of reintubation and ventilation be necessary, deep endotracheal suctioning should be avoided, because it stimulates more pulmonary secretions. Diuretics and morphine may be required, but digoxin and steroids are not indicated.[29] The patient usually improves within minutes of therapy, and extubation is often accomplished soon thereafter. The patient should be admitted to a hospital for at least 24 hours of observation.

Pulmonary Embolism

Pulmonary embolism is another complication that rarely occurs as a direct result of an ambulatory surgical procedure, although many at-risk patients may be in the ambulatory population. Most symptomatic episodes of pulmonary embolism are caused by thrombus formation; however, other substances such as air, amniotic fluid, fat (bone marrow), tumor, and foreign material (e.g., catheters) may travel through the pulmonary circulation and obstruct pulmonary blood flow. Pulmonary embolus from thrombus formation usually originates with thrombophlebitis of the deep veins in the calf, thigh, or pelvis.[31]

Predisposing Factors. A patient with hypercoagulability, altered integrity of blood vessel walls, or venous stasis is at increased risk for pulmonary embolism.[23] Table 11–4 lists factors that predispose a patient to an embolic event.

Prevention. The multiple approaches to prevention of pulmonary embolism involve addressing the appropriate predisposing factor. Probably most notable in an ambulatory surgery setting is the need for frequent movement of extremities. Intraoperatively, a patient undergoing a lengthy plastic surgery procedure or an ear, nose, and throat procedure should have pneumatic compression devices applied to the lower legs or periodic passive range of motion exercises for the legs. Postoperatively, active and passive exercises should be encouraged for patients who are and will be immobilized, and elevation of the legs should be used to promote venous return. Adequate hydration prevents increased viscosity of the blood or platelet clumping.[9]

A patient who will be recuperating at home with an immobilized leg should be given instructions about exercises such as isometric muscle contraction. The patient should know the symptoms of a thrombus or embolus and should be instructed to report them to the phy-

Table 11–4. **Factors Predisposing to Thrombus Formation**

HYPERCOAGULABILITY	ALTERATIONS IN VESSEL WALL	VENOUS STASIS
Malignancy	Trauma	Prolonged bedrest/immobilization
Oral contraceptives high in estrogen	Varicose veins	Obesity
Fever	Diabetes mellitus	Advanced age
Sickle cell anemia	Atherosclerosis	Burns
Polycythemia vera	Pregnancy	Postpartum period
Abrupt discontinuance of anticoagulants	Inflammatory process	Congestive heart failure

From Parrish N: Congestive heart failure, pulmonary edema and pulmonary embolus. In Parker J (ed): Emergency Nursing: A Guide to Comprehensive Care. New York: John Wiley & Sons, 1984, p 118.

sician immediately. Symptoms include pain and tenderness in the calf, sudden onset of chest pain, and others described later.

Symptoms. The type and severity of symptoms depend on a number of variables, including the size, number, and location of emboli; the amount of circulation impaired by the emboli; and predisposing factors.[32] Typical signs of a moderate-sized embolus include unexplained and sudden dyspnea, cough, nonspecific chest or abdominal pain that may be severe, hypotension, tachycardia, tachypnea, diaphoresis, and anxiety. Bronchoconstriction may lead to rales, wheezing, and diminished breath sounds. If pulmonary infarction accompanies an embolism, hemoptysis and pleuritic chest pain can also occur.[23] Profuse diaphoresis, cyanosis, pupillary dilatation, and death may ensue.

Treatment. Nursing intervention is based on the severity of symptoms and includes (1) providing a calm atmosphere; (2) interventions aimed at support of the vital signs; (3) elevation of the patient's head; (4) oxygen therapy, sometimes with IPPB or intubation and ventilation; (5) cardiac monitoring; and (6) administration of IV medications to alleviate pain, support circulation, and treat arrhythmias. Fibrinolytic medications such as urokinase or streptokinase may be given to dissolve the embolus and original thrombus, and anticoagulant therapy is instituted to prevent additional emboli. Embolectomy may be necessary.[22]

Traumatic Pneumothorax

Predisposing Factors. Pneumothorax results from the accumulation of air in the pleural space with a subsequent loss of normal negative (intrapleural) pressure. Partial or total collapse of the lung occurs when the pressures inside and outside of the pleural space are equal. Pneumothorax differs from hemothorax, a condition usually associated with severe accidental trauma in which blood collects in the intrapleural space (see Fig. 11–1). Some of the invasive procedures performed in ambulatory surgery facilities can result in pneumothorax, for instance, insertion of central lines for chemotherapy, interscalene or intercostal nerve blocks, stellate ganglion block, brachial plexus block, and surgical interventions such as breast needle localization, breast augmentation, and esophageal or neck procedures.

Prevention. The most important aspects of prevention of pneumothorax involve concentration, caution, and accuracy on the part of healthcare providers who perform invasive procedures.

Symptoms. The severity of symptoms depends on the amount or percentage of lung that has collapsed and the patient's ability to compensate. Shortness of breath, pain, and inability to catch the breath are typical symptoms. If the pneumothorax is significant, the pain is often sudden and severe and is accompanied by air hunger, anxiety, diminished or absent breath sounds on the affected side, unequal chest expansion, hyper-resonance on percussion, tachycardia, enlarged neck veins, and cyanosis. Chest radiographs and arterial blood gas values confirm the diagnosis.

A tension pneumothorax is a condition in which air enters the pleural space. With every inspiration air does not escape, and the intrathoracic pressure progressively increases—collapsing the lung on the affected side and causing a mediastinal shift. This eventually compresses the heart, great vessels, trachea, and uninjured lungs toward the unaffected side of the chest. Venous return is decreased, and ultimately cardiovascular and respiratory collapse occurs unless intervention relieves the intrathoracic pressure.[33]

Treatment. The patient should be kept calm and reassured. A small pneumothorax usually resolves spontaneously and often requires only oxygen therapy and bedrest. Initial nursing interventions include raising the patient's head and administering oxygen.

Cases in which the patient is acutely symptomatic require the insertion of a chest tube to remove air from the pleural space.[34] A chest tube is attached to an underwater sealed drainage system or to a flutter valve that allows air to pass in one direction only, away from the pleural cavity. After the chest tube has been properly placed, the patient should be encouraged to cough and deep-breathe to facilitate re-expansion of the lung. Sterile technique is essential when handling a closed-chest drainage system to prevent infection. An occlusive bandage and hemostat should be available at the bedside in case the chest tube becomes dislodged or disconnected. The need for hospitalization is obvious.

A patient with severe, sudden cardiovascular and respiratory compromise as a result of a rapidly evolving tension pneumothorax requires immediate relief of intrathoracic pressure to avert cardiopulmonary arrest. A 16-gauge or larger needle is inserted over the top of the 5th rib at the anterior axillary line or over the top of the 3rd rib at the midclavicular line on the affected side. If no relief is noted, the same procedure is done on the other side of the chest. When the tension is relieved, the patient's condition should improve immediately; a chest tube is then inserted.[34]

Acute Hypertension

Predisposing Factors. Hypertension in the healthy ambulatory population can be due to many factors, such as respiratory problems (hypoxia/hypercapnea), pain, anxiety, endotracheal intubation, bladder distention, or stressful anesthesia emergence.[35] Fluid overload, shivering, and the effects of intraoperative anesthetic agents and medications are also implicated. Patients with a history of hypertension, particularly those who have omitted their usual antihypertensive medications, are likely candidates for an episode of perioperative hypertension. In addition, patients with untreated essential hypertension frequently demonstrate labile episodes of hypertension throughout the perioperative course. Many patients who have experienced hypertensive episodes tend to deny their hypertension. Therefore, healthcare providers need to direct their preoperative questions to include: "Have you ever had a high blood pressure reading, even though it was only once?" This type of questioning is imperative to prevent the sequelae of hypertensive crisis. In the PACU, the possibility of hypoxia as a cause is significant, and respiratory interventions are often the most important preventive and therapeutic measures for hypertension.

Prevention. Innumerable methods to prevent hypertension are directed toward a wide variety of potential causes. These methods include the following:

1. Maintain the patient's optimal respiratory function.
2. Provide a calm atmosphere and accurate information to reduce stress.
3. Catheterize a patient who will be under general anesthesia for a prolonged procedure.
4. Inject local anesthesia at incision sites and provide adequate analgesia.
5. Have patients take their prescribed blood pressure medications up to and including the morning of surgery.

Symptoms. Elevated blood pressure readings should be evaluated in relation to the patient's normal level. Obtain the preadmission testing blood pressure when possible in order to monitor trends in the patient's hemodynamic status. Definitive numeric levels cannot be identified that relate to all people; however, a systolic reading of greater than 160 mm Hg and a diastolic reading of greater than 90 to 100 mm Hg are often cited. A mean arterial pressure of 130 mm Hg is considered significant. With diastolic readings of 120 to 140 mm Hg, a patient often suffers from visual disturbances, papilledema, and headache. The most significant effects of hypertension are on the eyes, brain, heart, and kidneys.[20]

Treatment. The therapeutic management of hypertension should be aimed at the cause and may include analgesics or sedatives for the management of pain and anxiety, respiratory support, or emptying of the bladder. Not all episodes of elevated blood pressure are or should be treated, because many are self-limited. Often the only treatment needed is time away from the stress of the OR or a period of active emergence. Vasodilators may be necessary in some cases; however, they are usually contraindicated if the hypertension is due to hypoxia, because vasodilatation could result in profound hypotension by counteracting the body's compensatory vasoconstriction.[36] Severe hypertension can produce postoperative bleeding, myocardial ischemia, heart failure, or intracranial hemorrhage.

Treatment of hypertension in the perianesthesia setting is focused on vasodilatation or depressing the myocardium (Table 11–5).[37] The purpose of using the vasodilating calcium channel blocking drugs, such as those in the nifedipine family, is 2-fold: to reduce afterload of the heart by vasodilatation while at the same time having a prompt, effective action. These medications, such as nitroglycerin or nitroprusside, are short-acting agents and can be given by IV bolus or infusion for prolonged or severe hypertension.[37] β-Blockers are also used in reducing cardiac output. However, one must remember that the β-adrenergic antagonists may potentiate bronchoconstriction of the smooth muscle and should be used cautiously in patients with compromised respiratory function.[37] Other antihypertensive drugs are presented in Table 11–5.

The nurse should assess the blood pressure frequently while observing for signs of untoward sequelae associated with the treatment protocol or with the hypertension itself. Symptoms of severe hypertension include visual disturbances, headache, dizziness, chest pain, or palpitations. If left untreated, severe hypertension can lead to stroke.

***Table 11–5.* Treatment Modalities for Postoperative Hypertension**

DRUG	DOSE RANGE	BETA HALF-LIFE
β-Blockers		
Propranolol (Inderal)	0.5–1 mg IV	2–4 hr
Labetalol (Trandate, Normodyne—mixed α and β)	Initial: 20 mg IV; additional dosages of 20–80 mg at 10 min intervals up to 300 mg	4–6 hr
Esmolol (Brevibloc β_1)	500 μg/kg/min (over 1 min) IV may be followed by infusion 50–200 μg/kg/min	9 min
Metoprolol (Lopressor B_1)	5–25 mg IV increments	2.5–4.5 hr
Smooth Muscle Vasodilators		
Hydralazine (Apresoline)	2.5–5 mg IV increments	4–6 hr
Nitroglycerin	5 μg/min initially; increase gradually as needed	1–4 min
Calcium Channel Blockers		
Nifedipine (Procardia)	10–20 mg PO	4–6 hr
Nicardipine (Cardene)	2.5 mg IV	6 hr
ACE Inhibitor		
Enalapril (Vasotec)	2.5 mg IV	4–6 hr

ACE, angiotensin-converting enzyme; IV, intravenous; PO, per os; SL, sublingual.
From Twersky RS: The Ambulatory Anesthesia Handbook. St. Louis: Mosby–Year Book, 1995.

Cardiac Arrhythmias

Predisposing Factors. Arrhythmias range from benign extrasystoles to life-threatening ventricular fibrillation. Patients with pre-existing cardiovascular disease or arrhythmias are more likely than others to experience arrhythmias in the perioperative period. The generally healthy ambulatory population is not at unusually high risk for major arrhythmias; however, anesthetic agents and sedatives may depress respirations and result in hypoxia, causing arrhythmias. Also, many anesthetic gases and drugs can directly affect the heart. For these reasons, all patients who have been given anesthesia should be considered at potential risk for drug-induced arrhythmias. Other potential causes of arrhythmias include anxiety or pain that stimulates the sympathetic nervous system, electrolyte imbalance, and hypoxemia or hypovolemia that results in decreased oxygen supply to the heart.

Prevention. Thorough preoperative assessments should identify people at risk for arrhythmias. Patients on long-term antiarrhythmic therapy usually continue those medications until several hours before surgery. Perioperative nurses should be able to identify aberrant rhythms in cardiac monitor patterns so that early treatment or prophylaxis can be instituted, if necessary.

Careful titration of sedative and anesthetic dosages is important in avoiding cardiac side effects. Effective oxygenation and ventilation must be maintained, particularly for a patient with pre-existing cardiac disease who poorly tolerates any reduction in myocardial oxygen supply.

Symptoms. Arrhythmias have many possible origins, and their symptoms are equally disparate in nature. For example, bradycardia can result in fatigue, syncope, mental confusion, hypotension, and convulsions; tachyarrhythmias such as supraventricular tachycardia can produce palpitations, hypotension, precordial pain, signs of congestive heart failure, and anxiety. Life-threatening arrhythmias such as ventricular tachycardia (VT), profound bradycardia, and complete heart block cause decreased cardiac output with hypotension and decreased perfusion to vital organs, including the myocardium, lungs, and brain. Cerebral ischemia and stroke may result. Other life-threatening arrhythmias, including ventricular fibrillation, asystole, and pulseless electrical activity, are discussed under Cardiopulmonary Arrest.

Treatment. Maintaining adequate circulation, restoring the normal cardiac cycle, and correcting the precipitating factors are the primary considerations in treating dysrhythmias. Continuous perioperative cardiac monitoring should be conducted. Emergency drugs and resuscitation equipment must be immediately available. IV access should be secured and maintained on all patients throughout their ambulatory surgery stay.

ACLS includes drugs and protocols indicated for the treatment of arrhythmias. Recommended protocols[38] for suppression of ventricular ectopy include the following steps:

1. IV lidocaine 1 to 1.5 mg/kg; if not effective—
2. Repeat lidocaine 0.5 to 1.5 mg/kg every 5 to 10 minutes up to 3 mg/kg or until ectopy is suppressed; if still not effective—
3. Procainamide (Pronestyl) 20 to 30 mg/min, up to a maximum of 17 mg/kg or until ectopy is suppressed; if still not effective—
4. Administer bretylium tosylate (Bretylol) 5 to 10 mg/kg in 50 ml D5W over 8 to 10 minutes or consider overdrive cardiac pacing. The reader is referred to the many available cardiac nursing texts for a detailed discussion.

External cardiac pacing is considered the mainstay of treatment for symptomatic bradycardia and heart blocks refractory to medications until a transvenous pacer is inserted. A plan for emergency insertion of a temporary pacemaker should be in place. This situation is somewhat more complicated for a freestanding surgery center than for a hospital-based unit.

A patient who experiences symptomatic arrhythmias should be observed for an extended period after treatment. Hospitalization may be indicated, dependent on the severity of the arrhythmia and the response to treatment.

Cardiopulmonary Arrest

Predisposing Factors. Cardiopulmonary arrest may occur as a result of progressive arrhythmias, allergic reactions to drugs, respiratory inadequacies, acute MI, pre-existing coronary artery disease, and other conditions. The most important factor predisposing a patient to cardiac risk in the immediate perioperative period is a history of previous MI.[39] Administration of depressant drugs and the potential for alterations in tissue oxygenation due to hypovolemia or hemorrhage may be contributing factors as well. It is important to remember that in 80% to 90% of cases, sudden death is due to ventricular fibrillation (VF).

Prevention. Prompt treatment is important in preventing potentially lethal arrhythmias that lead to cardiac arrest. Medications must be given with discretion, and the patient closely observed for untoward or allergic reactions. A sedated or postanesthesia patient should be encouraged to deep-breathe and cough to maintain adequate oxygenation, and supplemental oxygen should be given until the patient maintains adequate respiratory depth and rate. Arrhythmias, which are typically prodromal to VF or asystole, should be treated aggressively. VT, frequent PVCs or those occurring on or close to the T wave (repolarization) of the ECG cycle, supraventricular tachyarrhythmias with rapid ventricular response, and progressive heart block may require immediate intervention.

Symptoms. Patients experiencing cardiopulmonary arrest have an abrupt cessation of the pulse and respirations, with the ECG pattern VF, asystole, or pulseless electrical activity (PEA). Blood pressure and lung and heart sounds are absent; the patient is or rapidly becomes unconscious and may have a convulsion. VF is the most common rhythm associated with cardiopulmonary arrest in adults. VF is manifested as a coarse, chaotic waveform on the ECG.

If the cardiac arrest is secondary to acute MI, the arrest may be preceded by restlessness, hypotension, an expressed feeling of impending doom, chest or arm pain, and ECG changes. The hallmark ECG signs in the progression of MI include inverted T waves during periods of ischemia; ST elevation of 2 mm or more when muscle injury occurs; and eventually, when necrosis occurs, the appearance of a Q wave that is at least 0.03 second in duration and is one fourth the height of the total QRS complex.[40] Changes in various leads of the ECG after MI are identified in Table 11–6.

Treatment. Survival of an adult victim of cardiopulmonary arrest is influenced by a number of factors. The cardiac rhythm is significant. Asystole and PEA present a graver outcome than cardiac arrest secondary to VT or VF. The elapsed time from arrest to initiation of CPR and ACLS measures is another factor influencing survival, along with the duration of the resuscitative efforts. The best outcomes occur when CPR is initiated within 4 minutes of arrest, when advanced treatments occur within 10 minutes of arrest,[41] and when efforts are effective in restoring a viable rhythm within 15 to 20 minutes.[42]

Defibrillation for VF (the most common arrhythmia in an arrest) should be instituted rapidly; otherwise, it may be ineffective, especially in an elderly patient. The American Heart Association (AHA) recommends that immediately after identifying VF or pulseless VT, one should deliver the first shock at 200 joules (J).[43] If no conversion occurs, deliver the second shock at 200 to 300 J and the third shock at 360 J. Then administer compressions, ventilations, and drugs as recommended.[44] Definitive interven-

Table 11–6. **Relationship of Site of Myocardial Infarction to Leads with Characteristic Pattern Changes**

SITE OF MYOCARDIAL INFARCTION	LEADS	CHARACTERISTIC CHANGE
Inferior wall	II, III, AVF	ST segment elevation; pathologic Q wave; T wave inversion
Posterior wall	V_1, V_2, V_3	Tall R wave; upright T wave
Anterior wall	V_2, V_3, V_4	ST segment elevation; pathologic Q wave; T wave inversion
Septal wall	V_1, V_2	ST segment elevation; pathologic Q wave; T wave inversion
Anterolateral wall	I, AVL, V_5, V_6	ST segment elevation; pathologic Q wave; T wave inversion

Adapted from Grauer K, Whitney C: Clinical Electro-Cardiography: A Primary Care Approach. Malden, MA: Blackwell Science, 1993.

tions such as adequate ventilations, CPR, intubation, epinephrine, and antiarrhythmics are subsequently and sequentially instituted.

Protocols are often used by the nurse to initiate life-saving interventions until the physician arrives. The nurse must immediately summon assistance and have the appropriate physicians notified. CPR may be preceded by a precordial thump in a witnessed arrest using the hypothenar aspect of the fist to the center of the sternum from no more than a 12-inch height.[43] The AHA guidelines for management of cardiac arrest and life-threatening arrhythmias should be available and periodically reviewed in all ambulatory surgery settings.

The nurse further assists with drug administration, intubation, and defibrillation or insertion of a pacemaker. Figure 11–2 illustrates a flow sheet for documentation during an emergency code. Figure 11–3 is used for a follow-up critique or evaluation of the code process. This provides an excellent opportunity to review the code team's response as a quality improvement method and at the same time affords a critical debriefing process for the staff.

Myocardial irritability is treated most often with IV lidocaine or with procainamide or bretylium if lidocaine is ineffective.[45] If IV access is lost and cannot be readily re-established, certain emergency drugs can be administered via the endotracheal tube (2 to 2.5 times the peripheral IV dose) and flushed with 10 ml of normal saline. The mnemonic LEAN identifies those drugs by the first letters of their names: lidocaine, epinephrine, atropine, and naloxone. Positive-pressure ventilation with hyperventilation after drug administration is necessary to promote adequate delivery and ultimately absorption into the circulation.[42]

The acid-base imbalance of most cardiac arrest patients is respiratory in origin, and treatment should be directed to the respiratory system, such as hyperventilation with high-flow oxygen. Sodium bicarbonate should be considered only after 10 minutes of arrest in patients with pre-existing acidosis, hyperkalemia, and refractory VF. The recommended initial dose of sodium bicarbonate is 1 mEq/kg. Subsequent doses are one half of the first dose, given no more than every 10 minutes, based on the patient's arterial blood gas levels.[46] It is important to prevent overtreatment, which could result in alkalosis, which is extremely difficult, if not impossible, to correct.

Studies have not demonstrated calcium administration to be beneficial during resuscitative efforts unless hyperkalemia, hypocalcemia, or calcium channel blocker overdose exists.[42] When so indicated, the IV dosage for an adult is calcium chloride 500 to 2000 mg (maximum 30 mg/kg; do not exceed rate of 1 ml/min[46]) or calcium gluconate 5 to 8 ml.[47]

Initial treatment of asystole includes CPR, administration of epinephrine, and external cardiac pacing. Atropine may restore normal atrioventricular nodal conduction and initiate electrical activity. Use of an external pacemaker may be the only effective means of restoring a viable rhythm and should be considered early in the resuscitation.

PEA is a rare entity that occurs when the electrical activity of the heart continues while the pumping action is absent, rendering no cardiac output. Thus, an ECG pattern is present, but the patient has no pulse. Treatment is aimed at the underlying cause of the arrhythmia; for example, profound hypovolemia is treated by rapidly infusing IV fluids, tension

CARDIOPULMONARY RESUSCITATION FORM

Date:

Name	Age	Sex	ED Number	Time Arrived In ED:	Mode of Arrival	Approximate Time of Arrest:	Code Called:

Etiology of Arrest: ☐ Respiratory ☐ Cardiac ☐ Other:

Time CPR Started:

Notification of: By:
Family @ ________ ________
Physician @ ________ ________
Chaplain @ ________ ________

☐ Yes Time:
☐ No

Initial Rhythm: ☐ V. Fibrillation ☐ Asystole ☐ Other:
☐ V. Tachycardia ☐ EMD Time: By:

☐ Witnessed ☐ Unwitnessed By: Monitor to Pt. @ Local Physician:

Respiratory Management

Method	Time	By
Airway		
Oxygen		
Mouth-to-Mouth		
Ambu/Mask		
Ambu/ET		

Intubation

Tube Size:	Time:		
By:			
Placement			
Checked*			
Time			

*Breath Sounds

Circulatory Assistance

Time			
Method			
By			
Pulse Check			

Prehospital Care
☐ None ☐ BCLS @ ________
☐ ACLS @ ______ ; Meds,
I.V.s, etc.: ________

Lab	Time
X-ray	Time

Blood Gases

Time			
Site			
By			
O_2 Con			
pH			
$PaCO_2$			
PaO_2			
Base Ex			

Precordial Thump: ☐ No ☐ Yes Time: ________ Response: ________

Defibrillation or Cardioversion

Dysrhythmia							
Time							
Watts/Sec							
Response							

Intravenous Therapy

Solution & Amount	Site	Needle	Time Started	Rate	Medications Added	Amt Rec	By

History/Prior Condition:

Medications

Medication									
Epinephrine	Dose/Rt								
	Time								
Sodium Bicarb	Dose/Rt								
	Time								
Calcium Chloride	Dose/Rt								
	Time								
Atropine	Dose/Rt								
	Time								
Isoproterenol	Dose/Rt								
	Time								
Lidocaine Bolus	Dose/Rt								
	Time								
Lidocaine Drip	Dose/Rt								
	Time								
Bretylium Bolus	Dose/Rt								
	Time								
Pronestyl	Dose/Rt								
	Time								
Dopamine Drip	Dose/Rt								
	Time								
Dobutamine	Dose/Rt								
	Time								
Levophed	Dose/Rt								
	Time								
Verapamil	Dose/Rt								
	Time								
	Dose/Rt								
	Time								
	Dose/Rt								
	Time								

Comments:

Vital Signs

Time							
BP							
Pulse							
Resp							
Temp							
Pupils							

Procedures

Procedure	Time	Size	By
NG tube			
Foley catheter			
Pacemaker			

Neurologic Status by Glasgow Coma Scale

Time		
Eyes Open		
Best Verbal Response		
Best Motor Response		
Total Score		

Outcome: Time CPR Stopped: ________
☐ Survived
Disposition: ________
Time of Transfer: ________
Condition @ Transfer: ________

Disposition of Valuables: ________

Total Time of Resuscitation: ________
(Attach representative EKG strips to back.)

☐ Expired @ ________
Autopsy Requested: ☐ Yes ☐ No
Medical Examiner Notified:
☐ No ☐ Yes Time: ________
By: ________
Organs Donated: ☐ Yes ☐ No
Consent Signed: ☐ Yes ☐ No
Physician Summary/Impression: ________

CPR Team:
MD in Charge: ________
Others: ________

Signatures:

Recorder ________ Nurse ________ Physician ________

Figure 11–2. Cardiopulmonary resuscitation form. (Reprinted with permission. © Judith Young Bradford, RN, CEN, MSN, Waveland, MS.)

OUTPATIENT CENTER
Evaluation of Code Process

Date: ______ **Locale:**__________________ **Scenario:** ____________________ pg. 1

___ **Actual** ___ **Mock**

Center Name: ______________ **Evaluation of response of team:**

Write in times:	Functions:	PEOPLE RESPONDING/HELPING W/CODE
	Patient found	
1.	Code called	
2.	1st responder arrives	
3.	Code cart arrives	
4.	Code "leader" role fulfilled	
5.	ACLS &/or nurse arrives	
6.	Physician arrives	
7.	Code called "complete" - all assignment card roles fulfilled and paging stopped	

Evaluation of Patient Assessment: **COMMENTS**

8.	Establish unresponsiveness	
9.	Call for help	
10.	Reposition if necessary	
11.	Airway	
12.	Breathing	
13.	Circulation	
CART AVAILABLE, CODE TEAM ARRIVES		
14.	Apply monitor, check rhythm	
15.	Vital signs	
16.	IV access	
17.	ACLS protocols	
18.	Critical thinking verbalized	
	Responders performed roles	

Total Criteria = 26 **Criteria not met**______ **Total Score:** __/26__ (see next page)

Figure 11–3. Outpatient center evaluation of code process. (Reprinted with permission of Morton Plant Mease Trinity Outpatient Center, New Port Richey, FL.)

Evaluation of Code Assignments: **CODE LEADER:** ______________________

ROLE	DUTIES	NAME & EVALUATION OF PERFORMANCE
19. AIRWAY	☐ respirations maintain/establish airway oxygen administration rescue breathing prn Ambu prn	
20.CIRCULATION	☐ pulse compressions prn ☐ BP	
21. RECORDER	Fill out Code Blue sheet Info back to code team provides algorithm sheets assist ACLS leader	
22. PT. HISTORY	get chart if available fill out history form call pt's own physician	
23. TRAFFIC CONTROL	move other people away communicate/calm others inform other depts - status	
24. GO-FERs	respond to team request	
25. ACLS LEAD	assessment rhythm ID Directs Meds and defibs	
26. NURSE or PHYSICIAN	IV start/ give meds intubate as able shocks prn	

NOTES:____

____

____

****

CRITIQUE WITH TEAM:

____

____

____

____

PROCESS CHANGES IDENTIFIED & IMPLEMENTED:

____

____

____

____

Evaluated by :______________________________ CODEEVAL

Figure 11–3 *Continued.*

pneumothorax by inserting a needle thoracostomy, cardiac tamponade by performing a pericardiocentesis, or severe acid-base disturbance by giving sodium bicarbonate. The prognosis is usually grave.

Hemorrhage

Predisposing Factors. The most obvious cause of hemorrhage is surgical trauma. Bleeding can occur at the time of surgery, soon after, or later in the recuperative period. Intraoperatively, a perforated viscus or a lacerated major vessel may cause sudden and severe hemorrhage, requiring immediate intervention. Appropriate sterile instruments must be ready at all times. There may be concealed bleeding intraoperatively that becomes evident only in the postoperative period. Bleeding also can be triggered by postoperative restlessness, activity, or hypertension. Patients with primary bleeding disorders, chronic alcoholics, those with vitamin K deficiency, and people taking anticoagulant medications are at increased risk for bleeding.

Prevention. Preoperatively, the nurse should question the patient about any history of bleeding tendencies. Anticoagulants, including over-the-counter nonsteroidal anti-inflammatories and aspirin, are generally discontinued before elective surgery. Bleeding and clotting studies may be ordered to ascertain a patient's status before surgery. Foremost, a surgeon's precision is necessary to prevent accidental puncture of a viscus or vessel and to ensure that all bleeding points are thoroughly ligated or cauterized intraoperatively.

After surgery, patients should be monitored closely for symptoms of bleeding and kept calm and comfortable, particularly those at increased risk for bleeding. Sedation may be indicated, particularly after tonsillectomy and other ear, nose, and throat procedures, to prevent postoperative nausea, vomiting, and retching.

Symptoms. Hemorrhage can be as blatant as visible blood on the dressing or at the surgical site. Concealed bleeding is more difficult to assess. Symptoms depend on the type and site of the procedure. For instance, intra-abdominal bleeding from a liver biopsy or after a laparoscopy may present insidiously as restlessness, increased girth, and increased abdominal pain and rigidity. Other signs and symptoms of hemorrhage include frequent swallowing, hemoptysis, vomiting of blood, swelling or hardness at the surgical site, asymmetry of the body, hematuria, increased vaginal flow, or passage of clots.

If bleeding is significant, peripheral vasoconstriction develops and systemic physiologic symptoms become evident. The patient may show signs of cerebral hypoperfusion, hypoxia, and acidosis that may be exhibited as restlessness, anxiety, and inability to lie still. An awake patient may express feelings of uneasiness or fear. The skin becomes cool and moist as the pulse speeds and the blood pressure falls. If the bleeding goes unchecked, respirations become labored and the patient becomes "air hungry." Progressive decline in blood pressure and cardiac output leads to increased pallor, changes in level of consciousness, decreased urinary output, and extreme weakness. Hypovolemic shock is present when the circulating blood flow is inadequate and vital organs are denied or unable to use oxygen and nutrients.[48]

Treatment. Stopping any active bleeding and supporting the circulation are the priorities in managing hemorrhage. If possible, the nurse should apply direct pressure and elevate the site of bleeding. Sometimes ice may be used to promote vasoconstriction. The patient should be kept calm and warm, although excessive warming is avoided because it can cause peripheral vasodilatation that may add to hypotension. Analgesics or sedatives may be necessary to foster rest and promote cessation of bleeding. The patient should be kept recumbent and, if hypotension is present, a modified Trendelenburg's position should be used by elevating the legs.

IV fluid replacement usually involves the administration of crystalloids, such as lactated Ringer's solution. However, a patient with severe hemorrhage may require colloidal replacement because colloids remain in the vasculature more effectively. Colloids include blood, blood products, plasma, serum albumin, and plasma substitutes such as dextran.

A postoperative patient with significant or suspected bleeding should remain NPO in expectation of a return to surgery for definitive intervention. The nurse must carefully assess the progression of symptoms. In addition, the nurse should accurately report vital signs, surgical site, pain, airway patency (especially if the bleeding involves that area), and urinary output.

Compromise of Peripheral Circulation

Predisposing Factors. Circulation can be compromised if an encircling bandage, splint, or cast was applied too tightly at the time of surgery or if swelling occurs after surgery. Antiembolic hose should not be allowed if it causes constriction (by sagging or bunching around the knee, calf, or thigh). Another less frequent occurrence is the formation of a thrombus or embolus that can prevent blood flow in an artery or vein.

Prevention. Caution must be taken to avoid applying too tightly any dressing or immobilizing device, including wrist or arm restraints used to maintain an IV line. Initial assessment of circulatory status may be difficult if the patient's extremity was in a tourniquet intraoperatively, because the skin color may be flushed or pale for a while after deflation of the tourniquet. Frequent evaluations of the extremity must be continued in the postoperative period to ascertain the return of circulation to the extremity. An ultrasonic Doppler or pulse oximetry probe to the distal extremity when palpation is unsuccessful is a helpful assessment tool.

Instructions before discharge should include symptoms that the patient should report to the physician. Also important are methods to help avoid swelling in an extremity, thus reducing the chance of circulatory compromise from dressings and casts. Primarily, the patient should be told to elevate the extremity above the level of the heart.

Symptoms. Circulatory compromise includes color changes in the extremity distal to the bandage (flushed or bluish), swelling due to obstructed venous return, diminished pulses, and delayed or absent capillary refill. Subjective symptoms include numbness, prickling, and a feeling that the extremity is "asleep."

Treatment. Relieving the restriction to blood flow is the primary consideration. Loosening splints, Ace or other bandages, and tape is often sufficient to provide relief. If a cast is restrictive, it may need to be split and wrapped with Ace bandages to secure it. Treatment of peripheral circulatory compromise must be swift and definitive to provide adequate oxygenation to distal tissues.

Anaphylaxis

Predisposing Factors. Anaphylaxis and anaphylactoid reactions are immediate hypersensitivity responses that involve a systemic reaction to a specific antigen. Anaphylaxis is immunologically mediated through specific immunoglobulin E (IgE) antibodies and requires previous sensitization. The clinical severity ranges from mild to fatal. Anaphylactoid reactions, though clinically similar to anaphylaxis, are mediated by histamine—not IgE antibodies—and may follow a single exposure to an antigen. For example, a narcotic can activate the complement system and directly release histamine from the mast cells, resulting in a reaction such as the development of urticaria following high-dose morphine.[50, 51] The complement system, which acts as a mediator of inflammation, is activated by the classic pathway (requiring previous sensitization and an antigen/antibody response) and the alternative pathway (trauma, infection, sepsis, mast cell activation). Both pathways converge and develop into the terminal response or anaphylatoxin activation (anaphylactic/anaphylactoid response). Consequently, when patients experience anaphylatoxin activation, the smooth muscles contract in the arteries, trachea, and peripheral airways, which may cause an immediate life-threatening condition.

Prevention. Careful preoperative history taking helps identify patients at risk for an allergic reaction. Patients should be asked about allergy to shellfish, because the antigen involved (iodine) is found in contrast dyes and preparation solutions used in ASCs. Known allergies should be clearly documented on the medical record and referred to before administration of any drug in the ASC. A specific color-coded allergy identification bracelet should be worn by such patients, in addition to the admission bracelet, that lists the allergies and describes the reaction to each. If there is a question of possible allergic reaction, the nurse should have immediately available diphenhydramine, corticosteroids, and epinephrine.

Symptoms. The mechanism of this reaction involves the body's massive release of histamine and vasoactive mediators that act on blood vessels, with resulting capillary and arteriole dilatation. Erythema, hives, and wheals often occur initially. Capillary permeability increases, allowing fluid to shift from intravascular to interstitial spaces, with resulting hypovolemia.[35] Severe pulmonary or cerebral edema may develop owing to this fluid shift. In fact, massive upper airway edema is the most common cause of anaphylaxis-related death due to vasogenic shock.[50] Other symptoms may include bronchospasm due to smooth muscle contraction in the respiratory tract, gastrointestinal distress, diaphoresis, weakness, cardiac arrhythmias, ECG changes, hypotension, lightheadedness, urticaria, and apprehension or a sense of impending doom.

Treatment. Any substance causing an allergic reaction—antibiotics, blood, contrast dyes—must be discontinued immediately. Existing IV tubing should be changed if the allergen is being administered intravenously. Another priority is establishing and maintaining the airway, because obstruction may occur as a result of laryngeal edema. Epinephrine (0.1 to 0.5 mg of 1:1000) is usually given subcutaneously or intramuscularly and may be repeated 4 to 5 times at 3- to 5-minute intervals.[52] Diphenhydramine (Benadryl), an H_1-receptor antagonist, given intravenously, usually counteracts the body's histamine release. Rarely, an alternative H_2 blocker (H_2 antagonist) such as cimetidine or ranitidine may be used if diphenhydramine is not effective. IV fluids and vasopressors may be needed to support the circulation. Steroids and aminophylline may be required for persistent bronchospasm, and CPR may be necessary.

After any allergic episode, the patient should be given an explanation of what occurred, including the name of the causative agent and written instructions to avoid it in the future. The patient should be impressed with the importance of telling all future healthcare providers about the allergic reaction and should be encouraged to wear a MedicAlert bracelet.

Malignant Hyperthermia

Malignant hyperthermia, or malignant hyperpyrexia, is a potentially fatal pharmacogenetic complication of anesthesia.[53] This disorder of the skeletal muscle, due to an uncommon inherited cellular defect, is a rapidly progressive hypermetabolic state that is usually triggered by the administration of depolarizing muscle relaxants, such as succinylcholine and all volatile inhalation anesthetic gases except nitrous oxide. In addition, the hypermetabolic state causes increased CO_2 production and O_2 consumption, with resulting muscle membrane degradation. MH may have a subtle onset, or it may appear as a fulminant form, producing tremendous heat and rapidly increasing temperatures—as much as 1°C every 5 minutes—with temperatures exceeding 42°C (fever is usually a late sign).[54, 55] Other signs and symptoms of a crisis include tachycardia, dysrhythmias, hypercapnia, tachypnea, acidosis, cyanosis, mottled skin, and skeletal muscle rigidity. Laboratory findings reveal myoglobinuria and elevated serum calcium, potassium, and creatine kinase (drawn at 6, 12, and 24 hours after the event).[56] Previously, it was thought that stress, anxiety, pain, or heat could trigger an episode, but researchers currently acknowledge controversy over whether MH crisis is related to any of those factors.[57] Table 11–7 lists the known pharmacologic triggering agents.

Table 11–7. Malignant Hyperthermia–Triggering Agents

Succinylcholine (Anectine, Quelicin)
Potent inhalation anesthetics
Halothane
Enflurane
Isoflurane
Desflurane
Intravenous potassium when given rapidly
Possibly implicated agents
Phenothiazines
Chlorpromazine (Thorazine)
Prochlorperazine (Compazine)
Haloperidol (Haldol)
Nonpharmacologic (possible but unlikely triggers)
Stress
Heat stroke

Data from Malignant Hyperthermia Association of the United States: Understanding Malignant Hyperthermia. Sherburne, NY: MHAUS, 1997.

MH strikes all ages, sexes, and races but is more common in males after puberty. The reported incidence of MH in children is 1:7000 to 14,000 and in adults 1:50,000 to 120,000. In children, the higher incidence may reflect the misdiagnosis of MH in children with undiagnosed cardiomyopathies who suffer cardiac arrests following the administration of succinylcholine.[58]

Because MH is transmitted genetically, its prevalence may be significantly increased by the large groups of predisposed relatives living in certain communities and geographic areas. Mortality rates have dropped sharply (70% to 90%) since the introduction of dantrolene sodium in 1979, to about 7% in 1980. The current mortality rate is expected to be close to zero, owing primarily to the availability of a specific treatment agent and increased awareness of MH due in large part to the Malignant Hyperthermia Association of the United States (MHAUS).[59, 60]

Predisposing Factors. The underlying pathology in MH is a defect in the sarcoplasmic reticulum (SR), the area of muscle cells involved with the storage of calcium ions. Although the exact pathophysiology is not known, it is proposed that MH-triggering agents interfere with calcium re-entry into the SR. The calcium ion pumps run, releasing excessive calcium into the cross bridges of actin and myosin (contractile proteins), resulting in continuous contraction of the muscle fibers and the release of excessive amounts of heat. This causes the hypermetabolic state that consumes oxygen, releases carbon dioxide, and produces the classic muscle rigidity, fever, and acidosis. The body responds with increased sympathetic activity, resulting in cellular damage and metabolic derangements.[61]

Prevention. Careful preoperative screening is essential, including asking the patient or parents about previous MH episodes and thoroughly reviewing documentation of how the case was managed. In addition, it is important to inquire whether other family members have had adverse experiences related to general anesthesia.[55] Identification of MH-susceptible patients allows the anesthesia provider to plan an anesthetic that is free of MH triggering agents.

Drugs that are considered safe for use in a predisposed person are listed in Table 11–8. Many references cite amide anesthetics, such as lidocaine, among the triggering agents for MH, but recent evidence indicates that they are safe.[57, 58] In two separate studies on pigs that were inbred for high MH susceptibility, neither Harrison and Morrell[60] nor Wingard and Bobko[61] were able to induce MH with the administration of lidocaine or bupivacaine. Gronert notes that "based upon recent information, MH is unlikely to be precipitated by local anesthesia."[62] The advice of specialists in MH regarding the treatment of cardiac arrhythmias during a crisis is to use any antiarrhythmic drugs except calcium channel blocking agents.[63]

Preoperative identification of at-risk patients alerts all healthcare providers to a higher-than-normal probability of a crisis. The screening questionnaire in Table 10–5 is designed to help identify those people who may be at risk, but the only definitive test for a positive diagnosis of MH is the halothane-caffeine muscle contracture test. This test requires a skeletal muscle biopsy and is performed at only a handful of centers in the United States. These centers are listed in Table 11–9.

Many practitioners suggest that a patient at high risk for MH is not a candidate for ambulatory surgery and should be admitted to the hospital for postoperative monitoring and evaluation and often for a prophylactic preoperative course of oral dantrolene sodium. Some critics of that philosophy argue that if ambulatory surgery is considered safe for all the unknown MH-susceptible patients who may frequent the setting, it should be safe when the anesthesia has been purposefully designed to avoid triggering an episode in a known MH patient. Literature from the MHAUS states that a known MH patient undergoing outpatient surgery may be discharged on the day of surgery if the anesthetic has been uneventful. A minimum of 4 hours in the PACU is suggested.[63, 64]

Symptoms. An MH crisis usually occurs in the OR, particularly during induction, although occasionally the PACU may be the setting. In very rare situations, the crisis may develop hours after anesthesia has ended, but fulminant episodes occur close to the administration of the triggering agent. Early identification and treatment are essential for a positive outcome for the patient.

Often the presenting symptom of MH is rigidity of the jaw (masseter muscle rigidity, or MMR) after an initial dose of succinylcholine for intubation. When anesthesia and surgery are immediately averted and treatment instituted, a full-blown crisis may be avoided. Consider one 3-year-old child who developed MMR coupled with tachycardia of 170 beats/min during induction. Her end-tidal CO_2 was also noted to be elevated; this is considered to be the most sensitive initial physiologic indicator of MH. The case was canceled, and she was treated immediately with dantrolene. Her creatine kinase rose to 48,000 units (from a normal of <300), but she eventually had a full recovery.[63]

Unfortunately, the early alerting sign of rigidity may not occur, and the anesthesiologist may be unaware of any problem until there is unexplained tachycardia or the surgeon reports dark blood in the field. Ventricular arrhythmias are potentially dangerous signs and may occur secondary to potassium loss from cells and hypoxia due to the hypermetabolic state. The skin color changes, appearing flushed and then mottled; the color rapidly deteriorates to cyanotic mot-

***Table 11–8.* Agents Considered "Safe" for Malignant Hyperthermia–Susceptible Patients**

- Nitrous oxide
- Narcotics
- Barbiturates
- Droperidol (Inapsine)
- Propofol (Diprivan)
- Benzodiazepines
  - Midazolam (Versed)
  - Diazepam (Valium)
  - Lorazepam (Ativan)
- Etomidate
- Muscle relaxants (nondepolarizing)*
  - Pancuronium
  - Vecuronium
  - Atracurium
- Local anesthetics (amides and esters)

*The safety of curare is considered questionable.

From Malignant Hyperthermia Association of the United States: Malignant Hyperthermia: An Outpatient Anesthesia Concern. Sherburne, NY: MHAUS, 1997.

Table 11–9.* Directory of U.S. Malignant Hyperthermia Muscle Biopsy Centers

CENTER	CONTACT
Bowman Gray School of Medicine of Wake Forest University Winston-Salem, NC 27157	Thomas E. Nelson, PhD (919) 716-4285
Cleveland Clinic Foundation Cleveland, OH 44106	Glenn E. DeBoer, MD (216) 444-6331 Hiroshi Mitsumoto, MD (216) 444-5418
Allegheny University of the Health Sciences, MCP ♦ Hahnemann School of Medicine Philadelphia, PA 19102	Henry Rosenberg, MD (215) 448-7960
Mayo Clinic Rochester, MN 55901	Denise Wedel, MD (507) 255-5601
Northwestern University Medical School Chicago, IL 60611	Steven Hall, MD, or Silas Glisson, PhD (312) 908-2541
Uniformed Services University of the Health Sciences, F. Edward Hébert School of Medicine Bethesda, MD 20014	Sheila Muldoon, MD (301) 295-340
University of California, Davis, School of Medicine Davis, CA 95616	Gerald A. Gronert, MD (916) 752-9469
University of California, Los Angeles, UCLA School of Medicine Los Angeles, CA 90024	Jordan D. Miller, MD (213) 825-7850
University of Massachusetts Medical School Worcester, MA 01605	Barbara E. Waud, MD (508) 856-3160
University of Minnesota Medical School–Minneapolis Minneapolis, MN 55455	Paul A. Laizzo, PhD (612) 624-9990
University of Nebraska College of Medicine Omaha, NE 68105-1065	Dennis F. Landers, MD, PhD (402) 559-7405
University of South Florida College of Medicine Tampa, FL 33612	Julius Bowie, MD (813) 251-7438

*These centers have complied with the standardization protocol for the caffeine-halothane contracture test.
Reprinted with permission from Malignant Hyperthermia Association of the United States, Sherburne, NY, January 1994.

tling. Muscle rigidity affects the entire body, and tachypnea occurs as the body attempts to eliminate the rapid buildup of carbon dioxide and reverse the severe acidosis.

Only late in the crisis does the fever for which the syndrome is named occur. The temperature may rise as much as 1°F every 3 to 5 minutes, up to 42°C.[54, 55, 65] Although fever is usually a late symptom, continuous temperature monitoring is advocated for all patients during general anesthesia as one means of identifying an occurrence of MH. Generalized bleeding and heart failure are other late signs. If MH is left untreated, death usually ensues. Succinylcholine should be avoided in children owing to the potential for MH, but also because of the possibility of cardiac arrhythmias in children with undiagnosed cardiomyopathies.

Treatment. The initial response of the team must be to immediately stop all anesthesia and triggering agents. The surgeon closes the incision as rapidly as possible. The rubber or polyvinyl tubings and canisters on the anesthesia machine are changed or another ventilator is used so that lingering volatile gases are not being administered from the anesthesia machine. To respond to the body's increased oxygen needs during this hypermetabolic state, the patient must be hyperventilated with 100% oxygen. Many people are needed to respond to the rapid metabolic deterioration the patient faces, and summoning help early in the course is essential.

Dantrolene sodium (Dantrium) is the only specific treatment for MH. Administration must begin without delay when the diagnosis of MH is made or suspected. The recommended dosage ranges from 1 to 10 mg/kg, with an initial dose of 2 to 3 mg/kg being standard. Maximal dosage is 10 mg/kg,[58] although in some instances that dose is exceeded.

Dantrolene is known to have minimal effects on the blood pressure, heart rate, and cardiac output,[66] but it may affect intracardiac conduction.[67] Great caution should be taken when administering dantrolene to a person who is taking verapamil, a calcium channel blocker, because the combination can significantly depress cardiac function and elevate potassium to dangerous levels.[68] Because dantrolene is the only specific treatment for a life-threatening MH crisis, it must be given regardless of whether the patient is taking calcium channel blockers. In such an instance, cardiac function and serum potassium levels must be monitored closely. Serious cardiac depression is generally treated with infusion of fluids[69] and appropriate medications. Because dantrolene is a skeletal muscle relaxant, patients may experience profound subjective weakness, including a sense of respiratory inadequacy.

Reconstitution of dantrolene is time-consuming and requires several people for its rapid preparation. The powdered drug dissolves slowly and requires 60 ml of diluent added to each vial. Taskalos[70] suggests the use of a semiautomatic syringe that attaches with special IV tubing to a 500-ml glass, partial-fill bottle of a 1000-ml bag of nonbacteriostatic, sterile water for injection. This method greatly shortens the time needed to reconstitute dantrolene when compared with that required when using individual vials of diluent. Because of the large volume of diluent used to reconstitute a full course of the drug, diluents should not contain bacteriostatic agents.

All equipment and medication should be available for immediate use in the operating suite and perioperative areas and should be given hands-on attention during mock drills. Outdated dantrolene is nonreturnable for credit. Rather than discarding the vials, actual reconstitution of the outdated drug is an excellent form of practice for staff members.

Standard MH treatment protocol also includes:

1. Correction of acidosis with sodium bicarbonate (1 to 2 mEq/kg IV initially and then as necessary, based on blood gas analysis)
2. Administration of dantrolene
3. Aggressive cooling of the body (surface, cavities, and intravenously)
4. Treatment of ventricular arrhythmias with standard antiarrhythmic drugs, except calcium channel blockers (e.g., procainamide at a loading dose of 15 mg/kg IV over 10 to 60 minutes,[70] or lidocaine at standard doses—see Table 11–1)
5. Insertion of monitoring devices (arterial and central venous lines, Swan-Ganz catheter, temperature probe, ECG monitor, Foley catheter)
6. Aggressive IV fluid administration
7. Mannitol and furosemide to promote diuresis because the end products of cell breakdown can cause kidney failure
8. Diagnostic tests such as blood gases, serum potassium, creatine kinase, and urine myoglobin

Some sources also advocate the use of 50% dextrose and 10 U of regular insulin to provide glucose for metabolism and to treat hyperkalemia.[71] After the initial crisis has been managed, oral dantrolene sodium is initiated (1 to 2 mg/kg 4 times a day for 1 to 3 days).

Patient and Family Education. In the American Society of Perianesthesia Nurses' (ASPAN's) Competency Based Orientation and Credentialing Program, Snodderly and Younger discuss the need to instruct the patient in the immediate post-MH period about potential post–dantrolene therapy symptoms such as nausea, diarrhea, generalized muscle weakness, double vision, dizziness, and lightheadedness.[72] The patient should not engage in any hazardous activity, drive an automobile, or operate heavy equipment. ASPAN focuses on the following formal discharge teaching:

- Familiarizing patients with the signs and symptoms of a hypermetabolic state
- Instructing patients to obtain medical identification bracelets and to inform healthcare providers and healthcare settings about their MH susceptibility
- Explaining the autosomal dominance of the disease and the need to test blood relatives
- Informing patients of additional support and resources

More information about malignant hyperthermia can be obtained from several sources. MHAUS (P.O. Box 1069, Sherburne, NY 13460-1069; telephone 800-986-4287) is a vital resource for physicians, nurses, patients, and families. It supports education and research and maintains a 24-hour hot line (800-644-9737) and Internet site (MHAUS@norwich.net). A healthcare provider can call the hot line and speak with an anesthesiologist or other physician who is experienced in handling an MH crisis. The nonprofit MHAUS also supplies a variety of literature and information for health professionals as well as for patients suffering from MH and their families.

Procter and Gamble Pharmaceuticals, Inc., the manufacturer of Dantrium, also provides educational materials or sessions for healthcare facilities. Contact can be made through a local representative or the Director of Professional Services, Procter and Gamble Pharmaceuticals, Inc., 17 Easton Avenue, Norwich, NY 13814-0231; telephone 207-674-7901.

Healthcare providers are asked to report all episodes of MH to a registry for the purpose of tracking and research. A form for this report can be obtained from North American MH Registry, Pennsylvania State University, College of Medicine, Department of Anesthesia, P.O. Box 850, Hershey, PA 17033-0850; telephone 717-531-6936.

SUMMARY

The clinical safety of any facility depends on the collaborative efforts of the clinical, administrative, and financial leaders to plan and prepare for emergencies in the perianesthesia unit. In an ambulatory surgery setting, three basic components combine to contribute to an acceptable level of emergency preparedness. First, patients must be screened and prepared to avoid as many emergencies as possible. Second, adequate equipment and supplies must be on hand for use in an emergency. Finally, personnel, particularly nurses, must be personally responsible for remaining knowledgeable about their roles and responsibilities in urgent and emergency situations and must demonstrate clinical competence in recognizing and responding to any potential changes in cardiac or respiratory status that could lead to life-threatening events.

References

1. DeFazio-Quinn D: Ambulatory surgery. Nurs Clin North Am 32:377–386, 1997.
2. Williams G: Preoperative assessment and health history interview. Nurs Clin North Am 32:395–416, 1997.
3. American Society of Perianesthesia Nurses: Standards of Perianesthesia Nursing Practice. Thorofare, NJ: ASPAN, 1998.
4. Malignant Hyperthermia Association of the United States: Preventing Malignant Hyperthermia: An Anesthesia Protocol. Sherburne, NY: MHAUS, 1997.
5. Beck CF: Malignant hyperthermia: Are you prepared? AORN J 59:367–378, 1994.
6. Tobias J, Morgan W, Holcomb G, et al: Hyperthermia during repair of pectus excavatum. AANA J 65:68–71, 1997.
7. Bauman N, Sandler A, Schmidet C, et al: Laryngospasm induced by stimulation. Laryngospasm 104:209–214, 1994.
8. Murray-Calderon P, Connolly MA: Laryngospasm and noncardiogenic pulmonary edema. J Post Anesth Nurs 12:89–94, 1997.
9. Litwack K: Core Curriculum for Post Anesthesia Nursing Practice. Philadelphia: WB Saunders, 1995.
10. Drain CB: The Post Anesthesia Care Unit: A Critical Care Approach to Post Anesthesia Nursing. Philadelphia: WB Saunders, 1994.
11. Meyer-Pahoulis E: Pediatric postanesthesia care. Plast Surg Nurs 14:92–98, 1994.
12. Litwack K: Post Anesthesia Nursing Care, 2nd ed. St. Louis, CV Mosby, 1995.
13. Warner M: Risks and outcomes of perioperative pulmonary aspiration. J Post Anesth Nurs 12:352–357, 1997.
14. Dripps R, Eckenhoff J, Vandam L: Anesthesia: The Principles of Safe Practice, 8th ed. Philadelphia: WB Saunders, 1993.
15. Borland LM, Woeflel SK, Saitz EW, et al: Pulmonary aspiration in pediatric patients under general anesthesia: Frequency and outcome. Anesthesiology 83:A1150, 1995.
16. Ong B, Palahniuk R, Cumming M: Gastric volume and pH in outpatients. Can Anaesth Soc J 25:36, 1978.
17. Haines M: Fasting trends: Aspiration—prevention—control. AANA J 63:389–396, 1995.
18. Maree SM: Aspiration prophylaxis: An update. Curr Rev Nurse Anesth 16:223–232, 1994.
19. Beards S: Aspiration. Care Crit Ill 10:198–202, 1994.
20. Brooks-Brunn J: Postoperative pulmonary complications. Heart Lung 24:94–115, 1995.
21. Ingram RH, Braunwald E: Dyspnea and pulmonary edema. In Harrison's Principles of Internal Medicine, 13th ed. New York: McGraw-Hill, 1994, pp 175–187.
22. Brunner L, Suddarth D: Textbook of Medical-Surgical Nursing, 7th ed. Philadelphia: JB Lippincott, 1993.
23. Muntz J: Perioperative DVT and pulmonary embolus: Diagnosis, management, and treatment. Orthop Nurs J Suppl 3–4:25–29, 1997.
24. Beland I, Passos J: Clinical Nursing Pathophysiology and Psychosocial Approaches, 7th ed. New York: Macmillan, 1997.
25. Reed C: Care of the postoperative patient with adult respiratory distress syndrome. J Post Anesth Nurs 11:410–416, 1996.
26. Taff R: Pulmonary edema following naloxone administration in a patient without heart disease. Anesthesiology 59:576–577, 1983.
27. Prough D, Roy R, Bumgarner J, et al: Acute pulmonary edema in healthy teenagers following conservative doses of intravenous naloxone. Anesthesiology 60:485–486, 1984.
28. Deisering L, Douglass D: Post-laryngospasm pulmonary edema. J Am Assoc Nurs Anesth 56:246–248, 1988.
29. Mamaril ME, Zeltt KE: Care of the arthroscopy patient with noncardiogenic pulmonary edema. Orthop Nurs 16:2, 63–66, 1997.
30. Guertler A: The clinical practice of emergencies. Emerg Clin North Am 15:303–313, 1997.
31. Emergency Nurses Association: Emergency Nursing Core Curriculum, 4th ed. Philadelphia: WB Saunders, 1994.
32. Moser KM: Pulmonary thromboembolism. In Harrison's Principles of Internal Medicine, 13th ed. New York: McGraw-Hill, 1994, pp 1214–1220.
33. Well-Mackie J: Chest trauma. In Parker J (ed): Emergency Nursing: A Guide to Comprehensive Care. New York: John Wiley & Sons, 1993, pp 422–427.
34. Light RW: Pneumothorax in the ICU. J Crit Illness 12:77–84, 1997.
35. Morgan G, Mikhail M: Clinical Anesthesiology, 2nd ed. Norwalk, CT: Appleton & Lange, 1997.

36. Clark A: Complications and management of diabetes: A review of current research. Crit Care Clin North Am 6:723–734, 1994.
37. Twersky RS: The Ambulatory Anesthesia Handbook. St. Louis: Mosby–Year Book, 1995.
38. Zeigler V: Postoperative rhythm disturbance. Crit Care Clin North Am 6:227–235, 1994.
39. Grauer K, Whitney C: Clinical Electro-Cardiography: A Primary Care Approach, 2nd ed. Malden, MA: Blackwell Science, 1993.
40. Jacobson C: 12 lead ECG changes of ischemia, injury and infarction. Presentation to the Louisiana Association of Post Anesthesia Nurses' 8th annual seminar, New Orleans, June 1, 1991.
41. McCabe E: Code team hazards. Nurs Management 28:48K–48L, 1997.
42. Case J: Are you ready for a code? Nursing 94 24:32C–32F, 1994.
43. American Heart Association: Textbook of Advanced Cardiac Life Support. Dallas: American Heart Association, 1994.
44. Biggers VT: Codes for a code. Am J Nurs 92:57–61, 1992.
45. Meltzer L, Pinneo R, Kitchell J: Intensive Coronary Care: A Manual for Nurses, 6th ed. Bowie, MD: Brady, 1993.
46. Ehrhardt BS, Glankler DM: Your role in a code blue. Nursing 96 26:34–39, 1996.
47. American Medical Association: Standards and guidelines for cardiopulmonary resuscitation and emergency cardiac care. JAMA 268:2171–2302, 1992.
48. Brunner L, Suddarth D: Textbook of Medical-Surgical Nursing, 7th ed. Philadelphia: JB Lippincott, 1993.
49. Randall B: Reacting to anaphylaxis. Nursing 86 16:34–39, 1986.
50. Atkinson T, Kaliner M: Anaphylaxis. Med Clin North Am 76:841–854, 1992.
51. Barrows J: Dealing with anaphylaxis STAT. Nursing Life May/June:33–40, 1985.
52. Anaphylaxis: Five steps for fast treatment. Nursing 83 13:16V, 1983.
53. Katz D: Current understanding of malignant hyperthermia: Genesis, prevention, and treatment. CRNA: The Clinical Forum for Nurse Anesthetists 3:54–63, 1992.
54. Kaus SJ, Rockoff MA: Malignant hyperthermia. Pediatr Clin North Am 41:221–237, 1994.
55. Williams GD: Preoperative assessment and health history interview. Nurs Clin North Am 32:395–416, 1997.
56. Malignant Hyperthermia Association of the United States: What Is Malignant Hyperthermia? Sherburne, NY: MHAUS, 1996.
57. Viscusi ER: Malignant hyperthermia update. Presentation to the annual meeting of the Pennsylvania Association of Anesthesiologists, Baltimore, MD, April 19, 1997.
58. Rosenberg H: The HOTLINE in the communicator. Newsletter of the Malignant Hyperthermia Association of the United States 8:2–3, 1990.
59. Greenberg C: Hyperthermia in the postanesthesia care unit. In Shapiro G (ed): Post Anesthesia Unit Problems. Anesth Clin North Am 8:377–397, 1990.
60. Harrison G, Morrell D: Response of MHS swine to IV infusions of lidocaine and bupivacaine. Br J Anaesth 52:385–387, 1980.
61. Wingard D, Bobko S: Failure of lidocaine to trigger porcine malignant hyperthermia. Anesth Analg 58:99–103, 1989.
62. Golinski M: Malignant hyperthermia: A review. Plast Surg Nurs 15:30–58, 1995.
63. Malignant Hyperthermia Association of the United States: Managing Malignant Hyperthermia: A 1997/1998 Clinical Update. Sherburne, NY: MHAUS, 1997.
64. Meyer-Pahoulis E: Pediatric postanesthesia care? Plast Surg Nurs 14:92–98, 1994.
65. Malignant Hyperthermia Association of the United States: What Is Malignant Hyperthermia? Sherburne, NY: MHAUS, 1996.
66. Murphy JM: Astute assessment by perioperative nurse in an expanded role saves patient from malignant hyperthermia. AORN J 66:146, 1997.
67. Ellis R, Simpson P, Tatham M, et al: The cardiovascular effects of dantrolene sodium in dogs. Anaesthesia 30:318–322, 1975.
68. Hilton G: Case history: Malignant hyperthermia. Int J Trauma Nurs 1:41–46, 1995.
69. Rivera PH, Worley C: This looks like malignant hyperthermia! J Post Anesth Nurs 10:265–276, 1995.
70. Barker EM: A hereditary defect that complicates anesthesia. RN 57:70–71, 1994.
71. Donnelly AJ: Malignant hyperthermia: Epidemiology, pathophysiology, treatment. AORN J 59:393–400, 1994.
72. Management of malignant hyperthermia: You've only got a few minutes. Educational poster. Norwich, NY: Norwich Eaton Pharmaceuticals, 1995.

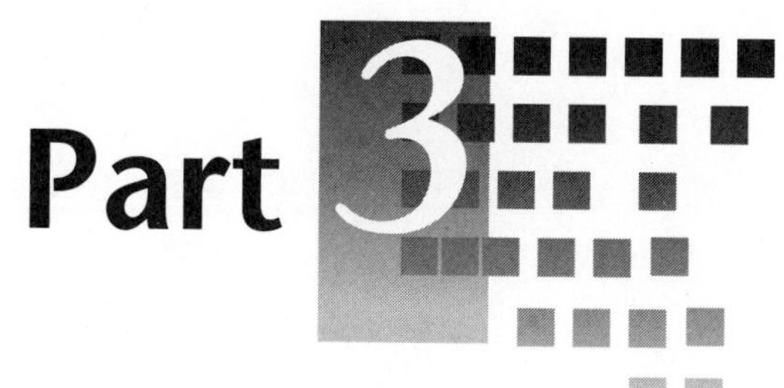

Anesthesia and Sedation for Ambulatory Procedures

Chapter 12

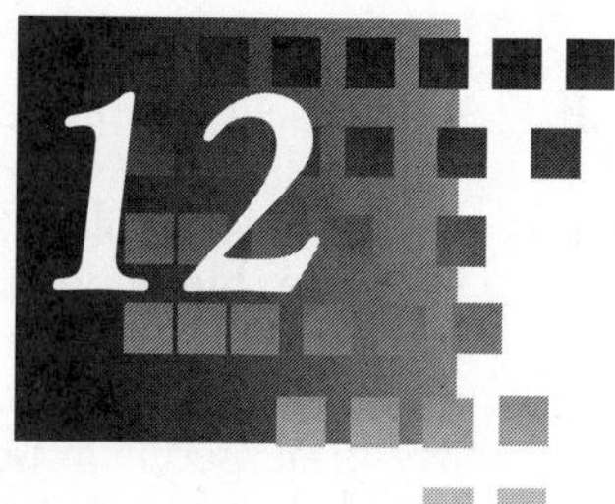

Anesthesia Management

Sujit K. Pandit

Safe anesthesia, absence of anesthetic complications and side effects, and prompt and complete recovery from anesthesia are the three cardinal prerequisites for successful outpatient surgery. A successful surgical outcome can be assured only when the surgeon, the anesthesia provider (anesthesiologist or nurse anesthetist), and the perioperative and perianesthesia nurses work as a team with the single-minded goal of providing the best possible care for the patient in the most cost-effective manner. Positive outcomes require careful consideration of a variety of factors that impact each surgical situation. These factors range from patient selection to complete recovery. This focus makes outpatient surgery and anesthesia safe, as a large retrospective study from a well-known medical center in the United States recently confirmed.[1] Many of the issues that affect outpatient surgery are presented elsewhere in this text; this chapter provides an overview of the provision of safe anesthesia in the outpatient setting.

ANESTHETIC CONSIDERATIONS FOR OUTPATIENT SURGERY

Selection of Patient and Procedure

The surgeon and the anesthesia provider must agree on the appropriate selection of patients and surgical procedures for outpatient operations. Patient safety is the primary focus and requires consideration of the physical status of the patient, the patient's age, and the procedure to be performed.

Physical Status of the Patient

The American Society of Anesthesiologists (ASA) Classification of Physical Status (Table 12–1) is the most convenient and most commonly accepted method of patient evaluation and selection for ambulatory anesthesia. In the 1970s and 1980s, when modern-day ambulatory surgery was just beginning, only patients with ASA physical status 1 or 2 were accepted as candidates for outpatient surgery. This has changed with experience, and currently patients with well-controlled and stable ASA physical status 3 (or even 4) are safely undergoing outpatient surgery. The crucial qualification here is *well-controlled and stable*. The main considerations in these choices are risk-benefit issues. For example, an immunologically compromised patient with ASA physical status 3 or 4 who

Table 12–1. **American Society of Anesthesiologists' Classification of Physical Status**

STATUS	DESCRIPTION
1	A normal healthy patient
2	A patient with mild systemic disease
3	A patient with severe systemic disease that limits activity but is not incapacitating
4	A patient with an incapacitating systemic disease that is a constant threat to life
5	A moribund patient not expected to survive 24 hours with or without an operation
6	A brain-dead patient being used as an organ donor

A suffix "E" should be used to denote emergency operation.

needs a minor procedure will benefit more if the operation can be done as an outpatient, thus avoiding the risk of nosocomial infection in the hospital.

Patient Age

Medically, there is no upper age limit for outpatient surgery, provided medical conditions are well controlled. For elderly patients, however, certain social issues must also be considered. Foremost is the level of care required during the important first 24 hours following the operation. Many elderly patients live alone or have an equally elderly spouse who may not be able to provide needed care. When this occurs, options for continuing care must be explored and confirmed before the day of surgery. Depending on the patient's procedure, general health, and postoperative care needs, admission to an observation unit after the operation (e.g., a 23-hour observation unit) may be an option. Community agencies or social service organizations can be contacted to locate home assistance for patients requiring companionship or nursing care or to provide respite care for family members.

Similarly, except for the first 2 weeks after birth, when normal physiologic adjustments (e.g., closure of patent ductus arteriosus) take place, normal full-term infants can be candidates for outpatient surgery in a facility where pediatric surgery is routinely done (e.g., a children's hospital). Caution should be exercised before selecting patients younger than 6 months of age for outpatient surgery in a facility where pediatric surgery is only occasionally done. Additionally, infants who were premature (ex-preemies) are at a higher risk for postoperative apnea after general anesthesia. Infants with a conceptual age of less than 50 to 60 weeks or infants with history of apnea are usually not accepted for outpatient anesthesia or surgery.[2] After an operation, they should be admitted and monitored overnight for apnea. Ex-preterm infants with a family history of sudden infant death syndrome (SIDS) or bronchopulmonary dysplasia should also be monitored postoperatively.

Procedures

Various technologic advances in surgery such as endoscopies (e.g., laparoscopy, arthroscopy, thoracoscopy), lasers, and shock wave therapies have made previously complex procedures safer and more acceptable for the outpatient setting. Conversely, there are still procedures that require admission. For example, procedures that involve major physiologic consequences (e.g., excessive blood loss; large fluid shifts; major intrathoracic, intracranial, or intra-abdominal procedures) should be done on an inpatient or day-of-surgery admission basis. Operations that are likely to result in severe postoperative pain are also best done as day-of-admission procedures. The duration of the operation by itself is not a serious consideration, although there are indications that the longer the operation, the greater the likelihood of postoperative complications.[3]

Preoperative Evaluation

The ASA and the Joint Commission on Accreditation of Healthcare Organizations (JCAHO) require that each candidate for outpatient surgery be evaluated by the operating surgeon and the anesthesia provider. Providing the preanesthetic evaluation has become a challenge for the anesthesia provider, because the patient and anesthesia provider may not meet until the day of the procedure, unlike in years past, when patients were admitted before the operative day. As a result, the major responsibility for screening patients falls to the surgeon. Based on a comprehensive history of medical and social conditions and a thorough physical examination, the surgeon must decide (1) whether the patient should be referred to a preanesthesia clinic (PAC) or testing unit for evaluation by an anesthesia provider; (2) whether a consultation from an internist is indicated; and (3) which laboratory or diagnostic tests, if any, must be ordered. Therefore, surgeons and anesthesia providers must clearly understand and agree to institutional policies about preanesthetic evaluation, consultations, and required laboratory or diagnostic tests. Before the operation, required preoperative documentation must be completed for every patient scheduled for an outpatient procedure (Table 12–2). A completed medical record or chart that includes this documentation should be available to the anesthesia provider for review before the operative day.

Preanesthesia Clinic or Evaluation Unit

Ideally, every patient scheduled for outpatient surgery, even those with ASA 1 and 2 physical status, should be referred to a PAC or evaluation unit managed by the anesthesiology department. Currently, referral of outpatient candi-

***Table 12–2.* Preoperative Documentation Requirements Before Arrival at the Surgery Facility**

History and physical evaluation by the surgeon
Completed health questionnaire by the patient, if used
Internist's consultation note, if necessary
Notes from preanesthesia clinic or evaluation unit, if used
Laboratory test results (e.g., ECG) when indicated
Informed consent for surgery and anesthesia

dates to a PAC or evaluation unit is becoming more common, but there are often logistic, financial, and practical considerations that preclude the visit.

The patient's visit to the PAC allows the anesthesia provider to complete a thorough preoperative evaluation of the patient (including a physical examination), obtain an informed consent for anesthesia, and accomplish any necessary laboratory tests and consultations with the internist. During the visit, the patient and the family have a chance to discuss anesthetic options and their associated risks with the anesthesia provider. Prescriptions for medications that may be necessary preoperatively may be given to the patient. Anesthesia providers consider the PAC visit an excellent opportunity to develop the crucial caregiver-patient rapport before the day of the procedure.

With changes in reimbursement and patient convenience and satisfaction issues, fewer patients are able to visit the PAC or evaluation unit before their scheduled operative procedures. Other means of evaluating the patient's physical status and anesthesia requirements continue to be developed to provide optimal care during the perioperative period. The method of patient preoperative evaluation chosen depends on the patient population served, facility needs, and cost issues such as reimbursement and staffing and space needs.

Health Questionnaire for Preoperative Evaluation

A health questionnaire, which is completed in the surgeon's office or at the PAC or evaluation unit, expedites the process of preoperative evaluation. The questionnaire can be a pencil-and-paper version or a computerized method (e.g., "HealthQuiz," Nellcor Incorporated, Pleasanton, CA). For patients with language or literacy difficulties, the questions can be asked verbally and the patient's verbal responses recorded. These questionnaires flag any positive findings for the clinician and may be preprogrammed to suggest the appropriate laboratory tests to order (Fig. 12–1). These records become a permanent part of the patient's chart. A copy may be transmitted to the anesthesia provider for review before the operation or before a telephone interview.

Telephone Interview

In the absence of face-to-face contact, a telephone interview with the patient before the operation gives the anesthesia provider an opportunity to ask relevant medical and social questions, to briefly discuss the anesthesia options, and to initiate rapport with the patient. For the telephone interview to be most beneficial, the anesthesia provider must be able to review the patient's chart and the completed health questionnaire before making the call. The drawbacks to this evaluation method are that it is time consuming, the contact rate is low, and it does not allow for a physical examination. On the positive side, problems may be identified during the interview that might result in cancellation or delay of surgery. Such problems include recent upper airway infection and exacerbation of pre-existing or new medical conditions. Thus, the telephone interview can be useful in reducing cancellation and delay rates on the day of surgery.[4]

Regardless of the type of preanesthetic evaluation used, a perianesthesia nurse usually telephones each patient within a few days of the scheduled procedure to review patient learning needs and give final instructions to the patient.

Evaluation on the Day of Operation

Final evaluation by the anesthesia provider on the day of the operation is the mainstay of preanesthetic evaluation in the majority of outpatient surgery facilities. For patients with ASA physical status 1 or 2, this may be the first direct contact with the anesthesia provider. During the evaluation, the anesthesia provider reassures the patient; develops rapport with the patient; reviews the medical and surgical conditions, including drug sensitivities and allergies; reviews the laboratory values and diagnostic test results; performs the necessary physical examinations; discusses the anesthetic options; gets an informed consent if that has not been done; and, if necessary, gives pharmacologic premedications.

UNIVERSITY OF MICHIGAN HOSPITALS
PATIENT INFORMATION REPORT

BIRTHDATE
NAME
CPI No.
SEX: M F VISIT No.

1. Please complete the following form, answering the questions to the best of your ability
2. If you then have questions, or do not understand an item, leave the section blank.

AGE:	WEIGHT:	HEIGHT:	
DATE:	DATE OF SURGERY:	HOME PH: ( )	WORK PH: ( )

PLEASE PLACE AN "X" IN THE BOX THAT APPLIES FOR EACH QUESTION BELOW — YES / NO / DON'T KNOW

1. Are you:
   a. Male and 40 years of age or older? ☐ ☐
   b. Female and 50 years of age or older? ☐ ☐
   c. If yes, are you also 70 years of age or older ☐ ☐
2. Do you take any of the following medications?
   a. Diuretics ("Water Pills") ☐ ☐ ☐
   b. Anticoagulants ("Blood Thinners") ☐ ☐ ☐
   c. Insulin ☐ ☐ ☐
   d. Digitalis (Digoxin, Lanoxin) ☐ ☐ ☐
3. Do you have or have you had any of the following heart-related conditions?
   a. Heart Disease ☐ ☐ ☐
   b. Family History of Heart Disease? ☐ ☐ ☐
   c. Heart Attack within the last 6 months? ☐ ☐ ☐
   d. Angina (Chest Pain) ☐ ☐ ☐
   e. Irregular Heartbeat ☐ ☐ ☐
   f. Heart Failure ☐ ☐ ☐
   g. Hypertension ☐ ☐ ☐
4. Do you have or have you ever had any of the following?
   a. Symptomatic Rheumatoid Arthritis ☐ ☐ ☐
   b. Hiatal Hernia or Reflux (Heart Burn) ☐ ☐ ☐
   c. Kidney Disease ☐ ☐ ☐
   d. Liver Disease ☐ ☐ ☐
   e. Blood Disease ☐ ☐ ☐
   f. Diabetes ☐ ☐ ☐

5a. Do you get short of breath when you lie flat? ☐ ☐ ☐
5b. Are you currently on oxygen treatment? ☐ ☐ ☐
5c. Do you have a chronic cough that produces any discharge or fluid? ☐ ☐ ☐
5d. Do you have lung problems (wheezing)? ☐ ☐ ☐
5e. Do you smoke? ☐ ☐ ☐

6. *If you answered yes to any of 3, 4 & 5 above:*
   a.) Do any of these problems significantly limit your daily activities? ☐ ☐ ☐
   b.) Do you feel tightness or chest pressure with activity? ☐ ☐ ☐
   c.) Are you seeing a cardiologist or another physician for any of these medical problems? ☐ ☐ ☐
   (Please continue in next column)

PLEASE PLACE AN "X" IN THE BOX THAT APPLIES FOR EACH QUESTION BELOW — YES / NO / DON'T KNOW

6c. (Continued)
If yes, complete below:

Date of last visit:
Physicians Name:
Phone No. ( )

d.) Have you had any changes in your symptons since that last physician visit? ☐ ☐

7a. Have you had any operations? ☐ ☐
7b. Were any of the operations conducted at the University of Michigan Hospitals? ☐ ☐
7c. Have you ever had a problem with any anesthesia other than nausea? ☐ ☐ ☐
7d. Has any blood member of your family had problems with anesthesia? ☐ ☐ ☐
7e. If yes, who:
7f. Do you have any allergies to medications? ☐ ☐

Medications:	Reactions:

8. Are you currently taking any medications? If yes, please list medications below.

Medications:	Dose:

8. If female, might you be pregnant? ☐ ☐

Please list date of last menstrual period:

For Physicians Use Only:

IP-2060592/PP Rev. 5/96 — University of Michigan Medical Center — PATIENT INFORMATION REPORT

Figure 12–1. University of Michigan Hospitals preoperative assessment checklist. (Reprinted with permission of University of Michigan Health System, Ann Arbor, Michigan.)

UNIVERSITY OF MICHIGAN HOSPITALS
PREOPERATIVE ASSESSMENT CHECKLIST

BIRTHDATE
NAME
CPI No.
SEX: M F VISIT No.

Please order the test(s) and/or studies as indicated below:

AGE:	WEIGHT:	HEIGHT:	
DATE:	DATE OF SURGERY:	HOME PH: ( )	WORK PH: ( )

1a. ECG	
1b. ECG	
1c. ECG & Preoperative Anesthesia Clinic Visit	
2a. Electrolytes	
2b. PT/PTT	
2c. ECG	
2d. ECG/CXR	
3a. ECG & Preoperative Anesthesia Clinic Visit	
3c. ECG & Preoperative Anesthesia Clinic Visit	
3d. ECG & Preoperative Anesthesia Clinic Visit	
3e. ECG & Preoperative Anesthesia Clinic Visit	
3f. ECG & Preoperative Anesthesia Clinic Visit	
4a. Cervical Spine X-RAY's & Preop. Anesthesia Clinic Visit	
4c. Elec.,Cret., BUN,CBC	
4d. SGOT/ALK,PT/PTT	
4e. PT/PTT,PLT,CBC	
4f. ECG & Preoperative Anesthesia Clinic Visit	
5a. CXR, ECG; Preoperative Anesthesia Clinic Visit	
5b. CXR, ECG, ABG; Preoperative Anesthesia Clinic Visit	
5c. CXR; Preoperative Anesthesia Clinic Visit	
5d. CXR; Preoperative Anesthesia Clinic Visit	
6b. ECG & Preoperative Anesthesia Clinic Visit	

6d. Preoperative Anesthesia Clinic Visit	
7c. Preoperative Anesthesia Clinic Visit	
8. Pregnancy Test	

In addition, please order the test(s) indicated below:

IP-2060592/PP Rev. 5/96		University of Michigan Medical Center	PREOPERATIVE ASSESSMENT CHECKLIST

Figure 12–1 *Continued*

Preoperative Laboratory Tests and Informed Consent

ASA supports the concept that no *routine* laboratory or diagnostic screening tests are necessary for preanesthetic evaluation of the patient.[5] JCAHO and the Accreditation Association for Ambulatory Health Care (AAAHC) are in agreement with this concept. All tests, with the exception of an electrocardiogram for male patients older than 40 years of age and for female patients older than 50 years of age, should be ordered only if indicated by the preoperative history and physical examination. A thorough clinical examination (history and physical examination) is more cost-effective for diagnosing pre-existing medical conditions than the use of a battery of routine laboratory screening tests.[6]

In addition to the huge cost of the unnecessary laboratory tests, false-positive and false-negative results may present unnecessary risk to the patient. It is estimated that in the United States, abolition of routine and often unnecessary preoperative screening tests would save the healthcare industry several billion dollars a year. Medical staff of each facility must formulate a policy regarding required tests that are acceptable to all professionals practicing at that facility. In most institutions, a laboratory test result obtained 3 to 4 weeks earlier is still accepted on the day of surgery if there has been no change in clinical symptoms.

For quick turnover of cases and to avoid delays on the day of operation, surgical informed consents should be obtained ahead of time at the clinic or office. Similarly, if the patient visits the PAC, informed consent for anesthesia is obtained at that time. Institutional policies vary, but an informed consent for surgery and anesthesia obtained 6 months before the operative day is usually accepted as valid on the day of operation at most facilities.

Preoperative Preparation and Instructions

Well-constructed and formalized preoperative instructions are the basis for good outcomes and patient satisfaction after outpatient surgery.[7] Because patient compliance with these specific instructions is so vital, the same instructions are often given by different professionals (e.g., clinicians and nurses). As a result, patients get their preoperative instructions not only at the surgeon's office and the PAC or evaluation unit but also in a phone call from a perianesthesia nurse at the facility. Unfortunately, the multiple instructions given by different professionals can create confusion for patients and their companions. Development of a multiuser evaluation form (for nurses, anesthesia provider, and surgeon) may decrease unnecessary repetition of questions and instructions. This is why it is vital to formulate institutional policies that are accepted by all professionals.

Preoperative instructions are given both verbally and in writing. They are often provided in the form of a brochure or a videotape in some facilities. The purposes of preoperative instructions are to educate and reassure the patient and to remind the patient and the family about:

- The scheduled time of surgery and the time to arrive at the facility
- The necessity of wearing loose and comfortable clothing
- The need to have a responsible adult (two in the case of a child or developmentally disabled patient) to escort the patient home after the operation
- What to bring (e.g., insurance card, hospital card, eyeglasses case, emergency medications that are normally taken)
- What not to bring (e.g., large amounts of cash, jewelry)
- Preoperative fasting guidelines
- Instructions about current medications

Those medications needed to maintain the patient's physiologic homeostasis should be continued on the day of surgery. Such medications include antihypertensives, antiarrhythmics, antianginal medications, anticonvulsant medications, bronchodilators, and antidepressants.

Preoperative Fasting Guidelines

The traditional preoperative fasting guideline (i.e., nothing by mouth after midnight before the day of surgery) has recently been challenged. Several studies have shown that prolonged preoperative fasting does not reduce the gastric volume and acidity and thus the risk of pulmonary aspiration.[8, 9] Instead, fasting was found to cause thirst, hunger, irritability, headache, and noncompliance; in children particularly, it may produce hypovolemia and hypoglycemia. A majority of facilities now allow clear liquids 2 to 3 hours before elective operations.[10]

Guidelines for preoperative fasting for elective operations state that no solid food is allowed on the day of surgery. This is because it takes solids 6 to 8 hours to clear from the stomach after ingestion, as they must first be broken down into small particles before they can leave the stomach via the pylorus. Cow's milk is considered a solid food. Human breast milk cannot be considered equivalent to clear liquid, but it is cleared faster than cow's milk.[11] Clear liquids leave the stomach comparatively quickly (the maximum time is 2 hours). A new guideline by the American Society of Anesthesiologists would allow clear liquid 2 hours, human breast milk 4 hours, a light breakfast (like toast and tea) 6 hours, and solid food 8 hours before an elective surgery (Table 12–3).[12]

Premedication

In the 1970s and 1980s, when outpatient surgery started to rise in popularity, it was recommended that no pharmacologic premedication be given before surgery. The concern was that the effects of the sedative premedicants would extend into the postoperative period and delay recovery. With experience and after many clinical studies with new short-acting antianxiety medications, this view has changed. Currently, it is common practice to premedicate the patient before outpatient surgery.

Purposes of Premedication

The primary purpose of premedication is to reduce preoperative anxiety. Secondary purposes are to provide sedation and amnesia; to ensure hemodynamic stability during induction of anesthesia; to prevent acid aspiration, postoperative nausea and vomiting, and allergic reactions; and to provide postoperative pain control. In younger children, premedication is often used to reduce separation anxiety from the parents.

***Table 12–3.* Preoperative Fasting Guidelines for Elective Operations**

Solid food: 8 hours
Light breakfast: 6 hours
Human breast milk: 4 hours
Clear liquid: 2 hours before the scheduled time of surgery

Common types of clear liquids allowed (children and adults) include water, apple or other clear juice, carbonated beverages, broth, tea and coffee without cream or milk. Light breakfast consists of nonfatty, nonmeat products like toast and tea.

Nonpharmacologic Methods of Anxiety Relief

Although preoperative anxiety is almost universal for both adults and children, it can be reduced to a great extent by several nonpharmacologic methods. These methods include patient education, reassurance, rapport with the surgeon and anesthesia provider, a preoperative facility tour, relaxation techniques, and, for children, play-based education (e.g., a puppet show depicting the operating room environment) and the presence of a parent during induction of anesthesia.[13] Although these nonpharmacologic methods of anxiety relief are obviously more cost-effective and have fewer side effects, they are time consuming and, at times, logistically difficult, but they should be considered.

Pharmacologic Premedicants for Anxiety Relief

Although nonpharmacologic methods of anxiety relief should be encouraged in all patients, pharmacologic means should not be denied to anxious patients. In fact, judicious use of pharmacologic premedicants, especially medications with a short elimination half-life (e.g., intravenous or oral midazolam), has become a fairly common practice before outpatient surgery. There are enough data to suggest that small doses of premedicants do not prolong recovery after outpatient anesthesia.

A short-acting water-soluble benzodiazepine (midazolam) is the most common premedicant in the United States for both adults and children. Its advantages include quick action (1 to 2 minutes after intravenous use), short elimination time (2 to 4 hours), water solubility, no pain on injection, and optional routes of administration (e.g., intravenous, intramuscular, oral, intranasal, or rectal). However, midazolam is somewhat expensive at $3.40 for a 2-mg vial. Diazepam, the prototype benzodiazepine, has a long elimination half-life (12 to 20 hours) and is painful on injection because of its diluent, propylene glycol, yet many advocate its use for outpatient premedication. It is much less expensive than midazolam ($0.02 for a 10-mg diazepam tablet) and is an effective anxiolytic. Temazepam, in a soft capsule formulation given orally, is the most common premedicant in Europe. Questions about the safety of temazepam have recently prompted withdrawal of this drug in some countries. Table 12–4 shows the comparative pharmacology of midazolam, diazepam, and temazepam. Table 12–5 shows the common premedicants for children.

Table 12–4. **Common Antianxiety Premedicants for Outpatient Anesthesia**

VARIABLE	DIAZEPAM	MIDAZOLAM	TEMAZEPAM
Distribution half-life (min)	37–78	5.7–10	21–98
Elimination half-life (hr)	20–40	2–4	7–33
Volume of distribution (L/kg)	0.71–1.5	0.53–2.9	0.57–2.8
Clearance (ml/kg/min)	0.25	6–12	0.59–2.5

Premedicants for Prophylaxis of Acid Aspiration

Several recent surveys and studies of healthy ASA 1 or 2 patients concluded that the incidence of pulmonary aspiration during outpatient operations is exceedingly low (about 1:30,000).[14] Clearly, routine prophylaxis against acid aspiration would not be cost-effective, so it is necessary to screen for conditions that put patients at high risk for this complication (e.g., obesity, pregnancy, diabetes, history of hiatal hernia, difficult tracheal intubation). A common practice with high-risk patients is to use a prophylactic H_2 blocker (ranitidine, famotidine, nizatidine), a gastrokinetic agent (metoclopramide), or a nonparticulate antacid such as sodium citrate (Bicitra) before induction of anesthesia. Of the H_2 blockers, oral nizatidine is the most cost-effective at $0.12 for a 150-mg tablet, compared with ranitidine at $1.04 for a 150-mg tablet.

Prevention of Postoperative Nausea and Vomiting

Postoperative nausea and vomiting (PONV) and postoperative pain are common after outpatient surgery and often are causes of patient discontent and delayed recovery.

Table 12–5. **Common Premedicants in Children**

MEDICATION	ROUTE	DOSE (mg/kg)
Midazolam	Oral	0.5
	Nasal/transmucosal	0.2
	Rectal	1
Methohexital	Rectal	25
Ketamine	Oral	6
	Rectal	3
	Intramuscular	2
OTFC (Oralet, fentanyl "lollipop")	Transmucosal	0.005–0.015

The incidence of PONV is higher after certain types of operations (e.g., eye; ear, nose, and throat; gynecologic laparoscopy) and among certain patient populations (e.g., young patients, females, patients with a history of previous PONV or motion sickness, and menstruating patients). Because PONV invariably delays discharge time, irrespective of the treatment given in the postanesthesia care unit (PACU), it makes more sense to prevent PONV with prophylactic antiemetics in at-risk patients. Unfortunately, the available antiemetics either have a potential for side effects (e.g., sedation, excitement, dysphoria, extrapyramidal effects) or are expensive. For example, the new serotonin $5HT_3$ inhibitor agents such as ondansetron or any of the other derivatives are effective antiemetics with minimal side effects, but they are expensive. Ondansetron costs $18.56 for 4 mg. However, it has been estimated that prophylactic ondansetron may be cost-effective when the risk of PONV is more than 33%.[15, 16] Droperidol in low doses (10 to 20 μg/kg) remains the most cost-effective prophylactic antiemetic for general use.[17, 18]

Prevention of Postoperative Pain

Postoperative pain is the most common cause of delayed recovery and unexpected hospital admission.[19]

Besides causing suffering, untreated pain may cause PONV, which by itself is a cause of delayed recovery. Because excessive use of narcotic analgesics in the PACU may cause prolonged sedation, dizziness, nausea, and vomiting, prophylactic use of analgesics, especially those with longer durations of action, is encouraged. The most common analgesics used to prevent postoperative pain are acetaminophen and the nonsteroidal anti-inflammatory drugs (NSAIDs).

Among the NSAIDs, the commonly used agents are ketorolac, diclofenac, indomethacin, and naproxen (these agents are used cautiously in patients with renal dysfunction). Any of these agents can be given either just before or just after induction of anesthesia. The route of administration can be oral, intramuscular, intravenous, or rectal. α_2-Agonists such as clonidine or dexmedetomidine are being used to reduce analgesic requirements during the postoperative period. However, because of the potential for side effects such as bradycardia or hypotension, their use is limited in outpatient surgery. Infiltration of the surgical wound with long-acting local anesthetic agents (e.g., bupivacaine) by the surgeon or use of nerve blocks (e.g., caudal block) by the anesthesiologist are very effective methods of postoperative pain control.

Selection and Conduct of Appropriate Anesthetic Technique

Anesthesia for outpatient surgery, including general anesthesia, regional anesthesia, and so-called monitored anesthesia care (MAC), which is also called monitoring and pharmacologic support (MAPS), is described in Chapters 13–15. Obviously, the availability of safe and short-acting general anesthetic agents (e.g., propofol, desflurane, sevoflurane) and anesthetic adjuvants (e.g., new muscle relaxants, synthetic narcotic analgesics) has made general anesthesia safer and more predictable for outpatient surgery.[20]

The use of fine and noncutting pencil-point spinal needles (e.g., Whittacre, Sprotte) for spinal anesthesia has reduced the incidence of postdural puncture headache to a minimum. As a result, this technique has become quite acceptable for outpatient surgery, even for young patients. Regional anesthesia (central neuronal blocks or peripheral nerve blocks) is often more cost-effective and is a safe technique for outpatient surgery. Regional blocks (e.g., caudal block in children, interscalene block for shoulder surgery, femoral and genitofemoral nerve blocks for saphenous vein stripping) and infiltration blocks (e.g., ilioinguinal, iliohypogastric, and penile block) to control postoperative pain after outpatient surgery are an important advance.[21] Local and regional anesthesia techniques are discussed in Chapter 14.

Postanesthesia Care

Postanesthesia care after outpatient surgery in the phase I and phase II PACU has recently undergone remarkable changes that make outpatient surgery safe and the outcomes more predictable. Because prophylaxis for PONV or postoperative pain is not always fully effective, contingency plans to treat these symptoms promptly in the PACU should be agreed on by both the anesthesia provider and the PACU nurse. For treatment of PONV, ondansetron or one of its analogues, droperidol, prochlorperazine, and metoclopramide are most commonly used (Table 12–6).

For initial treatment of postoperative pain, a quick-acting synthetic analgesic such as fentanyl in increments of 25 to 50 μg intravenously, repeated as necessary, is most effective. Currently, longer-acting narcotic analgesics are being advocated.[22] Intramuscular or intravenous ketorolac (an NSAID) is another agent commonly used. Ketorolac has less potential for respiratory depression and nausea and vomiting.[23] However, it is expensive, costing $6.16 for 30 mg versus $0.26 for 100 μg of fentanyl.

If a patient is expected to experience continued pain, either acetaminophen or an oral NSAID (e.g., ibuprofen, ketorolac, naproxen) with or without codeine or a codeine analogue like hydrocodone should be given as soon as the patient can swallow and retain oral medication. Patients should be encouraged to get an analgesic prescription filled before they leave the surgery facility, so that when pain becomes apparent during transport or at home, the medication is immediately available (Table 12–7). Patients may resist taking analgesics because of fear or concern over side effects. The patient may feel better and recover more quickly with adequate pain relief.

Safe Discharge Home (Home Readiness)

Rapid turnover of cases to maintain a constant flow of patients into and out of the PACU is often essential to maintain cost efficiency; however, discharging a patient home after outpatient surgery is an issue that must be thoroughly addressed at each surgery facility. Pri-

***Table 12–6.* Common Medications, Doses, and Cost to Prevent or Treat Postoperative Nausea and Vomiting**

MEDICATION	USUAL ADULT DOSE (mg)	COST (US$)
Droperidol	0.6–1.2	0.48/2.5 mg
Ondansetron	4–8	18.56/4 mg
Prochlorperazine	5	0.76/10 mg
Metoclopramide	10	0.20/10 mg
Ephedrine	25	0.78/50 mg

Table 12–7. Common Medications to Treat Postoperative Pain

MEDICATION	UNIT DOSE	COST (US$)
Fentanyl	100 μg	0.26
Morphine	10 mg	0.41
Meperidine	50 mg	0.35
Acetaminophen	500 mg	0.19
Ibuprofen	600 mg	0.05
Diclofenac	50 mg	0.76
Indomethacin	375 mg	0.17
Ketorolac	30 mg	6.16

mary concerns surrounding discharge are patient safety, economic, and medicolegal issues.[24]

The JCAHO stipulates that institutional discharge criteria that have been approved by the medical staff of the facility must be met before a patient can be discharged from the facility.[25] As long as the prescribed criteria are met, an experienced PACU nurse can safely discharge the patient. It is required, however, that the name of the licensed independent practitioner (LIP) who authorized the discharge be recorded. It is also required that an LIP who is trained in advanced cardiac life support be physically present in the facility until all patients are "medically" discharged from the PACU. Furthermore, the JCAHO expects that a staff member who is certified in cardiopulmonary resuscitation will be present at the facility until the last patient is "physically" discharged.

The AAAHC stipulates that patients who receive anesthesia must be evaluated by the operating surgeon or dentist and the anesthesia provider after recovery from anesthesia. This is a sound medical practice. Discharge requirements, discharge instructions, and the reasons for unanticipated hospital admission are discussed in further detail in Chapter 22.

Regardless of the discharge criteria, should there be a minimum stay in the phase II PACU before the patient is allowed to go home? Usually the answer is no; in some special situations, however, this may be necessary. For example, many institutions require that the patient be observed for bleeding for a minimum of 4 hours after a tonsillectomy or adenoidectomy. Or patients who have experienced laryngospasm may be required to stay a minimum of 2 hours following the episode. Usual medical causes of prolonged PACU stay include:

- Prolonged unconsciousness or drowsiness
- Respiratory complications (airway complications, respiratory depression)
- Hemodynamic problems (hypo- or hypertension, arrhythmias)
- Uncontrolled postoperative pain or nausea and vomiting
- Surgical complications (e.g., bleeding)
- Extended period of drowsiness, dizziness, headache, muscle weakness, or visual disturbances (diplopia)
- Inability to ambulate and void

The other major reason for prolonged PACU stay and delay in discharge is the unavailability of a responsible adult escort at the time of discharge.

The medical personnel working at the outpatient surgery center as well as the patient and the responsible adult companion must know the exact meaning of the term *home readiness*. It means that *the patient is now ready to be escorted home to continue to recover in the home environment for the next 24 or 48 hours*. The patient and the responsible adult companion must understand that during this time the patient's psychomotor and cognitive functions are not yet normal, and the patient should not be allowed to drive an automobile, operate complicated machinery, cook with open fire, consume alcohol or nonprescription drugs, or make important legal decisions. In other words, the patient is not "street fit."

The instructions given to the patient and the responsible adult companion at the time of discharge are very important. Instructions must be given verbally, and a written list must be provided to the patient and responsible adult companion. The written instructions are important because the patient's memory functions may not be fully restored at the time of discharge, especially in older patients. Most surgery facilities ask the patient or the responsible adult companion to sign a document stating that discharge instructions have been provided. Such instructions should include:

- A list of restricted activities, as mentioned earlier
- Medications to take and to avoid
- Care of the surgical wound
- What side effects to expect
- When to ask for medical help

The instructions should also include two or three contact telephone numbers, including the surgeon's office and the surgery facility. There should be clear instructions to go to a nearby emergency department if necessary.

Complete Recovery (Street Fitness)

Complete recovery takes place slowly over time. In general, complete recovery may take from 24 hours to 3 to 4 days, depending on the type of operation, the type of anesthetic used, and the patient's personality. The patient progressively regains psychomotor and psychological functions such as short-term memory, reasoning, concentration, and discrimination. Only then can the patient safely resume normal daily activities, including driving an automobile, operating complicated machinery, and making important legal decisions. The end-point of complete recovery may be called street fitness.

The assessment of complete or long-term recovery is difficult following outpatient surgery. This is not only because the patient is physically inaccessible to medical personnel for clinical assessment (i.e., the patient is at home) but also because a simple and reliable test of complete recovery has yet to be devised.

References

1. Warner MA, Shields SE, Chute CG: Major morbidity and mortality within one month of ambulatory surgery and anesthesia. JAMA 270:1437–1441, 1993.
2. Malviya S, Swartz J, Lerman J: Are all preterm infants younger than 60 weeks post conceptual age at risk for postoperative apnea? Anesthesiology 78:1076–1081, 1993.
3. Chung F: Recovery pattern and home readiness after ambulatory surgery. Anesth Analg 80:896–902, 1995.
4. Patel RI, Hannallah RS: Preoperative screening for pediatric ambulatory surgery: Evaluation of a telephone questionnaire method. Anesth Analg 75:258–261, 1992.
5. American Society of Anesthesiologists: Statement on routine preoperative laboratory and diagnostic screening. Approved by the House of Delegates on October 14, 1987, and last amended October 13, 1993. Park Ridge, IL: ASA, 1993.
6. Roizen MF: Preoperative evaluation. In Miller RD (ed): Anesthesia. New York: Churchill Livingstone, 1994, pp 827–882.
7. Green CR, Pandit SK: Preoperative preparation. In Twersky RS (ed): The Ambulatory Anesthesia Handbook. St. Louis: CV Mosby, 1995, pp 171–202.
8. Maltby JR, Sutherland AD, Sale JP, et al: Preoperative oral fluids: Is a five-hour fast justified? Anesth Analg 65:1112–1116, 1986.
9. Agarwal A, Chari P, Singh H: Fluid deprivation before operation: The effects of a small drink. Anaesthesia 44:632–634, 1989.
10. Green CR, Pandit SK, Schorck MA: Preoperative fasting time: Are the traditional guidelines changing? Anesth Analg 83:123–128, 1996.
11. Cavell B: Gastric emptying in infants fed human milk or infant formula. Acta Paediatr Scand 70:639–641, 1981.
12. Warner MA, Caplan RA, Epstein BS, et al: Practice guidelines for preoperative fasting and the use of pharmacological agents to reduce the risk of pulmonary aspiration: application to healthy patients undergoing elective procedures. Anesthesiology 90:896–905, 1999.
13. Hannallah RS: Who benefits when parents are present during anesthesia induction in their children (Editorial)? Can J Anaesth 41:271–275, 1994.
14. Federated Ambulatory Surgery Association: FASA special study I on incidence of pulmonary aspiration. Alexandra, VA: FASA, 1986.
15. Watcha MF, White PF: New antiemetic drugs. Int Anesthesiol Clin 33:1–20, 1995.
16. Watcha MF, Smith IL: Cost-effectiveness analysis of antiemetic therapy for ambulatory surgery. J Clin Anaesth 6:370–377, 1994.
17. Pandit SK, Kothary SP, Pandit UA, et al: Dose-response study of droperidol and metoclopramide as antiemetics for outpatient anesthesia. Anesth Analg 68:798–802, 1989.
18. Tang J, Watcha M, White PF: A comparison of costs and efficacy of ondansetron and droperidol as prophylactic antiemetic therapy for elective outpatient gynecologic procedures. Anesth Analg 83:304–313, 1996.
19. Chung F: Recovery pattern and home readiness after ambulatory surgery. Anesth Analg 80:896–902, 1995.
20. Pandit SK, Green CR: General anesthetic techniques. Int Anesthesiol Clin 32:55–79, 1994.
21. Pandit SK, Pandit UA: Regional anesthesia for outpatient surgery. Ambulatory Surg 2:125–135, 1994.
22. Claxton AR, McGuire G, Chung F, Cruise C: Evaluation of morphine versus fentanyl for postoperative analgesia after ambulatory surgical procedures. Anesth Analg 84:509–514, 1997.
23. Green CR, Pandit SK, Kothary SP, et al: Intraoperative ketorolac has narcotic sparing effect after diagnostic laparoscopy but not after laparoscopic tubal ligation. Anesth Analg 82:732–737, 1996.
24. Pandit SK, Pandit UA: Phases of recovery period. In White PF (ed): Ambulatory Anesthesia and Surgery. Philadelphia: WB Saunders, 1997, pp 457–464.
25. Joint Commission on Accreditation of Healthcare Organizations (JCAHO): Accreditation Manual for Ambulatory Healthcare. Oakbrook Terrace, IL: JCAHO, 1992.

Chapter 13

General Anesthesia

Deborah Dlugose

For some must watch while some must sleep . . .
(Shakespeare: Hamlet III.ii)

OVERVIEW OF GENERAL ANESTHESIA

Anesthesia care has advanced from the technical delivery of inhalational agents within a short window of time to an emphasis on the entire perianesthetic period. This includes the preanesthetic evaluation and optimization of physical status as well as consideration of postoperative analgesia and other comfort factors as part of the anesthetic plan. Ambulatory surgery nursing's continuum includes anesthesia care. Therefore, nurses who care for patients during the ambulatory surgical experience must be familiar with anesthetic medications, techniques, and emergency interventions. This knowledge allows nurses to function effectively as members of the anesthesia care team as well as to provide appropriate education for patients and families.

Because of the wide range of patient conditions and surgical requirements, appropriate preoperative evaluation and preparation of each patient must occur. Choices of technique and medications for general anesthesia must be formulated into a coherent plan that provides for rapid induction, prompt awakening, and minimal postanesthetic effects. This chapter is a broad overview of the elements of general anesthesia.

Although the unique considerations of ambulatory surgery care affect choices made for anesthetic technique, the standards for evaluation and care remain the same as those for inpatient care. Rapid discharge places a higher burden on anesthetic planning because postoperative care at home does not include the range of nursing care available to inpatients. The use of new shorter-acting agents with fewer side effects[1] is complemented with a variety of other medications to provide for patient comfort and safety. Some of these medications include antiemetics, analgesics, antibiotics and medications for autonomic stability.

The Ideal Anesthetic

Ambulatory surgical care has been a driving force for the development of agents that facilitate rapid recovery and discharge. The ideal anesthetic for ambulatory surgery is short acting, easily controllable, and free of side effects.[2] These factors are desirable both for healthy patients and for those with medical or surgical conditions requiring extra consideration. The development of "clean" drugs (those with minimal or no side effects) has decreased the risk of undesirable side effects, such as histamine release, tachycardia, and hypotension, which may be dangerous for certain patients.

Other characteristics of the ideal anesthetic for ambulatory procedures include rapid, smooth onset of action; intraoperative amnesia and analgesia; absence of toxic metabolites; high margin of safety; technical ease of administration; and usefulness for all ages. Many centers are now assessing the cost-effectiveness of agents and techniques[3–5]; medications also should be water soluble, with long shelf lives and stability in solution. The concept of "value-based anesthesia care," defined as the best patient outcome at a reasonable cost, is widely discussed.[6] Because no single agent meets all these criteria, a "balanced technique," which uses smaller amounts of a variety of drugs, is commonly seen in ambulatory anesthesia.

Forethoughts essential for the ambulatory postoperative course are also part of anesthesia care. These include such considerations as prevention of nausea and vomiting, pre-emptive analgesia, pain relief, and maintenance of appropriate fluid balance. Failure to plan for these considerations may prolong stay, increase costs, and diminish patient satisfaction.[7]

Safety considerations for the preservation of vital functions and the prevention of injury have high priority in anesthesia care. Maintenance of homeostasis (airway-breathing-circulation) is an essential element of anesthesia care. Warming strategies aim to prevent heat loss, and careful positioning with ongoing observation prevents injury.

General Anesthesia: A Definition

General anesthesia is a medication-induced, controlled state of unconsciousness that includes hypnosis (sleep), analgesia, muscle relaxation, and immobility, as well as control of the autonomic nervous system. The anesthetic plan must be adapted to existing medical conditions, such as cerebrovascular disease, coronary artery disease, reactive airway disease, and specific hazards of other systemic disorders. Loss of protective airway reflexes under general anesthesia is an important consideration for patient safety. Other factors, such as airway anomalies, may complicate airway management and must be considered.

Adjunct Medications

Anesthesia providers often administer medications that are not directly related to the anesthetic technique. Surgeons may request administration of antibiotics, steroids for reduction of inflammation, intravenous dyes to allow examination of anatomic structures, and other medications, such as oxytocics to improve uterine tone. Implications for drug interactions must always be considered.

AIRWAY MANAGEMENT AND VENTILATION TECHNIQUES

Airway maintenance is paramount. Anesthesia providers select the type of airway management from various techniques on the basis of patient factors, surgical factors, and preferences. Preinduction airway assessment allows the identification of potential airway difficulty to ensure planning for the safest airway management technique and avoidance of the dangerous "lost-airway" scenario.

Choice of Airway Technique

Some anesthetic care may be handled appropriately with a natural airway and facemask anesthesia.[8] Mask anesthesia is most commonly used in short cases with peripheral surgical sites for patients who do not have risk factors for aspiration of gastric contents. Adjuncts such as oral and nasal airways may be required for the maintenance of airway patency in light of soft tissue relaxation, which occurs under general anesthesia. Anatomic features may make mask ventilation difficult or impossible in some patients, who thus require endotracheal intubation, even for short cases.

Endotracheal intubation is often planned as part of the anesthetic technique. It is essential for situations in which patients are at risk for aspiration, surgery is in or near the airway, or neuromuscular blockade is being planned, or for long cases in which the anesthesia provider chooses not to maintain a mask airway. Readiness for immediate intubation is always essential during mask anesthesia as well as during other techniques in which unanticipated airway emergencies may arise. Orotracheal intubation is the most common route, although the nasotracheal technique is often chosen for certain intraoral procedures.

Laryngeal mask airways (LMAs) are gaining popularity for peripheral superficial cases in which spontaneous or assisted ventilation can be maintained (Figs. 13–1 and 13–2).[9, 10] The LMA, first used in Britain in 1983, is designed as an airway device that is more convenient than the facemask yet is less invasive to the patient's airway than an endotracheal tube (ETT).[11] A lower incidence of sore throat has been reported with the LMA than with the ETT. It is also less stimulating to cough reflexes and hemodynamic responses than the ETT.[12] The LMA is inserted blindly into the oropharynx of the unconscious patient, and the cuff is inflated to "mask" the larynx itself. Although the airway may be se-

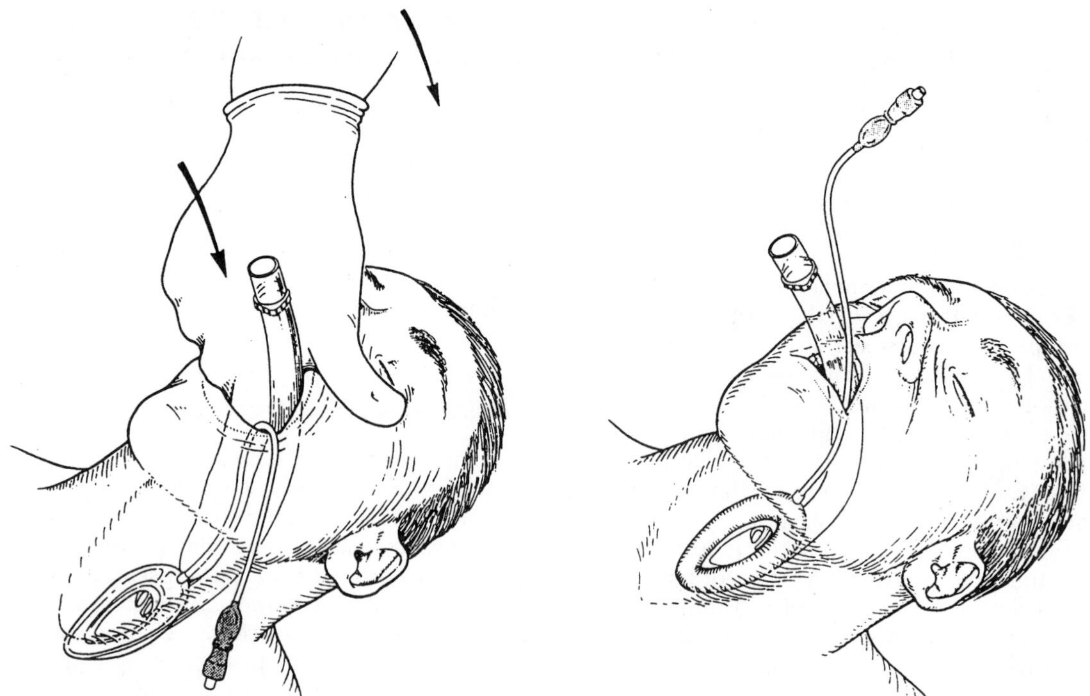

Figure 13–1. The laryngeal mask airway (LMA) masks the larynx rather than the nose and mouth. It is inserted blindly, as shown. (From Gensia Automedics, 9360 Towne Centre Drive, San Diego, CA 92121.)

cured effectively with the LMA, it does not provide as much protection against gastroesophageal reflux as the inflated cuff of an ETT, and it may actually increase risk of reflux.[13] Its blind insertion technique may provide an advantage in the difficult intubation situation in which loss of airway control occurs.[11]

The airway in an unconscious, apneic patient that cannot be secured by facemask or endotracheal intubation may be quickly secured by placing the LMA and then using it as a guide for a tube changer or a flexible fiber optic bronchoscope to place an ETT. This application is part of the American Society of Anesthesiologists difficult airway algorithm (see Fig. 13–5).

Ventilation Techniques

Under general anesthesia, ventilation may be accomplished by several techniques. Patients may breathe inhalational agents spontaneously via facemask, LMA, or ETT. However, because anesthetic agents are respiratory depressants that allow $PaCO_2$ to rise, ventilation is typically assisted manually by the anesthesia provider. Overzealous assistance may lower the CO_2 enough to depress central respiratory drive, resulting in apnea. Controlled ventilation is extremely common in intubated patients, whether or not the patient is paralyzed with neuromuscular blockers. Ventilation may be controlled manually by squeezing the breathing bag or by connecting the ETT to the automatic ventilator. Capnographic monitoring is the accepted standard of care, which allows the practitioner to maintain the patient's end-tidal CO_2 at levels consistent with physiologic safety. It also confirms continued proper placement of the ETT or LMA.

Airway Assessment

Certain characteristics have been associated with difficult tracheal intubation, including obesity, limited mouth opening, protruding upper teeth, receding mandible, short thick neck, and limited temporomandibular joint or neck range of motion.[14] Assessment of pharyngeal structures may provide clues to potential difficulty with intubation.

Mallampati's classification is now commonly used to estimate the degree of anticipated difficulty with intubation (Fig. 13–3).[15]

After careful assessment, the choice of an appropriate airway management technique is made. Uncertainty about the ability to visualize the vocal cords and to place an ETT by stan-

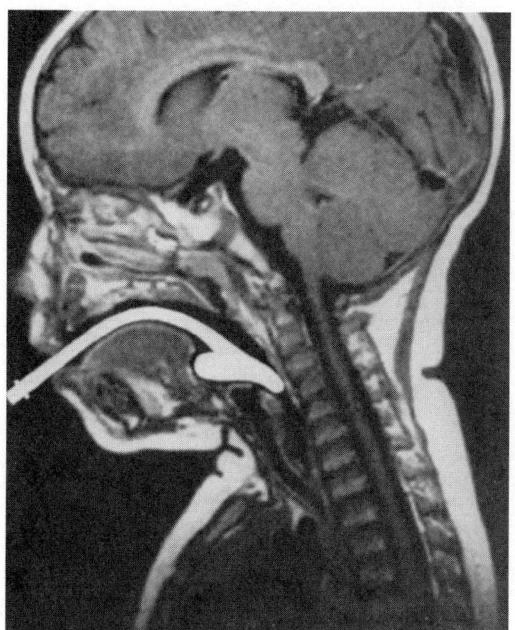

Figure 13–2. Magnetic resonance image (MRI) shows the laryngeal mask airway in place (*shown in white*). (From Rogers MC, Tinker JH, Covino BG, Longnecker DE [eds]: Principles and Practice of Anesthesiology. St. Louis: Mosby–Year Book, 1993, p 1030. Courtesy of NG Goudsouzian, MD.)

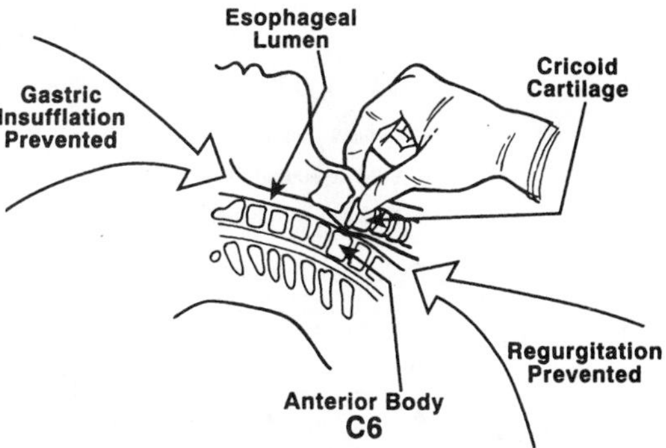

Figure 13–4. Sellick's maneuver. Sellick's maneuver is cricoid pressure held during the intubation process. Nurses should be familiar with the landmarks and techniques to provide properly applied cricoid pressure, including maintenance of the maneuver until tracheal intubation is confirmed. (From Cicala RS, Grande CM, Steve JK, et al: Emergency and elective airway management for trauma patients. In Grande CM [ed]: Trauma, Anesthesia, and Critical Care. St. Louis: CV Mosby, 1993, p 748.)

dard direct laryngoscopic technique necessitates a plan for other techniques. These may include awake (sedated) intubation by blind technique, direct visualization, or flexible fiberoptic bronchoscopy. The entire surgery team should be prepared to participate in emergency actions that accompany failure to secure the airway.

Nurses often assist at intubation by applying cricoid pressure for patients at risk for aspiration of gastric contents. These patients require rapid-sequence induction with Sellick's maneuver (cricoid pressure) (Fig. 13–4).[16] Familiarity with the landmarks of the anterior neck and the proper technique for cricoid pressure is essential. Cricoid pressure must not be released until the laryngoscopist indicates that (1) tracheal intubation is verified, usually by observing the CO_2 waveform on capnograph and auscultating bilateral breath sounds and (2) the ETT cuff has been inflated.

The American Society of Anesthesiologists Difficult Airway Algorithm

Inability to manage difficult airway problems is associated with a significant percentage of the

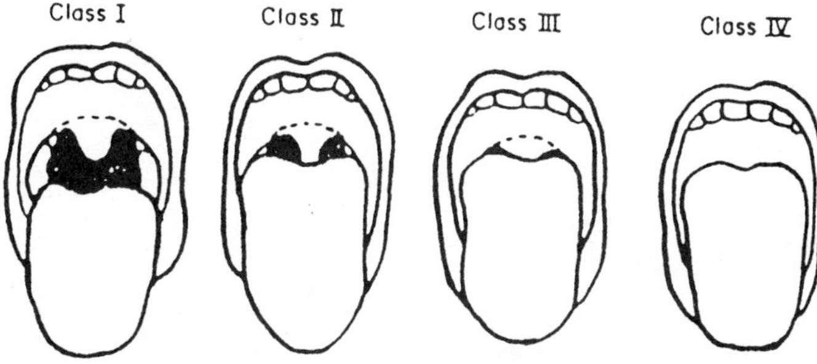

Figure 13–3. Mallampati's classification of oropharyngeal structures. A higher classification indicates greater likelihood of difficult intubation. Careful preanesthetic evaluation and planning reduces the risk of unanticipated airway management difficulty and potential for catastrophic airway emergencies. Classification of views of the pharynx is done according to Mallampati and associates. In class I, the soft palate, fauces, tonsillar pillars, and uvula are seen. In class II, all of the aforementioned structures (except the tonsillar pillars) are visible. In class III, only the base of the uvula is in view. In class IV, none of the aforementioned structures is visible. (From Samsoon GLT, Young JRB: Difficult tracheal intubation: A retrospective study. Anaesthesia 42:487, 1987).

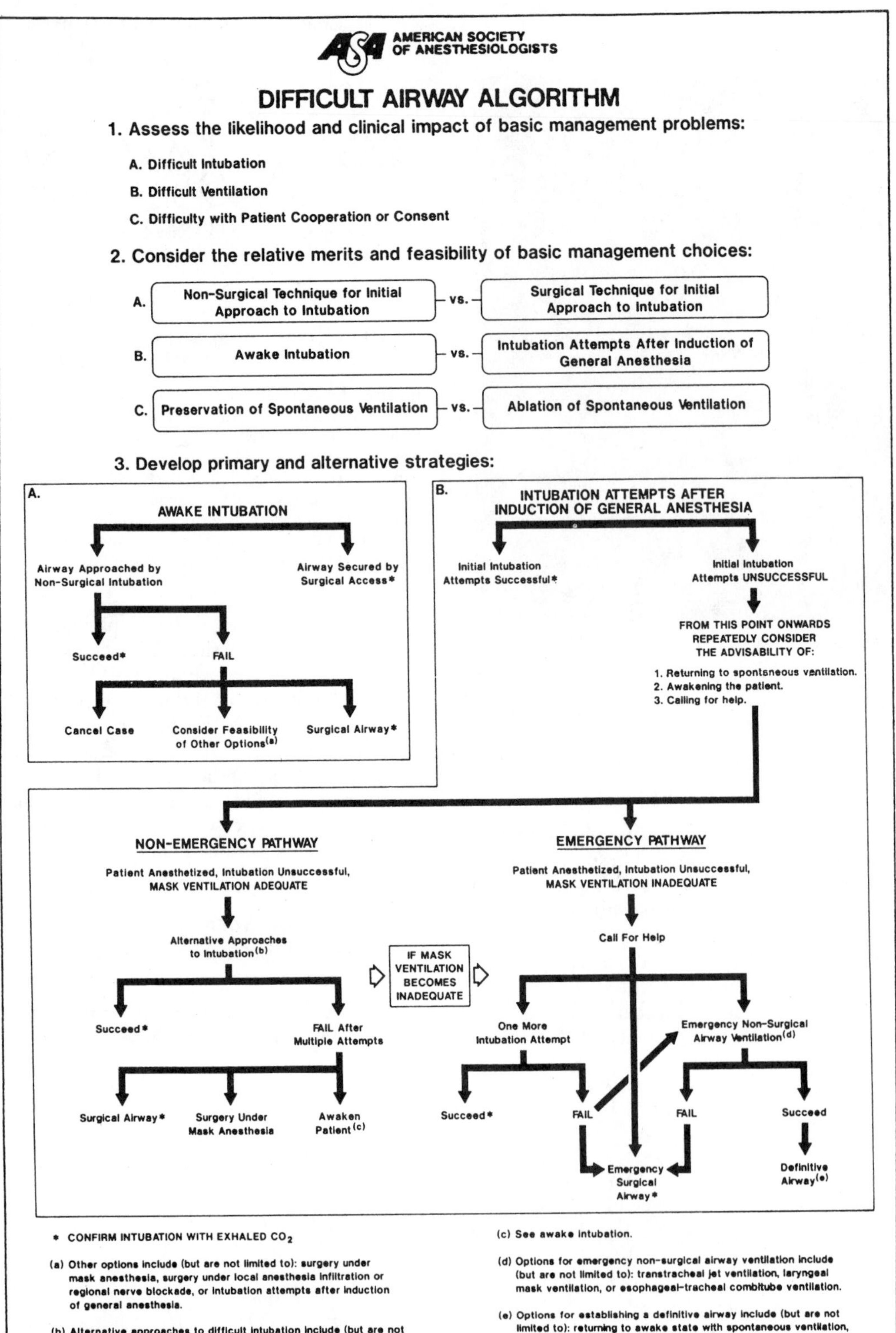

Figure 13–5. ASA difficult airway algorithm. All team members should be familiar with the steps and equipment described in this algorithm. Nurses' assistance in the situation of difficult airway management is critical. (From Benumoff JL [ed]: American Society of Anesthesiologists Task Force on Management of The Difficult Airway: Practice guidelines for management of the difficult airway: A report. Anesthesiology 78:597, 1993.)

deaths directly attributable to anesthesia alone. The American Society of Anesthesiologists has developed an algorithm to aid decision-making in this emergency scenario (Fig. 13–5). All team members should be familiar with options in this algorithm, focusing on location and use of various types of equipment and techniques. A dedicated "difficult airway cart" is ideal. Nurses should be familiar with devices such as specialized laryngoscopes and their assembly, ETT guides and specialized stylets, light wands, fiberoptic intubation equipment, LMAs, and esophageal-tracheal Combitubes. They should also be familiar with the equipment and actions necessary for cricothyrotomy and transtracheal jet ventilation. Teamwork and equipment preparedness are essential during this critical event.

Monitoring Breathing

Because anesthetic agents interfere with patient physiology and ability to maintain oxygenation and ventilation (removal of CO_2), anesthesia providers continuously monitor oxygen saturation and end-tidal CO_2. Chest motion alone is not evidence of breathing; capnography allows breath-to-breath measurement of expired CO_2 and confirms a patent airway. Assisted and controlled ventilation by the anesthesia provider is adjusted to maintain normal CO_2 levels.

Monitoring Circulation

Because most anesthetic agents have marked effects on the cardiovascular system, these drugs are titrated on the basis of the patient's vital signs. At the same time, vital signs may be manipulated with vasoactive medications to keep them within safe ranges to allow adequate anesthesia and amnesia while maintaining safety and homeostasis.

Electronic monitors used during anesthesia care are extensions of the anesthesia provider's sensory abilities. The importance of vigilant monitoring of all parameters as well as commonsense observation of the patient and surgical field cannot be overemphasized. Nurses' awareness of the significance of each monitoring parameter and expected activities during abnormal situations is an important function on the anesthesia care continuum.

Monitoring cardiovascular parameters, such as pulse, blood pressure, and electrocardiographic tracing, has long been a standard part of the art and science of general anesthesia. Within the past decade, noninvasive techniques, such as beat-to-beat monitoring of oxygenation with the pulse oximeter, increase safety. The addition of capnography (end-tidal CO_2 measurement) as a monitor of ventilation has further enhanced safety.

Other Monitoring Considerations

Temperature monitoring has also become standard. The subtle hazards of hypothermia and the serious potential hazard of malignant hyperthermia require the use of continuous temperature monitoring for all but the briefest of procedures under general anesthesia. Problems associated with reduced body temperature include (1) dramatic increase in oxygen consumption associated with shivering, (2) central nervous system depression, (3) prolongation of neuromuscular blockade, and (4) coagulation disorders. Decreased metabolism associated with hypothermia decreases drug doses required to maintain the level of surgical anesthesia and prolongs medication effect.

Monitoring of neuromuscular blockade is also essential in the ambulatory surgery situation, in which prompt emergence is important. Careful titration of neuromuscular blockers on the basis of the nerve stimulator's results allows optimum dosing and increases patient safety when adequate reversal of blockade is being assessed (Fig. 13–6).

Monitoring Patient Safety

Careful positioning of the patient is an essential safety consideration.[17] Anesthetized patients have no ability to protect themselves from noxious stimuli; they cannot express positioning discomfort, which may reflect the beginning of bodily injury by stretch, pressure, or compression. All members of the ambulatory surgery team are obligated to ensure that these safety considerations are met. Changes in position of the operating table or addition of factors such as a leaning surgeon require ongoing vigilance and intervention. Frequent rechecks of positioning are essential. Existing neurosensory deficits should be documented before surgery to allow for definitive postoperative comparison.

Eye protection[18] may be as simple as taping the patient's eyes closed during a short case. For longer cases, sterile ophthalmic ointment or saline eye drops may be placed. Laser cases usually require special protective goggles for both personnel and patients. Prone or lateral positions require measures to ensure that there is no pressure on eyes, ears, or facial structures.

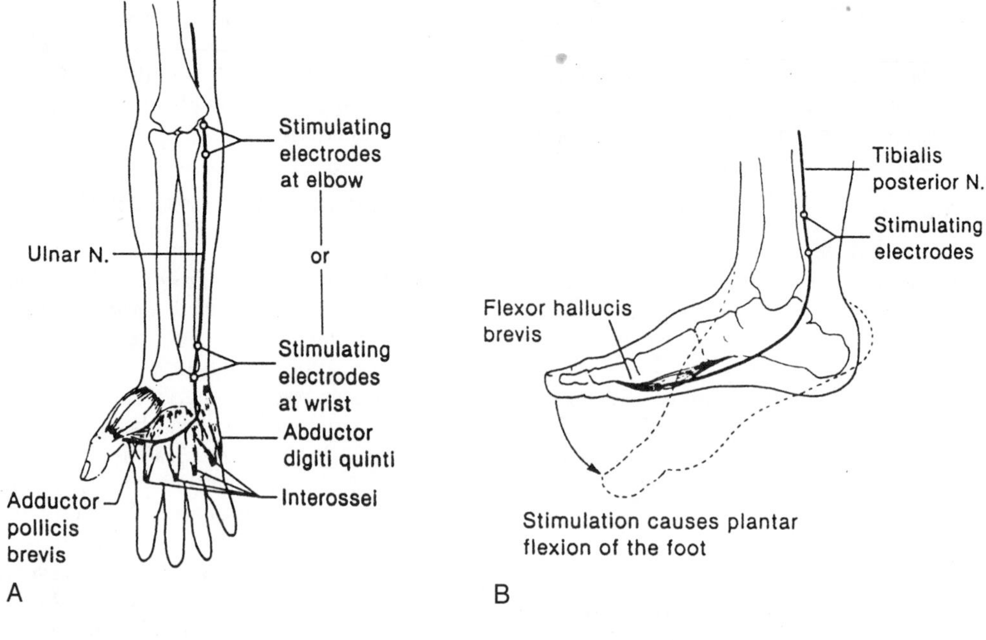

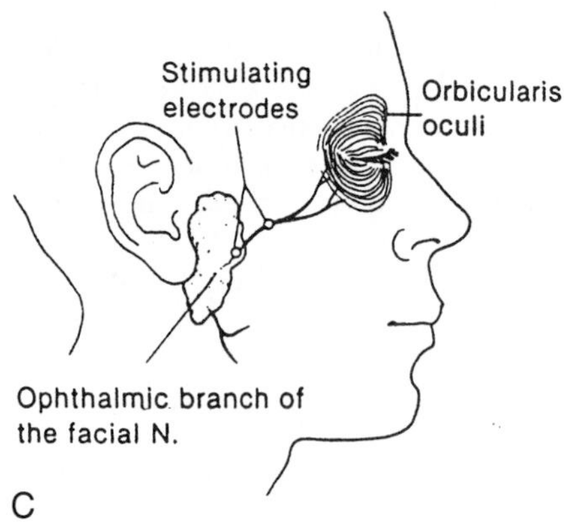

Figure 13–6. Placement of peripheral nerve stimulators (PNS). PNS may be placed on a variety of nerve sites to monitor the level of neuromuscular blockade and to confirm the return of neuromuscular function. (From Benumoff JL [ed]: American Society of Anesthesiologists Task Force on Management of The Difficult Airway: Practice guidelines for management of the difficult airway: A report. Anesthesiology 78:597, 1993.)

Use of limb tourniquets requires care in placement and attention to duration of use and degree of compression or pressure elevation.[19, 20] Surgeons should be notified of tourniquet time every 30 minutes, and their acknowledgment should be documented. Two hours is usually considered a safe tourniquet time. The tourniquet effect of automatically cycled blood pressure monitors should also be considered when their settings for automatic readings are selected. Radial nerve palsy has been associated with the use of these devices.[21]

Natural and artificial teeth may be damaged during airway manipulations. Preservation of the patient's dental status is more than cosmetic.[22] Broken teeth may be life threatening if they are aspirated into the tracheobronchial tree. Thus, careful preoperative and postanesthetic assessment of teeth must occur. Devices such as dental guards may be helpful but provide no guarantee.

Although patients traditionally come to the operating suite with all prostheses and clothing removed, the ambulatory surgical environment may allow flexibility regarding removal of cosmetic or functional items that enhance patient dignity. Each situation must be individually evaluated, with safety as the prime consideration. Dentures may actually facilitate mask airway management and then be removed for laryngoscopy and intubation. Allowing patients to retain wigs or prosthetic eyes may be an important psychosocial consideration; however, allowing contact lenses under general anesthesia is likely to be unsafe because of reduction in tear production during anesthesia. Children who are undergoing peripheral procedures, such as myringotomy, may feel less threatened in their own clothes, and even adults feel more secure if they are allowed to wear undergarments appropriate to the surgery. Concern for infection control may allow the substitution of surgical scrub trousers for underwear. Staff commitment to patient modesty should be apparent.

MEDICATIONS FOR ANESTHESIA

Historically, general anesthesia has been referred to as the inhalation of volatile anesthetic vapors. Today's general anesthesia is most likely to be a variable combination of intravenous and inhalational agents, with infiltrated local anesthetics added for pre-emptive analgesia in certain procedures. Balanced anesthesia is the use of multiple agents and medications, allowing for desired effects while limiting side effects from any individual agent.

Intravenous Induction

Intravenous induction agents cause rapid and predictable onset of sleep, without breathing of "smelly vapors."[23] These sleep-inducing agents do not have full anesthetic or analgesic qualities; thus, other techniques and drugs must follow the induction of sleep to provide surgical anesthesia. All doses are reduced when used in combined techniques with narcotics and sedatives as well as in elderly or debilitated patients.[7]

Propofol

During the 1990s, propofol (Diprivan) established itself as a valuable agent for many ambulatory surgery anesthetics.[2, 24, 25] Propofol is a unique nonbarbiturate sedative-hypnotic with a very short half-life. It is delivered in an intralipid emulsion, which includes soy, egg phosphatide, and glycerol; allergies to these substances should be identified.[26] It is considered safe for patients with allergy to egg albumin, not to the phosphatide.[27] Propofol's formulation requires strict aseptic technique; because it is a breeding ground for microbial growth, syringes must be used within 6 hours of drawing up. Septicemia and death have been attributed to problems with aseptic technique and handling of propofol.[28]

Propofol's short duration of action also facilitates delivery via continuous infusion for maintenance of general anesthesia, allowing close control of depth of anesthesia followed by rapid emergence. When compared with other induction and maintenance agents, propofol provides notable postanesthetic clear-headedness (sometimes euphoria) in most patients.[2, 29] Reduction of anesthetic "hangover" is highly desirable for ambulatory surgery patients. Propofol is also notable for its low incidence of postoperative nausea and vomiting (PONV). Current research indicates that it may be protective against PONV, and some centers are studying its use as a direct antiemetic agent in subhypnotic doses.[30] Its antiemetic action outlasts its sedative effect.

One disadvantage of propofol is pain on injection into small veins.[27] This discomfort may be reduced by administering a prior dose of intravenous lidocaine, by adding a small amount of intravenous lidocaine to the propofol syringe, or by selecting a larger vessel, such as the antecubital vein.

Because propofol is a vasodilator and myocardial depressant,[25] reduced dosage is necessary for patients who are elderly or for those with cardiovascular disease. The combination of propofol and any of the fentanyl analogues or succinylcholine may result in profound bradycardia.[29] Doses used to induce sleep commonly produce brief apnea. Anaphylactoid reactions to propofol, which have symptoms similar to these of anaphylaxis but are not mediated by immunoglobulin E, have been reported.[31]

Other reported effects of propofol that make it useful in ambulatory surgery include reduced postoperative shivering[32]; bronchodilation by relaxation of bronchial smooth muscle, similar to its action on vascular smooth muscle[33]; antiseizure effect,[34, 35] although there have been reports of delayed seizures after propofol[36]; and conversion of supraventricular tachycardia.[37] Propofol does not trigger malignant hyperthermia.[25]

Although propofol is more expensive per dose than thiopental or methohexital (which are available in generic formulations), its rapid emergence profile and antiemetic effect may reduce the cost of recovery time and nursing care. Patient satisfaction and feeling of well-being after propofol are also difficult to quantify in terms of dollars.

Other Induction Agents

Thiopental (Pentothal) is an ultra–short-acting barbiturate. For more than half a century, it set the standard for smooth induction of general anesthesia.[7] However, thiopental has some disadvantages. Large or repeated doses may cause prolonged somnolence, which conflicts with the goal of rapid patient discharge.[24] Thiopental may also contribute to increased incidence of PONV. Its highly alkaline pH (10 to 11) may cause tissue necrosis if the drug extravasates from a vessel.

Because generic thiopental is inexpensive, some practitioners are now studying a one-to-one mix of thiopental and propofol.[38] This combination appears to present a clinical profile similar to that of propofol alone, and the highly alkaline pH of the thiopental may contribute to the antibacterial protection of the propofol.

Methohexital (Brevital) is another ultra-short-acting barbiturate that is similar to thiopental. It may be cleared from the body more rapidly than thiopental. Methohexital may cause excitatory effects on induction, such as tremor, hypertonus, involuntary muscle movements, and hiccups.[24] In children, methohexital has been used for rectal induction of sleep before full general anesthesia has been established,[39] although it may have a slower recovery profile. Vigilance for maintenance of airway patency and oxygen saturation is essential with this technique.[40]

Etomidate (Amidate) is a nonbarbiturate induction drug that has a wider margin of cardiovascular safety than barbiturates and propofol.[41] Its use is commonly limited to patients with serious cardiovascular compromise. Studies have shown that it may suppress adrenal function, even after a single dose.[24] The clinical significance of this effect has not been determined. Injection of etomidate may also be associated with pain and myoclonic movements. It is associated with PONV,[29] especially if it is used for both induction and maintenance.

Ketamine (Ketalar) is a phencyclidine derivative (cousin of lysergic acid diethylamide [LSD] and phenylcyclohexyl piperidine [PCP]) that produces a dissociated mental state as well as profound analgesia.[29] Nystagmus, vocalization, and myoclonic movements may also occur.[24] Ketamine supports the cardiovascular system and causes bronchodilation.[24] Although ketamine may cause less reduction of protective airway reflexes than other induction agents, aspiration of gastric contents may occur in patients with unprotected airways. Increased oral secretions may require a drying agent, such as glycopyrrolate.

Depending on the dosage, ketamine can be used as an induction agent or as a sedative agent for peripheral procedures, such as painful dressing changes. Ketamine is also suitable for intramuscular induction of general anesthesia in patients who are unable to cooperate with intravenous or inhalational inductions. Recovery time after a single dose is usually less than 30 minutes.

Ketamine is well known for emergence dysphoria, which includes postoperative agitation, unpleasant dreams, and hallucinations, especially when given to adults. These effects may persist into the home recovery period after ambulatory surgery. Although this problem is reduced by concurrent administration of benzodiazepines, these effects clearly limit ketamine's usefulness for ambulatory procedures.[7] Postanesthesia care should include care in a quiet room (perhaps darkened) without a reduction in monitoring. Postdischarge telephone surveillance after ketamine should include reassurance about these psychological effects; patients with ongoing reactions should be referred to the anesthesia providers for follow-up.

Midazolam

Although best known as an intravenous sedative, higher-dose midazolam (Versed) can be used as an induction agent, especially in patients with cardiovascular compromise. However, longer recovery times must be expected.[29] Lower doses are used in a coinduction technique, combining it with another induction agent at reduced doses to improve the recovery time. The benzodiazepine antagonist flumazenil (Romazicon) is available if prolonged somnolence or respiratory depression occur. Antagonist effect may dissipate within 1 hour, requiring vigilance for return of somnolence or respiratory depression. Use of potent amnestics may interfere with the patient's ability to recall teaching about postoperative care,[25] making written and verbal instructions to patients and responsible adults essential.

Inhalational Induction

Although intravenous induction is the most commonly used technique, there are circumstances in which the intravenous route is not available. Small children or adults with limited mental capability or extreme needle shyness may not tolerate line placement well. Although the addition of EMLA (eutectic mixture of local anesthetics) cream may improve the chances of starting an intravenous line, sleep is often induced with inhalational technique, in which the patient breathes agents through a facemask until loss of consciousness occurs. For brief peripheral surgeries, such as myringotomy, an intravenous line may not be started at all; for most cases, the line is started after the agent has induced sleep and analgesia.

The inhalational agents are potent volatile liquids that are vaporized in agent-specific vaporizers on the anesthesia machine and carried to the patient's airway by carrier gases, which include oxygen, nitrous oxide, and air, in various combinations for selected clinical scenarios.

For the past few decades, inhalational inductions have been typically carried out with halothane (Fluothane), which was the least pungent volatile agent available. Other agents, such as isoflurane (Forane) and desflurane (Suprane), are airway irritants that may cause coughing, gagging, or laryngospasm when breathed for induction. The arrival of sevoflurane (Ultane) on the US market in 1995 brought another airway-acceptable agent, which also has the advantage of rapid onset and offset of anesthesia. Sevoflurane has replaced halothane in many ambulatory surgical centers.

The ideal inhalation agent is insoluble in body fluids and tissues.[42] Low-solubility agents, such as nitrous oxide, desflurane, and sevoflurane, provide quick onset and rapid emergence. Highly soluble agents, such as diethyl ether, have very slow onset and slow emergence as a result of their solubility and slow release from body tissues. Halothane and isoflurane have intermediate solubility. Although low-solubility agents may provide the most rapid emergence, discharge may be delayed by other factors, such as use of narcotics or sedatives.[43]

Minimum alveolar concentration (MAC) is a commonly used term that describes the potency for each inhalational agent.[44] (This abbreviation has no relationship to the other MAC commonly used in anesthesia care, which stands for monitored anesthesia care). Minimum alveolar concentration is the percent of anesthetic agent breathed that prevents movement in 50% of subjects in response to a standard surgical incision. Because it is not desirable for half of a patient population to move in response to incision, concentrations of 1.5 to 2.5 MAC are commonly delivered. MAC varies with age; it is slightly higher in children than in adults, and then it decreases with advancing patient age. MAC is only a general guideline for dosage; every anesthetic is titrated for the individual patient for each moment.

Stages of Anesthesia: Use of the Term

Stages of general anesthesia are mostly a historical concept.[42] These stages were described for the inhalation agent diethyl ether. Because of ether's slow onset, physical signs and progressive loss of consciousness were clearly notable as the patient underwent induction by breathing the agent. At emergence, patients progressed back toward consciousness in reverse order. These stages are blurred (or nonexistent) with rapid-acting intravenous agents in use today. However, the concept of stage II remains important in the rare situation in which a pure inhalational technique is given. This stage of physiologic "excitement" lies between the initial analgesia associated with mask induction and the desirable stage III of "surgical anesthesia." Gagging, coughing, airway obstruction, and laryngospasm are possible during this brief period, both at induction and at emergence. Extra vigilance and rapid intervention for these problems are essential. The addition of narcotics, sedatives, or muscle relaxants obscures this stage.

Parents who are present for induction of anesthesia (or emergence in the postanesthesia care unit [PACU]) should be taught about stage II and reassured that the agitation is a normal effect of inhalational agents for a brief period. Although patients may move vigorously, they are amnestic during stage II. Nursing vigilance for signs of airway obstruction and care for patient safety during agitation are essential.

Carrier Gases

The potent inhalational agents are delivered in small percentages that vary with each agent (Table 13–1). Because a minimum of 21% oxygen is a physiologic requirement, oxygen is the most important carrier gas for the potent volatile agents. Flowmeters on the anesthesia machine indicate the quantities of carrier gases being used (in liters per minute) to deliver the percentage of volatile agent selected on the calibrated vaporizer.

Inhalational agents are almost always delivered with oxygen as a carrier gas. One exception is laser-airway procedures in which medical air replaces the oxygen carrier gas to provide 21% oxygen ("room air") to reduce the danger of flammability in case of airway fire associated with laser ignition of the ETT or its cuff.

Nitrous oxide (N_2O) is an analgesic gas that is often used as a carrier (along with oxygen) for the potent inhalational agents. Its rapid onset and additive analgesic qualities potentiate the effects of the volatile agents and reduce their doses. This quality assists with smooth induction. Use of nitrous oxide remains controversial for many procedures because it may be

Table 13–1.* Highlights of the Inhaled Anesthetics

GENERIC NAME	TRADE NAME	TYPICAL RANGE OF INSPIRED CONCENTRATION	ONSET TIME	RECOVERY TIME	POSITIVE ASPECTS	NEGATIVE ASPECTS
Halothane	Fluothane	0.5–1% (induction: 2–3%, up to 5%)	Slow	Slow	Provides smooth inhalational induction	Slow uptake and elimination Cardiac depression and dysrhythmias (especially with epinephrine) Linked to hepatic necrosis in adults
Enflurane	Ethrane	0.75–1.5%	Intermediate	Intermediate	Good muscle relaxation Stable heart	Seizure activity on EEG Pungent odor
Isoflurane	Forane	0.5–1.5%	Intermediate	Intermediate	Good muscle relaxation Stable heart	Airway irritation, coughing
Desflurane	Suprane	2–8%	Rapid	Rapid	Rapid onset-offset Minimal metabolism	Airway irritation Tachycardia with rapid increase in dose
Sevoflurane	Ultane	1–2%	Rapid	Rapid	Smooth, rapid inhalational induction	? effect of breakdown products
Nitrous oxide	None	40–70%	Very rapid	Very rapid	Analgesia Minimal cardiac or respiratory depression	PONV Diffusion hypoxia Expands closed air spaces Requires high concentrations (limits increased FIO_2)

*Dosages are approximate. The art of anesthesia requires individual titration of dose. Each agent has other actions and side effects. Anesthesia drug manuals and pharmacology texts provide more information.
EEG, electroencephalogram; PONV, postoperative nausea and vomiting.

associated with an increased incidence of PONV,[43] perhaps related to gastrointestinal distention or increased middle ear pressure.[29] It diffuses easily into closed body spaces, where accumulation may dramatically increase pressures. This phenomenon is undesirable in patients such as those undergoing tympanic procedures, in which increased middle ear pressures can displace surgical grafts[29]; those undergoing retinal surgery, in which precisely sized bubbles of gas are placed into the globe of the eye; those with bowel obstruction, in which intestinal gas accumulates; and those at risk for pneumothorax, the size of which may be increased by nitrous oxide.

Nitrous oxide's historical place as the "light anesthetic" maintained at the end of procedures while dressings are placed may be supplanted by the rapid-offset agents desflurane and sevoflurane. Because of high inspired concentrations of nitrous oxide used (60% to 70%), the rapid diffusion of nitrous oxide out of the bloodstream at the end of anesthesia can contribute to immediate postoperative hypoxemia. As large quantities of N_2O are eliminated via the lungs, alveolar oxygen levels may be diluted.[45] This diffusion hypoxia is one reason for the administration of supplemental oxygen in transport from the operating room and in the PACU.[7]

Effects of Potent Inhalational Agents

Potent inhalational agents used today include halothane, isoflurane, desflurane, and sevoflurane. All inhalational agents have some common effects on major systems of the body. The most obvious site of action is the central nervous system, in which the agents "put the brain to sleep," blocking consciousness and certain noxious stimuli. This mechanism of action has not yet been completely defined, nor is it always complete. Certain autonomic stimuli may persist under general anesthesia (e.g., parasympathetic and sympathetic activity). A very small percentage of patients may also experience some level of awareness under general anesthesia, although this is usually associated with the use of neuromuscular blockers, which may mask the signs of too-light anesthesia. Inhalational agents are cerebral vasodilators, which can increase intracranial pressure; however, they also decrease cerebral metabolic oxygen requirements.

Spontaneous ventilation diminishes under inhalational agents, changing to rapid shallow breathing, which allows $PaCO_2$ to rise, unless ventilation is assisted or controlled by the anesthesia provider. Intercostal muscle function is reduced, leading to a rocking-boat appearance of ventilation in which the chest collapses and the abdomen protrudes during inspiration. The inhalational agents also cause bronchodilatation, which is ideal for patients with reactive airway disease. Loss of airway tone occurs with loss of consciousness; this situation has implications for the management of a patent airway. Functional residual capacity also decreases, perhaps related to compression atelectasis.[43]

All inhalational agents except nitrous oxide decrease blood pressure in a dose-related manner. Halothane decreases cardiac output by direct myocardial depression and slowed heart rate. Isoflurane decreases systemic vascular resistance. Isoflurane and desflurane increase heart rate, also in a dose-related fashion. Halothane increases cardiac irritability to catecholamines. The combination of halothane and injected epinephrine can produce severe ventricular dysrhythmias. All of these agents decrease electrical transmission through the heart's sinoatrial node. Junctional rhythms are common and usually have no effect on blood pressure.

Decreased blood flow to kidneys that is associated with inhalational anesthesia can decrease urine output. However, inadequate intravascular volume is a more common cause of perianesthetic oliguria. Normal expected urine output is 1 ml/kg/hr; a reduction to 0.5 ml/kg/hr under inhalational anesthesia may be acceptable.[46] Because this oliguria is directly related to the presence of the inhalation agents in the bloodstream, the postoperative patient who is awake should have the normal expected amount of urine output. Inadequate fluid replacement may delay the return of this function. Although selected patients may be discharged to home without having a postoperative void, discharge instructions should include a time for calling the physician if spontaneous urine output has not occurred.[47]

All inhalational agents potentiate nondepolarizing muscle relaxants; therefore, dosages are reduced and titrated depending on the clinical effect and peripheral nerve stimulator. Inhalational agents also cause uterine relaxation; this effect has implications for pregnant patients, in whom the agents decrease tone and inhibit contractions, although studies do not show a decrease in incidence of preterm labor.[46] In newly postpartum patients uterine relaxation may increase bleeding. Today's rapid-offset agents minimize this problem.

Specific Inhalational Agents

Halothane was developed in the 1950s as a "cleaner" alternative to diethyl ether. Halothane is nonexplosive and provides a more rapid onset and fewer side effects than ether. As the least pungent inhalational agent, halothane maintained its role for 4 decades for pediatric inhalational inductions because it had less chance for airway irritation, gagging, coughing, and laryngospasm. Halothane is well known for causing ventricular dysrhythmias in the presence of increased catecholamine levels, such as the scenario in which a surgeon infiltrates epinephrine to reduce bleeding. Hypercarbia also increases catecholamine levels and the risk of these dysrythmias. Halothane is a direct myocardial depressant and a potent cerebral vasodilator. Approximately 10% to 20% of the inhaled molecules are metabolized rather than being exhaled unchanged. This increases the chance of organ damage, especially to the liver. Halothane's solubility is higher than that of newer agents, leading to slower emergence from anesthesia.[29]

Isoflurane was introduced in the early 1980s, gaining rapid acceptance because of its low rate of metabolism (<1%).[48] Its onset and emergence are more rapid than halothane's. Although it is a potent respiratory depressant, it may produce less cardiac depression than halothane. Tachycardia may occur when the dose is increased. Isoflurane is too pungent for inhalational inductions. It does not sensitize the myocardium to catecholamines.[49]

Desflurane arrived on the market in late 1992, rapidly gaining popularity in outpatient anesthesia because of its rapid onset and recovery, which make recovery significantly faster than isoflurane.[29] It is the least soluble inhalational agent available now; this characteristic allows rapid adjustment of depth of anesthesia as well as prompt emergence.[50] Tachycardia may develop with rapid increases in the dosage delivered. Like other inhalational agents, desflurane causes dose-related cardiovascular and respiratory depression. Its degree of metabolism by the liver is almost nil. Desflurane's physicochemical structure requires storage in pressured bottles and delivery to the patient via a specialized heated vaporizer.[49]

Sevoflurane was introduced in the United States in late 1995. It is a little less soluble than desflurane, which provides rapid induction and emergence from sevoflurane. Because it has very little pungency, it provides smooth, rapid inhalational inductions. This major advantage and its low solubility may make it the agent of choice for short procedures.[49]

Sevoflurane is degraded by soda lime in the anesthesia machine's breathing circuit, with breakdown compounds whose potential neurologic and pulmonary toxicities remain under evaluation.[45] Metabolic breakdown products in patients include inorganic fluoride, which has been associated with renal failure. However, studies have not shown renal dysfunction in volunteers who were given sevoflurane.[29] Sevoflurane has been widely used outside the United States without significant problems.[51] Its lack of pungency and rapid on-off profile may change ambulatory surgery practice.

Total Intravenous Anesthesia

Although inhalational agents provide the typical foundation of general anesthesia, total intravenous anesthesia has its proponents. In this technique, the inhalational agent is replaced with precision-pump intravenous infusion of a sleep drug, such as propofol.[52] Muscle relaxants, narcotics, and amnestics are added to provide complete anesthesia. New short-acting agents and computerized infusion devices facilitate this application but also raise cost. However, it may be the ideal anesthetic method for patients who are susceptible to MH or for those in whom airway surgery may preclude the administration of volatile inhalational agents.[29]

Analgesics and Antagonists

Narcotics

The dose of an inhalational agent can be reduced by the administration of narcotics or non-narcotic analgesics at the same time. Appropriate well-timed doses should not delay patient discharge, yet should provide some residual analgesia for the postoperative period.[7] Without intraoperative intravenous analgesics, patients who have eliminated enough inhalational agent to be awake are likely to be in pain, requiring larger analgesic doses, which may delay discharge.

Older narcotics such as morphine and meperidine, are not "clean." Despite good analgesic effect, they have undesirable side effects, such as PONV, urinary retention, increased somnolence, and respiratory depression, which may contribute to prolonged patient stay. Nevertheless, morphine is still used in many centers for its better quality of analgesia.[53] Small doses of meperidine are valuable to suppress postoperative shivering, although the mechanism of effect has not been identified.[54]

Although any narcotic may be selected to provide analgesia, the ambulatory anesthesia plan is likely to involve the short-acting fentanyl analogues, which are easily titratable. The synthetic narcotic fentanyl (Sublimaze) has been a mainstay in anesthesia practice for 3 decades. Fentanyl and its analogues provide excellent analgesia with rapid onset, relatively short duration, and minimal histamine release, which allows cardiovascular stability.[7] However, the profound (and possibly prolonged) respiratory depressant effects of these drugs must be appreciated.[7] In addition to simple respiratory depression, all fentanyl analogues may cause "board chest," muscular rigidity of the thorax and neck muscles[54] to the point that ventilation is impossible. A small dose of muscle relaxant may be required to allow ventilation. This problem is usually related to higher doses and rapid speed of intravenous injection, although it has been reported for common clinical doses of fentanyl (1 to 2 μg/kg). Fentanyl's peak effect occurs within 5 minutes. Doses of 1 to 3 μg/kg generally provide an hour of analgesia; as dosages are increased and repeated, the drug's effects become cumulative.[55]

Alfentanil (Alfenta) is an ultra–short-acting narcotic with very rapid onset and offset, which makes it suitable for continuous infusion or intermittent intravenous boluses when a short duration of action is important.[7] Its peak effect may be seen in less than 2 minutes, and its duration is about 15 minutes.[55]

Sufentanil (Sufenta) is the most potent opioid now available. Theoretically, its greater potency increases its opioid effects while reducing the likelihood of side effects.[7] Its duration and action are similar to those of fentanyl, but its greater potency makes cautious dosing essential. Small doses of sufentanil appropriate for ambulatory surgical procedures may cause prolonged analgesia in the PACU, but patients may experience more symptoms that require antiemetic treatment.[29]

The newest synthetic narcotic is remifentanil (Ultiva), introduced in 1997, which is ultra–short-acting with a high margin of safety. Its half-life of about 3 to 10 minutes makes it ideal for continuous infusions, which can provide intense analgesia for variable levels of surgical stimuli yet can allow rapid recovery. Its unique characteristic is breakdown by body esterase enzymes rather than reliance on the liver or kidney. Remifentanil's short duration of action is likely to require other medications or techniques to provide postoperative analgesia.[56] Current research will decide remifentanil's place in ambulatory surgery.

Narcotic Agonist-Antagonist Agents

Pure narcotic agents bind to μ-receptors to produce analgesia, respiratory depression, and euphoria. Agonist-antagonist agents, such as butorphanol (Stadol), nalbuphine (Nubain), and dezocine (Dalgan), can provide analgesia as they bind to μ-κ- and σ-receptors with varying levels of activity at each receptor.[55] They are used most frequently as supplemental analgesic agents because their agonist activity may be weak with a "ceiling effect," in which increasing dose does not increase analgesic effect.[55] These drugs are sometimes used to reverse respiratory depression caused by pure opioid agonists without reversing analgesia.

Non-Narcotic Agents

Nonsteroidal anti-inflammatory drugs such as ketorolac (Toradol) have been shown to exhibit narcotic-sparing effect.[57] Although studies show that ketorolac is inadequate as a sole analgesic for surgery, it may allow reduced narcotic doses, thus minimizing undesirable narcotic side effects. Nonsteroidal anti-inflammatory drugs do not affect opiate receptors, producing no respiratory depression or PONV. Peak analgesia from IV or intramuscular administration occurs in 30 to 45 minutes,[54] and the duration of action is 6 to 8 hours. This time frame and the lack of opioid-type side effects make ketorolac a valuable adjunct to minimize postoperative pain.

Ketorolac's side effects may be significant in certain patients. Because it increases bleeding time, it must be avoided in patients with coagulation disorders, as well as in those with a risk of cerebrovascular or gastrointestinal bleeding. Risk of renal failure precludes its use in patients with reduced renal function, hypovolemia, or concurrent nephrotoxic medications.[54]

The usual dosage of ketorolac is 30 mg IV or intramuscularly. Reduced dosage (to 15 mg) is essential for elderly patients and small adults (<110 pounds). Although it is desirable for ketorolac's analgesic effect to peak at the time of emergence from general anesthesia, surgical hemostasis must be ensured before intraoperative doses are administered near the end of the case. Hypersensitivity reactions, such as bronchospasm and anaphylaxis, have been reported. Ketorolac must also be avoided in patients who are allergic to aspirin and other nonsteroidal anti-inflammatory drugs.

Neuromuscular Blockade

"Muscle relaxants" used in anesthesia are paralyzing drugs. Their advantages include profound relaxation to allow tracheal intubation, assurance of immobility during delicate surgical procedures, and maintenance of general anesthesia with lesser amounts of anesthetic drugs, thus contributing to more rapid emergence. Their disadvantages include undesirable effects on vital signs, such as tachycardia and hypotension, with certain neuromuscular blockers. Use of neuromuscular blockade prevents patients from maintaining their natural airways and breathing capabilities, which may contribute to lost airway emergencies. There are also reports of awareness in patients who have received neuromuscular blockade with inadequate anesthesia. (Paralysis is not anesthesia!)

Neuromuscular Transmission

Acetylcholine is the key to neuromuscular transmission.[58] Muscle contraction occurs after nerve transmission causes release of acetylcholine at the synapse between nerve and muscle (the neuromuscular junction). Acetylcholine then occupies a receptor, which causes the muscle unit to contract. If the receptor is already occupied by the neuromuscular blockade, contraction cannot occur, and the muscle is paralyzed. This blockade effect occurs only on skeletal muscle, not cardiac muscle or smooth muscle; however, neuromuscular blockers have other side effects on cardiovascular, gastrointestinal, and respiratory systems. Acetylcholine that has been "blocked" at its receptor remains in the synaptic cleft to be broken down by the enzyme acetylcholinesterase.

The characteristics of the ideal muscle relaxant for ambulatory anesthesia are the same as those for inhalational anesthesia: rapid onset (within 60 seconds), short duration of action (titratable by infusion for maximum control), and no side effects ("clean"). The ideal agent has not yet been developed. The two pharmacologic classes of neuromuscular blockers include depolarizing and nondepolarizing agents.

Depolarizing Agent

Succinylcholine is the only depolarizing neuromuscular blocking agent in clinical use in the United States. When it occupies the receptor at the neuromuscular junction, it causes depolarization of the muscle unit. The overall effect of the multiple depolarizations that occur can be seen as waves of small muscle contractions (fasciculations), which typically start in the facial area and sometimes extend to full-body muscle activity for a few seconds. Fasciculations may be reduced by prior injection of a very small dose of a nondepolarizing muscle relaxant. After onset of succinylcholine effect and fasciculations, the muscle cannot repolarize and contract until the succinylcholine has been broken down by the circulating enzyme plasma pseudocholinesterase, which generally occurs within 3 to 5 minutes. There is no reversal agent for succinylcholine. Succinylcholine is not a clean drug. Its many side effects are listed in Table 13–2.

Table 13–2. Side Effects of Succinylcholine

- Slight histamine release
- May cause bradycardia and asystole, especially on repeat dose and in children
- Hyperkalemia and cardiac arrest in certain patients
  - Myopathies
  - Burns
  - Neurologic lesions such as paraplegia and quadriplegia
  - Major multiple trauma
- Muscle fasciculations (at time of depolarization) may cause
  - Increased ICP
  - Increased intraocular pressure
  - Increased K^+ release
    - Avoid in patients who have undergone trauma and those with burns or renal disease
  - Postoperative muscle pain
    - Fasciculation may be reduced by small dose of nondepolarizer before succinylcholine, especially in ambulatory patients
- Trigger agent for malignant hyperthermia
- Possibility of prolonged blockade
  - Atypical or inadequate pseudocholinesterase
    - Prolonged blockade may occur with longer administration time by infusion (phase II block).

ICP, intracranial pressure.

Muscle pain after succinylcholine has been commonly reported, especially in ambulatory patients, even in those who did not exhibit fasciculations when succinylcholine was administered. In some patients, fasciculations may be blocked by pretreatment with a small dose of a nondepolarizing muscle relaxant, intravenous lidocaine, or atropine.[59]

Succinylcholine's major advantages are related to time because its onset is rapid, occurring within 60 seconds. Its short duration of action (3 to 5 minutes) makes it ideal for intubation. In the case of inability to control the airway by mask or inability to intubate the trachea, the patient resumes spontaneous ventilation fairly quickly.

However, in some patients, succinylcholine does not have a short duration of action. Patients with the genetic problem of atypical pseudocholinesterase may show prolonged paralysis with succinylcholine. Prolonged paralysis may also occur in some patients with reduced plasma pseudocholinesterase levels, which may occur in pregnancy, cirrhosis, cancer, burns, or dehydration. Patients who take anticholinesterase medications for glaucoma or myasthenia gravis may also have this prolonged drug effect.[59] This paralysis may persist for 3 to 5 hours, but paralysis lasting as long as 48 hours has been reported.[58] Mechanical ventilation with supplemental amnestic and analgesic agents is required until the drug's effect ceases.

In patients who have a history of prolonged paralysis after succinylcholine in themselves or in blood relatives, a blood test called the dibucaine number identifies whether the patient has the disorder. The dibucaine number reflects the quality of the plasma pseudocholinesterase (not the quantity). A normal dibucaine number is 80, a number from 40 to 60 predicts prolonged succinylcholine blocks, and a number of 20 predicts greatly prolonged paralysis. A dibucaine number of 20 is estimated to occur in about one of 3200 people.[60]

Patients who are diagnosed with atypical pseudocholinesterase and their families should be counseled and given written information about the implications of the enzyme deficiency.

This is valuable information to future anesthesia providers. A medical alert bracelet can be helpful, especially if the patient is unable to recall the drug's name or if he or she becomes a trauma victim.

There is now a strong warning about succinylcholine's routine use in children and adolescents as a result of case reports of hyperkalemic cardiac arrest in children with undiagnosed myopathies.[61] Although this contraindication is controversial in the anesthesia community,[62] its publication should increase vigilance for the possibility of serious complications when the drug is administered. All members of the surgical care team should be aware that cardiac arrest after succinylcholine requires rapid, aggressive treatment for hyperkalemia with calcium chloride, sodium bicarbonate, and glucose/insulin mixture. Prolonged resuscitative efforts may be required.

Nondepolarizing Muscle Relaxants

Nondepolarizers occupy receptors at the neuromuscular junction to prevent transmission of acetylcholine, but no depolarization occurs. Because they compete with acetylcholine, they may be displaced from receptors when antagonist agents are given. This process, commonly known as "reversal," is discussed in the next section.

Older nondepolarizers, such as curare (*d*-tubocurarine), pancuronium (Pavulon), and metocurine (Metubine), have longer durations of action and more undesirable side effects than agents used most commonly in ambulatory surgery today. Intermediate-duration neuromuscular blockers now used include atracurium, vecuronium, and rocuronium. Each agent has certain advantages.

Atracurium (Tracrium) was introduced in the early 1980s as an intermediate-acting alternative to previously used relaxants. Its unique Hofmann elimination process[58] causes breakdown of the drug at body pH and temperature, thus minimizing reliance on the liver or kidney. Nonspecific plasma esterase enzymes are also involved in its elimination. Although atracurium has a low level of histamine release, susceptible patients may show such symptoms, especially with rapid injection or large doses.[61]

Cisatracurium (Nimbex) was introduced in 1996. It is an isomer of atracurium that also provides neuromuscular blockade of intermediate duration[61, 63]; however, it does not cause histamine release.[64] Like atracurium, it has the advantage of Hofmann elimination.

Vecuronium (Norcuron) was introduced in the early 1980s as an intermediate-acting relaxant. It is noted for its cardiovascular stability and lack of histamine release.

Rocuronium (Zemuron) is a mid-1990s analogue of vecuronium with similar hemodynamic stability and duration. Its advantage is more rapid onset, which may provide intubating conditions within 60 to 90 seconds, compared with 2 to 3 minutes for other relaxants.[29] Thus, it is a nondepolarizing agent that is useful for intubation, replacing succinylcholine in certain patients. Its use for intubation is limited to patients whose airways can be controlled by facemask, in case intubation cannot be accomplished. Its intermediate duration requires about 30 minutes (after an intubating dose) before reversal can take place. Thus, although it has a rapid onset, it is not appropriate for short cases.

Mivacurium (Mivacron) is an analogue of atracurium that was introduced in 1992. It is shorter acting than other nondepolarizers, but its action is not as brief as that of succinylcholine. Histamine release is related to dose and speed of injection.[58] There are reports of delayed metabolism in patients with pseudocholinesterase deficiency.[65, 66] Mivacurium's short duration may not require administration of reversal agents. Because reversal agents such as neostigmine may contribute to postoperative nausea and vomiting,[67] an agent such as mivacurium, which may require no reversal agents, may decrease the chance of PONV. Anesthesia providers must ensure complete return of neuromuscular function before deciding to avoid using a reversal agent.

Reversal of Neuromuscular Blockade

Although *reversal* is the commonly used term, *accelerated recovery* is a more precise description.[68] Nondepolarizing blockade is described as "competitive," meaning that if the amount of acetylcholine enzyme in the synaptic cleft of the neuromuscular junction can be greatly increased, it will displace the neuromuscular blocker from receptor sites because both enzyme and blocker compete for the receptor site. The molecule in highest concentration "wins" the receptors. Thus, return of acetylcholine to the receptors ends paralysis as acetylcholine transmission resumes and neuromuscular function returns.

The only way to increase acetylcholine level in the synaptic cleft is to prevent its breakdown. Accelerated recovery is accomplished by giving a drug that inactivates acetylcholinesterase to prevent its breakdown of acetylcholine. Less cholinesterase availability allows acetylcholine concentration to increase and displace the muscle relaxant that competes for receptor sites. Certain amounts of the neuromuscular blockers are also metabolized and excreted over time.

Anticholinesterase drugs include neostigmine (Prostigmin), edrophonium (Tensilon), and pyridostigmine (Mestinon, Regonol). These anticholinesterases cannot be given alone, because they cause bradycardia, bronchoconstriction, increased gastrointestinal peristalsis, and increased secretions. Therefore, a protective anticholinergic drug must be given along with the anticholinesterase.

Atropine and glycopyrrolate (Robinul) are the available anticholinergic agents. Atropine may cause tachycardia and dysrhythmias. Because it crosses the blood-brain barrier, it may contribute to postanesthesia agitation. Glycopyrrolate produces less dysrhythmia and tachycardia, and it does not cross the blood-brain barrier.[58] A premixed combination of edrophonium plus atropine (Enlon Plus) is available commerically.

Monitoring Neuromuscular Blockade

The degree of neuromuscular blockade is monitored with a peripheral nerve stimulator (Table 13–3). Although any peripheral nerve site may be chosen for monitoring, the most convenient sites include the ulnar nerve at the forearm and the seventh cranial (facial) nerve at the temporal area. (see Fig. 13–6).[69]

Clinical assessment by more than one parameter is essential before it can be determined that neuromuscular blockade has been reversed.[70] The patient should show enough strength to demonstrate all of the following:

Eye opening and evidence of consciousness
Tongue protrusion
Strong hand grip strength
Head lift sustained for at least 5 seconds
Adequate oxygen saturation and end-tidal CO_2 values

Ability to sustain head lift for 5 seconds is considered the most reliable clinical sign. Endotracheal intubation and assisted ventilation must be maintained until there is evidence of complete reversal of neuromuscular blockade by both peripheral nerve stimulator and clinical correlation. Giving reversal drugs does not guarantee that full recovery of neuromuscular function has occurred or will be maintained. Attentive postanesthesia observation must continue beyond the time of reversal to identify the possibility of "re-curarization." Adjuncts for airway control, oxygenation, and administration of reversal agents should be instantly available in the PACU for this rare situation.

MAINTENANCE TECHNIQUES AND SPECIFIC CONSIDERATIONS

Although each patient's unique physiologic, pharmacologic, and surgical considerations re-

Table 13–3. Information Provided by the Peripheral Nerve Stimulator (PNS)

The PNS delivers small electrical impulses to the nerve being monitored. Each impulse is seen as a muscle twitch on the patient.

A single *twitch* stimulus (Tw) does not provide much information except the presence or absence of twitch and a possible crude visual estimate of its size compared with that of an earlier twitch.

Train of Four (TOF) stimulation is more helpful to estimate the level of blockade. The TOF provides 4 electrical stimuli within 2 seconds. The twitches are counted along, and whether they are all apparently equal or whether there is a difference in size (fade) between the first and fourth twitches.

Degree of blockade may be estimated by

4 of 4 twitches present	= no blockade
3 of 4	= 75% blockade
2 of 4	= 80% blockade
1 of 4	= 90% blockade
0 of 4	= 100% blockade (not reversible until drug effect starts to spontaneously wear off, shown by return of at least 1 twitch on the TOF)

Tetanic Stimulation is Chosen in Two Situations

- **If there is no twitch response at TOF,** a tetanic stimulus will release a burst of acetylcholine. A TOF stimulus is then given immediately. If there is a TOF response after tetanic stimulus, then some acetylcholine is still available for transmission, and the first of the 4 TOF twitches should return fairly soon, depending on blocker dose given.
- **At the time of reversal of neuromuscular blockade,** after full TOF has been demonstrated, a tetanic stimulation should be given. If full reversal has occurred, the muscle sustains tetanic contraction without fade. If tetanic contraction fades, reversal is not complete, and the patient is at risk for respiratory depression or apnea.

Table 13–4. A Typical Sequence of General Anesthesia Induction

- Place monitors. Baseline vital signs. *(Vigilant monitoring of all parameters continues at all times during the anesthetic.)*
- Administer preoxygenation by facemask while preinduction medications are given, which may include
  Benzodiazepine tranquilizer
  Small-dose nondepolarizing muscle relaxant to diminish fasciculations if succinylcholine will be used
  Narcotic
  IV lidocaine (to diminish hypertension and tachycardia at intubation)
- Administer sleep dose of induction agent.
- Check ability to ventilate by facemask.
  In a *rapid-sequence induction,* no mask ventilation occurs.
  The sequence is
  - Administer sleep dose
  - Apply cricoid pressure
  - Administer succinylcholine
  - Wait 45–60 seconds
  - Place endotracheal tube, inflate cuff, confirm tracheal placement
  - Release cricoid pressure

  Goal: to diminish the chance of aspiration of gastric contents in patients who are considered to have a full stomach.

  - Not NPO
  - Pregnant
  - Obese
  - Pain and trauma
  - Severe diabetes
  - Extreme anxiety
  - Noncompliant—unreliable historians
- Administer intubating dose of succinylcholine or nondepolarizer.
- Apply mask ventilation (with O_2 + agent) for 1–2 minutes (until muscle relaxant takes effect).
- Perform direct laryngoscopy and visualization of cords.
- Place ETT between cords and position in trachea (versus esophagus), confirmed by
  Presence of end-tidal $CO_2 > 30$ on capnograph
  Bilateral equal breath sounds
  Chest rising and falling
  Negative gastric auscultation
- Turn on inhalation agents (oxygen + nitrous oxide + potent agent).
- Secure ETT. Eyes lubricated and taped closed. Orogastric tube may be passed.
- Check peripheral nerve stimulator to see that paralysis from succinylcholine is gone—then give dose of nondepolarizer to provide surgical relaxation.
- Ensure that patient positioning is safe.

Maintenance

- Maintain appropriate level of anesthesia for procedure with combinations of inhalational agents, intravenous agents, narcotics, muscle relaxants, and other adjuncts.
- Monitor blood loss and provide appropriate fluid replacement.

Emergence

- Keep in mind that anyone can put patients to sleep; emergence is a highly refined art. Agents must be discontinued and reversed at the appropriate time.
- When procedure is complete and patient meets extubation criteria, extubate and give facemask oxygen.
- Transport to PACU, with oxygen and monitors as indicated.
- Report to PACU nurse to serve as foundation for postanesthetic nursing care.

IV, intravenous; NPO, nothing by mouth; ETT, endotracheal tube; PACU, postanesthesia care unit.

quire individualization of the anesthetic plan, a typical general anesthetic may be described (Table 13–4). Every aspect of the plan is continually monitored, and adjustments are made for variations that arise. Nurses should seek information about each procedure's common patient and surgical factors that affect induction, maintenance, and emergence plans. Anesthesia providers should share unique patient considerations for which extra teamwork may be required. Such considerations include management of airway difficulties; anticipation of crises, such as onset of malignant hyperthermia; position constraint posed by body habitus or disease; unique psychosocial factors; and unusual physiologic factors, such as the presence of implanted medication pumps, cardiac pacemakers, and automatic defibrillators. These few examples can only hint at all the special factors that must be identified for individual patients. Well-choreographed teamwork and commitment to complete communication set the stage for positive perioperative outcomes.

EMERGENCE FROM GENERAL ANESTHESIA

Emergence technique is an art that results in a patient who is awake and stable at the proper time when surgery ends. The technique includes reducing the concentration of inhalational agent, reversing neuromuscular blockade (and perhaps other medications), and delivering 100% oxygen. Returning the patient to consciousness also requires ongoing attention to airway, breathing, and circulation. Any of these parameters may deteriorate during emergence, requiring rapid intervention. An ideal emergence leads to an awake patient who is lucid and comfortable enough to move himself or herself to the stretcher with minimal assistance.

Reversal for Other Agents

Individual patient variability and selected doses of drugs may occasionally require antagonist agents for narcotics or benzodiazepines. If the patient remains apneic after adequate reversal of neuromuscular blockade and elimination of inhalational agent, a narcotic antagonist, such as naloxone (Narcan), may be slowly titrated in intravenous increments of 20 to 40 μg to raise the respiratory rate. Large doses should be avoided because they may reverse analgesia, perhaps leading to severe hypertension or pulmonary edema.[71] Because narcotic action may outlast naloxone's effect, repeat doses of naloxone may be necessary.

Flumazenil is a specific benzodiazepine antagonist that reverses the sedative effect of medications such as midazolam and diazepam.[24] Because benzodiazepine ventilatory effects are extremely variable, sedative effects may reversed without reversal of all of the ventilatory depression.[72] Flumazenil is titrated intravenously in 0.1-mg increments with close monitoring and readiness for repeat doses. Because midazolam's half life is 2.5 hours and flumazenil's half-life is 1 hour, vigilance for resedation is imperative.[29] Patients who take benzodiazepines long term may be at risk for withdrawal symptoms if they receive flumazenil; the reversal drug may precipitate tremors, profuse sweating, and hypotension. Seizure activity may occur in patients who take benzodiazepines for seizure control and are given flumazenil.

Underlying disease may also contribute to prolonged somnolence. Diabetic patients may have consciousness delayed by hypoglycemia, and hypertensive patients may be at risk for cerebrovascular accident. Such considerations should be investigated in patients who are slow to awaken.[73]

Central Anticholinergic Syndrome

Anticholinergics, such as atropine and scopolamine, may cause the central anticholinergic syndrome,[7] in which the patient is agitated, showing anxiety, disorientation, hallucinations, and hyperactivity. Autonomic muscarinic signs, such as dry mouth, large pupils, and flushed skin, may be apparent. The syndrome is treated with physostigmine (Antilirium), with caution being used for its adverse effects: nausea and vomiting, bradycardia, and convulsions with rapid injection.

Oxygen at Emergence

Delivery of 100% oxygen is an essential part of emergence. Its high concentration provides physiologic reserve in case of airway, breathing, or circulation problems. Some anesthesia providers may feel comfortable with a decision to transport selected healthy patients to the PACU without supplemental oxygen; this decision is based on the patient's condition at the moment as well as on contributing surgical considerations and underlying medical conditions. However, most patients require supplemental oxygen, which should always be available for transport.

PERIANESTHETIC PROBLEMS

Airway Problems

The airway is paramount because all other physiologic parameters depend on oxygen and ventilation. Unanticipated loss of airway control may occur at any point during induction, maintenance, or emergence. Patients with any evidence of airway obstruction require 100% oxygen. Tonsil-tip suction must also be at hand.

The tongue is the most common cause of airway obstruction in unconscious or semiconscious patients. A simple chin lift or jaw thrust often solves the problem. Nasopharyngeal airways (well-lubricated with a water-soluble gel and placed carefully to avoid nosebleeds) are usually well tolerated by patients who are ob-

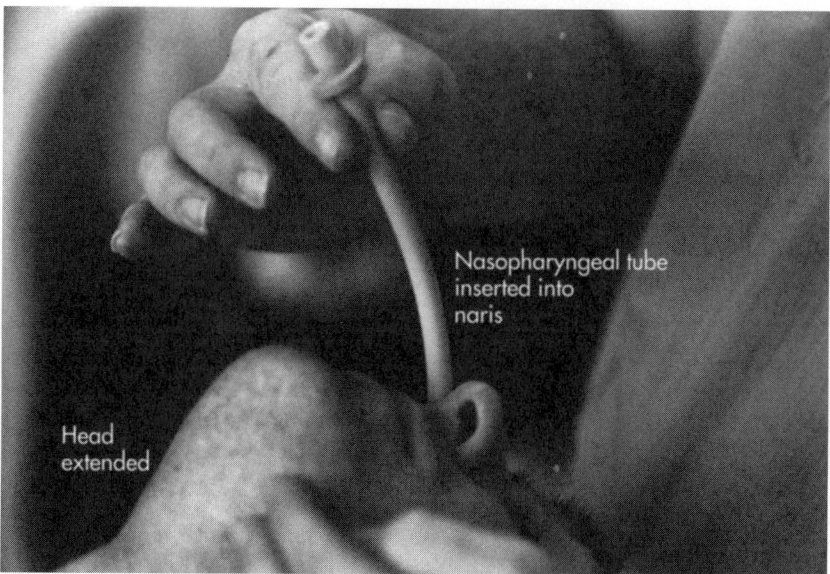

Figure 13–7. Technique for insertion of a nasopharyngeal airway. The airway is oriented concave to the hard palate and inserted straight back. Gripping the airway near the top allows the tube to bend if resistance to passage of the airway is extreme. If it is gripped close to the naris, sufficient force can be transmitted to shear off a turbinate. (From Benumoff JL [ed]: American Society of Anesthesiologists Task Force on Management of The Difficult Airway: Practice guidelines for management of the difficult airway: A report. Anesthesiology 78:597, 1993.)

tunded enough to need them. Size 8 to 9 nasopharyngeal airways are chosen for large adults, size 7 to 8 for medium-sized adults, and size 6 to 7 for small adults. Figure 13–7 describes the insertion technique for nasopharyngeal airways. These airways are not commonly used in children, because of the possibility of displacing enlarged adenoidal tissue with the tube.

Oropharyngeal airways are suitable only for unconscious patients; placing oral airways in a semiconscious patient may precipitate laryngospasm. An 80-mm oral airway is chosen for small adults, and 90- and 100-mm airways are used for medium-sized and large adults. Improper size or placement technique may worsen obstruction (Fig. 13–8).

The criteria for extubation should be documented (Table 13–5). Some postanesthesia nurses are assuming responsibility for extubation of selected patients. However, in the ambulatory surgery setting and patient population, extubation in the operating room before transfer to the PACU is the most common and appropriate process. Nurses must maintain current competency in airway management and must ensure that reintubation equipment is immediately available.

Although airway difficulties can occur at any

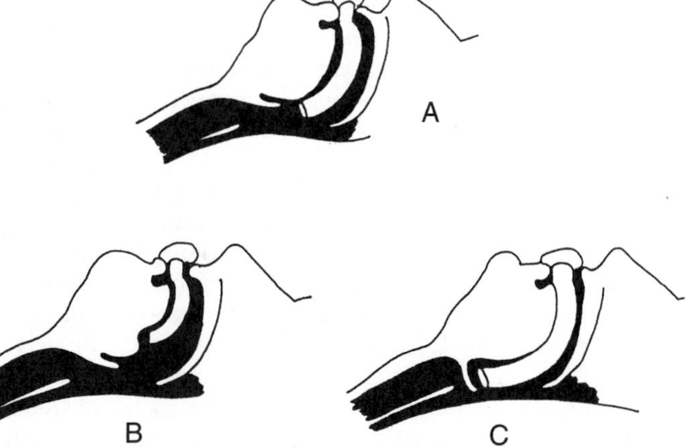

Figure 13–8. Oral airways are valuable adjuncts for maintaining airway patency in unconscious patients. Placement in semiconscious patients may precipitate a laryngospasm. An incorrect size may worsen the obstruction. Oral airway: *A*, Appropriate size; *B*, Small size causes obstruction to the airway by displacing the tongue into the oral cavity; *C*, Large size obstructs the airway by pushing the epiglottis against the glottic opening or laryngospasm. (From McIntosh LW: Essentials of Nurse Anesthesia. New York: McGraw-Hill Health Professionals Division, 1997, p 152. Reproduced with permission of the McGraw-Hill Companies.)

Table 13–5. Extubation Technique

Criteria for Extubation

- Has strong spontaneous ventilation at adequate respiratory rate.
- Is awake and responsive.
- Shows strength indicating reversal of neuromuscular blockade (sustained headlift for 5–10 seconds).
- Has no factors that may cause airway obstruction, especially if patient has had mouth or neck surgery.

Before extubation, carefully assess patients who are known to have experienced difficult intubations.
Never extubate a patient unless you are confident that you (or someone nearby) can immediately reintubate the patient.

Preparation and Equipment

- Stable vital signs.
- 100% oxygen via ETT. Pulse oximeter functioning.
- If NG tube present, suction it out completely.
- Facemask and positive-pressure breathing bag at hand.
- Nasopharyngeal airways and lubricant.
- Yankauer (tonsil-tip) suction with strong vacuum.
- 10-ml syringe to deflate cuff.
- Head of bed up to facilitate ventilation; be prepared to drop head of bed to flat position if airway control becomes necessary.
- Facemask to apply after extubation.
- Know location of nearest provider who can reintubate.

Technique

1. 100% oxygen.
2. Oropharyngeal suction. Use a Yankauer tip to suction oropharyngeal secretions on top of the balloon cuff.
3. Have patient inspire deeply. At peak of inspiration, deflate cuff and pull tube gently. The patient will exhale and cough up any secretions that were in the larynx. Oral suction may be necessary.
4. Provide facemask oxygen and close monitoring.

ETT, endotracheal tube; NG, nasogastric.

time, difficulties associated with emergence from general anesthesia include airway obstruction resulting from soft tissue changes or laryngospasm. Stridor or postintubation croup may develop. In the postoperative airway, foreign bodies, such as aspirated teeth, oral or nasal packing, and pieces of instruments, have been reported. Rapid diagnosis and intervention to remove such obstructions are essential.

Laryngospasm

Laryngospasm is airway obstruction by the forced closure of the vocal cords by muscles of the larynx[71] caused by such factors as blood or secretions on the vocal cords, too-light anesthesia (pain), and inhalation of irritant gases. It is more common in children.

Laryngospasm must be treated immediately with 100% oxygen and positive-pressure ventilation, with end-expiratory pressure being maintained to try to open the cords. Oropharyngeal suction may remove secretions that precipitated the spasm. If laryngospasm does not break quickly and hypoxemia ensues, a small dose of intravenous succinylcholine should relax the cords. Controlled or assisted ventilation may be necessary, and the patient may need reintubation.

Postobstructive pulmonary edema, also called noncardiogenic pulmonary edema, may develop after laryngospasm, especially in children.[74] It probably arises from hypoxia and inspiratory efforts against an obstructed airway, which changes the hydrostatic pressure gradient between the bloodstream and the alveoli.[75] The resulting pulmonary edema may require treatment with 100% oxygen, intubation, and mechanical ventilation with positive end-expiratory pressure. Noncardiogenic pulmonary edema has been reported as late as 2 hours after arrival in the PACU.[76] Anesthesia providers must inform PACU nurses about the occurrence of laryngospasm or other airway obstruction so that an appropriate nursing assessment plan can be instituted. Postoperative surveillance should continue for at least 2 hours.

Assessment for postintubation damage to teeth and soft tissues should be routine. Hoarseness or pharyngitis is extremely common and usually has a benign brief course. Unusual or extreme presentations of these symptoms after intubation or LMA should be thoroughly evaluated and documented, out of concern for such complications as dislocation of laryngeal cartilages.[75] For most patients, increased fluids and warm saline gargles help relieve sore throats. Patients should be instructed to report severe or prolonged symptoms.

Breathing Problems

General anesthesia may be associated with hypoxemia or hypercarbia. Several factors contribute to postanesthesia hypoventilation and rise in end-tidal CO_2. Continuous intraoperative measurement of end-tidal CO_2 allows anesthesia providers to use controlled or assisted ventilation to keep end-tidal CO_2 in a normal range. However, in the postoperative period, end-tidal CO_2 may rise significantly for various reasons, including inadequate ventilatory drive related to residual effects of anesthetics or lack of stimulation, altered ventilatory mechanics by increased airway resistance (obstruction) or decreased compliance related to obesity or fluid overload, and the possibility of residual neuromuscular blockade. The resulting hypercarbia may cause hypertension, tachycardia, dysrhythmias, and reduced level of consciousness. Thus, treatment is aimed at reducing end-tidal CO_2 rather than at treating the isolated symptom. This treatment may be as simple as frequent reminders for the patient to breathe deeply or as complicated as use of reversal agents for respiratory depressants and possibly reintubation and controlled ventilation in certain cases. Nurses should be aware that patients may experience hypercarbia, even with an oxygen saturation of 100%, if supplemental oxygen is being delivered.

Pulse oximetry's value lies in its ability to track oxygenation. The most likely cause of postoperative hypoxemia is mismatch of ventilation and perfusion associated with loss of functional residual capacity. The functional residual capacity is reduced by lying flat, especially in obese or asthmatic patients.[71] Further impingement on functional residual capacity may occur with any position or procedure that reduces thoracic excursion. Other causes of perioperative hypoxemia include increased tissue extraction of oxygen, which occurs with shivering or sepsis, and low cardiac output, which reduces mixed-venous oxygen values. Critical physiologic events, such as aspiration of gastric contents, pneumothorax, and pulmonary embolus, must also be considered. Patients with preoperative pulmonary dysfunction are at increased risk for such problems. Pulse oximetry allows continual observation of oxygenation to allow rapid intervention with 100% oxygen while causes of the problem are sought.

Circulation

Circulation problems associated with general anesthesia include hypotension, hypertension, and cardiac changes in rhythm, myocardial blood flow, and myocardial function. The care team must always be prepared for possible deterioration to full cardiopulmonary arrest; the rarity of such events must not lull caregivers into a false sense of security. Serious circulation abnormalities require delivery of 100% oxygen and aggressive intervention to support the circulation.

Hypotension

Hypotension is a symptom of another abnormality in the patient's physiology. It is treated symptomatically while the cause is being sought. The most common cause of hypotension is hypovolemia related to inadequate fluid replacement. Arterial hypoxemia, myocardial ischemia, cardiac dysrhythmias, pneumothorax, cardiac tamponade, and pulmonary edema must be considered. Although spurious readings from the wrong size cuff or an artifact in the noninvasive blood pressure monitor may occur, the first obligation must be assessment and treatment of the patient (not the monitors). Administering 100% oxygen and raising the bed's foot can be quickly accomplished as rapid assessment starts. If appropriate, the intravenous fluid rate should be increased. Rapid-acting vasopressors, such as ephedrine and phenylephrine, may be given to support blood pressure until definitive treatment is complete.

Hypertension

Hypertension may reflect uncontrolled preoperative blood pressure status. Even if the patient received a usual dose of antihypertensive medication on the morning of surgery, perioperative stressors may raise blood pressure beyond desirable levels. However, other causes must be considered so that the hypertension can be treated appropriately. Relief of pain may lower blood pressure. Hypoxemia and hypercarbia must also be considered as possible causes. Blood pressure may be elevated as a result of a full bladder or another distended viscus. In some patients, elevated blood pressure may be associated with the phenomenon of arousal, and may settle back to normal levels fairly quickly; this is particularly true when patients awaken with the ETT still in place.

If other causes of hypertension have been eliminated, high blood pressure may be treated with rapid-acting β-blockers, such as labetalol (Normodyne, Trandate) and esmolol (Brevibloc), or other medications, such as intravenous hydralazine (Apresoline). Side effects of these medications are hypotension, bradycardia, bronchospasm, and tachycardia.

Cardiac Abnormalities

Dysrhythmias

Perianesthesia dysrhythmias may be asymptomatic electrocardiographic abnormalities, such as junctional rhythms, which usually resolve spontaneously, or they may be warnings of other problems associated with general anesthesia. Underlying cardiac disease, metabolic imbalances, and medication toxicity must always be considered.

Bradycardia

Bradycardia shows increased parasympathetic nervous system activity associated with surgical stimulation or medications, such as opioids, anticholinesterases, and β-blockers. Serious underlying problems associated with bradycardia include development of heart block or onset of hypoxemia. Bradycardia in children is almost always due to hypoxemia, which requires immediate and aggressive intervention with airway control and 100% oxygen. Atropine is necessary only if the heart rate does not increase with airway support and 100% oxygen. Symptomatic bradycardia that does not respond to medications may require cardiac pacing, which is now available through externally placed devices.

Tachycardia

Tachycardia shows increased sympathetic nervous system activity, which may reflect pain or increased catecholamine levels related to exogenously administered sympathetic stimulators, such as epinephrine and cocaine. Hypercarbia also causes tachycardia. Because tachycardia dramatically increases cardiac workload, heart rate should be lowered with opioids, β-blockers, or increased minute ventilation as appropriate. Control of heart rate is particularly important for elderly patients or for those with coronary artery disease or valvular disease. Tachycardia with hypotension may reflect hypovolemia. The possibility of occult blood loss in cases such as laparoscopy should always be suspected in the tachycardic, hypotensive patient. Other possibilities, such as pneumothorax and congestive heart failure, should also be ruled out.

Nurses should be familiar with the range of normal heart rates for infants and children, lest their tachycardias be unnecessarily treated. Anesthesia providers should inform nurses of agents such as atropine and glycopyrrolate that may produce postoperative tachycardia. Unexplained tachycardia that persists despite treatment may herald the development of MH.

Ectopy

Premature contractions on the electrocardiogram may be benign atrial premature beats or they may be life-threatening ventricular dysrhythmias. Protocols for the treatment of dysrhythmias have been established by the American Heart Association's advanced cardiac life support algorithms; caregivers should be familiar with these decision trees.

In the patient under general anesthesia, ventricular dysrhythmias may indicate light anesthesia, hypercarbia, or development of MH. Ischemic cardiac dysfunction, electrolyte abnormalities, and drug interactions (e.g., between halothane and epinephrine) should also be considered.

Changes in ST Segment

Although traditional electrocardrographic monitoring has focused on rate, rhythm, and ectopy, changes in the ST segment should also be monitored to allow early identification and rapid intervention for coronary ischemia, especially because perioperative ischemia may be associated with increased risk for myocardial infarction.[77] New monitors provide analysis and trend capability for changes in the ST segment. Because patients under general anesthesia cannot express feeling the typical anginal chest pain associated with myocardial ischemia, ST segment monitoring serves as a marker. Significant changes in ST segment elevation or depression mandate investigation and treatment, especially in patients at high risk for ischemic events.[78]

Consciousness Problems

Some patients may not awaken in the ideal fashion associated with a smooth rapid emergence. Delayed emergence may reflect individual patient variability, residual drug effect, or other problems, which may be serious: hypoxia, hypercarbia, central nervous system injury, chemical abnormality (hypoglycemia or electrolyte imbalance), and hypothermia. These abnormalities should be ruled out; reversal agents for sedatives and narcotics may be given, and consultation with a neurologist may be necessary.

Patients may awaken with delirium and agitation as a result of a wide variety of causes. Several drug classes may contribute to this phenomenon; these include anticholinergics, barbiturates without narcotics, ketamine, dopamine receptor antagonists, and pure inhalational techniques. Nondrug causes for emergence agitation must be sought. These include factors such as pain, anxiety and separation, hypoxemia and hypercarbia, viscus distention of bladder or bowel, hypotension causing cerebral ischemia, and hypothermia or hyperthermia. Many other factors may be involved. Diagnostic and treatment challenges for agitation are enhanced by the importance of maintaining patient and staff safety.

UNIQUE EMERGENCY CONSIDERATIONS

Advances in technology have created new techniques that require special mention in relation to general anesthesia. These include procedures in which gas is insufflated into body cavities and surgical techniques that involve lasers in the airway.

Gas Insufflation Procedures

Laparoscopy has created a new set of anesthetic challenges. Postoperative nausea and vomiting are the most common complication of laparoscopy, occurring in 20% to 40% of patients.[79] Anesthesia providers must monitor for physiologic changes associated with pneumoperitoneum, such as hypoventilation, hypotension, hypertension, and dysrhythmias. Other potentially catastrophic complications require awareness and preparation for emergency action by all members of the surgical care team. These complications include hemorrhage, perforated viscera, pneumothorax, pneumomediastinum, and gas embolism.[80] Although the incidence of such serious complications is very low, the potential for cardiovascular collapse and arrest is real.

Myalgias are common after laparoscopy, independent of muscle relaxant used (depolarizing versus nondepolarizing). Thus, procedure factors, such as abdominal distention and manipulation, residual intraperitoneal gas, and intraoperative position, must contribute.[29] Residual intraperitoneal gas is cited as a cause of the postoperative shoulder pain commonly seen after laparoscopy.

Lasers in the Airway

Laser surgery for tracheal and laryngeal lesions carries the unique risk of fire in the airway.[81] Besides the obvious effect of flame on tissue, ignition of an ETT produces gases that are noxious to the lungs. The laser beam may ignite ETTs, cuffs, lubricants, or sponges. Other hazards are included in Table 13–6. Specialized, less-flammable "laser tubes" have been developed that may reduce this risk, although it cannot be completely eliminated. Conventional ETTs may be wrapped with special metallic tape, with care taken for tissue trauma from tape edges; the vulnerable cuff should be filled

Table 13–6. Hazards and Precautions for Laser Surgery of the Airway

Eye Damage

Post warning sign outside door to show that laser is in use.
All personnel must wear goggles specific for the wavelength light of the laser being used.
Use moistened gauze eye patch for the patient.
Nonreflective (matte finish) instruments help disperse the beam.
Laser should be in standby mode when not being used.

Fire Hazard

The lowest possible F_{IO_2} (21–40%) should be selected.
Oxygen and nitrous oxide support combustion.
Specialized endotracheal tubes designed to minimize the risk of combustion should be used.
The cuff may be filled with blue-dyed saline. Dye in the airway warns the surgeon that the cuff has been hit by the laser; the fluid absorbs heat and quenches a fire.
Water-soluble ointments are necessary; oil-based ointments are flammable.
Drapes must be kept away from the field.
Surgeon should use lowest possible power setting on intermittent mode to prevent heat buildup.
Ongoing team communication and readiness for fire are essential.
Stop oxygen flow, clamp tube, and remove.
Provide airway control by facemask.
Perform reintubation and bronchoscopy to evaluate airway damage.
Drapes and electrical equipment may ignite; water and carbon dioxide fire extinguishers should be present.

with blue-dyed saline to provide rapid identification of a leak or ruptured cuff.

Staff should rehearse for rapid management of an airway fire. Each team member should be prepared for instant action because airway fires may appear suddenly. Stopping oxygen flow and ventilation is the first step, followed by quick clamping, tube removal, and airway control by facemask. Bowls of water must be instantly available, as well as water and carbon dioxide fire extinguishers, because the fire may involve drapes as well as electrical equipment. Thorough airway evaluation by reintubation and bronchoscopy must follow.[82] Plans for transfer and observation in an intensive care unit should also be in place.

Malignant Hyperthermia

Every general anesthetic may carry the potential for development of MH. MH is a genetically transmitted disease that is triggered by succincylcholine and potent inhalational agents. MH is a fulminant hypermetabolic state, which may be fatal if untreated. Although careful preanesthesia evaluation may identify some patients with a personal or family history suggestive of MH, anesthesia providers must always be alert for the development of MH signs and symptoms in order to intervene rapidly. Unexplained tachycardia and rising end-tidal CO_2 are the first warning signs; rise in body temperature occurs later. All members of the surgical care team must also be familiar with the syndrome and treatment modalities to function effectively in this life-threatening situation. This is discussed fully in Chapter 11.

FORETHOUGHTS FOR THE POSTOPERATIVE PERIOD

With the philosophy that anesthesia care extends beyond the period in the operating room, practitioners are developing perioperative techniques that contribute to postoperative comfort and safety in pain management as well as control of PONV. Individualized anesthesia care aims to minimize postoperative development of these problems.[83]

Pain Management and Pre-Emptive Analgesia

Postoperative analgesia and comfort are now considered part of the anesthetic plan, especially when patients are discharged to home. This follows a 1994 report by the American Society of Anesthesiologists Task Force on Pain Management (Acute Pain Section) (Table 13–7).[84] In addition, the Agency for Health Care Policy and Research has published guidelines defining the problems of acute postoperative pain management and addresses a variety of treatment options.[85] Attentive analgesic care is now part of the entire perioperative care plan.

Interest in the phenomenon of pre-emptive analgesia is generating research into techniques to minimize postoperative pain. This research seems to indicate that tissue injury such as that resulting from surgery can trigger prolonged excitability in central nervous system function. This excitability influences responses that occur with later stimuli.[86, 87]

Nociception is the physiologic process that senses or transmits pain messages. Pre-emptive analgesia prevents nociceptors or nociceptive mechanisms from sensitizing central neurons and causing central nervous system "wind-up."[88] This wind-up results in hyperalgesia, which is a biologic amplification of pain stimuli. As a result, patients may show amplified reflex responses, increased subjective pain ratings, and exaggerated pain behaviors. Prevention of wind-up may produce pre-emptive effects that outlast the duration of action of drugs used.[89]

Although this sounds as simple as "an ounce

Table 13–7. Proactive Management of Pain for Ambulatory Surgery

The increasing trend toward ambulatory surgery poses special problems in perioperative pain management. One of the most common causes for unanticipated hospital admission is inadequate pain control . . . Analgesic techniques must provide safe, adequate pain relief for patients who quickly leave the supervised hospital environment. Techniques such as epidural analgesia and IV PCA . . . are not suitable for such patients but others such as local anesthetic wound infiltration and oral nonsteroidal anti-inflammatory drugs may be very effective.

Recommendations: Anesthesiologists who care for ambulatory surgery patients should proactively plan therapeutic strategies appropriate for them, recognizing that they are expected to leave the facility within a few hours after the completion of surgery.

Proactive analgesic care has been addressed by the American Society of Anesthesiologists. Nurses' participation in this aspect of patient care is crucial, both in patient education and planning as well as in appropriate dosage and timing of medications.

From American Society of Anesthesiologists: Practice Guidelines for Acute Pain Management in the Perioperative Setting. A Report by the American Society of Anesthesiologists Task Force on Pain. Anesthesiology 82:1071–1081, 1995.

of prevention is worth a pound of cure," complicated pain phenomena and wide patient variations make the issue difficult to quantify. Many factors are now being researched, including mechanisms of pain transmission and the natural course of hyperalgesia after surgery as well as possible drug combinations and appropriate doses. The optimal pain treatment is one that is applied perioperatively to prevent the establishment of pain hypersensitivity. The development of reliable multimodal pre-emptive analgesic techniques for all procedures and all patients has positive implications for ambulatory surgery patients.[90]

Many (but not all) studies in which analgesia was provided continuously in the entire perioperative period have shown pre-emptive analgesic effect. Examples of pre-emptive analgesia include long-acting local anesthetics administered by nerve block or infiltration,[91] preoperative administration of nonsteroidal anti-inflammatory drugs[92] and opioids,[89] and use of α_2-agonists, such as clonidine,[93] and dexmedetomidine.[93–95]

Current research in these techniques will determine whether potential side effects outweigh the value of pre-emptive analgesic effects.

Thus, planning for analgesia is part of the anesthetic care plan. This plan is one aspect of the overall concept of attentive analgesic care that combines preoperative education, preparation, and planning as well as perioperative analgesia and physiologic stabilization. All members of the ambulatory surgical care team (including the patient and the responsible adult) are involved in this effort.

Future possibilities for postoperative pain management include delivery of medications by transdermal and transmucosal routes as well as development of slow-release narcotics and local anesthetics that are encapsulated in liposomes.[96] At this time, questions about the safe delivery of potent medications to unmonitored patients at home have not been answered.

Postoperative Nausea and Vomiting

Postoperative nausea and vomiting has been identified as the most common anesthetic complication.[83] Its present occurrence in 10% to 40% of patients[97] is considerably lower than that of the ether era. However, it still remains the most common anesthetic-related cause of unexpected hospital admission after outpatient surgery. It also interferes with pain management plans that aim to move patients quickly from parenteral to oral analgesics. Thus, the problem has important economic considerations as well as psychological and physiologic implications. Discharge may be delayed after ambulatory procedures as a result of prolonged PONV or somnolence related to treatment medications. Other problems associated with PONV include dehydration, electrolyte imbalance, tension on suture lines, venous hypertension, and increased bleeding under skin flaps, as well as increased risk of aspiration if airway reflexes are depressed.

The multifactorial nature of PONV complicates treatment. Patient factors, such as female gender, younger age, obesity, menstrual cycle days 4 and 5, previous history of PONV or motion sickness, anxiety, and pre-existing gastroparesis are all important.[98] Some surgical procedures have a higher risk of PONV; these include laparoscopic techniques, strabismus surgery, orchiopexy, and ear surgery. Certain anesthetic techniques also contribute to an increased incidence of PONV: inhalational agents and opioids are well known for their association with this problem. Nitrous oxide's contribution to PONV is not clear.[99]

Thus, anesthesia providers must identify risk factors for PONV for individual patients to choose an anesthetic technique that is less likely to increase the problem. This includes avoidance of certain medications that have higher emetogenic incidence; for the most severe cases, inhalational agents may be omitted completely, substituting a propofol-based total intravenous anesthetic, because propofol may be "protective" again PONV. Reversal agents for neuromuscular blockade (e.g., neostigmine and edrophonium) may also increase PONV. Anesthesia providers may opt to use short-acting mivacurium, which may not require a reversal agent. Optimal timing of antiemetic doses is also under evaluation.[100]

A proactive anesthetic plan acknowledges the problem of PONV pre-emptively rather than trying to treat it after the fact. Incidence of PONV has been reduced (but not eliminated) by the recent development of a clean class of antiemetics, the serotonin antagonists such as ondansetron (Zofran), granisetron (Kytril),[101] and dolasetron (Anzemet).[102] Generous intravenous hydration, delay of postanesthetic oral intake, slow movement of patients, and nursing comfort measures, such as verbal reassurance and warm blankets, may also help. Other prevention and treatment strategies include psychological, physical, and pharmacologic maneuvers. Unfortunately, the multifactorial nature of the problem has prevented its complete elimination.

CONCLUSIONS

This chapter's brief overview has provided information about techniques, monitoring, medications, problems, and interventions in the delivery of general anesthesia. These highlights are guidelines to assist nurses who care for patients along the anesthesia continuum. Understanding the language, equipment, and techniques of general anesthesia contributes to patient safety, education, and comfort as well as clear communication among all healthcare providers.

References

1. Kapur PA: Controversy: What are the best drugs for ambulatory surgery? 1995 Review Course Lectures. Cleveland: International Anesthesia Research Society, 1995, pp 98–102.
2. Shlugman D, Glass PSA: Intravenous sedative-hypnotics and flumazenil. In White PF (ed): Ambulatory Anesthesia and Surgery. Philadelphia: WB Saunders 1997, pp 332–348.
3. Warner MA: Cost containment in anesthesia. 1995 Review course Lectures. Cleveland: International Anesthesia Research Society, 1995, pp 48–53.
4. Kopman AF, Lichtenstein A: Economic issues in recovery from neuromuscular block. Research Triangle Park, NC: Burroughs Wellcome, 1995.
5. Greenberg CP, Brown AR: Cost containment: Utilization of technique, personnel, equipment and supplies. In White PF (ed): Ambulatory Anesthesia and Surgery. Philadelphia: WB Saunders, 1997, pp 636–647.
6. Orkin FK: Moving toward value-based anesthesia care. J Clin Anesth 5:91–98, 1993.
7. Apfelbaum JL, Kallar SK, Wetchler BV: Adult and geriatric patients. In Wetchler VB (ed): Anesthesia for Ambulatory Surgery, 2nd ed. Philadelphia: JB Lippincott, 1990, pp 197–307.
8. Gravenstein JS, Kirby RR: General anesthesia: induction, maintenance and emergence. In Kirby RR, Gravenstein N (eds): Clinical Anesthesia Practice. Philadelphia: WB Saunders 1994, pp 588–596.
9. Springer D, Jahr J: The laryngeal mask airway: Safety, efficacy, and current use. Am J Anesthesiol 66:65–69, 1995.
10. Wat LI, Lynch ME, Hamamura RK: Cost effectiveness of the laryngeal mask airway in day surgery. In Leading The Way. Society For Ambulatory Anesthesia 10th Annual Meeting, 1995.
11. Joshi GP, Smith I, White PF: Laryngeal mask airway. In Benumof JL (ed): Airway Management: Principles and Practice. St. Louis: Mosby, 1996, pp 353–373.
12. Cork RC, Depa RM, Standen JR: Prospective comparison of use of the laryngeal mask and endotracheal tube for ambulatory surgery. Anesth Analg 79:719–727, 1994.
13. Owens TM, Robertson P, et al: The incidence of gastroesophageal reflux with the laryngeal mask: A comparison with the face mask using esophageal lumen pH electrodes. Anesth Analg 80:980–984, 1995.
14. Mallampati RS, Gatt SP, et al: A clinical sign to predict difficult tracheal intubation: A prospective study. Can Anaesth Soc J 32:429, 1985.
15. Mecca RS: Management of the difficult airway. In Kirby RR, Gravenstein N (eds): Clinical Anesthesia Practice. Philadelphia: WB Saunders 1994, pp 921–954.
16. Cicala RS: The traumatized airway. In Benumof JL (ed): Airway Management: Principles and Practice. St. Louis: Mosby, 1996, pp 736–759.
17. Martin JT, Warner MA (eds): Positioning in Anesthesia and Surgery, 3rd ed. Philadelphia: WB Saunders 1997.
18. Warner MA: Positioning the neck and head. In Martin JT, Warner MA (eds): Positioning in Anesthesia and Surgery, 3rd ed. Philadelphia: WB Saunders, 1997, pp 223–233.
19. Nakata DA, Stoelting RK: Positioning the extremities. In Martin JT, Warner MA (eds): Positioning in Anesthesia and Surgery, 3rd ed. Philadelphia: WB Saunders, 1997, pp 199–222.
20. Britt BA, Joy N, Mackay MB: Anesthesia-related trauma caused by patient malpositioning. In Gravenstein N, Kirby RR (eds): Complications in Anesthesiology, 2nd ed. Philadelphia: Lippincott-Raven, 1996, pp 365–389.
21. Schaer HM: Peripheral nerve injury and automatic blood pressure measurement. Anesthesiology 75:381, 1991.
22. Herlich A, Garber JG, Orkin FK: Dental and salivary gland complications. In Gravenstein N, Kirby RR (eds): Complications in Anesthesiology, 2nd ed. Philadelphia: Lippincott-Raven, 1996, pp 163–173.
23. Gravenstein JS, Kirby RR: General anesthesia: Induction, maintenance and emergence. In Kirby RR, Gravenstein N (eds): Clinical Anesthesia Practice. Philadelphia: WB Saunders 1994, pp 588–596.
24. Drain C: Nonopioid intravenous anesthetics. In The Post Anesthesia Care Unit. Philadelphia: WB Saunders 1994, pp 205–225.
25. Siler J: Propofol reduces prolonged outpatient PACU stay. Anesthesiol Rev 21:129–132, 1994.
26. Goldberg M: The allergic response and anesthesia. In Gravenstein N, Kirby RR (eds): Complications in Anesthesiology, 2nd ed. Philadelphia: Lippincott-Raven, 1996, pp 605–637.
27. Chung DC, Lam AM: Essentials of Anesthesiology, 3rd ed. Philadelphia: WB Saunders 1997, pp 11–27.
28. Veber B, Gachot B, et al: Severe sepsis after intravenous injection of contaminated propofol. Anesthesiology 80(3):712, 1994.
29. Philip BK: General anesthesia. In Twersky RS (ed): The Ambulatory Anesthesia Handbook. St. Louis: Mosby, 1995, pp 203–237.
30. Borgeat A, Wilder-Smith OHG, et al: Subhypnotic doses of propofol possess direct antiemetic properties. Anesth Analg 74:539–541, 1992.
31. Laxenaire MC, Mata-Bermejo E, et al: Life-threatening anaphylactoid reactions to propofol. Anesthesiology 77:275–280, 1992.
32. Singh P, Harwood R, et al: A comparison of thiopentone and propofol with respect to the incidence of postoperative shivering. Anaesthesia 49:996–998, 1994.
33. Conti G, Dell'Utri D, et al: Propofol induces bronchodilation in mechanically ventilated COPD patients. Acta Anesthesiol Scand 37:105–109, 1993.
34. Borgeat A, Wilder-Smith OHG, et al: Propofol in the management of refractory status epilepticus: A case report. Intensive Care Med 20:148–149, 1994.

35. Pitt-Miller PL, Elcock BJ, Maharaj M: The management of status epilepticus with a continuous propofol infusion. Anesth Analg 78:1193–1194, 1994.
36. Finley GA, McManus B, et al: Delayed seizures following sedation with propofol. Can J Anaesth, 40:863–865, 1993.
37. Hermann R, Vettermann J: Change of ectopic supraventricular tachycardia to sinus rhythm during administration of propofol. Anesth Analg 75:1030–1032, 1992.
38. Rashiq S, Gallant B, et al: Recovery characteristics following induction of anesthesia with a combination of thiopentone and propofol. Can J Anesth 41:1166–1871, 1994.
39. Bell C, Kain ZN: Pre-Medication in The Pediatric Anesthesia Handbook. St. Louis: Mosby, 1997, pp 21–33.
40. Audenaert SM, Montgomery CL, et al: A prospective study of rectal methohexital: Efficacy and side effects in 648 cases. Anesth Analg 81:957–961, 1995.
41. Koska J: Intravenous agents. In Kirby RR, Gravenstein N (eds): Clinical Anesthesia Practice. Philadelphia: WB Saunders 1994, pp 602–603.
42. Drain C: Inhalation anesthesia. In the Post Anesthesia Care Unit. Philadelphia: WB Saunders 1994, pp 190–204.
43. Stevens WC: Inhalation Agents. In Kirby RR, Gravenstein N (eds): Clinical Anesthesia Practice. Philadelphia: WB Saunders 1994, pp 606–620.
44. Longnecker DE, Miller FL: Pharmacology of inhalational anesthetics. In Rogers MC, Tinker JH, Covino BG, Longnecker DE (eds): Principles and Practice of Anesthesiology. St. Louis: Mosby, 1993, pp 1053–1086.
45. Nagelhout J: Inhalation anesthetics. In Mclntosh LW (ed): Essentials of Nurse Anesthesia. New York: McGraw-Hill, 1997, pp 71–78.
46. Dull DL: Recovery management of the healthy patient. In Rogers MC, Tinker JH, Covino BG, Longnecker DE (eds): Principles and Practice of Anesthesiology. St. Louis: Mosby, 1993, pp 129–147.
47. Chung FC: Discharge requirements. In White PF (ed): Ambulatory Anesthesia and Surgery. Philadelphia: WB Saunders 1997, pp 518–525.
48. Hawkins JL: Anesthesia for the pregnant patient undergoing nonobstetric surgery. In 1996 Annual Refresher Course Lectures. Park Ridge, IL: American Society of Anesthesiologists, 1996, p 156.
49. Fredman B, Jedeikin R: Volatile anesthetics and nitrous oxide. In PF White (ed): Ambulatory Anesthesia and Surgery. Philadelphia: WB Saunders 1997, pp 368–379.
50. Ghouri, A, et al: Recovery profile after desflurane-nitrous oxide versus isoflurane-nitrous oxide in outpatients. Anesthesiology 74, 419–424 1991.
51. Young C, Apfelbaum JL: Inhalation agents: Desflurane and sevoflurane. In Leading The Way. Society for Ambulatory Anesthesia 10th Annual Meeting, April 27–30, 1995, pp 1–7.
52. Koska J: Intravenous agents. In Kirby RR, Gravenstein N (eds): Clinical Anesthesia Practice. Philadelphia: WB Saunders 1994, pp 597–605.
53. Claxton AR, McGuire G, et al: Evaluation of morphine versus fentanyl for postoperative analgesia after ambulatory surgical procedures. Anesth Analg 84:509–514, 1997.
54. Rosow CE: Opioid and non-opioid analgesics. In White PF (ed): Ambulatory Anesthesia and Surgery. Philadelphia: WB Saunders 1997, pp 380–394.
55. Rosow C: Pharmacology of opioid analgetic agents. In Rogers MC et al (eds): Principles and Practice of Anesthesiology. St. Louis: CV Mosby, 1993, pp 1155–1181.
56. Philip BK: Remifentanil compared with alfentanil for ambulatory surgery using total intravenous anesthesia. Anesth Analg 84(3):515–521, 1997.
57. Souter AJ, Fredman B, White PF: Controversies in the perioperative use of nonsteroidal anti-inflammatory drugs. Anesth Analg 79:1178–1190, 1994.
58. Drain C: Muscle relaxants. In The Post Anesthesia Care Unit. Philadelphia: WB Saunders 1994, p 226–250.
59. Abbas TH: Succinylcholine. In Roizen MF, Fleisher LA (eds): Essence of Anesthesia Practice. Philadelphia: WB Saunders 1997, p 546.
60. Caldwell MA: Pharmacology of intravenous agents. In McIntosh LW (ed): Essentials of Nurse Anesthesia. New York: McGraw-Hill, 1997, pp 57–78.
61. Basta SJ: Muscle relaxant and reversal agents. In White PF (ed): Ambulatory Anesthesia and Surgery. Philadelphia: WB Saunders, 1997, pp 393–405.
62. Fisher DM: Pediatric ambulatory anesthesia: Controversies with muscle relaxants. In Leading The Way. Society for Ambulatory Anesthesia 10th Annual Meeting, April 27–30, 1995.
63. Belmont MR, Lien CA, et al: The clinical neuromuscular pharmacology of 51W89 in patients receiving nitrous oxide/opioid/barbiturate anesthesia. Anesthesiology 82:1139–1145, 1995.
64. Lien CA, et al: The cardiovascular effects and histamine-releasing effects of 51W89 in patients receiving nitrous oxide/opioid/barbiturate anesthesia. Anesthesiology 82:1131–1138, 1995.
65. Bevan D: Prolonged mivacurium induced neuromuscular block. Anesth Analg 77:4–6, 1993.
66. Naguib M, El-Gammal M, et al: Human plasma cholinesterase for antagonism of prolonged mivacurium-induced neuromuscular blockade. Anesthesiology 82:1288–1292, 1995.
67. King MJ, Milazkiewicz R, et al: Influence of neostigmine on postoperative vomiting. Br J Anaesth 61:403–406, 1988.
68. Savarese J: Choice of muscle relaxants. In 1994 Annual Refresher Course Lectures. Park Ridge, IL: American Society of Anesthesiologists, 1994, p 165.
69. Brull SJ: Monitoring of neuromuscular function. Sem Anesth 13:297–309, 1994.
70. Fontenot HJ, Gerner P: Neuromuscular junction monitoring and nerve stimulation. In Kirby RR, Gravenstein N (eds): Clinical Anesthesia Practice Philadelphia: WB Saunders, 1994, pp 412–413.
71. Rosenfeld BA: Postanesthesia care unit. In Rogers MC, et al (eds): Principles and Practice of Anesthesiology. St. Louis: CV Mosby, 1993, pp 2359–2386.
72. Greenberg CP, DeSoto H: Sedation techniques. In Twersky RS (eds): The Ambulatory Anesthesia Handbook, St. Louis: CV Mosby, 1995, pp 301–359.
73. Chung DC, Lam AM: Essentials of Anesthesiology, 3rd ed. Philadelphia: WB Saunders, 1997, pp 252–262.
74. Hoffman WD, Natanson C: Pulmonary complications of anesthesia. In Rogers MC, Tinker JH, Covino BG, Longnecker DE (eds): Principles and Practice of Anesthesiology. St. Louis: Mosby, 1993, pp 2401–2410.
75. Bainton CR: Complications of managing the airway. In Benumof JL (ed): Airway Management: Principles and Practice. St. Louis: CV Mosby, 1996, pp 886–899.
76. Glasser SA, Siler JN: Delayed onset of laryngospasm-induced pulmonary edema in an adult outpatient. Anesthesiology 62:370–371, 1985.

77. Hindman BJ, Tinker JH: Cardiovascular complications related to anesthesia. In Rogers MC, Tinker JH, Covino BG, Longnecker DE (eds): Principles and Practice of Anesthesiology. St. Louis: Mosby, 1993, pp 2411–2435.
78. Mangano DT, Roiz MF: Myocardial ischemia. In Roizen MF, Fleisher LA (eds): Essence of Anesthesia Practice. Philadelphia: WB Saunders, 1997, p 227.
79. Palahniuk RJ: Clinical pearls: The patient for 'oscopy surgery. In 1995 Review Course Lectures. Cleveland: International Anesthesia Research Society, 1995, pp 103–105.
80. Chan S: Laparoscopy, gynecologic. In Roizen MF, Fleisher LA (eds): Essence of Anesthesia Practice. Philadelphia: WB Saunders, 1997, p 408.
81. Neufield GR: Fires and explosions. In Gravenstein N, Kirby RR (eds): Complications in Anesthesiology, 2nd ed. Philadelphia: Lippincott-Raven, 1996, pp 73–78.
82. Kirk GA: Anesthesia for Ear, Nose and Throat Surgery. In Rogers MC, Tinker JH, Covino BG, Longnecker DE (eds): Principles and Practice of Anesthesiology. St. Louis: Mosby, 1993, pp 2262–2265.
83. Pasternak LR: Outpatient anesthesia. In Rogers MC, Tinker JH, Covino BG, Longnecker DE (eds): Principles and Practice of Anesthesiology. St. Louis: Mosby, 1993, pp 2275–2324.
84. American Society of Anesthesiologists: Practice Guidelines for Acute Pain Management in the Perioperative Setting: Report by ASA Task Force on Pain. Anesthesiology 82:1078–1079, 1995.
85. Agency for Health Care Policy and Research, Acute Pain Management: Operative or Medical Procedures and Trauma Clinical Practice Guideline. US Department of Health and Human Services, AHCPR Pub. No. 92-0032, Rockville, Maryland, 1992.
86. Pavlin D: Outpatient anesthesia. Clin Anesth Updates 4:1–18, 1993.
87. Cousins M: Postoperative pain management: State of the art. In Annual Refresher Course Lectures. Park Ridge, IL: American Society of Anesthesiologists, 1994, p 331.
88. Golinski MA, Fill DM: Preemptive analgesia. CRNA 6:16–20, 1995.
89. Bridenbaugh P: Preemptive analgesia: Is it clinically relevant? Anesth Analg 78:203–204, 1994.
90. Frey K: Multimodal approach to postoperative pain management in patients undergoing ambulatory anterior cruciate ligament (ACL) repair. In Leading the Way. Society of Ambulatory Anesthesia 10th Annual Meeting, April 27–30, 1995.
91. Szabo MZ, Tetzlaff JE, et al: Intraarticular injection for pain relief after outpatient arthroscopic knee surgery. In Leading the Way. Society for Ambulatory Anesthesia 10th Annual Meeting, 1995.
92. Souter AJ, Fredman B, White PF: Controversies in the perioperative use of nonsteroidal anti-inflammatory drugs. Anesth Analg 79:1178–1190, 1994.
93. Green CR, Pandit SK: Preoperative preparation. In Twersky RS (ed): The Ambulatory Anesthesia Handbook. St. Louis: Mosby, 1995, pp 171–202.
94. Ellis JE, Drijvers G, et al: Premedication with oral and transdermal clonidine provides safe and efficacious postoperative sympatholysis. Anesth Analg 79:1133–1140, 1994.
95. Aho M, Scheinin M, et al: Intramuscularly administered dexmedetomidine attenuates hemodynamic and stress hormone responses to gynecologic laparoscopy. Anesth Analg 75:932–939, 1992.
96. Duncan L, Wildsmith JAW: Liposomal local anaesthetics. Br J Anaesth 75(3):260–261, 1995.
97. Cohen MM, Duncan PG, et al: The postoperative interview: Assessing risk factors for nausea and vomiting. Anesth Analg 78:7–16, 1994.
98. Kapur PA: Postanesthesia recovery care and management. In Twersky RS (ed): The Ambulatory Anesthesia Handbook. St. Louis: Mosby, 1995, pp 399–430.
99. Everett LL, Kallar SK: Postoperative complications. In White PF (ed): Ambulatory Anesthesia and Surgery. Philadelphia: WB Saunders, 1997, pp 487–495.
100. Sun R, Klein KW, White PF: The effect of timing of ondansetron administration in outpatients undergoing otolaryngologic surgery. Anesth Analg 84:331–336, 1997.
101. Mikawa K, Takao Y, et al: The antiemetic efficacy of prophylaxis granisetron in gynecologic surgery. Anesth Analg 80:970–974, 1995.
102. Graczyk SG, McKenzie R, et al: Intravenous dolasetron for the prevention of postoperative nausea and vomiting after outpatient laparoscopic gynecologic surgery. Anesth Analg 84:325–330, 1997.

Chapter 14

Local and Regional Anesthesia

Michael Kost

Regional anesthesia is often an excellent choice for the ambulatory surgery setting. Regional anesthesia techniques may be as simple as the application of topical anesthetic solutions or as complex as continuous epidural administration of anesthetic agents for prolonged periods. The major routes of administration are topical, local infiltration, nerve block, subarachnoid (spinal), epidural, and intravenous (Bier block). Regional anesthesia can be arbitrarily subdivided into major (central) and minor (peripheral) categories. Central blocks are administered by the subarachnoid and epidural routes. Peripheral approaches include many types of extravascular nerve blocks and intravenous (IV) regional anesthesia (Bier block). The word *minor* is deceiving, however, because no invasive approach is without the potential for complications.

The various types of regional anesthesia have a number of generic similarities, yet there are inherent problems and advantages specific to the site and method of administration. This chapter presents some of the more frequently administered blocks and the nursing care associated with each procedure.

Nurses in all departments of an ambulatory surgery center (ASC) may be asked to participate in the administration of regional anesthesia and in the care of patients who have received central or peripheral blocks administered in the preprocedure admission area or in the postanesthesia care unit (PACU) before being transferred to surgery. A list of central and peripheral nerve blocks is presented in Table 14–1. Spinal, epidural, intercostal, local infiltration, and IV blocks are generally performed in the operating room (OR) suite or in a designated preinduction area near the OR suite. The phase II area, which in many hospitals is synonymous with the ASC as a whole, may be the site for administration of topical and infiltration anesthetics for procedures performed within the unit.

Nurses should be knowledgeable of the techniques, expected responses, and potential complications that can occur during and after the administration of local and regional anesthesia. Nurses must be prepared to assist with the procedure and to intervene when emergency situations arise. A nurse who does not participate or assist in the actual administration of regional anesthesia may provide vital preoperative patient education to prepare the patient for the operative experience. Firsthand knowledge is an exceptionally helpful teaching tool.

PHYSIOLOGY OF NERVE CONDUCTION AND LOCAL ANESTHETIC ACTION

Nerve conduction is dependent on the movement of sodium through channels in the permeable lipoprotein membranes of individual nerve cells. The depolarization of the membrane allows for rapid influx of sodium ions from the extracellular fluid compartment, which triggers a sequence of the same action along the nerve, resulting in the conduction of an impulse. This response is an all-or-nothing phenomenon and

***Table 14–1.* Central and Peripheral Nerve Blocks**

HEAD AND NECK REGIONAL BLOCKS
Trigeminal
Cervical plexus
Ophthalmic
Superior laryngeal
Translaryngeal
Glossopharyngeal
Accessory nerve (11th cranial)
Sphenopalatine ganglion
Occipital nerve
UPPER EXTREMITY BLOCKS
Brachial plexus
Interscalene
Supraclavicular
Perivascular
Subclavian perivascular
Infraclavicular
Median nerve
Ulnar nerve
Radial nerve
Ring block
Lateral antebrachial cutaneous
LOWER EXTREMITY BLOCKS
Femoral nerve
Obturator nerve
Sciatic nerve
Tibial nerve
Common peroneal
Saphenous
Posterior tibial
Sural
Superficial peroneal
Deep peroneal
Saphenous
TRUNK BLOCKS
Intercostal
Interpleural
Thoracic paravertebral
Lumbar paravertebral
Ilioinguinal, iliohypogastric
Intraperitoneal
Cave of Retzius
Sacral root
NEURAXIAL BLOCKS
Epidural
Spinal
Caudal

is depicted in Figure 14–1. The initiating trigger is either strong enough to overcome the resting cell membrane potential and causes a full depolarization of all cells in the fiber or is not strong enough to trigger any action. Once the initial cell has depolarized, all cells in the fiber will depolarize.

Local anesthetics work at the cellular level. They block the conduction of nerve impulses by interfering with the ability of nerve cell membranes to alter their permeability to the influx of sodium ions. Local anesthetics prevent the generation and the conduction of the nerve impulse by decreasing or preventing the large transient increase in the permeability of excitable membranes to sodium that normally is produced by depolarization of the membrane.[1]

To understand the mechanism of regional and infiltration anesthesia, one must understand the basic anatomy of the nervous system. The nervous system is a single entity but is often divided into two parts for discussion: the central nervous system (CNS) and the peripheral nervous system (PNS). The CNS includes the brain and spinal cord. The remaining PNS has two subdivisions: the 12 cranial nerves and the 31 pairs of spinal nerves. The cranial nerves link the body's sense organs to the brain. Somatic nerves allow the brain to sense and respond to impulses throughout the body.

The spinal cord has two functions. One is to link the brain with the body through long nerve fibers (white matter) that run along the full length of the spinal cord. The other function is to control reflex actions that occur within the gray matter of the cord without communication with the brain. Some of the large spinal nerves that originate along the spinal cord combine to form the cervical, brachial, lumbar, sacral, and coccygeal plexuses, or nerve networks. As the spinal nerves travel away from the central cord, they branch into ever smaller segments that make up the remainder of the peripheral nerve network. This somatic system controls voluntary skeletal muscle movement, sensation, and adjustments to the external environment.[2]

The autonomic, or involuntary, nervous system (ANS) also originates at the spinal cord. It links the brain with the internal organs, glands, and secretory cells. It is considered to be a motor pathway through which the brain sends signals to those effector organs. The function of the ANS is to maintain homeostasis of vital systems by controlling internal structures such as the heart, glands, and smooth muscles. It does so by a balanced activation of its opposing sympathetic and parasympathetic branches. The major functions of the ANS are described in Table 14–2. Under normal conditions, the autonomic system responds to changes in heart rate, blood pressure, stress, pain, and a multitude of additional factors.

The administration of local anesthetics blocks somatic nerve conduction of impulses controlling sensation and movement. Autonomic nerves also are affected by local anesthetics. In

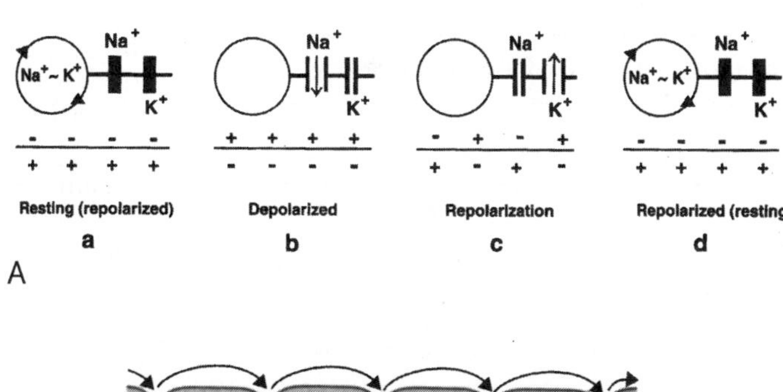

Figure 14–1. *A, B,* Sodium influx and the development of the action potential. (From Chung DC, Lam AM: Essentials of Anesthesiology, 3rd ed. Philadelphia: WB Saunders, 1997, p 81.)

fact, the thin, unmyelinated autonomic nerves are more readily affected by anesthetics than are the somatic nerves. With progressive increases in the concentration of local anesthetic agents, the autonomic, sensory, and then motor impulses are blocked.[3] Variations in the location, size, and myelination of nerve fibers allow the physician to localize nerve fibers and select local anesthetic solutions that will result in a particular intended effect.

When a local anesthetic agent is deposited near a nerve, impulses are blocked to and from the areas of the body innervated by that nerve. The intended effects include sensory blockade, elimination of pain, and immobility of a specific area during an operative procedure. Unfortunately, the unavoidable blockade of nearby sympathetic nerves sometimes produces undesirable effects. The order of fiber blockade is shown in Table 14–3. These effects include bradycardia, peripheral vasodilatation, and hypotension with resultant decreased systemic vascular resistance. These potential adverse reactions and complications require diligent observation and gentle movement of a patient who has received major regional anesthesia.

Tachyphylaxis, as it relates to local anesthesia, is a phenomenon in which there is a progressive

Table 14–2. **Comparison of the Sympathetic and Parasympathetic Branches of the Autonomic Nervous System**

SITE	SYMPATHETIC STIMULATION	PARASYMPATHETIC STIMULATION
General body effects	(Adrenergic) energizes, prepares for "fight or flight"	(Cholinergic) conserves/restores energy
Heart	Speeds and strengthens force of contractions	Decreases rate
Lungs	Bronchial dilatation	Bronchial constriction
Blood vessels	Constriction of skin and GI tract vessels; dilatation of coronaries and those supplying skeletal muscles	No effect on many
Iris	Dilates pupil	Constricts pupil
Adrenal medulla	Secretion of epinephrine and norepinephrine	No effect
Kidneys/urinary tract	Decreases urinary output	No effect
	Relaxes bladder	Contracts bladder
	Contracts sphincter	Relaxes sphincter
Liver	Increases breakdown of glycogen	No effect
Intestines/GI tract	Decreases motility by inhibiting muscle tone	Increases motility by increasing muscle tone
	Contracts sphincters	Relaxes sphincters
Pancreas	Decreases enzyme secretion	Increases enzyme secretion
Glands	Decreases tears	Increases tears
	Increases sweating	Stimulates salivation
Adipose tissues	Stimulates free fatty acid release from fat cells	No effect

Data from Stewart J: Clinical Anatomy and Pathophysiology for the Health Professional. Miami: MedMaster, 1997; and Jacob SW, Francone CA: Elements of Anatomy and Physiology. Philadelphia: WB Saunders, 1989.

Table 14–3. **Order of Fiber Blockade**

NERVE FIBER	MYELINATION	FUNCTION
A	Heavy	Motor
B	Light	Preganglionic, autonomic
C	Absent	Pain and temperature

Sequence of fiber blockade with central neuraxial anesthesia includes blockade of fibers C, B, and A after initial administration of spinal and epidural anesthesia.

decrease in response to a local anesthetic when repeated or continuous doses are administered. In other words, with repeated doses, more frequent and larger amounts of a drug are required to provide the same response. The mechanism appears to involve local pH changes occurring at nerve sites. A delicate pH balance is necessary for optimal effectiveness of local anesthetic action. Most local anesthetics are weak bases. With the phenomenon of tachyphylaxis, repeated injections tax the available buffering system so that an acidic form of local anesthetic builds up, leaving inadequate amounts of uncharged base available for neural penetration. This effect is most noticeable in areas with limited buffer reserves, for instance, in the cerebrospinal fluid (CSF).[4]

The pH of the tissues into which the agent is injected also influences the speed and extent of local anesthetic uptake. A low pH, such as that found in infected tissues, causes ionization of the drug. This change reduces the ability of the anesthetic to permeate cell membranes, thus decreasing the drug's effectiveness.

TYPES AND CHARACTERISTICS OF LOCAL ANESTHETIC AGENTS

Local anesthetics are chemically separated into two categories: esters and amides. Although chemically different, they have a similar membrane-blocking effect on neurons. Esters are rapidly metabolized in the plasma by pseudocholinesterase. In patients with a deficiency of plasma cholinesterase, esters are slowly converted in the liver and must follow a slower path of excretion. In this alternative and extended biotransformation, large amounts of the ester can build up in the plasma. A patient with this excessive plasma buildup is more likely to experience systemic toxic effects than is a patient with a normal pseudocholinesterase level.

Amide local anesthetic compounds are metabolized in the liver. Their clearance is more prolonged than that of the esters. Liver disease, low cardiac output, and advanced age can prolong the process of metabolism, increasing the likelihood of systemic toxicity because the drug remains in the bloodstream in an active state for a longer than usual period.[5] Owing to this longer metabolic process, the amide group is considered more likely to cause toxicity than are the esters. Lidocaine, in particular, is considered twice as toxic as procaine. Table 14–4 describes the characteristics of a variety of frequently used local anesthetics.

The potency, time of onset, and duration of action of local anesthetic agents are related to their inherent chemical properties and additional extrinsic factors. Usually a parallel relationship exists between the drug's onset and its duration of action. Drugs that rapidly cross the nerve cell membrane and thus have a rapid onset of action also diffuse out with ease, resulting in a short duration of action. In contrast, many drugs that have long durations of action require longer to become effective. Because of this characteristic, anesthesia providers often mix two agents together. Combining a rapid-onset local anesthetic with another one that has a slower onset but longer duration of action allows surgery to begin quickly while still providing adequate anesthesia and analgesia throughout surgery, as well as postoperative comfort.

The addition of a vasoconstrictor such as epinephrine to the anesthetic also influences its duration of action. Owing to the local vasoconstriction caused by epinephrine, local anesthetics are not readily absorbed into the bloodstream. The reduced absorption results in more profound penetration of the cell membranes and a longer duration of action.[6] The addition of epinephrine to local anesthetic solutions decreases the potential toxicity of an anesthetic agent by prolonging its uptake into the general circulation before metabolism.

Advantages of Regional Anesthesia

People react uniquely and have widely differing physical and emotional needs. Each patient must be carefully evaluated by the physician who will decide the type of anesthesia to be given. The anesthesia provider must consider the type and length of the procedure to be performed, the patient's past medical history and emotional state, and the patient's desires. The nurse may be the intermediary who relays patient concerns or reluctance to the anesthesia provider before the administration of the regional anesthetic.

Regardless of the mode of administration, regional and local anesthetic approaches offer some distinct advantages over general anesthesia. A significant benefit of regional anesthesia is avoidance of the complications associated with the administration of general anesthesia. This is particularly important for patients with significant past medical histories or those who physiologically may not tolerate the deleterious effects of general anesthesia. With an uncomplicated regional anesthesic, the patient remains conscious with no loss of protective reflexes and experiences a reduced incidence of embolic and pulmonary sequelae.

Postoperative nursing care and the recovery period are frequently reduced after the administration of regional anesthesia, particularly when compared with general anesthesia. Except after spinal and epidural blocks, patients often avoid the need for PACU care and may be reunited earlier with family and friends in a phase II PACU. Most patients are able to accept responsibility for some amount of self-care soon after the procedure is completed. Thus, regional anesthesia supports the concept of wellness encouraged by ambulatory surgery programs.

Another benefit is the usually lower cost associated with the supplies, equipment, and time required to administer regional anesthesia when compared with general anesthesia. Many regional techniques are quite simple and can be performed quickly. There is less staff exposure to potentially flammable, explosive, or physiologically harmful agents such as volatile anesthetic gases. There is the added benefit of having an awake patient who can cooperate with the surgeon's requests.

Another significant advantage for the ambulatory surgery patient is the postoperative sensory block that accompanies regional anesthesia. The sensory blockade frequently allows the patient to ambulate, travel home, and settle into a familiar environment before the onset of any significant pain. After arriving home, the patient may take oral analgesics without the gastrointestinal (GI) upset that is frequently associated with the ride home. Sometimes the duration and level of regional analgesia are such that the patient never experiences any significant postoperative pain.

Regional anesthesia is also beneficial for patients who have recently ingested food or beverages and must undergo urgent surgery. Successful regional techniques can eliminate the need for general anesthesia in these patients with full stomachs. However, slowed digestion and potential GI upset from preoperative anxiety, narcotics, or the complications of regional anesthetics still predispose the patient to vomiting and aspiration, particularly if the patient is sedated. Therefore, it is recommended that emergent procedures be performed after the administration of regional anesthesia with minimal or no supplemental sedation. Failed or incomplete blocks may require the administration of general anesthesia in order to complete a procedure. For these reasons, most anesthesia providers consider the risk-benefit ratio and patient safety when selecting an anesthetic technique for emergent surgical procedures.

Disadvantages of Regional Anesthesia

Disadvantages associated with regional anesthesia include increased anxiety and patient refusal based on the experiences of others who may have had regional anesthesia before the numerous refinements and advances in delivery. Patients often have doubts that the local anesthetic will truly provide anesthesia for the procedure. These concerns are often addressed by the anesthesia provider during a thorough preprocedure explanation, including the fact that sedation is also available. Sometimes even the most ardent anesthesia provider cannot convince a patient about the benefits of regional anesthesia. Regional anesthesia must not be considered for patients who refuse it. Continued efforts or the actual administration of regional anesthesia to patients who refuse it may result in charges of assault and battery.[7]

Local anesthesia may be impractical for some areas of the body because of the number and volume of injections required and the time consumed in providing an adequate block. Partial, incomplete, or failed blocks may require the administration of general anesthesia or cancellation of the case if the patient is physiologically unfit for the administration of general anesthesia. Difficulty in establishing a regional block or multiple attempts at administration are unpleasant for the patient as well as for the staff involved in patient care. Specific types of blocks are technically more difficult to administer than others and require more time, effort, and patient cooperation.

If a regional block becomes inadequate during surgery, the surgeon may attempt to supplement it with local anesthetic infiltration. If sup-

Table 14–4. Local Anesthetics

NAME OF DRUG (BRAND)	GROUP STRENGTHS (%)	DURATION OF ACTION (MIN)		MAXIMUM RECOMMENDED DOSES		POTENCY	ONSET OF ACTION	DURATION OF ACTION	NOTES
		Plain	*With Epinephrine*	*Plain*	*With Epinephrine*				
Cocaine	Ester 4, 10	10–55	Not added	200 mg 3 mg/kg	Not added	Low	Rapid	Short	Used topically, very useful in ear, nose, throat surgery Potent vasoconstrictor Highly addictive and highly toxic Difficult to make into sterile solution Causes apacity of cornea
Procaine (Novocain, Unicaine)	Ester 1, 2, 10	15–30	30–90	10 mg/kg	14 mg/kg	Low	Rapid	Short	No topical activity Not in wide use—short action and propensity to trigger allergic reactions
Chloroprocaine (Nesacaine)	Ester 1, 2, 3	15–30	30–90	800 mg 11 mg/kg	1000 mg 14 mg/kg	Low	Rapid	Short	Safest in terms of toxicity, used in continuous epidural but implicated in sensory/motor deficits when inadvertently injected into subarachnoid space—thought to be the preservative at fault
Tetracaine (Pontocaine)	Ester 0.5, 1	120–240	240–280	100 mg	200 mg	High	Slow	Long	High systemic toxicity Most commonly used for long-acting spinals 1–2% solution for topical use in trachea and pharynx Used for conjunctival anesthesia
Lidocaine (Xylocaine)	Amide 0.5, 1, 1.5, 2, 4, 5	30–60	60–120	300 mg 4 mg/kg	500 mg 7 mg/kg	Intermediate	Rapid	Intermediate	No local irritation, some topical use Relatively free of allergic reactions Cardiac depressant
Mepivacaine (Carbocaine, Polocaine, Cavacaine, Isocaine)	Amide 1, 1.5, 2	45–90	120–360	300 mg 4 mg/kg	500 mg 7 mg/kg	Intermediate	Intermediate	Intermediate	Minimal tissue reactions, no topical activity Not used for spinals 20% longer acting than lidocaine
Bupivacaine (Sensorcaine, Marcaine)	Amide 0.25, 0.5, 0.75	120–240	240–480	175 mg	225 mg	High	Intermediate	Long	Relatively high toxicity Cardiotoxic if given in large bolus
Ropivacaine (Naropin)	Amide 0.2–0.5	120–360	240–360	5–40 ml	40 ml	Moderate	Moderate	Moderate	Newly introduced amide local anesthetic for spinal, epidural, infiltration, and peripheral nerve block

Data from Drain C, Shipley C: The Recovery Room: A Critical Care Approach to Post Anesthesia Nursing, 3rd ed. Philadelphia: WB Saunders, 1994; Ivey D: Local anesthesia: Implications for the perioperative nurse. AORN J, 45:682–689, 1987; Philip B, Covino B: Local and regional anesthesia. In Wetchler B (ed): Anesthesia for Ambulatory Surgery. Philadelphia: JB Lippincott, 1985, pp 225–274; Wetchler B: Anesthesia for outpatients. In Mauldin B (ed): Ambulatory Surgery: A Guide to Perioperative Nursing Care. New York: Grune & Stratton, 1983, pp 111–157; Drain C: Postanesthesia Nursing. In Omoigui S (ed): The Anesthesia Drug Handbook, 2nd ed. St. Louis: Mosby, 1995; Chung D, Lam A: Essentials in Anesthesiology, 3rd ed. Philadelphia: WB Saunders, 1997.

plemental blockade proves insufficient, the anesthesia provider may administer heavy sedation or general anesthesia. The administration of general anesthesia may require an unexpected period of recovery in the PACU, which can be frightening to both the patient and family members. There may have been a different protocol used for preoperative medications, with less emphasis on prophylaxis of nausea and vomiting when a regional approach is planned. This, along with anxiety, can result in postoperative nausea and vomiting. Also, the patient now faces a recovery period without the benefit of the prolonged sensory block that was expected and may require more analgesics that further promote nausea and vomiting.

A concerted effort should be made by both the anesthesiologist and the nursing staff to reduce the negative impact of a failed block. First, a patient who is less anxious or upset generally has an easier and less stressful postoperative period. Second, it is a great disservice to allow a patient to harbor fear, anger, or other negative emotions about regional anesthesia, because future procedures or situations may demand the use of a regional approach. The patient should be encouraged to verbalize any thoughts or concerns, and a positive attitude should be used when discussing regional anesthesia. Individual approaches based on the patient's personality and the particular circumstances should be employed to elicit the desired level of patient satisfaction.

Other disadvantages of regional anesthesia include the potential for complications related to the actual injection technique, for instance, hemorrhage; nerve damage; pneumothorax; inadvertent intravascular injection or rapid circulatory uptake with related systemic toxicity; infection due to the introduction of microorganisms from the equipment, needles, or hands of the practitioner; other complications specific to the approach, such as puncture of a vessel or viscus; rarely, allergic reaction; and pain and other complications from the use of an extremity tourniquet.

Intraoperative sights, sounds, and conversations can be disconcerting even to the bravest and calmest of awake patients. The sounds of drills, instrument movement, and other noises can be magnified or distorted in an unsedated patient. To avoid some of these environmental noises, it is best to complete the room setup before the patient is brought into the OR. Methods to diminish these effects intraoperatively include diversion of the patient's attention through conversation or music played through headphones and the administration of sedative medications.

The entire staff must be cognizant of conversations within the hearing of awake patients. Irrelevant and inappropriate conversations can make the patient feel isolated, frightened, and unimportant to the operating team. Casual conversation should be kept to a minimum, particularly in the presence of an unsedated or lightly sedated patient.

During and after regional anesthesia, a concerted effort should be made to provide emotional support for each patient. The patient may feel intimidated or be afraid to speak up to report pain during a procedure. This fear often outweighs the amount of discomfort being experienced. Thus, patients must be monitored for objective symptoms of discomfort and permitted, instructed, and encouraged to speak up if anything is bothersome or painful during a procedure. Often the anesthesia provider or registered nurse holds the patient's hand and provides needed human contact, particularly for a patient whose head or face is covered with surgical drapes for the procedure. When a frozen section report from the pathologist is being awaited by the surgeon, particular care must be taken to avoid frightening or potentially misunderstood technical conversations that may occur within the hearing of the patient. A speaker telephone should never be used to relay a pathology report to the surgeon in the presence of an awake patient.

Sometimes minor procedures that usually would be amenable to a local anesthesia approach may be scheduled for general anesthesia to spare the patient emotional or physical distress. One example of this is when a physician strongly suspects a malignancy before performing a breast biopsy. Another example is a patient with limited or painful flexibility who will have difficulty lying still or maintaining a certain position throughout the surgical procedure.

Postoperatively, some patients experience a great deal of anxiety when they are unable to control anesthetized portions of their bodies, resulting in fear and even panic. The patient may become exhausted while trying to move an anesthetized area, even with repeated admonitions by the nurse about the futility of the effort. Explanations, assurances, and patient education are required to reassure the patient that the anesthetic block is not permanent. When prolonged anesthesia is exceptionally upsetting to a patient, sedation may be required until the effects of the block dissipate. At this point, the nurse should continue to reinforce the numerous positive aspects of prolonged sensory block and postoperative pain reduction.

Postoperatively, there is also the potential for inadvertent injury or abuse of the anesthetized area with continued sensory blockade. An example of inadvertent injury is a podiatry patient who is pain free and walks about at home after discharge, causing swelling and additional complications. Thorough postoperative instructions and explanations about the nature of regional anesthesia and methods to avoid injury are required as part of the patient's postprocedure education by the nurse before discharge. It may be helpful to use the explanation that pain is the very symptom that limits the patient's activity so that healing can take place. The absence of surgical pain allows a false sense of normalcy for a short time, so the patient must consciously refrain from activity that could cause harm to the incision or surrounding tissues and should visually inspect the area periodically while sensation is diminished. Protective devices such as slings, braces, casts, and bulky dressings help protect areas affected by regional anesthesia.

Adverse Effects of Regional Anesthesia

Several factors contribute to the adverse effects of regional anesthesia, including drug toxicity, allergic reactions, the addition of adjunctive agents, and the patient's anatomic and physiologic status, which may predispose to untoward reactions. Errors resulting from techniques of administration may also play a part. It is important to realize that more than one factor can be involved in the development of an untoward reaction.

Systemic toxicity and allergic reactions are related to the types of agents used, the speed and volume of the injection, and the patient's individual tolerance of that agent. There is often confusion about the difference between toxicity and allergy to local anesthetic solutions. Toxicity implies the response to an overdose of local anesthetic agent. Symptoms result when the amount of active drug in the patient's circulation is greater than the recommended maximal dose for the patient's weight and physical condition. True allergic responses to local anesthetics are rare. However, when a local anesthetic allergic reaction occurs, it is accompanied by histamine release, which triggers the ensuing allergic response. This is an idiosyncratic response to a foreign substance. Table 14–5 outlines the symptoms and treatment protocols for toxicity and allergic reactions.

***Table 14–5.* Symptoms and Treatment Protocol for Local Anesthetic Reactions**

SYMPTOMS
Feeling of uneasiness or doom
Agitation
Numbness of the tongue and mouth
Visual disturbance
Tinnitus
Restlessness
Slurred speech
Bradycardia
Hypotension
Cardiac arrest
Circulatory collapse
TREATMENT
Stop injection if current
Administer oxygen
Support airway and ventilation
Administer benzodiazepines or barbiturates
Support circulation (volume expansion)
Administer vasopressors and inotropes

Toxic Reactions

Toxic reactions are related to a rising plasma level of local anesthetics in the bloodstream. They can occur when an anesthetic agent is not metabolized or is injected directly into a blood vessel, or they may be secondary to excessive administration (overdose) of the local anesthetic agents being used. Toxic reactions most often follow (1) overdose of an agent in a single bolus or through repeated injections, (2) inadvertent deposit into the vasculature by direct needle puncture, or (3) rapid absorption into highly vascular areas. Interestingly, intra-arterial injection is less likely to cause toxic effects than intravenous injection; because arterial blood is just beginning its circulation through the vasculature, there is more time for the drug to be diluted and partially hydrolyzed in the plasma before it affects the CNS.[8] Another mechanism of undesirable drug release into the general circulation can follow a Bier block when the extremity tourniquet is deflated too soon or too rapidly after the injection.

There is wide variation in symptoms associated with local anesthesia toxicity. Ranging from minor and transient to life-threatening sequelae, these complications are usually related to the cardiovascular system and the CNS.[9] Toxic doses of local anesthetics initially stimulate the

CNS while causing medullary depression. It is essential that minor symptoms not be overlooked, because they can be precursors to a more serious reaction.

Early symptoms associated with local anesthetic toxicity include anxiety, excitement, euphoria, drowsiness, lightheadedness, tinnitus, nausea, a metallic taste, and blurred vision.[10] Tingling or numbness of the lips (circumoral numbness) and surrounding tissues is a common early sign of local anesthetic toxicity. Patients also can exhibit slurred speech, muscle tremors and twitching, confusion, and nystagmus. Stimulation of the medulla can cause hypertension, tachycardia, tachypnea, nausea, and vomiting. These symptoms may occur during or after administration of the anesthetic. Less frequently, they may become evident only after completion of the procedure.

If toxic symptoms occur, appropriate nursing care of the patient consists of continuous observation and monitoring of the patient, including electrocardiogram (ECG), blood pressure, and oxygen saturation. Maintenance and protection of the airway, administration of oxygen, and attentive reassurance are required for patients exhibiting signs and symptoms of local anesthetic overdose. The physician must be informed immediately at the first signs of toxicity, and the nurse must observe the patient closely and prepare to intervene if more serious complications ensue. Sometimes patient complaints are quite vague and limited to a feeling of "discontent" or "not feeling quite right."

At higher blood levels, more advanced symptoms of toxicity can involve frank convulsions, tonic-clonic seizure activity of the muscles, and coma. Respirations may become impaired owing to seizures, and hypoxia may follow. Hypoxia and hypercarbia generally result in hypertension and cardiovascular depression.[11] Profound peripheral vasodilatation and depression of the sinus and atrioventricular nodes further compromise the cardiovascular system. Anticonvulsant drugs such as diazepam or thiopental may be required to attenuate convulsions. Nurses must be prepared to administer cardiopulmonary resuscitation as indicated, including intubation, ventilation, defibrillation, and vascular support with IV fluids and potent vasopressors.

Allergic Reactions

An allergic reaction is an idiosyncratic response of the body to a foreign chemical that causes massive release of histamine with resulting capillary and arteriole dilatation, changes in vessel permeability, and an eventual shift of fluid from the vasculature into interstitial compartments. Hypotension associated with allergic reaction can be profound. Although allergic reactions to local anesthetic solutions are rare, the nurse must be prepared to respond and to assess, diagnose, and intervene when local anesthetics are administered.

Reactions are manifested by early signs of pruritus, rash, erythema, urticaria, and skin wheal formation. Symptoms may progress to wheezing, bronchospasm, and cardiovascular collapse. Besides the generic application of resuscitative measures, treatment also includes the administration of an antihistamine (H_1-receptor antagonists) such as diphenhydramine (Benadryl). An H_2 blocker such as ranitidine (Zantac) or famotidine (Pepcid) may be effective in treating histamine-related symptoms. Medical management for severe bronchospasm includes the use of β_2-adrenergic agonists, aminophylline, and IV corticosteroid therapy.[12]

Esters are somewhat more likely to produce true allergic reactions than are amides. This propensity may be attributed to the chemical para-aminobenzoic acid (PABA), which is a metabolite formed in the breakdown of esters.[13] Amide-induced allergies are extremely rare, and there is no cross-sensitivity between reactions to amides and esters. For instance, a patient with an allergy to the ester procaine (Novocain) would not necessarily have a related allergy to amides such as lidocaine (Xylocaine) or bupivacaine (Marcaine, Sensorcaine). Additives (preservatives) to prolong shelf life, such as methylparaben, may be implicated in allergic reactions rather than the local anesthetic itself.

Complications Related to Adjunctive Agents

Sedative, analgesic, and hypnotic agents may be administered during the infiltration of local anesthetics as well as during surgery to reduce patient anxiety and discomfort. Side effects related to a wide variety of agents must be considered. Decreased sensorium, predisposition to aspiration, loss of protective reflexes, and nausea and vomiting are potential complications associated with the use of adjunctive agents. The role of the anesthesia provider or nurse during conscious sedation or straight local procedures is to monitor the patient's status during the administration of local anesthesia and throughout the procedure.

Vasoconstrictive drugs are frequently added

to local anesthetic solutions to reduce bleeding at the surgical site and to slow absorption, which results in more prolonged anesthesia and reduced systemic toxicity. Epinephrine is frequently used in spinal anesthesia to prolong sensory blockade. Epinephrine, the most widely used vasoconstrictor, is generally mixed with a local anesthetic in concentrations of 1:200,000 (5 μg/ml) or 1:100,000 (10 μg/ml). When used with local anesthetic infiltration techniques, the addition of epinephrine causes vasoconstriction to decrease surgical bleeding and prolongs the duration of local anesthetic action. Systemic side effects of epinephrine include hypertension, tachycardia, and cardiac dysrhythmias.[14] These side effects are magnified with inadvertent IV administration.

Reactions attributed to local anesthetic drugs may actually be side effects of epinephrine. These symptoms may be markedly pronounced during the administration of dental anesthesia owing to the unusually high concentration (up to 1:50,000) of epinephrine used. Many patients incorrectly report reactions to local anesthetic infiltration at the dental office as an allergic reaction when, in essence, the reaction is simply a normal response to the absorption of epinephrine. Contraindications to epinephrine include digital blocking secondary to constriction of the terminal arteries with resultant ischemia and gangrene.[15] As a result, epinephrine with local anesthesia is contraindicated for areas such as the nose, penis, fingers, and toes.

Preservatives may be added to prolong the shelf life of local anesthetics and may cause neurotoxicity or allergic responses. Methylparaben, an antifungal additive, has already been mentioned as an allergen. Sodium bisulfite is another frequently used preservative; its concentration has recently been reduced in some local anesthetics to lower potential toxicity. A preservative-free drug is chosen by the anesthesia provider when introducing medication intrathecally or epidurally.

Complications Related to Predisposing Anatomic and Physiologic Factors

Factors that predispose patients to complications may contraindicate the use of a regional anesthetic. Anticoagulated patients, infection or abscess at the site of injection, increased intracranial pressure, platelet counts below 100,000, and other blood dyscrasias are contraindications to specific local injection techniques. Additional relative contraindications include uncooperative patients, anemia, and hypovolemia.

The patient's physical and emotional state before the injection of local anesthesia influences the physiologic response to the block. Anxious or frightened patients may exhibit hypertension, palpitations, tachycardia, and diaphoresis secondary to catecholamine release. A person with advanced liver disease or reduced cardiac output metabolizes local anesthetic agents slowly, which predisposes to toxicity and prolonged local anesthetic action. As outlined earlier, a deficiency of plasma pseudocholinesterase predisposes a patient to toxicity secondary to the alternative path of metabolism required.

Anatomic anomalies may lead to unexpected puncture of the vasculature or viscera during injection of local anesthetic solution. Parkinsonism and neuromuscular diseases that increase involuntary movements enhance the chance of technical error during injection. Anatomic deviation can result in an inability to obtain a complete block when anesthetic solutions are deposited but nerve branches are not in their expected positions.

An additional consideration is the potential for drug interactions secondary to the wide variety of medications that patients use. It is essential that the nurse and physician obtain an accurate medication history from each patient for both prescribed and over-the-counter medications.

Patients medicated with aspirin, nonsteroidal anti-inflammatory agents, vitamin E, or heparin may be predisposed to hemorrhage. Therefore, patients are generally instructed to omit these medications before the scheduled procedure to avoid the potential for hematoma formation. Preprocedure instructions range from 48 hours to 1 week of abstinence, depending on which anticoagulant is being used by the patient. The serious nature of some conditions may require consultation with the patient's medical physician before giving instructions to omit anticoagulant medicines.

Specific antidepressant medications deplete the sympathomimetic amines in nerve endings. This depletion causes an unpredictable response to indirect-acting vasopressor medications such as ephedrine. Hypotension in these patients is treated with direct-acting vasoactive drugs such as phenylephrine. Because many drug interactions are potentially harmful or would nullify the effects of local anesthetics, a complete medication history is a vital prerequisite to the administration of regional anesthesia.[16] Medication compatibility and considerations associated with the use of local anesthetics are featured in Table 14–6.

NURSING RESPONSIBILITIES

There are numerous nursing responsibilities associated with the administration of regional anesthesia. These nursing responsibilities include (1) preparing the patient physically and emotionally, (2) securing appropriate supplies and equipment, (3) positioning and supporting the patient during a procedure, (4) assisting physicians with technical aspects as needed, (5) monitoring and evaluating the patient's response during and after the procedure, and (6) maintaining emergency skills and equipment for immediate response to untoward reactions.

In addition to preparing the patient for regional anesthesia, the nurse must be attentive during the actual administration of the block. The basic principles of ABCD (airway, breathing, circulation, and drugs) must be foremost in the nurse's plan of care. Profound reactions can occur that may render the patient susceptible to cardiopulmonary depression within moments. Whenever regional anesthetics are administered, there should be appropriate monitoring equipment, oxygen, suction, and a full stock of emergency equipment and drugs available. A registered nurse should be present to assist and to continually assess the patient for complications.

Guidelines have been approved by the Association of Perioperative Registered Nurses (AORN) regarding monitoring a patient having local anesthesia without the involvement of anesthesia department personnel.[17] These recommended practices outline the OR nurse's responsibilities for monitoring the patient, documenting care, and developing and following written protocols.

The following discussion presents a chronologic listing of general nursing responsibilities before, during, and after regional anesthesia. Depending on the individual facility, some of the nurse's duties discussed may overlap with those of the anesthesia provider. The nurse does not administer local anesthetics, but other duties surrounding preparation and patient support may be assumed by either the nurse or anesthesia personnel, according to individual facility policies.

Preparations for the Administration of Regional Anesthesia

A variety of factors combine to ensure a safe setting for the administration of local or regional anesthesia, regardless of the department. Before any patient-related contact, the ambulatory surgery nurse should learn the types and properties of anesthetic agents, administration techniques, and potential complications related to each technique. Emergency protocols should be reviewed periodically, and a policy should be in place that ensures the constant availability of equipment, supplies, and personnel to respond to any emergencies.

To accurately assess patient parameters during and after regional anesthesia, a preanesthesia baseline must be established that includes the patient's preoperative health status and a physical assessment. This assessment should include at least the following:

Normal blood pressure, pulse, and respiratory ranges
Preoperative oximetry range when possible
Laboratory values as appropriate
Skin condition at the intended site of injection and overall skin appearance
Extremity circulation: color, temperature, pulses
Mental status that might indicate pre-existing mental confusion or drowsiness
Medical history, including diseases and previous anesthesia experiences
Problems of mobility or flexibility that might complicate or prevent proper positioning
Allergies and current medication protocol

If potential problems are identified or pre-existing conditions exist, the nurse must notify the appropriate physician before the block. Before the administration of any block, the patient must be identified verbally and by checking the name band, and the operative site must be verified. The procedure must be reaffirmed, and the operative consent should be reviewed for completeness. The anatomic site should be inspected for inflammation or infection, which would likely contraindicate the administration of regional anesthesia in the area. The area should be assessed for cleanliness. Shaving or clipping of long hair may be indicated. Clothing that could interfere with the anesthesia or with the surgical procedure must be removed.

All necessary supplies should be assembled before administration of the local anesthetic. Once the regional blockade is established, the nurse should not need to leave the room. As items are assembled, the nurse ensures their proper sterility and completeness. Equipment must be maintained in proper condition so that it is always ready for use, and a protocol should be in place to ensure adequate replacement of disposable supplies. The nurse reinforces any

***Table 14–6.* Potential Drug Reactions with Local Anesthetics or with Adjunctive Drugs Used with Local Anesthetics**

DRUG	INTERACTION	EFFECTS
Anticoagulants	Interfere with coagulation	Bleeding, hematoma at injection site
Furosemide, steroids High-dose aspirin Anti-inflammatories	Interfere with platelet adhesiveness	Bleeding, hematoma at injection site
Antihypertensives: *Rauwolfia* alkaloids (reserpine [Regroton], hydrochlorothiazide)	Deplete norepinephrine stores	Alters response to vasopressors, which may be used to treat hypotension secondary to major regional anesthesia
Antihypertensives: Quanethidine (Ismelin, Esimil) Methyldopa	Sensitize postsynaptic effector sites to norepinephrine	Exaggerated response to direct-acting sympathomimetics such as phenylephrine (Neo-Synephrine) and methoxamine (Vasoxyl) Decreased response to indirect-acting sympathomimetics such as ephedrine
β-adrenergic drugs (propranolol, pindolol [Visken], nadolol [Corgard], metoprolol [Lopressor])	Decrease ability to increase heart rate, decrease myocardial contractility and vasoconstriction of blood vessels	Decreased or no automatic response to hypotension occurring with major block
β-adrenergic drugs	Increase number of β-receptors	Runaway hypertension in combination with epinephrine in blocks
Propranolol and cimetidine	Either compete for same hepatic metabolic enzymes or decrease cardiac output and hepatic blood flow	Decrease rate of plasma clearance of lidocaine, thus increase systemic toxicity effects
Tricyclic antidepressants (amitryptyline [Elavil, Triavil], imipramine [Tofranil])	Inhibit norepinephrine uptake at postganglionic neurons	Exaggerated response to epinephrine and unpredictable response to indirect vasopressors (ephedrine) that may be given to treat hypotension, with extreme hypertension or hypotension possible
Monoamine oxidase inhibitors (phenelzine sulfate [Nardil], tranylcypromine sulfate [Parnate])	Increase body stores of epinephrine, norepinephrine, and serotonin	Exaggerated response to epinephrine and indirect vasopressors (ephedrine) that may be given to treat hypotension, with extreme hypertension possible Combine unfavorably with adjunctive narcotics, especially meperidine, with severe and sometimes untreatable hypertension and tachycardia
Antiparkinson drugs Levodopa (Larodopa, Sinemet)	Antagonized by droperidol Used for supplementation	Exacerbation of parkinsonian symptoms
Droperidol	Do not use epinephrine to treat hypotension	Further hypotension can occur
Echothiophate eye drops for glaucoma Insecticides containing organophosphates Chemotherapeutics such as nitrogen mustards and cyclophosphamide	All decrease plasma pseudocholinesterase used in metabolism of ester anesthetics	Increased duration of block with esters (chloroprocaine [Nesacaine], tetracaine [Pontocaine], procaine [Novocain])
Phenothiazines (prochloroperazine [Compazine], chlorpromazine [Thorazine], thioridazine [Mellaril], trifluoperazine [Stelazine]) and butyrophenones (haloperidol [Haldol], droperidol, fentanyl [Innovar])	Reduce or reverse pressor effects of epinephrine	Decreased response to direct-acting vasopressors
Sulfonamides	React with para-aminobenzoic acid, the metabolite of chloroprocaine (Nesacaine) and tetracaine (Pontocaine)	Action of sulfonamides inhibited

Data from Omoigui S: The Anesthesia Drug Handbook, 2nd ed. St. Louis: Mosby, 1995; Rice T: The Physician's Desk Reference, 51st ed. St. Louis: Mosby, 1997; Roisen M, Fleisher L: The Essence of Anesthesia Practice. Philadelphia: WB Saunders, 1997.

patient teaching that was provided by the anesthesiologist and answers questions that are within the scope of nursing in clear, lay terms.

As the patient is being prepared for regional anesthesia, the nurse should explain what is being done, why, and what is expected of the patient. The patient should be told what position will be required and given an approximation of the length of time it will take for the anesthetic to be administered. An atmosphere that encourages the patient's involvement and questions should be maintained. The nurse is a vital support for the patient, who may be anxious and frightened or sedated and unable to respond quickly to questions or to changes in the environment. Explaining the steps of the procedure as they occur can help alleviate the patient's anxiety and keep a heavily sedated patient in touch with the surroundings.

It is important for the nurse to ensure a safe environment in the immediate patient surroundings. Side rails should be up whenever possible, and padding should protect exposed areas of the body and bony prominences from pressure on hard parts of the stretcher or bed. Wheels should be locked at the anesthesia provider's direction. The following items should be available in the immediate vicinity of the block: oxygen and suction; crash cart with emergency medications, supplies, and defibrillator; ECG monitor; pulse oximeter; blood pressure equipment; emergency call bell; and telephone.

Before the administration of regional anesthesia, IV access is established for administering adjunctive sedation or emergency medications. Facility policies differ greatly in the requirement for an IV line when a patient is having a simple local infiltration without the involvement of the anesthesia team. In most institutions, the decision is made individually by each physician, but in some facilities, there may be a policy that applies to all patients having unsupplemented or "straight" local anesthesia.

Even minor local infiltration carries the potential for an untoward patient reaction. Not only can a toxic or allergic reaction occur, but the patient is often not premedicated and may be very anxious. It is not uncommon to have a frightened patient exhibit GI upset or experience a vasovagal response with accompanying faintness, bradycardia, and hypotension.

In one freestanding ASC, after several intraoperative occurrences that required the unexpected involvement of the anesthesia department, the medical director and nursing personnel approached the medical advisory board to establish guidelines that would direct the admitting nurse to secure an IV access on all local anesthesia patients. At first, some surgeons objected to the policy as too aggressive. When the reasoning and historical perspective were discussed in depth, however, the physicians agreed to the guidelines. The nursing personnel at the facility carefully explain to patients that the IV is a safety precaution, and no patient has refused or complained about having a venipuncture when approached in that manner.

Before receiving anesthesia, the patient may receive one or more sedative drugs. The nurse should be familiar with the expected and untoward effects of such sedatives and should explain the intended effects of any medications to the patient. Many people expect to be "totally asleep" as a result of the preoperative medication and are concerned when this "sleep" does not occur. Ongoing cardiorespiratory assessment and monitoring is also required until all discharge criteria are satisfied.

Nursing Responsibilities During Regional Anesthesia

A registered nurse often assists anesthesia personnel with a regional block. The anesthesia provider is frequently absorbed in the technical aspects of the regional technique or is positioned in a manner that may preclude general observation of the patient. Thus, the nurse is required to assist as a primary monitor of the patient's overall status. The patient's sensorium, skin color, vital signs, cardiac rate and rhythm, and respiration pattern must be continuously assessed. Diaphoresis, flushing, faintness, tinnitus, and additional subjective symptoms may herald a complication that can be reduced by astute observation and early intervention.

Patients are frequently sedated or may be anesthetized briefly during administration of a regional block. This is especially important when sensitive areas or multiple injections are required. Nurses engaged in the administration of sedative medications must follow hospital or office policy on which medications they are allowed to administer and the monitoring parameters required. Thiopental (Pentothal), propofol (Diprivan), and methohexital (Brevital) are IV anesthetic agents often used when unconsciousness is desired during administration of a regional block. These drugs are given by the anesthesia provider while another practitioner administers the regional anesthesia. Hypotension, respiratory depression, and prolonged somnolence are complications associated with the administration of these medications. Oxygen is given during the administration of the regional block and until the patient is awake.

As the anesthesia provider begins a regional anesthetic, the nurse ensures that the patient is in the proper position and helps the patient maintain that position by either physical support or verbal encouragement. It is reassuring for the patient to have visual contact with the nurse during the procedure. Maintenance of direct communication and emotional support, such as calm reassurance and hand-holding, are also appreciated. The nurse should remember that the patient is not asleep and, if necessary, remind others to limit conversation to a minimum.

The nurse may act as an intermediary between the patient and the anesthesia provider during positioning or draping. The nurse may need to relay subjective responses from the patient to the anesthesia provider such as wincing, crying, facial changes, and verbal complaints. The nurse also may repeat the anesthesia provider's directions and explanations if they are not audible to the patient.

The patient's privacy and dignity must be protected at all times. Physical comfort can be enhanced with warm blankets and appropriate pillows and padding to support the body, particularly when the patient is required to remain in an awkward position for a long period. Warming of skin preparation solutions can help the patient avoid the shock of a cold solution. The nurse also assists the physician as necessary by securing supplies, holding the patient, moving the light source, opening sterile supplies, and performing various other tasks.

Major complications (hypotension, bradycardia, seizures, respiratory depression) can be devastating. The fact that such occurrences are not common should not cause staff members to become complacent in their preparation and mental readiness. Additional complications include pleural puncture, hemorrhage from an arterial penetration, and cardiac arrest from direct vascular injection. Emergency preparedness is an essential component of nursing care during the administration of regional anesthesia.

Nursing Responsibilities After Regional Anesthesia

After the regional anesthetic has been administered, the patient must be observed closely for expected and untoward reactions. Vital signs should be monitored and the patient's sensorium and level of consciousness assessed. The nurse assisting the patient should move the patient gently and slowly when positioning for surgery, especially after subarachnoid or epidural anesthesia. Anesthetized areas of the body must also be protected from injury, because the patient may have little or no control over the affected extremity. Padding of pressure points is required for surgical procedures, as is protection of the limbs after the procedure until the effects of the sensory blockade have dissipated.

Total sensory loss may be deceiving. The patient appreciates verbal confirmation that the anesthetic has been completed or that the procedure is under way or finished. Some patients who react emotionally may require sedatives or constant verbal reassurance and attention until the effects of the block have dissipated. Music may be a way to distract the patient's attention from intraoperative sounds that can be disturbing. Music has also been shown to soothe patients who are awake during operative procedures, and it has been reported to help reduce self-preoccupation and imagined exaggeration of symptoms.[18]

After surgery has been completed, the affected extremity is assessed periodically for neurovascular status. Assessment parameters include visual inspection, palpation of pulses, skin temperature, and ascertaining motor and sensory abilities. A pulse oximeter or Doppler stethoscope may be useful assessment tools when attempting to determine the adequacy of peripheral blood flow. A more complete discussion of postoperative care for patients who have completed surgery under regional anesthesia can be found in Chapters 20 and 21.

ROUTES OF ADMINISTRATION

Many areas of the body can be anesthetized with local anesthesia. This section presents a variety of regional approaches and the specific nursing care related to these techniques. When administering regional anesthesia, the anesthesia provider employs an intimate knowledge of anatomy, techniques of administration, and pharmacologic actions of the drugs being used and is cautious not to exceed the recommended maximal doses (see Table 14–4). Likewise, the nurse should understand the basic anatomic, physiologic, and pharmacologic factors involved with each approach to provide truly knowledgeable patient care.

Topical Administration

Topical application of anesthetics may be used on skin surfaces, mucous membranes, conjunctiva, the peritoneum, and even on fallopian tubes during tubal banding procedures. Topical cocaine is often used for nasal surgery because of its inherent vasoconstrictive properties. Topical administration techniques can be complicated by rapid absorption of the agent into the circulation; therefore, toxicity must be considered even with this seemingly benign mode of administration. Nursing concerns involve close observation for return of the gag and cough reflex and swallowing after oropharyngeal application. After reflexes have returned, small sips of water should be the first oral fluid permitted under direct observation of the nurse.

Local Infiltration

This simple anesthetic approach involves the injection of a local anesthetic solution into tissues surrounding the operative site. Aspiration should precede any injection to prevent intravascular injection. This approach is frequently adequate as the sole anesthetic for many surgical and diagnostic procedures. Injection at the conclusion of the procedure also offers significant postoperative anesthesia and analgesia. This is especially useful after hand, anorectal, inguinal hernia, and penile procedures.

Epinephrine is generally limited to a concentration of no more than 1:200,000 (5 μg/ml), because stronger solutions can cause necrosis of the skin edges due to profound vasoconstriction. As previously mentioned, it is reduced or omitted in blocks of the digits and penis because of the potent arterial constriction and resultant ischemia and necrosis.

Intravenous (Bier) Block

The intravascular regional approach involves the injection of a local anesthetic into the empty vasculature of an extremity. This is a relatively simple procedure that results in excellent anesthesia for extremity surgery. The drug is held within the confines of the arm or, less often, the leg, by means of a tourniquet and diffuses out of the vasculature to effectively block nerve endings throughout the limb. It is rapidly effective and is usually complete, or "set," within 15 minutes. This block is performed in the OR, primarily because of the equipment required.

The technique is somewhat limited by the large volume of local anesthetic required to adequately fill the vasculature, especially of legs. Another limitation is the restricted time for surgery when the extremity tourniquet must be released to re-establish circulation to the limb. Usually the upper limit of acceptable tourniquet time is considered to be 90 minutes. If a single-cuff tourniquet is used, significant pain can occur intraoperatively at the cuff site, so a double-cuff technique is suggested.[18] With this technique, the inflated cuff is placed over an anesthetized portion of the limb.

For a Bier block, a peripheral vein is cannulated as far distally as possible on the limb to be anesthetized, as illustrated in Figure 14–2. With the patient in a comfortable supine position, a double-cuffed pneumatic tourniquet is placed on the upper arm. The limb is raised above the patient's head and wrapped snugly with an Esmarch bandage from the fingers toward the axilla or from the toes to the upper thigh. This forces the blood out of the limb. With the Esmarch still in place, the proximal cuff of the pneumatic tourniquet is inflated to 50 or 100 mm Hg over the patient's systolic pressure.[19] The Esmarch bandage is removed, and the limb is lowered to rest on the bed.

A relatively large volume of anesthetic agent without epinephrine is injected into the distal vein, and the venous catheter is then removed. Lidocaine is the most frequently used agent for IV regional anesthesia. Other drugs are effective, but several are contraindicated because of complications associated with their use; chloroprocaine has been implicated in thrombophlebitis and bupivacaine in cardiotoxicity and cardiac arrest.

After injection, the anesthetic diffuses from the venous system into the surrounding tissues. Once anesthesia of the limb has been obtained, the distal tourniquet cuff is inflated over the newly anesthetized area and the proximal cuff is deflated. The double-cuff technique helps prevent pain at the cuff site and allows the patient

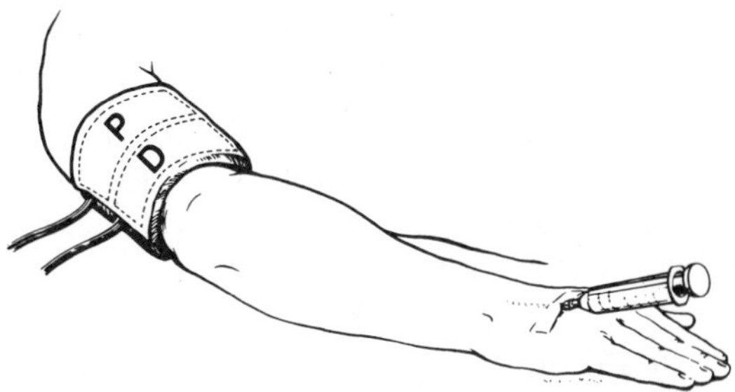

Figure 14–2. Bier block—intravenous regional anesthesia. Intravenous regional anesthesia of the upper extremity using a double arterial tourniquet. P is the proximal cuff, and D is the distal cuff. (From Chung DC, Lam AM: Essentials of Anesthesiology, 3rd ed. Philadelphia: WB Saunders, 1997, p 240.)

to tolerate the surgical period more comfortably. In addition, the anesthesiologist may administer a cutaneous block under the cuff to decrease or prevent pain related to the tourniquet.

Not only does the extremity tourniquet maintain the anesthetic in the limb, it also eliminates arterial blood flow into the limb and creates a bloodless surgical field. When the surgical procedure is complete, the tourniquet is deflated, re-establishing circulation to the extremity. At this point, bleeding may occur at the operative site if surgical hemostasis has not been adequate. Generally, there are 5 to 10 minutes of analgesia remaining after cuff deflation, during which time the surgeon can attend to any small areas of bleeding.

Although it does not produce as lengthy a period of postoperative analgesia as a nerve blockade, IV regional anesthesia is a relatively safe option for extremity surgery. The main complication associated with a Bier block is toxicity from the release of metabolically active drug into the general circulation with premature deflation of the tourniquet. This deflation may be purposeful, after completion of a short procedure, or it may be due to mechanical failure of the tourniquet cuff. To prevent a bolus of active anesthetic drug from entering the systemic circulation, the tourniquet should not be deflated until at least 25 minutes after the initial injection, even if the procedure is finished before that time.

Nursing implications involve careful handling and protection of the affected extremity. After a Bier block of the arm, the patient may be able to move the shoulder and upper arm muscles while forearm control remains poor or nil. If a supine patient attempts to move that arm, it can fall and hit the patient's face. Injury to the face or nose can occur, particularly if a cast has been applied to the arm. The patient should be warned about this possibility, and the nurse should ensure that the patient's arm is supported until neurologic control returns. This is particularly important when the patient moves from one surface to another. A sling is often used once the patient is out of bed to provide needed support and elevation of the arm.

Plexus Block

A plexus is a network of nerves that converge in one area. These nerves originate from the anterior branches, or ventral roots, of spinal nerves; therefore, they innervate motor impulses to effector organs.[21] A number of plexuses exist throughout the body, and a few are amenable to anesthetic block for surgical anesthesia.

The most common nerve plexus blocked is the brachial plexus for upper extremity surgery. Less common are anesthetic blocks of the sciatic and femoral plexus or the lumbar plexus for lower extremity surgery. These are more difficult procedures, because the nerve bundles are not as compactly positioned as those in the brachial plexus.

Brachial Plexus Block

Enclosed in a sheath, the brachial plexus originates from four cervical (C5-8) and the first thoracic (T1) spinal nerves. It runs between the scalene muscles in the neck and supplies innervation to the arm and shoulder. The subclavian artery runs along the same axis as the brachial plexus, making inadvertent vascular injection a real threat. Distally, this fascia sheath becomes the axillary sheath, which encases the axillary artery along with the median, radial, and ulnar nerves. The various branches of the brachial plexus nerves can be blocked using a number of different approaches, for instance, axillary, infraclavicular, supraclavicular, and interscalene approaches (Fig. 14–3). The choice of approach depends on the patient's anatomy, the expertise and comfort level of the practitioner, and the exact anatomic area of anesthesia required for the procedure.

Interscalene

The interscalene approach blocks the nerves most medially, thus providing anesthesia to the shoulder and upper arm. The injection site is in the lateral neck at the approximate level of C6 lateral to the sternocleidomastoid and anterior scalene muscles. Complications of this injection include arterial or venous puncture, accidental subarachnoid injection, phrenic nerve palsy, and the rare potential for pneumothorax.[22]

During administration, the supine patient may be asked to turn the head to the side opposite the block. The chin is tilted slightly upward, and the patient may be asked to reach for the knee[21] or lift the head off the bed against resistance.[23] These maneuvers can help the physician identify the sternocleidomastoid muscle. A nurse can be instrumental in helping the patient to maintain an acceptable position for the block. For the anesthesiologist to be sure that the plexus has been correctly located, a paresthesia is obtained. The patient should be previously

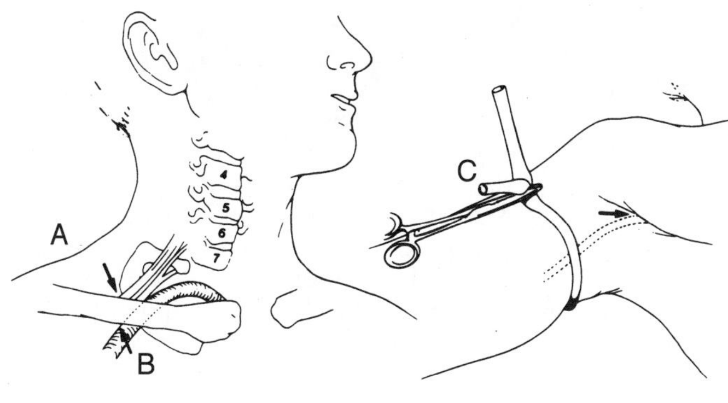

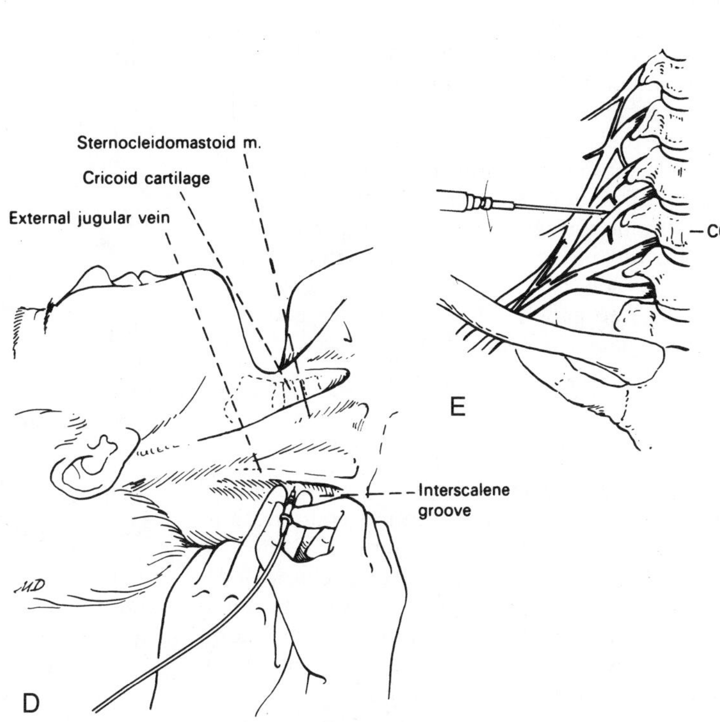

Figure 14–3. Four approaches to brachial plexus block. *A*, Supraclavicular approach. *B*, Infraclavicular approach. *C*, Axillary approach. (*A–C*, adapted from Chung DC, Lam AM: Essentials of Anesthesiology, 3rd ed. Philadelphia: WB Saunders, 1997, p 242.) *D* and *E*, Interscalene approach. (From Bonica J: The Management of Pain, Vol 2, 2nd ed. Philadelphia: Lea & Febiger, 1990, p 1908.)

informed of the sensations to be experienced. The nurse should be supportive if the patient is distressed by sudden, abnormal sensations such as tingling, prickling, pain, or numbness of the arm. The location of this injection site can cause significant anxiety, because the patient may understandably fear having an injection in the neck.

Axillary

The axillary route is the most frequently used approach and is particularly appropriate for procedures on the hand, forearm, and elbow. The lateral aspect of the arm is not blocked using this approach. This is a technically easier approach in which the anesthesiologist inserts the needle in the axilla just proximal to the axillary artery, which is being compressed with the physician's other hand. The supine patient's arm should be supported in an abducted angle of slightly greater than 90 degrees. Some practitioners use a tourniquet on the upper arm to help spread the anesthetic agent upward.

While slowly advancing the needle, the anesthesiologist identifies the appropriate placement by eliciting a paresthesia that radiates to the wrist and hand. A nerve tracking device using the process of electrolocation may be employed to ensure that the needle is positioned close to the nerve. Such a device emits a weak electrical current that causes twitching of the hand and fingers when proper placement is achieved near the nerves. The sensation can be unpleasant but is not usually painful. A volume of approximately 30 to 40 ml of local anesthetic is injected between periodic aspirations to ensure that no vascular injection occurs. The anesthetic is often a mixture of short- and long-acting drugs to provide both rapid onset and prolonged analgesia.

One disadvantage of this approach is the potential failure of the anesthetic to spread out sufficiently to provide adequate block of the nerves. After the injection of local anesthetic, pressure is maintained on the axillary artery for 2 minutes, and the arm is placed at the patient's side.

Complications of the axillary approach are usually related to inadvertent vascular injection. The potential for pneumothorax is less than with other approaches to the brachial plexus, which makes this a particularly popular approach. Onset of action may be prolonged for up to 30 minutes. Therefore, this block is frequently performed in the admitting area or in a dedicated induction room to avoid needless time in the OR while awaiting an effective block. The patient's blood pressure and pulse should be evaluated and documented periodically after this anesthetic block.

Supraclavicular

The supraclavicular approach is considered more likely than others to cause complications and is a less commonly used route. It is effective for procedures of the upper arm, elbow, forearm, and radial aspect of the hand. The technique involves identification of the intersection of the brachial sheath and the first rib. With the patient lying supine and the head turned to the side away from the block, the subclavian artery is depressed and the needle inserted behind the artery. Approximately 20 to 25 ml of anesthetic is injected after a paresthesia is elicited. Motor blockade is observable within 5 minutes in 90% of successful supraclavicular blocks. Because sensory fibers lie within the core of the sheath at this point, motor blockade precedes sensory losses.

The most obvious complication is pneumothorax, particularly if the patient coughs during the injection. Complaints of shortness of breath or objective signs of dyspnea, tachypnea, or aspiration of air into the syringe should alert the practitioner to immediately stop the injection and observe the patient for respiratory complications. A chest radiograph confirms the pneumothorax, which can be self-correcting with bedrest or may require insertion of a chest tube with underwater sealed drainage. Other complications include inadvertent block of the phrenic nerve, which can cause temporary elevation of the diaphragm, and Horner's syndrome with its hallmark ptosis of the eyelid, hoarseness, miosis (pupillary constriction), and dryness of the facial skin on the affected side.[24]

Nursing interventions include assisting the patient to maintain proper positioning and, for some patients, frequent reminders to lie quietly and not cough. Because of the high potential for pneumothorax, appropriate emergency supplies for chest tube insertion should be immediately available.

Infraclavicular

The final approach to the brachial plexus is infraclavicular, another less commonly used technique that also predisposes the patient to pneumothorax. After lateral palpation of the subclavian artery, the anesthesiologist inserts the needle 1 inch inferior to the midclavicular line, directing the needle laterally. As with other brachial plexus blocks, a paresthesia must be elicited for a successful block. Approximately 20 to 30 ml of anesthetic is injected. After the block, the nurse helps the patient maintain a supine position with arms in a neutral position.

Ilioinguinal and Iliohypogastric Nerve Block

This regional block may be used as the sole anesthetic for inguinal herniorrhaphy or as a supplement to general anesthesia for postoperative analgesia after inguinal herniorrhaphy or orchiopexy. Both pediatric and adult patients can benefit from the postoperative analgesia provided, with significant reduction in subjective complaints of pain and use of analgesic medications. Injections in children are accomplished after the induction of general anesthesia. For both adults and children, the block may be performed at the beginning of the procedure to lessen the patient's general anesthetic needs or at the end of the case solely for postoperative analgesia.

With the patient supine, the physician injects an area approximately 1 inch medial to the anterior superior iliac spine on a line with the umbilicus. About 8 to 10 ml of anesthetic agent is injected in a fan-shaped pattern.[25] Bupivacaine 0.5% is most often used in doses up to 2 mg/kg, although a more dilute concentration of 0.25% may be used in an attempt to lessen the potential for complications. There is a manufacturer's caution regarding the use of bupivacaine in children, although many ambulatory anesthesia practitioners are comfortable using it, provided it is administered appropriately.

Although complications are rare, the possibility of inadvertent anesthesia of the femoral nerve presents a problem for postoperative ambulation. Weakness of the affected leg may occur, precluding weight-bearing until resolution of the block. It is essential for the nurse and the patient to be prepared for that possibility upon the patient's first attempt to stand and walk.[26]

Intercostal Nerve Block

Intercostal nerve blocks may be used as supplements to general anesthesia or alone to produce anesthesia of the abdominal or chest wall. The intercostal spaces to be blocked are chosen based on the desired site of action. The patient is placed semiprone with the affected side uppermost. The patient is asked to raise the arm above the head to elevate the scapula. The artery, vein, and nerve are located under the rib's inferior border. After palpating landmarks, the physician injects approximately 3 to 4 ml of local anesthesia under each desired rib along the inferior margins.

Complications of intercostal blockade include the potential for pleural puncture with resulting pneumothorax, inadvertent spinal injection, or hemorrhage from a vascular puncture. Because multiple injections are involved when blocking a number of intercostal levels, the patient may be sedated for this procedure and, therefore, is also predisposed to respiratory depression. During the procedure, the nurse carefully observes the patient's responses, because the physician has only a limited view from behind the patient.

Eye Block

A number of approaches are used to anesthetize the eye for ophthalmic surgery, depending on the personal preferences and expertise of the practitioner. Examples are retrobulbar, peribulbar, the Van Lint and O'Brien techniques, and topical solutions. The first two, which are most common, are illustrated in Figure 14–4. The latter two are supplemental blocks that are infrequently used to prevent patients from squeezing their eyelids intraoperatively. Recently, topical application of local anesthesia has become common for certain ophthalmologic procedures.

Cataract extractions and, to a lesser degree, retinal procedures are common ambulatory surgical procedures, and the use of these blocks is widespread. Depending on facility policy and medical practices of the community, the anesthesiologist, the surgeon, or another person designated by the surgeon may perform the blocks. Facility policy and reimbursement practices dictate whether the patient is monitored during surgery by the registered nurse or by the anesthesia practitioner.

Before anesthetizing the eye, the correct eye must be identified with absolute certainty. Many ophthalmology patients are elderly and often sedated; some may be confused or slow to respond to queries regarding the side of surgery. Before any sedation, all consents should be verified, and the patient should be asked to physically point to the eye on which surgery is to be performed. This eye should be marked in some consistent manner to facilitate proper eyedrop instillation and block. Any discrepancy in the side of surgery requires immediate and thorough investigation before any sedation, eye drops, or anesthesia is given.

When the patient is awake for the local block, the practitioner may begin by raising a skin wheal of local anesthetic before any deep injections. Many people are given a short-acting IV anesthetic such as methohexital or propofol or a brief inhalation of nitrous oxide and oxygen[27] to reduce anxiety and discomfort during the injection.

The intent of any local eye block is to eliminate sensation and movement of the eye for surgery, not necessarily to obliterate vision by a block of the optic nerve. Some anesthetic solution may come in contact with the optic nerve, however, so all or part of the patient's vision may be temporarily diminished during the active phase of the block. The patient may continue to see light and images intraoperatively.

Retrobulbar block involves injection of the anesthetic behind the globe of the eye. The needle may be inserted through the skin of the lower lid, or the lid may be retracted to allow subconjunctival entry without a skin puncture. An awake patient may be asked to look upward and inward during the injection. This maneuver facilitates injection behind the globe but exposes the nerves and other structures that are posterior to the globe to potential damage from the needle. Retrobulbar hemorrhage, penetration of the globe, and optic nerve damage are serious sequelae that can occur secondary to retrobulbar block.

The nerves that control the eye muscles, and thus movement of the eye, may be anesthetized with as little as 2 to 3 ml of solution; however,

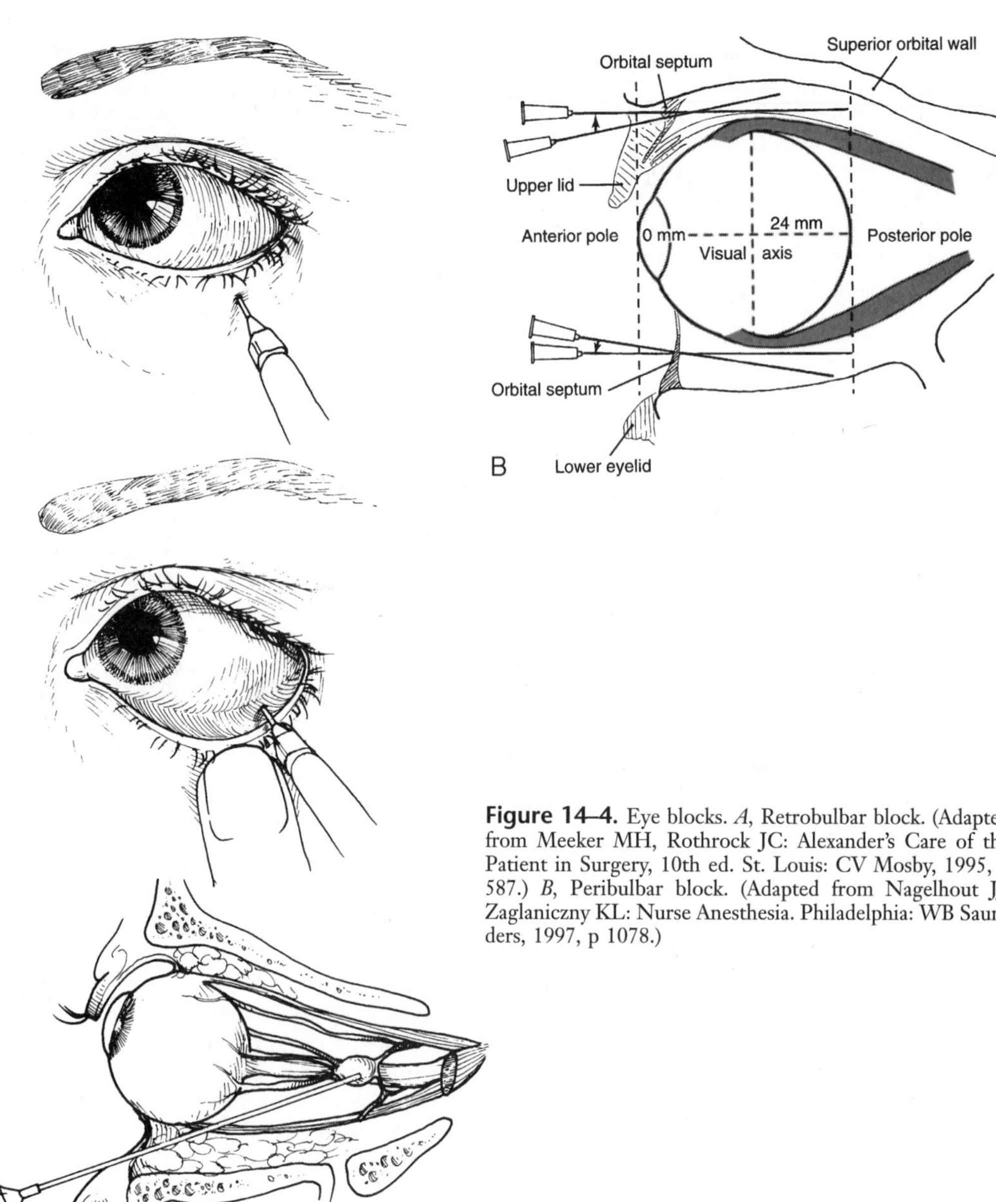

Figure 14–4. Eye blocks. *A*, Retrobulbar block. (Adapted from Meeker MH, Rothrock JC: Alexander's Care of the Patient in Surgery, 10th ed. St. Louis: CV Mosby, 1995, p 587.) *B*, Peribulbar block. (Adapted from Nagelhout JJ, Zaglaniczny KL: Nurse Anesthesia. Philadelphia: WB Saunders, 1997, p 1078.)

it is the depth of the needle that is the most critical factor in a successful block. For a retrobulbar injection, a needle measuring 3.5 cm from hub to tip is inserted to its full depth. A longer needle increases the potential for complications related to technique.[28]

With a peribulbar technique, the local anesthetic solution is deposited beside the globe rather than behind it. Nerves are affected more peripherally with this approach, eliminating or reducing the likelihood of complications resulting from needle trauma behind the eye. The potential for complications is reduced by limiting both the depth of needle penetration and the amount of solution injected. A large volume of solution is a potential source of damage, because it can place excessive pressure on the optic nerve and surrounding structures. A blunt needle is often favored to reduce the chance of cutting a nerve or blood vessel with its tip. The angle of the injection is in a more lateral direction, with the tip of the needle directed toward the bony lateral wall of the orbit.

The peribulbar block is quite effective, and

although the onset of block is slower than with the retrobulbar approach, it has become the favored approach with many physicians. It has few associated complications, although perforation of the globe has been reported.[29] Ecchymosis of surrounding tissues is not uncommon.

Both adjunctive sedation and the inherent effects of the retrobulbar or peribulbar block can cause cardiorespiratory sequelae. Apnea progressing to respiratory arrest that requires intubation and ventilatory support has been reported, as has full cardiopulmonary arrest.[30] Reflex bradycardia may occur as a result of the block or from compression of the eye with a pressure device such as a Honan cuff or a rubber ball used to reduce intraocular pressure before surgery. To reduce the chance of complication, such pressure devices should be used only after anesthetizing blocks have been completed.

Eye blocks are generally performed at least 15 minutes before surgery. If they are done before transfer to the OR, the patient may remain in the care of the preoperative nurse while awaiting surgery. Cardiac monitoring during and after the block is standard protocol in most facilities because of the potential for cardiopulmonary sequelae. Nursing responsibilities in this period include close evaluation of vital signs, respiratory adequacy, and level of consciousness. The nurse should remember that there is a rare possibility of brain stem anesthesia should the anesthetic mix migrate along the optic chiasm to the brain.

After peri- or retrobulbar injection, the patient does not have a blink reflex. It is imperative that the anesthetized eyelid remain closed to protect the cornea from drying effects of the air and from direct pressure by any device or gauze covering the eyelid. It is a good policy to tape the upper lid closed after an eye block until the time of surgery, particularly if eye drops are being instilled periodically after the block. Frequent removal and reapplication of the pressure device creates more opportunity for the lid to be inadvertently left fully or partially open.

Comfortable supine positioning can be enhanced using one or more pillows placed under the patient's knees to help reduce back strain. A warm blanket is often appreciated by these usually older adults. The patient's head must be positioned absolutely horizontally under the operative microscope, so neck and head supports should be arranged to effect that position and to provide as much comfort as possible for the patient, who must remain very still during surgery.

It is not unusual for the patient to have visual perceptions of images and light during surgery, although normal vision is usually blunted. Patients who have not been told of this possibility may become fearful that something is wrong or that the block will not be adequate to eliminate sensation. Patients need reassurance that it is normal to be unable to open the eyelid of the affected eye.

Because ophthalmic surgeries are most often performed under a microscope, movement of the patient's head or bed is magnified and is detrimental to the surgeon's progress. Therefore, the patient's head is usually taped intraoperatively to reduce the chance of movement. The patient should understand that the tape is purely a reminder not to move. This may make the patient feel less restrained and more in control. The patient is also told not to talk during the procedure, because even slight movement of the face or head affects the surgical field. Throughout surgery, the patient should be given verbal reassurance and some means of communicating. Often this includes hand-holding by the nurse or anesthesia provider.

Although retrobulbar and peribulbar blocks are usually very effective, the possibility remains that an incomplete block could result in the patient experiencing pain during the surgery. Without implying that the block may fail, the nurse should explain that the patient can use a hand signal if there is any discomfort during the procedure. Topical anesthetic drops or IV analgesia may be used as a supplement should this occur. Patients sometimes tolerate operative pain because they are afraid or embarrassed to speak up. Objective symptoms of tachycardia, hypertension, clenched fists, or restlessness may alert the anesthesiologist or nurse of the patient's discomfort.

Postoperatively, a patient who has had an O'Brien block of the facial nerve may experience lingering but temporary facial palsy, with drooping of one corner of the mouth. Swallowing can be affected, so nourishment must be given cautiously until the nurse determines that the patient is able to chew and swallow without problems. The patient must be cautioned to eat and drink carefully for the next several hours until the effects of the O'Brien block have completely dissipated. Such a patient also needs reassurance that the effect is temporary. This block is no longer commonly used.

Subarachnoid (Spinal) Anesthesia

Injection of a local anesthetic into the subarachnoid space constitutes a major invasion of the CNS and must be undertaken with great caution by a skilled practitioner. The technique is relatively simple, but it is very effective in producing surgical anesthesia of the lower torso and extremities.

A clear understanding of the anatomy of the spinal column and the relationship of the spinal cord, nerves, and CSF helps explain the concept of spinal, or intrathecal, anesthesia. The spinal cord originates at the base of the brain and is encased within the vertebrae. The vertebral column is made up of 7 cervical, 12 thoracic, and 5 lumbar vertebrae plus 5 fused sacral segments that constitute the sacrum and 4 fused coccygeal vertebrae called the coccyx.

Although there is some variation, in adults, the cord is approximately 17 inches long, has the diameter of a finger, and extends to the interspace between the first and second lumbar vertebrae (L1-2).[31] The 31 pairs of spinal nerves that exit along various levels of the cord control many reflex actions and carry impulses between the brain and the rest of the body.[32] The cord is covered by three layers of meninges, the outermost being the tough dura mater. This membrane is continuous with the inner meningeal layer of the intracranial dura and extends below the distal end of the cord to approximately the second sacral vertebra (S2). Beneath the dura lies the arachnoid membrane, separated by a potential space called the subdural space. A minute amount of liquid lubricates between these layers. Closest to the spinal cord and brain is the delicate, vascular pia mater.

The subarachnoid space between the arachnoid and pia mater contains the CSF and is the space into which the spinal anesthetic is injected to contact the nerve roots that exit through this space. Figure 14–5 illustrates both spinal and epidural needle placement and the relationship of the epidural and subarachnoid layers.

Subarachnoid injection of local anesthetic must be planned so that the intended nerve roots are bathed with the anesthetic solution. Common injection points for lower torso or extremity surgeries are at the L2-3, L3-4, or L4-5 intervertebral spaces, all of which are distal to the spinal cord, which ends at the disk space between L1 and L2 in most adults. An L4-5 injection is called a saddle block, which, as the name implies, anesthetizes the structures that would contact a saddle.

Spinal nerves are numbered, as are the vertebrae. In the thoracic and lumbar areas, the spinal nerve number coincides with the number of the vertebra above it. There is a variation in the cervical spine, where there are 8 spinal nerves and 7 vertebrae. Thus, C1 through C7 nerves are above the C1 through C7 vertebrae, but the C8 nerve is below C7 and above T1 (Fig. 14–6).

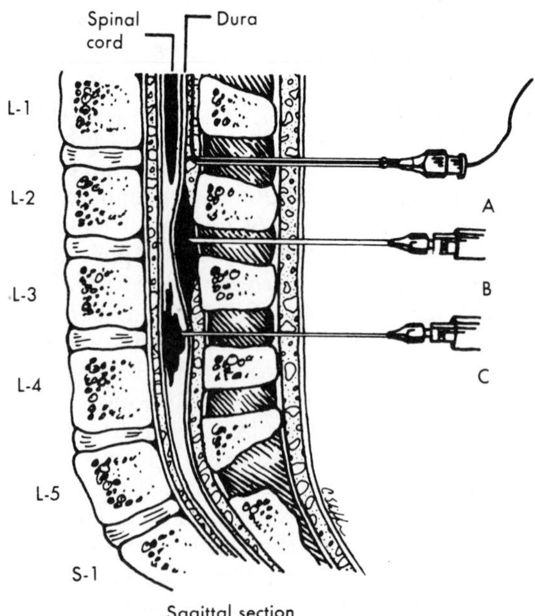

Figure 14–5. Subarachnoid (spinal) and epidural anesthesia needle placement. Location of needle point and injection of anesthetic in relation to the dura. A, epidural catheter; B, single injection epidural; C, spinal anesthesia injection. Interspaces most commonly used are L4-5, L3-4, and L2-3. (Adapted from Meeker MH, Rothrock JC: Alexander's Care of the Patient in Surgery, 10th ed. St. Louis: CV Mosby, 1995, p 169.)

Extending below the end of the cord is the cauda equina, a continuation of the lumbar and sacral nerve roots. These spinal nerves exit the vertebral canal through various openings (foramina) at the lower lumbar, sacral, and caudal levels. Because the subarachnoid space extends beyond the cord, a spinal needle can be inserted below the cord level, thus avoiding direct trauma to the cord, as some patients fear may happen. This is an important point of explanation, especially for fearful patients.

As a spinal needle is advanced, the following structures are encountered: skin, fat, subcutaneous tissues and muscle, the interspinous ligament, the ligamentum flavum, the epidural space, the dura arachnoid, and the subdural (subarachnoid) space. Upon entry into the subarachnoid space, a small droplet of CSF should return to the hub of the spinal needle, indicating proper needle position within the subarachnoid space for the injection. The anesthesiologist ensures this placement and the absence of blood before injection of the local anesthetic.

The CSF bathes and protects both the spinal cord and the ventricles of the brain, so great caution must be taken to avoid introduction of any pathogen or chemical that could injure these vital central nervous structures. Preservative-free solutions are used, and great care is taken to perform this block under sterile conditions.

The position in which the patient is maintained for the few minutes during and after the injection helps determine the nerves that will be affected and thus which areas of the body will be anesthetized. Figure 20–5 illustrates the areas, called dermatomes, innervated by individual spinal nerves. The local anesthetic is usually mixed with another solution, often dextrose, to make it hyperbaric, or heavier than the CSF. Gravity can then be used to great advantage in making the solution move to the intended area, for example, by placing the patient in a side-lying position or by having the patient remain sitting for diffusion of solution to the lower nerve roots. Hypobaric solution causes the opposite reaction—a rising block. This solution is rarely used but might be needed for a patient who will be in a jack-knife position for rectal surgery.

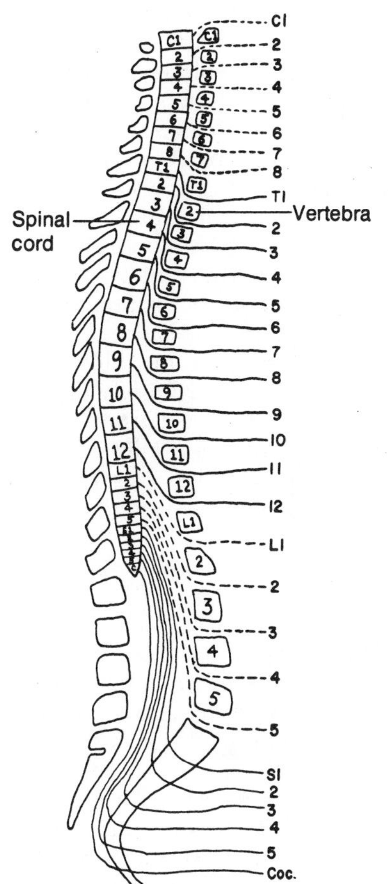

Figure 14–6. Location of spinal nerves. (From Goldberg S: Clinical Anatomy Made Ridiculously Simple. Miami: Med Master, 1997, p 6.)

As with all local anesthetic blocks, the duration of action is determined primarily by the drug used. The choice of agent is a particularly important decision for ambulatory surgery patients, who are expected to be discharged in a reasonable length of time after surgery. Tetracaine is a popular choice for many spinal anesthetics because it is a potent and long-lasting agent that provides anesthesia for procedures up to 150 minutes. Occasionally, it may used in an ambulatory setting if the patient is scheduled early in the day for a relatively long procedure, but most ambulatory surgical procedures do not require that long a duration of action.

Lidocaine is often the drug of choice for spinal anesthesia in the ambulatory surgery setting. It provides approximately 45 to 60 minutes of surgical anesthesia and up to 90 minutes if epinephrine is added.[9] This is generally sufficient time for the type of cases performed, and lidocaine allows the rapid postoperative recovery of sensation, movement, strength, and autonomic control.

Anything that increases intra-abdominal pressure affects the spread of a spinal anesthetic. Pregnancy, intra-abdominal pathology with ascites or tumors, marked obesity, or intestinal obstruction can raise the intravascular pressure in the abdomen, which in turn causes pressure on the subarachnoid space. These situations demand that less solution be used to obtain an effect similar to that in a person with normal intra-abdominal pressure.

In addition, other events occurring at the time of the injection can affect the level of spinal anesthesia obtained. Unexpected coughing, retching, moving, or straining by the patient can increase intra-abdominal pressure and result in a high block that affects the upper torso and extremities. Too fast an injection or too much solution also can result in a higher-than-expected block.

In extreme cases, breathing and consciousness may be affected as well. With a high or total spinal, the local anesthetic reaches near or into the brain. Typical symptoms include hearing or visual problems, unconsciousness, or apnea. Any ensuing respiratory inadequacy is treated with mechanical ventilation until the block dissipates. Although this rare occurrence is a treatable and transient situation, it is frightening to the patient and family, so the nurse must provide special emotional support and ongoing reassurance that the situation is temporary. Sedation may be needed to help the patient tolerate ventilatory support.

Other complications can occur. A traumatic puncture can result in irritation of the meninges, infection, bleeding with hematoma formation, or actual nerve root damage. Repeated injection attempts are often the cause of such sequelae. Neurologic deficits can be temporary or permanent.

A more common complication that follows spinal injection results from the sympathetic effect of the spinal anesthesia. Because autonomic nerves are affected by the anesthetic, profound hypotension can occur due to the body's inability to vasoconstrict the vasculature of the lower body. This is especially true when the level of block reaches T5 or above. Levels only to T10 (umbilicus) are usually not associated with significant reduction in blood pressure.

Hypovolemia significantly increases the potential for related hypotension and complicates its treatment. Because the vasculature is temporarily expanded due to the vasodilating effects of the spinal anesthesia, sufficient intravascular volume is necessary to maintain normotension. Thus, IV therapy is an essential adjunct to spinal anesthesia. Often, healthy patients are hydrated with 500 ml or more of IV fluid before the block. Significant hypotension is treated with increased fluid replacement and a vasoconstrictor such as ephedrine or phenylephrine.

Many patients fear the possibility of post–spinal anesthesia headache because of frightening stories they have been told by friends or family members. The anesthesiologist and the nurse play significant roles preoperatively in helping to mold the patient's positive expectations. The occurrence of postdural puncture headache (PDPH) is most frequently attributed to the slow loss of CSF at the puncture site.

Current technology involves the use of very small-gauge needles with minor propensity for such leakage, as well as needles that are designed to split through fibers of the dura rather than cut them. The size of the needle is considered by some to be the single most important factor in determining the occurrence of headache.[32] Meningeal irritation or infection is another possible, but rare, cause of headache. True PDPH is postural, with increased severity evident when the patient sits up. Treatment of this occurrence is discussed in more detail in Chapter 20, along with other details of nursing care for the patient after spinal and epidural anesthesia.

Nursing responsibilities during the administration of spinal anesthesia include helping the patient to maintain a proper position. Most often this is a side-lying position in which the patient draws up the knees, lowers the chin, and assumes a fetal position. This position effectively separates the vertebrae to facilitate insertion of the needle into the interspace. Patients with osteoarthritis or other diseases that affect mobility and flexibility may find it difficult or impossible to reach or maintain such an extreme position, so they will need encouragement and sometimes physical assistance.

The patient may be in a sitting position for the spinal anesthetic. A stool placed under the feet is helpful in maintaining a curled posture, as is a padded overbed table for the patient to lean against. In the OR setting, these props may not be available, so the nurse may provide physical support for the patient who is sitting on the edge of the OR bed. Occasionally, the patient may experience a transient shooting pain or sensation of electrical shock down the leg when the needle or solution is deposited close to a nerve. Emotional support is important, with reassurance that the sensation is not serious.

After a successful block, positioning for surgery should be done gently and slowly to avoid increasing the level of spinal blockade or decreasing the patient's blood pressure. The nurse ensures that the patient is in proper body alignment, avoiding undue pressure on skin surfaces. An awake patient may need ongoing reassurance of the effectiveness of the block. Adjunctive sedation helps decrease anxiety and awareness during surgery. The nurse also must assure the patient's safety with side rails and safety belts and should be prepared to assist the anesthesiologist with problems involving the airway or respirations.

Epidural Block

An epidural block produces similar effects to those of spinal anesthesia but allows more control of drug dosage, because a catheter may be left in the epidural space for ongoing injections throughout the surgical procedure and afterward. This technique not only allows the physician to control the duration and strength of the block but also allows smaller initial anesthetic doses.[33] Divided doses can reduce the incidence of hypotension, which can occur after a single, larger dose of spinal anesthetic. A single-injection epidural technique is also used. An epidural approach is technically more difficult than a spinal one, but it is a successful alternative mode of anesthesia for pelvic, lower abdominal, perineal, and lower extremity procedures. It has been used for laparoscopy, although it may be ineffective in eliminating shoulder pain secondary to insufflation of the abdomen with gas during the procedure.[9]

With the patient placed in one of the positions described for the spinal approach, an epidural needle of a larger bore than that for spinal procedures is inserted between the vertebrae. This is most often at the lumbar or caudal segment. Because the nerve roots exit through the epidural space, the results of local anesthetic block are similar to those of a subarachnoid (spinal) block. With a lumbar approach, a single 10- to 20-ml injection may be given, after which the needle is removed, or a small catheter may be threaded through the lumen of the needle and left in place. A lower, more caudal site usually requires a larger amount of solution, up to 20 to 30 ml. Chloroprocaine is often used for procedures lasting under 1 hour, and lidocaine, mepivacaine, and prilocaine are effective for 1 to 2 hours. Epinephrine added to the solution significantly prolongs the duration of action and the resulting recovery time.

Complications similar to those described for spinal anesthesia are possible with epidural anesthesia, hypotension being the most common. The epidural space ends cervically and has no natural communication with the CSF or the brain, so the potential for spinal headache is not a consideration with an uncomplicated epidural approach. There is, however, the potential for inadvertent dural puncture with entry into the CSF. Should this occur with a large-bore epidural needle, the possibility of PDPH increases. When an inadvertent dural puncture occurs, the practitioner may inject saline into the epidural space to create pressure that is intended to inhibit the leakage of CSF. Further treatment modalities are discussed in Chapter 20.

Several other infrequent complications of epidural anesthesia are possible. Intravascular injection can result in a sudden toxic reaction. A second devastating possibility is hemorrhage, with the rare occurrence of an epidural hematoma that could exert pressure on the spinal cord or nerve roots. Patients with coagulation defects or those who have been taking anticoagulants are at greatest risk. All reported cases have been associated with the rapid onset of neurologic deficits and severe back pain.[34] This complication can manifest itself with prolonged or returning numbness or other neuromuscular deficits in the postoperative period. An epidural hematoma requires immediate surgical intervention to relieve the pressure. Surgical treatment should occur within 12 hours of the onset of symptoms to be effective in avoiding permanent neurologic deficits.

Nursing responsibilities during the administration of an epidural anesthetic are the same as those for spinal anesthesia. It is also important to help educate the patient regarding the general concepts and effects of epidural anesthesia, particularly stressing the reduced potential for spinal headache with this approach.

CONCLUSION

Nurses throughout an ASC are responsible for the care of many patients undergoing regional anesthesia. By understanding the concepts, anatomy, physiology, and pharmacology of various local anesthetics and techniques, the nurse is better prepared to respond to the patients' needs before, during, and after these procedures.

Some ASC nurses, by virtue of the department in which they work or the practice of the facility, may not be directly involved in the actual administration of regional anesthesia. However, these nurses are often important contacts for the patient before and after surgery. As a result, these nurses' attitudes have an important influence on patients who may or may not be enthusiastic about having a regional anesthetic. One of the ways in which nurses can show enthusiasm for a particular technique is to observe or take part in the administration of all types of regional anesthetics and to gain a personal knowledge of the actual procedures and the effects of each approach. In this way, the nurse can gain both technical knowledge and an understanding of patients' actual experiences.

There are a number of ways in which the nurse can encourage a patient to have a positive attitude about regional anesthesia. First, the nurse should try to ascertain any specific fears or reservations the patient may have. A direct question often encourages patients to verbalize specific fears, which may or may not be what the nurse imagined was bothering them. The patient may need clarification or reinforcement of an explanation that was provided by the anesthesiologist. Many people need to hear that the incorrect and frightening accounts they have heard from friends or acquaintances are not true.

A number of specific fears are common. One is the misconception that the patient is able to see the surgery taking place, so it is helpful for patients to understand that there will be drapes blocking their view. Also, they should know that having a regional anesthetic does not mean being completely awake and that sedation is available and will be provided. Without emphasizing the idea that a regional block may fail, it is also important to encourage the patient to speak up intraoperatively if anything is uncomfortable or if the patient becomes anxious or afraid.

Fear of being left alone without someone to talk to is also common, and the patient should be told that the anesthesia provider will remain at the head of the OR bed within the patient's sight. Along with these explanations, more encouragement can be provided by explaining the many benefits of regional anesthesia, for instance, prolonged postoperative analgesia, maintenance of self-control, retention of normal thought processes and consciousness, quicker reunion with the family, and more rapid return to home.

The nurse plays many essential roles in the care of ambulatory patients undergoing regional anesthesia. Besides completing accurate and thorough physical assessments and providing nursing care related to the effects of the anesthetic, the nurse is constantly providing emotional support during a time that can be fraught with fear, anxiety, and sometimes discomfort for the patient.

References

1. Hardman J (ed): The Pharmacological Basis of Therapeutics, 9th ed. New York: McGraw-Hill, 1996.
2. Weinberg G: Basic Science Review of Anesthesiology. New York: McGraw-Hill, 1997.
3. Miller R (ed): Anesthesia, 4th ed. New York: Churchill Livingstone, 1994.
4. Brown D: Regional Anesthesia and Analgesia. Philadelphia: WB Saunders, 1996.
5. McLeskey C (ed): Geriatric Anesthesiology. Baltimore: Williams & Wilkins, 1997.
6. Conklin K: Pharmacology of local anesthetics. J Am Assoc Nurs Anesth 5:36–44, 1987.
7. Dornette W: Legal Issues in Anesthesia Practice. Philadelphia: FA Davis, 1991.
8. White P: Anesthesia for Ambulatory Surgery. Boston: Little, Brown, 1994.
9. Yao F, Artusio J: Anesthesiology: Problem Oriented Patient Management. Philadelphia: JB Lippincott, 1993.
10. Kost M: Manual of Conscious Sedation. Philadelphia: WB Saunders, 1998.
11. Morgan G, Mikhail M: Clinical Anesthesiology, 2nd ed. E. Norwalk, CT: Appleton & Lange, 1996.
12. Kost M: Anesthetic Management of the Asthmatic Patient. Philadelphia: JB Lippincott, 1993.
13. Omoigui S: The Anesthesia Drug Handbook, 2nd ed. St. Louis: Mosby, 1995.
14. Duke J, Rosenberg S: Anesthesia Secrets. Philadelphia: Hanley & Belfus, 1996.
15. Stoelting R, Miller R: Basics of Anesthesia, 3rd ed. New York: Churchill Livingstone, 1994.
16. Burden N, Iyer J: Local anesthesia: Not always benign. J Post Anesth Nurs 2:45–50, 1987.
17. Association of Operating Room Nurses: Recommended Practices for Managing the Patient Receiving Conscious Sedation/Analgesia. AORN Standards, Recommended Practices, and Guidelines, 1997, pp 149–154.
18. Chandler C: Hypoanesthesia and analgesia. J Am Assoc Nurse Anesth 48:241–244, 1980.
19. Brown D: Atlas of Regional Anesthesia. Philadelphia: WB Saunders, 1992.
20. Chung DC, Lam A: Essentials of Anesthesiology, 3rd ed. Philadelphia: WB Saunders, 1997.
21. Netter F: Atlas of Human Anatomy, 2nd ed. East Hanover, NJ: Novartis Pharmaceuticals, Ciba Geigy, 1997.
22. McIntosh L: Essentials of Nurse Anesthesia. New York: McGraw-Hill, 1997.
23. Brown D: Regional Anesthesia and Analgesia. Philadelphia: WB Saunders, 1996.
24. Kirby R, Gravenstein N: Clinical Anesthesia Practice. Philadelphia: WB Saunders, 1994.
25. Scott B: Techniques of Regional Anaesthesia. E. Norwalk, CT: Appleton & Lange, 1989.
26. Barasch P: Clinical Anesthesia, 2nd ed. Philadelphia: JB Lippincott, 1992.
27. Lichtiger M, Wetchler B, Philip B: The adult and geriatric patient. In Wetchler B (ed): Anesthesia for Ambulatory Surgery, 2nd ed. Philadelphia: JB Lippincott, 1985, pp 175–224.
28. Nagelhout J, Zaglaniczny K: Nurse Anesthesia. Philadelphia: WB Saunders, 1997.
29. Kimble J, Morris R, Witherspoon C, Feist R: Globe perforation from periobulbar injection. Arch Ophthalmol 5:749, 1987.
30. Shirsky C: Complications of Regional Anesthesia. CRNA Clinical Forum, Vol 4. Philadelphia: WB Saunders, 1993.
31. Solomon E, Phillips G: Understanding Human Anatomy and Physiology. Philadelphia: WB Saunders, 1987.
32. Ellis H, Feldman S: Anatomy for Anaesthetists, 6th ed. Oxford: Blackwell Scientific Publications, 1993.
33. Curran M: Epidural anesthesia: Practical considerations. Curr Rev Nurs Anesth 22:170–175, 1988.
34. Patt R, Kaleka L: Recovery from regional anesthesia. In Frost E (ed): Post Anesthesia Care Unit Current Practices, 2nd ed. St. Louis: CV Mosby, 1990, pp 106–117.

Chapter 15

Conscious Sedation/ Analgesia

Jan Odom

Administration and monitoring of the patient receiving conscious sedation (termed *sedation* and *analgesia* by the American Society of Anesthesiologists) have emerged as important practice issues for the ambulatory surgical registered nurse (RN). The practice of RN-administered conscious sedation has become routine with the advent of increased cost-effectiveness initiatives and the ever-increasing responsibilities of the RN. The proliferation of local anesthesia with the use of sedatives and analgesics has become common practice in many areas of the hospital/ ambulatory system. Conscious sedation is being used in the emergency department; endoscopy unit; radiology department; labor and delivery; cardiac catheterization laboratory; critical care unit; operating room; areas for special procedures, such as the postanesthesia care unit (PACU) and holding room; ambulatory surgery facilities; physician offices; dentist offices; and telemetry units for elective cardioversion.

Practice issues must be addressed with any type of new responsibility and practice area for RNs. This chapter deals with those practice issues, addresses the role of the RN in administration and monitoring of conscious sedation, and discusses the pharmacology of commonly used sedatives and analgesics. Quality-of-care issues associated with the administration of conscious sedation also are addressed, as well as certain legal issues. The development and administration of a hospital-wide conscious sedation program also is reviewed.

DEFINITION OF CONSCIOUS SEDATION

The American Dental Association Council on Dental Education was one of the first entities to define conscious sedation as a "minimally depressed level of consciousness that retains the patient's ability to independently and continuously maintain an airway and respond appropriately to physical stimulation and verbal commands, produced by a pharmacologic or a nonpharmacologic method, or a combination."[1] The goal of conscious sedation is not to produce a loss of consciousness, but to adequately sedate the patient to alleviate anxiety, provide relief from pain, produce intraprocedure amnesia, and ultimately to achieve adequate sedation with minimal risk.[2] The patient must maintain protective reflexes and respond to verbal or physical stimulation to adhere to the definition of conscious sedation. Intravenous (IV) conscious sedation is produced by the administration of pharmacologic combinations.

Sedation progresses on a continuum. The following definitions show that continuum:

Light sedation. The administration of oral medications for purpose of reducing anxiety. Normal respirations, normal eye movements, and intact protective reflexes are present.[3]

Conscious sedation. A medically controlled state of consciousness that allows protective reflexes to be maintained, retains the patient's ability to maintain a patent airway, and per-

Table 15–1. Responsibilities of the Registered Nurse

State board of nursing guidelines
National position statements or standards
Specialty organizations position statements/guidelines
Hospital/ambulatory facility policy and procedure
Additional education
Competency

mits response by the patient to physical or verbal stimulation.[3]

Deep sedation. A medically controlled state of depressed consciousness or unconsciousness from which the patient is not easily aroused. There may be a partial or complete loss of protective reflexes. The patient is unable to maintain a patent airway independently or respond to physical stimulation or verbal command.[3]

PRACTICE ISSUES

All states have a nurse practice act that defines the practice of nursing for that state. None of the current state nurse practice acts specifically address the issue of administration or monitoring of patients receiving IV conscious sedation.[4] The issue is addressed by some states as a position statement from the state board of nursing. Table 15–1 summarizes the responsibility of each RN whenever a new practice evolves.

Boards of Nursing

The board of nursing in each state has the responsibility of regulating the practice of nurses in that state. The state board of nursing should be contacted any time a new practice evolves for the RN. Some state boards of nursing specifically address each new practice to define the scope of practice for the RN (Fig. 15–1). Other boards of nursing have a decision-making tree that allows the RN to follow through and reach a conclusion based on the answers to certain questions. Some boards of nursing do not issue specific scope-of-practice statements but instead have a generic statement that for each new practice the nurse must meet appropriate educational goals and demonstrate competency. Other state boards have not addressed the issue of conscious sedation at present.

National Position Statement

The American Nurses Association (ANA) moderated a meeting of representatives from

The appropriately prepared Registered Nurse may administer intravenous nonanesthetic agents for the purpose of conscious sedation during medical procedures provided the following occur:

1. The medication must be ordered by a physician.
2. The physician must be present ("present" means that the physician is either in the room or is in the immediate unit and not otherwise involved in another procedure and is readily available to respond immediately).
3. The patient must be adequately monitored according to currently recognized standards of practice.
4. Whether or not the Registered Nurse actually administers the medication, the Registered Nurse is responsible for monitoring and assessing the patient receiving conscious sedation throughout the diagnostic or therapeutic procedure.
5. The Registered Nurse must not accept or be assigned additional responsibilities that would interfere with patient monitoring activities.
6. The institution must have a policy that addresses: (1) The maximum dosage that may be administered by the Registered Nurse for the purpose of conscious sedation during medical procedures; and (2) resources that must be immediately available, including, but not limited to, resuscitative equipment and resuscitative personnel.

It is incumbent upon the Registered Nurse to participate in this procedure only if:

1. Competency is maintained.
2. Necessary resources are immediately available.
3. The procedure is according to currently accepted standards of practice.

Although the determination of medication dosage and the patient's medical status is a medical decision, the Registered Nurse has the right and the obligation to question orders or decisions that are contrary to acceptable standards and to refuse to participate in procedures that will result in harm to the patient.

Approved 6-20-91/MBN
Reviewed 4-22-93; 12/3/97
Revised 8/19/94

Figure 15–1. Mississippi Board of Nursing: Statement on the role of the registered nurse in administration and monitoring of conscious sedation. Reprinted with permission from the Mississippi Board of Nursing.

several nursing specialties whose members are involved in some way with conscious sedation. A position statement on the role of the RN in the management of patients receiving IV conscious sedation for short-term therapeutic, diagnostic, or surgical procedures was written by those specialty organizations in 1991 and disseminated by the ANA. Twenty-three nursing organizations, including the American Society of PeriAnesthesia Nurses (ASPAN) and the Association of periOperative Registered Nurses (AORN), have endorsed this position statement. The position statement addresses the definition of IV conscious sedation, management and monitoring of patients, and additional guidelines that contain other specific criteria (Fig. 15–2).

Specialty Organizations

In addition to the position statement disseminated by the ANA, specialty organizations also have dealt individually with the issue of IV conscious sedation. ASPAN adopted the aforementioned position statement in its entirety.[5] Other organizations, such as the Association of periOperative Registered Nurses (AORN),[6] the American Association of Nurse Anesthetists (AANA),[7] and the Emergency Nurses Association,[8] have developed recommended practices on monitoring the patient receiving IV conscious sedation based on the ANA position statement. The American Society of Anesthesiologists (ASA)[9] also has developed practice guidelines for sedation and analgesia by nonanesthesiologists, and the Anesthesia Patient Safety Foundation (APSF)[10] has published recommendations for safe administration of sedation and analgesia.

Common elements for the national standard of practice for the patient receiving IV conscious sedation are:

1. Physician or anesthesia provider orders the medication(s).
2. Guidelines for patient management, including emergencies, are in place.
3. The RN managing the care of the patient has no other responsibilities that leave the patient unattended.
4. The RN has received appropriate education and demonstrated competency in the practice.
5. IV access must be maintained continuously in the patient.
6. Minimal monitoring for the patient are respiratory rate, oxygen saturation, blood pressure, cardiac rate and rhythm (electrocardiogram [ECG] monitor), and patient's level of consciousness.
7. Each room must have suction, bag-valve-mask device, oxygen, and nasal/oral airways available.
8. An emergency cart with a defibrillator must be immediately accessible.
9. A protocol has been established for appropriate backup in an emergency situation.[4–11]

Policy and Procedure

In addition to any required protocols, a written policy and procedure governing the practice of RNs involved in administering and monitoring the patient receiving conscious sedation is necessary. Hospital or ambulatory facility policy and procedure should follow any stipulations required by the state board of nursing, standards already set by specialty organizations, and any other national standards and protocols for care. The policy and procedure requires support of administration and should reflect actual practice of the institution. All RNs have a responsibility to know what the policy and procedure for the particular facility states before administering medication and monitoring the patient requiring conscious sedation.

Any policies and procedures should be consistent throughout the hospital or ambulatory facility so that any patient who enters the facility receives the same care, regardless of location within the facility.

Education and Competency

Because administration and monitoring of the patient receiving conscious sedation is an advanced skill not taught in nursing school, the RN is responsible for acquiring the necessary knowledge base and skills required for the task. The hospital or ambulatory surgery facility is responsible for ensuring that the RN who is assigned this responsibility has documentation of appropriate knowledge and is competent to perform the assignment.[11]

The RN who monitors the patient during conscious sedation should be able to demonstrate acquired knowledge in the following areas: anatomy and physiology, pharmacology of drugs, cardiac dysrhythmia interpretation, complications related to the use of IV conscious sedation, principles of oxygen delivery and transport, and respiratory physiology.[6]

One hospital that has an ambulatory surgery service in the hospital and a free-standing am-

A. Definition of IV Conscious Sedation

Intravenous (IV) conscious sedation is produced by the administration of pharmacologic agents. A patient under conscious sedation has a depressed level of consciousness but retains the ability to independently and continuously maintain a patent airway and respond appropriately to physical stimulation and/or verbal commands.

B. Management and Monitoring

It is within the scope of practice of a registered nurse (RN) to manage the care of patients receiving IV conscious sedation during therapeutic, diagnostic, or surgical procedures provided that the following criteria are met:

1. Administration of IV conscious sedation medications by nonanesthetist RNs is allowed by state laws and institutional policy, procedures, and protocol.
2. A qualified anesthesia provider or attending physician selects and orders the medications to achieve IV conscious sedation.
3. Guidelines for patient monitoring, drug administration, and protocols for dealing with potential complications or emergency situations are available and have been developed in accordance with accepted standards of anesthesia practice.
4. The RN managing the care of the patient receiving IV conscious sedation shall have no other responsibilities that would leave the patient unattended or compromise continuous monitoring.
5. The RN managing the care of patients receiving IV conscious sedation is able to:
   a. Demonstrate the acquired knowledge of anatomy, physiology, pharmacology, and cardiac arrhythmia recognition and complications related to IV conscious sedation and medications.
   b. Assess total patient care requirements during IV conscious sedation and recovery. Physiologic measurements should include, but not be limited to, respiratory rate, oxygen saturation, blood pressure, cardiac rate and rhythm, and the patient's level of consciousness.
   c. Understand the principles of oxygen delivery, respiratory physiology, transport and uptake, and demonstrate the ability to use oxygen delivery devices.
   d. Anticipate and recognize potential complications of IV conscious sedation in relation to the type of medication being administered.
   e. Possess the requisite knowledge and skills to assess, diagnose, and intervene in the event of complications or undesired outcomes and to institute nursing interventions in compliance with orders (including standing orders) or institutional protocols or guidelines.
   f. Demonstrate skill in airway management resuscitation.
   g. Demonstrate knowledge of the legal ramifications of administering IV conscious sedation and/or monitoring patients receiving IV conscious sedation, including the RN's responsibility and liability in the event of an untoward reaction or life-threatening complication.
6. The institution or practice setting has in place an education/competency validation mechanism that includes a process for evaluating and documenting the individual's demonstration of the knowledge, skills, and abilities related to the management of patients receiving IV conscious sedation. Evaluation and documentation of competence occur on a periodic basis according to institutional policy.

C. Additional Guidelines

1. IV access must be continuously maintained in the patient receiving IV conscious sedation.
2. All patients receiving IV conscious sedation will be monitored continuously throughout the procedure as well as the recovery phase by physiologic measurements including, but not limited to, respiratory rate, oxygen saturation, blood pressure, cardiac rate and rhythm, and the patient's level of consciousness.
3. Supplemental oxygen will be immediately available to all patients receiving IV conscious sedation and administered per order (including standing orders).
4. An emergency cart with a defibrillator must be immediately accessible to every location where IV conscious sedation is administered. Suction and a positive pressure breathing device, oxygen, and appropriate airways must be in each room where IV conscious sedation is administered.
5. Provisions must be in place for back-up personnel who are experts in airway management, emergency intubation, and advanced cardiopulmonary resuscitation if complications arise.

Endorsed by:

American Association of Critical Care Nurses
American Association of Neuroscience Nurses
American Association of Nurse Anesthetists
American Association of Spinal Cord Injury Nurses
American Association of Occupational Health Nurses
American Nephrology Nurses Association
American Nurses Association
American Radiological Nurses Association
American Society of Pain Management Nurses
American Society of Plastic and Reconstructive Surgical Nurses
American Society of Post Anesthesia Nurses
American Urological Association, Allied
Association of Operating Room Nurses
Association of Pediatric Oncology Nurses
Association of Rehabilitation Nurses
Dermatology Nurses Association
NAACOG, The Organization for Obstetric, Gynecologic, and Neonatal Nurses
National Association of Orthopaedic Nurses
National Flight Nurses Association
National Student Nurses Association
Nurse Consultants Association, Inc.
Nurses Organization of Veterans Affairs
Nursing Pain Association

11-1-91

Figure 15–2. Position statement on the role of the registered nurse in the management of patients receiving intravenous conscious sedation for short-term therapeutic, diagnostic, or surgical procedures. Reprinted with permission of the American Nurses Association.

bulatory surgery facility chose to meet the educational needs of RNs who would be responsible for administering and monitoring the patient receiving conscious sedation by offering a 4-hour workshop at the hospital. A clinical nurse specialist knowledgeable in conscious sedation and the director of education met and developed a format for the workshop.

The clinical nurse specialist was chosen to lead the workshop based on education and experience. The format chosen for the workshop was a 3-hour lecture with 1 hour set aside for a test (to confirm required knowledge of conscious sedation) and hands-on demonstrations at three work stations. The test has a required passing score and can be repeated as necessary. The work stations are pass/fail, with the clinician prepared to teach hands-on knowledge as necessary.

The lecture consists of information based on the objectives of required competencies listed in the ANA position statement (see Fig. 15–2). The nurse attendees receive a packet of information that includes the class schedule, handouts containing information on conscious sedation, and a test to study.

The work stations consist of an airway station, cardiac dysrhythmia station, and pulse oximetry station. At the airway station, the following competencies are demonstrated: chin tilt, jaw thrust, insertion of oral airway, insertion of nasal airway, and use of bag-and-mask device.

The cardiac dysrhythmia station uses a monitor with a simulator to display dysrhythmias that usually are related to respiratory depression. The rhythms that must be recognized are normal sinus rhythm, sinus tachycardia, sinus bradycardia, premature ventricular contractions, ventricular tachycardia, and ventricular fibrillation.

The pulse oximetry station gives the RN an opportunity for hands-on experience. The nurse demonstrates the ability to set high and low alarms and how to troubleshoot the monitors.

The mandatory workshop is offered every 6 months for any new employees or for RNs who may have transferred to the units who administer conscious sedation. The workshop is a requirement before an RN can administer medication or monitor conscious sedation to a patient.

Some ambulatory facilities have decided that the best route of education for the RNs is the self-learning module. The modules contain all the information that the RN needs to know, usually in a format that includes a pre- and post-test.

Ideally, any didactic information regarding conscious sedation is followed with clinical application by participants. The best way to apply new knowledge in the clinical setting is by use of a clinical preceptorship. The participant is assigned to deliver conscious sedation with an RN who is already familiar with the process. The participant observes and then actually begins to administer medication and monitor the patient under the watchful eye of an experienced RN.

ROLE OF THE REGISTERED NURSE

Patient Assessment and Education

Before the procedure, whether invasive or noninvasive, a baseline patient history and physical examination should be obtained. Proper attention to patients' histories and physical findings reduces the risk of an adverse outcome.[9]

Information that should be obtained includes:

- Current medications
- Adverse drug reactions and allergies
- Underlying medical problems, diseases, or disorders
- Family history of diseases or disorders
- Social history
- Height and weight
- Baseline vital signs and oxygen saturation level
- Airway assessment
- Pulmonary and cardiac assessment
- Last food intake (fasting history)
- Anxiety level

A detailed explanation of preoperative nursing assessment is found in Chapters 17 and 18.

Patients who will be undergoing sedation/analgesia during their procedures should have a focused physical examination that includes auscultation of the heart and lungs and evaluation of the airway. Patients with pre-existing diseases of the respiratory or cardiovascular system may need reduced doses of medication for sedation and analgesia because of the risk of depression.[10] An examination of the airway may help predict the patients at risk for airway obstruction should respiratory depression occur, and also may predict those patients who will be more difficult to manage should airway obstruction, hypoventilation, or apnea occur[10] (Tables 15–2 and 15–3).

The Mallampati scale is one tool that can be used to predict those patients who may be predisposed to difficult intubation.[12] The patient's airway is assessed by asking the patient to open his or her mouth and protrude the tongue maximally while in the sitting position.

Table 15–2. Example of Airway Assessment Procedures for Sedation and Analgesia

Positive pressure ventilation, with or without endotracheal intubation, may be necessary if respiratory compromise develops during sedation/analgesia. This may be more difficult in patients with atypical airway anatomy. Also, some airway abnormalities may increase the likelihood of airway obstruction during spontaneous ventilation.

Factors that may be associated with difficulty in airway management are:

- History
  - Previous problems with anesthesia or sedation
  - Stridor, snoring, or sleep apnea
  - Dysmorphic facial features (e.g., Pierre-Robin syndrome, trisomy 21)
  - Advanced rheumatoid arthritis
- Physical examination
  - Habitus
    - Significant obesity (especially involving the neck and facial structures)
  - Head and neck
    - Short neck, limited neck extension, decreased hyoid-mental distance (< 3 cm in an adult), neck mass, cervical spine disease or trauma, tracheal deviation
  - Mouth
    - Small opening (< 3 cm in adult); edentulous; protruding incisors; loose or capped teeth; high arched palate; macroglossia; tonsillar hypertrophy; nonvisible uvula
  - Jaw
    - Micrognathia, retrognathia, trismus, significant malocclusion

From American Society of Anesthesiologists Task Force on Sedation and Analgesia by Non-Anesthesiologists: Practice guidelines for sedation and analgesia by non-anesthesiologists. Anesthesiology 84:459–471, 1996, with permission.

The airway is assessed for visibility of pharyngeal structures (facial pillars, soft palate, and base of uvula), and the degree of concealment is rated. Patients assessed as a Class 3, in which only the soft palate can be visualized, are at risk for a difficult intubation because of poor visualization of the larynx[12] (Fig. 15–3).

Patient Selection

The patient should have a preoperative or preprocedure assessment based on selection criteria that the facility has adopted to assure suitable patients for nurse-administered conscious sedation.

Conscious sedation is appropriate for the patient who has understood the explanation of the technique and willingly agrees to undergo the procedure with conscious sedation. It is also suitable for the patient who has a fear of general anesthesia for appropriate procedures.[13] Conscious sedation may not be appropriate for a patient who is mentally impaired or is uncooperative. The patient who has a profound fear of pain or fears any view of the procedure also may not be a suitable candidate. The physician may decide that these persons are better candidates for general anesthesia.[13]

Possible candidates for nurse-administered conscious sedation must be screened using preset criteria based on medical history. A current frequently used assessment tool is the ASA Physical Status Classification (see Table 12–1). ASA Class 1 or Class 2 patients are always

Table 15–3. Patient Evaluation Findings and Nursing Implications

FINDINGS	NURSING IMPLICATIONS
Pre-existing cardiovascular or pulmonary disease	Reduce amount of medication because of risk of depression
Hepatic or renal abnormalities	Reduce amount of medication because of impaired drug metabolism and excretion
Patient smokes	Increased risk of bronchospasm, cough, or increased airway irritability
Patient is a substance user (alcohol, prescriptive or illicit)	Increased requirements of sedatives or analgesics for required effect
Previous adverse outcome with sedation or general anesthesia	Increased risk for complications during sedation and analgesia

Data from Anesthesia Patient Safety Foundation: Recommendations for Safe Administration of Sedation and Analgesia (Conscious Sedation). Pittsburgh: APSF, 1996.

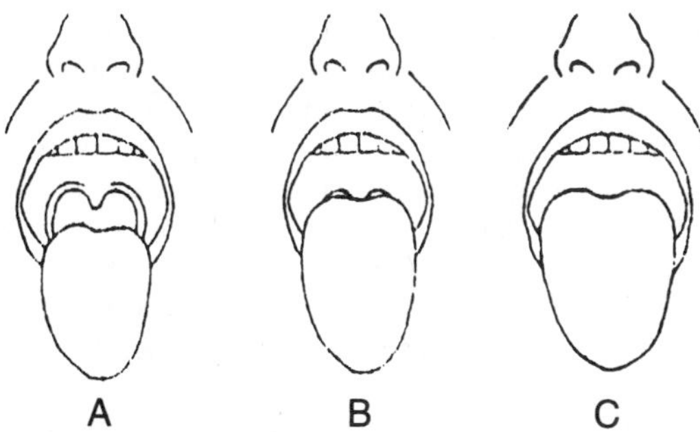

Figure 15–3. Classification of airway. *A*, Class 1: uvula, facial pillars, soft palate visible; *B*, Class 2: facial pillars, soft palate visible; *C*, Class 3: only soft palate visible. (From Mallampati S, Gatt S, Gugino L, et al: A clinical sign to predict difficult intubation: A prospective study. Can Anaesth Soc J 32[4]:429–434, 1985; with permission.)

appropriate for nurse-administered conscious sedation. Class 3 patients may be appropriate but should be assessed on an individual basis. Class 4 and 5 patients usually are not appropriate for nurse-administered conscious sedation.[14] Individual hospitals may have exceptions if the setting is controlled, if the RNs are comfortable and competent with the situation, and if patient outcome is not affected. An example of an exception may be the endoscopy nurse who travels to the intensive care unit (ICU, a controlled setting) with a gastroenterologist to perform a procedure on a patient who is categorized higher than a Class 3. This same patient would not be an appropriate patient for nurse-administered conscious sedation in the endoscopy setting. Exceptions should be monitored carefully and screened for appropriate use. Most patients in the ambulatory setting are Classes 1 and 2, and occasionally Class 3.

Some hospitals and ambulatory surgical facilities have had difficulty deciding which healthcare provider should be responsible for classifying the patient before the procedure or surgery. It is appropriate for the RN responsible for administering the medication and monitoring the patient to classify the patient. The ASA classification system is easy to learn and can be adapted easily for use during the preprocedure or preoperative assessment. The anesthesia department of the hospital or ambulatory facility can serve as a resource.

Patient Education

Conscious sedation can begin the moment the patient enters our environment. It is imperative that we begin immediately to allay anxiety and provide proper information. The patient should be assessed for their understanding of the procedure. Learning needs should be assessed and a plan for education of the patient formulated.

This is also an appropriate time to begin patient and companion education regarding discharge instructions. Some of the medications used during conscious sedation can cause varying levels of amnesia, notably the benzodiazepines. Therefore, after the procedure, the patient is very likely to forget any detailed discharge instructions and must rely on information from the responsible adult and any written discharge instructions. Information given to the patient before the medication is administered usually is retained by the patient.[15] Hopefully, this information, as well as support from the responsible adult, will aid in compliance to the postprocedure regimen prescribed by the physician. See Chapters 17, 18, 22, and 23 for detailed information on discharge teaching.

Informed Consent

Patients who receive sedation and analgesia should be informed of the benefits, risks, and limitations of this therapy, and alternative treatment should be discussed.[9, 16, 17]

Most importantly, the risks of sedation should be outlined specifically during the consent process. The consent form can be a separate form specifically for conscious sedation or a component of an anesthesia or procedure form.

Intraprocedure

Intravenous Access

IV access is a requirement for any patient who receives IV conscious sedation. For patients who receive sedation by non-IV routes, the advisability of establishing IV access should be determined on a case-by-case basis.[9]

Starting the IV line for the patient receiving IV conscious sedation may be the responsibility of the admitting nurse or the nurse in the procedure room. The patient may have IV fluids in place, but at the very minimum, the patient should have a capped accessible IV catheter (heparin lock) in place before the procedure begins. An intradermal injection of lidocaine may be used to numb the area before establishing venous access with a catheter. Buffered lidocaine is available and can be injected with no stinging. A mixture of lidocaine and prilocaine (EMLA) is also available in cream form that can be used before venipuncture, especially for children. However, the mixture must be placed on the skin 1 hour before the puncture and covered with clear plastic dressing. The dose must be measured for the size of the child to prevent a toxic amount. Refer to individual facility policies regarding the use of lidocaine and prilocaine for venipuncture.

Administration of Medication

The medication, which has been ordered by the physician, is given in increments until signs of sedation are present. Commonly accepted signs of sedation include:

- Patient is physically comfortable.
- Patient is slurring words.
- Patient is slightly sleepy.
- Respirations are normal and rhythmic, no less than 12.

If the patient is not responding to verbal or physical stimulation, carefully flick the patient's eyelashes. If there is no response, the patient has moved into deep sedation. At this point, no further sedatives or analgesics should be given. The patient must be vigilantly monitored and observed for patent airway until there is a response.

Patient Monitoring

The RN responsible for monitoring the patient should have no other duties that would leave the patient unattended.[3, 5, 6, 11] National standards require that the RN continuously monitor the patient's respiratory rate, oxygen saturation, blood pressure, cardiac rate and rhythm, and level of consciousness.[3, 5, 6, 11] Initial baseline measurements should be taken before the procedure begins for comparison during the procedure.

Ventilatory Function

The primary cause of morbidity associated with conscious sedation is respiratory depression caused by the sedatives and analgesics. Monitoring the ventilatory function of a patient during conscious sedation reduces the risks of adverse outcomes.[9, 10, 18] Ventilatory function can be monitored by observing depth and rate of respirations or auscultation of breath sounds.[16]

Pulse oximetry is used as an adjunct to clinical assessment to detect hypoxemia. Pulse oximetry also can be used to observe how medical and nursing interventions affect the oxygen saturation of the patient. Hinzmann and colleagues[19] studied the relationship of oxygen saturation and timing of nursing interventions in effecting positive patient outcomes during endoscopic procedures. Data revealed a clinically significant relationship between knowledge of oxygen saturation and timing of nursing interventions.

There should be a clear view of the patient's face. The RN is responsible for observing the airway and monitoring oxygen delivered by nasal prongs or facemask. McKee and associates[20] conducted a study of 100 sedated patients undergoing colonoscopy. Fifty-four percent of the patients became hypoxemic (oxygen saturation <90%) and required supplemental oxygen. Even low-flow nasal oxygen has been shown to reduce the risk of hypoxemia in patients receiving conscious sedation for upper and lower gastrointestinal endoscopy.[18, 21] This supplemental oxygen can increase the reserve of oxygen in the functional residual capacity of the lungs and delay the onset of hypoxia in patients who are hypoventilating or apneic. This can provide an extra margin of safety during which appropriate interventions, such as verbal stimulation, insertion of an airway, positive pressure ventilation, or pharmacologic reversal, can be instituted to correct the situation.[18] Many institutions and ambulatory facilities have chosen to provide supplemental oxygen during conscious sedation for these reasons.

Circulation

Circulation is monitored by assessing and documenting heart rate and rhythm by use of a stethoscope and cardiac monitor. Blood pressure and heart rate should be documented during the procedure every 5 to 10 minutes. Simon and associates[22] studied 730 endoscopic examinations performed using meperidine and midazolam intravenously for sedation. They concluded that use of meperidine and midazolam was safe and provided adequate sedation with proper monitoring of oxygen saturation, pulse rate, and cardiac rhythm in a patient with routine supplemental nasal oxygen.

Medications administered during conscious sedation may directly depress cardiac function or impair the ability of the autonomic nervous system to compensate for hemodynamic changes.[10] Monitoring heart rate and blood pressure at frequent intervals allows any changes to be detected early and treated if needed.[10, 16] A noninvasive blood pressure monitor is important to proper care. Experts differ on the importance of continuous electrocardiographic monitoring. The national nursing standard is to use the electrocardiographic monitor on all patients undergoing conscious sedation.[5, 6, 11]

The practice guidelines promulgated by the ASA suggest that this monitoring should be used in patients "with significant cardiovascular disease as well as during procedures in which dysrhythmias are anticipated."[9] Most ambulatory facilities and nurses who administer conscious sedation consider it wise to use continuous electrocardiographic monitoring on all patients rather than distinguish which patients may or may not need it.[16] Continuous electrocardiographic monitoring allows rapid detection and intervention in the event of dysrhythmias.

Level of Consciousness

The level of consciousness of the patient should be assessed continuously during the procedure. Preprocedure status should be known for effective comparison and assessment during the procedure. Terminology that can be used to describe the spectrum of consciousness may include: alert and awake, sedated and cooperative, asleep and easily arousable, asleep and slow to arouse to name, arousable only to pain, and not arousable at all.[23]

Sedation scores have been developed to quantify assessment of the level of sedation. Most sedation scales were created for assessment of patients in the critically ill setting and not for use with IV conscious sedation. Clark[24, 25] created a sedation scale specifically for use with patients undergoing conscious sedation.

The objectives of conscious sedation have been condensed into five parameters to be assessed: emotional affect, level of consciousness, physical reaction to discomfort or pain, variation in vital signs, and degree of amnesia. The scoring mechanism reflects three degrees of sedation: under, over, or optimal; scoring can range from 0 (oversedation) to 10 (optimal).[24] A pilot study was conducted to determine content validity and reliability of the Conscious Sedation Scale (CSS).[25] Content validity was established, but insufficient reliability was indicated, which means that further refinement of the tool is necessary.[25]

Beth Israel Deaconess Medical Center uses a simplified sedation scoring system[26] (Box 15–1). No sedation scale is perfect, although the scales available can be helpful adjuncts. Ongoing assessment of the patient undergoing conscious sedation is imperative.

Other Responsibilities

In addition to administering the medication, other duties of the responsible RN include:

- Observing for adverse reactions (e.g., reactions to the medication)
- Monitoring the patient's overall response to the procedure
- Acting as the liaison between the physician and the patient
- Monitoring and administering IV fluid
- Assisting with positioning of the patient
- Providing dignity and privacy for the patient during the procedure
- Protecting the patient from environmental harm

Table 15–4 lists a number of appropriate nursing interventions to help reduce the effects of anxiety and fear. These measures contribute to conscious sedation in a nonpharmacologic manner.

Emergency Equipment

Emergency equipment should be easily accessible. An emergency cart with a defibrillator should be available, as well as a positive pressure breathing device, suction equipment, and appropriate nasal/oral airways.

Backup personnel who are experts in airway management, including intubation and advanced cardiopulmonary resuscitation (CPR), must be available should complications occur.[6, 9–11, 17] This is especially important in the freestanding ambulatory setting, where the resources easily available in a hospital setting are not present. Emergency provisions must be in place to safely administer conscious sedation.

Box 15–1. BIDMC SEDATION SCORING SYSTEM

0:	No sedation, patient awake
S:	Sleepy, normal to rouse
1:	Mild sedation, occasionally sleepy, easy to rouse, responds to verbal stimuli
2:	Moderate sedation, frequently drowsy, responds to gentle shake
3:	Severe or deep sedation, somnolent, difficult to arouse, responds to sternal rub

Courtesy of Beth Israel Deaconess Medical Center: Guidelines for Sedatives and Analgesic Use. Boston, MA, 1995; with permission.

Table 15–4. **Adjunctive Nursing Measures to Support the Objectives of Conscious Sedation**

OBJECTIVE	ADJUNCTS TO IV MEDICATION
Reduced anxiety	Preprocedure education, explanations Open communication between patient, nurse, and physician Attendance of nurse-monitor within patient's visual field Touch, closeness, encouragement of caregiver Encouragement to patient to express needs during procedure Decreased environmental sounds and visual stimuli Soothing music, headphones No inappropriate conversation within patient's hearing Warm and private environment
Reduced pain and discomfort	Encourage use of topical or local anesthetics Comfortable positioning, good body alignment No external pressure on body—sheets, heavy equipment, leaning or resting on patient by caregivers Communication (warning) before potentially uncomfortable or painful portions of procedure
Reduced physical risks	Appropriate electronic and nurse monitoring of body systems (ECG, BP, respirations, pulse oximetry) Continuous assessment of level of consciousness Constant vigilant assessment of cardiovascular and respiratory systems Constant attention to airway and reflexes Maintenance of safe physical environment

BP, blood pressure; ECG, electrocardiogram; IV, intravenous.

Data from Zelcer J, White P: Monitored anesthesia care. In White P (ed): Outpatient Anesthesia. New York: Churchill Livingstone, 1990, pp 243–262; Scamman F, Klein S, Choi W: Conscious sedation for procedures under local or topical anesthesia. Ann Otol Rhinol Laryngol 94:21, 1985; and Rothrock J, Meeker M: Alexander's Care of the Patient in Surgery, 10th ed. St. Louis: CV Mosby, 1995.

These provisions should be delineated clearly in the conscious sedation/analgesia policy of the ambulatory facility.[16] See Figure 15–4 for a basic emergency algorithm.

Postprocedure

Postprocedure monitoring depends on type and amount of sedation administered, procedure performed, and institutional policy. The patient is monitored during the recovery phase using the same parameters that were used during the procedure: respiratory rate, oxygen saturation, blood pressure, cardiac rate and rhythm, and patient's level of consciousness. Other assessment factors may depend on the type of invasive or noninvasive procedure that was performed. This assessment may include condition of dressings or suture lines, patency and type of drainage tubes, catheters, receptacles, and the patient's level of comfort.

Criteria should be established for discharge that are consistent throughout the facility for all conscious sedation patients. Patients are monitored until all approved discharge criteria are met. There should be no time limitations, but objective parameters. See Chapter 22 for a detailed explanation of discharge criteria. The same criteria should apply to all patients who have received conscious sedation.

MEDICATIONS

Opioid analgesics and sedatives are the medications commonly used to provide conscious sedation. The RN who administers sedatives and analgesics should be knowledgeable about the manufacturer's directions for usual and maximal dosages, drug incompatibilities, the expected desirable effects, the potential side effects, and the treatment for adverse reactions.

Only an anesthesia provider should perform the administration of an anesthetic agent. The delineation between an anesthetic agent and an intravenous sedative may not always be clear. The only difference may be dose related. Drugs such as methohexital, thiopental, propofol, and ketamine are defined clearly as anesthetic agents and are not commonly considered appropriate for administration by RNs. The RN should contact the state board of nursing for any necessary clarification.

Sedatives and opioid analgesics frequently are given to help the patient tolerate unpleasant or painful procedures and to provide amnesia. The degree of sedation provided can be suited to the

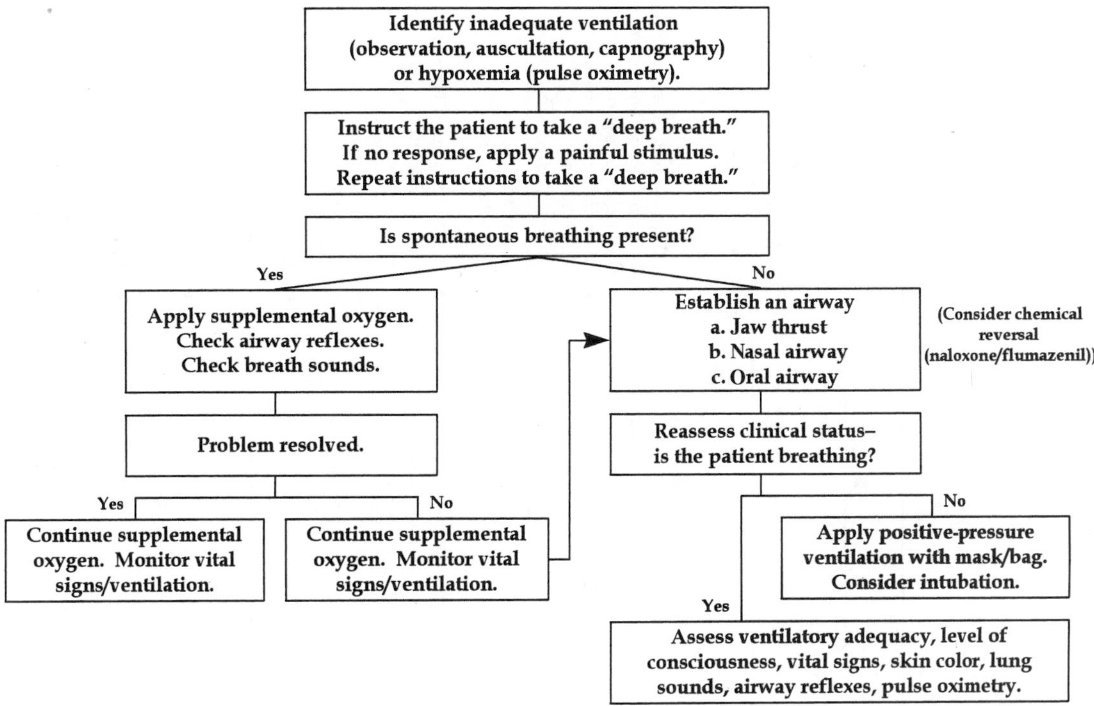

Figure 15–4. Emergency algorithm. (From American Patient Safety Foundation: Recommendation for safe administration of sedation and analgesia [Conscious Sedation]. Pittsburgh: APSF, 1996.)

needs of the individual patient and the type of procedure or surgery being performed.[2]

Sedatives do not inhibit perceptions of pain. They block sensory input but should not be used as the sole agent in a painful procedure.[27] Analgesic agents that cause sedation as a side effect also are not effective alone in a painful procedure. Combining the different agents can produce an effect not possible with each agent alone. These combinations enhance desired responses, but they must be used with caution because of enhanced adverse effects.[27] See Table 15–5 for dosing guidelines on commonly used medications.

Benzodiazepines

Benzodiazepines are used for sedation and amnesia during various procedures. The most commonly used benzodiazepines are diazepam and midazolam. Both drugs can cause anticonvulsant, muscle relaxant, sedation, amnesia, and antianxiety activity.[28] The mechanism of action of benzodiazepines is not clearly understood. They are thought to depress the limbic system and amygdala, where fear, anxiety, and apprehension are generated.[14] Benzodiazepines facilitate gamma-amino-butyric acid (GABA) neurotransmissions, which produce the sedative and anticonvulsant effects. Benzodiazepines also act on glycine inhibitory pathways to produce muscle relaxation and antianxiety effects.[28]

Contraindications are hypersensitivity to benzodiazepines, acute narrow-angle glaucoma, and untreated open-angle glaucoma. Also, concomitant use of cimetidine causes delayed clearance of benzodiazepines.

Midazolam

Midazolam[29–31] is a newer water-soluble benzodiazepine that does not produce pain on injection. It is three to four times as potent as diazepam but has an elimination half-life shorter than diazepam. Midazolam decreases the ventilatory response to hypoxia, and apnea is the most reported adverse effect.[32] Therefore, midazolam should be used intravenously only in appropriately monitored settings that provide for continuous monitoring of respiratory and cardiac function. Resuscitative drugs and equipment and personnel educated in their use should be immediately available.

Other adverse reactions include respiratory depression, apnea, and fluctuations in blood pressure. Hiccoughs, nausea, and vomiting, which can precipitate an irritable airway, have

Table 15–5.* Adult Dosing Guidelines for Conscious Sedation/Analgesia

DRUG	DOSE	ONSET OF ACTION/DURATION OF EFFECT	HALF-LIFE	POSSIBLE SIDE EFFECTS	COMMENTS
Narcotics					
Fentanyl	0.5–2 μg/kg or 25–100 μg IV titrated in increments to patient response	1–5 min/30–60 min	1.5–6 hr	• Respiratory depression • Chest wall rigidity (related to rate of administration) • Hypotension, especially if patient has pre-existing hypovolemia • Nausea and vomiting • Bradycardia	• 100 μg equivalent to morphine 10 mg or meperidine 75 mg • Histamine release rare • Contraindicated in patients taking MAOIs • Prolonged effect with elderly
Morphine	0.03–0.1 mg/kg or 2–10 mg IV titrated in increments to patient response	1–5 min/4–5 hr	1.5–2 hr	• Respiratory depression • Hypotension, especially if patient has pre-existing hypovolemia • Nausea and vomiting • Pupillary construction	• Decreased dose in liver dysfunction • Decreased dose in elderly • Contraindicated in bronchial asthma, respiratory depression, hypersensitivity
Meperidine	0.25–1 mg/kg or 25–100 mg IV titrated in increments to patient response	1–5 min/2–4 hr	3–4 hr	• Same as morphine • CNS stimulation effects including seizures related to metabolite, normeperidine	• Decreased dosage in elderly • Contraindicated in patients on MAOIs • Use with caution in patients with renal impairment
Benzodiazepine Sedatives					
Midazolam	25–100 μg/kg or <60 y: 1–2.5 mg initially over ≥2 min to a suggested maximum of 5 mg; >60 y, debilitated, chronically ill: 1.0–1.5 mg initially over ≥2 min to a suggested maximum of 3.5 mg	1–5 min/<2 hr	1.5–4 hr	• Respiratory depression, especially if given in conjunction with narcotics	• Decreased dosage in elderly • 3–4 times as potent as diazepam • Water soluble • Do not administer by rapid or single bolus administration • Contraindicated in narrow-angle glaucoma

Diazepam	50–150 μg/kg or 2.5–10 mg titrated in increments to patient response to a maximum of 20 mg	1–5 min/3–4 hr	20–50 hr	• CNS depression • Respiratory depression • Vertigo	• Do not dilute or mix • Irritating to veins—do not use small veins • Decreased dose in elderly, debilitated, chronically ill • Prolonged duration in hepatic dysfunction • Contraindicated in narrow-angle glaucoma
Opiate Antagonist Naloxone	0.1–0.2 mg titrated @ 2–3 min intervals (can dilute 0.4 mg/l ml in 9 ml NS and titrate 0.04 mg (1 ml) as needed	1–3 min/30–60 min (depends on dose and route of administration)	30–60 min	If abrupt reversal (med not titrated): • Nausea and vomiting • Diaphoresis • Tachycardia • Increased blood pressure • Pain • Tremulousness	• Repeated doses may be needed
Benzadiazepine Antagonist Flumazenil	0.2 mg over 15 sec; repeat every 1 min up to 1 mg/20 min; may be repeated at 20 min intervals Maximum 3 mg/1 hr	1–2 min/30–60 min	60 min	• Benzodiazepine withdrawal-induced seizures • Abnormal vision • Agitation • Dry mouth • Dyspnea • Fatigue • Headache • Nausea • Hot flashes • Hyperventilation • Palpitations • Insomnia	• Resedation with hypoventilation may occur and require repeated doses

CNS, central nervous system; IV, intravenous; MAOI, monoamine oxidase inhibitor; NS, normal saline.

*These dosing guidelines may require modification for individual patients. Lower doses may be needed if these medications are administered in combination.

Data from Batson VD: Conscious sedation: Implications for perioperative nursing practice. Semin Periop Nurs 2: 49, 1993; Berkowitz CM: Conscious sedation: A primer. RN 60:35, 1997; Gelman CR, Rumack BH, Hess AJ (eds): Drugdex® System. Englewood, CO: MICROMEDEX Inc (edition expired 8/31/97); Golembiewski J: Comparison of selected agents for conscious sedation. University of Michigan Medical Center. Unpublished; Holzman RS, Cullen DJ, Eiborn JH, et al: Guidelines for sedation by nonanesthesiologists during diagnostic and therapeutic procedures. J Clin Anesth 6:273, 1994; Krikorian SA: Intravenous conscious sedation. Pharmacist 22:HS–29, 1997; Somerson SJ, Husted CW, Sicilia MR: Insights into conscious sedation. Am J Nurs 95:30–31, 1995; Twersky RS: The Ambulatory Anesthesia Handbook, St. Louis: Mosby, 1995, p 317.

been reported. Other reactions include coughing, headache, and drowsiness. Less common side effects include laryngospasm, bronchospasm, confusion, and combativeness.

If confusion and combativeness result from the administration of midazolam, the drug should be discontinued, hypoxemia ruled out as the cause of the behavior, and another nonbenzodiazepine drug substituted. A reversal drug, flumazenil, may have to be administered if the symptoms persist after the benzodiazepine is discontinued.

Dosage must be individualized and titrated to patient needs without use of a rapid or single bolus injection. For use in IV conscious sedation, the 1-mg/ml solution is preferred to the 5-mg/ml solution.

Diazepam

Diazepam,[29–31] a lipid-soluble benzodiazepine was one of the first drugs used in conscious sedation.[32] Respiratory and cardiovascular depression from diazepam is minimal, but when used in conjunction with narcotics, depressant effects are potentiated.

Diazepam is poorly soluble in water and is solubilized in propylene glycol ethyl alcohol, benzoic acid, and benzyl alcohol. For this reason, the major disadvantage associated with IV administration of diazepam is pain and venoirritation at the injection site. Venous thrombosis and phlebitis also have been reported. Diazepam should be injected slowly, taking at least 1 minute for each 5 mg given to reduce the possibility of venous thrombosis, phlebitis, local irritation, swelling, and vascular impairment. Larger veins should be used, and diazepam should not be mixed with other solutions or drugs.

Common reported side effects of diazepam are drowsiness, fatigue, and ataxia. Other adverse reactions that have been reported less frequently are confusion, headache, nystagmus, respiratory depression, and laryngospasm.

Diazepam has an elimination half-life of 24 to 48 hours. It is metabolized in the liver to produce desmethyldiazepam and oxazepam, active metabolites that contribute to prolonged effects of diazepam, especially in the presence of liver or renal dysfunction. The introduction of shorter-acting benzodiazepines has diminished its use in the ambulatory setting.[18, 32]

Opioids

Opioids are used frequently in conjunction with sedatives for pain relief. All opioids interact with opioid receptors to produce analgesia and sedation. This interaction with the opioid receptors produces a state of decreased pain sensation and a decrease in general awareness.[27]

The level of comfort of the patient should be assessed continually during and after the procedure. The patient may be able to express the need for more pain relief. Objective signs of pain also may be seen, such as tearing of the eyes, grimacing, agitation, increases in blood pressure or respiration, or muscle rigidity.[33]

With all narcotics, there is a risk of respiratory depression that can progress to apnea. The risk increases with the dose and rate of administration. Common side effects associated with most opioids include hypotension, nausea, vomiting, constipation, increased pressure in the biliary tract, urinary retention, dizziness, mental clouding, dysphoria, and pruritus. All opioids are metabolized in the liver.

Fentanyl

Fentanyl[29–31] can be used as a supplement to local/regional anesthesia or postoperative pain or as an anesthesia adjunct. The dosage used determines the indication. Because fentanyl is lipophilic and crosses the blood-brain barrier quickly, the onset of the analgesic action of fentanyl occurs within 2 minutes of IV administration. Fentanyl lasts up to 1 hour, after which 99% of fentanyl is cleared from the body. However, the duration of the respiratory depressant effect of fentanyl may last longer than the analgesic effect.

Advantages of fentanyl include less emetic activity than either morphine sulfate or meperidine. Fentanyl also causes no significant histamine release. Contraindications to fentanyl are hypersensitivity, cardiac bradyarrhythmias, head injury or increased intracranial pressure, hepatic function impairment or cirrhosis, and respiratory impairment.

The adverse reactions associated with fentanyl include respiratory depression, apnea, bradycardia, and muscle rigidity. Muscle rigidity usually involves chest wall rigidity that includes the muscles of respiration. When this rare phenomenon occurs, anesthesia assistance should be sought because it is very difficult and sometimes impossible to ventilate the patient. At that point, backup in airway management must be initiated. The patient may be intubated at that time, or a dose of succinylcholine may be given with the patient ventilated by mask. The rigidity is a temporary condition that dissipates as the medication is cleared from the body. The muscle rigidity is a rare but life-threatening reaction that usually is associated with rapid administration of the medication. Other side effects noted have been hypertension, hypotension, dizziness, blurred vision, nausea, emesis, laryngospasm, and diaphoresis.

Meperidine and Morphine Sulfate

Meperidine and morphine sulfate[28–31] are used for treatment of pain and as an adjunct to anesthesia or conscious sedation. Both opioids are hydrophilic and therefore pass into the central nervous system more slowly than fentanyl. Maximal analgesic and respiratory depressant effects occur after several minutes. Morphine is the prototypical opioid analgesia agent. Morphine sulfate 10 mg is equivalent to meperidine 100 mg and fentanyl 100 μg.[34] Meperidine is a synthetic opioid analgesic. Advantages of morphine sulfate are its reduction of left ventricular work index and decreased anxiety.

Morphine sulfate is metabolized in the liver to its major metabolites, morphine-3-glucuronide, which is inactive, and morphine-6-glucuronide, which is pharmacologically active, more potent than meperidine, and has a slightly longer half-life than morphine. If renal compromise occurs, this metabolite can accumulate and lead to prolonged sedation.

Meperidine is metabolized to its major metabolite, normeperidine, which has a half-life of 15 to 20 hours, a longer half-life than meperidine. Normeperidine also can accumulate in renal failure or hepatic failure. Accumulation of normeperidine has been associated with tremors, muscle twitches, dilated pupils, hyper-reactive reflexes, and seizures. The elderly are especially susceptible to these effects.[35]

Contraindications include patients receiving monoamine oxidase (MAO) inhibitors and patients who have had severe allergic reactions. These opioid medications should be used with caution in patients with acute asthma and chronic obstructive pulmonary disease because they decrease respiratory reserve and with patients experiencing supraventricular tachycardia and atrial flutter because a possible vagolytic action may produce an increase in ventricular response rate. These medications also may aggravate pre-existing convulsions.

The most serious side effect of any opioid is sudden respiratory depression. The effects of any opioid can be potentiated when given in conjunction with sedatives.[33] Other adverse effects may include nausea and vomiting, urinary retention, blurred vision, and diaphoresis. Histamine release may produce vasodilatation, leading to hypotension, especially in the presence of hypovolemia, and allergic reactions, leading to an irritable airway.

Reversal Agents

Immediate accessibility to reversal agents is necessary to ensure patient safety if respiratory depression associated with IV conscious sedation develops. Daneshmend and colleagues[36] discovered that severe hypoventilation was the most frequently reported adverse outcome after conducting a nationwide survey on sedation for upper gastrointestinal endoscopy.

Naloxone

Naloxone[28–31] is a semisynthetic opioid antagonist that has an affinity for all three opioid receptor sites and competitively binds at those sites. Naloxone is indicated to reverse sedation and respiratory depression caused by opioid drugs. The only contraindication is a hypersensitivity to naloxone. If respiratory depression occurs, other resuscitative measures should be initiated as well as administration of naloxone.

Importantly, naloxone must be titrated when administered to the patient. The object is to reverse enough of the opioid to alter the respiratory depression but not so much that there is no pain relief. Desirable reversal results in alertness and adequate ventilation without discomfort.[33]

The duration of action is shorter than the opioids, so the patient should be observed for any further respiratory depression. If respiratory depression reoccurs, the patient may need additional reversal. The chance of reoccurrence seems to be opioid dose related. When naloxone is administered too quickly or in high doses, the patient may experience hypertension, emergence delirium, vomiting, tachycardia, and pain on reversal. The patient then is unable to experience any pain relief for a designated period of time that may last up to 1 hour. Naloxone also has been implicated in naloxone-induced noncardiogenic pulmonary edema.[37]

Flumazenil

Flumazenil[28–30, 32, 38] is a specific benzodiazepine antagonist that reverses central effects of benzodiazepines by competitively inhibiting the GABA receptor sites. Flumazenil reverses sedation and hyponosis without reversing amnesia and anxiolysis. Depression of ventilatory response to carbon dioxide (CO_2) and to hypoxia also may not be reversed completely. Therefore, the initial treatment for hypoventilation should be assisted ventilation. Hypoventilation may improve at times after flumazenil simply because the patient is awakening.

Use of flumazenil is contraindicated when hypersensitivity to benzodiazepines or flumazenil is present, when benzodiazepines have been given to control potentially life-threatening conditions, and in patients who show signs of serious cyclic antidepressant overdose. The most serious side effect noted with flumazenil has been seizures. Seizures, however, are most frequent in patients receiving benzodiazepines for long-term sedation and patients showing signs of serious cyclic antidepressant overdose. More frequently associated adverse effects include dizziness, pain at the injection site, diaphoresis, headache, and abnormal or blurred vision.

A patient can become resedated up to 2 hours after the initial respiratory depression, so an ambulatory patient should not be discharged prematurely. Nursing vigilance is required to observe the patient for resedation and ensure that the patient has met discharge criteria and leaves in the presence of a responsible adult. The reoccurrence of resedation seems to be dose related.

COMPLICATIONS

Common complications or emergencies that can occur with conscious sedation include respiratory depression causing hypoxia or hypercarbia, respiratory obstruction, cardiovascular complications such as dysrhythmias, hypotension, hypertension, and allergies or toxicity reactions to the medications. The RN should be knowledgeable in the management of these complications, and back-up assistance for emergencies should be spelled out in the hospital policies and procedures. See Chapter 11 for further detailed information on management of complications.

QUALITY ISSUES

Joint Commission on Accreditation of Healthcare Organizations

The Joint Commission on Accreditation of Healthcare Organizations (JCAHO) has been looking specifically at conscious sedation issues for the past several years. The issue of sedation versus anesthesia has been at the forefront.

JCAHO wants to see consistency in the care of all patients who receive conscious sedation. Every patient who enters a healthcare organization to receive conscious sedation should receive the same care preprocedure, intraprocedure, and postprocedure. Ideally, the healthcare organization/ambulatory facility has only one policy and procedure in place for all patients who are to receive conscious sedation.

Conscious sedation in every facility needs to be clearly defined. JCAHO states that, "Because conscious sedation is a continuum, it is not always possible to predict how an individual patient receiving sedation will respond."[3, 39, 40] JCAHO goes on to say that each organization should have specific protocols governing the care of the patient undergoing sedation. They expect a multidisciplinary approach to establishment of these protocols, and further specify that those protocols should address the areas of sufficient qualified personnel, appropriate equipment and monitoring of vital signs, documentation, and monitoring of outcomes[3, 39, 41] (Box 15–2).

Quality Improvement

Any areas that administer or monitor patients who have had conscious sedation also should have quality monitors in place to determine the quality of care or to improve the existing care. Monitors can include complications during the procedure, adherence to policy and procedure, infiltration of IV fluid, and discharge teaching. Other monitors may include selection of appropriate patients and amounts of medication administered. One important outcome monitor is to determine the percentage of patients who undergo procedures under conscious sedation who inadvertently become deeply sedated. The indicators to use in the study would be based on the definition of conscious sedation as main-

Box 15–2. JCAHO REQUIREMENTS FOR CONSCIOUS SEDATION/ANALGESIA

- Sufficient qualified personnel
- Appropriate equipment for care and resuscitation
- Appropriate monitoring of vital signs and oxygenation
- Outcome monitoring

taining protective reflexes and maintaining ability to respond to verbal or physical stimulation. Information can be obtained from the patient charts (retrospective), documentation as it occurs (prospective), and postprocedure telephone follow-up calls.

PEDIATRIC CONSIDERATIONS

The definition of the pediatric patient varies from younger than 13 years to younger than 18 years to those patients younger than 21 years of age.[42, 43] The specific age of the "pediatric patient" in each facility can be defined by that facility.

Criteria of selection for conscious sedation for the pediatric patient are nearly the same as for the adult. The differences involve age, weight, and cooperation. The facility may have a policy that defines the age at which various procedures may be performed under conscious sedation. For example, one pediatric gastroenterologist will perform an upper endoscopy on a child older than 7 years of age and a lower endoscopy on a child older than 7 to 10 years of age based on the length of the procedure.[44] Depending on the procedure to be performed, size of anatomic structures may be important. For example, in upper endoscopy, small children are not good candidates because the endoscope compresses the trachea, leading to airway obstruction and respiratory compromise.

Ability to cooperate is obviously an important criterion. The child's level of maturity and ability to understand play an important role in cooperation, regardless of age, sex, or procedure. The level of cooperation can be improved with proper patient preparation and help of the parents.[44]

Communication and Rapport

Rapport should be built with the pediatric patient before the procedure. Some guidelines for communicating with children include assuming an eye-level position, speaking in a quiet, unhurried manner, using simple words and short sentences, allowing children time to feel comfortable, and avoiding sudden or rapid advances that may be seen as threatening. Be honest with children and offer choices only when a choice exists.[45]

Explain the procedure to the child using the child's name. Preparing the child for a procedure decreases anxiety and promotes cooperation.[45] Explain all the noises that the child will hear in the room, such as the cardiac monitor, and allow the child to have a security object during the procedure. The child also may be assigned a task such as watching the numbers on the monitor. Other coping strategies can include relaxing, breathing, counting, squeezing a hand, or singing.[45]

If the parents will be present during the procedure, explain what to expect before the procedure, and tell the parent exactly what to do during the procedure. The parent may be given a task, such as sitting next to the child's face and talking to the child. Avoid using the parent for any type of restraint.

Patient Assessment

Monitoring requirements for the pediatric patient are the same as for the adult. Minimal monitoring requirements include respiratory rate, oxygen saturation, blood pressure, cardiac rate and rhythm, and level of consciousness. However, any change from baseline can be significant in the pediatric patient. The pediatric patient does not have physiologic reserves of the adult, and the physiologic status can deteriorate two or three times faster than that of the adult.[42]

Airway management is critical in the pediatric patient. During sedation, the head and neck position and chest movement should be assessed as well as other requirements previously described for the adult. It also may be important to determine whether these children have been exposed regularly to environmental tobacco smoke (ETS). Massand[46] reported that almost half of children exposed regularly to ETS needed oxygen therapy after surgery with general anesthesia compared with 1 in 20 children not exposed to ETS. Also, children exposed to ETS may be at greater risk for laryngospasm. If restraints are in place, frequent observation is necessary to assess circulation in the extremities. The patient also may be at risk for airway compromise and chest restriction with a restraint.

All monitoring equipment should be sized correctly for the pediatric patient and any alarm parameters set for the patient's age. All emergency equipment also must be size and age appropriate and immediately available, including the defibrillator, which should have pediatric paddles.

Thermoregulation is an important issue when caring for a sedated child. The younger child may have a greater heat loss than an adult. A neutral thermal environment and frequent monitoring of temperature should be maintained during the procedure.[47] Other goals of pediatric patient assessment include: guarding the patient's safety and welfare, maximizing amnesia, providing analgesia to decrease the negative psychologic responses, controlling the patient's behavior, and returning the patient to baseline health status.[43]

Medication for the Pediatric Patient

Appropriate relief of pain and anxiety for the pediatric patient is one of the goals of sedation and analgesia. The need for appropriate relief of pain and anxiety in the pediatric population is even more significant because of exaggerated responses.[27] See Table 15–6 for dosing guidelines for the pediatric patient.

Klooster and colleagues conducted a study to determine the age-related dosage range of midazolam in children. The authors concluded that the dosage of midazolam varies as a function of age similar to diazepam. They discovered that adolescents have dose requirements similar to adults. However, children 2 to 6 years of age require the highest doses to achieve sedation.[48]

Discharge Criteria

Objective, specified discharge criteria must be met before a child who has received conscious sedation/analgesia can be discharged. These discharge criteria should include stable respiratory and cardiovascular function, patient is easily arousable (can talk and sit up, if appropriate), and state of hydration is adequate.[43]

Parents or the responsible adult should receive verbal and written instructions. The responsible adult also must understand the importance of having another person sit with an infant/toddler on the drive home and monitor for adverse effects. Three deaths or neurologic devastations that occurred in a car on the way home have been reported.[49] These deaths or devastations possibly could have been prevented if specific discharge instructions had been given about residual effects of the medication and maintenance of a good head position to avoid airway obstruction.[49]

A detailed description of the pediatric patient is available in Chapter 26.

GERIATRIC CONSIDERATIONS

The geriatric population is defined legally as persons older than 65 years of age.[42] In terms of conscious sedation, some patients may be younger, have a multitude of diseases, and have aged more quickly than chronologic age indicates. There are also very healthy, robust older persons in their 70s. By the year 2000, 13% of the population consists of persons older than 65

Table 15–6. Pediatric Dosages

DRUG	DOSAGE	ROUTE
Meperidine	0.5–1 mg/kg (maximum dosage 2 mg/kg)	IV/IM
Morphine	0.05–0.1 mg/kg (maximum dosage 0.2 mg/kg)	IV/IM
	0.3 mg/kg	PO
Fentanyl	1–2 μg/kg (maximum dosage 4–5 μg/kg)	IV/IM
	5–15 μg/kg	PO (Oralet)
Diazepam	0.1–0.3 mg/kg (maximum dosage 10 mg)	IV
Midazolam	0.05 mg/kg every 5–10 min to a maximum of 0.1 mg/kg	IV
	0.5 mg/kg	PO
	0.2 mg/kg	Nasal
	1 mg/kg	Rectal
Chloral hydrate	25–50 mg/kg (small infants up to 12 mo)	PO
	25–75 mg/kg (children older than 12 mo)	
Naloxone	10 μg/kg (repeat at 2- to 3-min intervals to reversal)	IV/IM/SC
Flumazenil	10 μg/kg	IV

IM, intramuscular; IV, intravenous; PO, per os (by mouth); SC, subcutaneous.

Data from Acute Pain Management Guideline Panel: Acute pain management in infants, children, and adolescents: Operative and Medicare procedures. AHCPR Pub. NA. 92 - 0020. Rockville, MD: AHCPR, Public Health Service, U.S. Dept. of Health and Human Services; Gelman CR, Rumack BH, Hess AJ (eds): Drugdex® System. Englewood, CO: MICROMEDEX Inc (Edition expired 8/31/97); Golembiewski J: Comparison of selected agents for conscious sedation. University of Michigan Medical Center. Unpublished; Hill KJ, Anderson C: Pediatric pain management: Clinical aspects for the nineties. Semin Anesthesiol 16:142, 1997; Sacchetti A, Schafermeyer R, Gerardi J, et al: Pediatric analgesia and sedation. Ann Emerg Med 23:241, 1994; Twersky R: The Ambulatory Anesthesia Handbook, St. Louis: Mosby, 1995, pp 149, 163, 348–349.

years of age, and by the year 2030, it is projected to be 17%.[42]

Care of the geriatric patient during conscious sedation is of significance because of the physiologic changes that occur during later years. Disease processes that have afflicted the patient play a very important role in increasing the risk of IV conscious sedation. The patient should be assessed for a history of cardiovascular disease, including hypertension, congestive heart failure, and myocardial infarctions. The older patient also should be assessed for respiratory disease processes, such as chronic obstructive pulmonary disease and renal and disease processes.

Onset of IV agents is slowed, and an increased duration of action occurs because of decreased cardiac output and resulting decreased circulation times. The respiratory system is affected by advancing age, leading to increased secretions and airway resistance. Increased susceptibility of the older person to central nervous system side effects of drugs is the result of atrophic changes that interfere with the basic neuronal process. Decreased glomerular filtration rate and renal blood flow cause decreased drug clearance and increased drug half-life and duration. The geriatric patient is also susceptible to fluid overload. There is a reduction in the biotransformation actions of the liver, which leads to increased drug half-life and duration of action.[42] According to Darling:

"Elderly patients have an increased variability of drug response.
Elderly patients have a decreased requirement for most anesthetic drugs.
Elderly patients have a prolonged redosing interval."[50]

Clinically, the RN responsible for administering and monitoring the older patient receiving conscious sedation should be prepared to use smaller dosages of medications, as ordered by the physician, and titrate these medications very slowly. A decreased clearance rate and increased duration of effect of the medication should be expected.

Monitor oxygen saturation closely. Keep the head of the bed elevated, if possible, and encourage deep breaths as often as possible. Maintain normothermia to aid in drug clearance. The normal thermoregulatory system is impaired with age. The elderly patient cools more quickly and rewarms slower than the younger adult. Complications with hypothermia can include myocardial or cerebral ischemia, respiratory acidosis, and hypoxia.[50] Monitor the older patient for hypertension and hypotension and be prepared to intervene quickly to restore blood pressure to normal levels. Monitor the urinary output along with the amount of fluid administered to the patient. Speak loudly and clearly if the patient has hearing loss.[42] Refer to Chapter 27 for detailed discussion of the older adult in the ambulatory setting.

RISK MANAGEMENT/LEGAL ISSUES

Risk management is aimed at prevention of injuries and minimizing losses when injuries do occur.[51] The risk management process for use with sedation/analgesia is familiar to nurses: assessment, planning, intervention, and evaluation. This process must be applied continuously and consistently at all times during the period of sedation. As Dlugose says, " . . . it is almost impossible to separate risk management from good patient care."[52]

In a discussion of risk management or legal issues, one invariably returns to the practice issues discussed at the beginning of the chapter. Each nurse must know state regulations issued by the state board of nursing. The RN also should be aware of any national standards and become knowledgeable of the standards, policies, and procedures of the nurse's facility. Professional organizations that represent nursing specialities that deal with conscious sedation also may have guidelines and standards.[53]

When dealing with risk management issues, St. Paul Fire and Marine Insurance Company recommended to more than 1000 of its insured hospitals that risk management efforts concentrate on services in which conscious sedation is used. The recommendation suggested focusing on four issues during risk assessment: trained staff, knowledge and use of the drug, established protocols and patient selection criteria for conscious sedation, and quality assurance monitoring.[54] See Table 15–7 for areas of liability for the nurse during conscious sedation/analgesia and methods to prevent liability from occurring.

CURRENT CONTROVERSIES

Administration of Anesthetic Agents

In most states, the state board of nursing does not permit the administration of anesthetic agents, such as ketamine, propofol, and methohexital. The controversy that exists is caused by the apparent sedative effect, as opposed to

***Table 15–7.* Risk/Liability Issues and Methods of Prevention**

Medication administration
- Titration of drugs to prevent deep sedation
- Availability of antagonists for reversal if needed
- Constant monitoring to prevent/quickly treat respiratory depression

Emergencies
- Immediate availability of emergency equipment
- Equipment must be maintained in good, working condition
- Immediate availability of competent, educated staff to respond
- Intravenous access

Discharge criteria
- Objective assessment parameters
- Verbal/written instructions

Communication
- With patient
  - ⇒ Assessment of response to verbal communication
  - ⇒ Demonstrate an attitude of care and competence
- With physician—any change in patient's condition

Documentation
- Of all nursing care during the course of the sedation/analgesia
- Will reduce cost of adverse event, should it occur

Monitoring of patient
- Nursing vigilance
- Early identification of problems and rapid intervention will help circumvent a crisis[52]

Appropriate patient selection
- Objective criteria for selection
- Consultation with anesthesia and other specialties when appropriate

Policies and procedures
- Written with multidisciplinary approach
- Nurse knows and follows policy and procedure for sedation/analgesia
- Are consistently applied throughout facility
- Follows policy of state board of nursing

anesthetic effect, of low doses of these medications. Some states have begun to address this issue and have composed practice statements addressing these medications. The Maryland Board of Nursing addresses conscious sedation in one ruling,[55] and addresses RN administration of medications classified as anesthetic agents for the purpose of sedation or analgesia[56] in a separate ruling. This trend may continue and carry to other states as experience and research allows us to determine which medications may be given safely by the RN during sedation and analgesia.

Unlicensed Assistive Personnel

The use of unlicensed assistive personnel (UAP) to administer sedation/analgesia is a controversial but important issue in the ambulatory setting. It is likely in some settings (e.g., dental offices, physician offices) that persons responsible for administering the medication are UAP. Some states address this issue, but each state has a different approach. In one state, the Nurse Practice Act mandates that the RN cannot delegate administration of a medication to UAP. Another state has dealt with the issue by issuing a statement to the public to warn against administration of medication by unlicensed persons.[16] Some malpractice insurance providers have requirements that prevent the physician or dentist from assuming total responsibility for the actions of unlicensed persons.[16]

JCAHO has no standard that requires the administration and monitoring be performed by a licensed nurse. The only requirement is that the assistant is judged to be competent by the mechanism in place at the hospital or ambulatory facility.[3, 39, 40] The expectation is simply that documentation of preparation is available. Kobs[40] notes that "JCAHO will not survey competency of those people involved when such agents are given." She then continues, "Although . . . numerous literature sources do call for a qualified nurse or registered nurse, JCAHO has no mandate for the types of caregivers involved."[40]

All professional nursing organizations that have written practice statements and most hospitals (at present) believe that the use of professional judgment is what sets RNs apart from "sedation technicians" whose training would be inadequate to provide safe patient care.[52] Consistent application of the nursing process (assessment, planning, intervention, evaluation) is integral to safe practice during sedation/analgesia.

Providing safe patient care during sedation requires the RN to apply critical-thinking skills, in which information is synthesized and applied to the individual clinical situation.[52] Rapid recognition of complications, quick planning, and definitive intervention is required of the RN. The safe administration and monitoring of the patient receiving conscious sedation/analgesia cannot occur with a technician whose skills lie in knowing how to insert the needle in the tubing and insert the medication. Safe administration requires a professional whose role is assessment and intervention during the preprocedure, intraprocedure, and postprocedure period and who has the knowledge and skills to assess the patient appropriately for discharge readiness.[16]

SUMMARY

The administration and monitoring of patients who receive conscious sedation is a skill that has been assimilated into the practice of the ambulatory surgery nurse. The ambulatory surgery nurse is in an excellent position to add this skill to his or her repertoire. Additional skills in the current healthcare environment can add to the desirability of the nurse as an employee. Conscious sedation is also a practice that has proven to be safe to patients who receive quality care in the hands of the educated and prepared nurse.

References

1. McCarthy FM, Soloman AL: Conscious sedation: Benefits and risks. J Am Dent Assoc 109:546, 1984.
2. Smith I, White PF: Use of intravenous adjuvants during local and regional anesthesia. Curr Rev PACN 14:46–51, 1992.
3. Joint Commission on Accreditation of Healthcare Organizations: Comprehensive Accreditation Manual for Hospitals 1997. Oakbrook Terrace, IL: JCAHO, 1996.
4. Murphy E: OR nursing law: Monitoring IV conscious sedation, the legal scope of practice. AORN J 57:512–514, 1993.
5. American Society of Post Anesthesia Nurses: Standards of Perianesthesia Nursing Practice. Thorofare, NJ: ASPAN, 1995.
6. Association of Operating Room Nurses: Recommended practices for managing the patient receiving conscious sedation/analgesia. AORN J 65:129–134, 1997.
7. American Association of Nurse Anesthetists: Position statement: Qualified providers of conscious sedation. Park Ridge, IL: AANA, 1991.
8. Emergency Nurses Association: Position statement: Conscious sedation. Park Ridge, IL: ENA, 1994.
9. American Society of Anesthesiologists Task Force on Sedation and Analgesia by Non-Anesthesiologists: Practice guidelines for sedation and analgesia by non-anesthesiologists. Anesthesiology 84:459–471, 1996.
10. American Patient Safety Foundation: Recommendations for safe administration of sedation and analgesia (conscious sedation). Pittsburgh: APSF, 1996.
11. American Nurses Association: Position statement on the role of the registered nurse (RN) in the management of patients receiving IV conscious sedation for short-term therapeutic, diagnostic, or surgical procedures. Washington, DC: ANA, 1991.
12. Mallampati SR, Gugino LD, Desai Sukumar P, et al: A clinical sign to predict difficult tracheal intubation: A prospective study. Can Anaesth Soc J 32:429–434, 1985.
13. Kallar SK: Conscious sedation for outpatient surgery. Wellcome Trends Anesthesiol 9:3–9, 1991.
14. Watson DS, James DS: Intravenous conscious sedation: Implications of monitoring patients receiving local anesthesia. AORN J 51:1512–1522, 1990.
15. Ghoneim MM, Dembo JB, Block RI: Time course of antagonism of sedative and amnesic effects of diazepam by flumazenil. Anesthesiology 70:899–904, 1989.
16. Odom J: Conscious sedation in the ambulatory setting. Crit Care Nurs Clin North Am 9:361–370, 1997.
17. Holzman RS, Cullen DJ, Eichhorn JH, et al: Guidelines for sedation by nonanesthesiologists during diagnostic and therapeutic procedures. J Clin Anesth 6:265–276, 1994.
18. Blouin RT, Gross JB: Ventilation and conscious sedation. Semin Anesth 15:335–342, 1996.
19. Hinzmann CA, Budden PM, Olson J: Intravenous conscious sedation use in endoscopy: Does monitoring of oxygen saturation influence timing of nursing interventions? Gastroenterol Nurs 15:6–13, 1992.
20. McKee CC, Ragland JJ, Myers JO: An evaluation of multiple clinical variables for hypoxia during colonoscopy. Surg Gynecol Obstet 173:37–40, 1991.
21. Gross JB, Long WB: Nasal oxygenation alleviates hypoxia in colonoscopy patients sedated with midazolam and meperidine. Gastrointest Endosc 36:26–29, 1990.
22. Simon IB, Lewis RJ, Satava RM: A safe method for sedating and monitoring patients for upper and lower gastrointestinal endoscopy. Am Surg 57:219–221, 1991.
23. Dlugose D: IV conscious sedation and local anesthesia: Perioperative nursing issues. AORN/ASPAN Joint Ambulatory Symposium, San Diego, CA; Sept 1993.
24. Clark BA: A new approach to assessment and documentation of conscious sedation during endoscopic examinations. Gastroenterol Nurs 16:199–203, 1994.
25. Clark BA: Development of the conscious sedation scale: Establishing content validity and reliability. Gastroenterol Nurs 20:2–8, 1997.
26. Bryan RJ: Administering conscious sedation: Operational guidelines. Crit Care Nurs Clin North Am 9:289–299, 1997.
27. Sacchetti A, Schafermeyer R, Gerardi M, et al: Pediatric analgesia and sedation. Ann Emerg Med 23:237–250, 1994.
28. Krikorian SA: Intravenous conscious sedation. Pharmacist 22:HS26–HS36, 1997.
29. United States Pharmacopeial Convention Inc: USPDI: Drug Info for the Health Care Professional Vol I, 16th ed. Rockville, MD: United States Pharmacopeial Convention Inc, 1996.
30. Arky R (Consultant): Physicians' Desk Reference. Montvale, NJ: Medical Economics Co, 1999.
31. Shields RE: A comprehensive review of sedative and analgesic agents. Crit Care Nurs Clin North Am 9:281–288, 1997.
32. Greenberg CP, De Soto H: Sedation techniques. In Twersky RS: The Ambulatory Anesthesia Handbook. St. Louis: Mosby, 1995, pp 301–359.
33. Somerson SJ, Husted CW, Sicilia MR: Insights into conscious sedation. Am J Nurs 95:26–32, 1995.
34. Golembiewski J: Comparison of selected agents for conscious sedation. Ann Arbor, MI: University of Michigan Medical Center, 1996. Unpublished.
35. Pasero CL, McCaffery M: Managing postoperative pain in the elderly. Am J Nurs 96:39–46, 1996.
36. Daneshmend TK, Bell GD, Logan RFA: Sedation for upper gastrointestinal endoscopy: Results of a nationwide survey. Gut 32:12–15, 1991.
37. Odom JL: Airway emergencies in the post anesthesia care unit. Nurs Clin North Am 28:483–491, 1993.
38. Claussen DW: Endoscopy nursing education competency: Romazicon. Gastroenterol Nurs 17:121–123, 1994.
39. JCAHO: 1996 Comprehensive Accreditation Manual for Ambulatory Care. Oakbrook, IL: JCAHO, 1995.

40. Kobs A: "Conscious sedation" questions about the anesthesia continuum. Nurs Manage 28:14, 17, 1997.
41. O'Sullivan C: Setting new standards: IV conscious sedation. Nurs Spectrum (FL ed) 7:6–7, 1997.
42. Drain CB: The Post Anesthesia Care Unit: A Critical Care Approach to Post Anesthesia Nursing, 3rd ed. Philadelphia: WB Saunders, 1994.
43. American Academy of Pediatrics Committee on Drugs: Guidelines for monitoring and management of pediatric patients during and after sedation for diagnostic and therapeutic procedures. Pediatrics 89:1110–1113, 1992.
44. Preud'Homme DL: Conscious sedation in pediatric patients undergoing endoscopic procedures. AORN Dayton, Ohio Chapter Seminar, Dayton, OH; Oct 1, 1994.
45. Wong DL: Whaley & Wong's Nursing Care of Infants and Children, 5th ed. St. Louis: Mosby, 1995.
46. Anonymous: Notes from the ASA annual meeting: Secondhand smoke hinders children's recovery from surgery. J PeriAnesth Nurs 12:115, 1997.
47. Zeigler VL, Brown LE: Conscious sedation in the pediatric population. Crit Care Nurs Clin North Am 9:381–394, 1997.
48. Klooster MJ, Logan LA, Grill BB: Developmental variation in midazolam dose used for sedation in pediatric endoscopy. Pediatr Res 25 (Part 2):68A, 1989.
49. Coté CJ: Monitoring guidelines: Do they make a difference? (Commentary). AJR Am J Roentgenol 165:910–912, 1995.
50. Darling E: Practical considerations in sedating the elderly. Crit Care Nurs Clin North Am 9:371–380, 1997.
51. Odom JL: The emerging role of risk management. J Post Anesth Nurs 5:120–123, 1990.
52. Dlugose D: Risk management considerations in conscious sedation. Crit Care Nurs Clin North Am 9:429–440, 1997.
53. Mannino MJ: Conscious sedation: Legal issues. CRNA: Clin Forum Nurs Anesth 2:31–33, 1991.
54. Newman PW: IV conscious sedation: Nursing issues. Spec Nurs Forum 2:1, 4–5, 1990.
55. Maryland Board of Nursing: Registered Nurse Administration of Conscious Sedation for Short Term Therapeutic, Diagnostic, and Surgical Procedures. Declaratory Ruling 96-1. Revised January 1996, Baltimore, MD.
56. Maryland Board of Nursing: Registered Nurse Administration of Medications Classified as Anesthetic Agents for Purpose of Sedation and/or Analgesia. Declaratory Ruling 95-2. December 19, 1995, Baltimore, MD.

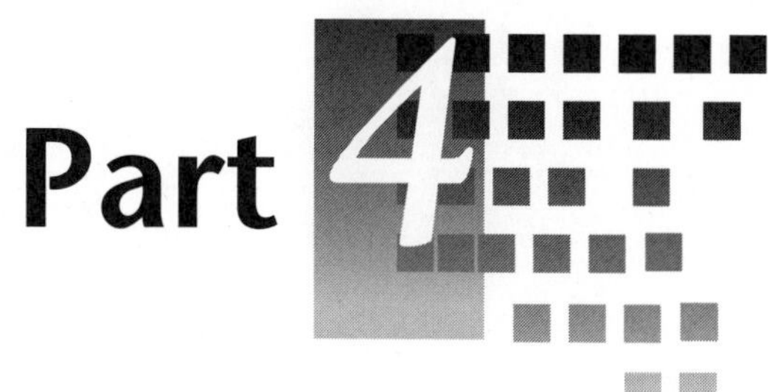

Part 4

Patient Care Issues: A Continuum

Chapter 16

Nursing Care of the Ambulatory Surgical Patient

Nancy Burden

STANDARDS OF NURSING PRACTICE

The nurse in an ambulatory surgery setting provides comprehensive and intense nursing care, emotional support, and patient education in a compressed time frame. Simultaneously, the nurse directs the patient toward self-care and independence and includes the patient's support unit of family or friends. Providing the right balance of physical, emotional, and educational support requires a nurse to be intelligent, observant, self-motivated, efficient, and caring.

Professional nursing practice and effective application of the nursing process in any setting require the competent use of a broad knowledge base coupled with technical skills, good judgment, and experience. These characteristics are some of the practice tools that nurses use to assist the ambulatory surgical patient back to health and independence. A number of issues specific to ambulatory surgery require patient care decisions to be made in a short time frame. These include early ambulation, patient education needs, infection control, antiemetic and analgesic administration, intravenous therapy, and nutrition and elimination needs. Nursing decisions have far-reaching implications into the home setting, where patients and families cope with lingering effects of sedation, anesthesia, and surgery. Sound nursing judgments and actions are essential.

Nurses involved in all phases of perioperative care require a broad knowledge base, which includes many aspects of medical-surgical and critical care nursing. They need specialized knowledge about the actions and side effects of general and local anesthetic agents, sedatives, narcotics, cardiovascular agents, and other drugs. The nursing process is the basis for patient care; thus, the nurse must be prepared to assess, plan care, intervene, and evaluate the patient's responses in myriad situations. Perianesthesia care nurses should have strong clinical backgrounds with experience in airway maintenance, respiratory management, arrhythmia identification and treatment, and certification in basic cardiopulmonary resuscitation. Advanced life support certification or its institutionally approved substitute is considered appropriate for a phase I postanesthesia care unit (PACU) nurse.[1]

Nurses must be capable of meticulous assessments; they are frequently called on to make judgments concerning patient care management. Critical nursing decisions regarding the effectiveness of respiratory effort, circulatory adequacy, or subtle symptoms of bleeding are necessary in the early stages of postanesthesia recovery. Rapid changes in patients' physical conditions require nurses to think clearly and to act confidently on the decisions they make. Ambulatory surgical nursing care is not limited to isolated actions. Although the application of independent nursing judgment is essential, likewise professional collaboration with nursing peers, anesthesia providers, physicians, other healthcare providers, and business personnel is integral to the patient's total care needs.

Ultimate patient outcomes for the ambulatory surgery population are greatly affected by nursing decisions such as the timing of initial attempts to ambulate or raise the patient's head, the timing and type of oral intake allowed, and the choice between several types or routes of medications ordered. Beyond this necessary attention to the patient's physiologic needs, the nurse should recognize and address the patient's emotional, cultural, and spiritual needs and promote the patient's dignity and privacy at all times.

The fact that there is no nurse "on the next shift" when a patient returns home requires an exacting thoroughness from the nurse in the ambulatory surgery facility. That often means spending a significant amount of time providing instructions to the patient and family and being involved in the details of the patient's transportation and home support needs. For a plan of care to be most effective, it should be implemented before the procedure. This early assessment provides a baseline of patient and situational information and allows early nursing interventions to prepare the patient and family as fully as possible for the procedure and recovery process. Despite competent medical and nursing interventions, complications sometimes do occur. The plan of care that is dynamic and interactive provides the basis for addressing unexpected occurrences and prepares the patient and family for such interventions during the home recovery period.

The nurse's role encompasses risk management and marketing functions in tandem with clinical care. Just as in any nursing setting, a patient may express concern or displeasure over an incident or situation. Concerned follow-up of complaints by the appropriate nursing, administrative, and medical staff members helps to defuse negative reactions and communicates a positive image of the facility and staff.

Ambulatory surgery programs, whether hospital based or freestanding, are governed by both internal and external standards. Licensing bodies require that nursing care be provided in a manner consistent with certain basic standards. Standards of nursing practice define the scope of nursing, identify appropriate actions for specific areas of practice, and serve as a model against which nurses are measured in their practice settings and in courts of law.

One type of practice standard that governs nurses is a state nurse practice act, which defines professional nursing practice in each state. Nurses should be aware of the content and meaning of their state's nurse practice act. This is particularly important in specialty areas like ambulatory surgical nursing, in which there can be a fine line between the parameters of nursing, anesthesia, and surgical care.

National nursing associations and organizations also establish practice standards. Clearly, the practicing nurse should be an active member in appropriate national specialty organizations. Whether the nurse chooses to maintain professional membership or not, that nurse's clinical practice continues to be judged on the national standards. Both the American Society of Perianesthesia Nurses' and the Association of Operating Room Nurses' standards address the individual patient's perioperative needs through the format of the nursing process. This approach is a way to ensure that all patients receive thoughtful and comprehensive nursing care based on recognized nursing standards.

The Joint Commission on Accreditation of Healthcare Organizations and the Accreditation Association for Ambulatory Health Care also impose standards on facilities choosing to undergo the voluntary accreditation process. These various standards involve the facility's physical environment as well as the policies and practices of both the nursing and the medical professions. Successfully passing this accreditation process attests to the high standards of all departments in the facility.

A more complete discussion of nursing standards can be found in Chapter 6. Internet Web sites for various associations and organizations are listed in Chapter 1 in Table 1–1. These Web sites provide an abundance of information as well as links to other associated sites.

HUMANITY OF CARE

Another aspect of nursing care is the interest, empathy, and concern that the nurse focuses on the patient's physical, social, and emotional needs. These issues are not necessarily essential to the physical acts of anesthesia, surgery, and recovery, but they bring humanity to the patient's world. Professional behavior demands that nurses treat all patients with courtesy, concern, and human kindness. Emotional support offered by nurses is an essential intervention that helps patients learn and believe in their own abilities. When applicants for a position have similar technical skills, the person with the strongest interpersonal skills is usually the best choice. These attributes are not mere niceties but are germane to the essence of ambulatory surgical nursing.

Sincerity, eye contact, respect for the patient's privacy and belongings, appropriate use of humor, and upholding of the patient's right to express emotion or to cry are ways that demonstrate a caring attitude. Others include minimizing patient and family waiting periods, providing explanations for any delays, and reuniting the patient with family or friends as quickly as possible. The ambulatory surgical patient also appreciates a nurse who provides support without judgment or criticism, particularly when faced with an emotionally charged issue, such as termination of pregnancy, sterilization, alternative insemination, and cosmetic surgery. Other issues frequently encountered include differences in sexual orientation, sexually transmitted diseases, body piercing, and tattooing.

Addressing the patient respectfully entails using an adult's formal name unless otherwise directed. Older adults, in particular, appreciate this courtesy and usually let the nurse know whether they prefer to be called by their first names. Using pet names is inappropriate, and referring to a patient as a disease, a number, or a procedure is inexcusable. During an initial patient contact, the nurse should ascertain any special preference that the patient may have and communicate it to other healthcare providers. Likewise, documenting a preferred nickname or the pronunciation of a difficult name allows the entire staff to address the patient in the manner that he or she prefers. Children respond positively to the familiar, so their nicknames are generally preferred.

Ambulatory surgery patients are generally healthy, more aware, and less sedated than other surgical patients. As a result, they are more physically and emotionally able to engage in and appreciate the interest and time that nurses invest in their care.

Touch is one of the most powerful resources available in nursing. The power of touch is available in the broad sense not only through the nurse's hands but also through the nurse's eyes, voice, body position and movements, apparel, and attitude. The comfort of the nurse's physical touch is a caring gesture that reassures patients that they are not alone and that any needed help is close and available. Conversely, the nurse should be aware of and respect the wishes of those who prefer not to be touched.

Taking time with a patient is very important. In addition to the opportunity it gives the nurse to comprehensively assess the patient, spending time with the patient and answering questions, both spoken and unspoken, can be more therapeutic than a preoperative medication. The demands of a busy ambulatory surgery unit often rob the nurse and patient of that luxury, but even a few seconds of sincere eye contact, a smile, and words of understanding are reassuring. The nurse needs to develop sensitivity to the importance of time. Time spent waiting can seem very lengthy for the patient and may enhance feelings of anxiety, fear, or loneliness.

The nurse who is able to master the fine art of being hurried without looking harried conveys to patients an attentive quality. Methods to project the appearance of calm include

- Avoiding rapid movements (the "hustle and bustle" look)
- Changing sheets, washing stretchers, and restocking supplies out of view of patients and families
- Maintaining a pleasant and smiling demeanor and voice
- Completing routine activities as efficiently as possible to avoid duplication of effort

Conversations with patients can be therapeutic or distressing. The nurse's overall communication skills have a profound effect on how a patient feels and responds. The nurse should take into account both verbal and nonverbal forms of communication. Nonverbal components of communication can be more important than words. Eye contact, facial expressions, body orientation and movements, gestures, and posture all communicate their own messages. Patients can perceive sincerity and gain a sense of self-importance when the nurse maintains good eye contact during conversations, dresses and acts in a professional manner, and indicates concern and interest with pleasant facial expressions. Vocabulary and grammar indicate a level of education and intelligence and can inspire or discourage the patient's confidence in the nurse. In every contact, the nurse is communicating in a multitude of parameters beyond the actual words being spoken.

Both the content and the interpretation of conversations are extremely important. The nurse's instructions, the physician's explanations about the outcome of surgery, and the wording of questions and other dialogue should be expressed clearly and purposefully with a sensitivity to the potential for misinterpretation. The staff should avoid using medical jargon that the patient cannot understand or may misinterpret. The content of any discussion has the ability to evoke a wide range of emotions; it can soothe, anger, frighten, irritate, offend, or amuse patients.

Listening is the other side of communication. Active, attentive listening is a sensitive nursing action. Not only does it provide clues to the patient's physical status and emotional needs but it also is essential to the patient's physical well-being. It provides the nurse with information for evaluation and proper planning of nursing actions.

The nurse's sincerity has a major impact on a patient's attitude. Given the short-term contacts made between patients and nurses in an ambulatory surgery setting, establishing bonds of trust can be a challenge. Some specific ways in which the nurse can inspire the patient's trust include being truthful, following through on promises, treating the patient respectfully, providing clear and accurate explanations, showing concern for family members or other waiting companions, exhibiting professional behavior, and demonstrating clinical excellence. Acting in a manner that encourages trust helps the patient to have confidence in the nurses and physicians who are providing care.

ATTRACTING NURSES TO AN AMBULATORY SURGERY SPECIALTY

Nurses are drawn to the ambulatory surgery setting for many reasons. Many arrive as an alternative to demanding critical care units, such as intensive care and cardiac care units and mainstream PACUs. Often, the lure is to work predetermined hours with no "on call" time and less or no evening or night hours. Others are drawn by the challenge of a new setting or the opportunity for expanding nursing practice arenas and experiencing new types of nurse-patient interactions.

The medical-surgical nurse brings a varied experience that can be readily applied to the needs of ambulatory surgery patients. A critical care background also offers an ideal basis for ambulatory surgical nursing practice, where emergency situations are always possible. Many of today's patients have systemic illnesses and are elderly people with an increased potential for complications. Invasive monitoring, code situations, and critical illnesses are not the norm but may occur throughout the perioperative period. The nurse with corresponding expertise is well prepared to respond to the unexpected.

Both the most experienced critical care nurse and the general duty nurse face challenges when they enter an ambulatory surgical nursing setting. They must learn and practice the philosophy of encouraging patient wellness and self-care and must see the patient as a partner in, rather than a recipient of, healthcare. They interact intensely on an integrated social and family level, more than in many other nursing specialty settings. Teaching skills must be honed to allow accuracy and clarity in a short time frame. The nurse is in a visible and public role with patients and family members who are acutely aware of, and dependent on, the nurse's knowledge, skills, and caring attitude.

What does the ambulatory surgery setting offer to the nurse in return? Foremost, it is an excellent opportunity to experience the complete cycle of patient care from beginning to end. The nursing process comes alive, beginning with the preadmission assessment of the patient's individual needs and ending with a postdischarge telephone evaluation of the patient's condition and the effectiveness of the planned and actual nursing interventions. The satisfaction of being a key player in the patient's safe and generally pleasant surgical experience is very rewarding. But with the reward comes an intense responsibility for accuracy and completeness in patient assessment, both before and after surgery. This accuracy is an integral part of the plan of action for the patient's surgical experience and home course.

This specialty allows the nurse to cultivate teaching skills and to practice and maintain acute care skills in a setting that is purposefully targeted to promote social and emotional warmth. There are also opportunities for nurses to experience expanded roles. This is particularly evident in a freestanding unit, where the nurse may act as a marketing agent, in-service director, quality improvement coordinator, purchasing agent, and initiator of budgetary, educational, and patient-flow issues. In the hospital setting, the ambulatory surgical nurse can promote the needs of the ambulatory care unit and its patients by serving on facility-wide committees and task forces. The facility and patients benefit from these expanded nursing roles, but no one benefits as much as the nurse. The challenges and growth involved in researching, planning, understanding, and initiating change add to the nurse's professional expertise and personal advancement.

NURSING ACCOUNTABILITY

Regardless of the practice setting, nurses must be accountable for their clinical and professional actions. This accountability exists on many levels. Professional regulatory departments set minimal requirements for nursing practice within each state. For instance, all nurses must maintain current licensure and must conform to their state's nurse practice act or face disciplinary action or possible revocation of license. Contained within nurse practice acts are the guidelines for professional conduct and practice that direct and protect nurses professionally, ethically, and legally.

Accountability exists at other levels as well. By virtue of their employment, nurses are held accountable to nursing superiors and ultimately to the administrators of the facilities where they work. Clinical actions and judgments, economic and fiscal practices, educational goals and actions, and professional loyalties are all subject to the scrutiny of managers. Nurses are accountable to physicians (surgeons, anesthesiologists, and others) in the context of carrying out actions in a particular patient's care, as directed by the physicians involved. The nurse must also report significant symptoms or variances to the physician in a timely manner.

The professional nurse also has personal accountability to nursing colleagues, patients, and their families or friends, despite the lack of formal lines of authority. Dependability, reliability, and trustworthiness are a few of the basic values that contribute to fulfilling both peer and nurse-patient relationships. This accountability exists on many levels—professional, ethical, legal, moral, and humanitarian.

Unfortunately, nurses sometimes are accountable to the court system as well. In that situation, nurses are judged on their individual practices compared with the generally accepted standards of the facility (policies and procedures), the surrounding community (nearby hospitals and surgery centers), and the broader nursing community (specialty organization standards, nurse practice acts, and legal precedents). The courts ask whether the nurse did what a reasonable and prudent nurse would have done in a similar situation.

Although accountability implies legal risks, the nurse can lessen those risks by engaging in careful practice. Some of the areas of care that are most likely to be implicated in legal matters include thoroughness of the preoperative assessment and assurance of an adequate informed consent on the medical record before medicating the patient for surgery. Other areas of legal culpability involve inadequate observation or documentation of postoperative complications and discharge assessments, wrong site of surgery, inadequate teaching before discharge, and inadequate evidence of an evaluation of the patient's capability to follow those instructions.

The responsibility for obtaining surgical consent belongs to the physician. In the perioperative setting, the anesthesia provider is just as responsible as the surgeon for supplying the patient with information and an opportunity to ask questions. During the preprocedure assessment it is the nurse's obligation to ascertain whether the patient has received adequate information from the physician with which an informed decision can be made. Patient misunderstanding, reservations, or concerns regarding the upcoming procedure should be documented and reported to the physician before surgery or sedation. As the patient's advocate, it is the perioperative nurse's responsibility to facilitate an additional physician-patient contact for clarification of the patient's concerns.[2]

A good resource to help patients remember 12 key questions (Table 16–1) to ask their physicians can be accessed via the Internet at www.ahcpr.gov/consumer/surgery.htm. This site provides the booklet "Be Informed: Questions to Ask Your Doctor Before You Have Surgery." The document also provides the names of other agencies and sites that provide similar information.

Although the various sources of accountability provide the external regulations aimed at ensuring quality professional practice and superior patient care, day-to-day accountability is actually driven by internal values. The professional nurse practices self-accountability in daily clinical and ethical decisions. For instance, no one except the nurse really knows whether an unobserved operating room nurse has contaminated a sterile field or whether a PACU nurse has falsified vital signs on the record or given an incorrect medication. Responsibility and

Table 16–1. Be Informed: Questions To Ask Your Doctor Before You Have Surgery

1. What operation are you recommending?
2. Why do I need the operation?
3. What are the alternatives to surgery?
4. What are the benefits of having the operation?
5. What are the risks of having the operation?
6. What if I don't have this operation?
7. Where can I get a second opinion?
8. What has been your experience in doing the operation?
9. Where will the operation be done?
10. What kind of anesthesia will I need?
11. How long will it take me to recover?
12. How much will the operation cost?

From Be Informed: Questions To Ask Your Doctor Before You Have Surgery. Consumer brochure #95-0027. Agency for Health Care Policy and Research. Rockville, MD. Available at: http://www.ahcpr.gov/consumer/surgery/htm. January 1995.

ownership come from within in the form of a professional conscience.

Attainment of specialty certification is a visible way to demonstrate professional excellence. Perianesthesia certification from ASPAN can be obtained in two venues: certified ambulatory perianesthesia nurse and certified postanesthesia nurse. Operating room nursing certification results in a certified nurse in the operating room designation, and gastroenterology specialists are certified as certified gastroenterology registered nurses. Table 16–2 provides details regarding these certifications.

The ambulatory surgical nurse frequently assumes the important responsibility of directing and evaluating the ability of the patient and the family to assume the demands of home care almost immediately after a surgical intervention. This professional responsibility must be embraced if the patient is to receive safe, high-quality care. Thus, the nurse must provide appropriate instructions and act on any indication that the patient's home situation may not be adequately supportive.

It is self-accountability that drives an individual nurse to always strive to provide the most comprehensive and personal care possible, rather than merely to provide what is noticed and recorded by others who are observing and evaluating that nurse's performance. The ambulatory surgical patient is particularly vulnerable in the sense that an omission or a casual approach by the nurse can spell disaster after discharge, when the patient and family must function independent of professional assistance.

FOSTERING TEAMWORK

Frequent collaboration with physicians, certified registered nurse anesthetists, and other nurses requires that the ambulatory surgery center (ASC) nurse is able to effectively interact with other professionals as well as with patients. Physicians provide medical orders for the patient's care but expect that the nurse will use discretion and good judgment in the subsequent application of those orders. Should a patient's condition affect the appropriateness of an order, the nurse should contact and provide the physician with a current evaluation of the patient's status. The nurse's ability to give an accurate and efficient accounting to the physician helps to build a mutually respectful professional relationship.

The nurse should foster communication among nursing departments in the ASC regarding both departmental issues and individual patients. Comprehensive reports should be expected and provided when a patient is transferred between departments. On transfer from the procedure or operating room, both the transporting nurse and the anesthesia provider should report all necessary information about the patient before the receiving nurse accepts responsibility for that patient.

The ASC staff also nurtures professional contacts with other facility departments. The laboratory, radiology, social services, dietary, and other departments provide valuable collaborative services. Coordination of these services, which are essential for the smooth working of

***Table 16–2.* Nursing Certifications Related to Ambulatory Surgery Specialties**

ACRONYM	CERTIFICATION	ORGANIZATION	WEB SITE	CONTACT INFORMATION
CPAN	Certified Postanesthesia Nurse	ABPANC—American Board of Perianesthesia Nursing Certification, Inc.	www.cpancapa.org	ABPANC 475 Riverside Drive, 7th Floor New York, NY 10115-0089 Telephone: (800) 6ABPANC FAX: (212) 367-4256
CAPA	Certified Ambulatory Perianesthesia Nurse	ABPANC—American Board of Perianesthesia Nursing Certification, Inc.	www.cpancapa.org	ABPANC 475 Riverside Drive, 7th Floor New York, NY 10115-0089 Telephone: (800) 6ABPANC FAX: (212) 367-4256
CNOR	Certified Nurse in the Operating Room	CBPN—Certification Board of Perioperative Nursing	www.certboard.com	2170 South Parker Road, Suite 295 Denver, CO 80231 Telephone: (888) 257-2667
CGRN	Certified Gastroenterology Registered Nurse	CBGN—Certifying Board of Gastroenterology Nurses and Associates, Inc.	www.cbgna.org	3525 Ellicott Mills Drive, Suite N Ellicott City, MD 21043-4547 Telephone: (410) 418-4808 FAX: (410) 418-4805

the surgery process, is enhanced through mutually effective communication skills.

NURSING PROCESS AND OUTCOMES MEASUREMENT

Components of the nursing process—assessment, planning, implementation, and evaluation—are clearly identifiable throughout the ambulatory surgical process. Nurses use this ongoing approach to provide comprehensive perioperative care for their patients. The Joint Commission on Accreditation of Healthcare Organizations requires that a multidisciplinary plan of care be in place for each patient, although this does not necessarily mean a separate "care plan" in the traditional sense.[3] A care plan can be an effective means to provide the basis for care; however, policies, procedures, and written action plans are appropriate substitutes. Figure 1–1 illustrates a patient recovery plan in a format also called a care map, yet another method of planning for care and assessing outcomes against a predetermined norm.

The Joint Commission provides standards for assessment, followed by care decisions, care delivery, reassessment, and eventually a change in the care setting (discharge) when no further care is needed.[4] Nursing diagnoses pertinent to the patient's actual or potential problems and needs are identifiable as part of the nursing process. Nursing diagnoses focus on the patient's response to health problems, unlike medical diagnoses that identify pathology and disease processes.

In many nursing communities, considerable attention is being given to nursing care planning that reflects patient outcomes rather than, or in addition to, the process of nursing diagnoses. Outcomes must be identifiable and measurable in order to be properly evaluated. Figure 1–1 provides an example of the use of outcomes in the ambulatory surgery setting. The nurse evaluates patient outcomes through physical, emotional, and social assessments, including subjective input from the patient. Some evaluations are completed during the postdischarge telephone contact.

Through this process of outcome standards, it is possible to show that nursing care has resulted in positive patient outcomes. Objective measurements through nursing observations and the patient's subjective descriptions help to compare the patient's actual experience with the desired outcomes. The United States Agency for Health Care Policy and Research, established in 1989, is responsible for developing and updating guidelines that will be used to manage clinical conditions. Clearly, the nursing community must continue to develop strategies to demonstrate that nursing care results in optimal healthcare outcomes.

In addition to encouraging appropriate patient results related to healthcare and nursing interventions, outcome standards may have other far-reaching implications. For example, as nurses strive for direct third-party reimbursement for services, they must be able to show that their interventions result in high-quality, cost-effective healthcare that leads to positive patient outcomes.[5] Table 16–3 lists clinical, financial, quality of life and satisfaction outcomes affecting patients, families, facilities, and staff. Applied to the ambulatory surgical setting, many of these outcomes can translate into target goals and quality improvement indicators for individuals and facilities.

It is vital for the nurse to use all possible resources to complete a comprehensive assessment in a relatively short time frame. Assessment of the patient before, on, and after the day of surgery is an ongoing process. The patient presents a variety of needs and potential problems while progressing from the preanesthesia stage through surgery and on toward discharge. The parameters to be addressed encompass physical, mental, intellectual, spiritual, emotional, and social factors, with a particularly strong emphasis on the patient's educational needs.

The nursing and medical professions have begun to investigate the value of applying a widely used generic health status survey, the SF-36, in the ambulatory surgical setting. The SF-36 is a medical outcomes study questionnaire that queries how a person perceives his or her health to have changed after a certain event or time. The tool is "patient based and obtains the patient's assessment of his or her behavioral functioning, subjective well-being, and perceptions of health."[6] Data can be compared with those of other patients undergoing similar procedures or with similar conditions. Limitations of this tool include the time required for adequate completion of the form and possible difficulties in understanding in aged or less educated patients.

With the rapid turnover of cases, assessment, planning, and implementation are accomplished almost simultaneously. It is vital that information is communicated among nurses and departments. Care then continues to be based on data pertinent to the individual patient and the actual

Table 16–3. **Classification of Outcomes**

CLASSIFICATION	PATIENT/FAMILY-RELATED OUTCOMES	HEALTH CARE AGENCY–RELATED OUTCOMES
Clinical	• Improved patient care outcomes, such as reduced pain, morbidity, and mortality • Reduction in signs, symptoms, and degree of progression of the disease • Prevention of adverse effects of treatments and complications of illness • Reduction in practice variation	• Standardization of care processes (establishing standards of care) • Streamlined care processes and delineation of responsibilities • Improved turnaround time of tests, treatments, and procedures • Increased compliance with standards of care of regulatory agencies such as the Joint Commission on Accreditation of Healthcare Organizations and the National Council for Quality Assurance
Financial	• Optimal and appropriate use of resources and services • Provision of care in appropriate setting(s) • Maximal coordination of care among providers • Streamlining of diagnostic and therapeutic tests and procedures	• Appropriate changes in staff mix/skill mix • Reduced cost (e.g., reduction in length of stay, reduction in (or elimination of) fragmented and duplicative services • Improved reimbursement and revenue • Reduction in denials of claims • Improved communication among providers and payers (e.g., hospitals and managed care companies)
Quality of Life	• Improved/maximized physical abilities and level of independence • Improved psychological, physiological, and social functioning • Improved state of well-being • Improved perception of health status • Enhanced self-care abilities • Enhanced knowledge of health care needs	• Prevention of inappropriate hospitalizations • Reduction in inappropriate utilization of emergency department services • Provision of a safe environment of care • Provision of programs that meet patient and family needs • Improved accessibility to care
Satisfaction	• Increased patient/family satisfaction with care • Improved continuity of care • Improved patient-nurse and family-nurse relationships	• Improved staff satisfaction • Reduced rates of burnout, turnover, attrition, and absenteeism • Enhanced states of communication, collaboration, and teamwork among providers and disciplines (interpersonal, interdisciplinary, and interdepartmental)

From Flarey DL: Nurse case managers' responsibilities toward patient care outcomes. Semin Nurse Manag 6:101, 1998.

situation at hand. With evaluation and reassessment comes the opportunity to adjust the plan as needed. Thus, the process is a continuing cycle addressing patient needs that change rapidly and extend into the home setting. Ultimately, positive patient outcomes are the result of adequate planning, comprehensive evaluations, and appropriate interventions.

In addition to the Internet resources listed in Table 1–1, others exist that are more specific for outcomes management information. An article by Pelletier in the *Journal of Nursing Care Quality*[7] provides more specific information about the Internet resource sites listed in Table 16–4.

CRITICAL THINKING

The professional nurse should apply the principles of critical thinking in the daily planning and execution of patient care. Critical thinking about a problem, situation, or question requires the nurse to call on a wide variety of sources while considering various issues. The object is to think of further questions, to identify and challenge current assumptions, and to make connections with other information and issues. With this type of thinking, the nurse broadens the scope of possible solutions and avoids being trapped into predetermined paths.

Critical thinking is essential to finding creative solutions to specific patient or unit related concerns and for the advancement of individual professional growth. This process requires an open mind, inquisitiveness, thinking "outside the box," a willingness to invest the time in sufficient investigation, a measure of skepticism, and well-developed cognitive and problem-solving skills. Critical thinking challenges the status quo and requires the nurse to apply knowledge, experience, and intuition while examining the context and environment of the issue at hand.[8] When issues are discussed in a group setting or with a peer, it is imperative that a supportive climate permits the nurse to verbalize all possible scenarios without the fear of criticism, ridicule, or loss of respect.[9]

The application of critical thinking skills in an ambulatory surgical setting might look like this. The nurse goes to the waiting room to admit a 5-year-old boy for surgery and finds the child running and screaming while throwing toys. The mother appears to be ignoring the activity. Both the child and the parent are wearing worn, stained clothing. Their hair is unkempt, and the child's bare feet are dirty. On the child's shirt and on his chin are what appear to be chocolate stains. Immediately, the astute nurse begins an inner conversation of critical questions:

1. Has this child been appropriately prepared for surgery?
2. Does the mother have the ability and resources to understand and implement the preoperative instructions we provided? What nurse spoke with this parent? Maybe that person has some history or insights that can help me with a course of action.
3. Is the reason that this child is out of control

***Table 16–4.* Outcomes Management Internet Resources**

WEB SITE ADDRESS (ALL BEGIN WITH http://www.)	AGENCY NAME	COMMENTS
ahcpr.org	Agency for Healthcare Policy and Research	Part of US Department of Health and Human Services—charged with supporting research designed to improve the quality of healthcare, reduce its cost, and broaden access to essential services.
asqc.org	American Society for Quality	Dedicated to the ongoing development, advancement, and promotion of quality concepts, principles, and techniques.
ahsr.org	Association for Health Services Research	National membership organization formed exclusively to promote the field of health services research and to increase the contribution that health services research makes to improving the healthcare system and health status of Americans.
best4health.org	Best Practices Network	This network promotes information sharing in healthcare by nurses, physicians, and other healthcare professionals. It facilitates the exchange of ideas, encourages collaboration in results-oriented problem solving, and enables health professionals to learn from one another.
facct.org	Foundation for Accountability	This not-for-profit organization is dedicated to helping Americans make better healthcare decisions.
henryfordhealth.org	Henry Ford Health System	With over 1000 studies now underway, this foundation supports research to investigate better ways to diagnose and treat disease and illness.
kff.org	Henry J. Kaiser Foundation	Independent philanthropic foundation (not associated with Kaiser Permanente or Kaiser Industries) that focuses on health policy, reproductive health, HIV policy, and health and development in South Africa.
ihqi.com	Institute for Healthcare Quality	Provides practical solutions to issues of healthcare quality and costs by use of advanced technology, international expertise, quality price management databases, & CQI.
outcomes-trust.org	Medical Outcomes Trust	Nonprofit public service organization dedicated to improving health and healthcare by distributing standardized, high-quality instruments that measure health and outcomes of medical care.
nahq.org	National Association of Healthcare Quality	Leading US professional organization for healthcare quality professionals.
rand.org	RAND (acronym for research and development)	Nonprofit institution that helps improve policy and decision making through research and analysis.
rwjf.org	Robert Wood Johnson Foundation	Nation's largest philanthropic organization devoted solely to health and healthcare.

HIV, human immunodeficiency virus; CQI, continuous quality improvement.
Data from Pelletier LR: Outcomes management Internet resources. J Nurs Care Qual, 1998.

hyperactivity, poor discipline, or something else? What do we need to do to calm the child before induction?
4. Has the child been continually monitored this morning to ensure that he has not eaten or had anything to drink. Should I consider that he might not have fasted?
5. What are these stains? Should I be questioning whether they are fresh or from the previous day? What is the best way to ask this question to be nonconfrontational and to elicit a truthful response from the child or the mother? Will the mother know whether the child drank chocolate milk or ate candy this morning?

For most nurses, this type of self-talk goes on continually and subconsciously during nursing activities. Purposefully and consciously developing such critical thinking skills encourages professional growth and provides the nurse with expert assessment skills in different situations.

ETHICAL DILEMMAS

Daily, the professional nurse is presented with situations that call for judgment and decision-making. Often, situations have an ethical overtone that makes a decision more challenging than others. Ambulatory surgery settings are no different. The nurse, as a patient advocate and as a member of a multidisciplinary team, must choose among options and know when to compromise and when to stand firm on an issue.

Ethical considerations in healthcare have three basic principles in common. First is the principle of autonomy. The patient has a right to make decisions for himself or herself, and clinicians must honor those decisions. Second is beneficence, the obligation of the healthcare provider to do good and to prevent harm. Third is the principle of justice, that all people receive a fair share.[8] These principles are and will continue to be encountered in the ambulatory surgical setting with increasing frequency as healthcare becomes more complex technologically, financially, and medically.

Examples of ethically demanding decisions surround informed consents. Does the patient truly understand the implications of the procedure at hand? Have the risks and alternatives been provided in a way that the patient can comprehend? Managed care and its increasingly rigid controls on access to care present some of the most demanding ethical dilemmas in healthcare. Other tough questions the ASC nurse may face include

- Should we reuse single-use items to reduce cost and should the patient be told?
- How far do we go in providing adequate pain control for the person addicted to narcotics?
- Do I join the light banter in the lunchroom that may inadvertently disclose a patient confidentiality?
- What should I do when I believe that a peer is acquiring controlled substances but I am not sure?
- Is it so wrong to document unsubstantiated research data that proves the point that we want to make if it will help push change that is good for patients and staff alike?
- Does my patient understand that advance directives are not applied in this ASC or in the operating room?
- Is making 50 personal copies on the photocopier considered wrong?
- If I accidentally contaminate an expensive sterile item, should I charge the patient for it along with the subsequent one I use for care?

These challenges may seem to have only one answer—the most ethical one. However, nurses are continually faced with situations in which the answers are not always clear. Conscience, professionalism, and honesty often conflict with peer pressure, the status quo, and the pressures of getting through the day's assignments. The right choice is not always the easy choice.

NURSING RESEARCH: A PROFESSIONAL OBLIGATION

As one of the newer subspecialties in healthcare, ambulatory surgery has not been widely studied using the scientific process. Often, studies in similar specialties are relied on for answers about patient care. For instance, the emergency department often discharges patients after procedures and sedation, so can the research about that setting be applied to the ASC? Can studies of patients undergoing surgery that requires hospitalization be applied to those people who are being discharged on the same day?

Research is a diligent, systematic inquiry or investigation to validate and refine existing knowledge and generate new knowledge. It is planned and organized investigation that is undertaken to address specific questions being posed. Nursing research must be consistent with nursing's existing holistic philosophy that takes the entire person into consideration.[10]

Fetzer[11] expands on that basic description of research to include the following purposes. She points out that research

- Validates interventions used by ambulatory perianesthesia nurses
- Defines the unique contribution of the ambulatory perianesthesia nursing specialty
- Uncovers perianesthesia phenomenon not previously realized
- Develops and tests theories
- Substantiates the unique contribution of ambulatory perianesthesia nurses as healthcare providers

Every day, the nurse encounters situations that pose excellent research questions. Enthusiasm and a team focus on improving care are basic catalysts for entering into research studies. The nurse who is not educationally prepared to design a valid study can bring ideas for study topics to the table and can remain an active participant under the guidance of the primary study investigator or investigators.

DOCUMENTATION

Comprehensive documentation provides accurate information on which care can be based. Accurate charting of nursing actions and interventions has multiple purposes. First, it is an ongoing description of the patient's condition that is communicated to other personnel, so it documents and drives actual care. It also provides an accurate reference of the care given in the event of chart audit or legal action. In particular, instructions for aftercare in the home setting and the nurse's assessment of the patient's understanding should be painstakingly documented in the ambulatory surgery setting. Finally, documentation of care must comply with predetermined standards set forth by third party payers for reimbursement purposes.

Common documentation inadequacies involve many areas, including: (1) documentation of a discharge plan or provision for follow-up care, (2) patient education and responses, (3) inadequate laboratory testing or reports not available at the time of surgery or on the medical record, (4) actions taken related to abnormal laboratory reports, and (5) inadequate or missing history and physical or progress note by the physician.

All nursing documentation should support the policies and standards of the facility and of the profession and regulating bodies. The needs of the ambulatory surgery unit may require development of forms specific to the setting, such as preadmission and postdischarge telephone tools and discharge instruction sheets. Adaptation of forms that are used in other areas in a hospital setting may be possible, but the specific standards of the ASC must be maintained in the revisions. For instance, the main PACU record may need revision for use in the dedicated ambulatory unit's PACU by removing such headings as "arterial lines," "thoracotomy tube," and "ventilator settings."

The facility-wide list of accepted abbreviations in a hospital should include those appropriate to the ambulatory unit. If it does not, revision of the list should be considered. Abbreviations that nurses use must be appropriate, unambiguous, communicated to the entire staff, and incorporated into the standard policy of the facility.

As in all nursing documentation, certain standards always apply. The nurse must ensure that all entries are signed and that the note and signature are legible. Grammar and spelling should be correct. An entry should never be obliterated so that it cannot be read, nor should a note be squeezed between lines or in margins. Rather, it should be entered and labeled as a "late note," charting the time of the entry and the time of the actual occurrence or observation. The nurse should chart promptly to allow accurate recall of the specific details of care.

Finally, charts should not reflect judgments. Rather, they should include the patient's subjective statements: "Patient states that the pain in her right knee is intolerable and asks for pain medication," and the nurse's objective assessments: "Patient moves restlessly, holds her left knee with her hands and is moaning." It is inappropriate to chart that "the patient has pain in her right knee," because there is no way that the nurse can know what the patient is feeling or thinking.

Consistency of charting practices should be reflected from one nurse to another and from one department to another. Appropriate inclusions and acceptable abbreviations should be discussed at staff meetings. Time keeping is important in a setting where patient conditions change rapidly from one minute to another, so clocks in various departments should be synchronized. Quality improvement audits should address issues of completeness and consistency.

The shortened time frame in which patients are admitted, prepared, treated, recovered, instructed, and discharged in the ASC demands charting that allows rapid yet comprehensive inclusion of all necessary data with minimal time involvement. The amount of documentation and monitoring seems to be escalating in the face of standards required by licensing and accrediting bodies and third party payers, and in response to the ever-increasing potential for litigation. Although this situation appears to threaten the original premise of streamlined, cost-effective nursing documentation, creative nurses develop forms that allow comprehensive yet efficient charting practices. Checklists and areas to fill in with content rather than narrative-type documentation help to decrease charting time. Various forms of this type are presented as samples in appropriate chapters throughout this text.

Comprehensive documentation in all phases of care is an essential form of communication as the patient travels from one department to another. The chart should reflect the patient's status and all interventions that have been instituted so that each nurse is able to build on the previous nurses' care and assessments.

Interventions to ensure appropriate documentation by physicians may seem to be beyond the scope of nursing practice. However, in most settings, the nurse is a facilitator of physician documentation. Making the paperwork as simple and as streamlined as possible encourages physician compliance. Facility policies that clearly outline charting requirements for physicians must be communicated and supported by the governing board. It is helpful when nurses in each area of the ASC consistently draw attention to current signature and documentation needs. This practice not only encourages complete records during the patient's stay but also helps prevent an accumulation of incomplete charts in the medical records department.

Electronic records are becoming more common as facilities computerize more processes. Integrating records from one service to another allows the nurse to reduce duplicated entries of demographics. In addition, the electronic record entered at the bedside encourages immediate, rather than delayed, entries.

Physician compliance in completing required documentation, such as the history and physical (H & P), demands a united front by all nursing personnel. Strict adherence to the requirement that it be on the chart before surgery enhances the comprehensive care of patients; thus, a patient should not be taken into the procedure room without the H & P actually documented in the medical record. This requirement is very clearly addressed by accrediting bodies such as the Joint Commission on Accreditation of Healthcare Organizations and by regulatory agencies such as the Health Care Financing Administration.

The content of the H & P is another area of concern that is ultimately addressed by the physician governing body, via quality improvement and medical peer review chart audits. Before the procedure, the nurse must have the H & P to match to the patient's signed consent and the scheduled procedure. Any inconsistency among any of those three documents requires immediate investigation before further action related to the patient's procedure is taken.

The responsibility for providing complete H & Ps and other physician documentation lies in the hands of physicians to supply comprehensive information and to encourage their peers to do likewise. However, nursing personnel and management can support the effort by suggesting or providing forms that allow the physician to document a comprehensive H & P with little time involvement. A preprinted outline that includes body systems, allergies, medications, family and individual significant histories, presenting symptoms, preoperative diagnoses, and planned surgical procedures is one method that allows physicians to complete a form quickly. Some facilities provide checklists of "normals" that allow physicians simply to mark appropriate responses. Others streamline physician documentation by combining various forms on one sheet.

THE CHALLENGE

Nursing in an ambulatory surgery setting offers the opportunity for intensive hands-on interactions with patients and families. The environment is punctuated by patients with widely divergent nursing care needs. Each patient travels a continuum from the time of scheduling to the time of home recuperation. Before surgery, the patient requires emotional support and information. Soon, that same patient requires a highly technical intraoperative and critical PACU focus and then progresses to a period of supportive, social, and educational needs. Even after discharge, the patient often looks to the ASC nurse to provide emotional support and technical information during the follow-up telephone contact. Nurses are constantly accommodating these diverse patient needs and levels of care each day.

Nurses with backgrounds in postanesthesia care and operating room practice are often able to broaden their experience to include areas previously outside their respective practices. Establishing home health support, making telephone contacts, and providing preoperative and postoperative family instructions are responsibilities that have rarely been part of the operating room or PACU nurse's daily routine before the development of ambulatory surgery programs. The ASC provides this opportunity for nurses who want to expand their roles.

Cross-training of nurses to work in all areas of the ASC is a controversial concept and one that often precipitates heated arguments between proponents of the system and those who feel that expertise remains more defined in nurses who specialize in one particular area. On one hand, cross-training allows utilization of staff members wherever the need is greatest on a given day. This is especially helpful in smaller or freestanding units with limited staff. The system also helps nurses to gain new knowledge from peers and to understand and become familiar with staff members in other areas, promoting rapport and teamwork. For some, it provides a break in the monotony of working in a single-practice setting and may help to avoid professional "burnout" for those nurses who desire diversity.

On the other hand, the technology and knowledge involved in today's nursing require nurses to specialize in an area if they are to become true masters of it. That is not to say that the skills necessary for working in various areas of the ASC cannot be learned, but most nurses migrate to practice settings that interest them and where they are comfortable and competent. Many prefer to stay in those areas as a matter of personal choice. Whatever the policy is regarding cross-training in a given ASC, the staff members should have a forum to discuss their feelings about the system, both approval and grievances.

The ASC nurse builds a special environment where patients can learn about, experience, and recover from ambulatory surgery. The building blocks include excellence and adaptability in clinical nursing practice, caring and concern about each patient as a person, emphasis on wellness and the patient's self-responsibility, and encouragement of family involvement in care. Surgery in the ASC may take only a portion of a day, but it has an impact on the patients' lives.

Nurses in busy ASCs must deal with extremes of caseloads in a demanding and often frustrating setting. In that sometimes frantic pace, the nurse who truly cares about the patients and who has a sincere desire and an ability to communicate with people emerges with the power and the responsibility to contribute significantly to those people's lives.

The best intentions cannot stand alone without knowledge. The following chapters present a body of information to assist the ambulatory surgical nurse in understanding many aspects of the patient's nursing needs. However, to keep knowledge current, the nurse must continually read, study, and investigate the many and varied sources of nursing-, anesthesia-, and surgery-related information available. With both desire and knowledge, the ambulatory surgical nurse can provide the type of nursing care that reflects the very highest standards of professional practice.

References

1. American Society of Perianesthesia Nurses: Standards of Perianesthesia Nursing Practice, revised ed. Thoroughfare, NJ: Published by Author, 1998.
2. Hartgerink BJ, McMullen P, McDonough JP, et al: A guide to understanding informed consent. CRNA Clin Forum Nurse Anesth 9:128–134, 1998.
3. Official dispels myths about revised nursing care standards. Hosp Peer Rev 15:138, 1990.
4. The Joint Commission on Accreditation of Healthcare Organizations: 1998–99 Comprehensive Accreditation Manual for Ambulatory Care. Oakbrook Terrace, IL: Published by Author, 1998.
5. Smith C: At last: A common language for nursing? Breathline: Newsletter of the American Society of Perianesthesia Nurses. 11:1, 1991.
6. Shapiro ET, Richmond JC, Rockett SE, et al: The use of a generic, patient-based health assessment (SF-36) for evaluation of patients with anterior cruciate ligament injuries. Am J Sports Med 24:195–200, 1996.
7. Pelletier LR: Outcomes management Internet resources. J Nurs Care Qual 1, 1998.
8. Luckmann J (ed): Saunders Manual of Nursing Care. Philadelphia: WB Saunders, 1997.
9. Harris R: Critical thinking. Executive Excellence 3:8, 1996.
10. Burns N, Grove S: The Practice of Nursing Research: Conduct, Critique and Utilization, 2nd ed. Philadelphia: WB Saunders, 1993.
11. Fetzer SJ: Nursing research. In Defazio-Quinn DM (ed): American Society of Perianesthesia Nurses Ambulatory Surgical Nursing Core Curriculum. Philadelphia: WB Saunders, 1999, pp 16–26.

Chapter 17

Preoperative Preparation of the Ambulatory Surgery Patient

Gwen D. Williams

BENEFITS OF A PREOPERATIVE PROGRAM

Proper preoperative preparation and assessment contribute to favorable outcomes for the ambulatory surgery patient. By initiating discharge planning before the procedure, patient needs are identified and referrals are initiated as appropriate. The keys to a successful preadmission program are flexibility and education. This includes educating ambulatory surgery center (ASC) users regarding the benefits of a preadmission program. The users include surgeons, the surgeons' office staff members, patients, and their families.

Some benefits of a preadmission program include performing a cost-effective patient evaluation and gaining improvements in operating room efficiency, patient safety, and patient satisfaction.[1]

Cost-Effectiveness

Currently patients are no longer subjected to routine laboratory or diagnostic screening as part of the preanesthetic evaluation. Testing should be based on specific clinical indicators or risk factors, such as age, pre-existing disease, and magnitude of the surgical procedure being performed. A multidisciplinary team, including members from nursing, administration, and anesthesia, should develop guidelines for appropriate preanesthetic screening tests. Consideration should be given to the probable contribution of each test to patient outcome.[2] An estimated $20 to $30 billion could be saved each year from the national healthcare bill by replacing multiphasic screening with assessments that ask patients about their health problems before surgery.[3] Chapter 12 provides a further discussion of anesthesia management.

Preoperative assessment also contributes to improved operating room efficiency by reducing the amount of time the patient spends in the preoperative holding area before going into the operating room and by reducing cancellations or procedure delays because of the ability to anticipate specific patient needs, such as the need for special equipment or consultations.

Patient Safety

A comprehensive preprocedural evaluation is designed to identify potential anesthetic-related difficulties, such as a difficult airway, poorly managed medical conditions, previous anesthetic complications, or family/patient history of malignant hyperthermia. With such information, the anesthesia provider is better able to formulate an individualized plan of action before anesthetic agents are administered.

Communication of identified areas of potential risk with nursing staff in all areas of care allows the staff to prepare for the patient's individual safety needs throughout the continuum of care.

In addition, preoperative assessment permits appropriate and timely consultations with the surgeon, anesthesiologist, and other physicians involved in the care of the patient. If necessary, modifications in the patient's plan of care can be made before the day of surgery. Proper preoperative preparation can reduce patient anxiety and may reduce the need for preoperative medication.

Patient Satisfaction

The patient benefits from knowing what to expect not only on the day of the procedure, but also what modifications and care will be necessary after discharge. Preoperative preparations done before the day of surgery can be reviewed and reinforced by the preoperative professional registered nurse (RN) on the day of surgery. In addition, cancellations and delays on the day of surgery are minimized, thereby avoiding disruption of the patient's or the caregiver's schedule.[4]

THE PREADMISSION ASSESSMENT

The current fiscal challenges facing ambulatory surgery programs are forcing nurses to reevaluate the preadmission assessment process. In some settings processes have been altered to reduce the amount of time spent interacting with patients prior to the day of surgery, relying more on information secured from and given to the patient by the surgeon's office. Financial realities are forcing such changes, whether or not this approach is in the best interests of patients and reflects the most comprehensive nursing process. Nurses, then, are challenged to provide the most individualized assessment and education possible in an age of shrinking resources and time compression. A discussion follows about a variety of approaches to preadmission preparation of patients and represents the ideal.

Timing of the preoperative assessment should be far enough in advance of the procedure so that postponement of the procedure, if necessary for further evaluation, will not increase procedure-related costs or place the patient at increased potential risk. Conversely, it should not take place so far in advance that the patient forgets what has been taught. In general, evaluating the patient at least 1 week in advance allows for identification of problems requiring additional preoperative testing and consultation. This provides sufficient time to obtain and evaluate additional test results to determine whether to proceed with the surgery. If it is necessary to cancel or reschedule the procedure, the patient has sufficient notification. Also, there is time for the center to schedule another procedure and prevent time gaps in the operating room schedule.

During the preanesthesia assessment, the nursing role focuses on preparing the patient both physically and emotionally for the surgical experience. A professional registered nurse assesses the patient and develops a plan of care to meet the patient's preprocedural needs.

Assessment factors include, but are not limited to:

1. Relevant preoperative status, including:
   - History of cardiac or respiratory problems
   - Radiologic findings, if relevant
   - Laboratory values, if relevant
   - Vital signs, height, weight
   - Oxygen saturation
   - Allergies, to include history of latex sensitivity or allergy
   - Medication history, to include over-the-counter drugs, prescriptions, transdermal patches, herbal therapy, and vitamins
   - Disabilities
   - Substance abuse
   - Physical or mental impairment
   - Mobility or communication limitations
   - Prosthetic or assistive devices
   - For pediatric patients, a birth history, developmental stages and parent/child interactions, nickname, favorite toys, feeding information and immunization status
2. Relevant preoperative, emotional, safety, and psychological needs and individual coping mechanisms
3. Anesthetic history, patient and family, with and without complications
4. An understanding of the proposed procedure
5. An understanding of the proposed anesthesia
6. Availability of accompanying responsible adult
7. Availability of safe transport home
8. Responsible adult help at home after discharge
9. An understanding of preprocedural teaching and discharge instructions

10. Reading level and ability to comprehend information provided
11. Activities of daily living—independent, requires assistance, totally dependent[5]

Preoperative preparation of the patient and the family can be accomplished in various ways: an in-person interview, telephone interview, patient/family completed questionnaire, preoperative seminars, assessment and education in the home, off-site preadmission clinics, computers, or a combination of methods.[5]

To facilitate in-person preparation, patients may be assigned appointments at specified times. This works well for patients scheduled well in advance. To accommodate patients who are added to the operating room schedule close to the day of surgery, regular patients may be scheduled far enough apart to allow for unscheduled patients.

In many facilities, the anesthesiologist or nurse anesthetist also sees the patient during the preadmission interview to evaluate and educate the patient, build rapport, and provide the opportunity for questions. This approach enhances the value of the preadmission program by providing another parameter of early intervention. It also allows specific anesthesia care planning, including ordering appropriate preoperative tests.

An on-site interview may not be accommodating for some patients given the busy lifestyle of the current population. Patients may believe that they already are inconveniencing their employer by taking time off from work to have surgery. An additional request for time off for the preadmission interview may pose a problem. This is especially true for patients who are undergoing minor procedures, where they will be off from work for several more days. Furthermore, elderly or physically challenged patients and those with transportation concerns may find the extra trip to be difficult.

For the patient who is unable to come for a preadmission interview, telephone screening permits appropriate data collection and patient education (e.g., medications to be taken or held before surgery, nothing by mouth [NPO] requirements). When considering telephone interviews, certain rules of courtesy should be followed. When making a telephone call, first inquire whether it is a convenient time for the patient to talk and whether the patient feels he or she can appropriately answer some very personal questions about medical history. If not, find out when would be a better time to call. A patient who does not have access to a private telephone in the workplace may be reluctant to answer health-related questions. If the nurse determines that the patient's privacy cannot be assured, alternative arrangements should be made to conduct the telephone interview at a more convenient time.

Telephone interviews are appropriate for patients with minor or well-managed medical problems. If a problem is encountered during the screening or the screener believes that a face-to-face evaluation is necessary, an appointment can be scheduled and a more detailed preoperative assessment can be performed in person.

When deciding which patients are healthy enough to be screened by telephone, two factors merit consideration—the physical status of the patient and the degree of invasiveness of the surgical procedure. The scheduling office should be able to provide this information. Generally, for any significantly invasive procedure:

- American Society of Anesthesiologists (ASA) PS-1 (Physical Status 1) patients may undergo evaluation via telephone.
- PS-2 patients should be screened via telephone and seen in the facility if potentially serious problems or questions arise.
- PS-3 or higher patients are best served with an in-person evaluation.

If a less invasive surgical procedure is planned (i.e., cataract surgery or chronic venous access implantation), even patients with more severe physical problems can be evaluated safely by telephone because the risks of the surgical procedure and the anesthetic method needed for the procedure are low.[4]

Patient-completed questionnaires may make the patient and family feel more comfortable in answering questions of a personal nature (i.e., drug or alcohol use, sexually transmitted diseases, bowel function). When developing the questionnaire, use familiar terms. The form should include the following:

- Reason for surgery (to ascertain the patient's general understanding)
- Current and past medical problems
- Surgical history (including childhood, dental)
- Any anesthesia complications
- Family history of anesthetic complications
- Medication use (including vitamins, over-the-counter medications, prescriptions, herbal preparations, or recreational drug use)
- The physical environment of the home (stairs, bathroom accessibility)

- Family situation (primary caregiver, lives alone with no available help)
- Nutritional status (special diet, loss of appetite, unexplained weight loss or gain)
- Current functional status (independent, assistance, total care)

If the patient is a child or is mentally challenged, a developmental assessment should be included. Figure 17–1 shows a sample preoperative questionnaire.

It is important to know whether the planned care will jeopardize or interfere with the patient's religious or cultural beliefs and practices. Inquiries of this nature could be interpreted as intrusive or could be embarrassing or difficult for the interviewer as well as for the patient. Thus, they should be asked in a manner that is nonjudgmental. One way to phrase such a question might be as follows: "Is there anything in your culture or religion that would affect your care before, during, or after your surgery that you would like to share with us?"

In many facilities, the preadmission clinic program provides intake care for inpatients as well as outpatients. Group education is another method of preoperative preparation. Preoperative seminars may be feasible for high-volume and complex procedures. Most often, these are directed at in-patient surgical procedures. These sessions should be multidisciplinary, bringing in all services that could be of assistance to the patient. Once the general information has been covered, smaller groups may form to discuss specific procedures. Team members should include representatives of the following departments or services: admissions, social services, preadmission nurses, financial services, and case managers. Other departments that may be involved include anesthesia, therapies, dietary, wound care, and others. Involvement of the team members helps to facilitate the admission and assessment process.

For pediatric patients, setting up group tours works well. Parents, the child, and siblings are invited to come to the facility, usually during evening hours. After an overview of what to expect on the day of surgery, a tour of the facility occurs. Children get a chance to enter the operating room, handle some equipment, and ride on a stretcher. Afterward, while enjoying refreshments, parents and children get an opportunity to have any unanswered questions addressed by the clinical staff. This process allows the children to actually see where they will have their surgery. In addition, by meeting with the clinical staff beforehand, they are more relaxed when they see that familiar face on the day of surgery.

There are other alternatives for preoperative teaching. One is to perform an in-home assessment. An in-home assessment program may be more conducive to learning and affords the nurse the opportunity to evaluate the home environment. However, this method is labor intensive and may be reserved best for more complex in-patient procedures, such as joint replacement, spinal fusion, or osteotomy surgery.

Another possibility is to provide off-site admission clinics. These can be of benefit if the facility draws from an extended geographic area. The volume of cases from an area determines the frequency and location of off-site clinics.

The use of a computer for preoperative education has several advantages.

1. Consistency—quality and content is standardized.
2. Individualized instruction—patients proceed at their own pace and can repeat and review information.
3. Privacy—only the patient sees incorrect answers, avoiding embarrassment over incorrect answers.
4. Time efficiency—reduces professional time spent presenting information common to most patients.
5. Accessibility—it can be used at any time, for inpatients as well as outpatients.

Some disadvantages may include patient reluctance to use a computer and the necessity of medical staff involvement because, ideally, instruction should start in the surgeon's office as soon as the need for surgery is identified.[6] In addition, language barriers and illiteracy must be taken into consideration. However, with widespread use of the Internet in so many homes, it is feasible to expect to see electronic preadmission interactions taking place in the future.

PREOPERATIVE TEACHING

Before developing a teaching plan, the general characteristics and specific attributes of the adult learner should be considered. In addition, consideration should be given to individual cognitive processes that may have an impact on the teaching and learning interaction. The professional registered nurse should provide a comfortable, relaxed environment with adequate time to answer questions. Open-ended ques-

Please answer the following questions and return the form in the envelope provided. This questionnaire will be used to evaluate your medical status and assist the anesthesiologist in planning your anesthesia. If you are not sure of an answer, write it anyway and your anesthesiologist will discuss it with you. For children, the parent should fill out the questionnaire. All information you provide will be confidential.

Patient's Last Name		M.I.	First
Date of Birth	Age	Height	Weight
Telephone number: Home:		Work:	
Can we call you at work to discuss your upcoming surgery? Yes ☐ No ☐ Best time to call: ____________			
Date of scheduled surgery			
Reason for surgery			

Please list previous operations	Approximately what year?	Type of anesthesia (if known)	Any complications or problems (if known)

CHECK EACH QUESTION YES OR NO. IF YES, PLEASE EXPLAIN

☐ **Yes** ☐ **No** 1. Are you allergic to anything? If yes, what?____________

☐ **Yes** ☐ **No** 2. Are you being treated for any medical problems, or had any recent illnesses? If yes, please explain: ____________

☐ **Yes** ☐ **No** 3. Have you ever had any of the following? (please circle):

Arthritis	Convulsions	Heart Disease	Kidney Disease	Sickle Cell Anemia
Asthma	Depression	Hepatitis	Motion Sickness	Thyroid Disease
Bronchitis	Diabetes	High Blood Pressure	Muscle Weakness	Yellow Jaundice

☐ **Yes** ☐ **No** 4. Are you taking any medicine, injections, or pills? If yes, please explain:

PRESCRIPTION, OVER THE COUNTER, AND HERBAL MEDICATIONS	DOSE	HOW MANY TIMES A DAY

☐ **Yes** ☐ **No** 5. Have you or any blood relative had a reaction to an anesthetic? If yes, please explain: ____________

☐ **Yes** ☐ **No** 6. Do you smoke? If yes, how long and how many packs per day? ____________

☐ **Yes** ☐ **No** 7. Do you have a physical impairment which limits the motion of joints, back, arms, or wear a device such as a hearing aid, glass eye, or artificial limb? Please explain: ____________

☐ **Yes** ☐ **No** 8. Will your surgery impact on your ability to get around in your home environment? (Stairs, accessibility to bathroom? Please explain: ____________

☐ **Yes** ☐ **No** 9. Will you have someone available to be with you when you go home and for the first night? Explain:____________

Figure 17–1. Sample preanesthesia questionnaire.

tions are used to promote/facilitate feedback and to assess the patient's understanding of the information. Verbalization of questions or concerns enables the nurse to help alleviate fears and decrease anxiety. Chapter 18 provides further detailed information about patient education techniques and issues.

Factors such as age; general, physical, and mental condition; attitude toward ambulatory surgery; and the existing social and family situation may influence a patient's ability to learn. Personal traits, including past experiences, education, gender, and cultural or religious orientations and practices, can contribute to the success of the instructional encounter. Assessment of the patient's reading level and ability is imperative.

The educator in the preadmission setting evaluates the patient who will undergo surgery using a participative, nonthreatening, and constructive manner. Building on the knowledge gained, the nurse educator is able to formulate an individualized and comprehensive teaching plan that addresses physical/clinical, emotional, social, and procedural issues. Skillful questioning can reveal the patient's knowledge base about the diagnosis and the proposed procedure. Questions may include the following:

- Have you ever been in the hospital as a patient?
- Have you ever had a surgical procedure, and if so, what do you remember about the surgery?
- What is the reason for this surgery?
- What has the doctor told you to expect from this surgery and about your recovery?
- In the past, if you had pain, what helped to relieve the pain?
- If you are in pain now, how are you treating it?

To assess a patient's coping strategies, asking questions such as the following can provide insight:

- What do you usually do when faced with a stressful or unpleasant situation?
- What activities have you found to make a difficult situation easier for you?
- What do you do for relaxation?
- Do you prefer to be made aware of what will happen, or does this make you worry more?
- How do you feel about this surgical preparation teaching?
- Will you have financial concerns as a result of having this surgery?

The person undergoing an ambulatory surgery procedure is discharged home before he or she is fully able to resume normal functions. A review of the patient's home routine will assist in discharge planning. Some questions to elicit information regarding the patient's home environment include:

- Do you live alone, and if so, do you have someone to help when you go home?
- Are you the primary caregiver for children or for an elderly or incapacitated person, and if so, have you made arrangements for someone to help until you are able to do so again?
- Have you used a home healthcare agency or received social services in the past?
- Do you know if you will need any medical equipment at home?
- Are there any barriers at home that may cause problems, such as stairs or small door openings?
- Will you be able to make arrangements for your follow-up visits to the doctor?
- Do you have any worries or concerns that have not been covered?

The nurse should provide a telephone number so that the patient may contact the preadmission clinic if questions arise.

Written instructions, pamphlets, or brochures are effective means to reinforce verbal information only if the patient is able to read and comprehend what is provided. An easy way to assess reading skills is to ask the patient if he likes to read, watch television, or engage in other activities to relax. Asking if he or she enjoys the daily newspaper, and which parts he or she enjoys most, may provide clues to his or her abilities.

Current Internet Web sites address a multitude of medical issues, and many provide consumer information that is applicable to ambulatory surgery and anesthesia. The ASA is one that has online copies of commonly asked questions and other helpful anesthesia related information for patients and families (Table 17–1 and Table 1–1).

Successful teaching techniques include the following:

- Maintaining eye contact
- Providing a quiet, distraction-free environment
- Eliminating extraneous information
- Requesting feedback
- Using short sentences, simple words, and a conversational voice tone
- Using visual aids
- Progressing in the order that the information will be used

***Table 17–1.* Resources Regarding Surgery and Anesthesia**

ORGANIZATION/RESOURCE	WEB SITE	TELEPHONE	COMMENTS
American Society of Anesthesiologists (ASA)	www.asahq.org	847-825-5586	Public education section has information on many topics—such as: Anesthesia and You Anesthesia for Ambulatory Surgery Know Your Anesthesiologist Latex Allergy Links The Management of Pain The Senior Citizen as a Patient When Your Child Needs Anesthesia My Trip to The Hospital Coloring Book
American College of Surgeons (ACS)	www.facs.org	312-202-5000	Provides links to specialty surgery sites Click on Public Information to find: Information on Patient Choice When You Need an Operation Who Should Do Your Operation? Should You Seek Consultation? Giving Your Informed Consent What Will Your Operation Cost? Protecting Your Health
American Academy of Ophthalmology	www.eyenet.org	415-561-8500	
American Academy of Orthopedic Surgeons	www.aaos.org	800-345-AAOS	
American Academy of Otolaryngology—Head and Neck Surgery	www.entnet.org	703-836-4444	
American College of Gastroenterology	www.acg.gi.org	703-820-7400	Single topic patient information sheets to download
American College of Obstetricians and Gynecologists	www.acog.org		
American Society of Colon and Rectal Surgeons	www.facsrs.org	847-290-9184	
American Society of Plastic and Reconstructive Surgeons	www.plasticsurgery.org	847-228-9900	
American Urological Association	www.auanet.org	410-727-1100	
Society of American Gastrointestinal and Endoscopic Surgeons	www.sages.org	310-314-2404	
Society of Laparoendoscopic Surgeons	www.sls.org	800-644-6610	
Vascular Surgical Societies	www.vascsurg.org	Multiple	Links to several societies

- Using familiar words and phrases
- Showing respect for the learner

Formulate the teaching plan and modify it to meet the patient's needs and to overcome any sensory or language barriers. Include an overview of the following:

1. The preparation phase
2. Length of time in each phase of the perioperative period
   - Preoperative preparation
   - Operating room
   - Postanesthesia care unit (PACU) phase I
   - PACU phase II
   - Other areas, such as phase III
3. Other people who will be providing care
4. Environmental descriptions, such as sights, sounds, smells, equipment, and uniforms
5. Opportunity for questions related to the perioperative experience
6. Use of preoperative medications (if applicable) and management of postoperative pain and nausea
7. How the patient is likely to feel and look after the surgery
8. Necessity of postoperative exercises and activity limitations
9. Discharge criteria
10. Appropriate continuum of care services—that is, home health, rehabilitation therapies

11. Visiting policy
12. Location of family/responsible adult waiting area
13. What to bring to the hospital
14. Leave all money, valuables, jewelry, and expensive clothing/shoes at home.

Recent emphasis on pain and its treatment has led the Joint Commission to develop new standards that address not only pain management but also aspects of how patients are being taught about their rights to pain control, how pain will be assessed, and what their responsibility is in clearly communicating their needs relating to pain management.

Reviewing each area that the patient will visit allows the patient and the responsible adult to have a general idea of the perioperative routine. The amount of information provided should be directed to the individual's identified needs and responses. For some individuals, information increases their comfort level and that of the family. Other individuals may prefer not to know the details. It is best to determine the individual needs of each patient. The general preoperative orientation process outlines expectations and leads to a more positive perioperative experience for all concerned.

Home support/aftercare is essential to the safe recovery of the patient. Ideally, arrangements are made before the patient returns to the home environment. Clarification of the expectations of the patient and the responsible adult are addressed at this time.

Each patient should have a responsible adult available for transportation home after surgery. The institution should have a policy addressing the issue of patient discharge after administration of sedation/anesthesia. This issue is addressed best before administration of medications. If the patient does not have a responsible adult escort available for transportation home, the nurse should be knowledgeable about the options available. It is not uncommon for some facilities to cancel the case if proper transportation arrangements are not made. Other facilities work with the patient to find appropriate community resources to assist the patient.

Identified possible risks, such as the potential for malignant hyperthermia or latex allergy, for instance, are communicated to the healthcare team involved in the patient's care and documented in the patient's medical record. This, along with documentation of education and instructions provided, serves for legal and quality improvement purposes.[7]

PREOPERATIVE ASSESSMENT ON THE DAY OF SURGERY

On the morning of surgery, the RN is responsible for ensuring that the preoperative assessment is complete and that the patient's emotional needs are met. Patients with high anxiety levels may not comprehend the information that is given to them unless their immediate needs are satisfied. The nurse should determine the patient's immediate needs, ensure that they are met, and then continue with preoperative preparations.

On arrival to the ambulatory surgery center (ASC), the patient is greeted by a receptionist. The patient or guardian is required to complete the necessary admission paperwork. This usually includes consent forms, financial requirements, and other relevant paperwork. The patient then is taken to the preoperative unit, where they are asked to change into hospital attire. The patient's valuables then are placed either in a locker or under the patient's stretcher.

The nurse also should ensure that the patient's privacy is maintained at all times. In addition, if the patient needs emotional support, the nurse should assess who is best able to provide this. A family member or friend should be allowed to stay with the patient for as long as possible before transfer to the operating room suite. It is best to check with the patient first to ascertain whether they desire to have the family member or friend present. Often, it is best to wait until the interview is complete and personal information is obtained before bringing in the support person.

Children are particularly in need of the companionship of their trusted caregivers. Every consideration should be given to limit the amount of separation time for them. The parents/guardians of minors should be informed before the day of surgery that they are required to remain in the facility throughout the child's complete course of care. Additionally, the nurse should oversee parental interactions with the child patient and provide tactful guidance when necessary that is in the best interest of the child's physical, social, and emotional needs.

Some facilities allow patients to wear clothing into the operating room. For example, patients undergoing cataract surgery may have a hospital gown placed over their clothing, or pediatric patients undergoing myringotomy with tube placement may be allowed to wear their clothes or pajamas into the operating room. The patient usually is asked to wear clothing that buttons down the front so that his or her chest is easily accessible for cardiac electrode placement.

Once admission has occurred, the RN assesses the patient. If the history and physical examination were completed during the preadmission assessment, the RN verifies that the information is still accurate. If the patient did not go through a preadmission assessment interview, the nurse completes that step at this time.

In completing the preoperative assessment, the nurse determines the patient's understanding of the surgical procedure that he or she is about to undergo. If the patient expresses concern or verbalizes uncertainty with the procedure, the surgeon should be notified and preparations halted. The surgeon needs to speak with the patient to clarify any concerns before the surgical process continues. The nurse should record in the patient's medical record the fact that the patient verbalized questions; the surgeon was notified; the surgeon met with and explained the procedure to the patient; and the outcome as to proceed or cancel the procedure. The same process applies to anesthesia-related concerns and notification of the anesthesiologist.

If the patient was not seen for a preadmission assessment before the day of surgery, any necessary preoperative teaching specific to the surgical procedure needs to be completed and documented according to facility policy. It is best to ensure the patient's immediate needs are met before teaching. Patients with high anxiety levels or multiple questions may not be receptive to teaching. It may be best to answer the patient's specific questions before starting the teaching. Once teaching has been completed, check with the patient again to ensure that all of their concerns have been addressed adequately.

When dealing with parents, it may be best to address their concerns away from the child. Children often take cues from their parents. A parent who exhibits a high anxiety level can unknowingly transfer that anxiety onto the child. The nurse who exhibits a positive, caring attitude toward the parents and the child can assist in decreasing the anxiety level for both.

The nurse should review the medications that the patient has taken or held on the morning of surgery. This information needs to be documented in the medical record and passed on to the anesthesia team. In addition, NPO status must be verified. Current trends have seen leniency in the NPO requirements. Each facility, in conjunction with the department of anesthesia, must establish a policy regarding acceptable NPO requirements before surgery. Chapter 12 provides more detailed information about NPO status.

The nurse assesses the patient's vital signs before administration of any medications. The patient's pulse, respiratory rate, blood pressure, temperature, and oxygen saturation level are recorded. If the patient was seen during the preadmission interview and vital signs were recorded, the nurse needs to compare the data for variances. If substantial differences or abnormalities are noted, the anesthesia team needs to be notified.

Documentation of the nursing assessment can be accomplished using checklists, narratives, and other forms. Refer to the individual facility policy for specifics. Generally, the nurse assesses and documents the following information:

- Vital signs, including blood pressure, temperature, pulse, respiration, breath sounds, oxygen saturation, and height and weight
- Allergies
- Medications, including those taken, held, over-the-counter, and herbal preparations
- NPO status
- Emotional status
- Prosthetic devices, including those retained by patient, secured with patient belongings
- Unusual bruising, abrasions, especially at the proposed surgical site
- Loose or capped teeth
- Potential recent exposure to communicable diseases
- Responsible adult escort to provide transportation home
- Support person at home according to facility policy/recommendation
- Phone number where patient's relative/support person can be reached

If, during the course of the nursing interview, the nurse discovers significant changes in the patient's status as previously recorded during the preadmission interview, the surgeon and the anesthesia team must be notified. Patients presenting with respiratory infections, fever, nausea or vomiting, or breaks in skin integrity at the operative site need to be assessed and cleared for surgery. It is best to obtain clearance at this point rather than allow the patient to get further along in the system.

The patient also receives a visit from a member of the anesthesia team. The anesthesia plan of care is reviewed. Many facilities have instituted separate anesthesia consent forms. If required, this is completed by the patient and the anesthesia provider at the conclusion of the anesthesia interview. Preoperative medications may or may not be given to the patient preoperatively. The anesthesia provider determines what is best for the patient after the anesthesia assessment is complete. Preoperative medications may be given to accomplish the following goals:

- Decrease patient anxiety
- Reduce the incidence of postoperative nausea and vomiting
- Decrease oral secretions
- Decrease the potential for intraoperative or postoperative laryngospasm
- Prevent infection
- Decrease gastric acidity
- Encourage rapid recovery

After assessing the patient, the anesthesia provider determines whether preoperative medication is necessary. Based on the patient's history, the surgeon also may order antibiotics to be given preoperatively. If necessary, the patient may need to have an intravenous (IV) line inserted while in the preoperative holding area so that the required medications can be administered.

Once the assessments are complete, the patient is prepared for the operating room. Because specific procedures vary according to facility policy, the method and procedure for transport to the operating room vary. Some facilities allow the patient to ambulate to the operating room. Once in the operating room, an IV line is placed and surgical preparations begin. Other facilities place patients on stretchers in the preoperative holding area. An IV line may be inserted by the preoperative holding nurse once the assessment is complete. There is no right or wrong method to proceed; facilities need to decide what works best for them.

The patient's family or companion should be allowed to stay with the patient as long as possible before the patient is transported to the operating room. They should be instructed about where they can wait and the approximate length of time that they can expect to wait. Family members should not be forgotten during the perioperative process. If an unusually lengthy delay occurs in the operating room, the nurse should ensure that the family is notified. This is especially important if the patient is a child. Nurses should be constantly on the lookout for measures to decrease patient anxiety.

Families and companions are also under the nurse's care in many respects. The nurse is the liaison for information, emotional support, and encouragement. Providing a comfortable waiting area is one way to show concern and compassion, as is having a separate private area for physician/family discussions. The link to the family is not just a nice thing to provide but an essential part of providing family-centered, wellness-focused care that typifies outpatient care.

The nurse involved in the preparation of the patient before surgery is fulfilling an important role. Adequately preparing the patient before surgery results in a more positive perioperative experience for the patient. The patient experiences decreased anxiety levels, increased understanding of what to expect, and an overall increase in the level of satisfaction.

GERIATRIC PATIENTS

The term *geriatric* historically has been applied to a person older than 65 years of age, although more recent practice is to consider those older than 75 or even 85 years as the geriatric population. The older patient may experience a decline in sensory function, resulting in a lessened ability to assimilate new information, and increased time requirements for processing that information. When interviewing the geriatric patient, have the room at a comfortable temperature for the patient. Chairs should be easy to get into and out of, and there should be no obstacles in the path as barriers. Providing a well-lighted room, facing the patient during conversations, and speaking in a strong low-pitched voice are all appropriate accommodations. The older patient is discussed in greater detail in Chapter 27.

PEDIATRIC PATIENTS

The term *pediatric* is applied to any patient younger than 18 years of age. When assessing the pediatric patient, identify the child's age and stage of development, both of which directly affect the child's coping ability. In addition to the history obtained on all patients undergoing surgery, the following information should be included:

- Family status—parents' marital status, custodial parent, guardian, usual caregiver, siblings
- Developmental level
- Response to separation from parent or guardian
- Security objects or sleep-time ritual
- For infants and small children—usual feeding pattern
- Immunization status

- Recent exposure to communicable or infectious diseases
- Childhood diseases
- Previous hospitalizations
- Episodes of bradycardia
- Parents' reading level
- Parents' ability to reinforce teaching

Without accurate information, children may develop fantastic and distorted ideas about the upcoming surgery. Information and education provided during the preadmission visit help the child to retain independence and control.

An often-overlooked aspect of care for pediatric patients is confidentiality. The older pediatric patient should be interviewed by the RN in private, with the assurance that the information will only be shared with members of the healthcare team. Begin with less personal questions, progressing to inquiring about the use of alcohol, tobacco, or drugs, or the possibility of pregnancy or a sexually transmitted disease. Having the patient complete a written personal history questionnaire that includes questions about substance use and other high-risk activities may help the patient feel more at ease answering personal questions. If substance abuse, pregnancy, or sexually transmitted disease is suspected, the surgeon should be notified immediately; the issue needs to be addressed by the physician while maintaining the confidentiality of the patient. Know the policy of your facility regarding information gained from minors before the issue arises.[8] The pediatric patient is discussed in greater detail in Chapter 26.

PATIENTS WITH SPECIAL NEEDS

In addition to the many physical, emotional, social, educational, and nursing needs that all patients have, patients with special needs challenge nurses to provide care that encompasses myriad special issues. The following discussion addresses some of the more frequent special needs encountered in ambulatory surgery. Chapters 24 and 25 provide a more in-depth discussion of a variety of special needs of patients and their families.

The Mentally Disabled Patient

To prepare the mentally disabled patient for surgery, the nurse must establish what is normal for this patient and develop the plan of care based on the information obtained. Generally, the patient with an intelligence quotient (IQ) greater than 40 can verbalize feelings in some way. An in-person interview is preferable because nonverbal communication may be the only way the patient can communicate. Depending on the severity of the disorder, it may be best not to bring the patient in for an interview. Severely mentally disabled patients do not do well with changes in their daily routine. In these situations, it is probably best to schedule the preoperative assessment with the patient's parents or caregiver. Some techniques that may help in the surgical preparation and assessment include the following:

- Exhibit an attitude of patience, calmness, and acceptance.
- Materials and methods used with pediatric patients may be appropriate.
- Be sensitive to nonverbal communication.
- Use the name with which the patient is familiar.
- Speak slowly and clearly, but do not talk down to the patient.
- Come to the point quickly.
- Ask the patient to repeat important points.
- Demonstrate skills that need to be learned, and have the patient do a return demonstration.
- Include the family/caregiver in the preoperative preparations.
- Observe the interaction between the patient and the family/caregiver.[6]
- Consider that physical impairments and defects may coexist.

In addition to the assessment done for any patient undergoing surgery, the following assessments should be included:

- Level of impairment/ability (A pediatric-based assessment style may help to determine the patient's functional ability.)
- Cognitive ability
- Mental status
- Sensory function
- Method of communication
- Defects of the craniofacial area
- Joint deformities
- Differences in skin temperature may indicate a difficulty with temperature control
- Variations in appearance of skin color
  - Pallor may indicate anemia.
  - Uneven coloring and/or mottling may indicate poor neural functioning of the autonomic system.

Levels of mental impairment can range from mild to profound. Some characteristics include:

- Mild—The patient usually is a slow learner,

and rarely asks questions. The patient usually can function at the level of a 10 year old.

- Moderate—The patient usually has little or no speech, can understand and follow simple commands, and probably needs supervision to perform simple tasks. The patient usually can function at the level of a 2 to 6 year old.
- Profound—The patient can show a basic emotional response and may be able to perform simple self-care tasks with supervision. They usually are able to function at the level of up to a 2 year old.[1]

Malignant Hyperthermia

Malignant hyperthermia (MH) is a distinctive set of signs and symptoms that may occur in susceptible individuals after exposure to certain drugs used to produce general anesthesia or muscle relaxation during anesthesia. Once an episode has been triggered, it progresses, if unchecked, to death. When a person has been identified as MH susceptible and proper protocols are followed, the hazards of anesthesia essentially are reduced to those faced by any other patient undergoing anesthesia.

Some patients with certain muscle disorders are believed to be more susceptible to MH. Not all patients with these disorders are susceptible to MH, nor do all patients identified with MH have a muscle disorder. Some of the muscle disorders in which MH has occurred are:

- Duchenne's muscular dystrophy
- Central core disease
- Myotonia congenita
- Congenital muscular dystrophy
- Becker's muscle dystrophy
- Neuroleptic malignant syndrome
- King Denborough syndrome
- Schwartz-Jampel syndrome
- Osteogenesis imperfecta

MH is an inherited condition that places the patient at risk throughout his or her lifetime. Some patients who are MH susceptible have had surgery using potent triggering agents without incident, only to react during the next exposure to the triggering agent. Certain physical characteristics have been observed more frequently in the MH-susceptible patient. These include eye muscle abnormalities (droopy eyelids or crossed eyes), spinal deformities such as scoliosis or pigeon breast, or frequent joint dislocations.

Any patient who is to undergo general anesthesia should be asked specific questions as part of a medical history, such as the following: Is there a blood-relative with a history of MH? Have there been unexplained family deaths or complications resulting from anesthesia, including surgery in a dental office? Do you have any type of muscle disorder? Have you ever had unexplained dark or cola-colored urine after anesthesia? Have you had unexplained high fever after anesthesia?[6] The Internet web site for the Malignant Hyperthermia Association of the United States (MHAUS) provides consumer and professional information about the condition. Contact information is provided in Table 17–2.

If a patient is identified as being at risk for MH, the anesthesiologist and the perioperative team must be notified as early as possible to allow time for preparations. Pertinent findings and the communication of those findings to involved departments should be documented. The anesthesiologist will make the determination whether to proceed with the patient as an outpatient using nontriggering agents or to defer to hospitalization for the patient at risk for an MH episode. Chapter 11 provides more information about MH.

The Physically Impaired Patient

Physical impairments range from visual and hearing deficits, necessitating glasses or hearing aids, to quadriplegia. Persons with similar disabilities react in different ways, therefore, each person must be treated as an individual. After determining the method of coping and the functional ability of the patient, develop the plan of care based on individual needs. Some physical disabilities that may be encountered are sensory.

Visual impairment can range from limited vision or the ability to perceive light to total blindness. Unless the patient is hard-of-hearing, do not raise your voice. Provide a safe, well-lighted environment. Information provided may

Table 17–2. Malignant Hyperthermia Association Contact Information

Malignant Hyperthermia Association of the United States
39 East State Street
Sherburne, NY 13460-1069
800-98-MHAUS or 607-674-7901
FAX 607-674-7910
Web Site: www.mhaus.org

need to be in large print or even Braille. Providing a taped recording of the information for the patient to review at home may be helpful.

Hearing loss may range from slight to complete deafness. It is important to determine the patient's method of communication: hearing aid, lip reading, sign language, written messages, alphabet, picture, word or phrase board, or a combination of methods. A quiet, well-lighted, distraction-free environment is helpful. After getting the patient's attention, speak slowly and distinctly, sit or stand directly in front of the patient, and keep your mouth visible when speaking. Maintain a comfortable speaking voice volume; shouting distorts words and may make it more difficult for the patient to read your lips.

The patient who is visually or hearing impaired may need an interpreter. To avoid delays, this request should be made at the time the appointment for the preadmission visit is made. Assure the patient that the use of assistive devices will be allowed as long as possible preoperatively and returned as soon as possible after surgery. If an interpreter will be needed on the day of the surgery, arrangements should be made before the day of the surgery.

The Aphasic Patient

Aphasia affects the person's ability to communicate in one or more different ways. Speak to the patient naturally, using short and simple sentences, and encourage the patient to respond in whatever way he or she can. The patient probably can understand all or part of what is being said and should be included in discussions related to care. Having one person speak at a time can help minimize confusion. Ask questions that require one-word answers, and maintain a relaxed attitude. It may be easier for the patient to write responses or use gestures.[9]

The Patient with a Spinal Cord Injury

Spinal cord injury may be complete, manifested by total paralysis and loss of sensation below the zone of injury and resulting in quadriplegia or paraplegia. Or the injury may be incomplete, with the patient exhibiting partial preservation of function below the zone of injury.

In addition to information required for any patient anticipating surgery, additional specific information should also be obtained from the patient with prior spinal cord involvement. Ascertain the level and duration of the disability; coping strategies used by the patient and the family; and the willingness and ability of the family to participate in the preoperative preparation and postoperative care.

Other essential information includes any previous history of cardiac arrest or cardiac arrhythmias; episodes of orthostatic hypotension; and history of autonomic hyperreflexia that may be triggered by noxious stimuli, such as urinary calculi, severe bladder infections, and operative incisions. The patient's pain history should be discussed and documented preoperatively so that postoperative pain can be assessed adequately in relation to that baseline. Pain may range from mild tingling to severe and intractable or spasticity. The patient who requires frequent catheterization may be at increased risk for developing latex sensitivity or latex allergy; thus, latex precautions should be maintained in each care area. Orthostatic hypotension usually is associated with injuries above the level of T7. Autonomic hyperreflexia occurs only with an injury above the level of T6.[9]

The Patient with Multiple Sclerosis

Multiple sclerosis (MS) also is known as disseminated sclerosis and is a chronic, progressive, degenerative disease that affects the myelin sheaths and conductive pathways of the central nervous system. Symptoms of MS include:

- Sensory—numbness, anesthesia, paresthesia, pain, decreased proprioception and sense of temperature, depth, and vibration
- Motor—paresis, paralysis, dragging of the foot, spasticity, diplopia, bowel and bladder dysfunction (incontinence or retention)
- Cerebellar—ataxia, staggering, loss of balance and coordination, nystagmus, speech disturbances, tremors, vertigo
- Other—optic neuritis, impotence or decreased genital sensation, depression or euphoria, fatigue or decreased energy levels

Surgery, undue fatigue, overheating, excessive cold, or emotional stress may cause a relapse in the patient who has been in remission.

The preoperative interview should be conducted in person. Some factors to consider include allowing adequate time because the patient may become fatigued or may require extra time to formulate questions and responses. Inquire about the patient's previous response to physical and psychological stress and what events may have triggered a relapse. Determine the willingness, as well as the ability, of family members to participate in the preoperative preparation and postoperative care. Inquire about successful management techniques, sensory or motor deficits, and cerebellar disturbances. If the patient has bladder control problems requiring frequent catheterizations, latex precautions should be initiated.[10]

The Patient with Parkinson's Disease

Parkinson's disease is a chronic degenerative disease of insidious onset that is characterized by motor impairment. Symptoms include the following:

- Tremors that improve at rest and are absent during sleep
- Rigidity
- Bradykinesia (slowness in starting and completing voluntary muscle activity)
- Shuffling gait and a tendency to accelerate walking and falling
- Postural and reflex changes
- Mask-like facial features where the patient appears expressionless, stares straight ahead, and has decreased blinking of the eyes
- Imbalance and stooped posture
- Speech changes such that the patient may have difficulty initiating speech and coordinating expiration and articulation
- Autonomic symptoms—drooling, excessive perspiration, constipation, orthostatic hypotension, and dysphagia
- Changes in behavior and mental ability—dementia, depression, social withdrawal, and generalized apathy
- Generalized weakness and muscle fatigue

An in-person interview affords the opportunity to observe the patient's abilities and interactions with family members. Factors to consider during the preoperative visit include allowing adequate time for the visit; providing periods for rest; maintaining a calm, accepting attitude; and providing a safe environment. Do not leave the patient unattended, and provide assistance with ambulation. The patient with Parkinson's disease may be unable to stay still, so provision for space to move about may lessen the patient's apprehension. Speak to the patient, and encourage a response in whatever manner is possible. Determine the patient's functional capabilities, and develop a plan of care based on the individual's needs and abilities.[9, 11]

The Patient with Alzheimer's Disease

Alzheimer's disease is a chronic, neurologic disorder characterized by progressive and selective degeneration of neurons in the cerebral cortex and certain subcortical structures. The patient may have:

- Sensory-perceptual alterations such as memory loss, lack of concentration, confusion, lack of motivation, decreased problem-solving ability, depression, or the inability to recognize familiar objects (agnosia)
- Impaired motor function characterized by difficulty with balance, problems moving arms and legs, lack of coordination, spasticity, decreased muscle tone, the inability to carry out a skilled act (apraxia), and difficulty swallowing
- Impaired communication manifested as halting speech, the inability to remember the necessary word, or the inability to communicate (aphasia)

The patient may lack a support system because of personality changes, altered behavior patterns, depression, an inability to interact in an adult manner, delusions, or because of socially unacceptable behavior.

When planning care, assess the abilities and needs of the patient as well as those of the family or primary caregiver. Determine the patient's and family's successful management techniques and the willingness and ability of the family to participate in the preoperative preparation and postoperative care. Keep instructions and information simple, repeat information frequently, and ask the patient to repeat back the information provided.[12]

SOCIAL AND CULTURAL ASSESSMENT

Healthcare workers must respect the patient's personal beliefs, regardless of whether they understand or agree with them. Every effort should be made to accommodate the patient's beliefs or practices as long as safety is not compromised.[6] See Chapter 24 for additional information.

THE NEEDS OF THE CAREGIVER

Ambulatory care is, by its nature, intertwined with a strong family-oriented approach. Providing support and education for the patient's caregiver is essential, particularly during the preoperative time frame. In addition to needing emotional support before and during the procedure, the waiting family member who will be caring for the patient at home has real challenges to address. Caregivers are asked to assess and care for their loved ones, making judgments and decisions that a nurse or other healthcare worker would have been making in the past model of surgical care.

In addition to providing specific information about discharge instructions relating to the type of procedure, the nurse also should consider that caregivers appreciate the following:

- Information and updates as to the length and progress of surgery or recovery
- Information about the method of contacting the physician—when, why, how
- Suggestions about keeping a written list of questions as a reminder for upcoming physician discussions
- Methods that the caregiver can use to provide comfort, over and above pain medications
- Whether it is good for the patient to have visitors, and ways to limit and minimize fatigue from visitors—for the patient *and* caregiver
- An idea of which type of emotional responses the patient may exhibit and why
- Encouragement to help the patient to be as self-sufficient as possible
- Clear expectations about the level of oversight the patient will need at home—for instance, does the caregiver need to stay awake, sleep next to the patient's bed, or help the patient each time to the bathroom?
- How to protect themselves when lifting or moving the patient
- The importance of getting enough sleep and good nutrition to keep themselves strong and healthy
- Suggestions that they, themselves, may need help so as not to become exhausted, for instance, when their health is not good or they have physical or medical limitations

The astute nurse is trained to assess situations and patients quickly and accurately and to formulate a plan of action almost intuitively. This ability should be transferable to the family members who look to that nurse as the expert educator. Nurses are not fully executing their roles if they are not providing support, education, and concern for the family/friend who will be the caregiver when the patient is discharged.

SMOKING

Because smoking is associated with decreased gas exchange, decreased mucous production, decreased mucous clearance, and increased morbidity and mortality, the surgical candidate who smokes and who is to have a procedure requiring general anesthesia should be advised to stop smoking at once. Even if a local or regional anesthetic is planned, smoking should be stopped in the event that the anesthetic must be converted to a general anesthetic unexpectedly. Discontinuing smoking can produce dramatic changes within a relatively short time, as shown here:

- Within 20 minutes—blood pressure and pulse decreases to normal, and the temperature of hands and feet increases to normal.
- Within 8 hours—carbon monoxide level in the blood decreases to normal and oxygen level in the blood increases to normal.
- Within 24 hours—the chance of a heart attack decreases.
- Within 48 hours—nerve endings start regrowing and the sense of smell and taste is enhanced.
- Within 72 hours—bronchial tubes relax, making breathing easier; lung capacity increases.
- Within 2 weeks to 3 months—coughing, sinus congestion, fatigue, and shortness of breath decrease; cilia regrow in the lungs, increasing the ability to clean the lungs and decrease infection. The body's overall energy level increases.

When taking a patient's history, inquire about smokers in the household as well. Second-hand smoke also should be avoided.[4] Table 17–3 provides valuable contact information for resources to stop smoking. Chapter 25 provides further information on smoking as it relates to the perioperative experience.

DISCHARGE PLANNING

An important aspect of the preoperative visit is the initiation of discharge planning. The patient and the adult caregiver must understand that recovery is not complete at the time of discharge from the hospital or surgery center. After general anesthesia, sedation, or pain medications, the patient should not drive, operate complicated or dangerous machinery, cook with heat or flame, drink alcoholic beverages, use nonprescription drugs unless approved by physician, or make legal decisions or sign legal documents.

***Table 17–3.* Stop Smoking Resources**

ORGANIZATION/RESOURCE	WEB SITE	TELEPHONE	COMMENTS
American Cancer Society (ACS)	www.cancer.org/tobmenu.html	800-ACS-2345	National organization with local offices for assistance
American Lung Association (ALA)	www.lungusa.org	800-LUNG-USA	General lung health, including smoking issues
Students Against Drugs and Alcohol (SADA)	www.sada.org/tobacco.html	800-782-4062	Nonprofit organization founded in 1988 Addresses use of all types of substances, including tobacco
American Association for Respiratory Care (AARC)	www.aarc.org	972-243-2272	National association for respiratory care professionals General lung health, including smoking issues, in "patient" section
Quitnet	www.quitnet.org	NA	Free service of Boston University School of Public Health and Massachusetts Tobacco Control Counselors from ACS participate in Quitline Provides links to many other sites Note "The Big Quit" section
The Mining Company—Internet Web Guide	www.quitsmoking.miningco.com	NA	Collection of resources about quitting smoking and staying off tobacco
American Society of Anesthesiologists (ASA)	www.asahq.org	847-825-5586	Public education links has information on smoking and anesthesia

Other aspects that may be covered include restrictions and limitations, special diet, and equipment or supplies that may be needed after surgery. If the patient is to have surgery on the lower extremities, inquiries should be made about the need to climb stairs at home, work, or school. If so, it may be necessary to schedule a preoperative physical therapy appointment to teach crutch walking. In addition, the patient should be instructed to bring suitable clothing to wear home on the day of surgery. If the patient is a child or is mentally or physically incapacitated, two adults should be available to accompany the patient home. If the patient has received prescriptions for medication or will need special supplies postoperatively, these should be obtained before the day of surgery, whenever possible. Including discharge planning in the preadmission visit can reduce delays or confusion at the time of discharge.

SUMMARY

A preadmission program can provide many benefits. Identifying potential complications that can lead to cancellation of the procedure on the day of surgery is one of the major benefits. Providing patients with the opportunity to tour the unit and meet with the health professionals who will be involved in their care on the day of surgery is another benefit.

Each facility must decide how to set up its preadmission program to meet the needs of its unit. For a single specialty unit that deals primarily with a healthy population, the preadmission program may not be necessary. For a multispecialty unit that cares for a variety of patients, the preadmission program is essential.

To establish an effective program, a multidisciplinary team consisting of members from admissions, preadmission testing, postanesthetic care unit, operating room, anesthesia, and physician offices and surgeons should collaborate on the development of the program. This will ensure that the individual needs of each department are met.

References

1. American Psychiatric Association: Diagnostic and Statistical Manual of Mental Disorders, 4th ed. Washington, DC: American Psychiatric Association, 1994, pp 29–35.
2. American Society of Anesthesiologists Statement on Routine Preoperative and Diagnostic Screening. American Society of Anesthesiologists, Chicago, IL. Approved by the House of Delegates on October 14, 1987, and last amended on October 13, 1993.

3. O'Brien D: Notes from the American Society of Anesthesiologists Annual Meeting. J Perianesth Nurs 8:104–108, 1993.
4. Ault ML, Cooper SJ, Peruzzi WT. The preoperative assessment clinic: Its value and function. Anesthesiol Clin North Am 4:735–752, 1997.
5. American Society of Perianesthesia Nurses: Standards of Perianesthesia Nursing Practice 1998. Thorofare, NJ: The American Society of Perianesthesia Nurses, 1998, p 29.
6. Williams GD: Preoperative assessment and health history interview. Nurs Clin North Am 32:395–416, 1997.
7. American Society of Perianesthesia Nurses: Competency Based Orientation Credentialing Program, 1997 Ed. Thorofare, NJ: American Society of Perianesthesia Nurses, pp 239–240.
8. Tweed SH: Intervening in adolescent substance abuse. Nurs Clin North Am 33:29–45, 1998.
9. Mumma CM: Rehabilitation Nursing: Concepts and Practice, A Core Curriculum, 2nd ed. Evanston, IL: Rehabilitation Nurses Federation, 1987, pp 125–130, 228–230, 237–239, 249–253, 258–265.
10. Antel JP: Multiple sclerosis. Neurol Clin 13:1–2, 174, 191, 197–207, 1995.
11. Cedarbaum JM, Gancher ST: Parkinson's disease. Neurol Clin 10:471–475, 1992.
12. Hickey JV: Quick Reference to Neurologic Nursing. Philadelphia: JB Lippincott, 1984, pp 117–123, 341–342, 487–507.

Chapter 18

Patient Education: Enhancing the Potential of the Teacher and the Learner

Carol DiMura

OVERVIEW

There are many good reasons to provide patient and family education. The Nurse Practice Act and the Joint Commission on Accreditation of Healthcare Organizations (JCAHO) state that we have to teach, but research says that there are benefits far beyond meeting regulation standards. Patient and family education can result in decreased morbidity and mortality, decreased unpaid bills, increases in obtaining follow-up care, and increased compliance.[1] The achievement of any of these has the promise of a better outcome for the patient and also can contribute to the hospital and outpatient facility's viability by ensuring that patients do not have to come back.

Nurses are no longer in this venture of teaching alone; JCAHO has required all licensed personnel in hospitals and outpatient facilities to assist in patient and family education. Additionally, the physician is another primary educator, providing the specific information to patients regarding the intended surgical procedure, expected outcome, potential complications, and alternative care.

Ambulatory surgical nurses are challenged to assess a patient and family's needs and develop a plan of learning for each unique individual. Additionally, they are challenged to meet this task in a short period of time. Nurses are willing to meet this challenge because they know that the information they provide is going to increase the patient's chance of doing the right things while preparing for surgery and when they get home. There are some specific skills and a body of knowledge that nurses can develop to improve their teaching abilities.

Teaching and learning opportunities occur throughout the ambulatory surgical experience: preoperatively, intraoperatively, and postoperatively. These educational opportunities can take a variety of forms. The patient may require formal or structured teaching, such as a surgical specific teaching plan. Conversely, time may allow for only casual "at the bedside" type of teaching. A good method for this latter type of teaching is described later in the chapter as the "Five Minute Quickie." Learning can even be by example (of what the nurse does). Patients watch carefully as dressings are changed and catheters are emptied and also take note of facial expressions of the nurse. The ambulatory surgical nurse needs to discern which type of teaching best suits each patient. A good working knowledge of skills needed for effective teaching greatly benefits the nurse.

SKILLS NEEDED FOR EFFECTIVE TEACHING

What skills are needed to be an effective teacher? A working knowledge of the adult learning principles, teaching strategies for children, good communication skills, and Benjamin Bloom's three domains of learning (affective, cognitive, and psychomotor domains)[2] can enhance the teaching skills of the nurse and the learning potential of the patient. A review of how the nurse can incorporate the use of these three very important skills can be helpful to the ambulatory surgical nurse. Additionally, it is helpful to examine some of the barriers to teaching and even how construction of a teaching tool can contribute to better learning.

Adult Learning Principles: Patients Are a Virtue

One of the exciting and perplexing things about teaching patients is that the process is full of surprises and unexpected events. Principles have been developed for the specific purpose of helping educators better understand and prepare for some of the surprises the adult patient presents. In the field of education, there are many learning principles developed by various educators. Discussed in this section are the ones that can be particularly beneficial in the preadmission, day surgery, and ambulatory surgery areas.

Learning Principle 1

Learning is influenced by personal factors, such as past experience, culture, age, ability to learn, and beliefs about health.[3, 4] Each individual is a unique blend of experiences, and all those past experiences influence how he or she learns. For example, if you chose to draw an analogy to explain something, the analogy you would choose for the artist likely would be very different from the analogy you would choose for the engineer.

This means that the nurse must try to anticipate how the patient will view the educational information from his or her perspective. Table 18–1 is a tool that can be used to gain insight

Table 18–1. **Barbe Modality Checklist A Key to How a Patient Learns**

Listed below are incomplete sentences followed by three ways of completing each. Distribute 10 points among the three phrases. Divide the 10 points according to how strongly each phrase describes the student. The phrase that describes the student best would receive more points than the phrase that least describes the student. For instance, if you believe each phrase describes the student equally well, mark a 3 in two blanks and a 4 in the one which favors the student even slightly more. If the student is completely described by one of the phrases, mark a 10 by it and 0 by the other two. Remember you *must* use a total of 10 points for each.

A. Student's emotions can be interpreted by:	____facial expression.	____voice quality.	____general body tone.
B. Student's hobbies, outside interests include:	____reading, artwork, watching TV, movies.	____listening to music, playing instruments.	____sports, active handwork.
C. The part of school the student likes best is:	____reading and writing,	____talking, music.	____gym, art crafts.
D. When studying, the student prefers:	____working alone; underlining, highlighting books and notes.	____working with someone else, asking and answering one another's questions.	____working alone for short periods of time interspersed with breaks, rewriting notes.
E. When angry, the student:	____uses silent treatment, either glares or looks away.	____shouts, whines, turns up volume of TV or stereo.	____reacts physically, clenches fists, stamps out of room.
F. When explaining something, the student:	____describes in detail; sees color, size, shape.	____tells more than I ever knew before; repeats self.	____gives minimum information, information has to be pried out.
G. When examining something new, the student:	____moves closer to it, looks from every angle.	____asks questions about it.	____handles it, turns it over, wants to feel texture, weight.
H. In a social group, the student:	____watches others, ceases talking when several others begin.	____talks at the same time as others; talks louder as noise increases.	____puts hands on others, moves frequently, suggests doing something.
I. When excited, the student:	____demands my attention, some visible reaction; sentences get choppy.	____talks rapidly, gives little or no time for response.	____cannot stand or sit still, uses hand and arm movement.
J. When looking for encouragement or reward, the student:	____looks for a smile, must have me see accomplishment.	____needs verbal praise.	____needs a hug, a pat on the back.
Total	____VISUAL	____AUDITORY	____KINESTHETIC

***Table 18–1.* Barbe Modality Checklist A Key to How a Patient Learns** *Continued*

	MODALITY CHARACTERISTICS YOU CAN OBSERVE		
	Visual	*Auditory*	*Kinesthetic*
Learning Style	Learns by seeing; watching demonstrations	Learns through verbal instructions from others or self	Learns by doing; direct involvement
Reading	Likes description; sometimes stops reading to stare into space and imagine scene	Enjoys dialogue, plays; avoids lengthy description, unaware of illustrations; moves lips or subvocalizes	Prefers stories where action occurs early; fidgets when reading, handles books; not an avid reader
Spelling	Recognizes words by sight; relies on configuration of words	Uses a phonics approach; has auditory word attack skills	Often is a poor speller; writes words to determine if they "feel" right
Handwriting	Tends to be good, particularly when young; appearance is important	Has more difficulty learning in initial stages; tends to write lightly; says strokes when writing	Good initially, deteriorates when space becomes smaller; pushes harder on pencil
Memory	Remembers faces, forgets names; writes things down, takes notes	Remembers names, forgets faces; remembers by auditory repetition	Remembers best what was done, not what was seen or talked about
Imagery	Vivid imagination; thinks in pictures, visualizes in detail	Subvocalizes, thinks in sounds; details less important	Imagery not important; images that do occur are accompanied by movement
Distractibility	Generally unaware of sounds; distracted by visual disorder or movement	Easily distracted by sounds	Not attentive to visual, auditory presentation so seems distractible
Problem Solving	Deliberate; plans in advance; organizes thoughts by writing them; lists problems	Talks problems out, tries solutions verbally, subvocally	Attacks problems physically; impulsive; selects solution with greatest activity
Response to Periods of Inactivity	Stares; doodles; finds something to watch	Hums; talks to self or to others	Fidgets; finds reasons to move; holds up hand
Response to New Situations	Looks around; examines structure	Talks about situation, pros and cons, what to do	Tries things out; touches, feels; manipulates
Emotionality	Somewhat repressed; stares when angry; cries easily, beams when happy; facial expression is a good index of emotion	Shouts with joy or anger; blows up verbally but soon calms down; expresses emotion through changes in tone, volume, pitch	Jumps for joy, hugs, tugs, and pulls when happy; stamps, pounds when angry, stomps off; general body tone is a good index of emotion
Communication	Quiet; does not talk at length; impatient when extensive listening is required; may use words clumsily, uses words such as *see*, *look*, etc.	Enjoys listening but cannot wait to talk; descriptions are long but repetitive, likes hearing self, others; uses words such as *listen*, *hear*, etc.	Gestures when speaking, stands close; does not listen well; uses words such as *get*, *take*, etc.
General Appearance	Neat, meticulous, likes order; may choose not to vary appearance	Matching clothes not so important, can explain choices of clothes	Neat but soon becomes wrinkled through activity
Response to the Arts	Prefers the visual arts; tends not to voice appreciation of art of any kind, but can be affected deeply by visual displays; focuses on details and components	Favors music; finds less appeal in visual art but is readily able to discuss it; misses significant detail, but appreciates the work as a whole; is able to develop verbal association for all art	Responds to music by physical movement; prefers sculpture; touches statues and paintings; at exhibits stops only at those in which he or she can become physically involved; comments very little on any art form

into the type of learner being taught. The reader should score the tool as directed on the tool.

A basic tenet of critical thinking further complicates learning. "While it is important for us to look at how others think, we have this innate instinct to look at things from our own point of view."[5] The ability to look at how others think and learn can determine how, and even whether, the nurse connects with the patient. This connection is necessary for learning to take place.

The nurse's prejudices and life experiences can influence his or her ability to teach effectively. Imagine an ambulatory surgical nurse who experiences a miscarriage and whose coping mechanism is to talk about the experience. Our imaginary nurse could be assigned an auditory orientation, and verbal delivery of information would work well for her. The next time this nurse cares for a patient experiencing perinatal loss, she may assume that the patient also will feel better talking about it, whereas the patient may have a visual orientation and prefer to be given reading material. It would be good for the nurse to think ahead about issues, such as caring for the patient having an abortion, cultural biases, and even feelings about patients with certain disease entities such as acquired immune deficiency syndrome (AIDS). Strong feelings about these and other issues may result in a different standard of care or avoidance, which could change the amount of time spent with the patient.

Learning Principle 2

Students learn more when they perceive a need to learn and when they have a clear overview of the plan.[3, 4] Patients do a lot of informational reading during the preoperative period because they have a need to know. This is seen currently when the patient presents with a handful of papers they have printed from the Internet. This can be the most opportune time to teach because the patient has a need to know and may be able to listen while undistracted by the intensity of anxiety that accompanies the actual admission. Because of time constraints in the preadmission clinic, the tendency can be to focus on the medical assessment regarding fitness for surgery. Although this is an extremely important aspect of care, it does little to reduce the patient's anxiety. Presenting procedural information (i.e., what happens next, where to expect the incision site, where to get help if needed, and whom to ask for help) provides needed information and helps reduce the anxiety at a time when patients actually can synthesize the information.

Learning Principle 3

Learning is facilitated when the learner is accepted and respected as a person of worth in a mutually trusting relationship without fear of criticism or ridicule.[3] The teacher must listen and understand the patient's perceived need. "Listen" is the operative word. Listen with your eyes and your ears. For example, the nurse may want to talk about wound care, but the patient may want to go to the bathroom or may be gazing off and preoccupied with an entirely different issue. The teacher can advance the needed agenda by first taking a moment to understand and address the patient's agenda. Listening and applying this principle is very helpful in building the trust needed to facilitate learning and in the assessment of the patient's learning needs.

Learning Principle 4

People learn through their five senses: seeing, hearing, feeling, smelling, and tasting.[3, 4] Rorden describes how a wide variety of experiences contribute to one's resources for learning. Written materials, stick drawings, enlarged photographs, models, and videotape all are appropriate media for teaching patients in any part of the ambulatory surgery process. Encourage the patient to handle a leg bag, catheter, or walker. Give them a demonstration and then have them give a return demonstration so that they can absorb the information before surgery.

Learning Principle 5

Learning is facilitated when the student has knowledge of how well he or she is performing in a learning experience.[3, 4] Recognition and praise are easier for some teachers than for others, but everyone benefits. Table 18–2 provides a list of 100 ways to tell someone that they are doing a good job. Commonly recognized as effective for motivating employees, these ideas are equally applicable for praising learners.

Strategies for Teaching Children

A special set of guidelines applies when teaching children. Children learn through play. Children learn differently at each stage of their development, so the teaching must be adapted to appropriately fit the age. For children up to 2 years of age, education is directed to the par-

Table 18–2. **100 Ways to Say "Very Good"**

1. You're right!	51. You're learning fast.
2. Good work!	52. You certainly did well today
3. Well done.	53. I'm glad your approach is working.
4. You did a lot of work today!	54. Keep it up!
5. It's a pleasure to work with you.	55. I'm proud of you.
6. Now you have it.	56. That's the way.
7. Fine job!	57. You're learning a lot.
8. That's right!	58. That's better than ever.
9. Neat!	59. Quite nice.
10. Super!	60. You've figured it all out.
11. Nice going.	61. Perfect!
12. That's coming along nicely.	62. Fine!
13. That's great!	63. I'll sign the order.
14. You did it that time!	64. You've got it.
15. Fantastic!	65. You figured that out fast.
16. Terrific!	66. Very resourceful.
17. Good for you!	67. You are really improving.
18. Make it so!	68. Look at you go.
19. That's better.	69. You've got that down pat.
20. Excellent!	70. Tremendous!
21. Good job (name).	71. I like that.
22. Super fine!	72. I couldn't do it better myself.
23. That's good.	73. Now that is what I call a fine job.
24. Good going.	74. You did that very well.
25. That's really nice.	75. Impressive!
26. Wow!	76. Sharp!
27. Keep up the good work.	77. Right on!
28. Outstanding!	78. That's wonderful.
29. Fantastic!	79. You mastered that in no time.
30. Good for you.	80. Very nice!
31. What talent!	81. Congratulations!
32. Good thinking.	82. That was first class work.
33. Exactly right!	83. Sensational.
34. You make it look easy.	84. Right!
35. Yes!	85. You don't miss a thing.
36. Awesome!	86. You make our work fun.
37. Way to go.	87. You must have been practicing it.
38. Superb!	88. I'm glad I assigned this to you.
39. OK!	89. You came through again.
40. You're on target.	90. Dynamite!
41. I knew you could do it.	91. I knew I could count on you.
42. Wonderful!	92. You deserve a raise.
43. You're great.	93. How can I help you with this?
44. Beautiful work.	94. Go for it!
45. You've worked hard on this!	95. The best!
46. That's the way!	96. You have my complete support.
47. Keep trying.	97. Marvelous!
48. That's it.	98. Clever idea.
49. Let's tell the boss.	99. I'm glad you are on our team.
50. You're very good at that.	100. Thank you!

Reprinted with permission of Roger L. Firestien, Ph.D. PO Box 615, Williamsville, NY 14231-0615.

ents. If the parent is anxious, the child is likely to be anxious.[6] Take time to acquaint the child with the equipment by letting them play with the surgical mask, gloves, anesthesia mask, and other items. When teaching children 2 to 4 years of age, play therapy is best. They can benefit from becoming familiar with the equipment, and playing with puppets or dolls to simulate the procedure is suggested.

Patients 4 to 7 years of age can enjoy activities that involve any of the senses—seeing, hearing, smelling, tasting, and touching. If possible, provide some hands-on experience. Verbally explain to this age group why a procedure is being done and then demonstrate by using dolls. At this age, and sometimes even earlier, the child is very literal. Avoid phrases that can be misunderstood such as "put to sleep" because they often have their pets put to sleep. When the nurse describes how the patient receives "gas" as anesthesia, the child may think that someone is going to pour gasoline in the mask. A discussion about a "CAT" scan (computed axial tomography) may make the child think that cats will be walking around.

For patients 7 to 11 years of age, the teaching techniques are the same as for 4 to 7 years of age, but the older children have a longer attention span. This group often thinks that they are too old to cry, so it is a good idea to let them know that it is okay to cry. School-aged children also have a great fear of body mutilation.[6]

Adolescents still can benefit from knowing what they will see, hear, smell, taste, and touch, but they also want to know why something is being done. The teenager is able to understand more detailed information.[7] See Chapter 26 for more information on the teaching process and children.

Effective Communication Skills: The Gift of Being Simple

There are many nurses who are gifted teachers, and effective communication is challenging even to them. The development of both verbal and nonverbal skills is important in teaching both patients and their families. This skillful interchange of giving and receiving information is elemental to the success of the teaching process and can enhance learning potential. This section addresses verbal and nonverbal communication and active listening as it affects the ambulatory surgical nurse.

When using verbal communication, be sure to choose your words carefully. The interpretation of the spoken word lies in the learner, not in the spoken word. For example, when a patient asked the nurse to describe laparoscopic surgery, the nurse explained, "They put a tube in your belly and *blow it up* with a gas." The patient's eyes were filled with surprise. In another instance, a nurse was trying to assess the patient's knowledge about his surgery and asked the question, "What brought you to the hospital?" The patient replied, "The ambulance."

Proper terminology should be used. Nurses are prone to use jargon and acronyms to excess, such as *NPO*, *TIA*, *CPR*, and *PACU*. Healthcare jargon and acronyms are a great source of bafflement to both patients and families. Even nurses often use the same acronym to mean different things. Example: *SOB* means string of bottles for the genitourinary patient. The same acronym, SOB, means short of breath in the cardiac patient. This acronym used in the presence of the patient and family could be construed to be something embarrassing, depending on the patient's orientation. To achieve a clear understanding, state the full word or phrase.

Nonverbal communication sends messages before a word even is spoken. Facing the patient and maintaining eye contact helps in assessing the patient's understanding. Eye contact during teaching can prevent misunderstandings and misinformation. Often patients say that they understand and yet still have confused looks on their faces. The nurse who is looking down at paperwork misses this cue. Other nonverbal communication can have a negative effect on patients. Do not let the patient know you are in a hurry. Rolling your eyes or expelling a heavy sigh certainly is inappropriate, and even glancing at your watch may be interpreted by the patient as a sign of impatience or disinterest.

We communicate in lots of different ways, and one of the skills valuable to both the teacher and the learner is active listening. Listening is inexact for many reasons; for instance, the listener thinks he or she knows what the other person is going to say, or the speaker inundates the listener with words and the listener has a difficult time sorting through the words to find the intended point. Another problem can occur if something is spoken that triggers other thoughts in the listener's mind, so the listener tends to stay at that point until clarification is made. Active listening can clear up and even prevent communication problems.

In her book, *Tribal Warfare in Organizations*, Peg Neuhauser, an anthropologist and communication expert, suggests ways to stop making these listening mistakes.[8]

- Take notes to remember the speaking party's key points or to remember a point you want to address. You may want to explain the purpose of your note-taking to the patient before they begin speaking.
- Repeat key points that the patient makes, for clarification.
- A return demonstration and verbalization are acceptable ways to validate understanding. A good question to verify comprehension is, "What do you understand about . . . ? " This question is more likely to produce an accurate response than "Okay?" One never must assume that the written or spoken word is too clear.
- Look straight into the patient's eyes when

they are talking. This shows attentiveness and keeps the listener focused on the spoken word.[8]

Incidentally, the Neuhauser book can serve as a great communication resource to improve communication for teaching or to improve communication between departments.

Bloom's Three Domains of Learning: Be All That You Can Be

Benjamin Bloom,[2] an early learning theorist, devised (and Knowles[9] furthered the use of) three domains of learning that simplify the nurse's ability to individualize the approach to teaching and tailor the presentation to each patient's learning style.[3] The domains of learning not only help to distinguish the type of learning that is being addressed, but they also determine the best method of presentation to select depending on the particular domain being taught. The three domains of learning include the cognitive domain, the psychomotor domain, and the affective domain. Some simply define these learning domains as thinking (cognitive), doing (psychomotor), and feeling (affective). Elements of thinking, doing, and feeling can be found in most of what we teach, so it is important for us to understand each domain of learning.

The cognitive domain addresses the patient's understanding. This domain is used when the teacher is trying to create a new body of knowledge for the patient and often incorporates the use of facts, details, and information basic to intellectual learning. This domain is best taught with the use of multiple media. The more media the patient is exposed to, the better the understanding and retention of the information. An accepted maxim in the training industry[10] is that:

People remember . . .
10% of what they read
20% of what they hear
30% of what they see
50% of what they see and hear
90% of what they say and do.

The psychomotor domain addresses the teaching of a motor skill. This particular domain is best taught by demonstration and providing the student with a hands-on experience, including the opportunity to practice until the skill is perfected. The key to the success of this teaching method is ensuring that the student gives a return demonstration. Skills that merit observation include proper attachment of a leg bag, use of crutches, and changing of a simple dressing. The observation of the return demonstration provides an opportunity for intervention to correct any misunderstandings.

The affective domain addresses attitudes, beliefs, and feelings—that is, our values. This domain is best addressed with discussion and some exchange between the teacher and the patient, including presentation of facts. Lecturing is not very useful for effecting learning in this particular domain. This is the most difficult domain in which to effect learning because we hold our values so close. We can understand something intellectually, but to change our behavior, a change of values is often necessary.

Think about prudent heart living. Nurses all know that prudent heart living entails a low-fat diet, no smoking, getting plenty of rest, managing the stress in our lives effectively, and getting exercise at least three times a week. Yet who among us honestly can say that we live by the regimen of prudent heart living? We are certain that we are invincible. The untoward circumstance of heart problems could only apply to others, not us . . . until someone in our family or a friend close in age encounters some heart pathology. Then we are ready to listen. We are instantly able to incorporate our cognitive knowledge (facts and details) and make a change in our affective domain (attitudes and beliefs). Learning takes place.

The affective domain takes the longest to effect, but the ambulatory surgery nurse should not be too quick to dismiss this responsibility just because the time for perioperative teaching is brief. Nurses can be the start of something *big*! You can be the beginning of this long process. The nurse may be the reason that a patient sits up and takes notice of the need for a change in lifestyle.

The best learning takes place when multiple domains are incorporated. A courtroom scenario can be used to illustrate the active use of all three domains. An analogy can be created between the teaching of patients and the teaching of a jury in a courtroom setting. For the purposes of our analogy, the attorney would be the teacher (as is the nurse) and the jury would be the students (as are the patient and family). An attorney is faced with the task of imparting learning in a relatively short time span. The attorney understands that incorporating all three domains in a presentation increases the chance that the jury will understand the client's view of the occurrence. The jury then can make a decision that, hopefully, results in a favorable outcome for the client.

Take for example, the application of the three domains of learning to a famous trial with which most are familiar. Almost everyone has some familiarity with the O. J. Simpson trial. There were many instances in which the cognitive domain was taught, but the one that most audiences readily identified as key to the trial was the presentation of facts and details about DNA. The prosecuting attorneys first had to teach the jury about the relevance, the statistical accuracy, and even where to find DNA before their case could move forward. The psychomotor domain was used in the trial by the prosecution via the display of pictures and the trip to the crime scene. But the demonstration that is forever emblazoned on everyone's memory is the trying on of the glove. This powerful display brought gasps in the courtroom that day and even may have determined the outcome of the trial. A demonstration so powerful is difficult to erase from the jury's memory.

This could be equally important to remember in your patient teaching. The affective domain was the main hinge of the defense's case in this trial. To win this case, the defense attorneys were counting on the jurors' preformed opinions about Simpson: "He's an all American athlete, likeable celebrity, he would never do this." Remember, the mission in this example was not to try Simpson but to look at the powerful usefulness of these three domains. They can be used in any learning situation. Use them to your best advantage.

PERSONAL QUALITIES THAT ASSIST THE NURSE IN TEACHING

Nurses depend on their credibility with the patient to entice them to listen, just as attorneys depend on their credibility with the jury to win cases. Consequently, nurses can take lessons from a book called *Winning Trial Advocacy Techniques*, which teaches attorneys how to develop this credibility with their jury to win trials.[11] This book describes four dimensions of credibility that an attorney (a nurse teacher) can develop to ensure that the jury (the patient and family) will listen and be persuaded. These qualities are likeability, expertness, trustworthiness, and dynamism.

Likeability

The attorney knows that his or her greatest weapon is not the law or the facts, but his or her personal standing with the jury. Similarly, nurses recognize that an unwritten rule in malpractice insurance is that if the patient and family like them, the nurse is less likely to be sued. This likeability component is so important that *Winning Trial Advocacy Techniques* devotes half of its content to developing likeability.[11]

Expertness

Like the attorney, the teacher needs to build credentials to convey expertness. These credentials can include education or experience. With the advent of the Internet, patients are very sophisticated in their knowledge of healthcare issues. Nurses must stay current as well. Another feature of expertness is being organized. Think about your own assessment of the teacher who is shuffling papers or looks disheveled and disorganized.

Trustworthiness

To convey this quality, attorneys are told to be calm, gentle, sincere, friendly, and hospitable. Abraham Lincoln was described as not particularly learned in the law, and he spoke irritatingly slowly. So why did every railroad company want him to represent them? They were buying his personal qualities with the jury. Patients often are invited to preadmission testing areas for completion of their laboratory tests and some education. Many times, the portion of the invitation that they are most interested in is the education. If the department is busy and the nurse is brusque, not allowing time for questions, this can set a tone of dissatisfaction for the entire surgical experience. It could be inferred that patients would listen to your personal qualities as much as to your information.

Dynamism

This is described as the forcefulness of delivery and the energy of the presentation—Enthusiasm! This kind of drama convinces people to listen. Have you ever heard someone speak who sounded knowledgeable and convincing, but later you discovered that the person did not have a clue what he was talking about? That is the picture of dynamism. (A word of caution—the forcefulness and energy can be very entrancing to the patient but, if overdone, can result in a loss of likeability.) Taking the time to establish better credibility brings better learning opportunities for your patients and families.[12]

TIME-SAVING TIPS

An interview with various ambulatory surgical nurses reveals time as a barrier to effective patient teaching.[13] Because time also is cited as one of the most common barriers to documenting patient teaching,[14] the nurse must preserve as much of it as possible. It is valuable to look at a tool that can optimize the time spent teaching and to look at exactly what should be taught.

A great tool to maximize teaching in a brief time frame is the "Five Minute Quickie."[15] There are three steps to the "Five Minute Quickie":

Step 1: Give it a title. Make this clever or attention getting so that you grasp the patient's attention at the earliest possible moment. Humor also enhances the retention and desire for learning.

Examples 1. "I Am A Teapot" to teach the patient how to assess for bladder fullness.

2. "Waiting To Exhale" when teaching the patient the proper use of an incentive spirometer.

3. "The Jane Fonda Portion of Our Program" to teach postoperative leg exercises.

Step 2: Make only three points. Be selective.

Step 3: Review the three points.

Planning the salient points to be taught and inserting them into a "Five Minute Quickie" can add interest for the learner. Much of what is taught is repeated, so even the "Five Minute Quickie" can become a standardized teaching plan.

LEARNING ASSESSMENT

An assessment of learning needs actually can save the nurse time by identifying the patient's current knowledge base and using that as a starting point. Instead of imposing an assumed agenda on the patient, the assessment allows the nurse to investigate the patient's and family's current agenda in their quest for knowledge. The nurse then can begin teaching at that point. JCAHO places a special emphasis on assessment in the patient teaching standard.[16] Five areas must be assessed by nurses for every patient. These areas include readiness to learn, emotional intelligence, knowledge of disease or care management, functional barriers, and cultural or spiritual beliefs.

Readiness to Learn

Readiness to learn refers to the willingness or ability of the patient to accept any information taught. If the patient is asking questions, maintaining good eye contact, and generally participating in the conversation, this could be taken as an indication of readiness to learn. Similarly, if the patient is in tears, in pain, or is sedated postoperatively, these could be taken as an inopportune moments of readiness to learn. Readiness to learn must be an ongoing part of the assessment.

Emotional Intelligence

Daniel Goleman, in the book *Emotional Intelligence,*[17] describes how, after the delivery of such information as a serious diagnosis, the brain can experience a flood of chemical changes, causing the mind to experience an inability to accept any further information. Watching for nonverbal clues can be very helpful during the assessment of readiness to learn. The nurse must be attuned to the fluidity of the patient's ability or inability to receive information.

Knowledge of Disease or Care Management

Assessing the patient's knowledge of disease or care management gives the nurse insight into what the patient already knows. Can the patient or family explain the goal of this surgery or procedure? Do they know where to expect the incision? Ask questions such as: "What worries you most?" This can save the nurse and the patient the time of unnecessary explanation. The nurse also can be attuned to areas of misunderstanding and focus more education on this information.

Functional Barriers

Assessment of functional barriers helps the nurse to think about things that can get in the way of learning, such as language, reading ability, and sensory problems. In response to the identification of such barriers, many hospitals have devised tools to assist in addressing the problems. A language bank can be created easily by a survey of new employees on employment.

Reading ability can be assessed quickly and informally by handing the patient the desired written teaching sheet upside down and then pointing out a specific point and asking the patient to describe what it means to them. (If the patient continues to look at the piece upside down or if the patient cannot say what the point means to them, it may be an indication of inability to read or slowed reading ability.) This readability assessment helps the nurse identify those patients who require additional instruction time. Guard against that false sense of comfort that can accompany the complacent nod of the agreeable but "very hard of hearing" patient who has not heard a word.

Cultural or Spiritual Beliefs

The cultural or spiritual beliefs assessment recently has been acknowledged for its contribution to the improvement of the patient's wellness status. JCAHO currently requires this assessment, and there is ample research that shows this assessment's value. A study at San Francisco General Hospital is an example of such research.[18] This double-blind study compared the results of 393 coronary bypass patients who were divided into two groups (prayed for and not prayed for); for the purposes of the research, prayer was described as Judeo-Christian prayer. Ten months later, the results showed that the "prayed for" group had fewer patients with congestive heart failure (CHF) (8 vs. 20), used less diuretics (5 vs. 15), had fewer cardiopulmonary arrests (3 vs. 14), used fewer antibiotics (3 vs. 17), and were intubated less frequently (0 vs. 12). The results of this research were not unique. Of 146 studies in scientific journals at the National Institutes of Health, 112 showed that spirituality had a positive effect on health.[19]

JCAHO has placed a strong emphasis on this area of assessment. Nurses must work to develop a comfort level with assessing for the patient's cultural and spiritual beliefs. An excellent question for the nurse to pose might be: "Do you have any cultural or spiritual beliefs that we need to consider when planning your care?" Often, the patient's response is either the identification of a specific belief or a confused look. As long as the nurse is sure that the patient heard the question, the nurse should offer assurance that the patient would know whether they had any beliefs that needed to be identified. The nurse needs to have a resource available to interpret the requests or comments of patients who are able to identify need. This assessment has been deemed important enough in some hospitals to involve the pastoral care department in assembling a one-page synopsis of the various religions practiced in their particular county. This type of reference allows the nurse to quickly look up what it means to the patient's care when the patient says, "I'm Islamic." If the patient is Islamic and going into a procedure with a male doctor, you can expect a request for a female accompaniment because this is part of the Islamic culture.[20] A patient may state, "I'm Native American." The nurse may discover that in the Southwest, some Native Americans still believe in the curative powers of the medicine man—Curandero. The nurse should try to allow the patient's medicine man to have a part in the preparation for surgery, provided that it is possible without interference.

WHAT TO TEACH

Preoperative instruction results in better preoperative and postoperative compliance at home. The patient who is better educated can prepare the home for postoperative needs whether this takes the form of dietary needs for the healing patient or arranging for a ride home. The discharge chapter further discusses what to teach the patient before discharge. Information that can be useful to all surgical patients includes the following:

- Describe the diet to follow after discharge. For any surgical patient, a diet high in protein (4 ounces per meal), zinc, and iron assists in the growth of new cells needed for the wound to mend.[21] The patient may benefit from a reminder that vitamin E is a blood thinner and should be stopped when aspirin and other

***Table 18–3.* Web Sites Providing Nutritional Information**

ORGANIZATION	WEB SITE ADDRESS
International Food Information Council	http://ificinfo.health.org
American Diabetes Association's Gateway to Nutrition	http://www.eatright.org/healthorg.html
The Children's Nutritional Research Center	http://www.bcm.tmc.edu.cnrc
Food and Nutrition Information Center	http://www.nal.usda.gov/fnic
Networking Organization of Nutrition and Dietetic Professionals	http://www.dietetics.com

From Vitamins and Health: Nutrition Online. US Pharmacist 23:84, 1998.

The Healing Patient

Postoperative Nutrition

The Food Pyramid below contains the types and amounts of foods that are needed to maintain good health. Foods at the top are items that we should consume the least of because they do not contain many nutrients. Foods at the bottom of the pyramid are the foods that we should eat the most of. They are the foundation of a healthy diet.

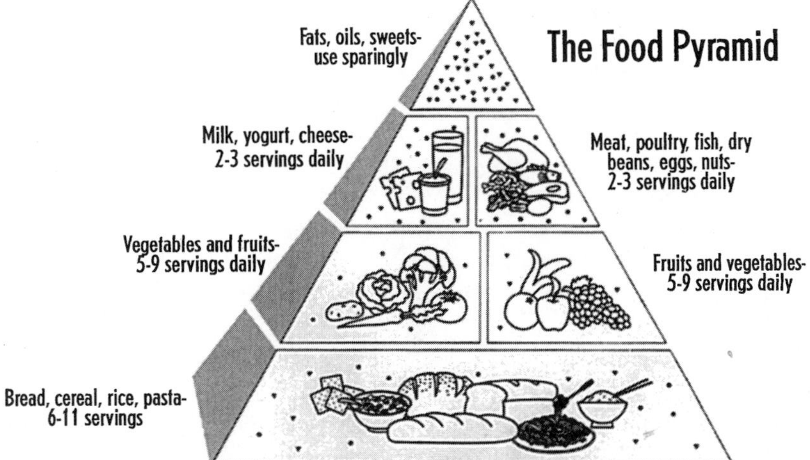

Some nutrient sources (and where to find them) can contribute to speed up your recovery, including:

Protein
Meat, poultry, seafood, eggs, dairy products, and peanut butter

Zinc
Seafood, meat and poultry (best source), whole grain cereals and breads, dairy products

Fluids
Water, juices and gelatin

Iron
Red meats, egg yolk, chicken, turkey

Calcium
Milk, yogurt, cheese, fortified orange juice

Vitamin A
Dark green, leafy vegetables, deep orange and yellow vegetables, and fruits (e. g., spinach, winter squash, carrots, sweet potatoes, melons, peaches, pumpkin, and apricots) milk and dairy products, liver, egg yolk

Vitamin C
Citrus fruits and juices, broccoli, green pepper, spinach, brussel sprouts, cabbage, strawberries, tomatoes, potatoes, cantaloupe

Figure 18–1. Good nutrition required for healing. (Reprinted with permission from Morton Plant Mease Health Care, Dunedin, FL.)

blood thinners are stopped. Although vitamin C assists with the absorption of iron, the tannin (not the caffeine) found in all teas interferes with the absorption of iron needed to nurture the new cells. See Figure 18–1 for a resource that can be provided to patients. This handout explains the nutrients needed for recovery and healing after surgery in simple-to-understand terms. Also, many Internet web sites are available that provide nutritional information (Table 18–3).

- State clearly the signs and symptoms that would merit a call to the doctor or nurse before the scheduled appointment. Give them permission to call. Patients are often reluctant, thinking it can wait until morning. At the end of the lesson, ask the patient to identify the symptoms that would signal the need for a call.
- Describe safe and effective medication use. A written handout can standardize the content that the patient is taught. Tell the patient what the medicine is supposed to do and how often and at what times it should be taken, if pertinent. Be sure to discuss any complication factors that can pose problems for the patient's

Information for Your Pain Management

We want to work with you to lessen or relieve pain after your procedure. **Keeping pain under control will help you get well faster.** You can return to your normal activities, do breathing exercises to prevent pneumonia, and regain strength more quickly.

The key to the best pain control is:
- Take pain medication as soon as the pain starts.
- Take pain medication before you start doing anything that will cause pain such as walking, dressing, or sitting. It is harder to ease pain once it has started.

Measuring Your Pain

To help us measure your pain, you will be asked to rate your pain before and after a dose of pain medication. Rate your pain on the 0 to 10 Pain Scale drawn below.

0 = no pain 5 = moderate pain 10 = the worst pain imaginable

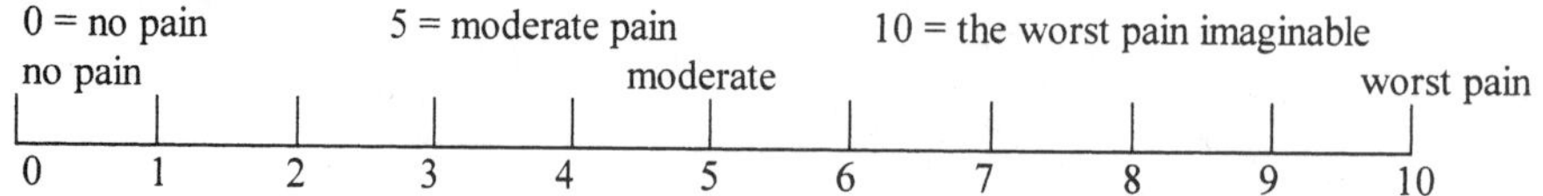

Tell your nurse if your pain is not relieved, if you have nausea, itching, difficulty passing urine or bowel movements, or if the pain relief wears off too quickly. Your pain medication and/or dose can be changed to best meet your needs. Getting hooked on pain medication should not be a concern. Studies show that this is very rare - unless you have a history of drug abuse.

Forms of Relief

There are several forms of pain control. Your doctor will choose which form best suits your needs.
- Some people will have orders for pain medication (pills, shots, or IV) to be given upon request.
- Others will have doctors orders that specify exact times that they will be given pain medication.
- Still others will be given Patient Controlled Analgesia (PCA).

When you begin to feel pain you press a button to inject pain medication. This can be through the IV tube (IV PCA), or through a small tube in your spine (Epidural PCA).

How to Use Your PCA Pump

Your nurse will show you how to use the pain control button on the pump to receive your pain medication. Only you are to press the pain control button. Sleepiness and the lack of desire to press the button is a sign that you are getting enough medication.

Figure 18–2. Pain management teaching tool. (Reprinted with permission from Morton Plant Mease Health Care, Dunedin, FL.)

particular type of surgery, such as how to avoid constipation caused by pain medications in the hernia patient. This is a great time to assess the feasibility of the patient getting the medications. It may be appropriate to refer them promptly to an outpatient social worker who can address various concerns, including cost in some instances.

- Review the physician's orders regarding medication use, in particular which medications are to be taken or omitted before the day of surgery.
- The patient is always particularly interested in anesthesia and pain control, and it is a responsibility of the nurse to provide information about pain to the patient prior to surgery. Figure 18–2 provides a teaching sheet that can be reviewed preoperatively. Not only does it provide specific information about pain management and what to expect, but it also opens discussions on the topic and helps to relieve anxiety associated with the fear of pain. A tool such as this one is developed appropriately by an interdisciplinary group of nurses, surgeons, anesthesiologists, and a pharmacist. It is important for patients to know that they have a right to pain management and that they should tell the nurse if they are in pain.
- Describe and demonstrate the leg exercises that will assist in the prevention of blood clots in the legs. Discuss activity that is acceptable for the patient's particular type of surgery.

The pump makes a "beep" sound when you press the button. This sound will let you know that the pump is working. The pump also has an alarm that might beep. If the alarm sounds, call the nurse.

Anesthesia Information

You may require one or more types of anesthetics for your procedure. You may have some discomfort specific to the different types of anesthesia.

General Anesthesia: (you will be asleep)

- You may have a sore throat. Use throat lozenges as needed.
- Drowsiness is expected for 24 hours after procedure.
- If you have nausea that does not go away, call your doctor.

Regional Block (specific body area will be numb)

- Feeling will begin to return in about 1 to 8 hours. When you start to have a tingling feeling, take oral pain medicine right away. Do not wait for all feeling to return or it will be hard to control the pain.
- Protect the numb area from injury until feeling and movement return fully.

Spinal / Epidural (from waist down will be numb)

- You will be with us for a longer period of time after your procedure because you must have full movement and bladder control before going home.
- If you have a headache when you stand up that goes away when you lie down, lie flat and call your doctor. This is a rare side effect.

Nondrug Pain Relief Methods

The following can be helpful for mild to moderate pain and to boost effects of pain medicine.

- Apply cold packs if ordered by your doctor.
- Practice slow rhythmic breathing for relaxation. Breath in and out slowly and regularly, at whatever rate feels good to you. Imagine that you are in a place that is very calming and relaxing for you. End with a slow deep breath! If you plan to do this for more than a few minutes try to get comfortable in a quiet place.
- Some areas have guided imagery cassette tapes available for you to listen to before and during your procedure. Ask about this if you are interested.

Once You Go Home

Know your pain control plan,

- You will be given a prescription for pain medication. If you are given a prescription in your doctor's office, get it filled before your procedure. Take it as ordered.
- Follow directions carefully. Some pain medications cause nausea if not taken with food. If you continue to have nausea, call your doctor.
- If your pain is not relieved or gets worse, call your doctor.
- When your pain lessens, you may switch to an over-the-counter pain medicine.
- Many prescription pain medications cause constipation. Increase your intake of water, fruits, and vegetables. To help reduce this side effect, try walking.

Figure 18–2 *Continued*

Figure 18–3 provides simple-to-follow illustrations that can be taken home for later reference. This tool will help the patient recall verbal instructions.

- Inform the patient of the general time frame in which they can expect the results of a pathology report and that they will receive this report from their physician.
- Allow time for any questions that the patient or family may have. Encourage patients to write their questions (and later your answers) down on paper before they arrive or while they are waiting. Making a list of questions accomplishes two things: (1) the patient prioritizes questions by importance and possibly even realizes that some are unnecessary and (2) the patient will not forget that "most important" question that he or she just knew they would remember. Having patients take the time to write down their questions in advance optimizes even the briefest encounter. The same suggestion can help the patient prepare questions for their physician visits.

Each patient's instructions must be individualized. The selected instruction must be based

1. Push the toes of both feet toward the foot of the bed. Relax. Pull the toes toward the chin. Relax. Repeat this three times.

2. Rotate the foot in a circular motion from the ankle. Move first to the right then to the left. Relax. Do this three times in each direction. Repeat the entire exercise for the other foot.

3. Bend the knee and bring toward the chin, raising the leg above the bed. Relax. Do this three times, and repeat the entire exercise for the other leg.

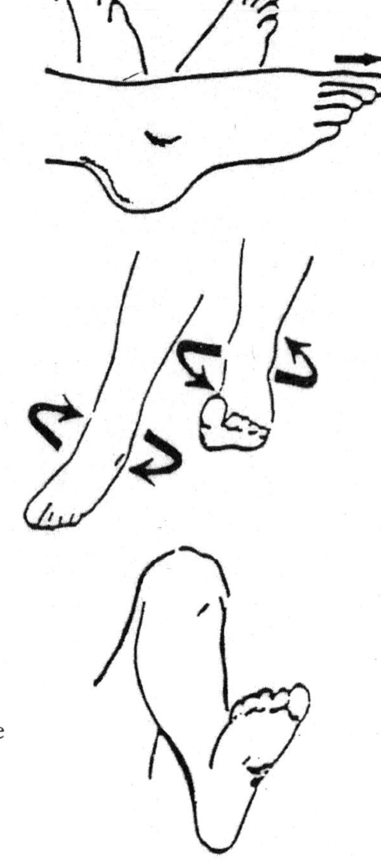

Figure 18–3. Leg exercises healing tool. Postoperative exercises to help prevent blood clots in the legs. Perform these exercises fairly slowly, but with strong muscle contractions. **For total hip and knee replacement patients, use only numbers 1 and 2.** (Reprinted with permission from Morton Plant Mease Health Care, Dunedin, FL.)

on the physician's orders, usual protocols, actual procedure being done, any complicating factors in the home setting, and the patient's support systems.

DEVELOPING THE TEACHING TOOL: THE GIFT OF BEING SIMPLE

There are many considerations to include in the creation of a teaching sheet. The content of the teaching sheet should include the items identified in the What to Teach section, but there are many more details than the content that must be considered in the creation of a teaching sheet. A prepublication checklist helps ensure that nothing is forgotten, such as physician approvals or who will pay for the printed piece. See Figure 18–4 for an example of a prepublication checklist.

Large print (size 12 font or larger) makes for ease of reading, particularly for the elderly or visually impaired. Any written information needs to be understood easily by the reader, so there needs to be a check system in place to ensure this. Figure 18–4 helps to identify the questions that should be resolved before a written piece is implemented. You may want to have a sampling of the target audience review the tool and make suggestions.

Readability of a teaching sheet is a major concern. The newspaper is written at an eighth-grade reading level,[22] but Doak and Doak recommend a fifth-grade reading level for teaching pieces in healthcare for a variety of reasons.[23] The fifth-grade skill level meets the reading needs of a broader audience. The patient often is dealing with issues that are private in nature and that have an emotional component. Even college-educated people can enjoy reading at a fifth-grade level because it allows them to assimilate information more quickly. Simpli-

MORTON PLANT MEASE HEALTH CARE
PATIENT EDUCATION

PRE-PUBLICATION CHECKLIST for PATIENT EDUCATION

All boxes must be checked before submitting for approval. Remember: The goal of writing for instructional or educational purposes is to *present information* that may be comprehended *easily and rapidly* by the intended audience.

Title of education piece: ______________________________ Initiation date:__________

Person submitting education for approval : ____________________ Deadline date:__________

Telephone: ____________________ Department: ______________________________

Planning Phase:

☐ Is this piece already in existence some place in the organization? ☐ Yes ☐ No (save duplication of work)

☐ Is this piece written in sixth grade language?

☐ Has this piece been written from the patient perspective? (In other words "Answers questions they have.") ☐ Yes ☐ No Has the piece been lay person tested? ☐ Yes ☐ No

☐ Who will be paying for the printing of this piece? ____________ Cost center # ______

☐ Who will use this form?______________________________

☐ How will it be used? ______________________________

☐ Have you met your learning objectives? (Examples available at Education/Staff Development)

☐ Is your content logically organized?

☐ Select proper format: (select one) ☐ Brochure (detailed info.)
☐ Take One (used at Health Fairs)
☐ Teaching Sheet (frequent use in acute care)

☐ Is there a need to inservice? ☐ Yes ☐ No Who should teach? ____________________
☐ Plan content

Writing Style:

☐ Have you employed "active voice" (personalized the sentence structure) wherever possible? (Examples available at Education/Staff Development)

☐ Are your words, sentences and paragraphs simple, short and concise?

☐ Have you used terminology that consistently avoids unfamiliar abbreviations and acronyms?

☐ Is your message positive and direct?

☐ YOU DIDN'T USE LOTS OF UPPERCASE LETTERING, DID YOU? (over) ☞

Figure 18–4. Prepublication checklist for patient education. (Reprinted with permission by Morton Plant Mease Health Care, Dunedin, FL.)

Illustration continued on following page

Visual Considerations:

☐ Are your illustrations simple and clearly related to the text?

☐ Do your main points stand out clearly?

☐ Do your headings clearly identify the content?

☐ If you use the following guidelines when typing on computer and save a copy on a 3 inch disk, you will save time with the publication. **Margins:** Top 2.75", Bottom .5", Left and Right .5", **Title Font:** Times New Roman Bold 28 pt., **Subtitle Font:** Times New Roman Bold 16 pt., **Standard Font:** Times New Roman 12 pt.

Feedback:

☐ Have you given anyone else a chance to critique this from a fresh perspective?

Who? Layperson: ______________ Clinician: ______________

☐ Have you made appropriate adjustments based on your pre-testing results?

Approvals Needed:

Signatures:

☐ Your department at other facilities:
Countryside ______________
Dunedin ______________
Clearwater ______________
or any of the outpatient facilities ______________

Additional Approvals:

__ Doctors' Section Meeting ______________
__ Pertinent Doctors ______________
____
__ Home Health ______________
__ Dietary ______________
__ Nursing ______________
__ Physical Therapy ______________
__ Respiratory Department ______________
__ Pharmacy ______________
__ Radiology ______________
__ Rehabilitative services (Speech, Audio, OT) ______________
__ Pharmacy/Therapeutics committee ______________

☐ Return with disc to Patient Education Coordinator to assign publication number.

☐ Patient Education Coordinator Signature ______________

(Submit draft with this completed form to the Patient Education Coordinator prior to going to Community Affairs for print.)

Figure 18–4 *Continued*

fying the reading level also makes good sense because it allows for a better opportunity of understanding.

A fifth-grade reading level can be achieved by selecting words that are two syllables or less. For example, the word "physician" can be replaced with the word "doctor"; the word "prescription" can be replaced with the word "order." This can be carried to the extreme. Obviously the word "schizophrenia" cannot be replaced with the word "schizo." In these instances, the long word must be defined in two-syllable words and used despite the increased reading level. Care must be taken to retain the original meaning in the content. Cecelia Doak adds that regardless of literacy skill, people remember better with a picture than with words. Thus, pictures also should be included when possible.[23]

A good test of the teaching tool might be a review by a group of fifth graders, or by using more formal methods such as the Gunning Readability Formula (Fog) or another test called the SMOG Readability formula (SMOG).[24] Although difficult to confirm in the literature, some sources describe the latter tool developed by Harold McGraw of Towson, Maryland, as an acronym for "Simple Measure of Gobbledygook."[25] Fog and SMOG are just two of the many readability formulas that are used to look at various aspects of written communication to determine a reading level grade. Fog looks at sentence length and the number of three-syllable words. SMOG looks at words of 3 syllables or more per 30 syllables. Both tools are available on computer.

Chapter 22 discusses some of the tools available to determine the reading level of the teaching tool. Some of these tools are available on prewritten software. Be cautious if the software provides substitute phraseology because it also may alter the meaning. Healthcare jargon also can complicate a computerized translation. Do not depend exclusively on software. The nurse, or even better, the patient should be the final measure of whether the message is communicated as intended.

PROFESSIONAL PREPARATION

The best teaching tool the nurse has is a prepared mind. The nurse needs to read to remain current in the profession. In school, reading is a forced march, so many new nurses fresh out of school are at the pinnacle of information about their profession. But after school, reading becomes a self-imposed activity. The patient's knowledge soon will surpass the nurse's if a routine of reading is not practiced. The patient is actively seeking the information because he or she has a need to know, so the nurse who wants cutting-edge knowledge also must do so.

Access to information about specific medical diagnoses is widely available. If a president becomes hospitalized, information regarding that particular diagnosis or surgery becomes newsworthy and the public's interest in learning about it is intensified. When George Bush was Vice President, the media taught the public about Graves' disease. When Ronald Reagan was President, the media taught the public about prostate cancer and colon cancer. When President Clinton fell down the stairs and injured his knee, the media taught the public about the anterior cruciate ligament. This has far-reaching implications for today's nurse. The patient has a need to know and will seek out this information. The patient may not be as discerning about the validity of the source, but the nurse must be. Healthcare information used by nurses must be from reliable and tested scientific sources, often research.

Information is everywhere. The patient need only go as far as the corner drugstore to find very informative pictures and descriptions in his or her favorite periodical. Many libraries and video stores carry a complete medical library. Patients are proficient at accessing information on the Internet, and a recent study indicated that 30% of the users of the professional Internet web sites are nonclinical.[25–27] An excellent example of a web site providing patient-related information pertinent to ambulatory surgery is that of the American Society of Anesthesiologists at http//www.ASAhq.org.

Increased use of the Internet could have profound significance to nurses who are teaching. Patients accessing clinical web sites on the Internet are potentially more knowledgeable than the average layperson; conversely, they may misunderstand or misinterpret what they read because they are accessing a professional web site on which healthcare jargon is used. Either scenario is an excellent case to prompt the nurse to seek cutting-edge knowledge about the types of patients being seen.

The ambulatory surgical nurse can have a profound effect on the patient's surgical outcome. The nurse has teaching responsibilities before, during, and after surgery. By cultivating the skills to be an expert educator, the nurse can be armed with the tools necessary to provide expert care.

References

1. Quirk Bourie P: Costing the nursing service of patient education. Nurs Manage 24:46–50, 1993.
2. Bloom B: Taxonomy of Educational Objectives: The Classification of Educational Goals. New York: David McKay Co, 1956.
3. Rorden JW: Nurses as Health Teachers: A Practical Guide. Philadelphia: WB Saunders, 1987.
4. Rorden JW: Discharge Planning Guide for Nurses. Philadelphia: WB Saunders, 1990.
5. LeFevre R: Critical Thinking in Nursing: A Practical Approach. Philadelphia: WB Saunders, 1995.
6. Cort-Johnson S: Making Sure Lessons Are Age-appropriate for Kids. Patient Educ Manage 2:129–144, 1995.
7. Gaster R: An Ambulatory Approach: Patient Education Priorities for All Ages. Moorhead: Minnesota Dakotas Society of Post Anesthesia Nurses, 1997.
8. Neuhauser PC: Tribal Warfare in Organizations. New York: Ballinger Publishing Co, 1988.
9. Knowles M: The Modern Practice of Adult Education: From Pedagogy to Andragogy. Chicago: Follett Publishing Co, 1984.
10. Patterson O (ed): Special Tools for Communication. Chicago: Industrial Audio-Visual Association, 1962.
11. Stern HG: Winning Trial Advocacy Techniques. New York: Harcourt Brace Jovanovich Publishing Co, 1986.
12. Redman BK: The Process of Patient Education, 7th ed. St. Louis: Mosby-Year Book, 1993.
13. Spencer KW: Patient Education in Practice Settings: A Candid Discussion with Plastic Surgical Nurses. Plast Surg Nurs 14, 1994.
14. Casey F: Documenting patient education: A literature review. J Continuing Educ 26:257–260, 1995.
15. Simpson N: Time-savers squeeze in quick education. Patient Educ Manage 2:120, 1995.
16. JCAHO: Folio Bound Use Info Base Automated Comprehensive Accreditation Manual for Hospital Use (Official JCAHO Handbook). Chicago: JCAHO, 1998.
17. Goleman D: Emotional Intelligence. New York: Bantam Books, 1995.
18. Byrd RC: Positive therapeutic effects of intercessory prayer in a coronary care unit population. South Med J 81:826–829, 1988.
19. Piscopo N: Healing power of prayer. St Petersburg Times Floridian Section D:1. April 23, 1996.
20. King F: Handbook of General Religious Beliefs and Practices. Clearwater: Morton Plant Hospital, November 1996.
21. Chima C, Barco K, Dewitt M, et al: Relationship of nutritional status to length of stay, hospital costs, and discharge status of patients hospitalized in the medicine service. J Am Diet Assoc 97:975–978, 1997.
22. Hollingsworth A: Can your patients read what you give them? Patient Educators Newsletter 1:1, 2, 7, 1994.
23. Doak LC, Doak CC, Root JH: Teaching Patients with Low Literacy Skills. Philadelphia: JB Lippincott, 1985.
24. Mumford M: A descriptive study of the readability of patient information leaflets designed by nurses. J Adv Nurs 26:985–991, 1997.
25. McLaughlin G: SMOG grading: A new readability formula. J Reading 12:639–646, 1969.
26. Anonymous: Patients can get caught in web without advice. Patient Educ Manage 4:29–30, 1997.
27. Dudley TE, Salvo DR, Poded RN, et al: The informed patient poses a different challenge. Patient Care 30:128–132, 134, 136–138, 1996.

Chapter 19

Intraoperative Care

Denise L. Geuder

INTRAOPERATIVE CARE

The intraoperative care of the surgical patient begins when the patient enters the operating room (OR) and ends when the patient is taken to the postanesthesia care unit (PACU) or discharge area of the facility. The responsibilities of the perioperative nurse begin in the planning and preparation that must occur long before the patient actually enters the OR. Careful set-up and preparation occur so that the focus of the intraoperative nurse is the patient and not the tasks associated with preparation of the room for surgery.

Intraoperative care of the ambulatory surgery patient is similar to that of traditional hospitalized patients. The nursing staff must be attentive to the needs of the patient in regard to education, patient identification, safety, consents, site preparation, positioning, equipment operation, emotional support, documentation, and various other actions based on the identified needs of the patient. In addition, the perioperative nurse working in the ambulatory surgery setting must assess and plan for the entire continuum of care for the surgical event. Although the ambulatory surgery center (ASC) has traditionally been used for shorter, rapid turnover, high-volume procedures and technologic advances in surgical technique (e.g., laparoscopic cholecystectomy and hysterectomy) are rapidly expanding the scope of services available in the ASC setting.

The high proportion of generally healthier patients in an ASC means fewer critical needs for life support and fewer patients with serious systemic illness. The typical ASC patient has been carefully screened and is generally healthy. However, as ambulatory surgery has become more routine, a higher-acuity patient population is being seen in hospital-based and freestanding centers alike. It is important to include the patient in all aspects of care, maintaining the concept of wellness and establishing the expectation before the procedure is performed that the procedure will go well and that the patient will be able to return home after the procedure.[1]

Nursing care of the ASC patient goes beyond the technical and the procedure-oriented realms. All nurses, including the intraoperative nurse, are actively involved in providing psychosocial care and support to the patient. The frequent use of local and regional anesthetics and the high volume of patients having little or no premedication result in more alert and anxious patients, increased nurse-patient interaction, and increased nursing responsibilities. Therefore, careful attention is necessary to ensure that the team is focused on the patient and to provide support and encouragement while maintaining a safe environment.

The perioperative nurse's goal is to implement each procedure as safely, efficiently, and compassionately as possible. One of those responsibilities is knowing and implementing appropriate and accepted standards of practice. The Association of Operating Room Nurses has developed nationally recognized standards and recommended practices that are considered the definitive basis of practice of perioperative nurses. They include specific recommended practice and core competency statements that provide the perioperative nurse with a firm basis for practice. Compliance is voluntary, but it is suggested that these recommendations be used to guide the nurse's practice and to update and refine the individual facility's policies and procedures.[2]

THE ENVIRONMENT

The surgery suite of the ASC is quite similar to that of hospital ORs in that each suite must conform to appropriate standards of space requirements, equipment needs, fire and electrical safety, restricted access, and asepsis. State and federal licensing agencies have specific standards that determine certain space requirements, lighting, air filtration, humidity, and temperature controls for intraoperative areas. Each facility should know its state's specific licensure requirements and ensure compliance with these standards. Contaminated, clean, and sterile work spaces should be separated. Access to sterilizers, a centralized area for administrative and scheduling needs, and adequate storage areas should also be a part of the work space.

Movement of patients, personnel, and equipment should reflect issues of safety, efficiency, and infection control. The design of an individual OR suite affects the traffic patterns within the unit. Most ORs are divided into three zones related to the level of restriction of access: (1) the public or unrestricted area, (2) the semirestricted area, and (3) the restricted area.

Each facility focuses either generally on a variety of procedures or targets specific procedures, such as plastics and ophthalmology. The disciplines from which procedures are most commonly performed in the ASC setting are ophthalmology, gastroenterology, gynecology, orthopedics, otolaryngology, and plastics, in that order.[3] Many facilities focus on a few high-volume procedures and require equipment that is specific to those particular types of surgery only. Whatever the type of procedures performed, it is important to plan for easy access, storage, proper electrical outlets, water supply, steam access, and possible drainage for particular types of equipment.

Traditionally, ASC rooms have been 20 × 20 feet (400 square feet) in size. With the introduction of more technical equipment, such as lasers and video equipment, many ASCs are planning for larger rooms. One common surgery that demonstrates this trend is laparoscopic cholecystectomy. This procedure was traditionally performed in hospital settings, requiring a postoperative stay of several days. Laparoscopic techniques have enabled the procedure to be performed in ambulatory settings; however, the extensive equipment requires more space.

An intercom telephone system, as well as an emergency call device, should be immediately available in all patient care areas. This call system should be audible throughout the unit or, in the case of a freestanding center, throughout the entire facility to summon needed staff members who may be outside patient care areas, in the lounge, or in the business office. Overhead paging is often restricted inside ORs to avoid loud distractions during anesthesia induction or emergence when extraneous sounds may become distorted and frightening. Also, potentially upsetting messages, such as pathology reports, should be given privately rather than by overhead paging or speaker telephone.

THE SURGICAL TEAM

The healthcare team that provides intraoperative care consists of a combination of the following: surgeons, first assistant (physician or nurse), anesthesiologist, nurse anesthetist, circulating nurse, scrub nurse or technician, and other unlicensed assistive personnel. Individual members of the team need to trust and respect each other for their valuable contribution to patient care. Each contributes specific knowledge and skill, which results in overall positive patient outcomes. All staff members should be involved in an ongoing quality improvement process and other programs that ensure safety and efficiency.

The composition of the team differs according to the procedure to be performed.[4] Factors such as type of anesthetic, complexity of the case, special equipment, and community norms all influence the composition of the team. One of the greatest successes of ASCs has been the cross-training that has occurred in order to increase the flexibility of the staff dedicated to these units. A true team approach to patient care is frequently seen in the most successful facilities that encourage cross-functional roles and job descriptions and foster a focus on the patient as the center of work instead of on specific job descriptions.[5]

Although there are few areas of overlap between the roles of scrub nurses and circulating nurses, the following discussion generally refers to the perioperative nurse in the context of the circulating nurse's role. This registered nurse has direct responsibility for the general well-being of the patient during surgery, sometimes alone and sometimes in combination with anesthesia personnel. As resources continue to be carefully scrutinized in the healthcare industry, the pressure will be for more cost-effective staffing patterns. When appropriate staffing is being determined, it is important to focus on the nurse's responsibility for the components of the nursing process, not on tasks.[6]

Perioperative nurses chosen to work with ambulatory surgery patients should possess a broad knowledge base because they are responsible for providing care to patients before, during, and after surgery. Because of the constant potential for any minor procedure to become major or for any patient to have cardiorespiratory or other serious complications, the perioperative nurse should have well-developed emergency skills, including cardiopulmonary resuscitation certification. Many seek advanced cardiac life support certification as well. The perioperative nurse's command of basic electrocardiographic interpretation, equipment procedure monitoring, principles of medication administration, and the effects and side effects of common anesthetic and sedating drugs is essential for providing a safe environment. It is especially important for those patients having local anesthesia who are primarily monitored by a registered nurse. See Chapter 15 for a complete discussion of the administration of conscious sedation.

The perioperative nurse who displays a positive attitude and a willingness to work closely with other nurses, physicians, and patients is a tremendous asset to the surgical team. The ability and willingness to work as part of a team is a skill that is integral to the surgical environment. This caring and supportive attitude facilitates the promotion of health and wellness, which begins before surgery with each patient. When such caring attitudes pervade the entire nursing staff, physicians, and ancillary personnel, the philosophy of the ambulatory approach is truly supported. With fewer staff in the ASCs than in the traditional hospital setting, cross-training and a team approach are essential.

Particularly in a freestanding ASC (FASC), the perioperative staff nurse may be expected to perform duties that are not typically considered staff nursing functions in many facilities. Some examples include ordering supplies and equipment from outside suppliers, meeting with vendors or physician office staff members, developing marketing literature, and coordinating health fairs or other marketing programs within the community. As in many ORs, various staff nurses often function as the department's infection control or quality improvement coordinators or as committee chairpersons for laser safety, staff development, or product review. These extended responsibilities beyond patient care add a dimension of professional growth for the individual nurse and are considered by many nurses to be both a privilege and an opportunity.

Careful and competent practitioners prudently follow safety rules when identifying, transporting, positioning, and monitoring patients. They understand and apply the concepts of electrical and mechanical safety, proper body mechanics, and infection control in order to provide each patient with a safe environment. Perioperative nurses' integrity regarding asepsis in the surgical field should be above reproach, and they must document all nursing actions thoroughly and accurately. It is imperative to remember that the current legal trend is to hold nurses responsible for their own actions. This personal accountability is a change from the many years of popularity of the "captain of the ship" doctrine, in which the surgeon was held responsible for the actions of every person in the OR.

Before the perioperative nurse can adequately provide quality care to individual patients, the general needs of the department as a whole must be addressed to ensure that the environment is safe and well prepared for individual cases. Nursing responsibilities involve implementation of policies and procedures related to the emergency preparedness of the unit, nursing staff development, maintenance of supplies and equipment, asepsis, safety of the environment, and continual efforts to improve the quality of care. A copy of the facility policies should be easily accessible to the staff for reference and for periodic review.

CASE MANAGEMENT

Case management is a model of patient care delivery that is widely used in healthcare facilities and that can be very beneficial to the intraoperative period of care for the ambulatory surgery patient. Although most of the case management models are being developed in acute care settings, the concepts of case management are also appropriate for use in the ASC. As a model of care delivery, case management integrates patient and provider satisfaction and consideration of cost factors. It is well suited to the ambulatory surgery environment in that it focuses on an individual's holistic health concerns rather than only on episodes of illness and intervention. The goals of case management are to optimize patient self-care, decrease fragmentation of care, provide quality care, enhance patients' quality of life, decrease length of stay, increase patient and staff satisfaction, and promote cost-effective use of scarce resources.[7]

Case management is a model of care delivery that brings various disciplines together to plan for the most cost-effective, highest quality of care possible for each patient. Many case management models use critical paths for planning the care of patients. The plans are actually paths or maps of what should occur in each phase of patient care. To be effective, they should be multidisciplinary and should set expectations for all members of the team, including physicians, nursing staff, and the patient. Most care paths focus on high-volume, high-cost procedures in order to make the most productive use of the resources dedicated to developing these paths.

Because most of the procedures performed in the ASC are fairly routine elective surgeries, the use of care paths or critical paths can be readily implemented in the ASC environment. These paths can be considered extensions of the traditional preference cards routinely used in intraoperative settings to prepare for each case. The cost associated with surgery makes the use of care paths a logical planning tool for surgical patient care. The use of the paths to clearly define expectations to all team members and the patient has proved to be an effective mechanism for communication and demonstrates the desired outcomes. The result is optimizing self-care, decreasing fragmentation of care, and increasing patient satisfaction.

Most acute care critical paths are set up in time increments of days in the hospital. Obviously, this is not the case in the ASC, so many perioperative plans are set up in terms of phases, such as admission to the facility, induction, procedure, transfer to the PACU, phase I recovery, phase II recovery, and then discharge from the facility. These phases can be set up to reflect significant aspects of the care of the patient populations in the ASC. Many facilities are providing patients with their own version of the path to define expectations for the patient of the procedure, and also as a teaching tool.

CONTINUOUS PERFORMANCE IMPROVEMENT

It is the responsibility of every perioperative nurse to participate in the facility's formal performance improvement program, as well as to address quality issues informally in every patient contact. The perioperative nurse is an essential resource for developing intraoperative indicators and for providing ongoing suggestions for improving the care on a continuous basis. Some examples of quality improvement indicators are listed in Table 19–1. The nurse's participation in improving the quality of care should be reflected in that nurse's periodic performance evaluations.

***Table 19–1.* Examples of Quality Improvement Indicators in the Perioperative Setting**

Delay of surgery
Cancellation of surgery
Improper consent
Procedure performed without valid consent
Incorrect site or side
Break in aseptic technique
Medication reaction
Anesthesia-related untoward event
Faulty equipment
Clinical complication
Case cancelled after admission to OR or after induction
Patient taken to OR without complete record, e.g., H & P laboratory results
Inappropriate radiation exposure
Break in confidentiality or privacy
Lost, contaminated, improperly prepared, or mislabeled specimen
Unplanned removal or repair of organ or structure
Retained instrumentation or sponge
Unresolved incorrect count
Improper or incomplete documentation
Unusual or incorrect technique by team member, physician, or other person
Emergency environmental occurrence
Injury to healthcare worker

OR, operating room; H & P, history and physical examination.

Ambulatory surgery centers that have implemented case management use the expected outcomes of the care paths or critical paths to track variances that indicate system problems to continually enhance performance in the facilities. This variance tracking is helpful because the information clearly identifies system problems that prevent staff, physicians, or patients from following the path and obtaining the desired outcomes.[8]

Quality issues in the OR may be related to administration, anesthesia, surgery, or nursing. In addition to reporting nursing-related occurrences, perioperative nurses may be expected to initiate reports regarding anesthesia or surgical occurrences because of the nurse's presence as the facility's representative during any happenings. Situations may involve actual or potential patient injury or other incidents that present the facility with possible legal risk, so the follow-up identifies not only quality care issues but also liabilities. In those instances, an incident or occurrence report usually accompanies any performance improvement reports. Any unexpected patient outcome or event should be reported to the manager or designated person responsible for risk management activities for the ASC. Equipment implicated in a patient incident should be secured immediately, along with all packaging from disposable supplies used with it in order to prevent tampering. An investigation of that equipment should be completed to assess the cause of the problem. This investigation can be essential to the legal defense of the facility.

The risk manager should be informed immediately of any occurrence that may have involved equipment in order to determine whether the incident must be reported under the guidelines of the Safe Medical Device Act of 1990. This act requires that facilities using certain devices communicate or report to the manufacturer problems or issues regarding the device that may have caused or contributed to a patient's death or serious illness or injury. Certain forms are required to be sent to the manufacturer, and in the case of death or serious illness or injury, a copy must be sent to the United States Food and Drug Administration's medical product reporting program. Every hospital or ASC should have a person designated to ensure compliance with the Safe Medical Device Act (see Chapter 3).[9]

A nurse reporting any occurrence should present objective information. The nurse's subjective interpretation of the occurrence or its preventability may be valuable to those who will investigate the occurrence, but great care should be taken to present only the objective details of any happening on a written report or the medical record. It is vital to follow through in reporting on the patient's condition as it relates to any occurrence and to ask questions that help identify the reason why the situation occurred, what could have been done to prevent it, and what can be done to prevent a similar situation in the future. This approach benefits the organization, the employee, and future patients.

EMERGENCY PREPAREDNESS

Both the department and the staff must be in constant readiness for emergencies. Some issues are basic, such as having the OR fully stocked at all times, requiring all staff members to know the location and operation of emergency equipment, and ensuring the proper function of an emergency power generator. This is particularly important in an FASC because a department of biomedical engineering may not be on site, and the staff must be knowledgeable about what to do in the event of a power failure. Appropriate surgical instruments and trays should be kept sterile and ready for immediate use in case an emergency procedure needs to be performed.

A fully stocked emergency cart must be quickly available for use. It should contain the drugs and supplies necessary for responding to cardiovascular or respiratory complications, malignant hyperthermia, and other medical emergencies (see Chapter 11). Appropriate emergency telephone number listings for access to code team, respiratory therapy, ambulance, or advanced cardiac life support response team should be available at each telephone. Personnel readiness depends on adequate orientation of nurses to the unit, hiring of adequately experienced nurses, periodic classes and drills that test staff response to possible emergency situations, and sharing of responsibility for ensuring adequacy of equipment.

During a cardiorespiratory emergency, restoring the patient's heartbeat and other vital functions obviously takes precedence over maintaining a sterile field. The scrub person generally steps back and remains in sterile attire, prepared to assist if rapid closure of the wound is required after the emergency has been resolved. The circulating nurse assigned to the case assumes the primary nursing responsibility for the patient during any emergency situation.

Not all emergencies are as dramatic or compelling as cardiorespiratory crisis. Some may be the result of intraoperative technique that causes potential or actual injury. Other occurrences may result from human errors or misjudgment. It is important that when untoward occurrences happen, immediate and proper action is instituted to correct or rectify the situation. Total candor is an essential character trait for the perioperative nurse.

Policies should be in place to address environmental emergencies, such as loss of electrical power, failure of equipment, electrical shock, fire, and sterilizer malfunction. Each facility should check applicable state or accrediting body regulations to ensure compliance with standards. Telephone numbers for emergency repair of equipment should be conspicuously posted, and flashlights should be stored in a consistent location within each OR. Emergency lights that automatically turn on during a power failure provide a measure of safety by illuminating exits. If these are not available or if they malfunction, strips of reflective tape that glow in the dark may be used to help the nurse locate the flashlight or the door in a dark OR. Because most ORs do not have windows, the darkness can be overwhelming.

The remote possibility that the surgeon or anesthesiologist could become suddenly incapacitated during a procedure demands that a contingency plan be in place. In a large institution, there is likely to be another physician available who could assist during such an emergency, but in an FASC, another mechanism for securing such support must be available. There also should be a plan for the availability of specialists during times of emergency need. For example, a thoracic or vascular surgeon might be needed to assist during a surgical complication or an internist or cardiologist may be needed during a medical crisis.

Certainly, the needs of an FASC are different from those of a hospital-based ASC. The backup contingency plans for an FASC must be carefully worked out and expectations clearly communicated to staff in the facility as well as to any staff, ambulance service, or physicians that would be expected to respond. Agreements for response to emergencies should be carefully negotiated and presented in written format, not just verbally, so that everyone involved clearly understands. Some of these arrangements may actually require letters of agreement to communicate in writing the expectations of both the facility and the responder. During a crisis is a poor time to determine that expectations were not clear. Periodic internal drills for each type of emergency are necessary to ensure that the plan actually works and appropriate systems are in place.

SUPPLY INVENTORY

Policies must be followed to ensure that the correct amount and types of supplies and medications are available when needed, are stored properly, and are used wisely. Well-established standards for stocking the OR include removing all supplies from outside cartons before they are placed in areas for clean and sterile packaged supplies, as well as rotating stock so that the oldest of any particular item is used first. Logical and efficient storage for supplies should be in close proximity to the ORs so that rapid retrieval of items is possible, with sterile and clean supplies stored separately. Physician preference cards should be continually updated to reflect the surgeon's current needs and requests. Changes in a surgeon's usual protocol should be communicated to all perioperative staff members and the person responsible for the inventory so that changes in the supply order can be made.

The ongoing issues with cost containment have focused the attention of ASC staff and management on supply cost and usage issues. This pressure will only intensify as the drive to be the lowest-cost, highest-quality provider continues. Physician preferences must be considered, but the days of stocking several different brands for each surgeon's particular preference are gone. Product standardization is a goal in order to achieve the best pricing possible; inventory items sitting on the shelf cost the facility money. Various supply handling options are available from many vendors, such as just-in-time inventory and consignment. One must be careful to weigh the options against the pricing because the vendors usually charge more for each individual supply item if these options are exercised (see Chapter 5).

Occasionally, an item must be borrowed from or loaned to another facility or department. Generally, this practice is mutually helpful because all centers occasionally find themselves in need of a reciprocal agreement to secure items quickly. A policy should be in place that identifies the proper protocol for such exchanges. Both parties should clearly understand what is to be loaned; how and when it will be returned, replaced, or paid for; and who is the responsible party on each end, both loaner and borrower. A stock transfer sheet or other method should be used to document the transaction.

When a piece of equipment is loaned, the facility's name should be marked on it for identification. All parts should be clearly identified and documented as present when it is loaned and when it is returned. An accompanying form that lists all the parts to be returned is helpful. Packaging should be appropriate in order to avoid damage in transit. The equipment's proper function should be ascertained each time it is transferred in order to immediately identify any problems, missing parts, or breakage. It may be unwise to transport delicate equipment to and from other facilities or departments because of the potential for damage or misalignment, particularly in the case of delicate equipment, such as lasers and microscopes.

The transfer of sterilized items brings up serious quality concerns, regarding both the ultimate patient user and the legal protection of the loaning institution. Handling and maintaining sterility of an item during transit cannot be guaranteed or, in many instances, monitored. The loaning party has no control over the storage and use of an item in the recipient facility.

This situation could lead to liability if a patient injury was traced to the item in question. Any break in technique that contaminated the item could well have occurred before, during, or after transit, and either facility could have difficulty defending its position.

MAINTENANCE OF EQUIPMENT

The variety and the complexity of the various equipment used in the OR can be overwhelming to even the experienced perioperative nurse. The basic equipment for one OR can include monitors, anesthesia machines, electrocautery unit, mechanical or electrical bed, and other equipment, such as lasers, video monitors, and microscopes. Each piece of equipment must be cared for respectfully and according to manufacturer's recommendations. Before any staff member operates a piece of equipment, it is imperative that proper training and assurance of competency have been completed before that individual participates in the care of patients requiring that equipment. Before being placed into use, and periodically thereafter, equipment must be safety checked by an appropriately trained and credentialed person, such as a biomedical engineer. Careful records of the repair and maintenance of each piece of equipment must be kept in order to document that preventive maintenance has occurred on the equipment.

Each time a piece of equipment is used, the nurse should inspect all parts to identify breakage or frayed areas. Standard checks should be carried out to ensure that the equipment is in proper working order before the patient is brought into the OR. Any piece of equipment with the slightest hint of damage should be labeled and removed from service immediately until it can be inspected and repaired. Preventive maintenance should be provided routinely for all equipment, both medical and environmental, such as air conditioners, filters, refrigerators, and sterilizers. Alarm systems should be tested according to predetermined intervals.

Equipment should be appropriately disassembled and cleaned after each use, then covered for storage. Clear plastic covers allow rapid identification in the storage areas. Items used infrequently require extra cleaning before patient use. All clean parts should be stored together with the main unit in clearly labeled packages or drawers. A notation of the whereabouts of any sterilized parts that may or may not be stored in a separate area should be attached to the machine for quick retrieval. Items such as shavers, ophthalmoscopes, Doppler pulse monitors, and defibrillators may require that batteries be recharged periodically or continually. Sterilizers also require specific documentation of testing of function and performance; thus, one or more staff members should be assigned to ensure that proper testing of these various pieces of equipment is carried out and documented according to the facility's policies.

MAINTENANCE OF ASEPSIS

Staff members should maintain a constant awareness of their actions and attitudes that could contribute to the spread of infection in patients and staff members. The natural barrier to infection is violated by an incision or puncture of the skin or by a break in the mucous membrane, for instance, with catheter insertion, nasal or oral surgery, or intubation of the trachea. These situations significantly reduce the patient's resistance to infection, thus the OR environment must be as free from microbial contaminants as possible.

The sterility of items used at the surgical site and the actual technique of the surgical team members are primary concerns in the OR, but many other issues must be addressed to make the environment safe in terms of infection control. These include: (1) the health and hygiene of personnel, (2) limited access to the OR by authorized and appropriately clothed personnel, (3) traffic patterns that discourage the frequent cross-over of personnel between restricted and nonrestricted areas, and (4) keeping doors to procedure rooms closed. During procedures, doors should be opened slowly if at all, and movement of personnel should be minimal to discourage turbulence that causes the air to become laden with bacteria from the floor or the adjoining corridors.[2]

In the ambulatory surgery setting and particularly in freestanding units, patient, families, OR staff members, and business office employees often share common areas. The delineation of restricted, semirestricted, and nonrestricted areas is somewhat less clear than in more traditional OR suites in a hospital. It is sometimes difficult to identify who should wear scrub apparel. Upholding the facility's predetermined standards of practice regarding apparel in this setting is sometimes challenging. Further concerns related to infection control are discussed in Chapter 4. For a thorough presentation of sterilization techniques, the reader is referred to texts devoted to this complex subject.

SAFETY ISSUES

Many inherent environmental hazards exist in the OR, so nurses must be continually alert for potential dangers. These may be electrical, infectious, or accidental, depending on the equipment used and the type of work being performed. Other dangers result from working closely with anesthetic waste gases and toxic chemicals. The types of hazards are diverse, but the perioperative nurse can help decrease these potential dangers and contribute to a safe environment. Consideration of these dangers should be included in the facility's ongoing performance improvement and risk management programs.

The ever-expanding technology in the surgical environment has increased the possibility of patient and staff exposure to injury from electrical shock.[10] If the operator of a piece of equipment or the patient inadvertently acts as the pathway for stray electricity to reach the ground, the damage to that person can be anything from tingling in the limbs with muscle damage to burns and irreversible cardiac arrest. Electrical current flows more readily through wet skin, so a dry environment is essential when electrical equipment is in use. Improper grounding and faulty insulation of equipment are common causes of operator injury.

Electrocautery units are among the most frequently found electrical devices in the OR. The unit generates a high-frequency current to cut tissue and coagulate blood vessels at the surgical site. Appropriate grounding of patients is essential to provide for safety of the staff and patients whenever an electrocautery unit is used. After the patient has been positioned, the connection is made between the patient and the electrocautery unit by use of a dispersive pad. This pad should be placed close to and on the same side of the body as the operative site. The best placement for the pad is on intact skin that is clean and relatively free from hair, preferably over a large muscle mass, such as the thigh or buttocks of the patient.[11] It is important that the condition of the skin under the pad be assessed and documented before placement and after removal of the pad. The current from the electrocautery unit is dispersed through the electrosurgical pencil. It travels through the patient's body and is directed back to the generator by the dispersive pad. Bipolar circuits in electrocautery units provide the safest type of cautery because their electrical output is isolated within the unit and there is little or no leakage of current. This type of coagulation device may be used in close proximity to organs and other structures where unipolar units would be hazardous. Bipolar cautery eliminates the need for a grounding plate.[12]

Practices that help to ensure that electrical shock or fire will not threaten the staff or patient include removing from service any equipment with frayed or broken wiring, broken prongs, or cracked insulation. Extreme caution must be employed when electrocautery or other equipment with powerful electrical voltage is used around drapes, flammable liquids, and other combustible materials. Cautery should be avoided around volatile liquids, such as acetone, collodion, and alcohol. Of particular concern is the use of alcohol-based skin prepping agents. Unless these skin preparations are allowed to dry thoroughly, the use of the cautery unit can quickly ignite a fire.

CASE STUDY

Elizabeth Stewart was scheduled for a diagnostic laparoscopy. During her preoperative preparation, she asked to speak to her surgeon about the removal of two small skin tags on her chest. The surgeon was notified and came to see Ms. Stewart. After assessing the skin tags, the surgeon agreed to take them off while Ms. Stewart was asleep. Because Ms. Stewart had not received any preoperative sedation, a permit was obtained for removal of the skin tags. At the completion of the laparoscopy, the surgeon asked that the two skin tags be prepped with the same type of solution used for the laparoscopy.

The circulating nurse prepped the two skin tags. The physician then picked up the electrocautery pencil to remove the skin tags, without allowing the prep solution to dry. At the activation of the pencil, the prep solution ignited into a flame and quickly set fire to the surrounding drape. The scrub person immediately pulled the drape off, and smothered the fire on the floor.

On examination, Ms. Stewart was found to have suffered second-degree burns at the site of the skin tags on the upper chest and following a line into the axilla, where the prep solution had dripped from the chest. The wound was dressed and the patient taken to the PACU. When Ms. Stewart was awake and alert, the physician explained the occurrence to her and her family. She was followed closely after surgery by the physician and required no further intervention other than routine burn care.

DISCUSSION

A performance improvement team was assembled to review the events and make recommendations to prevent recurrence of the situation. Analysis revealed that the prep solution used was alcohol based and was highly flammable unless it was allowed to dry thoroughly before contact with an electrocautery pencil. The facility had recently gone through an extensive emphasis on fire prevention and safety, making the staff in the room aware of the appropriate response. The staff's action to remove the drapes from the patient and quickly extinguish the drape fire on the floor prevented further spread of the fire. This event resulted in a facility-wide effort to educate staff and physicians on the selective use of alcohol-based prep agents and the necessary precautions.

The incidence of OR fires has been widely reported in the literature. The presence of an (1) oxygen-enriched environment; (2) combustible materials, such as drapes, gowns, and sponges; and (3) ignition source from electrical cords and cautery units make this a serious concern for all the OR team. A small spark can ignite quickly in the presence of the oxygen-enriched environment and can quickly engulf the drapes or gown, with a potentially fatal outcome. It is essential that every staff member know what to do in the event of a fire and that drills be carried on routinely. In the event of an actual fire, protection of the patient and staff takes priority over concerns regarding sterile technique. The fire should be covered with a wet towel or laparotomy sponge in order to smother the fire. Pouring solution on water-retardant drapes does not put out the fire; instead, it may cause the fire to spread. If the fire cannot be extinguished with the wet towel or sponge, the drapes should be immediately pulled off of the patient onto the floor, and the flames should be extinguished on the floor.

Accidents may result from faulty equipment or, more often, from an operator's failure to use it properly or safely. For example, lasers are dangerous when used improperly and have been implicated in fires when the beam was reflected off a shiny object or aimed, in error, at a flammable material. Equipment for the implementation of policies to protect the staff should be available, for example, goggles, gloves, and impervious sharps containers.

All patient waste should be disposed of in a manner that avoids contact with personnel. Any spills should be cleaned immediately to prevent falls and to avoid staff contact with potentially dangerous materials. Proper methods must be available for the disposal of substances such as caustic or harmful chemicals, biologic wastes and tissues, mercury, and radioactive agents. Enforcement of effective procedures and adequate environmental venting to avoid buildup of ambient anesthetic gases is another important safety measure.

The use of intraoperative x-rays and fluoroscopy poses the threat of ionizing radiologic exposure to the nurse and to other team members. Image intensifiers and radioactive implants and injections are also sources of exposure. Excessive radiation causes the molecular structure of the body's cells to change. Damage that could result from prolonged or extensive exposure includes cataracts, burns, bone marrow injury, and tissue necrosis. The effects of radiation may not manifest for years as a result of the extended latency period before the emergence of symptoms.[10]

The unit of measure for exposure is called a rem (roentgen equivalent for man) or a millirem (1/1000 rem). The National Council on Radiation Protection and Measurements recommends an acceptable annual radiologic exposure for health workers as follows:

Total dose equivalent, 5 rem
Lenses of eyes, 15 rem
Skin, extremities, and individual organs, 50 rem

Pregnant personnel should avoid exposure to radiation.

Recommended methods of reducing exposure to radiation include: (1) having all nonessential personnel leave the room; (2) using a lead shield, apron, or gloves when unavoidable exposure will occur; (3) utilizing cassette holders instead of hand-held films; and (4) turning off fluoroscopy equipment when it is not in use. A fifth method is maintaining adequate distance from the source of radiation. The nurse can apply the inverse square law to reduce personal exposure to radiation. This law states that by doubling the distance from the source of radiation, a person reduces exposure by one fourth.[12]

Lead aprons should be hung when not in use because folding them can cause cracks in the lead, making them ineffective barriers to radiation.[12] These aprons also require periodic x-ray studies to detect cracks in the lead that may allow employee exposure to occur. Dosimeters that monitor the amount of radiation received should be worn by personnel who will be working near radiologic equipment. These badges should be read and replaced periodically. Results of dosimeter readings should be used when assigning nurses to high- or low-exposure areas and should be included in the quality improvement program of the facility.

Exposure to anesthetic waste gases is another concern. Although current research regarding exposure to anesthetic gases is inconclusive, some suggest that long-term exposure to waste gases, especially nitrous oxide, can contribute to, or result in, cancers, renal hepatic disorders, and nervous system involvement. Greater attention has been placed on the effects on reproduction and spontaneous abortion, but thus far, studies present inconclusive evidence of any causal relationship between exposure to waste gases and the potential outcomes listed.[12]

Proper ventilation and safe anesthesia practices support reduction of anesthetic waste gases in the air. Besides the normal exhalation ports of anesthesia machines that are connected to scavenging systems for disposal of waste gases, other sources of gas escape are leaking endotracheal tube cuffs, leaks in the anesthesia system, and sometimes the technique used during anesthesia induction. Of note is the ambient anesthesia gas allowed to escape when anesthesia is induced with an open-mask technique in a child. Another source is the patient's expirations in the immediate postanesthesia period.

The National Institute of Occupational Safety and Health has determined a safe level of exposure to anesthesia waste gases to be 25 parts per million for nitrous oxide.[12] Specific recommendations to reduce exposure include checking the function of all waste gas disposal systems, ensuring proper fit of face masks on patients during induction, turning on anesthesia gas flow only when induction is begun and not before, emptying the ventilating bag into the scavenging device before removing it from the system, and continually monitoring equipment for cracks and other leaks.[13] Private companies are available to provide a periodic gas monitoring service.

Other sources of potential injury are the antimicrobial soaps that are used frequently in the OR setting. Side effects such as skin breakdown and irritation are commonly reported by individuals with sensitivity to ingredients in the soaps. Many varieties of antimicrobial soaps are currently available, and different brands should be tried until an acceptable one is found for use by individuals with sensitivity.

Another danger is exposure to ethylene oxide used for gas sterilization. Gas sterilization techniques have been used to sterilize delicate equipment that cannot withstand the high temperatures and humidity necessary for steam sterilization. It is considered one of the most hazardous chemicals because it is known to cause mutation and chromosomal damage in humans and it is highly flammable.[14] It affects reproduction and is shown to be carcinogenic in animal studies; this may also be true in humans.[12] Aeration chambers must be properly vented for employee protection against toxic fumes. Several alternatives to gas sterilization are available, although no one method has been able to totally replace gas sterilization.

Other sterilization processes, such as steam autoclaves and glutaraldehyde, also expose staff to risk. The heat and steam produced by steam autoclaves during the sterilization process can serve as a source of burns to staff in the handling and transportation of items from the autoclave. Glutaraldehyde is a chemical that is frequently used for cold sterilization or high-level disinfecting of equipment for endoscopy procedures. The Occupational Safety and Health Administration has set an exposure limit of 0.2 parts per million for glutaraldehyde. Symptoms experienced during exposure to this chemical include respiratory, eye, throat, skin irritation; headache; allergies; eczema; and asthma.[15] Periodically, a careful review of work practices and ventilation in areas of glutaraldehyde use helps limit employee exposure.[16] Many ASCs are limiting or eliminating the use of glutaraldehyde.

Formaldehyde is another dangerous chemical that is used for specimen fixation and sometimes for disinfection. Depending on the amount of exposure, formaldehyde can cause eye and upper respiratory irritation, allergic dermatitis, and, with repeated exposure, hives; symptoms may advance to coughing, headache, heart palpitations, and tightness in the chest. Extensive exposure can be fatal.[10] All efforts should be made to reduce or avoid exposure to this chemical. Prefilled specimen containers are preferred over those that must be filled. Both the Occupational Safety and Health Administration and the Joint Commission on the Accreditation of Healthcare Organizations have requirements for monitoring environmental exposure to formaldehyde.

Anesthetics, bone cement, chemotherapy agents, preservatives, cleaning and disinfecting agents, dyes used in lasers, and antiseptics are examples of other chemicals that can be hazardous to the intraoperative team. Their specific dangers are addressed in material safety data sheets that should be available in each unit for the employees' reference. These data sheets and Occupational Safety and Health Administration regulations regarding their availability are discussed in Chapter 3.

PREPARING FOR A CASE

Before a patient is transferred to the OR, the nurse prepares the room with appropriate supplies, medications, and equipment and ensures that all equipment, including suction, is in proper working order. The nurse also ensures that proper housekeeping procedures have been completed. Some centers use a daily checklist to document that specific items have been checked and that procedures have been completed before the OR is to be used. This checklist is similar to the type of equipment check that the anesthesia team completes on its equipment each day.

The nurse should never leave the patient unattended in the OR to secure additional supplies that were forgotten. Not only is the patient's safety at risk, but the delay increases OR time and costs. Data from several sources help the nurse to secure proper and complete items ahead of time. These include: (1) the surgery schedule, which identifies the procedure to be performed, the type of anesthesia planned, and the patient's age and gender; (2) the surgeon's preference card, which itemizes the usual supplies needed for the procedure; and (3) the patient's medical record and communication from other nurses who have secured and documented information of importance to the OR team—for instance, extremes of height or weight and other anatomic variances. Facilities that have implemented critical paths can also use these as tools to prepare for the case. Other special requirements may be communicated to the ASC staff by the surgeon's office personnel at the time of the booking—an arrangement that should be encouraged.

The perioperative nurse should review the patient's chart to ascertain any special needs before preparing the room. Needs might include (1) extensions or straps for the OR bed; (2) extra pillows, blanket rolls, and safety straps for special positioning; (3) substitutions for the usual solutions used for skin preparation, contrast dyes, or other alternative medications for patients with allergies; and (4) special padding for prevention of pressure injuries for elderly or debilitated patients.

The perioperative nurse also must ensure the availability of any needed prosthesis, hardware, or sizers before the patient is taken to the OR. Intraocular lenses, penile or breast prostheses, reconstructive implant devices, screws, and pins are a few examples of items that must be available in the correct size and must be sterile and ready for use. Also, a back-up supply should be available in the event of contamination or inappropriateness of the original item.

INTRAOPERATIVE NURSING ISSUES

The first exposure of the intraoperative nurse to the patient may occur in the preoperative waiting area, in a holding area, or at the door of the OR. Remembering that first impressions are lasting, it is important to greet the patient in a warm, open manner that communicates to the patient that he or she is the focus of the nurse's activity and attention. It is important that the perioperative nurse introduce himself or herself as the nurse who will be responsible for the patient's nursing care during the surgery.

The nurse should remove any facemask before the encounter so that the patient is able to see the nurse's face and expression. A warm and genuine greeting conveys the nurse's concern about the patient as an individual. A visible name tag should be worn by all personnel so that the patient knows the nurse's name and professional capacity.

Patients should be addressed respectfully, usually by title and last name unless permission has been granted to use a first name. Pet names should be avoided because they can convey a sense of familiarity that might be considered offensive at a time when the patient already feels vulnerable. The patient may fear alienating a caregiver by asking to be referred to in another manner. It is also important to remember that the effects of preoperative sedation can cloud the patient's ability to express opinions clearly.

Careful identification of the patient both verbally and by looking at the identification bracelet or other identification system is essential. Patients should be asked to repeat their name and the site of surgery rather than having the nurse supply the correct data and ask only for a "yes" or "no" verification. The site and the side of surgery should be checked very carefully with the patient, the surgery schedule, and the chart and consent form. Asking the patient to lift, mark, or point to the operative site is one way to help avoid confusion between left and right sides. The term "right" should not be used to mean "correct" when identifying the surgical side. The physician's office record may be consulted as a primary source of documentation if there is a question; however, the patient's insistence on a site other than the one documented should be heeded, and discrepancies must be resolved before the patient is transferred into the OR.

CASE STUDY

Catherine Koval was scheduled for a right knee arthroscopy at the ASC by Dr. Fisher's office. The nurse from the ASC called Ms. Koval 5 days before the surgery to perform a telephone assessment and to reinforce preoperative instructions as given by Dr. Fisher. When the nurse asked Ms. Koval to verify the procedure as being a right knee arthroscopy, Ms. Koval stated that the surgery was to be performed on her left knee. The nurse told Ms. Koval that the ASC staff would verify the procedure with Dr. Fisher's office. She then reinforced the time Ms. Koval should arrive at the ASC, the requirement for NPO (nothing by mouth) status, and for a responsible adult to transport her home and provide care for the first 24 hours after the procedure.

The morning of surgery, Ms. Koval arrived at the ASC as instructed at 10:00 AM. She was the fourth arthroscopy scheduled for Dr. Fisher that day. Dr. Fisher's office routinely worked closely with the ASC to facilitate the case flow by grouping all of the right-sided procedures and left-sided procedures together to enhance room set-up and prevent errors. On arrival, the admitting nurse verified that the permit was correct for an arthroscopy of the left knee to be performed by Dr. Fisher.

At the door of the OR, the circulating nurse asked Ms. Koval to state what procedure was being performed. Ms. Koval stated that an arthroscopy of her left knee would be performed by Dr. Fisher. Checking the permit against the printed OR schedule, the nurse noted that the schedule indicated that the procedure was to be performed on the right knee. The first three arthroscopies performed by Dr. Fisher in the room were on the right side. The nurse called Dr. Fisher to verify the correct side, in order to ensure that the confusion over the side was clarified. Dr. Fisher verified the procedure as being on the left knee with Ms. Koval and from his printed preoperative history and physical. The scrub person was notified of the error on the schedule, and the room was prepared to accommodate the left side. The procedure was completed, and Ms. Koval was discharged to home later that day.

The circulating nurse reported the near-incident to the staff member who chaired the ASC performance improvement committee. The committee reviewed the occurrence and the literature regarding verification of laterality in surgery. The occurrence was reviewed with both the physician's office staff and the involved staff at the ASC. Later that month, the event was discussed at the monthly staff meeting and used for a performance improvement educational opportunity. Improvement initiatives included a written mechanism to notify the scheduling clerk when the patient preoperative phone call revealed a difference in the patient's understanding of the procedure and the printed schedule. Also, the admitting nurse would begin to verify the permit against the printed schedule during the admitting process. The circulating nurse was commended for her identification of the discrepancy, and all staff expressed increased awareness of the potential for error in issues of laterality. The event was also used to create a scenario in the monthly ASC newsletter of the surgeons, their office staff, and the anesthesiologists.

DISCUSSION

The verification of right or left side is a critical indicator for perioperative services. The potential for error is easily seen in the aforementioned scenario, but the alertness of the circulating nurse prevented an unnecessary surgery for the patient. All staff and physicians share the responsibility to ensure that policies and procedures are in place to deal with the complex issues of verification of laterality.

The lack of proper consent becomes a significant problem at this point if the patient has been medicated and thus is legally unable to sign any documents. The facility's policy should clearly delineate the approved protocol for such an occurrence. It may be cancellation of the case, or, depending on the situation and the physician's previous conversations with the patient, the physician may choose to obtain consent from the next of kin. Another approach is to reschedule the patient for later in the day after the effects of the medication have worn off and the patient is lucid and able to sign the consent form. Obviously, prevention is the best remedy, and the admitting nurse should be sure that a valid consent form is signed before giving any preoperative medication. Fortunately, this occurrence has become less frequent because many ASC patients do not routinely receive preoperative sedation.

Before being taken to surgery, the patient should be given an opportunity to ask any questions or explain any special needs to the perioperative nurse. The patient should be made aware of the right to express any concerns and ask questions in the OR. Understanding that such conversation is encouraged, as well as knowing when it may not be appropriate to talk, can help the patient feel less isolated and frightened in the OR.

The perioperative nurse also reviews the patient's record, briefly assesses the patient, and receives a report from the admitting nurse who has recently evaluated the patient more fully. The perioperative and admitting nurses share the responsibility of ensuring that the medical record is complete before the patient is transferred to the OR. All necessary consents must be on the chart along with all other documentation that is required by facility policy, for instance, the history and physical examination, informed consent forms, diagnostic reports, and a notation about the patient's adult companion who will be responsible for postoperative transport and home support. If required documents are missing, facility policy may dictate that the patient is not transferred to surgery until the record is complete. Strict adherence to such a policy may be one way to gain physician compliance.

To develop a comprehensive plan for the intraoperative nursing care of the patient, the experienced perioperative nurse uses information gleaned from physical and psychosocial assessment, a report from the admitting nurse, and a review of the patient's chart to secure information before the patient goes to surgery. Information from the chart includes the physician's history and physical examination, the evaluation by the anesthesia provider, and the results of diagnostic tests, such as laboratory values, radiology reports, and electrocardiogram if ordered. However, many ASCs do not require any diagnostic testing if the patient meets certain criteria. Other information from the chart includes allergies, previous surgical experiences, current medications being taken, preoperative preparation, significant health problems, and host risk factors for nosocomial infection.

Patient assessment should be conducted in an efficient manner that provides privacy for the patient. The hall outside of the OR is not a place for conducting an in-depth physical assessment. Of particular importance to planning intraoperative care is assessment of skin condition, mobility of body parts, previous surgery, presence of internal and external prostheses, abnormalities, and injuries, all of which should be noted in the operative record. Any physical impairments that may affect positioning or communication with the patient, such as blindness and hearing deficits, should be noted and communicated to all members of the intraoperative team. For instance, the patient with a hearing impairment may require that hearing aids be left in place until the patient is asleep and taken to the PACU in order to allow for communication with the patient. Impairments that will affect the care of the patient in the PACU should be communicated by the perioperative nurse before arrival to the PACU. Any items that have accompanied the patient to the OR, such as dentures, hearing aids, glasses, and prostheses, should be labeled with the patient's name and placed in a safe area or returned to the patient's family for keeping.

Mobility of body parts is very important to the planning for intraoperative positioning. Patient's statements of difficulty with mobility should be verified with a range of motion assessment. Also important in positioning the patient is the presence of internal and external prostheses and implants. Previous surgeries, such as mastectomy, make placement of arms, intravenous lines, and blood pressure cuffs very important.

Routine assessment data, such as vital signs, skin color, edema, and respiratory, cardiovascular, and renal status, are all important in the care of the intraoperative patient. The patient's height and weight should be noted on the chart. Finally, the nurse should verify any preoperative instructions, such as NPO status, and whether routine medications, such as cardiac medications and insulin, were taken, particularly prescribed preoperative medications, such as antibiotics as ordered by the surgeon.

The psychosocial aspects of the patient are as important to the outcome of the surgical intervention as the physical assessment. It is important to assess the patient and family's perception of surgery in order to ascertain their understanding of the procedure, expected outcomes, patient plans, and expectations for postoperative care and recovery. Knowledge of the patient's normal coping mechanisms and ways to deal with stress and pain can help in reducing anxiety and controlling pain after surgery.

It is also important to assess the patient's level of knowledge concerning the actual surgical procedure and the expected postoperative course of events. Any philosophical or religious beliefs that could potentially affect patient care decisions should be documented, communicated, and used in planning. Presence of support personnel, such as clergy, and requests from patients to engage in personal prayer or reflection or to maintain religious medallions should be respected and planned for. Cultural practices should also be assessed and planned for in a similar fashion. The psychosocial aspects of assessment should be carefully documented and communicated to ensure awareness on the part of the entire intraoperative team.

PLANNING

To develop a comprehensive intraoperative plan, the experienced perioperative nurse uses a physical and sensory assessment, a report from the preoperative nurse, and a review of the patient's chart to secure information before the patient goes to surgery. The perioperative nurse assimilates the information from the patient's chart, diagnostic data, and physical assessment, along with the information about the procedure and the type of anesthesia planned. Combining this information with the nurse's knowledge base, the perioperative nurse establishes expected outcomes and nursing interventions to facilitate those desired outcomes. Table 19–2 illustrates an intraoperative care grid based on nursing diagnoses and patient outcomes.

When the patient is admitted to the OR, the circulating nurse has direct responsibilities to that patient and to the other members of the healthcare team involved in anesthesia and surgery. The principles of asepsis, patient and staff safety, efficient management of resources, patient monitoring, and psychological support are all incorporated into the establishment of the intraoperative plan of care based on the nursing diagnoses. Goals should be developed and individualized to each patient and situation on the basis of the assessment data. The goals should be realistic, attainable, and measurable for the surgical experience, including time frames for expected achievement of the goals.

The ability to plan care based on nursing diagnoses and patient outcomes is important in the provision of intraoperative nursing care. The identification of nursing activities to achieve the outcomes and established priorities for nursing actions are key components of care. The ability to organize nursing activities in a logical sequence leads to a smooth flow as the care is orchestrated with the entire team, surgeon, anesthesia provider, and nursing team members.

This organization often takes the form of a previously determined critical path or plan of care that directs the flow of the intraoperative activities for the entire team. The care path helps the nurse plan and coordinate the care of the patient. An important part of the planning for care is the anticipation of possible patient needs. This ability to anticipate demonstrates the perioperative nurse's knowledge of the care of intraoperative patients and is one of the most important skills that the perioperative nurse possesses. The role of the intraoperative nurse includes coordinating the team and assigning and delegating activities to appropriate team members based on their qualifications and patient needs.

IMPLEMENTATION

Ensuring Patient Safety

Patient safety during transport is addressed by constantly monitoring, using safety straps and side rails, locking the OR bed in position, placing the bed at the same height as the stretcher before moving the patient, and having a second staff member stand on the opposite side of the OR bed during transfer to prevent the patient from falling off that side. Patients who walk to surgery should wear nonskid slippers or shoe covers and should not encounter any wet floors or other environmental hazards in their path. The patient should be accompanied and assisted to accomplish a safe transfer from a standing position to the OR bed.

Protecting the patient from environmental dangers is a constant responsibility of the perioperative nurse. Careful electrical grounding around patients, use of nonflammable anesthetics, and maintenance of a proper humidity (at least 60%) to avoid static electricity all help to avoid explosions, burns, and shocks from electrical equipment. High-voltage equipment should be placed close to the operator and as far from the anesthesia machine as possible. Other concerns that help to avoid equipment-related injury include protection of the patient's eyes during laser procedures and shielding of the body during radiologic exposures. Finally, it is important to prevent the pooling of prepping solution under or around the patient. This helps prevent skin irritation and breakdown, and eliminates one source of fire if the solution is contacted by a cautery unit or laser because some prep solutions are flammable when wet.

Patient Teaching

Although much of the teaching of the patient occurs before and after the surgical intervention, the teaching aspect of patient care can and should continue as long as the patient is awake. An atmosphere should be created by the perioperative nurse and intraoperative team that encourages the patient to ask questions and allows for reinforcement of teaching.

Table 19–2. Patient Outcomes Grid: Intraoperative Phase

POTENTIAL AND ACTUAL PROBLEMS/NURSING DIAGNOSES	OUTCOME GOALS: THE PATIENT WILL BE ABLE TO	NURSING INTERVENTIONS AND EVALUATIONS	RESOURCES
Knowledge deficit R/T surroundings and processes	Explain perioperative routines concurrent with care in lay terms Freely express lingering questions or concerns Express reduced anxiety both verbally and nonverbally and display calm demeanor Express confidence in healthcare providers Maintain normal cardiovascular parameters	Assess patient's current knowledge base and understanding of procedure. Provide simple and concise explanations of process as care is rendered. Refer to surgeon or other staff as needed.	Patient-focused philosophy of care Patient record and consent form ASPAN Standards of Perianesthesia Practice AORN Standards and Recommended Practices Surgeon and anesthesia provider
Self-care deficit and risk of injury or disruption of integrity of skin or mucous membranes R/T environment, equipment, positioning, surgical procedure	Remain free from allergic reactions, burns, skin breakdown or pressure points, falls, nerve or joint injuries, and retained foreign bodies Show no symptoms of bruising, inflammation, or breaks in integrity of skin or mucous membranes Undergo complete surgical course having had correct procedure without surgical complications Identify the site of surgery that agrees with consent	Evaluate patient and consult patient record before transfer to OR; identify allergies and special needs. Identify patient, health status, and NPO time verbally and by ID band prior to OR transfer. Ensure that patient, medical record, surgical schedule, and consent are all in agreement regarding surgical procedure. Position patient according to acceptable standards of care and individual needs using proper body mechanics for staff and patient. Apply safety belt across patient's knees. Avoid pooling of prep solution on patient's skin. Enact electric, laser, and other equipment safety standards, including safety and operational checks. Lock stretcher and OR table before transfer of patient. Attend patient at all times. Keep only current patient's chart in room. Enact appropriate sharps, sponge, and instrument counts. Check emergency call bell system and emergency equipment periodically.	Patient record Competency-based nursing practice AORN Standards and Recommended Practices Equipment manufacturers' instructions for proper use Patient positioning guidelines Appropriate positioning supplies, e.g., pillows, padding, foam sheeting Ongoing program of preventive maintenance of equipment Policy on enacting Safe Medical Device Act

Table continued on following page

***Table 19–2.* Patient Outcomes Grid: Intraoperative Phase** *Continued*

POTENTIAL AND ACTUAL PROBLEMS/NURSING DIAGNOSES	OUTCOME GOALS: THE PATIENT WILL BE ABLE TO	NURSING INTERVENTIONS AND EVALUATIONS	RESOURCES
Loss of body temperature	Maintain normal body temperature	Keep patient covered as fully as possible. Increase OR temperature for patients at high risk for hypothermia (infants, frail elderly). Assist anesthesia provider in application of warming equipment.	AORN Standards and Recommended Practices Warming cabinets with blankets and solutions Forced warm air heating blankets Access to thermostat within OR
Risk of hemorrhage	Maintain blood volume at normal level	Ensure availability of all appropriate instrumentation, equipment, and solutions. Provide skilled circulating and scrub nursing interventions.	Electrocautery and laser equipment in good working order Blood bank contract and policies for rapid availability of blood products
Risk of infection	Remain free from symptoms of infection, e.g., fever, wound inflammation, and dehiscence Display uncomplicated postoperative course of recovery Avoid skin cuts R/T preoperative hair removal Avoid extraneous breaks in skin or mucous membranes	Maintain strict aseptic technique and proper skin preparation, ensure proper decontamination and cleaning of room, instruments, and equipment before and between cases. Monitor environment and personnel, including physicians, for any breech of aseptic technique and intercede to correct errors. Restrict healthcare personnel with contagious diseases from OR. Prepare skin with clipper prep as close to time of surgery as possible. Maintain safe environment that avoids breaks in integrity of skin or mucous membranes.	AORN Standards and Recommended Practices Access to, and knowledge of, principles of aseptic technique Monitoring system for postoperative surveillance of patients to identify potential nosocomial infections Policy encouraging clipper preps rather than shaving of surgical site Approved, effective disinfectants Effective sterilization methods and equipment

Anxiety R/T unfamiliar surroundings and sedative medications	Freely express lingering questions or concerns Express reduced anxiety both verbally and nonverbally Display calm demeanor Express confidence in healthcare providers Maintain cardiovascular parameters within normal range	Use active listening to identify verbal and nonverbal cues of anxiety. Give ongoing explanations of processes, equipment, procedures, and expectations of patient. Provide appropriate social, physical, emotional, and pharmacologic interventions. Assess vital signs and emotional status. Introduce self and others providing care. Describe activities and implications for patient. Appropriately apply tactile, verbal, and visual contact while patient is awake.	Patient-focused philosophy of care Warm blankets or other warming devices for skin and solutions Apparatus to measure vital signs Staffing patterns allowing one-to-one nursing at patient bedside
Risk of impaired circulation	Maintain adequate peripheral and central circulation Maintain adequate tissue perfusion	Position appropriately with no constriction of periphery. Assess patient for pressure points, compromise of circulation R/T positioning. Assist anesthesia personnel in supporting fluid maintenance as necessary.	AORN Standards and Recommended Practices Patient positioning guidelines and adequate supplies
Risk of impaired respiratory effort	Maintain adequate respiratory effort and oxygenation	Assist anesthesia personnel in supporting respiratory effort as necessary, e.g., during patient's intubation, induction, and emergence.	Basic references in airway management, intubation and extubation techniques Oxygen and airway management equipment
Potential for pain and discomfort	Remain free of pain and discomfort Tolerate positioning and any changes	Observe and evaluate verbal/nonverbal cues of awake patients. Communicate and intercede on behalf of patient with physician provider.	Collaboration with anesthesia provider and/or attending surgeon regarding pain management techniques
Potential untoward reactions to medications	Remain free of unexpected and untoward reactions to medications Maintain physiologic balance	Identify before OR any sensitivities or allergies. Observe for symptoms and communicate same to anesthesia providers.	Anesthesia and medication texts, patient's medical record

OR, operating room; NPO, nothing by mouth; R/T, related to; ID, identification; AORN, Association of Operating Room Nurses; ASPAN, American Society of Perianesthesia Nurses.

Obviously, any sedation or a high level of anxiety significantly affects the patient's ability to identify and express teaching needs and to retain any knowledge imparted by the intraoperative team. The time should be used to reinforce teaching about intraoperative expectations and anesthesia-related concerns of the patient. Although this can be an extremely busy time for the nurses as the case is being readied, the patient, not the preparation of the room, should remain the focus of the nurse's activity.

Patient Rights

Throughout the intraoperative period, the circulating nurse serves as the patient advocate to protect the patient's safety, dignity, and privacy. Healthcare providers should avoid inappropriate laughter, confusion, and loud or unrelated conversations in the OR. This is especially important during induction of general anesthesia, when sounds and sensations can be distorted and frightening. It is vital to remember that the patient may hear what is said in the OR even while anesthetized. Conversations that should not be held in front of an awake patient should be avoided near an anesthetized patient as well.

Over the years, many patients have reported the ability to hear while under general anesthesia. Derogatory remarks about obesity or lifestyle are particularly common topics of recall that patients report, along with comments regarding pathology reports and surgical techniques. Such experiences can leave patients with permanent psychological and emotional trauma and are avoidable if the climate within the OR is respectful and conscientious about the possibility of patient awareness. Several approaches are used to limit patient hearing of staff activities and conversation during surgery. In addition to avoiding inappropriate conversation and overhead paging, the facility may provide earplugs or music through earphones to the patient.[17]

The nurse and other team members should communicate with awake patients before induction of general anesthesia and throughout those cases being performed under local or regional anesthesia. Awake patients need reassurance that their fears and individual needs are being considered. In order to help reduce anxiety for the patients, it is important to remember that the OR environment, which is so familiar to the staff, is quite foreign and often frightening to the patient. Certainly, music remains an acceptable and appreciated diversion for some patients.

It is important that the planning and implementation of the care being provided intraoperatively considers and ensures patient rights. Of great importance is the issue of maintaining and respecting the patient's privacy. The OR bed should be positioned in the room for maximal privacy of the patient during surgery. Windows to the OR are often covered when a patient's body must be exposed during a procedure, and the patient's body should not be exposed for longer than necessary. Only personnel who are directly involved in the procedure should be allowed in the OR, and visitors should be limited to those approved by the patient. Photography requires the prior consent of the patient, although photography through laparoscopic, endoscopic, and arthroscopic instruments is considered a fundamental element of these procedures.

Confidentiality is a patient right that the perioperative nurse should uphold at all times. The surgical schedule should be treated as a confidential document and should not be displayed in the lounge or in other public areas. Patients awaiting interviews or laboratory work should not have access to the schedule. Any discussion regarding a patient or a procedure should be kept within the confines of the surgical suite and should be limited to appropriate, health-related topics. Physicians and nurses who are not involved in the surgery, office personnel, and ancillary staff members are not automatically entitled to information about perioperative occurrences of all patients and should not be privy to such conversations. The staff lounge is an inappropriate site for discussions about patients.

Ambulatory surgery units occasionally receive patients who request total anonymity for a variety of reasons. Such a request should be honored whenever possible. In no situation should a patient's experience be discussed outside of the surgery center without that person's permission.

Comfort Measures

To promote the patient's physical comfort, warm blankets and pillows or other support for the patient's joints, neck, and back are appreciated. Overhead spotlights should be turned off or away from the patient's eyes. Many awake patients are afraid or unsure if they are allowed to talk during surgery, and they should be instructed to tell the nurse or anesthesia personnel of any discomfort or concerns during the procedure. This grants them the permission to communicate. Patients who are awake and who are requested not to talk for a period of time should have some other form of communication available (e.g., a hand to squeeze).

Many anesthesiologists allow patients to wear dentures until the time of induction or throughout surgery. Religious medals, a child's favorite toy or blanket, medical alert jewelry, wedding rings, hearing aids, and eyeglasses are other personal items that may find their way into the OR, particularly in the patient-centered atmosphere of the ASC setting. The safety of such items should be ensured by the use of consistent practices based on the facility's policy and procedures.

INTERACTING WITH THE ANESTHESIA TEAM

The perioperative nurse has a joint responsibility with the anesthesia team for the general well-being of the patient and serves as a direct assistant to anesthesia team members during induction of general anesthesia or during regional anesthetic procedures. One of the nurse's important functions, as attested to by many patients, is holding the patient's hand during induction. This is the patient's link to humanity at a frightening time.

The anesthesiologist or the certified registered nurse anesthetist (CRNA) directs and oversees the patient's medical care. Monitoring devices, such as cardiac monitor, noninvasive blood pressure cuff, pulse oximeter, and some form of temperature monitor, are attached. If intravenous access has not been secured before admission to the OR, a venipuncture is performed as soon as monitoring devices are in place. The patient is usually preoxygenated before receiving an intravenous induction agent, such as thiopental sodium (Pentothal), propofol (Diprivan), and methohexital (Brevital).

A calm, quiet environment should be established while the circulating nurse assists with induction and intubation. The unconscious patient's airway is established and maintained by the anesthesiologist, sometimes with positioning only or with an oral or nasal airway under an anesthesia mask. If the patient is to be intubated, a short-acting muscle relaxant, like succinylcholine (1 to 1.5 mg/kg) is generally given to facilitate relaxation of the vocal cords and to allow gentle insertion of the tube. A laryngoscope is used to visualize the cords for placement of the tube.

This period of time marks one of high risk while a competent airway is being established. Concurrently, the patient must be protected against the potential aspiration of stomach contents. The nurse may be asked by the anesthesia provider to apply cricoid pressure (Sellick's maneuver) during the intubation attempt. This pressure, when applied correctly, occludes the esophagus by compressing it with the cricoid cartilage between the trachea and vertebrae. Because the cricoid cartilage is a complete ring, its compression does not occlude the trachea or interfere with the intubation attempt. Proper hand placement is essential to avoid lateral movement of the trachea or injury to other structures. The nurse's thumb and second finger are placed on lateral sides of the cricoid cartilage and the index finger on the anterior, one finger width below the thyroid cartilage, as illustrated in Figure 19–1. The nurse may provide support under the patient's neck with the other hand while applying the pressure. Neither the thyroid nor the tracheal cartilages should be compressed. Both are incomplete rings, and pressure to either could cause occlusion of the trachea or damage to the cartilage.[18]

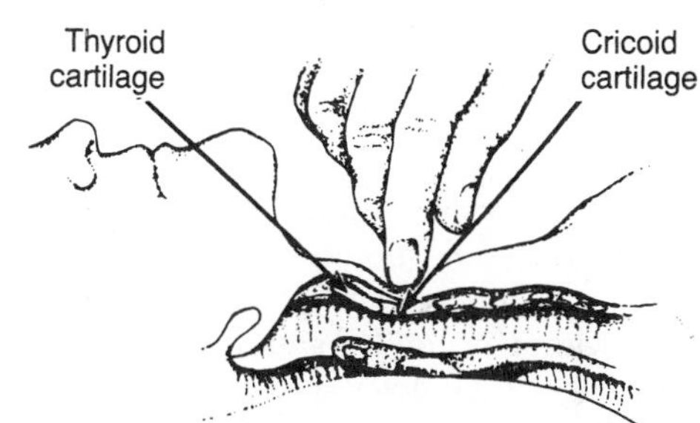

A Using the index finger to displace the cricoid cartilage posteriorly, thus obstructing the esophagus.

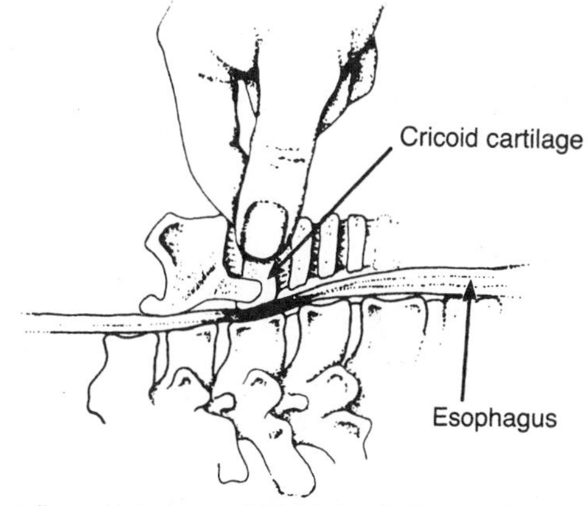

B Two-finger technique, which obstructs the esophagus between the body of the sixth cervical vertebra and the cricoid cartilage.

Figure 19–1. Application of cricoid pressure or the Sellick maneuver. (From Ethicon: Nursing Care of the Patient in the OR, 2nd ed. Somerville, NJ: Ethicon, 1987, p 23.)

Patients for whom cricoid pressure is indicated are those at high risk for vomiting and aspiration, including patients with active nausea and vomiting; those with esophageal reflux; pregnant women; and patients with full stomachs (those who have recently eaten). In particular, ambulatory patients may have questionable compliance with NPO status or may require an emergency return to surgery after postoperative nourishment has been allowed. Also, outpatients have been shown to have a higher stomach volume with a lower pH than hospitalized patients.

It is essential that the nurse not release cricoid pressure until instructed to do so by the anesthesiologist or CRNA performing the intubation. Criteria for release of pressure include the placement of the endotracheal tube, inflation of the cuff, and confirmation of proper position of the tube by auscultation of the chest. If the intubation attempt is unsuccessful, the nurse continues to hold pressure on the cricoid cartilage to prevent the patient from vomiting and aspirating. Should the patient begin to vomit while cricoid pressure is being maintained, pressure is released while the patient is turned to the side and the airway is suctioned. Otherwise, esophageal rupture may occur because of the pressure of forced vomiting against a closed esophagus.

After a successful intubation, the nurse may be asked to inflate the endotracheal cuff. The tube is secured by the anesthesiologist or CRNA with tape or by another method, and the patient is then given an anesthetic gas or a balanced technique that combines gas, sedatives, muscle relaxants, and opioids to maintain surgical unconsciousness. At this point, the anesthesiologist monitors inspired oxygen and expired carbon dioxide along with the other previously monitored parameters. When anesthesia personnel indicate that the patient's condition is stable, the circulating nurse turns primary attention to completing the preparations for the procedure. The patient is positioned; the site is prepared and draped; the sterile field is created; equipment is brought to the bedside; and the surgery begins.[19]

Another technique for general anesthesia is the use of the laryngeal mask airway. The laryngeal mask airway has been widely used since it became available in the United States in December 1992. Placement of the laryngeal mask airway is considered to be simple and does not require laryngoscopy or muscle relaxation.[11] It is beneficial to use in difficult airway situations and is considered to be an alternative to face-mask or tracheal intubation in many clinical situations.[20]

When regional anesthesia is being administered, the nurse often assists in the procedure and continues to provide emotional support for the awake patient throughout the case. Nursing responsibilities during spinal, epidural, and regional blocks vary from one institution to another but often include positioning the patient and helping maintain that position, setting up a sterile field, securing local anesthetics and solutions for skin preparation, applying necessary extremity tourniquets, and monitoring the patient's general response and vital signs during the procedure.

The nurse must be attentive to patients receiving local anesthetic agents because they may be awake and anxious and because they can exhibit unexpected signs of allergic or toxic reaction to the agent injected. Symptoms might include diaphoresis, circumoral tingling, faintness, a feeling of doom, flushed or pale skin, erythema, bradycardia, tachycardia, cardiac dysrhythmias, and respiratory or cardiac arrest. Other complications directly related to the invasive techniques are also possible, for instance, pneumothorax, hemorrhage, ruptured viscus, and inadvertent subarachnoid puncture. The nurse must be constantly prepared to respond to these or other unexpected situations. A thorough discussion of the nursing responsibilities surrounding local and regional anesthesia is provided in Chapter 14.

The circulating nurse may assist the anesthesia team with administration of intravenous fluids and of medications such as antibiotics and intramuscular antiemetic or anti-inflammatory drugs. Another duty may be to obtain blood samples from the patient or, in rare instances, to secure blood for transfusion. The anesthesiologist, circulating nurse, and surgeon collaborate on issues such as estimated blood loss, fluid and electrolyte needs, patient temperature and warming or cooling needs, duration of the procedure, and times of intraoperative events. Accuracy of documentation by all parties is paramount.

PATIENT POSITIONING

The circulating nurse waits for a cue from the anesthesia provider before moving or positioning the patient after induction of anesthesia. Positioning is accomplished in combination with the anesthesia team, and the patient is moved gently and slowly to avoid injury or circulatory compromise or collapse. During positioning, the airway is attentively maintained by the anesthesiologist or CRNA, who again listens for breath sounds indicating proper endotracheal tube placement after positioning is completed.

Proper patient positioning ensures proper anatomic alignment and avoids compromise of respiration and circulation. The nurse considers the type of procedure and exposure required, necessary support and proper safety devices, and any modifications needed to meet the patient's unique needs and physical requirements. The operative site must be adequately exposed, and the anesthesia provider must have access to the patient's airway, monitoring devices, and intravenous lines. There should be no pressure on nerves and little on skin, particularly over bony prominences. Bony areas are particularly vulnerable to injury from rubbing and sustained pressure.[11]

Many variations of positions exist for specific procedures. Basic positions and potential pressure points are illustrated in Figure 19–2. Of special note are safety practices regarding positioning that help to protect the patient from injury during the procedure:

- Do not hyperextend an arm past 90 degrees to prevent damage to the nerves and blood vessels of the brachial plexus.
- Do not allow any parts of the body to extend over the edge of the OR bed.
- Do not allow unprotected body parts to touch any metal or unpadded surfaces.
- Use an arm board to support the arms and to protect the intravenous line site.
- When in a supine position, the patient's ankles or legs should remain uncrossed to prevent occlusion of blood vessels.
- When in a lateral position, the patient should have a pillow between the legs to prevent pressure on blood vessels and to prevent pressure sores on bony prominences.
- When the patient is prone, free chest movement should be ensured by positioning and supports along the lateral chest walls.
- The patient's legs are moved into and out of lithotomy simultaneously by two people.
- An unconscious patient is lifted, never pushed or pulled, except with the aid of devices expressly designed for such maneuvers.
- Sufficient personnel are needed to properly position an unconscious patient.
- If a patient's position is changed intraoperatively, the circulating nurse must ensure that such movement does not result in new pressure points or a position that might injure the patient.
- No team member should lean on the patient or place heavy instruments on the patient.
- The Mayo stand should not put pressure on the patient.

It is important that the OR nurse look objectively and critically at the patient's final position for surgery. The awake patient is asked to provide a subjective description of comfort. For the patient who is already anesthetized, the nurse must assume the responsibility of deciding whether the patient is in the anatomically correct position appropriate for the duration of the surgery. Perioperative nursing texts are available to provide more specific information regarding patient positioning.

SITE PREPARATION

The primary goal of skin preparation is decreasing the number of microorganisms at the operative site. Dirt and skin oils are removed with scrubbing action, and antimicrobial agents are used to reduce the number of bacteria present on the skin and to prevent further microbial growth.

Cleansing and antisepsis of the skin are accomplished by the circulating nurse, who wears sterile gloves and mask and uses a sterile field for the solutions and supplies. The choice of antimicrobial agent is generally made by the operating surgeon or physician, although facility policy also may affect the use of particular agents. More complete guidelines for preoperative hair removal and skin preparation should be consulted. Some general principles of skin preparation include:[21]

1. Maintain the dignity and privacy of the patient by exposing only the necessary areas of the body.
2. Assess skin before beginning the preparation. Breaks in the skin or symptoms of infection may preclude the surgery.
3. Check patient allergies before using any solution.
4. Use warm solutions and keep the patient well covered for comfort and to reduce the risk of hypothermia.
5. Scrub in a circular motion from the incisional site outward in an expanding circle. Discard each sponge when the periphery has been reached and start again in the center of the circle with a new sponge.
6. Never reapply a sponge to an area that has been cleansed because bacteria from adjacent skin can be introduced on the prepped area.

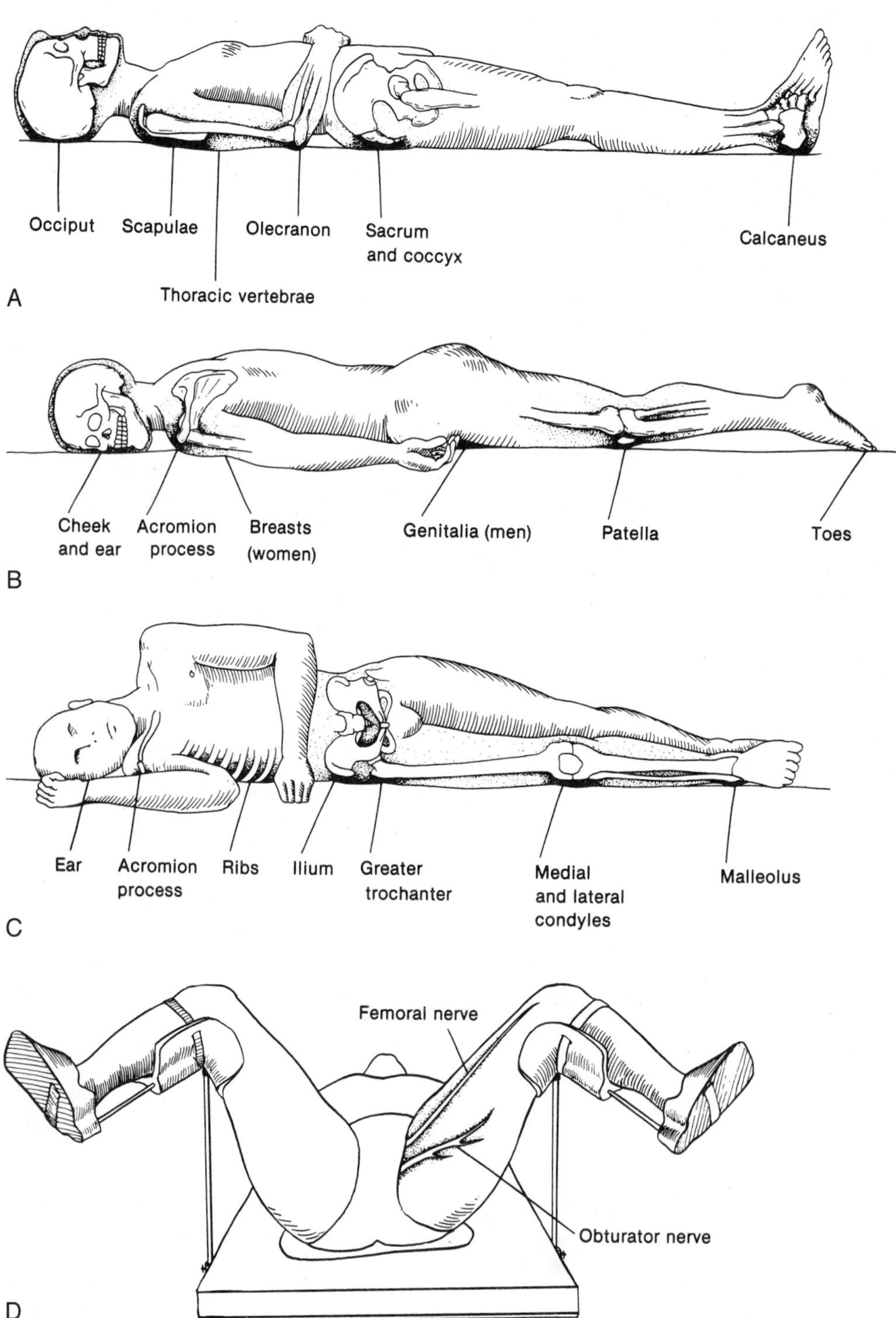

Figure 19–2. Potential pressure points related to patient positioning. (From Groah L: Operating Room Nursing: The Perioperative Role. Old Tappan, NJ: Reston Publishing Co., 1983, pp 265, 268, 269, 271, 273.)

7. Do not allow prep solutions to pool under the patient or under tourniquets, grounding pads, or electrodes because skin irritation or chemical burns can ensue.[22] This is particularly true for patients with fair or sensitive skin and for those who are placed on warming blankets during the procedure.
8. Always move from cleanest to dirtiest area and do not return. For instance, the vagina and rectum are cleansed after the surrounding skin for a perineal preparation. The axilla is prepared last during a shoulder preparation.
9. Limb preparation requires that the limb be held up by another person or device to allow the entire circumference to be prepared.
10. Cleansing is performed gently when a superficial malignancy is suspected so as not to spread potentially cancerous cells.
11. Flammable liquids like acetone and alcohol are not recommended, because remaining liquid or lingering fumes can create a spark when used in conjunction with electrocautery or lasers. If such liquids are used, drapes should not be applied until the area is totally dry.
12. Allow antiseptic paints to dry before applying drapes.

Draping the surgical site creates the surgical field. Sterile drapes are made of either reusable fabric or disposable synthetic material. Placement of these drapes isolates the prepared area from other parts of the patient's body and covers tables and work spaces. The goal is to decrease the spread of microorganisms from the patient's body, the surgical team, or the environment to the surgical site. Drape materials should resist soaking with blood or solutions and should be easily drapable and lint free.

Draping is performed by the surgeon and the scrub nurse or other surgical assistants who are appropriately gowned and gloved to assist during the procedure. Drapes should be handled as little as possible and should be taken to the OR bed while still folded. The persons applying the drapes should protect themselves from contamination on nonsterile areas of the sheets and surrounding pieces of equipment. During the draping process, all drapes should be kept above waist level because anything that drops below that level is considered contaminated. Once a drape is placed, it should not be moved, nor should personnel reach or lean across a nonsterile area to place a drape on the other side of the patient. The closest area to personnel is draped first, and the central areas near the operative site are draped before the periphery. As with all sterile supplies or equipment, if there is the slightest doubt about potential contamination of a drape, it should be considered nonsterile and discarded or covered appropriately.[11]

INTRAOPERATIVE RESPONSIBILITIES

Numerous nursing responsibilities occur throughout the procedure. One is ensuring that proper equipment is available and that all personnel are operating the equipment according to manufacturer's instructions and accepted policy. The nurse maintains constant awareness of the proceedings and ensures that any additional supplies, including emergency supplies, are secured when needed. The nurse also ensures a correct needle and sharps count, assesses urinary output, and helps monitor the amount of blood loss and intravenous fluid status. Patients undergoing extended procedures may require passive exercises of the extremities intraoperatively, another responsibility for the circulating nurse.

If a procedure extends over the projected time because of length of case or prior delay, the circulating nurse should communicate information to waiting family members. Surgeons scheduled for subsequent cases that may be delayed should be notified of the projected start time.

THERMOREGULATION

The circulating nurse should maintain an awareness of the patient's temperature. Malignant hyperthermia is a rare, but potentially fatal, occurrence in the OR. The circulating nurse must be aware of its signs and symptoms and must be prepared to respond with the appropriate emergency protocol. Chapter 11 provides a detailed discussion of malignant hyperthermia.

Hypothermia, on the other hand, is a common occurrence that often can be avoided by proper attention to the patient's physical needs. Hypothermia contributes to the patient's subjective discomfort and can prolong recovery from general anesthesia because medications and anesthetic agents take longer to be metabolized when the body's metabolic rate is slowed during hypothermic periods. Normally, the body is in balance between heat production through metabolism and heat loss through convection, radiation, conduction, and evaporation.

Radiant and conductive losses through the skin account for most heat loss, but some is lost by evaporation through the skin and lungs and a small portion through urine and feces.

When faced with a decreased core temperature, the body normally responds in several ways to produce or conserve heat. Decreased perspiration and peripheral vasoconstriction reduce heat loss through the skin. Shivering increases body temperature through internal heat production. Perioperative shivering is a particularly unpleasant occurrence for the patient, and the resulting increase in metabolic activity and oxygen consumption can lead to cardiorespiratory sequelae, particularly in a patient with preexisting cardiac compromise. Perioperative shivering is not always related to hypothermia but is a common sequela of general anesthesia.

Anesthesia techniques often obliterate or reduce the body's normal thermoregulating mechanisms. General anesthesia has a depressant effect on the hypothalamus and causes vasodilatation of peripheral vessels. Muscle relaxants prevent the body from shivering to produce heat. Spinal and epidural anesthesia also produce vasodilatation distal to the block. Additionally, the OR environment assaults the body's temperature regulation in many ways, including cool room temperatures, exposure of the body and body cavity to infusions, and irrigation with cool solutions.

Awareness of the patient's temperature is the first step in preventing hypothermia, which is defined as a core temperature below 96.8°F (36°C).[23] Continuous monitoring of temperature is often accomplished by use of a skin sensor placed on the patient's forehead, neck, or elsewhere. Complex or lengthy procedures may require monitoring devices that more accurately reflect the body's core (internal) temperature, for instance, rectal, nasopharyngeal, esophageal, tympanic membrane, and bladder sensors.

Whenever possible, the patient's environment should be altered to reduce the opportunity for heat loss. OR temperature is usually kept low for the comfort of the gowned surgical team and to inhibit the growth of bacteria,[24] but if the room temperature is lowered past 68°F (20°C), the patient's core temperature often falls below 96.8°F (36°C). A room temperature of 72°F is suggested, with an increase to 80°F for infants or fragile elderly patients.[25]

All patients should be kept covered as much as possible. Automatic warming pads may be used for cases expected to extend past 1 hour. Cloth blankets from a warming cabinet are particularly pleasant for the awake patient and may help to reduce heat loss. Rewarming devices, such as a forced air blanket, may be employed. Covering the patient's head in the cold OR is especially helpful because a significant amount of heat is lost through the head. Warmed irrigating fluids and skin prep solutions help maintain body temperature; some facilities keep intravenous solutions in warming cabinets, particularly for patients undergoing general anesthesia. Manufacturer's instructions regarding warming should be followed for all solutions, and blood transfusions should be warmed in an approved warming device. Solutions, intravenous solutions, and blood products should never be warmed in a microwave oven. Anesthesia techniques to decrease heat loss through respirations are also used.

MONITORING ASEPTIC TECHNIQUE

The circulating nurse is charged with monitoring and maintaining aseptic technique to help protect the patient from infection. When the case is set up, all supplies must be inspected to identify potential breaks in packaging that could contaminate the contents. Sterility indicators must be present and checked when items are removed from the sterilizer or packages.

The circulating nurse must inform any team member immediately on observing a break in aseptic technique. There should be no question or argument on the part of that team member; caution is always preferred over casualness. The vehicle for documenting any break in aseptic technique varies from one facility to another but should be established by an approved, written policy. Examples of methods include a performance improvement or risk management transmittal tool or an OR log book.

Unnecessary body movement and practices, such as tossing linen or wastes, should be avoided in the OR. Gowns worn during the procedure should be removed before the gloves, and both must be discarded in the room before personnel leave. Physicians and their private scrub nurses or technicians are expected to comply with all facility policies.

SPECIMENS

The circulating nurse and scrub person often assume a dual responsibility for the proper fixation, identification, storage, and transport of specimens. The following practices should be employed when tissue specimens are handled:

1. Ensure the source of the specimen before labeling. Ask the physician if there is any doubt.
2. Place the specimen in the proper medium. Specimens for immediate evaluation by frozen section are left dry. Other specimens may be placed in formaldehyde or another preservative or in saline at the request of the pathologist and the surgeon. As a general practice, specimens are not sent to the laboratory on x-ray–detectable sponges, because this affects the accuracy of the sponge count at the completion of the procedure.
3. Cultures require special handling. The perioperative nurse should obtain information from the appropriate laboratory regarding specific techniques and mediums for viral, fungal, and bacterial specimens as well as for anaerobic and aerobic specimens.
4. Treat all specimens as potentially infectious; use the principles of standard precautions when handling all specimens.
5. Clearly label any known infectious tissue for the protection of pathology department personnel.
6. Label all specimens with the patient's name, facility or medical record number, date, and exact source of tissue.
7. Always label specimens before they are removed from the individual OR.
8. Tightly cover specimens to prevent spillage.
9. Clean the outside of the specimen container before its removal from the OR.
10. Send a properly completed requisition with each specimen in accordance with facility protocol.
11. Place all specimens in a predetermined, central location before transport to the pathology department. This area should be out of the view of patients and away from the usual traffic patterns used by staff members.
12. All specimens should be enclosed and labeled as biohazardous in transit between departments.

Frozen sections require special handling. A pathologist should be available at the appropriate time for the study. The surgeon often waits in the OR for the results of the frozen section because further surgical intervention may be indicated if a malignancy is found. It is best for the pathologist to give the report directly to the surgeon, but the circulating nurse may be responsible for taking a telephone report. The nurse should have a clear understanding of the content of the report. The report should be given to the physician before the telephone call is completed in case any questions arise. The nurse should document the conversation and the caller's name in the intraoperative notes.

PERFORMING SPONGE, SHARPS, AND INSTRUMENT COUNTS

It is a key responsibility of the intraoperative nurse to account for counted items to ensure that they are not retained in the patient. Institutional policies and procedures should be strictly adhered to in order to maintain compliance with this important aspect of intraoperative care. These policies should establish responsibility for counted items and should provide direction for items to be counted, how the count should be completed, and what to do in the instance of an incorrect count. Usually, the circulating nurse maintains responsibility for ensuring that counts are taken and are accurate and documented. The actual count is performed in cooperation with the scrub person, with each visualizing the items being counted and counting each item out loud so that both individuals participating in the count can hear. The accuracy of the count should be announced to the operative team at intervals as designated per facility policy. The assurance of a correct count signals the team that it is acceptable to proceed with closing the wound and completing the surgery.

Institutional policy should be clearly written to indicate what actions should be taken in the case of an incorrect count of any kind. Usually, the procedure involves notification of the team at the field so that the incision area can be thoroughly searched for any possibly retained item. If the search does not produce a correct count, institutional policy usually requires a radiographic examination to determine the presence of any retained item.

PREPARING THE PATIENT FOR TRANSFER FROM THE OPERATING ROOM

When the case has been completed, the circulating nurse helps to remove the drapes, turn off equipment, remove cords and machinery from the bedside, and cleanse the patient's skin to remove the disinfectant and soap from areas surrounding the dressing. Skin creases must be cleansed, as well as areas where solutions have dripped or pooled, to help prevent skin irritation. While the patient is being prepared for transfer from the OR, the dressing should be monitored to ensure that it is intact and that no significant bleeding or drainage has occurred before transfer.

At the direction of the anesthesiologist, the patient is placed back into a position that allows transfer from the OR bed to the stretcher. The anesthesiologist protects the patient's head during the transfer. A sufficient number of people must help in moving any anesthetized patient. This time from the end of surgery to the transfer to the PACU is a dangerous period for the patient. Stress is reduced because the procedure is finished and personnel tend to make light conversation and lessen their vigilance over the patient. Many tasks are necessary at this time, such as removing equipment, gowns, and gloves; moving overhead lights out of the way; ensuring the safe storage of specimens; and securing paperwork and signatures from the physician. It is essential that the circulating nurse maintain conscious responsibility for overseeing the patient's nursing care during this period.

The patient who has undergone regional anesthesia requires protection of affected body parts. The patient who is to walk to the postoperative area should be allowed to sit on the edge of the OR bed for a moment until any dizziness dissipates. If faintness or nausea occurs, the patient should be returned to a supine position and a stretcher obtained for the transfer.

Depending on the physical and administrative set-up of the facility and the type of procedure the patient has undergone, the perioperative nurse may assist in transporting the patient to the PACU or to another type of unit designed to receive patients after ambulatory surgery or special procedures. The nurse receiving the patient should be given a comprehensive report before the OR and anesthesia personnel leave the patient. Sometimes, those reports overlap, but the anesthesiologist or CRNA generally provides information about the patient's significant health history, anesthesia approach, agents and events, estimated blood loss, and whether the patient was intubated.

The perioperative nurse reports the actual procedure and any deviations from the procedure listed on the OR schedule or consent. The nurse also reports any allergies, medications given in surgery, type of dressing, presence of any drains or catheters, drainage that occurred since surgery, and any special orders or requests of the physician regarding postoperative care. If the patient had a tourniquet on an extremity during surgery, the accepting nurse should be informed. This knowledge allows the postanesthesia nurse to more accurately assess and interpret the color and temperature changes in that extremity. It is important that the postanesthesia nurse be made aware of any untoward or unexpected intraoperative occurrences or injuries to the patient so that proper observation, assessment, documentation, and follow-up are undertaken.

DOCUMENTATION OF CARE

Documentation of intraoperative nursing care should be ongoing during the patient's stay in the OR. It is important to document all occurrences, nursing interventions, and assessments because later recall of precise details is impossible in many instances. The names of all personnel involved in the care of the patient in surgery should be listed on the intraoperative notes, including those who relieve others for rest breaks. The nurses' notes, like those in other areas, must be legible, including the signature of the nurse.

Some overlap may occur in the documentation of the anesthesia team and the perioperative nurse, depending on facility policies. Nurses' notes should be designed for ease and speed of documenting care because many ambulatory surgical procedures are of short duration and require the almost constant attention of the perioperative nurse for actual patient care needs.

Some facilities provide separate forms for various special procedures, requiring that only pertinent data be documented. Suggestions for content follow; they reinforce the need for an efficient, yet comprehensive, way to include all necessary aspects of care and assessments in a short time. General intraoperative documentation often includes

- Patient's name, identification number, preoperative and postoperative diagnoses
- Procedure or procedures performed
- Intraoperative x-ray films taken
- Names of all persons involved in care, including those relieving for short periods of time
- Documentation of preoperative patient identification and mode
- Preoperative assessment of patient's physical and emotional status, including level of consciousness and anxiety level
- Presence and disposition of any sensory aids or personal belongings of the patient

- Mode of transportation, safety practices during transport (rails, straps)
- Names of persons transporting patient to surgery
- Times of patient transfer, start and finish times of anesthesia and surgery, and time out of room. These times should be coordinated with the anesthesia record to reflect no gaps in times.
- Operating room number or identification of the location of the procedure room
- Intravenous solutions and site, including condition of site (may be documented by anesthesia team)
- Position for surgery, including notes on padding, supports, devices, or special positioning needs
- Skin condition—general condition and at area specific to operative site
- Skin preparation
- Use of warming blanket
- Equipment used, including serial number or identifying number assigned to the equipment, including information appropriate to the type of equipment, for example
    - Electrosurgery unit: location of grounding pad, level of voltage used, cautery or coagulation setting, postoperative condition of the skin at the pad site
    - Operative tourniquet: pounds per square inch, location of cuff, padding used under cuff, actual times and length of time inflated, skin condition under cuff and distal to cuff before and after inflation
- Source, number, and disposition of specimens
- Prostheses implanted, including serial numbers and sizes if applicable. Attach any identifying labels if provided by the manufacturer. Some labels may be given to the patient, for instance, intraocular lens cards that identify the power of the lens implanted.
- Blood administered—autologous or donated, type, times of start and stop, amount infused, any untoward reactions, warming device used. The completed form that accompanies the unit of blood should be attached to the chart according to facility protocol.
- Medications given or dispensed by the registered nurse—local anesthetics, antibiotics, topicals, irrigating fluids
- Patient protection—shielding of eyes during laser treatment, the body during x-ray tests
- Urinary status if applicable, output if the patient is straight catheterized, Foley size and amount of solution in balloon, amount of urine output in OR, incontinence during procedure
- Dressing, drains, packings, splints, casts, and slings
- Sponge, needle, instrument, and sharps counts when applicable
- Any special complications, occurrences, all written objectively without speculation or subjective data
- Wound classification
- Persons accompanying during discharge transport
- Area of disposition—PACU, ASC, emergency department
- Name of the person receiving the patient
- Signature and title of person recording data

Intraoperative nursing documentation for a patient undergoing local anesthesia without the presence of an anesthesia team member requires further inclusions (see Chapter 14).

While the surgeon is still in the OR, the circulating nurse also should ensure that appropriate medical documentation is complete, in particular, a handwritten operative note that includes the procedure, the postoperative diagnosis, and the patient's condition. Postoperative orders should be written and signed. If verbal orders are given to the perioperative nurse during or immediately after the procedure, the nurse should ask the physician to write those orders or should personally write them and have the physician sign them before leaving the OR. The perioperative nurse should inform the physician of the whereabouts of the patient's family, if known.

AFTERCARE OF THE OPERATING ROOM ENVIRONMENT

Facility policies and the principles of standard precautions should be followed for disposal of wastes from the case. The process should protect personnel within the department and all people who may come into contact with that waste at a later time. Sharp or dangerous items should be placed in impervious containers. After all wastes are removed from the room, surfaces should be decontaminated using a suitable detergent/disinfectant, and the floor should be damp-mopped in areas visibly soiled.

Turnover time between cases is a constant source of discussion and debate in many facilities. Decreasing this time is desirable so that the OR can be used more efficiently and produce more revenue in any given period. Rapid turnover between cases is often a hallmark objective of the ASC's OR staff. The quick turnover combines with generally shorter cases to allow many procedures to be accomplished in a limited period. This efficiency is a focal marketing tactic for interesting physicians in the ambulatory facility, whether it is in a hospital or a freestanding center. However, safety should never be sacrificed for speed.

If turnover time is a source of discord, it is important to identify the actual problems contributing to the situation. Forces both outside and within the OR can contribute to delayed starts. Solutions to problems of prolonged turnover times require cooperation and understanding between the nursing, anesthesia, and surgery departments. It is rarely the problem of one department but rather a combination of the three that contributes to delays. Using the tenets of continuous performance improvement, a team approach to looking at the problem often reveals that no one discipline is responsible for delays on a consistent basis. An objective approach to looking at patient preparation and timely arrival time of patients, staff, and physicians often identifies process problems that can be resolved when all involved work together cooperatively.

CONCLUSION

Today's perioperative nurse must deal with an ever-increasing number of responsibilities. Advances in technology have brought complex equipment into the setting. Simultaneously, economic pressures have forced sicker and older patients into ambulatory surgery facilities. OR nursing care requires a combination of highly developed technical, social, and clinical skills. Efficiency in getting duties accomplished cannot overshadow the patient's need for a safe and caring environment. This has never been so true as in the current ambulatory surgery population, where more patients are awake and expected to be involved and responsible for self-care.

Inherent in the philosophy of care in the ASC is the provision of a caring, safe, and respectful environment. Patients expect that they will receive high-quality medical and nursing care and that their dignity and privacy will be maintained. The OR is one link in the patient's continuum of care. The patient must depend on the perioperative nurse to contribute appropriate knowledge, experience, technical skills, and concern to ensure that this link reflects the overall philosophy of the ASC as a whole.

References

1. Nash MG, Blackwood D, Boone EB, et al: Managing expectations between patient and nurse. J Nurs Admin 24:49–55, 1994.
2. Association of Operating Room Nurses: Standards and Recommended Practices. Denver: Published by Author, 1997.
3. Trendlines: National and Regional Trends in Ambulatory Care: Ambulatory Surgery. Chicago: Society for Ambulatory Care Professionals of the American Hospital Association, March, 1995.
4. Glover TL: Preliminary exploration of variables related to operating room staffing methods. Surg Serv Man 1:37–41, 1995.
5. Anderson A: Best Practices in Ambulatory Surgery. Dallas: Author, 1992.
6. Applegeet CD, Phippen ML: Differentiating perioperative practice. Surg Serv Man 1:32–36, 1995.
7. Girard N: The case management model of patient care delivery. AORN J 60:403–415, 1994.
8. Tahan HA, Cesta TG: Evaluating the effectiveness of case management plans. J Nurs Admin 25:58–63, 1995.
9. White GG: Getting involved in national post marketing surveillance. Surg Serv Man 1:44–51, 1995.
10. Phippen ML, Wells MP: Perioperative Nursing Practice. Philadelphia: WB Saunders, 1994.
11. Meeker MH, Rothrock JC: Alexander's Care of the Patient in Surgery. St. Louis: CV Mosby, 1995.
12. Roth RA: Perioperative Nursing Care Curriculum. Philadelphia: WB Saunders, 1995.
13. US Department of Health and Human Services, Centers for Disease Control and Prevention, National Institute for Occupational Safety and Health. NIOSH recommendations for occupational safety and health standards. HHS Publication No. (CDC) 85-8017, 1985.
14. Reichert M, Young JH: Sterilization Technology for the Healthcare Facility. Gaithersburg, MD: Aspen Publishers, 1993.
15. Conrad F: Should you monitor for glutaraldehyde exposure? Healthcare Hazardous Materials Man 5:7, 1992.
16. Clinical issues. AORN J 47:1159–1160, 1993.
17. Gaberson KB: The effect of humorous and music distraction on preoperative anxiety. AORN J 62:784–790, 1995.
18. Fezer S: Cricoid pressure: How, when and why. AORN J 45:1374–1377, 1987.
19. Stein RH: The perioperative nurse's role in anesthesia management. AORN J 62:794–804, 1995.
20. Pennant JH, White PF: The laryngeal mask airway: Its uses in anesthesiology. Anesthesiology 70:144–163, 1993.
21. Spry C: Essentials of perioperative nursing: A self learning guide. Rockville, MD: Aspen Publishers, 1988.
22. Franklin R: Skin injury in the OR and elsewhere. Health Devices 9:312–318, 1980.
23. Flacke G, Flacke W: Inadvertent hypothermia: Frequent, insidious and often serious. Semin Anesth 2:183, 1983.
24. Fallacaro M, Fallacaro N, Radel T: Inadvertent hypothermia: Etiology, effects and prevention. AORN J 44:54–61, 1986.
25. Dennison D: Thermal regulation of patients during the perioperative period. AORN J 61:827–831, 1995.

Chapter 20

Immediate Postanesthesia Care

Rose Ferrara-Love

A postanesthesia care unit (PACU) is the appropriate care setting for postoperative patients while they regain physiologic homeostasis. The primary purpose of a PACU is "the critical evaluation and stabilization of postoperative patients with emphasis on anticipation and prevention of complications resulting from anesthesia or the operative procedure."[1] Patients who have undergone general anesthesia, major regional anesthesia, or extensive sedation should be afforded this intensive PACU observation after their procedures. Moreover, any patient who has experienced a significant intraoperative complication or cardiovascular instability is also a candidate for PACU attention, whatever the type of anesthesia administered.

Whether the PACU is in the main surgical suite or is dedicated strictly to the care of ambulatory surgery patients, the foci of care remain the same:

To observe the patient's physiologic status and to intervene appropriately in a way that encourages uneventful recovery from anesthesia and surgery

To provide a safe environment for the patient experiencing limitations in physical, mental, and emotional function

To avoid or immediately treat complications in the immediate postanesthetic period

To uphold the patient's right to dignity, privacy, and confidentiality

To encourage a sense of wellness and self-confidence needed for early discharge.

Patient care should be provided according to the practice standards of the American Society of Perianesthesia Nurses. Specific nursing actions in a PACU involve attention to many issues; the patient's basic reflexes, airway, cardiovascular and respiratory status, level of consciousness, condition of the surgical site, orientation to surroundings, analgesia and other comfort measures, fluid and electrolyte status, and progressive ambulation. A perianesthesia nurse plans nursing care to avoid complications, such as aspiration, hypoventilation, nausea, vomiting, hypotension, hypertension, and pain.[2] The ultimate patient outcome is safe return to consciousness and resolution of the effects of major regional anesthesia without complications or untoward responses to drugs and treatments.

The ambulatory surgical patient may be cared for in the main PACU or in one exclusive to the ambulatory unit, depending on the facility. A PACU assigned to ambulatory surgery patients exclusively may enhance patient satisfaction by providing a generally less stressful setting than a mainstream PACU. Patients are often allowed a more rapid reunion with family or responsible others and are cared for by nurses who are attending strictly to their postanesthesia needs. The facility ultimately benefits when satisfied patients tell their physicians and other people in the community about their positive experiences.

Cost-effective advantages of having the ambulatory surgical patient mainstreamed into a primary PACU include more efficient use of personnel, space, and costly equipment.[3] Many physicians appreciate the convenience of having their recovering patients in one location. Although PACU staff in each unit may be equally educated and skilled, nurses in the main PACU are often more experienced in handling emergencies because emergencies occur more frequently in that setting. Also, the immediate availability of sophisticated equipment often kept in the mainstream PACU is an asset.[1]

On the other hand, the more awake and essentially healthy ambulatory surgical patient can find the mainstream PACU frightening. Ventilators, monitors, alarms, general traffic, and conversational noises can negatively affect alert PACU patients. Some facilities have addressed this problem by restructuring their PACUs so that outpatients are partially isolated from more critically ill patients.[2] Other measures may be instituted to decrease an ambulatory patient's contact with, or awareness of, potentially frightening surroundings.[4]

The ambulatory surgery patient requires the same sort of postanesthesia care as the hospitalized patient, although the focus of that nursing care is altered when the patient is expected to return home on the day of surgery (Table 20–1). Ambulatory surgery patients have special PACU nursing care requirements; for instance, heavy sedation is avoided because it could unduly prolong the period of recovery and could necessitate overnight hospitalization. All postoperative patients deserve multifocused methods to prevent and treat pain and nausea; these interventions must be particularly aggressive for the ambulatory patient because those complications are well known for causing delayed recovery and occasional hospitalization. Early ambulation is advocated, and an attitude of wellness and health is projected to promote the patient's self-confidence and to encourage self-care. Whenever possible, the patient's sensory aides, eyeglasses, dentures, and other personal items should be returned in order to encourage a sense of normalcy and dignity.

The PACU environment should address the emotional and social needs of patients. Beginning with the early moments of recovery from general anesthesia, the nurse should be actively suggesting wellness and relaxation to both unconscious and semiconscious patients. Even in the busiest unit, intangibles, such as eye contact, a smile, a touch to the brow, genuineness in conversations, provision of privacy for personal care, and use of the patient's proper name, take no extra time in patient care but help to maintain the patient's dignity and sense of importance.[4]

Early reunion with family or friends is also a hallmark of the recovery period for ambulatory surgery patients and should be provided when possible. This can be effected by allowing a family member into the PACU or by providing a timely discharge from the PACU to the phase II area. The decision should be based on the patient's actual condition rather than on predetermined, arbitrary, and antiquated time frames.

***Table 20–1.* Focus of Postanesthesia Care Unit Nursing Care for the Ambulatory Surgery Patient**

Primary
Maintain patent airway
Monitor and support respiratory and cardiovascular systems (e.g., oxygen, positioning, deep breathing, IV fluids, vital signs)
Prevent aspiration
Encourage return of consciousness and orientation
Protect patient from injury
Prevent or treat pain, nausea, and vomiting
Prevent or treat shivering
Provide for warmth and comfort
Prevent or treat emergence delirium
Provide care applicable to procedure
Monitor operative site
Specific for Ambulatory Patients
Place particular stress on preventing pain, nausea and vomiting
Encourage patient's sense of wellness
Promote self care
Avoid heavy sedation
Encourage ambulation
Encourage early family reunion and involvement in care
Applicable to all patients in PACU, but especially important for patients who will be discharged soon after anesthesia

IV, intravenous; PACU, postanesthesia care unit.

EQUIPMENT AND ENVIRONMENTAL CONCERNS

A PACU should be positioned close to the operating rooms (ORs). It should be a well-lighted area that encourages visibility of patients from all areas of the room. In a freestanding facility, there may be an access door from the PACU to the lobby area to allow the entry of family members. A hospital-based PACU is most efficiently situated between the OR suite and the phase II department of the ambulatory surgery unit to allow the efficient progression of patients from one area to the next. The American Society of Perianesthesia Nurses recommends that the PACU and phase II (for patients not given general anesthesia) areas be separate sections or rooms and that preoperative patients not be cared for in the same location as patients who are recovering from anesthesia.[5]

Certain amenities should be included in the PACU if ambulatory surgery patients will remain there for the full duration of their recovery. These include a bathroom and changing area, a bedside chair, room for one or more family members to visit, and appropriate diversionary materials.[4]

When an ambulatory surgery facility is being planned, it has been suggested that 1.5 PACU beds be available for each operating room. Consideration should be given to an individual facility's patient mix, the volume of cases per OR, and the type of anesthesia used, and the average anticipated length of PACU care.[1] Two PACU beds per OR may be a more workable number if the caseload consists generally of short procedures performed on healthy adults.[6] An emergency call system must be available for summoning outside help, and sufficient work space should be available for preparing and using patient supplies and documenting care. In addition to oxygen, suction, and monitoring equipment, emergency drugs and resuscitation equipment are essential in the PACU. A comprehensive list of recommended equipment and supplies is available in the ASPAN Standards of Perianesthesia Nurses, which can be ordered via www.ASPAN.org.

To promote the wellness philosophy associated with the ambulatory approach to surgery, many PACUs specializing in ambulatory care are transforming a clinical look to a decor that better enhances the sense of wellness. Wallpaper, printed draperies, greenery, windows, and wall decorations add to the visual appeal, and modern cabinets are designed to hide the clinical look of a unit's storage areas. This approach provides a less clinical atmosphere while maintaining the efficient, critical functions of the unit.

POLICIES, PROCEDURES, AND STAFFING

A policy manual that contains topics related to perianesthesia nursing care should be maintained in the PACU for reference and referral by the staff. Policies should address the broad range of nursing duties and administrative issues pertaining directly to PACU care. Staff nurses should be expected to document periodic (annual) review of the policy book, and a mechanism should be in place that encourages staff nurse participation in ongoing policy revisions. Additionally, nursing staff should prove technical knowledge and skills annually. The Joint Commission on Accreditation of Healthcare Organizations made competency a factor beginning with the 1994 surveys. In the *2000–2001 JCAHO Manual*

Section HR.3 states "the competence of all staff members is continually assessed, maintained, demonstrated, and improved.

HR.3.1 The organization encourages staff self-development and learning.

HR.4 New staff orientation provides initial job training and information, and assesses capability to perform job responsibilities.

HR4.1 Ongoing in-service or other education and training maintain and improve staff competence.

HR.4.2 Ongoing data collection about staff competence patterns and trends is used to respond to staff learning needs.

HR.5 Staff members' abilities to fulfill expectations of their job descriptions are assessed."[7]

The staffing ratio in PACU should conform to national guidelines for safe postanesthesia nursing care. Nurse-to-patient ratios for phase I PACUs recommended by the American Society of Perianesthesia Nurses are listed in Table 20–2. In some ASCs, the phase II area is next to the PACU, and nursing personnel move between the areas as patient flow requires. In the rare facility where ambulatory surgery patients are discharged to home directly from the PACU, staffing patterns must consider the time required for patient needs. Tasks such as dressing into street clothes, ambulating, dispensing verbal and written instructions, securing a responsible adult to accompany the patient home, and transferring to awaiting transportation take additional time. The presence of several debilitated, elderly, or pediatric patients on the schedule also increases staffing needs.

TRANSFER OF THE PATIENT TO A POSTANESTHESIA CARE UNIT

Whether the patient has been cared for in the OR, radiology department, or special procedures unit, the nurse and all anesthesia personnel transporting the patient to the PACU should give complete reports to the PACU nurse.[5] Transporting teams should remain at the patient's bedside in the PACU until the postanesthesia nurse accepts responsibility for the patient. Reporting and ensuring the immediate safety of the patient after transfer should be a team effort by the transporting and receiv-

Table 20–2. Nurse-to-Patient Ratios (Postanesthesia Care Unit Phase I)

Class 1:2 One Nurse to Two Patients Who Are

a. One unconscious, stable without artificial airway and over the age of 9 years; and one conscious, stable and free of complications
b. Two conscious, stable and free of complications
b. Two conscious, stable, 11 years of age and under; with family or competent support staff present.

Class 1:1 One Nurse to One Patient

a. At time of admission, until the critical elements are met
b. Requiring mechanical life support and/or artificial airway
c. Any unconscious patient 9 years of age and under
d. A second nurse must be available to assist as necessary

Class 2:1 Two Nurses to One Patient

a. One critically ill, unstable, complicated patient:

Two licensed nurses, one of whom is an RN competent in phase I postanesthesia nursing, are present whenever a patient is recovering in phase I.

From American Society of PeriAnesthesia Nurses: Standards of Perianesthesia Nursing Practice. Thorofare, NJ: Published by Author, 1998, p 27.

ing personnel.[5] Particularly important are the airway and the respiratory adequacy of the anesthetized patient who has been moved from the OR table, special procedures room bed or table to the transporting stretcher.

The nurse and the anesthesia provider who accompanies the patient to the PACU should provide a comprehensive report as a baseline for the PACU nurse to begin comprehensive assessment and planning for care. The immediate postanesthesia period is a dangerous time for patients, who may experience such untoward complications as airway obstruction, respiratory depression, cardiac arrest, circulatory collapse, aspiration, hemorrhage, and renarcotization or reparalysis from inadequately reversed narcotics or muscle relaxants. Each patient deserves the transfer of complete information when care is being placed in the hands of a new provider. The patient's record should be consulted for information that is not provided in verbal reports.

Often, the PACU nurse is concurrently assessing the patient's vital functions while listening to reports. Anesthesia personnel and the OR nurse may attempt to provide information concurrently when both have pressing needs to return to their own practice areas for further cases. When the patient's condition is unstable (i.e., is unconscious, obtunded, dyspneic, or experiencing color changes), reports should wait until the accepting nurse completes the initial assessment of vital signs and airway patency. The patient is positioned, oxygen is applied, and the patient's immediate safety is ensured before or concurrently as the operative and anesthetic report is obtained.[5]

INITIAL PATIENT ASSESSMENT AND CARE PLANNING

Patients should have a complete systems assessment during the first few minutes of PACU care. Usually, a rapid initial appraisal is completed that focuses on vital functions, followed by a more thorough and comprehensive assessment. The 1998 Standards of Perianesthesia Nursing Practice, published by ASPAN, describe this assessment in detail. Subjective information regarding level of comfort and nausea from the awake patient is also solicited. The patient's alertness, lucidity, orientation, and motor abilities are assessed, with particular attention being paid to the return of sensory and motor control in areas affected by local or regional anesthetics.

With this information, the nurse can plan the appropriate care for the patient. The nature of the PACU period requires that the nursing plan be dynamic and frequently revised; minute-to-minute changes occur in the patient's level of consciousness, physiologic status, and comfort level. The postanesthesia nurse must be flexible and observant and must provide ongoing assessments and re-evaluations concurrently with nursing interventions.

Ongoing nursing assessment during the patient's dynamic and often rapid clinical changes requires the nurse to use highly developed, critical thinking skills to make frequent and essential judgements to differentiate between benign and ominous symptoms. Table 20–3 illustrates some of the differential diagnoses typical of the immediate postanesthesia period.

Sharing the patient's successful progress in the PACU can be a source of tremendous job satisfaction. A plan of nursing care must be dynamic, changing with the patient's usually rapid progress from dependency to a level of self-care that promotes discharge. This plan is formulated on the basis of the patient's history found in the medical record, the physical nurs-

Table 20–3. Differential Diagnoses of Postanesthesia Complications

Restlessness

Hypoxemia (↓ S_pO_2)
Pain
Hypotension
Bladder distention/urinary retention
Emotional response
Shivering/feeling of being cold
Hypercarbia (↑ CO_2)
Emergence delirium
GI distress/distention
Psychotropic effects of preoperative medications
↑ Intracranial pressure, intracranial event

Hypotension

Decreased preload
- Hypovolemia from prolonged fasting or inadequate fluid replacement
- Excessive urinary or third-space losses bleeding
- Peripheral vasodilation (↓ resistance); i.e., effects of major regional anesthesia

Effects of sedative and narcotic drugs
Decreased myocardial contractility
- Effects of anesthesia drugs
- Perioperative cardiac event, e.g., MI
- Pre-existing cardiac disease

Orthostatic effects of progressive ambulation

Hypertension

Pain, surgical stimulation
Hypoxemia (↓ SpO_2)
Bladder distention/urinary retention
Shivering, vasoconstriction due to hypothermia
Pre-existing disease, e.g., hyperthyroidism, essential hypertension, renal disease
Emergence delirium, emotional response
Hypercarbia (↑ CO_2)
Retching or vomiting
Fluid overload
Effects of medications, e.g., vasopressors, naloxone, ketamine, anticholinergics, cocaine, ephedrine, epinephrine

Dysrhythmias

Pain
Hypoxemia (↓ SpO_2)
Perioperative myocardial infarction
Catecholamine release
Metabolic changes, e.g., acidosis, alkalosis
Pre-existing disease
Hypercarbia (↑ CO_2)
Failure of artificial pacemaker
Side effects of perioperative medications
Electrolyte imbalance (potassium, calcium)

Tachycardia

Pain
Hypovolemia
Emergence delirium
Fever, e.g., malignant hyperthermia, sepsis
Hyperthyroidism
Effects of medications, e.g., atropine, glycopyrrolate

Bradycardia

Oculocardiac reflex
Stimulation of baroreceptors
Hypoventilation, especially in children
Cardiac effects of heavy athletic activity
Sedative, anesthetic drugs
Effects of medications, e.g., neostigmine, narcotics

Respiratory Depression

Inadequate airway
Splinting, secondary to pain
Pulmonary congestion
Positioning, especially in the obese
Prolonged neuromuscular blockade
Mechanical failure of equipment (ventilator, bag/valve/mask)
Pre-existing disease, COPD, reactive airway

SpO_2, oxygen saturation as measured by pulse oximetry; MI, myocardial infarction; COPD, chronic obstructive pulmonary disease; GI, gastrointestinal.

ing assessment, the reports of the intraoperative team, and the nurses' knowledge of nursing theory. A sample patient outcome grid for patients in PACU is found in Table 20–4.

As the patient progresses from a dependent state to an alert and ambulatory one, the nurse should combine appropriate instructions and emotional support with the physical aspects of care. Encouraging self-care when the patient is ready is indispensable to the ambulatory approach.

RESPIRATORY ADEQUACY

The patient who has received general anesthesia or a significant amount of sedation is in danger of respiratory inadequacy through many catalysts: airway obstruction and hypoventilation are the principal factors. Untreated, these mechanisms quickly lead to hypoxemia and ultimately to decreased tissue perfusion and inadequate cellular oxygenation. Patients at particular risk are the elderly, obese, or pregnant; those with pre-existing lung disease; and cigarette smokers.[1]

On admission to the PACU, the patient should have an immediate auscultation of breath sounds and assessment of chest expansion, ease and depth of respirations, use of accessory muscles, skin and mucous membrane color, and oxygen saturation level. Lack of chest movement or presence of paradoxical movement, or rocking between the thorax and chest without effective respiratory effort, are causes for aggressive intervention to reestablish a patent airway.

The alveoli are vesicles or sacs, and the normal breath sounds heard over them are soft, with a low pitch and a breezy characteristic. Total absence of breath sounds in the airways or lungs suggests apnea or complete airway obstruction. Stridor, wheezing, coughing, crowing, or other adventitious sounds can suggest partial obstruction, bronchospasm, or laryngospasm. Crackles or rhonchi indicate the presence of secretions and some degree of pulmonary congestion.[8] The nurse also auscultates the tracheal area to listen for unobstructed upper airway sounds. Normal tracheobronchial sounds are hollow sounding, high pitched, and loud.

Administration of oxygen is often considered standard practice after general anesthesia or heavy sedation and should be instituted as ordered on the patient's arrival in the PACU.[9] Respiratory problems occur with some frequency in the PACU, especially because general anesthesia agents and narcotics affect the respiratory system. Oxygen therapy is particularly important in the early minutes after inhalation anesthesia that has included a large proportion of nitrous oxide because of a phenomenon called "diffusion hypoxia." Nitrous oxide diffuses out of capillary blood into the alveoli very rapidly, inundating the alveoli and diluting the existing oxygen. Because the amount of nitrous oxide mixed with other inhalation agents is generally small and because hypoventilation is aggressively identified and treated, this occurrence is not as common as it may have been in the past.[10] Many anesthesia providers now do not advocate oxygen therapy for all patients; rather they use the oxygen saturation level and clinical status as determinants of the need for supplemental oxygen.

Shivering can increase the body's oxygen demand and consumption by 400% or more.[11] Thus, supplemental oxygen is continued to offset the increased demand until the patient is no longer shivering. This is particularly important for the patient with compromised cardiorespiratory reserves for whom an increased O_2 demand could result in acute myocardial ischemia or other sequelae. Patients with ischemic brain or kidney disease are also at particular risk.

Other factors besides shivering contribute to altered myocardial oxygen supply and demand. They include pain, hypoxia, hypercarbia, anxiety, hypotension, hypertension, rapid fluctuations in intravascular volume, intubation, dysrhythmias (especially tachydysrhythmias), hyperthermia, hypothermia, thromboembolic events, left ventricular failure, and catecholamine release.[7, 12]

Monitoring Equipment

In monitoring a patient's respiratory status, the nurse's eyes and ears are primary assessment tools. Armed with a stethoscope and astute powers of observation, the nurse uses auscultation, palpation, and observation to assess the gross parameters of ventilation. Modern technology has provided sensitive equipment that is extremely useful in assessing the finer parameters of respiratory adequacy. A respirometer is used to detect lung volumes (e.g., tidal volume, vital capacity). Most ambulatory surgery patients awaken from general anesthesia rapidly and do not remain intubated into the PACU period. In rare instances, uncertainty about muscle strength and ventilatory capacity requires continued intubation or the close assessment that a respirometer can provide.

Blood gas analysis provides valuable information but requires an invasive, and often painful, arterial puncture for obtaining a blood specimen. It is also time consuming when the patient's respiratory status needs immediate evaluation. Average arterial blood gas parameters considered normal for a normothermic patient breathing room air are

pH	7.35–7.45
PCO_2	35–45 mm Hg
HCO_3	22–26 mEq/L
PO_2	80–100 mm Hg
Base excess	0 ± 2

A pH below 7.20 or above 7.60 is rarely compatible with life.

Pulse oximetry is a noninvasive method for detecting the oxygen saturation or hemoglobin in the blood. It is particularly sensitive to changes in blood oxygen content and can herald a hypoxic event well before clinical signs appear. Oximetry is considered a standard of care monitoring tool in anesthesia and PACU settings.[13] Oximetry's main advantages include its simplicity and its noninvasiveness. Provision of a continuous display, sensitivity to changes in blood oxygen levels, ability to be applied to all ages, and comparatively low expense when compared with its value in preventing major hypoxic events are other advantages. Oximetry is continued for a time after discontinuation of oxygen therapy to assess the patient's response.

Oximetry measures the ratio of oxygenated hemoglobin to the total amount of hemoglobin and expresses it as a percent of saturation. A very simple explanation of its mechanism is that it analyzes the color of the blood with two light-emitting diodes (one red, one infrared) and a photodetector. Various wavelengths of light are detected with a sensor and are analyzed after they pass through a pulsating arterial bed in the patient's finger, hand, foot, earlobe, or nose; newer models allow for sensors to be placed on the forehead by use of a sweatband to maintain position. The oximeter then calculates the oxygen saturation of hemoglobin based on the light waves by use of Beer's Law.[13]

A 95% to 100% saturation is considered normal in an adult who is breathing room air. Pulse oximetry readings in the 70% to 100% range are considered to be accurate when compared with arterial blood samples. Many factors can interfere with the reliability of data obtained from an oximetry unit: motion at the sensor site, low perfusion of the arterial bed monitored (hypothermia, hypotension, large doses of vasopressors), significant dysrhythmias, carbon monoxide or methemoglobin in the blood, severe anemia with a hemoglobin level below 5 g/dl, venous pulsation (e.g., when the sensor is applied too tightly), interference from ambient or extrinsic light sources, electrical interference, and circulating intravenous dyes. When difficulty is experienced in obtaining a reading or when the accuracy of the reading is in question, moving the sensor to another digit or another part of the body may help solve the problem.[13]

Complications of pulse oximetry are rare but should be mentioned. Blisters and burns may occur on infants as a result of short circuits when a probe from one manufacturer is used with a base unit from another manufacturer. Pressure necrosis has occurred from the spring-clip finger probes.[13]

The relationship of hemoglobin oxygen saturation (SpO_2) to the partial pressure of oxygen in the blood (PaO_2), which is determined by arterial blood sampling, is represented graphically by the oxyhemoglobin dissociation cure illustrated in Figure 20–1. The values of PaO_2 and SpO_2 are not interchangeable. At a normal pH of 7.4, the following approximate relationships exist in the adult with a normal range of hemoglobin:

SpO_2 (%)	**PaO_2 (mm Hg)**
91	60
93	65
94	70
96	80
97	90–100
98	120

Cyanosis is a late sign of hypoxia; it requires an absolute value of 5 g/dl of reduced hemoglobin (hemoglobin without oxygen) before becoming visually apparent. This usually relates to a PaO_2 of 40 mm Hg and an SpO_2 of only 75% or lower if the patient is anemic.[13] The advantages of an oximeter as an early warning mechanism are obvious when one considers the significant level of hypoxia that is necessary to produce clinically apparent cyanosis.

Capnography involves the monitoring of exhaled carbon dioxide, or end-tidal CO_2. It has become the state-of-the-art technique for intraoperative monitoring of patients under general anesthesia and is being used more frequently for PACU patients, especially with the availability of single-patient-use capnography monitors. Generally, PACU use of capnography is confined to critically ill patients and is not often applicable to the ambulatory surgery population.[1]

Table 20–4. Patient Outcome Grid: Postanesthesia Care Unit

POTENTIAL AND ACTUAL PROBLEMS/NURSING DIAGNOSIS	OUTCOME GOALS: THE PATIENT WILL BE ABLE TO	NURSING INTERVENTIONS KNOWLEDGE BASE	RESOURCES
Ineffective airway clearance Potential for aspiration Ineffective breathing patterns, respiratory depression R/T Sedation Anesthesia Positioning Pain Increased respiratory secretions Vomiting	Maintain normal respiratory parameters (rate, depth, ease, clarity of breath sounds) Maintain clear airway Avoid aspiration Maintain adequate oxygenation of tissues Avoid symptoms of hypoxia Perform effective cough and deep breathing exercises	Knowledge of effects of anesthetics, analgesics, sedatives, and muscle relaxants and associated drug interactions Airway maintenance techniques, including suctioning Bag-valve-mask resuscitative techniques Apply stir-up regimen Administer oxygen per protocol Continuous assessment of respiratory status Timely report of untoward symptoms to anesthesiologist/surgeon Provide adequate hydration and safe positioning Identify pre-existing respiratory disease and individualize care appropriately	Physiologic monitoring equipment at each bedside Adequate staffing patterns to ensure proper nurse-to-patient ratio Immediate access to anesthesia provider Comprehensive anesthesia report before transfer of patient *ASPAN Standards of Perianesthesia Nursing Practice* Facility policies regarding interventions for cardiovascular/respiratory problems Oxygen and suction at each bedside Immediate access to emergency equipment Crash cart Resuscitator bag Ventilator Airway maintenance supplies Drugs
Potential alteration in tissue perfusion Cardiovascular instability	Maintain normal cardiovascular parameters, avoiding hypertension and hypotension Demonstrate expected postoperative arousal and mental status Demonstrate normal parameters of peripheral circulation	Assess all parameters of vital signs in ongoing fashion, including heart rate and rhythm, BP Assess mental status and progression Check peripheral pulses, color, and sensory adequacy in ongoing fashion Timely report of untoward symptoms to anesthesiologist/surgeon Maintain adequate fluid balance and hydration	
Altered skin integrity R/T surgical wound Potential for infection at surgical site	Experience appropriate and uncomplicated wound healing	Use aseptic technique Enhance circulation of surgical wound site Maintain adequate hydration Avoid constricting bandages at surgical site Assess surgical site throughout PACU stay	Standard precautions Personal protective equipment and sterile dressing supplies Intravenous fluids Antibiotics, if ordered

Altered skin integrity R/T pressure points, positioning	Avoid skin breakdown R/T pressure, tape, constricting bandages	Position patient using appropriate padding to avoid pressure points Encourage stir-up regimen Assess skin around tape for reaction—report to physician and/or change tape if necessary Avoid constricting bandages in PACU Assess full body throughout PACU stay	Frequent position changes, assessment of skin Nonallergic tape Padding, pillows, foam, and so on, for padding
Anxiety R/T unfamiliar surroundings, isolation from family or responsible adult, potential diagnosis or surgical outcome	Express reduced anxiety Display calm demeanor Verbalize needs R/T family, emotional support Maintain CV and R parameters within normal limits	Block sights and sounds of other areas of PACU whenever possible Encourage/allow family or RA presence in PACU Provide emotional support and answers to patient questions within boundaries of nursing	Policy allowing families/responsible adult to visit in PACU Cubicle curtains to reduce view of PACU Separation of ambulatory and critical care patients in PACU
Altered thought processes and/or memory loss R/T sedation/anesthesia	Display/verbalize appropriate orientation to surroundings and situations Avoid self-injury R/T altered thought patterns Rely on RA who understands nature of patient's temporarily altered thought patterns and responsibility for patient care	Provide frequent affirmations of orientation to time, place, and events Assess patient's orientation Monitor and oversee patient care while patient is vulnerable to environment	Pharmaceutical literature outlining effects of anesthesia and sedative medications Predetermined PACU discharge criteria that includes assessment of mental status *ASPAN Standards of Perianesthesia Nursing Practice*
Alterations in comfort: pain	Express acceptable comfort level Maintain normal CV and R parameters	Administer appropriate analgesics Position patient for comfort Apply cold therapy as ordered Provide positive reinforcements and encourage philosophy of wellness throughout process Encourage appropriate pace for increased activities	Physician's orders for analgesics Analgesic medications Knowledge of nursing interventions for comfort Positioning and support of body areas Breathing exercises Positive reinforcement of comfort
Alterations in comfort: nausea and vomiting	Express acceptable comfort level Avoid vomiting and retching	Encourage appropriate pace for oral intake of fluids Administer antiemetics as needed Provide positive reinforcement and encourage philosophy of wellness throughout process	Physician's orders/prescriptions for antiemetics Intravenous fluids Literature R/T reducing GI symptoms Appropriate food and beverages—avoid acid-producing juices, spicy, or difficult-to-digest foods

Table continued on following page

Table 20–4. Patient Outcome Grid: Postanesthesia Care Unit *Continued*

POTENTIAL AND ACTUAL PROBLEMS/NURSING DIAGNOSIS	OUTCOME GOALS: THE PATIENT WILL BE ABLE TO	NURSING INTERVENTIONS KNOWLEDGE BASE	RESOURCES
Self-care deficit	Display sufficient level of alertness and self-care for safe discharge to phase II PACU	Provide comprehensive nursing care modified to patient's abilities Assess patient for ability to turn, move, sit up, and call for assistance before transfer	PACU discharge criteria
Actual or perceived, loss of privacy or dignity	Express content at level of privacy provided Maintain dignity and sense of self-esteem	Support patient's right to privacy and dignity Promote unit philosophy that demands support of patient's right to privacy Explain and demonstrate to patient before surgery that privacy and dignity will not be invaded while patient is asleep or sedated Provide privacy Curtains Blankets Clothing that covers the patient Allow patient as much decision-making as is possible in the PACU setting	Surroundings that are friendly, family focused, private, and apart from view of other patients or staff Patient bill of rights Patient linens that provide adequate cover Cubicle curtains
Risk of hemorrhage	Maintain blood volume at normal level Avoid hypertension	Ensure availability of intravenous solutions Observe surgical site for signs of bleeding and report to physician Administer anxiolytic and/or antihypertensive medications as ordered	Blood bank contract and policies for rapid availability of blood products Antihypertensive agents Anxiolytic medications
Alterations in health that can complicate the postanesthesia course	Provide preoperative information about any medical factors present Have complied with instructions to optimize medical status before day of surgery Experience no complications R/T prior medical status	Encourage patient to provide accurate information regarding health status and practices before surgery Assess patient's physical status frequently Use active listening and observe for clues to patient's health status Review record and receive comprehensive report from anesthesia provider Individualize patient care R/T prior health status	Structured preoperative time frame for physical and historical assessment Books and literature on patient assessment and various medical conditions Primary care physician available to assist in optimizing patient health status before and after surgery

Risk of injury R/T environment, equipment, positioning, medications, emergence delirium	Remain free from allergic reactions, burns, skin breakdown or pressure points, falls, or nerve or joint injuries Complete PACU course without complications or injury	Position patient according to acceptable standards of care and individual needs using proper body mechanics for staff and patients Ensure that side rail remains in up position Lock stretcher while patient is on it and during transfers Observe patient at all times Keep only current patient's chart at bedside Check emergency call bell system and emergency equipment periodically Reinforce patient's orientation to time and place Identify symptoms of emergence delirium and appropriate actions, interventions	Patient record Competency-based nursing practice *ASPAN Standards of Perianesthesia Nursing Practice* Manufacturers' instructions for proper use of equipment Appropriate positioning supplies Pillows Padding Foam sheeting Ongoing program of preventive maintenance of equipment Policy on enacting Safe Medical Devices Act Gentle restraint policy
Hypothermia Discomfort R/T cold	Maintain normal body temperature Verbalize comfort with temperature Avoid shivering	Assess and document patient temperature on admission and periodically in PACU Keep patient covered as fully as possible, including head and neck areas Apply warm blankets or warm forced air warming equipment, especially on patients at high risk for hypothermia (infants, frail elderly)	*ASPAN Standards of Perianesthesia Nursing Practice* Warming cabinets with blankets and solutions Forced warm air heating blankets Thermometer
Discomfort R/T thirst	Express comfort	Nursing interventions to moisten mouth Water or ice orally as soon as possible postoperatively	Policy that encourages appropriate early interventions for thirst

CV, cardiovascular; R, respiratory; R/T, related to; PRN, as needed; PACU, postanesthesia care unit; GI, gastrointestinal; BP, blood pressure; ASPAN, American Society of Perianesthesia Nurses.

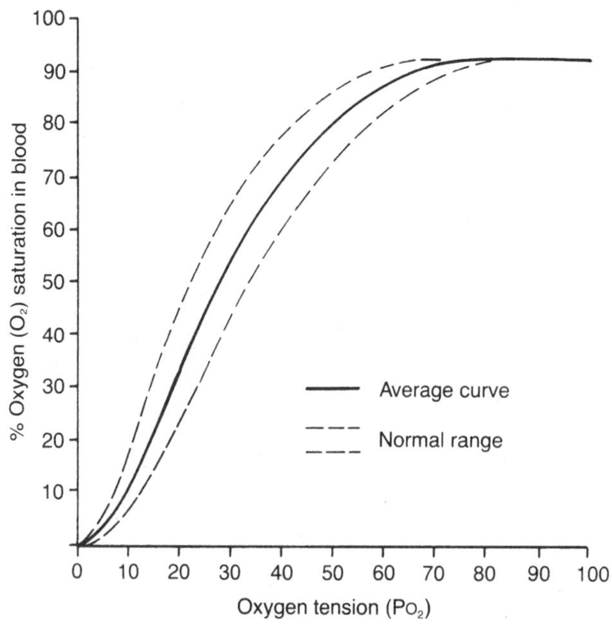

Figure 20–1. Oxyhemoglobin dissociation curve. This curve represents the relationship between the partial pressure of oxygen (Po_2) in the blood and the saturation of hemoglobin with oxygen (O_2). The relationship is shown as an S-shaped curve. At higher Po_2 tensions (above 90 mm Hg), the curve flattens, and the percentage of oxygen saturation does not rise as steeply. The flat portion of the curve is advantageous to the lung because despite significant decreases in the alveolar Po_2, the hemoglobin circulating through the pulmonary capillaries is almost saturated to full capacity with oxygen. The body's tissues benefit from the steep portion of the curve. As even a small decrease in the oxygen tension occurs, oxygen is rapidly released to the tissues by the hemoglobin. This is illustrated by the way that the curve drops off quickly as the saturation curve reflects the lower saturation of hemoglobin. The oxyhemoglobin saturation curve shifts upward to the left when conditions occur that cause oxygen and hemoglobin to bind more tightly, so that less oxygen is actually released to the tissues. The curve shifts down and to the right when conditions occur that cause hemoglobin to be released more readily to the tissues. (From Luckmann J, Sorensen K: Medical-Surgical Nursing: A Psychophysiologic Approach, 3rd ed. Philadelphia: WB Saunders, 1987, p 659.)

Airway Obstruction

Airway obstruction in an unconscious postanesthesia patient is generally the result of soft tissue displacement in the upper airway and mouth. The tongue is the most obvious and frequent offender, and its displacement against the posterior pharynx can generally be remedied by one or more of the following interventions: turning of the patient to the side, mandibular extension or jaw thrust (forward displacement of the jaw), insertion of an artificial nasal or oral airway, gentle backward tilt of the head, or, in persistent cases, manual tongue extension by use of a piece of gauze to grip the tongue. Sometimes, removing the pillow from under the head or placing a small towel roll under the shoulders provides enough neck extension to clear the airway (Fig. 20–2).

Lateral positioning is considered safest for prevention of aspiration if an unconscious or semiconscious patient vomits. Whenever an unconscious patient is moved or repositioned, the nurse must re-evaluate the patency and adequacy of the airway. Oxygen should be instituted when a general anesthesia patient arrives in the PACU. Gentle suctioning is indicated if secretions or blood is obstructing the airway or is copious in the mouth. Care should be taken not to irritate the posterior pharynx or trachea with deep suctioning unless absolutely necessary because coughing, gagging, or laryngospasm could result. If these interventions do not immediately improve or re-establish diminished or absent respiration, further assessment and alternative treatments are warranted.

Laryngospasm may be the cause of airway obstruction and resulting respiratory distress. Laryngospasm occurs when the muscles of the larynx contract and cause reflex closing of the vocal cords as a protective mechanism against foreign material entering the larynx and trachea. Symptoms include dyspnea, hypoxemia, hypercarbia, use of accessory muscles of respiration, suprasternal retraction, and either absent or crowing breath sounds.[8] The awake patient becomes agitated, anxious, and panicky.

Laryngospasm is often due to irritation of the

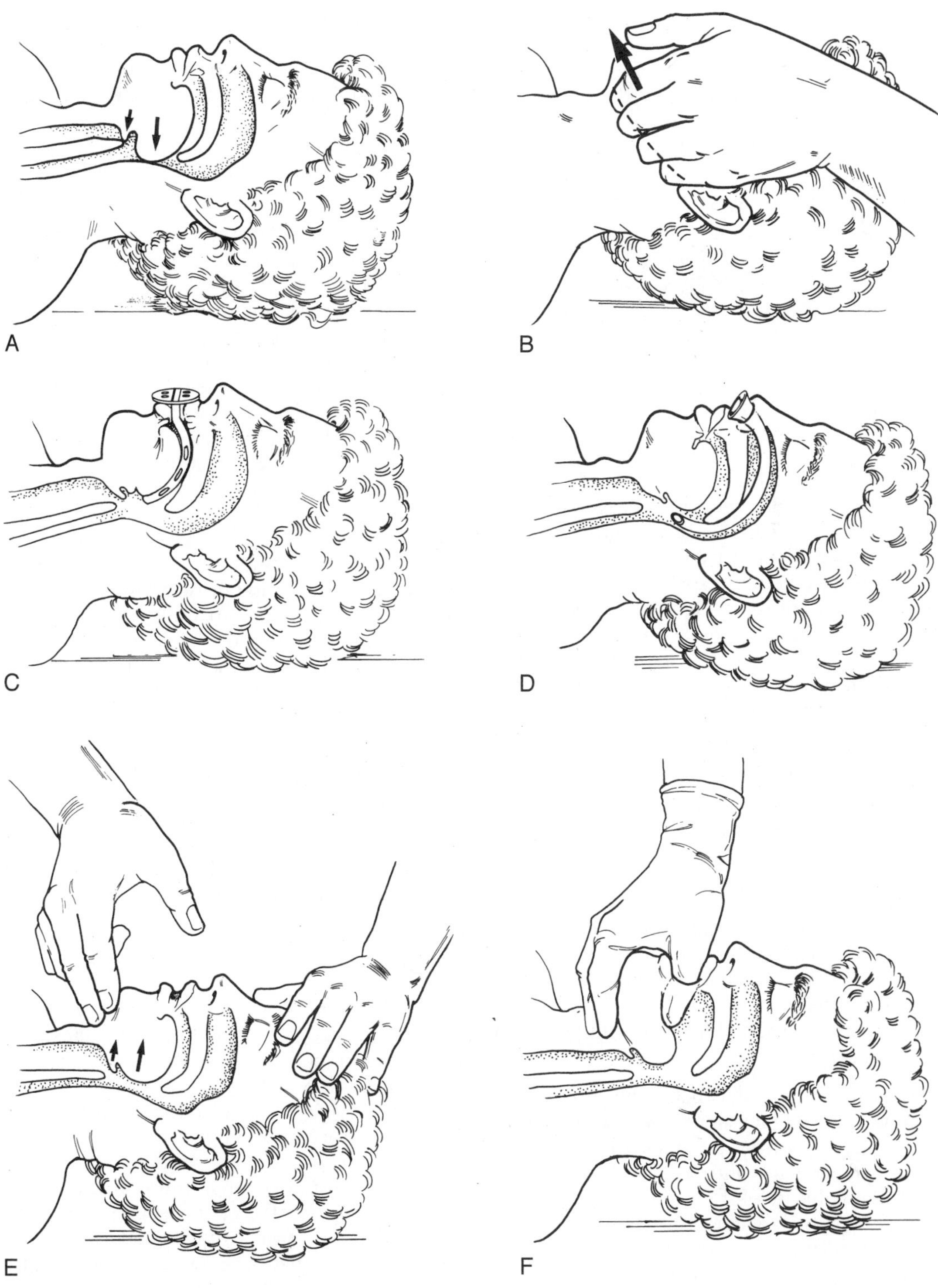

Figure 20–2. Maintaining the patent airway. *A*, Obstructed airway (the tongue against the pharynx); *B*, Manual jaw extension/jaw thrust (anterior displacement); *C*, Insertion of oral airway; *D*, Insertion of a nasal airway; *E*, Head tilt; *F*, Manual tongue extension.

Illustration continued on following page

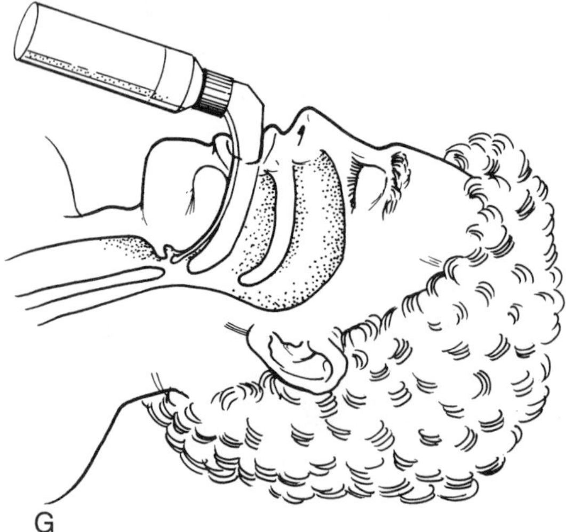

Figure 20–2 *Continued. G,* Intubation.

pharynx or larynx during the initial, or "twilight," period of emergence or during a light plane of anesthesia. Irritation also can come from airway secretions, artificial oral or nasal airways, blood, other foreign matter, or instrumentation in the airway.

Artificial oral or nasal airways in awakening patients may cause gagging or coughing. Removing or partially withdrawing them may eliminate the source of pharyngeal irritation and prevent laryngospasm. Other preventive maneuvers include

1. Extubating patients either while they are still deeply anesthetized or after they are completely awake and protective reflexes have returned
2. Reducing environmental stimuli for patients who are coughing or exhibiting signs of laryngeal irritation while emerging from general anesthesia
3. Administering humidified oxygen to moisten the upper airway

Some practitioners advocate the intravenous administration of lidocaine before extubation to prevent laryngospasm, although the usefulness of the practice is controversial. It is usually given in a bolus dose of 50 to 100 mg IV.[14]

Treatment of laryngospasm should be instituted immediately. The aggressiveness of intervention is based on the extent of the spasm and the patient's respiratory distress level. The nurse should

1. Summon anesthesia help
2. Remove any obvious irritant
3. Gently suction the mouth and upper airway, if indicated
4. Extend the neck; maintain anterior displacement of the mandible
5. Avoid unnecessary movement of the patient's head and neck to reduce stimulation of an already irritated airway
6. Administer humidified oxygen
7. Display a calm demeanor for the benefit of the semiconscious or awake patient

An awake patient experiencing a laryngospasm is usually terrified because of the inability to take a breath. Hearing calm and confident nurses and physicians who explain that breathing will rapidly improve and that the patient will not be left alone for any reason is especially helpful for an aware patient.[12] Even seemingly unconscious patients may be aware and can benefit from verbal reassurances.

Partial laryngospasm is usually self-limiting if it is treated in this manner, but for persistent or total laryngospasm, more aggressive interventions must be instituted. These include 100% oxygen under pressure (bag-valve-mask) and sometimes IV sedation or reparalysis with succinylcholine (Anectine) (0.5 mg/kg IV) by the anesthesiologist. Rarely, reintubation is necessary. A small dose of atropine may be given IV to decrease upper respiratory secretions that could cause further irritation.[11]

In the rare event that these measures do not provide a patent airway, the anesthesiologist should be prepared to use an alternate airway. A cricothyrotomy may be necessary until a surgeon is available to perform a tracheotomy. Equipment should be available in the PACU for such an emergency.

Aspiration

Although rare, aspiration is a dreaded and usually preventable complication of anesthesia. It can result in airway obstruction if the aspirate consists of large particles, or it can cause hypoventilation as a result of chemical irritation of the respiratory tract. Hypoxemia is the earliest and most consistent symptom of aspiration.[15] The postanesthesia nurse must maintain constant awareness of each patient's potential for aspiration and must institute practices that decrease or eliminate the opportunities for this to occur.

A full stomach increases the possibility of aspiration, however, critics consider lengthy preoperative fasting a ritual that causes anxiety, dehydration, and nausea and vomiting and believe that overnight fasting does not guarantee an empty stomach.[15] Newer studies have shown that clear liquids ingested up to 2 hours before elective surgery do not increase the risk of aspiration in healthy patients. Some surgical centers have adopted the following guidelines for healthy patients:

1. No solid food on the day of surgery
2. Unrestricted clear fluids up to 2 to 3 hours before surgery
3. Oral medications with 30 ml of water up to 1 hour before surgery
4. A histamine$_2$-receptor antagonist with clear liquids[15]

Other predisposing factors for aspiration include obesity, hiatal hernia, pregnancy, and nausea and vomiting in a semiconscious or unconscious patient. Presence of a nasogastric tube, a deflated or incompetent cuff on an endotracheal tube, and recent ingestion of alcohol, which slows the emptying time of the stomach, are also factors.

Prevention of aspiration is much preferred over treatment. Preventive measures should begin before admission, and careful instructions regarding the NPO restrictions and the avoidance of alcohol on the night before surgery should be provided. On the day of surgery, preventive measures may include preoperative administration of histamine antagonists, histamine$_2$-receptor antagonists and antacids, lateral positioning of unconscious patients, antiemetic therapy, and constant surveillance. Of the histamine$_2$-receptor antagonist therapy used, cimetidine at bedtime and a combination of cimetidine and metoclopramide the morning of surgery seemed most beneficial.[15] Intubated patients should have the endotracheal tube cuffs inflated until the time of extubation so that blatant or insidious aspiration of stomach contents does not occur around the tracheal cuff. The patient under general anesthesia who is not intubated is at risk for a "silent aspiration," or passive regurgitation of stomach contents, which can result in aspiration pneumonia or Mendelson's syndrome.

Symptoms vary depending on the extent of the aspiration. Clinical symptoms of mild aspiration include dyspnea, cyanosis of varying degrees, tachycardia, and abnormal lung sounds. Aspiration of large amounts of stomach secretions can result in immediate bronchospasm, hypoxemia, and respiratory or cardiac arrest.[11]

Treatment of aspiration depends on the severity of symptoms and the amount and pH of the aspirant. As little as 25 ml of aspirant can cause significant pulmonary involvement, and a pH of 2.5 and a volume of 0.4 ml/kg are considered the critical point of acidity that causes serious lung damage.[15] Oxygen should be administered immediately, and the physician should be notified.

Obvious aspiration secondary to vomiting should be aggressively addressed by lowering the head of the bed, laterally positioning the patient, administering oxygen, and suctioning the airway as needed. Reintubation may be required, along with administration of steroids and antibiotics. Chest radiography may be ordered to confirm the aspiration or to identify its extent; however, positive findings are absent in up to 10% of aspiration patients.[15] The patient is hospitalized for continued treatment after clinically significant aspiration.

Pulmonary Edema

Pulmonary edema is rare in the ambulatory PACU, but the potential remains. Some predisposing factors include laryngospasm, narcotics, administration of naloxone as a narcotic reversal agent, intravenous fluid overload, allergic reactions, pulmonary embolism, and of course, preexisting congestive heart failure.

Despite the cause (cardiogenic or noncardiogenic), pulmonary edema (PE) has common symptoms, including tachycardia, dyspnea, tachypnea, confusion, wheezing, and rales or crackles on auscultation. Noncardiogenic pulmonary edema is also called negative-pressure pulmonary edema. Signs specific for noncardiogenic pulmonary edema include normal blood pressure, decreased lung compliance, normal heart size, and no signs of cardiac failure on chest radiograph. In comparison, cardiogenic pulmonary edema presentation includes decrease in blood pressure, paroxysmal nocturnal dyspnea, cardiomegaly and upper lobe pulmonary veins on chest radiography, and increased jugular vein distention.[16]

Treatment of pulmonary edema is aimed at reducing the workload of the heart, reducing hypoxemia, and removing fluids through diuresis to reduce venous congestion. The nurse should place the patient in an upright position to aid respiratory effort, administer oxygen, suction the airway appropriately, and closely monitor the patient's vital signs during treatment. A more detailed discussion of pulmonary edema and its treatment is found in Chapter 11.

Hypoventilation

Hypoventilation may result from airway obstruction or from other causes. Residual effects of anesthetic agents, muscle relaxants, and analgesics are often the cause. Occasionally, a patient in pain may be splinting a wound to avoid painful expansion of the chest or abdomen so much that it interferes with respiratory effort. The latter scenario usually occurs in patients with extensive chest or upper abdominal wounds rather than in patients having ambulatory surgical procedures.

Immediate ventilatory support should be instituted for the patient with shallow or absent breathing. Intervention may be simply to administer oxygen and remind the patient to breathe deeply until the effects of sedation have lifted. Elevating the patient's head slightly may help to encourage chest movement, particularly for the patient who is obese or has pre-existing respiratory compromise. Raising the patient's head must be tempered in relation to the patient's cardiovascular stability.

The usual postanesthesia "stir-up" regimen of deep breathing, coughing, turning from side to side, and exercising the extremities is undertaken at least every 10 to 15 minutes to encourage respiratory effort and to increase circulation, and alertness. Left undisturbed, the postanesthesia patient doing the stir-up regimen even once may fall back into an obtunded or depressed state.

The patient who is apneic or exhibits signs of hypoxia requires aggressive ventilatory assistance to prevent cardiovascular and neurologic sequelae. Those signs, which may be masked by the effects of general anesthesia, can be any of the following: lethargy, confusion, restlessness, anxiety, dysrhythmias, cyanosis, decreased PaO_2, hypertension followed by hypotension, and decreased urinary output. Respiratory acidosis may follow if the situation is not corrected. Representative blood gas parameters and treatments for acidosis and alkalosis are presented in Table 20–5.

The specific treatment of anesthesia-related hypoventilation depends on the pharmacologic cause. Narcotics, muscle relaxants, inhalation agents, and other sedating drugs all have the potential to depress respirations. Other drugs are implicated as well, when they potentiate the effects of these agents.

Narcotic depression may be treated with an intravenous narcotic antagonist, such as naloxone (Narcan) in a dose of 0.4 to 2 mg IV, repeated every 5 to 10 minutes until ventilatory adequacy has been established.[10] Side effects of naloxone therapy include cessation of analgesia, agitation, hypertension, noncardiogenic pulmonary edema, atrial and ventricular dysrhythmias, and cardiac arrest.[10] These untoward effects can be diminished by administering small, incremental doses until desired effects have been reached. Slow injection is found to reduce the nausea and vomiting that sometimes follow a rapid bolus. Naloxone's 35- to 45-minute duration of action may be shorter than that of the original narcotic administered; thus, the patient should be observed for potential renarcotization for at least 1 hour after being given naloxone.

The phenomenon called negative-pressure pulmonary edema, which can occur after naloxone therapy or laryngospasm, even in the young, healthy patient, is uncommon. Its occurrence is particularly unexpected in an ambulatory surgery center (ASC), healthy patient population. Negative-pressure pulmonary edema is treated in much the same manner as pulmonary edema of cardiogenic origin, including administering oxygen, elevating the head, lowering the legs to a dependent level, and administering narcotic sedation, diuretics, and supportive care. Digoxin and steroids are not suggested in the treatment protocol.[16] The ambulatory surgical patient who experiences negative-pressure pulmonary edema requires overnight admission and observation.

Muscle relaxants may be implicated in postanesthetic hypoventilation. Succinylcholine, a depolarizing muscle relaxant, is a short-acting drug. It is rapidly metabolized in the plasma and is not pharmacologically reversed. Its action at the neuromuscular junction is self-limiting, so its effects usually dissipate from the body before the patient's admission to PACU. If large enough amounts of succinylcholine have been administered to cause what is called a phase II block, the effects can mimic the characteristics of nondepolarizing blockade and require pharmacologic reversal. This situation is uncommon, and succinylcholine is not considered to be a usual cause of postanesthesia respiratory depression.

One exception is the patient with a deficiency of normal plasma pseudocholinesterase, the agent that is responsible for the metabolism of succinylcholine. This deficiency may be genetic, secondary to chronic renal or hepatic disease, or the result of prolonged exposure to certain chemicals, such as organophosphate, which is found in pesticides, and echothiophate (Phospholine Iodide), which is used to treat glaucoma.[17]

The nurse should consider a diagnosis of pseudocholinesterase deficiency when a patient is admitted to PACU with hypoventilation and muscle weakness after receiving succinylcholine.

Table 20–5. **Acute, Uncompensated Acidosis and Alkalosis; ABG Parameters and Treatments (N = Normal)**

	pH	P_{CO2}	H_{CO3}	BASE EXCESS	CAUSES/TREATMENT
Respiratory acidosis	↓	↑	N	N	Causes: hypoventilation Treatment: improve ventilation Stimulate breathing Reversal agents Elevate head of bed Oxygen
Respiratory alkalosis	↑	↓	N	N	Causes: hyperventilation—may be due to pain, anxiety Overstimulation of the brain's respiratory center Treatment: oxygen, if hyperventilation due to hypoxia Sedate or provide analgesia Encourage slow, easy breathing
Metabolic acidosis	↓	N	↓	↓	Causes: excessive loss of NaH_{CO_3}, diabetes mellitus, hyperthyroidism infections with high fevers, renal diseases, loss of alkali—diarrhea Treatment: encourage deep breathing Monitor electrolytes Na bicarbonate, insulin Avoid overcorrection, which may be difficult to treat
Metabolic alkalosis	↑	N	↑	↑	Causes: excessive upper GI losses without adequate electrolyte replacement Treatment: maintain fluid and electrolyte balance Treat vomiting/diarrhea Avoid further GI irritation Support compensatory respiratory pattern

N, normal; GI, gastrointestinal.

Treatment is symptomatic, with ventilatory support until other modes of metabolic drug elimination from the body occur. The patient is typically frightened by this respiratory difficulty and needs special emotional support and often sedation. The waiting family should be informed of the reason for any extended PACU stay and should be provided with other appropriate information and support to help reduce their anxiety.

Later, when the patient is lucid and conversant, the anesthesiologist usually discusses the occurrence with the patient and family. The nurse should reinforce the need for the patient to discuss any enzyme deficiency or variance with the anesthesiologist before any future anesthetic is administered. Appropriate information should be written for the patient's later reference.

Definitive diagnosis is possible through blood testing. The test that is frequently performed to identify atypical pseudocholinesterase is the dibucaine number test. It has been found that genetically normal pseudocholinesterase responds to the local anesthetic dibucaine differently than does atypical pseudocholinesterase. A normal dibucaine number of 80 reflects the fact that dibucaine inhibits the normal enzyme by 80%. A low dibucaine number of approximately 20 is seen in patients with an atypical enzyme because dibucaine inhibits only 20% of it. This value does not reflect the amount of pseudocholinesterase present but reflects the quality of the enzyme. Thus, a patient may have a normal level of pseudocholinesterase but prolonged response to succinylcholine because much of the pseudocholinesterase is atypical.[17]

Nondepolarizing agents are the muscle relaxants that are most frequently implicated in respiratory depression caused by muscle weakness or reparalysis. Inadequate pharmacologic reversal of these drugs can result in return of muscle weakness in the PACU if the effects of the muscle relaxant extend beyond the effects of the reversal agent. This is called *reparalysis* or *recurarization.* Other factors besides inadequate amounts of reversal agents may cause prolonged muscle paralysis or make it difficult to reverse. These potentiators include

- General anesthetics
- Hypothermia
- Antidysrhythmics, such as quinidine, procainamide, and calcium channel blockers
- Respiratory acidosis or metabolic alkalosis, hypokalemia or hypocalcemia
- Local anesthetics, including lidocaine given as an antidysrhythmic by IV drip or bolus postoperatively
- Intravenous furosemide when given in doses of 1 mg/kg
- Dehydration
- Hyponatremia
- Antibiotics, particularly mycins and aminoglycosides (especially in patients with renal disease).

The aminoglycosides (e.g., neomycin, tobramycin, gentamicin, kanamycin, streptomycin, netilmicin, and amikacin) are associated with an inherent property that can cause neuromuscular blockade in rare instances.[1] It is essential that the nurse be aware of the increased potential for reparalysis if any of these potentiators is in effect in the immediate postanesthesia period.

Many types of ambulatory surgical procedures do not call for prolonged or extensive muscle paralysis with nondepolarizing agents. However patients who have received muscle relaxants, such as *d*-tubocurarine, gallamine (Flaxedil), pancuronium (Pavulon), atracurium (Tracrium), and metocurine (Metubine) must be considered at risk for reparalysis and should be observed closely in the immediate postanesthesia period.

Reversal of the effects of curare and similar drugs is accomplished with the administration of an anticholinesterase, such as neostigmine (Prostigmin), pyridostigmine (Mestinon), and edrophonium (Tensilon). Because of the vagal (muscarinic) effects of these reversal agents, severe bradycardia could accompany their administration. This undesirable effect is avoided by concurrently administering a vagolytic drug, such as atropine or glycopyrrolate (Robinul). A combination of neostigmine (0.035 to 0.07 mg/kg up to a maximum of 5 mg) and atropine (0.03 mg/kg up to a maximum of 2.4 mg) is commonly used. It is mixed in the same syringe and given intravenously as a bolus.[10] Reversal is usually seen within 5 minutes. Rarely, a second dose of reversal agents may be necessary in the PACU and is administered by anesthesia personnel, who may use a peripheral nerve stimulator to evoke muscle twitching to identify an effective reversal.

The postanesthesia nurse must identify signs of muscle weakness and assess a patient's recovery from a neuromuscular blockade thoroughly and accurately. Respiratory parameters that indicate return of muscle strength include tidal volume of at least 5 ml/kg, vital capacity of at least 15 to 20 ml/kg, and inspiratory force of 20 to 25 cm negative water pressure. Return of muscle strength is assessed clinically by the patient's ability to lift and hold the head off the stretcher for at least 5 seconds, sustain a strong hand grasp, protrude the tongue, open the eyes wide, and cough effectively.[18] These clinical signs are considered reliable indicators of the return of neuromuscular strength, particularly the ability to lift and hold the head off the bed. They should be assessed and met before any intubated patient is extubated and before oxygen therapy is discontinued after general anesthesia. Because of the serious implications of hypoventilation caused by muscle relaxants, it is essential for the patient to be observed for a long enough period to ensure that the potential for reparalysis has passed before the patient is discharged from the PACU.

Providing an appropriate period of observation after the administration of all types of reversal agents is important so that any episode of renarcotization or reparalysis is identified and addressed immediately. Besides a period of close observation, other practices accompany the administration of respiratory reversal agents. These potent drugs should be given in small, incremental doses to provide the desired respiratory effect while overstimulation, untoward side effects, and loss of analgesia are avoided. Reversal therapy should be combined with oxygen administration, physiologic monitoring, emotional support, and maintenance of a patent, unobstructed airway.

The Intubated Patient

The very nature of ambulatory surgery programs demands the administration of anesthetics that rapidly clear from the body and promote early recovery and ambulation. Rarely, a patient may remain in a depressed respiratory state that requires the presence of an endotracheal tube in the immediate postanesthesia period. Nursing care of the intubated patient includes

1. Providing constant nursing observation
2. Administering humidified oxygen to compensate for the bypassed upper airway that normally provides natural moisture to inspired air
3. Protecting the patient from aspiration by maintaining inflation of the cuff of the endotracheal tube, suctioning secretions from the mouth and airway above the cuff as needed before extubation, and properly positioning the patient
4. Ensuring the proper position of the endotracheal tube by periodically listening for bilaterally equal breath sounds
5. Maintaining the proper position of the tube by securely taping it and by keeping the patient from pulling on it
6. Providing emotional support and understandable explanations to the awakening patient about the presence of the tube, its use, and the projected length of time it will remain
7. Evaluating the patient for signs of sufficient recovery to allow a safe extubation

Controversy surrounds the decision about who should extubate a postanesthesia patient. Two distinct schools of thought exist. Many believe that the physician or certified registered nurse anesthetist who intubates should be responsible for extubating the patient, or that an equally prepared professional should do so. In many facilities, an experience postanesthesia nurse who has demonstrated clinical competency extubates patients on the basis of rigid criteria approved by the anesthesia department.

The patient must meet clinical indications of respiratory adequacy before extubation. The parameters previously discussed regarding return of strength after reversal of muscle relaxants all apply. The patient also should be awake, respond to questions with a nod or other method of communication, swallow and cough, and have a regular respiratory pattern with a rate of more than 10 breaths per minute.[18] A minimum SpO_2 level may be set by the anesthesia department. After extubation, the nurse should observe the patient closely for signs of hypoventilation because removal of the endotracheal tube may have eliminated the very irritant that was stimulating the patient to breathe adequately and remain awake.

CIRCULATORY ADEQUACY

Blood pressure, heart rate, rhythm, contractile strength, and fluid and electrolyte values all affect a patient's cardiovascular status. Many anesthetic agents exert a depressant effect on the heart and vascular bed, and thus careful evaluation of these parameters is essential during the immediate postanesthesia period. Volatile anesthetics and intravenous agents can promote vasodilation; decrease peripheral vascular resistance; decrease cardiac contractility; increase cardiac irritability; or cause sympathetic ganglion blockades, depression of the vasomotor center, and inhibition of the baroreceptor reflex.[2] Depression of the baroreceptor reflex inhibits vasoconstriction and tachycardia in response to a fall in blood pressure.[8] Table 20–6 identifies the cardiovascular and respiratory effects of various anesthetic agents and adjuncts. These effects may persist into the postanesthesia period and must be considered when nursing care is planned. Appropriate nursing actions aid in the reduction or elimination of untoward effects.

Blood Pressure

The blood pressure is a reflection of several factors that combine in a dynamic process. These factors include cardiac output, arterial blood volume, peripheral vascular resistance, viscosity of the blood, and elasticity of arterial walls. This is an ever-changing relationship that, for the ambulatory surgery patient, is affected by general anesthetic agents, regional anesthetics, changes in fluid status, individual factors about the patient's preoperative state of health, and the practice of early postoperative ambulation.

The goal of maintaining postoperative normotension is often elusive. Many factors affect the blood pressure and must be addressed individually. In particular, the patient's usual preoperative blood pressure range should be determined to establish the baseline for the postanesthesia goal. Normal ranges for systolic and diastolic pressure are generally 100 to 140 mm Hg and 60 to 95 mm Hg, respectively; however, these are arbitrary levels from which individual patients vary.

Preoperative blood pressure readings may reflect the patient's anxiety level. Blood pressure values may also indicate the effects of preoperative sedation or a state of dehydration, particularly in the elderly patient who has not had any recent oral intake. Other pertinent facts that

Text continued on page 437

Table 20–6. Cardiovascular and Respiratory Effects of Anesthesia Agents and Adjuncts

AGENT	CLASSIFICATION	SPECIAL NOTES	CARDIOVASCULAR EFFECTS	RESPIRATORY EFFECTS	CAUTIONS, CONTRAINDICATIONS
Alfentanil HCl hydrochloride (Alfenta)	Opioid	Onset of action: IV, 1–2 min; IM, <5 min; epidural, 5–15 min	Bradycardia, hypotension, dysrhythmias	Respiratory depression	Epidural alfentanil may cause pruritis, nausea and vomiting, urinary retention, and delayed respiratory depression up to 8 hr after single dose. It crosses placental barrier, use in labor may cause respiratory depression in neonates.
Atracurium besylate (Tracrium)	Nondepolarizing muscle relaxant	Onset of action: <3 min.	Hypotension, vasodilation, sinus tachycardia, sinus bradycardia	Hypoventilation apnea, dyspnea, bronchospasm, laryngospasm	Use with caution in patients with history of bronchial asthma and anaphylactoid reactions.
Diazepam (Valium)	Benzodiazepine sedative/hypnotic	Onset of action: IV, <2 min; rectal, <10 min; PO, 15 min–1 hr (shorter in children)	Bradycardia, hypotension	Respiratory depression	Contraindicated in patients with acute narrow-angle or open-angle glaucoma. Return of drowsiness may occur 6–8 hr after dose.
Droperidol (Inapsine)	Antiemetic, neuroleptic agent	Onset of action: IM/IV, 3–10 min.	Hypotension, tachycardia	Laryngospasm, bronchospasm	Contraindicated in patients with Parkinson's disease. Extrapyramidal reactions may consist of dystonic reactions, feelings of motor restlessness. Prolonged CNS depression may occur with neuroleptic analgesia.
d-Tubocurarine chloride (tubocurarine chloride)	Nondepolarizing skeletal muscle relaxant	Onset of action: <2 min.	Hypotension, vasodilation, sinus tachycardia, sinus bradycardia	Hypoventilation, apnea, bronchospasm, laryngospasm	Use with caution in patients with history of bronchial asthma.

Edrophonium chloride (Tensilon, Enlon, Reversol)	Short-acting anticholinesterase agent Reversal agent for nondepolarizing muscle relaxants	Onset of action: IV, 30–60 sec; IM, 2–10 min Duration: IV, 5–20 min; IM, 10–40 min.	Bradycardia, tachycardia, AV block, nodal rhythm, hypotension	Increased oral, pharyngeal, and bronchial secretions; bronchospasm; respiratory depression	Because of brief duration of edrophonium, neostigmine or pyridostigmine is generally preferred for reversal effects of nondepolarizing muscle relaxants. Contraindicated in patients with peritonitis or mechanical obstruction of the intestines or urinary tract. Use with caution in patients with bradycardia, bronchial asthma, cardiac dysrhythmias, or peptic ulcer disease.
Fentanyl (Sublimaze)	Opioid	Onset of action: IV, within 30 sec; IM, <8 min; Epidural/spinal, 4–10 min; transdermal, 12–18 hr; oral transmucosal, 5–15 min	Hypotension, bradycardia	Respiratory depression	Epidural, caudal, or intrathecal fentanyl may cause delayed pruritus, nausea and vomiting, urinary retention, and respiratory depression (up to 8 hr after single dose). Epidural, caudal, or intrathecal injections should be avoided in patients with septicemia, infection at injection site, or coagulopathy. Transdermal route is contraindicated in management of acute or postoperative pain, including outpatient surgery. Deaths have been reported with misuse.

Table continued on following page

***Table 20–6.* Cardiovascular and Respiratory Effects of Anesthesia Agents and Adjuncts** *Continued*

AGENT	CLASSIFICATION	SPECIAL NOTES	CARDIOVASCULAR EFFECTS	RESPIRATORY EFFECTS	CAUTIONS, CONTRAINDICATIONS
Flumazenil (Romazicon)	Benzodiazepine receptor antagonist	Onset of action: 1–2 min	Dysrhythmias (atrial, nodal, ventricular extrasystoles), tachycardia, bradycardia, hypotension, angina	None reported	Reversal of benzodiazepines may be associated with onset of seizures in certain high-risk patients. Monitor patients who have responded to flumazenil for up to 120 minutes for resedation, respiratory, depression. Do not use flumazenil until the effects of neuromuscular blockade have been fully reversed.
Hydromorphone hydrochloride (Dilaudid)	Opioid 7 times more potent than morphine	Onset of action: IV, almost immediately; IM/PO/SC, 15–30 min; rectal, 10–15 min; epidural 5 min	Hypotension, hypertension, bradycardia, dysrhythmias	Bronchospasm, laryngospasm	Epidural, caudal, or intrathecal route may cause delayed pruritus, nausea/vomiting, urinary retention, and respiratory depression up to 8 hr after single dose. Avoid in patients with septicemia, infection at injection site, or coagulopathy. Crosses placental barrier, use in labor may cause respiratory depression in the neonate.

Ketamine hydrochloride (Ketalar)	Dissociative anesthetic	Onset of action: IV, <30 sec; IM/rectal, 3–4 min	Hypotension, tachycardia, hypertension, dysrhythmias, bradycardia	Respiratory depression, apnea, laryngospasm	Emergence reactions (dreaming, hallucinations, confusion) are more common in adults, high doses, and rapid administration; reduced with premedication with benzodiazepines and droperidol. Patients with catecholamine depletion may respond with unexpected reductions in blood pressure and cardiac output. Use with caution in patients with severe hypertension, ischemic heart disease, or aneurysms; increased intracranial pressure; and in chronic alcoholics and acutely alcohol-intoxicated patients. Avoid use after topical nasal cocaine.
Meperidine hydrochloride (Demerol)	Opioid	Onset of action: PO, 10–45 min; IV, <1 min; IM, 1–5 min; epidural/spinal, 2–12 min	Hypotension, cardiac arrest	Respiratory depression, respiratory arrest, laryngospasm	Use with caution in patients with asthma, chronic obstructive pulmonary disease, increased intracranial pressure, and supraventricular tachycardia.

Table continued on following page

***Table 20–6.* Cardiovascular and Respiratory Effects of Anesthesia Agents and Adjuncts** *Continued*

AGENT	CLASSIFICATION	SPECIAL NOTES	CARDIOVASCULAR EFFECTS	RESPIRATORY EFFECTS	CAUTIONS, CONTRAINDICATIONS
Methohexital sodium (Brevital)	Ultra–short-acting anesthesia induction agent	Onset of action: IV, 20–40 sec; rectal, <5 min	Myocardial depression, dysrhythmias	Respiratory depression, laryngospasm, bronchospasm	Extravascular injection may cause necrosis; intra-arterial injection may lead to gangrene. Use with caution in patients with status asthmaticus. Incompatible with lactated Ringer's solution and other acid solutions (atropine sulfate, metocurine iodide, and succinylcholine chloride).
Metocurine iodide (Metubine Iodide)	Nondepolarizing skeletal muscle relaxant	Onset of action: <3 min	Hypotension	Hypoventilation, apnea, bronchospasm	Rapid IV injection may produce hypotension, tachycardia, and signs of histamine release. Contraindicated in patients with allergy to iodine.
Midazolam hydrochloride (Versed)	Benzodiazepine, sedative	Onset of action: IV, 30 sec–1 min; IM, 15 min; PO/rectal, <10 min; intranasal, <5 min	Tachycardia, vasovagal episode, premature ventricular complexes, hypotension	Bronchospasm, laryngospasm, apnea, hypoventilation	Respiratory depression and arrest may occur when used for conscious sedation. Patients with COPD are unusually sensitive to the respiratory depressant effects. Unexpected hypotension and respiratory depression may occur when given with opioids.

Mivacurium chloride (Mivacron)	Short-acting nondepolarizing skeletal muscle relaxant	Onset of action: <2 min	Hypotension, vasodilation, tachycardia, bradycardia	Hypoventilation, apnea, bronchospasm, laryngospasm, dyspnea	Prolonged blockade may occur in patients with low plasma pseudocholinesterase levels (severe liver disease or cirrhosis, burns, malignant tumors, infections, decompensated heart disease, peptic ulcer, pregnancy).
Morphine sulfate (MS Contin, Astromorph PF, Duramorph, Infumorph)	Opioid	Onset of action: IV, <1 min; IM, 1–5 min; SC, 15–30 min; PO, 15–60 min; PO slow release, 60–90 min; epidural/spinal, 15–60 min	Hypotension, hypertension, bradycardia, dysrhythmias, chest wall rigidity	Bronchospasm, laryngospasm	Contraindicated in patients with acute asthma, bronchitis. Opioid-induced biliary tract spasm may mimic MI symptoms.
Pancuronium (Pavulon)	Long-acting nondepolarizing skeletal muscle relaxant	Onset of action: 1–3 min	Tachycardia, hypotension	Hypoventilation, apnea, bronchospasm	Prolonged paralysis (days–months) may occur after long-term infections, renal failure, electrolyte imbalance, or concomitant corticosteroid and/or aminoglycoside use.

Table continued on following page

***Table 20–6.* Cardiovascular and Respiratory Effects of Anesthesia Agents and Adjuncts** *Continued*

AGENT	CLASSIFICATION	SPECIAL NOTES	CARDIOVASCULAR EFFECTS	RESPIRATORY EFFECTS	CAUTIONS, CONTRAINDICATIONS
Physostigmine salicylate (Antilirium)	Anticholinesterase neuromuscular blocking agent	Onset of action: IV/IM, 3–8 min	Bradycardia, palpitations	Bronchospasm, dyspnea, respiratory paralysis	High doses may cause tremors, ataxia, muscle fasciculations, and ultimately a depolarization block. Rapid IV administration may cause bradycardia, hypersalivation leading to respiratory problems, or possibly seizures. Use with caution in patients with epilepsy, Parkinson's disease, or bradycardia. Do not use in presence of asthma, diabetes, or mechanical obstruction of intestine or urogenital tract.
Pipecuronium bromide (Arduan)	Long-acting nondepolarizing skeletal muscle relaxant	Onset of action: <3 min	Hypotension, hypertension, bradycardia, myocardial infarction	Hypoventilation, apnea	Pretreatment doses may induce a degree of neuromuscular blockade sufficient to cause respiratory depression in some patients.
Rocuronium bromide (Zemuron)	Rapidly acting steroidal skeletal muscle relaxant	Onset of action: 45–90 sec Duration of action similar to that of vecuronium.	Tachycardia, dysrhythmias	Hypoventilation, apnea, bronchospasm, pulmonary hypertension	Rocuronium does not appear to trigger malignant hyperthermia.
Succinycholine chloride (Anectine, Sucostrin, Quelicin)	Ultra–short-acting depolarizing skeletal muscle relaxant	Onset of action: IV, 30–60 sec; IM, 2–3 min	Hypotension, bradycardia, dysrhythmias, tachycardia, hypertension	Hypoventilation, apnea, bronchospasm	Use with caution in patients with fractures, cardiovascular, hepatic, pulmonary, metabolic, or renal disorders. Abrupt onset of malignant hyperthermia may be triggered with succinylcholine.

Sufentanil citrate (Sufenta)	Opioid	Onset of action: IV, 1–3 min; intranasal, <5 min; epidural/spinal, 4–10 min 5–7 times more potent than fentanyl.	Hypotension, bradycardia	Respiratory depression, apnea	May produce dose-related rigidity of skeletal muscles.
Thipental sodium (Pentothal)	Ultra–short-acting barbiturate Induction agent	Onset of action: IV, 10–20 sec; rectal, 8–10 min	Circulatory depression, dysrhythmias	Respiratory depression, apnea, laryngospasm, bronchospasm	Shivering after pentothal anesthesia is a thermal reaction caused by sensitivity to cold. Contraindicated in patients with asthma. Use with caution in patients with hypertension, hypovolemia, ischemic heart disease.
Vecuronium bromide (Norcuron)	Intermediate-acting nondepolarizing skeletal muscle relaxant	Onset of action: <3 min	Bradycardia	Hypoventilation, apnea	
Desflurane (Suprane)	Volatile inhalation anesthetic agent	Changes in mental function may persist beyond the immediate postoperative period.	Hypotension, dysrhythmias	Respiratory depression, apnea	Use with caution in patients with stenotic lesions of aortic or mitral valves. May trigger malignant hyperthermia.
Enflurane (Ethrane)	Volatile inhalation anesthetic agent	Changes in mental function may persist beyond the immediate postoperative period.	Hypotension, dysrhythmias	Respiratory depression, apnea	Contraindicated in patients with seizure disorders. May trigger malignant hyperthermia.

Table continued on following page

Table 20–6. Cardiovascular and Respiratory Effects of Anesthesia Agents and Adjuncts *Continued*

AGENT	CLASSIFICATION	SPECIAL NOTES	CARDIOVASCULAR EFFECTS	RESPIRATORY EFFECTS	CAUTIONS, CONTRAINDICATION
Halothane (Fluothane)	Volatile inhalation anesthetic agent	Associated with hepatic dysfunction.	Hypotension, dysrhythmias, bradycardia	Respiratory depression, apnea	Not recommended for obstetric anesthesia except when uterine relaxation is required. Concomitant use with epinephrine, cocaine, or sympathomimetics may be associated with cardiac dysrhythmias. May trigger malignant hyperthermia.
Isoflurane (Forane)	Volatile inhalation anesthetic agent	Changes in mental function may persist beyond the immediate postoperative period.	Hypotension, dysrhythmias, tachycardia, coronary artery steal	Respiratory depression, apnea	May trigger malignant hyperthermia.
Nitrous oxide	Volatile inhalation anesthetic agent	Chief danger is hypoxia; at least 30% oxygen should be used. Increased risk of hepatic and renal disease has been reported by dental personnel.			
Hypotension, dysrhythmias	Respiratory depression, apnea, diffusion hypoxia	During first 5–10 min of recovery from anesthesia, nitrous oxide may displace alveolar oxygen, resulting in diffusion hypoxia. May trigger malignant hyperthermia.			
Sevoflurane	Volatile inhalation anesthetic agent	Changes in mental function may persist beyond the immediate postoperative period.	Hypotension, dysrhythmias	Respiratory depression, apnea	May trigger malignant hyperthermia.

IV, intravenous; IM, intramuscular; CNS, central nervous system; AV, atrioventricular; PO, orally; SC, subcutaneously; COPD, chronic obstructive pulmonary disease; MI, myocardial infarction.

should be recorded on the chart for reference include the patient's usual antihypertensive medication protocol and compliance with that protocol, the last dose of any vasoactive drugs, emotional makeup, and nutritional status.

Hypotension may be a result of fluid deficits from a prolonged NPO period, inadequate intravenous replacement, or blood loss. Some anesthetic agents cause cardiovascular depression and decreased peripheral vascular resistance, which can allow blood to pool in the extremities with a resulting drop in the central blood pressure. Halothane, enflurane, narcotics, barbiturates, droperidol, and curare are all potentially implicated in the hypotensive response.

Major regional anesthetic blockade also can result in vasodilation as a result of sympathetic nerve blockade. Significant areas of dilated vessels can lead to a drop in blood pressure. Patients who have undergone subarachnoid or epidural blocks should be moved gently and should receive supportive IV fluid therapy until the vasomotor (sympathetic) effects of the block have passed. In the immediate postoperative period, the patient who has recently been repositioned from lithotomy to supine position may also exhibit a drop in blood pressure caused by a rapid shift of blood volume into the legs. A gradual intraoperative position change from lithotomy and gentle transfer to the transporting stretcher should be implemented.

Treatment for hypotension depends on the cause but may include a combination of some or all of the following:

Continued oxygen therapy
Gentle movement of the patient
Supine positioning
Elevation of the legs
Infusion of IV fluids
Pharmacologic intervention in more persistent cases

Either vasopressors or anticholinergic drugs, such as atropine and glycopyrrolate, may be used. They are sometimes combined. Intravenous dosage ranges for several adrenergic drugs[10] given for hypotension are

Ephedrine	0.2–1.0 mg/kg
Phenylephrine (Neo–Synephrine)	1–10 μg/kg/min
Metaraminol (Aramine)	10–100 μg/kg
Isoprotenol (Isuprel)	0.01–0.2 μg/kg/min

Ephedrine, a potent sympathomimetic drug, is particularly useful for treating hypotension secondary to spinal or epidural anesthesia. It can be administered by intravenous bolus and is rapidly effective. Its effects are more pronounced on the heart than on blood vessels, and the increased heart rate and cardiac output affect the subsequent rise in blood pressure. Ephedrine also increases blood flow to the myocardium, brain, and muscles. The usual adult intravenous dose of ephedrine is 5 to 20 mg. Intramuscular dosage is 25 to 50 mg. For intravenous administration, the drug is diluted and given slowly. Adverse effects are often linked to higher doses; they include tachycardia, dysrhythmias, precordial pain, nervousness, vertigo, headache, palpitations, and diaphoresis. Nausea, vomiting, and dysuria may occur as well.

Hypertension is a blood pressure of 160/95 mm Hg or greater; a blood pressure of 140/90 to 160/95 mm Hg is considered borderline or labile hypertension and is a leading cause of morbidity and mortality after surgery.[11] Pinpointing the cause of postanesthetic hypertension is sometimes difficult. Often, the reason is sympathetic nervous system activity caused by catecholamine release in response to the stress of surgery and anesthesia.[19] Pain, discomfort, anxiety, or full bladder may be a sole predisposing factor, or any of these may accompany a more serious cause. Respiratory inadequacies may result in hypoxemia and hypercarbia, which affect aortic and carotid chemoreceptors and, in turn, cause peripheral vasoconstriction and consequent hypertension. Drug-induced hypertension may occur after the administration of ketamine, naloxone, pancuronium, oxytocin, and other intraoperative agents. Fluid overload is possible but is rarely a significant predisposing factor in the ambulatory surgical patient who has undergone a relatively short procedure. Other factors include the intense stimulation during extubation of an awake patient, emergence excitement, or an episode of retching or vomiting.

Hypertension may be the result of hypothermia because of the peripheral vasoconstriction that occurs as a mechanism to conserve body warmth. Shivering is another factor. The increased metabolism of the shivering muscles increases oxygen consumption and carbon dioxide production, with an inevitable increase in the cardiac workload.[2] As a result, hypertension often accompanies shivering.

Frequently, a hypertensive episode in a PACU is a reflection of the patient's pre-existing state of health. More than 37 million people in the United States are hypertensive.[8] Most of those

37 million people have essential hypertension, a sustained elevation of arterial blood pressure without known cause.[8] Although many anesthetic agents encourage a drop in blood pressure, the patient may return to a normal hypertensive state once the depressant effects of anesthetics have dissipated after surgery. Usually, the physician asks that patients continue taking their oral antihypertensive medications with a small sip of water until the time of surgery.

The cause of postoperative hypertension must be investigated. Often, it is self-limiting and does not require treatment, particularly if it reflects the preoperative pattern typical of the individual patient. Analgesics are often effective in reducing hypertension that occurs because of operative pain. Extremely high readings or prolonged episodes of elevated blood pressure may require administration of antihypertensives or diuretics and judicious reduction of intravenous fluid rates. After delicate surgeries (plastic, ophthalmic, or otolaryngoscopic) in which bleeding is a particularly undesirable complication, avoiding hypertension is especially important because it can further increase the risk of hemorrhage.

Several pharmacologic approaches are suggested to produce appropriate reduction of the blood pressure. Slow injection of the calcium channel blocker diltiazem (Cardizem) is one approach to reducing hypertension, but it should be avoided in the bradycardic patient. The sublingual administration of short-acting doses of nifedipine (often referred to as a "Procardia squirt") to quickly reduce very high blood pressure has never been an FDA-approved use of the drug. This practice has fallen out of favor because of the possible disastrous results of stroke, myocardial infarction, or other potentially fatal outcomes.[57] Wetchler[20] describes the IV use of hydralazine (Apresoline), a peripheral vasodilator, given in slow intermittent bolus doses of 2.5 mg to 5 mg, up to a total of 20 mg. For patients in whom the resulting increased heart rate (a secondary effect of hydralazine) is contraindicated, concurrent administration of IV propranolol (Inderal) may be appropriate. Sublingual nitroglycerine (0.4 mg) has been effective in reducing blood pressure as well.[10] Patients may be asked to take their usual oral medications when gastrointestinal (GI) status allows. Other agents that are effective in the postoperative period are calcium channel blockers, α- and β-blockers, and smooth muscle relaxants.

Data now suggest that tachycardia combined with hypertension is a particularly dangerous situation. With this combination, authorities recommend treating tachycardia first, often by restoring fluid volume or administering β-blocking agents. Any factor that is determined to be causing the tachycardia should be treated. Once the heart rate is reduced, the hypertension can be addressed. Labetalol (Normodyne, Trandate),[10] which has α- and β-blocking properties, is often the drug of choice in this situation. Esmolol (Brevibloc) is a short-acting, cardioselective β-blocking agent that can be helpful when hypertension is accompanied by supraventricular tachycardia or rapid ventricular response to atrial fibrillation of flutter. Although its primary indication is to reduce heart rate, esmolol often results in a reduction of coexisting blood pressure. In fact, the possibility of hypotension is a side effect that must be monitored. Because esmolol is such a short-acting drug (an elimination half-life of 9 minutes), it is ideal for the ambulatory surgery setting, where prolonged cardiovascular drug effects are undesirable. Esmolol should be used with caution in patients with a history of bronchospastic disease.

Ventilatory assistance, oxygen therapy, and reversal of narcotics or muscle relaxants are appropriate interventions that help lower blood pressure when hypoventilation is determined to be the causative factor. Peripheral vasodilators should not be used for hypertension caused by hypoxia, because they counteract the body's compensatory vasoconstrictive mechanism, which could lead to profound hypotension.

In its most profound state, hypertension is deemed a crisis. A diastolic reading more than 120 mm Hg is a medical emergency. Left untreated, it can result in damage to organs and even death. A disturbance in one or more of three physiologic mechanisms is implicated: (1) arterial baroreceptors, (2) fluid volume regulation, and (3) the renin-angiotensin system.[8] Perioperative causes of such a crisis include

- Vasoconstriction due to catecholamine release during pain or shivering
- Hypothermia
- Hypervolemia due to fluid overload
- Inadequate ventilation
- Withholding of the patient's usual antihypertensive medications
- Interactions with a monoamine oxidase inhibitor (MAOI) antidepressant, such as phenelzine (Nardil) and tranylcypromine (Parnate).[1]

Traditionally, the patient taking MAOIs was required to discontinue them for several weeks before elective surgery because of potentially dangerous interaction with anesthesia drugs.[21] Currently, it is thought that with proper anesthesia technique and selection, these patients can be anesthetized safely without discontinuing their usual medications. Because of a MAOI-induced catecholamine buildup, certain drugs must be given with caution in the perioperative period, and others should be totally avoided. In particular, meperidine and indirect sympathomimetic drugs are avoided. A meperidine/MAOI interaction can trigger a response that involves excitation, agitation, headache, hypertension or hypotension, rigidity, hyperthermia, convolutions, coma, and death. This is thought to be due to increased action of serotonin in the central nervous system.[22] Other narcotics are not absolutely contraindicated, but they may interact, causing increased or prolonged respiratory depression, hypotension, and coma. Special caution should be employed whenever analgesia is provided to patients taking MAOIs.

Other drugs given perioperatively must be used with caution in the patient taking MAOIs. One reason is the tendency of MAOIs to decrease the activity of hepatic enzyme systems that metabolize many drugs, thus prolonging the effects of those drugs. In combination with MAOIs, the following drugs may produce enhanced effects: barbiturates; direct-acting sympathomimetics, such as epinephrine, norepinephrine, isoproterenol (Isuprel), and phenylephrine; and succinylcholine when given with phenelgine. These drugs are not absolutely contraindicated for use in the patient taking MAOIs, but the patient receiving them should be observed very closely.

Table 20–7 lists several pharmacologic agents used for the treatment of hypertensive crisis. These, along with intravenous diuretics, such as furosemide (Lasix) and ethacrynic acid (Edecrin), are used to effect a rapid drop in blood pressure to normal or near-normal levels. Prevention, rather than treatment, of postoperative hypertension is the ultimate goal of any ambulatory surgery program.

Cardiac Status

Constant assessment of the patient's cardiac status, particularly identification of symptoms of myocardial ischemia and dysrhythmias, is of special importance. Elderly or ill patients with pre-existing cardiac disease must be managed carefully so that episodes of decompensated congestive heart failure or pulmonary edema do not occur. Physical assessment, historic information, and monitoring parameters guide the nurse in the evaluation of the patient's cardiac status.

The pulse should be assessed not only for rate and rhythm but also for amplitude as well. Weak, absent, or irregular pulses may reflect hypovolemia, decreased cardiac output, acute myocardial infarction (MI), cardiac dysrhythmias, or local pathology of the artery or extremity in question. A bounding pulse can denote excitement, hypertension, or fluid overload. Figure 20–3 illustrates arterial pulse sites. The nature of care in the PACU demands the use of cardiac monitoring. Alarm parameters should be established, and the alarm system should be activated.

Although any patient can experience decreased myocardial oxygenation, the patient with previously compromised cardiac status is at much higher risk for serious cardiac complications. Myocardial oxygenation cannot be measured definitively without sophisticated diagnostic equipment. However, symptoms indicative of it can be identified clinically, for instance, changes in the electrocardiographic (ECG) pattern, chest pain, changes in skin color, diaphoresis, and GI sequelae.

Heart disease accounts for a large proportion of perioperative complications. A previous MI is the single most important cardiovascular risk factor for the perioperative patient.[1] The relationship of elapsed time between a prior MI and surgery affects the morbidity for reinfarction. Perioperative morbidity has improved since 1972, probably because of imparted hemodynamic monitoring practices and myocardial muscle-sparing treatments during acute myocardial events. Although the risk has dropped considerably since the 1970s, delaying nonurgent surgery until at least 6 months after acute MI is widely recommended as a method of reducing perioperative morbidity.[1] Careful screening to identify these patients is essential because they are poor candidates for ambulatory surgery until their cardiac status is improved. Most ambulatory procedures are elective in nature and can be deferred for the cardiac patient in an acute or subacute illness. For procedures that cannot be delayed, the poor-risk patient is often admitted to the hospital after surgery.

The nurse must hold a high degree of suspicion for problems in the cardiac patient, even after a minor procedure. Anesthesia and related events contribute significantly to the myocardial oxygen supply and demand. Early signs of acute infarction or ischemia include ECG changes and subjective symptoms described by the patient.

Classic signs of impending MI are anginal pain, which is often constant; nausea; vomiting; and diaphoresis. All may be present, but it has been determined that only 25% of patients who have a MI in the postoperative period experi-

Table 20–7. Parenteral Antihypertensive Drugs

DRUG	DOSE	ONSET OF ACTION	ADVERSE EFFECTS	PREFERRED USE
Clonidine hydrochloride (Catapres)	IV 0.15–0.3 mg over 5 min	<5 min (hypotensive effect)	Drowsiness, dizziness, severe rebound hypertension Use with caution in patients with severe coronary insufficiency, recent MI, chronic renal failure	Essential, renal, and malignant hypertension
Diazoxide (Hyperstat)	IV bolus 1–3 mg/kg	Within 5 min of IV bolus	Headache, seizures, paralysis, cerebral ischemia, dysrhythmias	Hypertensive crisis
Enalaprilat (Vasotec IV) Enalapril maleate (Vasotec)	IV 1.25-mg infusion over 5 min	15 min after IV administration	Headache, dizziness, hypotension, chest pain	Hypertension
Hydralazine hydrochloride (Apresoline)	10–20 mg given slowly and repeated as necessary	Within 5 min of IV administration; unknown for IM use	Headache, tachycardia, angina, palpitations	Essential hypertension
Labetalol hydrochloride (Normodyne, Trandate)	200 mg diluted in 160 mg D5W infused at 2 mg/min until satisfactory response; alternately 20 mg IV bolus over 2 min	Within 2–5 min of IV administration	Orthostatic hypotension, dizziness, ventricular dysrhythmias, dyspnea, bronchospasm	Severe hypertension and hypertensive emergencies
Methyldopa (Aldomet)	250–600 mg diluted in D5W and infused over 30–60 min	Unknown	Sedation, decreased mental acuity, bradycardia, orthostatic hypotension, myocarditis, edema	Hypertension, hypertensive crisis
Metoprolol tartrate (Lopressor)	PO 100–450 mg/day in single or divided doses IV 5 mg q 2 min for 3 doses	PO <15 min IV almost immediately.	Fatigue, dizziness, bradycardia, CHF, hypotension, bronchospasm	Hypertension, acute MI, angina
Nitroprusside (Nipride, Nitropress)	50 mg diluted in 250, 500, or 1000 ml D5W infused at 0.3–10 μg/kg/min	Within 1 min	Headache, dizziness, restless, muscle twitching, diaphoresis, bradycardia, ECG changes, palpitations, hypotension	Hypertensive emergencies, reduced preload and afterload (may be used with or without dopamine)
Trimethaphan camsylate	500 mg diluted in 500 ml D5W, normal saline solution, or lactated Ringer's for concentration of 1 mg/ml; infuse at 3–4 mg/min	Immediate	Extreme weakness, severe orthostatic hypotension, tachycardia, angina, respiratory depression	Hypertensive emergencies
Verapamil hydrochloride (Calan, Isoptin)	PO 40–80 mg tid IV 2.5–10 mg (0.05–0.2 mg/kg)	PO 30 min IV 2–5 min	Transient hypotension, CHF, pulmonary edema, bradycardia, AV block, ventricular asystole, ventricular fibrillation	Hypertension, treatment of supraventricular tachydysrhythmias, angina
Esmolol hydrochloride (Breviblok)	25–100 mg (0.5–2 mg/kg); may repeat in 5 min if necessary	1–2 min	Hypotension, bradycardia, bronchospasm	Perioperative hypertension, supraventricular tachydysrhythmias

IV, intravenous; MI, myocardial infarction; D5W, 5% dextrose in water; IM, intramuscular; PO, orally; CHF, congestive heart failure; ECG, electrocardiographic; AV, atrioventricular.

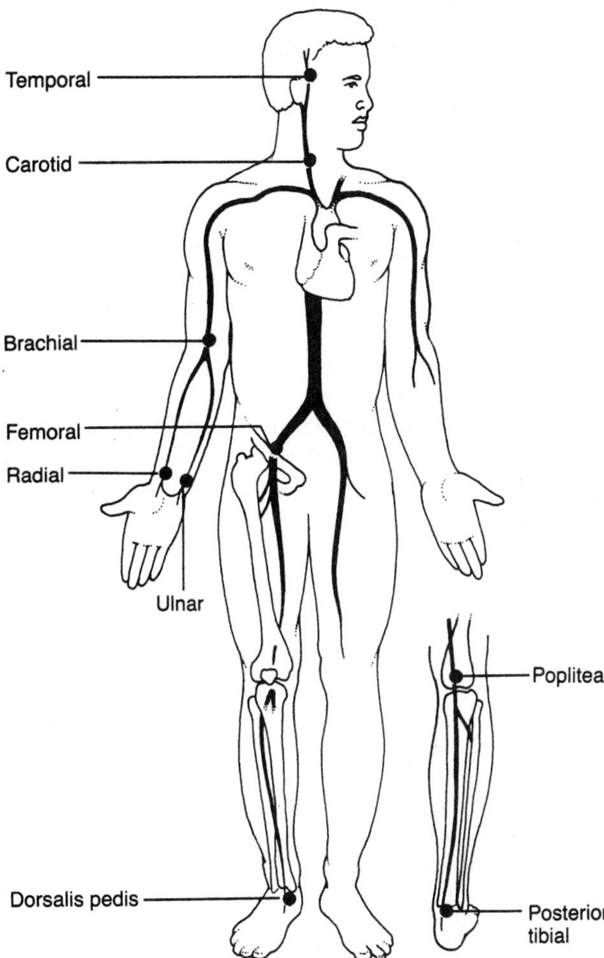

Figure 20–3. Peripheral pulse sites. (From Ignatavicius D, Bayne M: Medical-Surgical Nursing: A Nursing Process Approach. Philadelphia: WB Saunders, 1991, p 2096.)

ence typical anginal pain. Silent MI, one without the typical symptoms of heart-related pain, is most frequently seen in diabetic patients, the elderly, and people with hypertension.[8] Other symptoms of MI or impending MI that may or may not be present include psychological changes, including the fear of impending doom or dying. Anxiety and fear can further stimulate the autonomic nervous system, resulting in an undesirable increased catecholamine release, increased heart rate, and therefore, a heightened myocardial oxygen demand.

On the electrocardiogram, T wave inversion and ST segment depression of 1 mm or more below the baseline are indications of myocardial ischemia, although digitalis therapy, hypothermia, electrolyte abnormalities, and cardiac dysrhythmias can produce those changes as well.[23] ST elevation indicates actual myocardial injury, and the later appearance of a Q wave of 0.03 or more seconds is definitive for infarction and tissue necrosis. ST and T wave abnormalities on the cardiogram are not absolutely diagnostic of an acute MI; they should be considered as one parameter of the diagnosis, which supports clinical evaluations and diagnostic blood enzyme test results.

Lead II monitoring is typically used in the PACU because of its superiority for dysrhythmia detection. However, lead II provides no information about the inferior areas of the heart supplied by the right coronary artery and may fail to detect ischemia in lateral and anterior areas of the heart.[23] If a question arises regarding possible coronary ischemia, a 12-lead ECG should be obtained without delay so that all areas of the heart can be evaluated.

Immediate treatments include continued oxygen therapy, aggressive analgesia for cardiac pain, and maintenance of the intravenous access. Further specific treatment is directed at reducing cardiac workload, preventing further myocardial damage, and maintaining a stable cardiac rhythm. When an MI is definitively diagnosed, thrombolytic therapy to dissolve clots in the coronary arteries is likely to be instituted.

Dysrhythmias are also a threat in the postanesthesia period. Many are benign and self-limiting, but major dysrhythmias must be identified and treated before serious cardiovascular compromise occurs. The nurse in the PACU must be attentive to the cardiac pattern even on the young, healthy patient.

The impact of severe tachydysrhythmias or bradydysrhythmias lies primarily in two potential outcomes: (1) decreased oxygenation to tissues that ultimately occurs if the dysrhythmia is left untreated and (2) progression into life-threatening dysrhythmias. Some dysrhythmias (premature beats) reflect irritability of the myocardium, and others (heart block) indicate a problem with the heart's electrical conduction system. A current reference text on dysrhythmia interpretation and treatment should be available in the PACU.

Many anesthesia- and surgery-related factors predispose the patient to disturbances in cardiac rhythm. Anesthesia-related factors include pharmacologic factors (e.g., depressant drugs, reversal agents, epinephrine), alterations in oxygen supply and demand, pain, hypoxia, hypercarbia, acid-base or electrolyte imbalances, changes in blood volume and blood pressure, intubation and extubation. Surgery-related factors include manipulations and positioning in surgery (Trendelenburg's position), and abdominal insufflation for laparoscopic procedures. Pre-existing diseases (thyroid, cardiovascular), advancing age, anxiety, and medication protocols are factors as well.

Treatment depends on the cause, gravity, and effects of the dysrhythmia (Table 20–8). General supportive measures include continued monitoring of the electrocardiogram, oxygen therapy as indicated, emotional support, and a calm environment. Treatment should begin with an attempt to remove any identifiable cause of the dysrhythmia. A supply of antidysrhythmic drugs and monitoring and resuscitative equipment should be immediately available in each PACU. If a life-threatening dysrhythmia occurs during the patient's stay, hospitalization for observation and treatment is warranted.

FLUID AND ELECTROLYTE BALANCE

Most ambulatory surgical procedures are not associated with significant alterations in the fluid and electrolyte status, but various factors make the assessment of this parameter essential in the postanesthesia period. Many ambulatory surgery patients are young, healthy people who can readily compensate for fasting and intraoperative fluid losses. Small children and debilitated or elderly patients have less cardiovascular reserve and may not easily maintain their homeostatic fluid and electrolyte balance. Patients with pre-existing renal, GI, endocrine, and cardiovascular disease are at increased risk, as are those who are particularly thin or emaciated.

The average adult requires approximately 2000 to 2220 ml of fluid each day. When this is not provided orally, parenteral administration is substituted. Although many ambulatory surgery procedures are not associated with significant fluid or electrolyte loss, other factors related to surgery and anesthesia affect fluid and electrolyte balance. Stress and associated emotions, such as fear and anxiety, can cause a retention of both water and sodium. GI disturbances (e.g., vomiting, nasogastric suction, bowel preparation for endoscopy) can lead to potassium and sodium losses. Extensive bleeding can rapidly deplete fluid and electrolytes.

Blood Administration

Although the administration of blood products is not common in the ambulatory setting, it is a possibility. Blood may be administered to treat unexpected bleeding during or after surgery, and with procedures in which significant blood loss had been expected and, in fact, did occur. Suction lipolysis, or lipectomy, is one such procedure.

The practice of autologous blood donation before surgery has become so popular that more than 5% of blood donations are autologous.[24] The patient may be asked to donate several units of blood in the weeks before surgery for autologous transfusion on the day of surgery. Fresh, unfrozen blood can be stored for up to 35 to 42 days, depending on the policies of the blood bank. The last unit must be drawn by 72 hours before surgery to allow regeneration of the patient's blood volume. Other criteria for eligibility to donate autologous blood include

- Cardiovascular stability without significant cardiac disease, such as angina and recent MI
- Age between approximately 12 and 75 years
- History of no seizures in adult life
- Minimum hemoglobin level of 11 g/dl or 34% hematocrit
- No active infection
- No cancer of the bone marrow
- Availability of adequate venous access for blood collection.

Table 20–8. Causes and Treatments of Cardiac Dysrhythmias

RHYTHM AND CHARACTERISTICS	CONTRIBUTING/ PREDISPOSING FACTORS	CLINICAL SYMPTOMS AND SIGNS	TREATMENTS/NOTES
Sinus Tachycardia Normal complex sinus rate of 100–150 bpm. Usually secondary to factors outside the heart.	Exercise, fever, anxiety, hypovolemia	Palpitations, hypotension, signs and symptoms of congestive heart failure, decreased level of consciousness, persistent chest pain	Never treat tachycardia, treat the cause of it. Fluid/electrolyte replacement, analgesics, sedation, emotional support Dangerous to give drug therapy without determining cause because severe hypotension may occur. Propranolol if cardiac ischemia. Do NOT give digitalis unless cause is CHF.
Premature Atrial Contractions (PACs) Beat initiated by an ectopic atrial focus and appears early in the cycle (before the next sinus beat is expected). P waves differ in shape because the impulse is from a site other than the sinus node and the PR interval may vary.	May be indicative of atrial irritability from distention, stress, or heart disease. May initiate atrial tachydysrhythmias. Electrolyte imbalance, COPD, nicotine, anxiety, caffeine, drug toxicity.	Usually asymptomatic	Asymptomatic patients need no treatment. Occasionally procainamide, quinidine, propranolol, and digitalis are used.
Paroxysmal Supraventricular Tachycardia (PSVT)/ Paroxysmal Atrial Tachycardia (PAT) A re-entry phenomenon with abrupt episodes of tachycardia, usually between 150–250 bpm, averaging around 180 bpm. P waves may be abnormally shaped because of ectopic atrial site or may be buried in preceding T wave. May appear as VT if bundle branch block is present.	Wolf-Parkinson-White disease, chronic lung disease, digitalis toxicity, thyrotoxicosis. Anxiety, stress, caffeine, nicotine	Reduction in cardiac output, palpitations, dyspnea, faintness, CHF, hypotension	Vagal stimulation from a cough, Valsalva maneuver, or carotid message may terminate this. Adenosine, 6 mg IVP over 1–3 sec should be initiated if above measures are not effective; a second or third dose of 12 mg may be tried after 1–2 min. Verapamil, 2.5–10 mg IVP (up to 10 mg). Digitalis, procainamide, and β-blockers may be used. If not effective and symptoms of myocardial ischemia, CHF, hypotension, pulmonary edema are evident, consider cardioversion.

Table continued on following page

Table 20–8. Causes and Treatments of Cardiac Dysrhythmias *Continued*

RHYTHM AND CHARACTERISTICS	CONTRIBUTING/ PREDISPOSING FACTORS	CLINICAL SYMPTOMS AND SIGNS	TREATMENTS/NOTES
Atrial Fibrillation Very fast atrial rate arising from many ectopic foci. P waves are irregularly shaped, and ventricular response is irregular. Pulse rate is rapid (160–220 bpm) or slow, depending on ventricular response.	Sick sinus syndrome, hypoxia, increased atrial pressure, pericarditis, COPD, ASHD, pulmonary embolism, hyperthyroidism, CHF	CHF, hypotension, angina	Rate control is initial treatment: diltiazem, verapamil, β-blockers, or digoxin. Chemical cardioversion after anticoagulation can be achieved with procainamide or quinidine. Electrical cardioversion is the third alternative; however, in symptomatic patients with new onset of short duration (1–3 days), this is treatment of choice.
Atrial Flutter P waves have characteristic "saw-tooth" appearance. A result of re-entry circuit within atria. QRS usually regular with an AV block at 2:1, 3:1, 4:1 ratio.	Less common than atrial fibrillation. Anxiety, movement, and excitement can trigger this	Hypotension, CHF, decreased cardiac output, dizziness, faintness	Digitalis often used to decrease ventricular rate by blocking AV node. Synchronized cardioversion is treatment of choice in unstable patients.
1st Degree AV Block A delay in passage of impulse from atria to ventricles. PR interval is >0.21 sec.		Usually asymptomatic	No treatment except observation.
Mobitz Type I 2nd-Degree AV Block (Wenckebach's Block) PR intervals become progressively longer until a ventricular beat is missed, in a consistent pattern. PR interval is irregular and there are more P waves than QRS complexes.	Increased parasympathetic tone or drug effect (digitalis, propranolol, or verapamil). May be caused by inferior wall MI causing AV node ischemia	Usually asymptomatic	Treatment rarely needed unless symptoms are present.
Mobitz Type II 2nd-Degree AV Block Occurs below the AV node at either the Bundle of His (uncommon) or the bundle branches (common). Some beats are conducted while others are not, often in a ratio of atrial to ventricular beats of 2:1 or 3:1. Conducted beats have consistent PR interval; in blocked beats, there is a P wave not followed by a QRS complex.	Organic lesion in the conduction system; rarely the result of increased parasympathetic tone or drug effect	May be faint, weak, tired	Atropine is often ineffective. Artificial pacemaker is first line of therapy.

Table 20–8. Causes and Treatments of Cardiac Dysrhythmias *Continued*

RHYTHM AND CHARACTERISTICS	CONTRIBUTING/ PREDISPOSING FACTORS	CLINICAL SYMPTOMS AND SIGNS	TREATMENTS/NOTES
3rd-Degree AV Block/ Complete Heart Block No connection between atria and ventricles. Atrial rate is always equal or faster than ventricular rate. Rate depends on whether the heart is being driven by nodal (40–50 bpm) or ventricular (30–40 bpm) area.	Infranodal conduction system disease, atherosclerosis, extensive anterior wall MI	Hypotension, decreased cardiac output, weakness	Atropine, transcutaneous pacemaker, catecholamine infusions (dopamine or epinephrine). Isoproterenol is rarely indicated.
Premature Ventricular Contractions (PVCs) Sign of irritability in the ventricles. Appear as wide, bizarre QRS complexes, occurring early in the cycle and not preceded by a P wave. T wave is usually in opposite direction and followed by full compensatory pause (the duration of two cycles, including the PVC, is the same as the duration of two normal cycles). Unifocal PVCs originate from same site and have same configuration; multifocal PVCs arise from different sites and have different appearance from each other.	Hypoxia, cardiac disease, anxiety, pain, hypercarbia, mitral valve prolapse, nicotine, hypokalemia, halothane, succinylcholine, digitalis toxicity, irritation from endotracheal tube		Lidocaine is drug of choice. Procainamide and bretylium. Acute onset should be monitored for underlying cause. Chronic PVCs, usually related to underlying heart disease and producing no symptoms, do not require treatment
Ventricular Tachycardia (VT) Series of three or more consecutive PVCs occurring at a rate of 150–200 bpm	Myocardial irritability	Decreases cardiac output, may lead to ventricular fibrillation, especially if PVC falls on the T wave	In hemodynamically stable patient, treat with lidocaine bolus of 1–1.5 mg/kg. A second bolus may be given after 5 min for total of 3 mg/kg. Procainamide or bretylium are the next choices of treatment. In unstable patient with a pulse, synchronized cardioversion often suppresses VT.

Table continued on following page

***Table 20–8.* Causes and Treatments of Cardiac Dysrhythmias** *Continued*

RHYTHM AND CHARACTERISTICS	CONTRIBUTING/ PREDISPOSING FACTORS	CLINICAL SYMPTOMS AND SIGNS	TREATMENTS/NOTES
Ventricular Fibrillation (V-fib) Most common dysrhythmia in adult cardiac arrest. Uncoordinated, irregular, chaotic rhythm; no P wave, and QRS complexes are bizarre waves with no relationship to each other	Myocardial irritability R on T phenomenon	Pulseless state No cardiac output	Defibrillate with 200 J (watt-seconds) to start, increase to 300 and 360 J. Alternate defibrillation with drug therapy; epinephrine followed by lidocaine, procainamide and bretylium. Calcium and magnesium are given when a deficiency is suspected.
Asystole No electrical activity noted on cardiogram; may be slightly wavy line	Alfentanyl toxicity May be transient with 2nd dose of succinylcholine	Pulseless state **Must be verified in two ECG leads**	Initiate CPR. Apply pacemaker as soon as possible. Atropine and epinephrine are drugs of choice.
Pulseless Electrical Activity (PEA) Electrical conduction present but no mechanical action of the heart is detectable	Massive MI, drug overdose, pulmonary embolus, acidosis, tension pneumothroax, cardiac tamponade, hypothermia, hypoxemia, hyperkalemia, hypovolemia	No palpable pulse	Identify and treat initial cause. Initiate CPR. Epinephrine and atropine are first-line drugs.

bpm, beats per minute; CHF, congestive heart failure; VT, ventricular tachycardia; COPD, chronic obstructive pulmonary disease; AV, atrioventricular; MI, myocardial infarction; CPR, cardiopulmonary resuscitation.
Data from Cummins R (ed): Advanced Cardiac Life Support. Dallas, TX: American Heart Association, 1997.

Low body weight may prevent withdrawal of a full unit of blood at once, but it does not preclude autologous donation altogether. Before surgery, the ambulatory surgery center nurse should establish if and where autologous blood has been donated and should communicate this information to other healthcare providers.

Whether blood is autologous or allogeneic, the same vigilant observation and care should be provided for the patient during transfusion. Policies should clearly identify the proper methods for securing donated or autologous blood from the blood bank, identifying the patient, initiating the transfusion, monitoring the patient throughout, and responding to any untoward reactions. Two nurses or one nurse and another licensed professional should verify the typing and cross-matching of any unit of blood before it is administered.

The process of securing blood may be more complicated in a freestanding center that must have both a contract with a blood bank and a procedure in place for rapid procurement when needed. Transfer of the blood product from one location to another must be efficient to address emergencies.

Although they are self-donated, autologous units of blood are cross-matched. Chances of a clerical or handling error during processing make even autologous blood a danger. The possibility of serious sequelae resulting from an error in handling or administering blood must be a constant consideration.

Specific complications of blood transfusion include volume overload, bacterial contamination, and air emboli.[25] Hypotension has been reported and can occur because of bacterial contamination or venous emboli, hypocalcemia (citrate intoxication), or hypersensitivity to the plastics or stabilizers in tubings and bags.[8] Anaphylaxis and hemolytic reactions are other serious possibilities that require careful observation of the patient during transfusion therapy. Urticaria (hives), chest tightness or pain, dyspnea, hyperthermia, and wheezing are all symptoms that should prompt the nurse to discontinue the blood transfusion immediately, maintain a patent IV with new tubing and solution, notify the physician, closely monitor vital signs, and administer oxygen if necessary. Intravenous diphenhydramine (Benadryl) is the antihistamine of choice to counteract untoward allergic symptoms. Facility or blood bank protocol may require that a blood and urine specimen be obtained for analysis and that the tubing and bag of blood in question be returned to the blood bank.

Other sources of replacing blood loss exist including the addition of erythropoietin to enhance the autologous red blood cell yield and to "prime" bone marrow to increase erythropoietin production during autologous harvesting. During the operative procedure two techniques that may be used are intraoperative blood salvage and intentional intraoperative isovolemic hemodilution.

In intraoperative blood salvage, the blood lost by the patient is returned after processing usually by centrifugation and washing. It may reduce the transfusion requirements in procedures in which the blood loss is great or there is difficulty in obtaining autologous blood. Intraoperative blood salvage has also been used in Jehovah's Witness patients, provided that the blood is not processed outside the operating room.[25]

Intentional intraoperative isovolemic hemodilution involves preincisional withdrawal of whole blood to be returned to the patient later in the procedure. It is theorized that the blood loss in the surgical field is dilute, thereby conserving blood. However, this procedure is still highly controversial because of the lack of controlled studies.[25]

Nonblood Volume Substitutes

Occasionally, volume expanders, such as dextran and hetastarch (Hespan), may be used if blood components are not available. These are relatively inexpensive, are readily available, and carry no risk of disease transmission, although hypersensitivity reactions can occur.[1]

Dextran is a synthetic plasma substitute and is administered through standard IV tubing. Hypersensitivity reactions have been reported, usually in the first 30 minutes of infusion. Dextran may also interfere with platelet function and has been associated with a transient prolongation of bleeding time. Certain methods of typing and cross-matching of blood have been affected by use of dextran.[1]

Hetastarch is an artificial colloid. It is derived from a corn starch molecule that closely resembles human glycogen. It is available as a 6% solution in a 0.9% sodium chloride solution. Minimal coagulation effects and less likelihood to produce allergic reactions make hetastarch an economic and safe alternative to blood products.[1]

Oral Intake

An oral fluid intake is usually preferred by the patient over the intravenous route. Unless the type of procedure precludes it, oral fluids are allowed after the patient is sufficiently alert, has regained all protective airway reflexes, and is not nauseated. Raising the patient's head promotes easy swallowing without choking, although it may increase nausea in the early postanesthesia time frame. Care should be taken to choose appropriate types of fluid after general anesthesia, beginning with water or ice chips. Citrus juice and coffee are usually avoided to prevent nausea and vomiting and to limit the damage if aspiration occurs. IV therapy should continue until it is ascertained that the patient can tolerate oral intake.

Urinary Status

The types of surgery performed on an ambulatory basis usually do not severely alter urine production. An average daily output of 600 ml of urine is necessary to excrete the waste products of metabolism, although an optimal amount to ensure kidney function and adequate hydration is 30 ml/hour.[8] Hypovolemia, hypothermia, and the body's reaction to stress can decrease urine production.

Urinary retention may occur after anesthesia and surgery for several reasons. Controlled by sympathetic innervation, the bladder tone can be affected by spinal and epidural anesthesia, surgical manipulation, and use of local anesthetics in surrounding structures. The patient's bladder should be carefully assessed for distention, particularly after urinary procedures; inguinal herniorrhaphy, spinal or epidural anesthesia; and gynecologic procedures. Patients may be required to void before home discharge, but they may be discharged to phase II before voiding if they are not distended or uncomfortable.

Bladder distention is palpable in the lower pelvis and can be felt as a firm, domed area above the pubis. Other symptoms of bladder distention include restlessness, lower abdominal pain, hypertension, tachycardia, anxiety, tachypnea, and diaphoresis. Because many of these symptoms mimic those of hypoxia, a careful differential diagnosis must be made. If the patient is sufficiently recovered from anesthesia, using the bathroom rather than a bedpan or urinal is often enough to promote spontaneous voiding. If the patient remains distended or uncomfortable and unable to void, a physician's order for catheterization is indicated. When the patient has an indwelling catheter, the nurse should follow the basic principles of catheter care. The nurse should appropriately assess and document the patient's fluid intake and output.

TEMPERATURE REGULATION

Normothermia is a state of equilibrium between heat loss and heat production. The hypothalamus is the regulatory center of the body that maintains body temperature between 98.6°F and 99.5°F (36°C to 37.5°C). The major sites of heat production—a byproduct of metabolism—are the muscles, liver, and glands. Approximately 25% of the body's heat is produced by the muscles, 50% by the liver, and 15% by the brain.

Heat is lost through numerous mechanisms. These include (1) conduction of heat from the body to cold surfaces that it touches, (2) convection (heat loss to air current), (3) radiation (electromagnetic energy loss to colder objects in the room), and (4) evaporation from the skin during preps and through the respiratory system and urine. Radiation accounts for about 65% of heat loss.

Hypothermia

Temperature regulation is affected by many intraoperative events and factors. Often, these factors combine to produce hypothermia—core temperatures of less than 95°F or 35°C. Elements that affect body temperature during surgery include (1) patient weight (thin patients lose more heat and generate less heat than heavier counterparts), (2) amount of time and length of surgical exposure of the skin and internal structures, (3) site of surgery (peritoneal exposure significantly increases heat loss), (4) IV infusion of room-temperature fluids, (5) cool irrigants or skin preparation solutions, (6) ambient room temperature, and (7) old or very young age. Constant air circulation also increases the environmental effect of the cool room temperature.

The OR room temperature should be 75°F or higher to avoid hypothermia in the patient, although lower temperatures are often maintained. The average range is from 63°F to 79°F.[3] A lower room temperature is not only generally more comfortable to the gowned surgical team, it is believed to discourage the proliferation of microorganisms and may discourage bleeding and reduce drug requirements because the patient's metabolic rate is lowered.

Adjustments in room temperature must be made for the extremes of age. Small children and babies show greater heat loss because of their proportionately larger body surface area compared with their muscle mass. Children 6 months to 2 years of age should be cared for in an OR with the environmental temperature raised to 76°F. Temperatures should be even higher for newborns and premature babies.

Elderly patients also have problems with heat conservation. Their shrinking muscle mass and decreasing subcutaneous fat layer predispose them to hypothermia.[3] Although it is not a common practice to warm the OR for the elderly or debilitated patient, the idea should be given careful consideration because to do so would be helpful in preventing heat loss.

Anesthesia-related factors significantly affect heat loss as well as the ability of the body to regenerate heat. Many anesthesia agents depress the thermoregulatory center, and neuromuscular relaxants stop muscle activity, which is a method of heat production. Relaxants also prevent the shivering that increases body heat. Respiratory heat loss may occur if oxygen and gases are not warmed during delivery. Anesthesia agents, narcotics, and major regional anesthetics produce peripheral vasodilation, thus allowing for heat significant loss through the skin.

Intraoperative temperature monitoring is usually continuous. Measures should be instituted to prevent heat loss before and during the procedure. Methods include increasing room temperature; using warmed blankets and irrigating and prep solutions; using foil blankets to prevent radiation of the patient's body heat; employing intravenous fluid warmers; and using other external warming devices.[26] Respiratory circuits used to deliver anesthesia gases are primary targets for heat conservation because they are considered the best way to prevent and treat hypothermia. The patient's head should be covered in the OR and during the immediate postanesthesia phase because most heat loss occurs through the head. In one study, it was shown that almost 50% of the body's heat may be lost as radiation from the scalp.

The lowered metabolic rate associated with hypothermia is beneficial in one way—by decreasing the body's oxygen requirements, thus protecting the body tissues from the effects of hypoxemia. Conversely, the effects of medications are greatly enhanced in the hypothermic patient. When metabolism is slowed, active drug remains in the body longer, so it takes less medication to produce a desired effect in the cold person than in the normothermic one. When anesthesia is stopped, the thermoregulatory center in the hypothalamus begins functioning to increase the body temperature back to a normal range.

In the PACU, the patient's temperature should be included in the admission assessment. The hypothermic patient may exhibit cyanosis, particularly of the fingers and toes. Because of vasoconstriction of distal vessels, this occurrence is a physiologic response to conserve heat. Extensive vasoconstriction may preclude accurate oxygen saturation measurements by oximetry. Warming methods include radiant or forced air heat,[26] warmed blankets, warmed intravenous fluids, and covering of the patient's head and upper torso. Analgesic doses may need to be decreased as a result of their enhanced effects during a hypothermic period.

Because dysrhythmias can occur secondary to hypothermia, the patient should continue to be monitored. It is also important to understand that the patient who has been hypothermic and is rewarmed to a normal temperature range may exhibit the renewed effects of muscle relaxants. This can occur if the dosage of reversal agents that was effective in the hypothermic patient is no longer effective when the metabolic rate increases in response to the patient's warmer temperature.

Shivering

Shivering occurs both as a major mechanism for postanesthesia heat production and spontaneously without known cause in the normothermic patient. It is an uncomfortable and unpleasant occurrence for the awakening patient. It also carries a physiologic threat because of the potential for hypertension, self-injury to the operative site or teeth, and tremendously increased oxygen demands, which may rise to four to five times that of normal during shivering.

Oxygen therapy should be continued until shivering stops, and the patient should be closely observed for signs of associated hypoxia or its sequelae. Patients with ischemic heart, renal, and brain disease must be carefully monitored because of their increased sensitivity to further hypoxia to these organs. Economic costs related to the additional PACU time required, the expense of supplies and medications used in treatment, and the nursing time required for rewarming and supportive care of the shivering patient must also be considered.

Despite the lack of a constant or clear-cut correlation between hypothermia and postanesthetic shivering, attempts at reducing shivering in the PACU include rewarming the hypothermic patient. Even normothermic patients appreciate any palliative efforts to ease their discomfort when they are experiencing the intense sensation of cold and muscular discomfort that can accompany shivering. For these people, warm blankets or other external rewarming devices provide a welcome, if transient, sense of warmth. Several studies have found warmed blankets to be ineffective in relieving shivering, but radiant heat to the patient's chest and abdomen has been shown to reduce shivering within 1 to 2 minutes.[27, 28]

Medications have been used in an attempt to reduce shivering. Of the narcotics, meperidine has shown the most usefulness. An 80% effectiveness rate has been reported with 12.5- to 25-mg IV doses, with no resulting increase in nausea. Fentanyl and morphine have been ineffective.

Vogelsang and Hayes[28] initiated a classic study in 1989 in an attempt to discover the effectiveness of the opiate agonist-antagonist analgesic butorphanol tartrate (Stadol) in reducing or eliminating shivering. The authors studied 247 patients; of these patients, 20 experienced postanesthetic shivering. A 1-mg IV dose of butorphanol was effective within 5 minutes in 95% of those patients, and 60% of those patients experienced relief within 2 minutes. The authors also reported no nausea, vomiting, or respiratory depression after the administration of butorphanol.

The patient who has experienced shivering may have diffuse muscle aching for 1 or more days after surgery because of the intensity of muscle activity during the perioperative period. Shivering that is extreme or prolonged should be reported to the phase II nurse so that relevant information can be included with discharge instructions. In this manner, the patient can better understand postoperative myalgia related to the surgical site.

Hyperthermia

Rarely is the ambulatory surgery patient hyperthermic on admission to the PACU. The patient with an infectious process that would manifest itself in a fever in the immediate perioperative period is generally not a candidate for ambulatory surgery. Another rare state that would produce an elevated temperature in its late stages is malignant hyperthermia, a serious hypermetabolic state that is genetic in origin and can be triggered by certain anesthesia agents and muscle relaxants. This entity is described in detail in Chapter 11.

LEVEL OF CONSCIOUSNESS

In the immediate postanesthesia period, the nurse must obviously vigilantly assess the patient's level of consciousness. Until protective reflexes and cognitive abilities return after general anesthesia or heavy sedation, the patient is totally dependent on the nurse for protection against the environment. The unconscious patient should never be left unattended.

It is accepted that hearing is the first sense to return on awakening, and thus that sense should be employed to help orient and arouse the semiconscious patient. The nurse should use the patient's name and speak in a calm and low tone. Extraneous noises and laughter as well as unrelated or upsetting conversations should be avoided near the bedside during the arousal period because they can become distorted and confuse or agitate the awakening patient.

Periodic, frequent attempts to awaken the unconscious or semiconscious patient should continue until the patient responds, although exceptions exist. The semiconscious patient with signs of upper airway irritation, such as coughing and gagging, should be positioned to avoid aspiration, given oxygen, constantly attended, and allowed to awaken slowly without aggressive intervention so that the possibility of laryngospasm is decreased. Also, severe hallucinations and bad dreams can follow administration of ketamine, so the preferred nursing action for these patients is quiet vigilance. Vital signs should be taken, but other stimulation, noises, and bright lights should be kept to a minimum. Intravenous diazepam (5 to 10 mg) or thiopental (50 to 75 mg) is the usual treatment to reverse ketamine-induced delirium.[10]

Emergence Delirium

Occasionally, a phenomenon called emergence delirium, or emergence excitement, can occur during arousal from general anesthesia.[29] It manifests itself with behaviors such as restlessness, thrashing of extremities, combativeness, crying, moaning, screaming, irrational talking, and disorientation. Besides the general disruption that such behavior causes in the PACU, injury to the patient can occur, including straining or opening of surgical incisions, injury to limbs, and dislodging of IV lines and endotracheal tubes.

During such an occurrence, the patient requires constant nursing attention, often by several nurses and attendants. Gentle physical restraint to prevent self-injury may be indicated, but total restraint of the extremities or a rough physical grasp usually serves only to agitate the semiconscious patient further. Legally, such restraint also could be considered a form of battery. The safety of the nursing staff is also in question if the patient is physically combative.

Numerous factors influence the occurrence of this uncommon reaction. Barbiturates and scopolamine given before surgery are implicated as triggering events, as is the presence of pain, a full bladder, feelings of suffocation during arousal, and possible cerebral hypoxia. Several studies point to the importance of psychological preparation as a preventive tactic. Fear of surgery or disfigurement or threat to body image seems to predispose the patient, particularly the child or adolescent, to emergence excitement. It follows, then, that one preventive measure is comprehensive preoperative preparation to establish a rapport between the patient and the caregivers. This approach helps to reduce anxiety, encourage trust, and reduce the fears surrounding surgery.

Pharmacologic interventions for episodes of acute emergence delirium have also been studied in depth. Intraoperative use of meperidine, fentanyl with droperidol (Innovar), morphine, or methadone may reduce the incidence. The usefulness of physostigmine (Antilirium) as a reversal agent to end an episode of delirium is controversial.[10] Its usefulness is well established, however, in the reversal of symptoms caused by scopolamine or other anticholinergic drugs, so its use is not questioned when the drug is given to patients who have been given such agents. The recommended dosage is 1 mg in incremental doses given slowly IV and not exceeding 3 mg total. Higher doses or rapid administration can cause severe bradycardia, a cholinergic response.[10]

Delayed Awakening

Prolonged unconsciousness may result from the type and the amount of drugs given before and during anesthesia.[29] Preoperative drugs that may be implicated are benzodiazepines, neuroleptic agents, narcotics, and barbiturates. Most intraoperative inhalation agents, narcotics, and barbiturates may prolong recovery as well, particularly if the patient's metabolism, ventilation, or circulations are impaired. Other drugs that may delay arousal after general anesthesia include cimetidine, lidocaine, some antihypertensive agents, MAOIs, and depressant drugs that are self-administered by patients before anesthesia.

Other causes of delayed awakening include hypothermia, malignant hyperthermia, metabolic diseases, and cardiovascular pathology, such as hypertension, hypovolemia, and myocardial ischemia. Respiratory inadequacy that delays arousal may be narcotic induced or pathologic. Also, intracranial causes may be cerebral depression, a cerebrovascular accident, an undiagnosed intraoperative seizure, or embolism.[30] The anesthesiologist should be summoned to evaluate any patient who does not awaken in a reasonable period.

NEUROLOGIC FUNCTION

Motor and sensory return after general and regional anesthesia must be evaluated. Neurologic sequelae of skeletal muscle relaxants are assessed as previously discussed. Major regional anesthesia can produce long-lasting motor and sensory blockades.

Depending on the extent and the area of the body affected, the patient may be required to remain in a PACU until the neurologic effects of local anesthesia have dissipated. Blocks of the upper extremities often do not require a PACU stay because the relatively small area affected does not significantly effect the central circulatory status and does not interfere with ambulation. With the affected arm in a sling, the patient is often ready for immediate ambulation to a chair and usually goes directly from surgery to the phase II recovery area. Similarly, a field block of one or both feet is usually not a contraindication for ambulation to a chair. After spinal or epidural anesthesia, the patient requires PACU nursing care until the major effects have dissipated. A discussion of the specific nursing needs of the patient after regional anesthesia follows.

After a procedure with an inherent propensity to affect peripheral nerves, the function of those specific nerves should be assessed both before and after surgery. For example, the patient's ability to smile symmetrically should be evaluated after a rhytidectomy, eyelid closing should be ascertained after blepharoplasty, and the function of the fingers should be assessed after a carpal tunnel release. The usual period of motor loss typical for a local anesthetic is also considered.

POSITIONING

Until patients can move and position themselves, the nurse must ensure proper body alignment to provide comfort and safety and to promote cardiovascular and respiratory homeostasis. Lateral positioning is the safest for prevention of aspiration until the unconscious patient awakens and demonstrates adequate gag, cough, and swallow reflexes. The patient's head and neck should always be well supported, and the extremities should be positioned to avoid damage to nerves, tendons, and muscles. Hyperextension of joints beyond their normal physiologic positions can result in pain and physical damage to joint structures. Opposing skin surfaces should be separated with padding, pillows, or a blanket roll when appropriate. If the patient is unconscious or immobile for a prolonged period, the nurse should provide gentle, passive movement of extremities and should reposition the patient periodically to avoid lengthy pressure on any surface of the skin and underlying tissues. Awake patients should be encouraged to exercise their extremities actively and to change positions occasionally unless these measures are contraindicated by the type of procedure.

Some procedures require special postoperative positioning. Surgically affected extremities are usually elevated above heart level to prevent bleeding and edema, which can lead to pain or delayed healing. Often, the surgeon prefers that patients remain in Fowler's position after face, head, neck, or breast surgery for the same reasons. After ear and eye surgery, the surgeon is consulted for special positioning instructions. Position changes should be made slowly after anesthesia, particularly in the patient who has experienced cardiovascular instability or hypotension. Vital signs are assessed after each move. Pre-existing physical problems may limit mobility or require special positioning; a comprehensive explanation of those special needs should be relayed to the postanesthesia nurse by means of a verbal report and the medical record.

OPERATIVE SITE

Observations and nursing interventions pertinent to the operative site are as diverse as the many types of procedures performed in the ambulatory setting. All wounds or dressings should be assessed frequently for signs of bleeding, including frank bloody drainage, rapid filling of drainage collecting systems, bruising, and skin discoloration or swelling that could indicate hematoma formation. After ear, nose, and throat procedures, frequent swallowing or subjective complaints of drainage in the back of the throat may indicate active bleeding. Heavy vaginal flow or extensive hematuria can herald uterine or urinary hemorrhage.

Signs of intra-abdominal bleeding that may not appear until blood loss is significant include apprehension, hypotension, tachycardia, splinting, abdominal pain, tenderness and rigidity, pallor, and diaphoresis. Laparoscopic procedures place patients at particular risk for occult bleeding because of the potential for unidentified laceration or inadvertent burning of abdominal organs or vessels intraoperatively. Even a seemingly benign dilatation and curettage can result in a perforated uterus, particularly in elderly or recently parturate patients.

While summoning the physician to examine the bleeding patient, the nurse should take steps to reduce or stop any excessive bleeding, for instance, manual pressure and elevation of the site. Bleeding involving the airway requires constant nursing attention, appropriate patient positioning, and possibly gentle suctioning of the patient's mouth to remove blood or secretions. The suction catheter should not be placed near the source of the hemorrhage.

The following emergency procedures may be initiated, depending on the facility's standing emergency protocols: ice or cool compresses to the surrounding area or increased intravenous fluid infusion rates. On the specific orders of the physician, the anxious, restless, or hypertensive patient may require sedation to help reduce bleeding. Administration of pressor agents or replacement of blood volume with colloids or blood products may be necessary to combat hypotension. Oxygen therapy is also indicated if active bleeding is present to offset the body's reduced oxygen-carrying capacity related to lowered hemoglobin levels.

Resuturing an incision or packing a body cavity may be necessary, and sterile supplies should be readily available in the PACU for such emergency interventions. A sterile instrument set kept in the PACU can be used interchangeably for various needs: chest tube insertion, cutdown, bleeder or incision suturing, and tracheotomy. Associated disposables or other supplies should be stored in the same area, ideally in a common container for ease of transport. Sterile gloves, suture materials, gauze packings, sterile vaginal speculum, and antiseptic preparation solution are examples.

Bleeding may require a return to surgery. Should this occur, both the patient and the family are very often distraught. Their fears are founded because a second surgery is not without risks; they require particularly considerate emotional support. A calm environment not only helps to keep the patient psychologically tranquil but also can help to prevent increased bleeding. Any patient with signs of bleeding should remain NPO because of the possible need for a second general anesthetic. The anesthesiologist must be informed if the patient has had any oral intake before return to OR so that safe anesthesia can be planned.

In the often hurried situation of returning a patient to surgery a frequently forgotten consideration is that of surgical consent. Because the sedated patient is not able to sign a legal document at this point, an accompanying family member or one who is telephoned is often called on by the surgeon to sign the consent or to give verbal consent. In a true emergency, the surgeon may waive the need for consent.

Besides the primary operative site, any tubes, drains, and catheters must be inspected and changed or emptied appropriately. Frequent or continuous irrigations of urinary catheters may be necessary to maintain their patency, particularly if clots are present. If the origin of hematuria is prostatic, the physician may place tension on the Foley catheter by affixing it securely to the patient's leg. This tension should not be released without a physician's specific order. The nurse should follow universal standard precautions whenever caring for the operative site, drains, catheters, or body fluids for both self-protection and patient protection.

PERIPHERAL CIRCULATION

Peripheral circulation of a surgically involved extremity should be assessed frequently. Circulatory compromise can occur as a result of the constriction of an encircling bandage, elasticized wrap, or cast, which may require loosening to allow sufficient blood flow to the extremity. More serious causes could be occlusion of a vessel caused by a thrombus or embolus or internal pressure from bleeding within an encircling dressing. Peripheral pulses should be palpated bilaterally to ascertain their presence, strength, and symmetry. Pulses are generally described numerically as

0	Absent
1+	Weak and thready
2+	Normal
3+	Full and bounding

A pulse oximeter that provides a visual depiction of pulse strength may be placed on a digit of the operative extremity periodically to provide an indication of blood flow to the distal portions. Color of the skin and the nailbeds is an important parameter as well, but vasoconstriction in the hypothermic patient may produce cyanosis that mimics other, more dangerous, conditions. Blanching or redness of the skin may persist after the deflation of an intraoperative tourniquet; thus, the patient should be observed long enough to allow evaluation after the tourniquet-related symptoms have dissipated.

Capillary refill, indicated by the quick return of normal color to the nailbed or distal area of the skin blanched by pressure placed on it should occur within three to five seconds[8] after releasing that pressure. This is an especially helpful assessment when a large dressing on the foot or hand precludes all visual evaluation except at the tips of the digits. If a peripheral pulse is not palpable, the extremity should be repositioned and the pulse again sought. A Doppler ultrasound stethoscope is an alternative noninvasive method of assessing blood flow. This device is more sensitive than an ordinary stethoscope and does not depend on the hearing acuity of the practitioner. It uses the relationship of sound wave frequency to the relative motion between two sources to detect the movement of red blood cells in underlying vessels. It can detect flow to a depth of about 5 cm, so it is limited to the superficial vessels. Cyanosis or the absence or weakness of the pulse in an extremity may be due to pre-existing vascular disease. Thus, the patient's medical history is an important parameter of the complete assessment.

ANALGESIA

Nociceptors are free nerve endings found throughout the body. Pain is a complex phenomenon that generally results from the chemical, thermal, or, with surgery, mechanical stimulation of nociceptors. The stimulation causes impulses to be transmitted to the spinal cord through afferent nerve fibers and eventually to the brain, where pain is consciously perceived. Several of these circulating chemicals can either cause or decrease pain. These chemicals, along with other factors, can prevent some impulses from traveling to the brain. The complexity of this process makes pain an intensely personal experience that is variable between people and at different times in the same person.[31]

The physical and emotional impact of surgical pain on the patient is often intense, particularly for the person who is not prepared for the amount or the type of pain being experienced. Preoperative counseling should include a general description of what the patient can expect after surgery. Several investigators described a direct relationship between comprehensive preoperative education and patient encouragement and decreased analgesic needs, less fear, and earlier postoperative mobility. Before surgery, the patient should be told that some discomfort may be expected after surgery, but that medication will be given and home discharge will not be attempted without adequate pain relief.

The patient who is taught pain-relieving techniques before surgery avoids feelings of powerlessness after surgery. Deep-breathing and relaxation techniques, appropriate body mechanics, and positioning to help alleviate pain are ways in which the patient can actively decrease postoperative pain. Providing encouragement and expressing confidence in the patient's ability to handle the discomfort inherent in the procedure are often therapeutic and very reassuring.[32] Explaining the use of intraoperative injections of local anesthesia to reduce pain may be helpful if the physician routinely does so. With such information and preparation, the patient is more likely to arrive on the day of surgery with a positive attitude and less anxiety than if he or she is expecting the excruciating pain that a neighbor or acquaintance may have described.

The operative site and the patient's emotional makeup affect how much pain the patient experiences after surgery. For example, chest, abdominal, and rectal procedures cause more inherent discomfort than breast, scrotal, chest wall, or extremity procedures. The anesthesia technique plays a significant role as well, with regional anesthesia usually providing a longer period of analgesia than general anesthesia. Intraoperative narcotic administration and local anesthetic infiltration at the surgical site are also effective in reducing postoperative pain levels. Social issues affect pain perception and tolerance. Especially nervous or anxious people and those with particularly protective families may exhibit difficulty in managing pain, as do some people of certain ethnic or cultural groups.[33, 34]

Pain is a subjective experience. No one other than the patient really knows how much pain that person is experiencing. Objective observations of the patient's vital signs, restlessness, facial expression, splinting, posturing, mood, voice, and refusal to move or assist with repositioning can provide valuable clues to the discomfort level. However, these are only clues, not definitive indications, because every person reacts to pain individually.

It is not the nurse's place to judge the patient's pain. The nurse's role is to assess the patient thoroughly and to provide appropriate interventions to help relieve discomfort.[32] Along with objective observations, assessment also includes asking the patient about the location, intensity, and type of discomfort being experienced. Asking the patient to rate pain level numerically on a scale of zero to 10 may be helpful. This helps the nurse ascertain the patient's perception of the pain intensity and leaves little room for misinterpretation of terminology.[32]

Sources of pain other than the operative site include bladder distention; uncomfortable positioning; pain due to arthritis, gout, decubitus ulcer, or other pre-existing diseases; placement of the intravenous line, tubes, or catheters; and gastric distention. Postoperative complications, such as embolic events, myocardial or pulmonary ischemia, hemorrhage, and ruptured viscus, may cause pain as well.

The concept of ambulatory surgery is closely interwoven with wellness and caring. Providing adequate analgesia is part of that philosophy. Patients should expect that their analgesic needs will be met. The nurse's attitude, manner, and words can be important determinants of a patient's response to and perceptions of pain. Many ambulatory surgery centers discourage the use of the word "pain" and focus on the idea of "discomfort." The latter terminology has a significantly different connotation that fits into the philosophy of wellness of an ambulatory program. An exception is the patient experiencing obviously severe pain, to whom the use of the term "discomfort" could be construed as unfeeling or trite.

Besides providing symptomatic comfort, adequate analgesia promotes the general well-being of the patient. Many untoward physiologic responses can result from the experience of pain. Some of these include respiratory dysfunction due to wound splinting; shallow respirations that can lead to respiratory acidosis; tachycardia; hypertension; increased peripheral resistance, cardiac output, and myocardial oxygen consumption; gastric stasis and paralytic ileus; and endocrine and metabolic changes.[34] Treating pain helps the patient to avoid these potentially dangerous occurrences.

Oral analgesics were once believed to be the only appropriate postoperative pain medications for ambulatory surgery patients. With the increased complexity of procedures being performed in the ambulatory surgical setting, these are not always sufficient to alleviate pain. Providing the patient with immediate and effective pain relief is one of the most important aspects of postoperative care. Preventing severe pain is usually easier than controlling it once it has overtaken the patient's thoughts and focus. Pain also bears a distinct effect on the nausea and vomiting cycle, and eliminating one often helps prevent or eliminate the other.

In a PACU, the patients in need of analgesia are often awakening from general anesthesia. General anesthesia provides the poorest inherent pain relief into the postanesthesia period when compared with regional and local approaches. The semiconscious patient is often psychologically less able to handle pain that would otherwise be manageable during wakefulness and full control of coping capacity, and pain can seem magnified in the half-awake state of emergence. The restless or complaining patient may only need a few minutes to become more awake and able consciously to discern the source of discomfort.

An evaluation period before analgesics are administered in a PACU is important for several reasons. First, patient restlessness may be due to hypoxia rather than pain. Also, although rarely, the patient may have been given a reversal dose of naloxone at the end of the anesthetic. This narcotic antagonist causes reversal of both the analgesic and the depressant effects of intraoperative narcotics. It is vital that the anesthesiologist inform the postanesthesia nurse if a narcotic reversal agent has been given; otherwise, the nurse could administer further narcotics ordered by the surgeon to alleviate the patient's current complaints of pain. Once the stimulant effects of naloxone wear off, an additional analgesic dose could produce dangerous additive depressant effects when combined with any lingering intraoperative narcotics.

This scenario is one reason that justifies the practice of obtaining postanesthesia medication orders from the anesthesiologist who knows all the drugs given during the anesthesia and how the patient responded to those drugs. The anesthesiologist becomes the logical primary therapist for the patient's pain, nausea, and sedative needs during the PACU stay.

The challenge for the PACU nurse is to provide adequate pain relief without oversedation. The smallest effective dose should be given, and incremental administration is often favored over a single large dose of medication. Narcotics are the most frequently used and the most effective treatment instituted in the PACU for relief of postoperative pain. When narcotics are given in the early recovery period after general anesthesia or extensive sedation, the potential for cumulative, undesirable side effects is omnipresent. Respiratory depression is the most significant problem, and it can be accompanied by prolonged somnolence, nausea, and vomiting. Thus, a period of close observation should follow the administration of narcotics.

Calculation of individual doses is essential because patients vary significantly in weight, age, sensitivity to drug actions, and their personal need or desire for a certain level of analgesia. Medication history plays a significant role as well. The patient who rarely takes even an aspirin may require only small analgesic doses. On the other hand, previous or current heavy alcohol or drug use or heavy smoking may decrease the effectiveness of drug therapy for the patient after surgery through a mechanism called enzyme induction.

Metabolism, or biotransformation, pharmacologically converts active lipid-soluble drugs into water-soluble, usually pharmacologically inactive, metabolites. This transformation to a water-soluble state allows their eventual excretion through renal tubules. Hepatic microsomal enzymes are responsible for the metabolism of most drugs. Long-term use of substances such as alcohol, tobacco and cigarettes, barbiturates, analgesics, and other medications causes increased production of these hepatic enzymes over time. A long-term increase in circulating enzyme levels increases the rate of drug metabolism. That process leads to increased dose requirements for effective analgesia. Increased doses of drugs are needed to produce a therapeutic effect in patients who habitually use certain chemicals, including cigarettes.

Many analgesics are available and can be given by various routes. Oral, intravenous, intramuscular (IM), subcutaneous, and rectal are the most common routes for the ambulatory population. The choice of agent and route depends on the patient's individual pain experience and response. Research and clinical studies continue to report that transdermal and nasal agents[35] may have widespread application for ambulatory surgery. Epidural analgesia is popular for hospitalized patients but has not gained application for ambulatory surgery patients.

Fifty times more potent than morphine, fentanyl is an extremely effective, rapid-acting analgesic that is appropriate for the ambulatory surgical patent. Not only is it quick acting, it also produces minimal sedative hangovers. Like other narcotics, it should be given in small incremental doses when administered intravenously. Because of potential respiratory complications, intravenous fentanyl should be given only by those familiar with its actions and potency in a monitored environment. Personnel should be experienced in resuscitative techniques and should have appropriate equipment closely available. Although fentanyl does not evoke histamine release or cause significant cardiovascular changes, it can produce bradycardia and is usually avoided in the patient whose pulse rate is less than 50 beats per minute. A single IV dose of up to 50 μg (1 ml) is usually appropriate for the adult patient of average weight. Although fentanyl is rapid acting, it also has a short duration. Action lasts 3 to 60 minutes when administered IV and for up to 3 hours after IM injection.

Once the patient is awake and retaining oral fluids, oral analgesics are often given. Intravenous medication provides short-term analgesia until the oral medication produces effective serum levels. After some procedures, such as breast augmentation in which the prostheses are implanted under the muscles, the patient may respond favorably to the addition of a muscle relaxant drug to reduce surgical discomfort. Oral nonsteroidal anti-inflammatory drugs, such as ibuprofen and ketorolac (Toradol), may be ordered for mild pain relief, although gastric irritation and interference with the coagulation mechanism are complications associated with their use.[35] Patient-controlled analgesia by infusion pump is a method of IV postoperative narcotic pain control that may become more applicable to ambulatory patients as the types of procedures continue to become more complex. Manufacturers are now developing miniaturized, battery-operated, or completely disposable systems that can be used in the home setting.[36]

Some surgeons order IM narcotics for postoperative analgesia either intentionally or out of habit for hospitalized patients. The IM route may be incompatible with the goals of rapid analgesia, quick arousal, rapid ambulation, and discharge. Many studies have shown that one third of the postoperative patients given IM analgesics continue to experience moderate-to-severe pain. The peak action of an IM narcotic is accompanied by sedative effects and sometimes hypotensive and respiratory depressant effects. This requires that the patient be observed for a sufficient period, which may prolong or preclude discharge. The patient's home support, age, preoperative physical status, and current level of pain all affect the ability to tolerate IM analgesics and to be judged appropriate for discharge.

Despite the potential for sedation, if a procedure typically causes significant postoperative pain, IM medication with a longer-acting narcotic may be appropriate. Meperidine and morphine are two potent narcotics that may be administered either IV or IM in individually calculated doses. Typical dosage ranges for adults for morphine are 2 to 4 mg IV to 6 to 10 mg IM, and for meperidine are 10 to 15 mg IV to 50 to 100 mg IM. Doses in the higher ranges may significantly delay discharge due to sedation and/or resulting nausea and vomiting. A combination of IV and IM administration is often effective in producing both rapid and long-lasting analgesia. Morphine also can promote urinary retention and postural hypotension when the patient ambulates.

In an ambulatory setting, the titration of opioid agents in incremental IV doses seems more reasonable than the administration of larger one-time doses. A rapid onset of action and a rapid onset of side effects become apparent while the patient is being observed in the PACU. For instance, respiratory depression after morphine may occur up to 90 minutes after subcutaneous injection and 30 minutes after IM injection, but it is most frequently seen within 7 to 10 minutes of IV administration.[10]

Opioid agonist-antagonists, such as pentazocine (Talwin), butorphanol tartrate, and nalbuphine (Nubain), act to reduce pain in much the same manner as narcotics when given to the patient who has not had previous narcotics. When given in the presence of narcotics, however, their antagonistic characteristics can result in reversal of narcotic effects, resulting in pain, anxiety, and loss of sedation. They are contraindicated in the person with a long-term dependence on narcotics because severe withdrawal symptoms can occur with their use.

One parenteral nonsteroidal anti-inflammatory drug, ketorolac tromethamine, is ideal for many patients in the ambulatory surgical population. This IM preparation is administered in dosages of 30 to 90 mg, depending on the patient's weight and other variables. It has been shown to be as effective as 12 mg of morphine or 100 mg of meperidine.[10, 36] In clinical trials, postoperative analgesia also was shown to last longer with ketorolac than with meperidine and morphine.[36]

Ketorolac produces few side effects.[10, 36] Specifically, the incidence of nausea, dyspepsia, drowsiness, and GI pain ranges from 3% to 9%. Even less frequently observed symptoms include edema, diarrhea, dizziness, headache, tinnitus, peptic ulcer, sweating, and pain at the injection site. More important, respiratory function is not altered, and no significant cardiovascular effects are noted. It does not produce additive untoward effects, such as drowsiness when administered with narcotics and general anesthetic agents, and it is sometimes given concurrently with narcotics to obtain added analgesic benefits. Ketorolac does not have a potential for addictive abuse and is, therefore, ideal for use in the narcotic-addicted or drug-seeking patient. Metabolism occurs in the liver, and excretion is via the urine, with more than 50% of the drug being excreted unchanged. Caution is advised when it is administered to patients with kidney or liver dysfunction, and dosages should be reduced in the elderly.

After IM injection of ketorolac, the onset of action occurs at approximately 10 minutes. Analgesic effect peaks between 45 and 90 minutes, and duration is approximately 6 hours.[10, 35] Administering this drug in the operating room 45 to 60 minutes before the end of surgery, while the patient is under general anesthesia, prevents the patient from experiencing the pain of an injection. Effective pain relief is provided during the arousal period for many. It is not recommended for obstetric use before delivery because of its inhibitive action on prostaglandin synthesis.[10]

Other IM drugs that may be ordered with analgesic therapy are hydroxyzine (Vistaril, Atarax) or phenothiazine derivatives, such as promethazine (Phenergan). These drugs potentiate the effects of narcotics and enhance pain relief but should be used cautiously in ambulatory surgery patients because they may cause significant sedation. Both have antiemetic and anxiolytic properties.

Intraoperative supplementation of general anesthesia with local anesthetics is often beneficial in controlling postoperative pain. A regional blockade may be provided by the anesthesiologist at the beginning or the end of the case, or local infiltration may be administered by the surgeon. Adjunctive administration of local anesthesia before surgery leads to reduced general anesthetic needs and a resultantly shorter recovery period. The intraoperative instillation or injection of a long-acting local anesthetic, such as bupivacaine, at the end of the case is particularly helpful in providing analgesia into the postoperative period.

Many other types of injections that provide local or regional sensory loss and prevent painful stimuli in the early postoperative period are available. Intra-articular injections are often performed at the end of arthroscopic procedures. Local infiltration in tonsillar beds can produce significant pain relief in the immediate postoperative period, as evidenced by the ability to talk and swallow without discomfort. The pain of circumcision may be addressed with a dorsal nerve block; topical spray, jelly, or ointment; subcutaneous ring block; or caudal block. A field block of tissues surrounding an incision is also a very simple means of providing analgesia.

When these various local techniques are employed, a nurse can provide information and positive reinforcement about the projected length of analgesia to be expected. The patient should be instructed to avoid excessive activity during the time that the local anesthetic is effective and to begin using oral medications at home when the supplemental local anesthetic begins to wear off, as directed by the surgeon.

Nonpharmacologic interventions should not be discounted in the search for pain relief. Basic nursing actions, such as positioning, soothing conversation, hand holding, and massage, all have their place in the nurse's analgesic arsenal. The experience of pain is often exacerbated by anxiety and fear.

With patients who are sufficiently awake, other types of interventions are appropriate as well. Positive encouragement of relaxation may reduce pain in an anxious patient. This intervention requires an environment that allows the patient to focus on such relaxation techniques as counting, rhythmic breathing, or guided imagery. The latter technique involves having the patient imagine pleasant visions, sounds, and smells. A similar tactic is called "distraction," in which the patient's attention is focused on something besides the pain.[1] The effectiveness of these nonpharmacologic methods requires patient acceptance, nursing skills, and sometimes preoperative discussion and practice. Sullivan[32] emphasizes the benefit of preoperative preparation in reducing the amount of postoperative pain and points out that the rapport built between the patient and the caregiver is an important part of that process.

A transcutaneous electrical nerve stimulator (TENS) is another nonpharmacologic method of decreasing pain. It is based on stimulation of cutaneous afferent nerve pathways that inhibit the perception of pain. The actual mechanism of pain relief is unknown. One theory suggests that the electrical stimulation causes the release of endorphins that attach to opiate receptors and block the transmission of painful stimuli. It is primarily used for control of chronic pain, although there are postoperative applications. The device is easy to learn and to use and can provide analgesia without the unwanted side effects of narcotics.[1]

Still, TENS therapy has not been widely associated with ambulatory procedures. In one study by Wetchler,[37] some patients involved had bilateral inguinal hernia repairs performed 1 week apart and used the TENS approach for one, but not for the other, operation. The investigator reported a significant decrease in oral analgesic needs at home in the patients using TENS units. Contraindications to the use of transcutaneous electrical nerve stimulators are few: cardiac pacemakers (particularly demand types), recent or impending MIs or significant dysrhythmias, and first trimester of pregnancy. The TENS electrodes should never be placed over the carotid sinus nerves, the eyes, or the laryngeal or pharyngeal muscles.[1, 37]

Patients who are discharged with a TENS in place should have thorough written and verbal instructions about its use, potential problems, and troubleshooting techniques to correct those problems. One of the most common problems encountered is the need for periodic battery replacement. The patient should be supplied with extra batteries and taught how to change them at home. In particular, the amplitude setting should be lowered when changing to new batteries because fresh batteries are more powerful and can produce an unpleasant intensity of electrical stimulation at the setting that is appropriate for worn batteries.

NAUSEA AND VOMITING

The occurrence of nausea with or without vomiting is both an unpleasant complication and a potentially dangerous event leading to aspiration when it occurs in an unconscious or a semiconscious patient. The intensity and the duration of nausea and vomiting can vary significantly, and the patient is both physically and emotionally affected. Both the patient and the family are affected when the length of stay must be extended to treat significant nausea and vomiting.

Sometimes overnight hospitalization is necessary because of excessive vomiting or somnolence that results from pharmacologic treatment. Such situations are physically and emotionally difficult for the patient, economically undesirable for the patient and the healthcare system, and frustrating for the healthcare providers. The primary goal is to prevent rather than treat nausea and vomiting. Preoperative counseling, pretreatment with prophylactic histamine blockers and antiemetics, and use of anesthetic agents with low incidence factors are a few of the methods enlisted for aggressive prevention.

Nausea is a very subjective occurrence. It is often difficult for the patient to describe and is usually very unpleasant. It may or may not result in vomiting or retching. Vomiting is a complex occurrence that involves the skeletal muscles and the autonomic nervous system. It occurs from reflex or direct stimulation of the vomiting, or the emetic, center located near the dorsal nucleus of the vagus nerve in the medulla. Various physiologic and emotional mechanisms can encourage vomiting.

The vomiting center can be stimulated by the chemoreceptor trigger zone (CTZ) of the brain and via three primary afferent nerve pathways: the (1) cortical, (2) visceral, and (3) vestibular afferent pathways, in which causative reflexes may originate in the pharynx, GI tract, cerebral centers, or vestibular center, which controls the sense of balance.[38] In response to stimulation, the emetic center responds through efferent nerve pathways. Impulses are sent via the cranial and spinal nerves to the respiratory center and GI tract, particularly to the diaphragm and upper abdominal muscles, which control the actual act of vomiting.[38, 39] This process is illustrated in Figure 20–4.

Cortical afferent stimulation can be a result of emotional, organic, and sensory factors.[41] Stress, depression, and fear are a few of the many emotions that can result in nausea or vomiting. The effects of sensory pathways can be seen in the patient who is nauseated by the sights and smells of surgery or the PACU. Cortical input can also be organic and caused by hypoxia, pain, hypotension, or increased intracranial pressure. Hypovolemia is one of the most frequent causes, and aggressive fluid therapy is often an effective treatment. This is typically exemplified in the young, hypotensive woman who becomes nauseated when she sits up, whose nausea responds to hydration, the supine position, and possibly to a vasoconstrictive drug, such as ephedrine. Electrolyte imbalances and dehydration are also causes.[38]

Visceral afferent stimulation comes from both the viscera and the vagal nerve. It is often the result of delayed gastric emptying and abdominal distention. Typical causes include handling of the abdominal contents during surgery, primary GI disorders, and cardiac disease. Induced pneumoperitoneum for laparoscopic procedures contributes to visceral afferent stimulation and accounts, in part, for the increased nausea and vomiting typically seen in these patients.

Vestibular effects can be the result of tremors; motion; otitis media; ear, nose, and throat procedures; and anesthetics and narcotics that can sensitize the vestibular system. The pathway is from the auditory nerve to the cerebellum to the CTZ and to the vomiting center.[40] The patient with a strong history of motion sickness may have postoperative vomiting because of vestibular afferent activity.[38, 40]

Circulating drugs (in particular, narcotics) or decreased cerebral blood flow can affect the CTZ and the vomiting center directly to cause what is termed *central vomiting*. These drugs include many inhalation and IV anesthetic agents, narcotics, amphetamines, cardiac glycosides, ergotrates, nitrogen mustard, and other chemotherapeutic agents.

It is apparent that with this etiologic diversity, no single approach to prevention or treatment of nausea and vomiting is effective from one person to another. Many factors that can cause nausea and vomiting are closely related to the process of anesthesia and surgery. For example, laparoscopy, ovum retrieval, abdominal procedures, pediatric strabismus procedures or orchipexy, procedures involving the ear, and tonsillectomy or other procedures in which blood may enter the stomach are more likely than others to result in postoperative nausea and vomiting. Gagging due to the presence of artificial airways or nasogastric tubes or with suctioning can stimulate vomiting as well. Women experience postanesthesia nausea and vomiting two to three times more often than men. Hiatal hernia and anxiety also increase the incidence. Obesity is known to increase the incidence because of usually increased gastric volumes and sometimes related anatomic airway difficulties that can lead to air swallowing.

Notable for the ambulatory surgery patient, the presence of gastric contents is a major risk factor. Careful preadmission instructions that stress the importance of maintaining the approved length of fasting before surgery are essential. Some authorities consider the concept

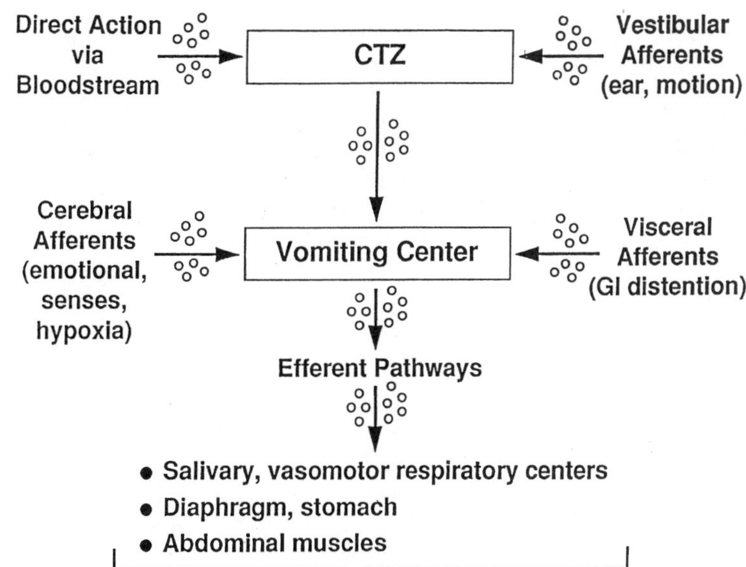

Figure 20–4. Multiple pathways to and from the emetic center.

of an empty stomach to be more myth than reality because gastric juices are always present. Also, gastric emptying can be significantly prolonged by anxiety or alcohol consumption, and undigested food can remain in the stomach for more than 24 hours.

Preoperative counseling combined with an appropriate medication program can be a significant deterrent to postoperative nausea and vomiting. Part of the success of preventive maneuvers stems from the positive attitude of staff members who can instill confidence in the patient before surgery and help to change or reinforce that person's expectations. Some issues that might be included in the preoperative discussion follow:

- The surgery center's low rate of nausea and vomiting
- The development of newer and better anesthetic agents with lower associated incidences of nausea and vomiting
- The fact that ether and similar drugs are no longer used
- The availability of highly effective antiemetic drugs
- The expertise of the anesthesia and nursing staffs in dealing with perioperative nausea and vomiting
- The aggressive manner in which that patient's medication protocol can and will be managed to prevent nausea and vomiting

A generic statement might be made about a previous patient who had described a strong history of GI symptoms but who did not experience any after surgery in the center. The nurse should avoid promising the patient that there will be no nausea or vomiting because this is an impossible guarantee.

The patient with significant history of motion sickness or previous nausea and vomiting related to anesthesia is often given a prophylactic antiemetic before or during anesthesia along with a well-chosen anesthetic agent. Narcotic techniques, on the other hand, are associated with increased postoperative nausea and vomiting by three mechanisms: (1) direct action on the CTZ, (2) decreased gastric emptying times, and (3) slowed gastric motility.[40]

Nitrous oxide traditionally has been implicated as a significant causative factor because of its inherent property to diffuse into air-filled chambers 34 times faster than air can escape from them. Resulting collection in the middle ear can affect the vestibular system and predispose the patient to nausea and vomiting. Nitrous oxide also gravitates to any air-filled areas of the stomach and bowel, increasing distention and pressure and thus potentially increasing nausea. The use of a combination of nitrous oxide and narcotics for anesthesia has been shown to increase the rate of postoperative nausea and vomiting when compared with an inhalation technique.[38–40]

As evidenced by the literature, nitrous oxide's use and its predisposition to cause nausea and vomiting remain controversial. Regional and local anesthetic approaches provide a much lower incidence of nausea and vomiting and are especially appropriate for people predisposed to these effects.

Propofol (Diprivan), a new anesthetic agent for induction and maintenance of anesthesia, has a low (1% to 3%) incidence of nausea and vomiting. One study has indicated that a 10-mg dose actually may be beneficial as an antiemetic agent.[39]

Nursing Interventions

The nurse's primary consideration in relation to nausea and vomiting in a PACU must be to protect unconscious or semiconscious patients' airways to avoid aspiration of stomach contents. As previously discussed, placing the patient in a side-lying position, suctioning as necessary, and removing mechanical airways quickly on arrival at the PACU are appropriate methods.

The factor causing the nausea and vomiting should be sought and eliminated whenever possible. Postanesthesia nursing interventions for the nausea-prone patient are as follows:

- Providing positive reinforcement to reduce anxiety
- Avoiding sights, smells, or conversations near the patient that could evoke nausea or vomiting
- Moving and ambulating the patient slowly
- Allowing the patient to awaken slowly without aggressive stimulation
- Maintaining cuff inflation on any endotracheal tube until extubation
- Providing adequate analgesia
- Ensuring a judicious oral intake with avoidance of citrus juice and coffee
- Limiting irritation of the upper airway to reduce gagging: limiting suctioning, removing artificial airways when possible, and positioning for drainage of oral secretions or blood resulting from procedures of the upper airway or GI tract

Patients who are vomiting should be provided with privacy from the view of others in the PACU. They often need reassurance because they may be more upset and embarrassed about bothering the nurse or other patients than about the physical discomfort of vomiting. An emesis basin kept nearby is usually a valued comfort to some patients, but to others, it can be a negative visual reminder that encourages more vomiting.

Too-rapid elevation of the patient's head after general anesthesia is a common factor in the onset of nausea. The mechanism may be the development of orthostatic hypotension with nausea triggered via the cortical afferent pathway. Another possible mechanism may be a response to the change in position in the middle ear. Hypovolemia is a particularly common factor. Aggressive IV fluid therapy is often effective in correcting nausea related to position changes or hypovolemia. Slow progress from a supine to a sitting position is preferred, with a temporary return to supine if nausea or vomiting occurs. If no GI symptoms occur after 5 to 10 minutes, the process of head elevation can be initiated again.

The topic of oral intake is a challenging one to address because each patient, anesthetic, operative procedure, and situation are different. Usually, oral intake should begin with small sips of water or ice chips. Potential aspiration of this type of liquid is much less dangerous than that of dairy-based products or other beverages. Some practitioners advise against ingestion of cold drinks or ice and provide only room-temperature beverages. However, there is no research to suggest that cold drinks and ice have initiated more episodes of nausea and vomiting than drinks at room temperature. Probably the best advice is for the nurse to find the approach that works best in his or her own clinical setting, given the types and the ages of patients who are typically seen and the types of anesthetics administered.

For some patients, avoiding all beverages is wise until the major effects of anesthesia or any nausea have passed, and oral intake may not be allowed until the patient has been transferred to the phase II area. The patient's desire for fluids is often the best measure of readiness. IV hydration is continued until the patient can drink and retain beverages.

Should these interventions fail at preventing or treating nausea and vomiting, pharmacologic interventions may be ordered, depending on the causative factors and the physician's preference. Antiemetic drugs have chemically diverse modes of action and may be chosen by their mechanism of action.

Antiemetic drugs that block the specific receptors responsible for the patient's symptoms would, theoretically, be the most effective. For example, chlorpromazine (Thorazine), trimethobenzamide (Tigan), and droperidol (Inapsine) are dopamine antagonists that may suppress CTZ activity.

If hypotension accompanies nausea, placing the patient supine, increasing IV fluid replacement, and administering oxygen along with 10 to 25 mg of ephedrine IV have been effective in restoring normotension and reducing nausea and vomiting.

Analgesic therapy is another method employed. Nausea and vomiting can be directly attributed to the use of narcotics, particularly meperidine, but pain is another well-established factor that has been found to contribute to nausea and vomiting.[39] Judicious use of analgesics to reduce pain can help eliminate the nausea and vomiting associated with pain. In a classic study of hospitalized patients, Anderson and Crohg[41] identified an 80% reduction of nausea with the use of IV narcotics to relieve pain in patients with both pain and nausea.

Antiemetic therapy should be designed to reduce GI symptoms without oversedating the patient. Droperidol is the most frequently used agent for treating nausea and vomiting in ambulatory patients. Given intravenously, it can reduce nausea and vomiting by exerting action on the CTZ. In an adult patient, 0.635 to 1.25 mg (0.25 to 0.50 ml) is an average IV dose, although doses as low as 0.25 mg have been effective.

Droperidol can cause drowsiness, potentiate narcotic-induced drowsiness, and prolong recovery when given in larger doses. The maximal total recommended IV dose is 2.5 mg (1 ml), but it is administered in small, divided doses and titrated to the desired effect. Other potential side effects include hypotension and tachycardia, which are usually self-limiting; anxiety; dizziness, chills and shivering; hallucinations; laryngospasm; and bronchospasm.

Extrapyramidal reactions that can be treated with antiparkinson drugs include dystonia (muscle spasms), akathisia (restlessness and agitation), and oculogyric crisis (paroxysmal fixation of the eyes in one position). IV diphenhydramine, 50 mg given alone or in combination with incremental diazepam to a total of 10 mg IV, has been effective in treating extrapyramidal side effects. Symptoms may occur hours after droperidol administration, thus after discharge.[10] Another unpleasant untoward effect of droperidol is a sense of dissociation between the mind and the body. It is more likely to occur when droperidol is administered without any other sedative or narcotic and is less likely to occur in the PACU than during the preoperative period.

Metoclopramide (Reglan) has been used as an antiemetic with some success in the postanesthesia period. It acts in two ways: (1) it increases the rate of gastric emptying, and (2) exerts an antiemetic effect that may be the result of antagonizing central and peripheral dopamine receptors. Dopamine produces nausea and vomiting by stimulation of the medullary CTZ, and metoclopramide blocks that stimulation.

Traditional antiemetic agents, such as the phenothiazines, prochlorperazine (Compazine), chlorpromazine, and promethazine (Phenergan), are used in various settings but must be carefully titrated to avoid the sedation that often accompanies their use. One advantage of their use is the variety of routes by which they can be administered. Rectal, oral, and IM routes each provide inherent benefits for individual situations.

The antiemetic agent ondansetron (Zofran), which is to treat GI symptoms after chemotherapy, is also used to treat postanesthesia nausea and vomiting. It is classified as a 5-hydroxytryptamine (5-HT_3) serotonin receptor antagonist, and its primary benefit is that of excellent antiemetic action without many of the side effects associated with other drugs, for instance, sedation, hypotension, and tremors. This low incidence of side effects makes it an excellent choice for outpatients. In a study of 71 young women who experienced nausea and vomiting after laparoscopic surgery, Bodner[42] compared ondansetron with a placebo. Only 51% of the patients treated with ondansetron had further symptoms, although 92% of the placebo groups were symptomatic.

Other drugs in the 5-HT_3 serotonin receptor antagonist category include granisetron, tropisetron, and dolasetron. Granisetron has been compared with droperidol. Doses are 20, 40, or 60 μg/kg, with 40 μg/kg (3 mg for a 70-kg person) being the optimal dose. When compared with droperidol, granisetron produced less postoperative sedation and drowsiness.[38]

Dolasetron in doses of 25, 50, 100, and 200 mg has been given 1 to 2 hours before surgery in clinical trials. When compared with a placebo, dolasetron 100 mg orally was found to be statistically superior to placebo (54% versus 29%).[38]

Table 20–9 lists most of the antiemetic agents and their properties. When administered with narcotics or central nervous system–sedating agents, the doses of both are often reduced to avoid additive sedative effects. As with all medications, doses must be calculated for each patient.

PROGRESSION OF CARE

The postanesthesia nurse does not merely observe but plays an active role in the patient's progress in recovery from anesthesia. The nurse

Table 20–9. Antiemetics

GROUP/DRUG	ACTION/USES	DOSAGE RANGES/ROUTES FOR ADULTS	SIDE EFFECTS/SPECIAL NOTES
Phenothiazines			
Prochlorperazine (Compazine)	Patantiemetic, anxiolytic Tranquilizer	PO 5–10 mg IM (deep) 5–10 mg Rectal 25 mg IV 5–10 mg **slowly**—use great caution to avoid hypotension	Caution with CNS depressants (reduce doses of both), drowsiness, dizziness, hypotension, restlessness, extrapyramidal symptoms. Depressed cough reflex can lead to aspiration.
Chlorpromazine (Thorazine)	Antiemetic, anxiolytic Decreases restlessness	IM (deep) 12.5–25 mg PO 10–25 mg	Caution with other CNS depressants (reduce doses of each). Use caution in cardiovascular or liver disease, asthma, emphysema, drowsiness, sedation, dizziness, faintness, decreased cough reflex, postural hypotension (keep flat for 1/2 hour after injection), extrapyramidal symptoms.
Promethazine (Phenergan)	Antiemetic, sedative, antimotion sickness, anticholinergic	IM (deep) 12.5–25 mg (reduce with CNS depressants)	Potentiates other CNS depressants, drowsiness, impaired thought patterns, tachycardia, bradycardia, hypotension, extrapyramidal symptoms, caution in patients with heart disease. **Never** give epinephrine to treat hypotension caused by promethazine because it could further lower blood pressure.
Others			
Trimethobenzamide (Tigan)	Antiemetic—depresses CTZ, sedative, weak antihistamine	PO 250 mg IM (deep) 200 mg, onset in 15 min, lasts 2–3 hr Rectal 200 mg	Drowsiness, sedation, blurred vision, hypotension, extrapyramidal symptoms, disorientation
Benzoquinamide (Emete-con)	Antiemetic Depresses CTZ	IM (preferred) 50 mg; onset in 15 min, peak 15 min, lasts 3–4 hr IV 25 mg **very slowly,** decrease dose if patient is taking pressor agent or epinephrine-like drug or in cardiac patient	Drowsiness, sedation, blurred vision, hypotension or hypertension, headache, dry mouth. Dysrhythmias (especially with IV route) include atrial fibrillation, PACs, PVCs. Elevated temperature. Flushing, hepatic metabolism.
Ondansetron (Zofran)	Antiemetic Depresses CTZ and 5-HT_3 receptor	PO 16 mg 1 hour before anesthesia induction IV 4 mg undiluted over 2–5 min	Headache, malaise, fatigue, dizziness, sedation. Constipation, diarrhea, abdominal pain. Musculoskeletal pain, chills, urine retention, hypoxia. Drugs that alter hepatic drug-metabolizing enzymes (phenobarbital or cimetidine) may alter pharmacokinetics, but no dosage adjustment is necessary.
Dolasetron mesylate (Anzemet)	Antiemetic Selective serotonin 5-HT_3 receptor antagonist	Prevention of postoperative nausea and vomiting: PO 100 mg within 2 hours prior to anesthesia induction IV 12.5 mg approximately 15 minutes before cessation of anesthesia Children (2–16 years) PO 1.2 mg/kg within 2 hours of surgery up to a maximum dose of 100 mg IV 0.35 mg/kg (up to 12.5 mg) approximately 15 minutes before cessation of anesthesia **(Injectable formula may be mixed)**	Headache, dizziness, drowsiness, arrhythmias, hypotension, hypertension, tachycardia Diarrhea, dyspepsia, abdominal pain, constipation, anorexia Oliguria, urinary retention Pruritus, rash Elevation of liver function tests, chills, fever, pain at injection site Drugs that prolong ECG intervals **Drug is not recommended for children under 2 years of age.**

***Table 20–9.* Antiemetics** *Continued*

GROUP/DRUG	ACTION/USES	DOSAGE RANGES/ROUTES FOR ADULTS	SIDE EFFECTS/SPECIAL NOTES
Droperidol (Inapsine)	Potent tranquilizer (neuroleptic agent), anxiolytic Potentiates narcotics and CNS depressants	IV 0.625–1.25 mg (reduce doses when given with narcotics or CNS depressants); onset, 3–10 min, peak 30 min, lasts 3–6 hr	Drowsiness, hypotension, anxiety, tachycardia, shivering/chills, extrapyramidal symptoms, laryngospasm, bronchospasm, hepatic metabolism.
Dimenhydrinate (Dramamine)	Antiemetic, anti–motion sickness Depressant action on hyperstimulated labyrinthine function	IM 50 mg IV (dilute) 50 mg in 10 ml slowly over at least 2 min IV infusion 50–100 mg in 500-ml solution	Drowsiness, dizziness, dry mouth, blurred vision, nervousness, restlessness, dysuria, or inability to void, thickened bronchial secretions, tachycardia.
Metoclopramide (Reglan)	Increases gastric motility (gastrokinetic agent) Dopamine antagonist in CTZ	IM 10 mg (range, 5–20), onset 0–15 min, lasts 1–2 hr IV **(slowly)** dilute 10 mg over at least 15 min; onset, 1–3 min, lasts 1–2 hr	Restlessness, drowsiness, fatigue, extrapyramidal symptoms, hypertension, hypotension. Contraindicated in epileptics, use with caution in hypertensive patients, hepatic metabolism.
Hydroxyzine (Vistaril, Atarax)	Antiemetic, anxiolytic Potentiates narcotics	IM (deep), 25–100 mg decrease up to 1/2 when given with CNS depressants (12.5–50 mg IV) **Do not give IV or SQ**	Potentiates narcotics, barbiturates and other CNS depressants. Drowsiness, dry mouth.
Diphenhydramine (Benadryl)	Anti–motion sickness Competes for H_1 receptor site	IM (deep) 10–50 mg IV 10–50 mg PO 25–50 mg	Sedation, hypotension, dizziness, disturbed coordination, thickening bronchial secretions, wheezing. Use with caution in patients with asthma. Increased intraocular pressure, CV disease.
Scopolamine (transderm Scōp)	Anti–motion sickness Antimuscarinic activity Acts on vestibular pathway and directly on vomiting center	1 patch behind the ear 4 hr before surgery, delivers 0.5 mg over 72 hours.	Dry mouth—most common side effect. Dizziness, mydriasis (dilated pupil), blurred vision, drowsiness, confusion/restlessness, bradycardia, photophobia. Avoid in people with glaucoma. Wash hands well after application to avoid getting in eyes. Instruct patient on removal and side effects if discharged with patch in place.

PO, orally, IM, intramuscular; IV, intravenous; CNS, central nervous system; CTz, chemoreception trigger zone; PAC, premature atrial contraction; PVC, premature ventricular contraction; 5-HT_3, serotonin; H_1, histamine$_1$; CV, cerebrovascular.

is the external source of encouragement, information, and appropriate practices involving ambulation and other physical aspects of activity. The nurse also monitors the progress of the patient's vital signs, reflexes, ability to move, and level of consciousness. It is expected that these parameters will consistently progress toward the patient's normal preoperative state. The operative site and any involved areas are monitored for complications. Regression in any of these areas during the immediate postanesthesia period must be aggressively evaluated and reported to the appropriate physician.

Movement and ambulation are gradual: first, elevation of the patient's head and exercise of extremities; then, sitting on the stretcher or in a recliner; eventually, ambulation. With each level of movement, the patient should be assessed for untoward effects, including hypotension, nausea, faintness, and dizziness. Should any of these occur, progress is slowed or reversed until symptoms subside.

The patient may require frequent explanations and orientation to the surroundings after receiving general anesthesia or sedating drugs. The postanesthesia nurse provides that link with reality and is integral to aiding the return of the patient's cognitive abilities and clear thought patterns. Intelligent and judicious use of analgesics and other depressant drugs is essential to avoid prolonging the period of sedation and confusion.

The nurse appropriately assesses and attends to the operative site, institutes appropriate treatments as ordered, and maintains a safe environment for the patient, including the use of universal precautions. Although most structured patient education is provided in phase II, beginning to explain postoperative instructions to the awake patient in the PACU is never inappropriate. Instructions and explanations given in this early period to people who have had sedating drugs must be repeated or reinforced in the phase II area, where the patient is more lucid and a family member or a responsible adult is available to join the discussion.

Often, the postanesthesia nurse is called on to answer questions, although the awakening patient will obviously not remember the conversation, let alone the answers. Although the nurse's response may not be remembered for the long term, a short, direct answer may relieve the patient's concerns and fears momentarily and help to reduce anxiety and fear and facilitate a smooth period of emergence.

EMOTIONAL AND PSYCHOLOGICAL SUPPORT

The patient recovering from any type of surgery and anesthesia needs the understanding and patience of a compassionate nurse. The postanesthesia nurse is the first experience with normalcy after an often frightening experience. Besides the typical fears regarding the pathology or the outcome of the surgery or because of the desire to have a parent or loved one near, the patient may be dealing with other fears related specifically to the ambulatory surgical approach: fear of going home, where, there is no nursing or medical attention; concern about the ability to handle pain at home; and apprehension about the family's ability to be supportive of postoperative needs. The nurse with an awareness of such fears can encourage a patient to express them. The patient who expresses fear of saying or doing something embarrassing or incriminating after surgery needs reassurance that the behavior was proper and will be kept confidential.

Even in the early minutes of arousal and recovery, the nurse should use the positive language and suggestions of wellness and self-sufficiency that began when the patient was being prepared for ambulatory surgery. Early family involvement is generally desirable for ambulatory patients, but the PACU may not be an appropriate place for the reunion, particularly in the main hospital PACU. Nevertheless, one way that the nurse can encourage the family approach is by drawing the family, friends, or home setting into conversation. This helps to remind the patient of home and facilitates return to normalcy, rather than focusing on the surrounding hospital environment. Fiorentini[43] studied the effects of parental visitation on children in the PACU. She found that the negative comments from families who were allowed to visit all involved the lack of space in the PACU. Although the incidence of reduced narcotic needs and length of stay were not statistically significant, a reduction in patient stress was indicated by a decrease in crying by the child.

Allowing the entire family into the PACU to remain at the bedside is not practical, but a short visit from one family member or significant other is both physically and psychologically beneficial to the patient.[44] It has been suggested that reducing the patient's anxiety and stress level enhances wound healing, and length of stay is reduced, thus reducing patient cost.[45]

Discharge from the PACU should be based first on the patient's physical recovery and safety, with consideration given to emotional and social needs. Rather than stringent adherence to the clock as an indication of patient readiness, the patient's actual physical and emotional status should be used to determine discharge time. Should the PACU stay be prolonged, a message to any waiting family or friends can help alleviate their worry about the patient's condition and, simultaneously, can relieve the patient of worry that the family is overly concerned or frightened. Some PACUs, especially those in the main hospital, use cordless phones to allow patients to speak with their family or friends if discharge is prolonged. When visitation is allowed in the PACU, other patients' privacy must be maintained.

SPECIAL NEEDS OF PATIENTS AFTER LOCAL AND REGIONAL ANESTHESIA

Depending on the individual facility's protocol, the patient who has undergone a brachial plexus, IV, periorbital, or other regional block may be cared for in the PACU.[46] It is more likely, however, that the person is transferred directly from the OR to the phase II recovery area. Most of the care for patients having these types of regional approaches is provided in the phase II area, although patients who experience complications relating to anesthesia, surgery, or exacerbation of a pre-existing medical condition are admitted to a PACU for a time. Some examples of such cases include allergic or toxic reactions to the local anesthetic, chest pain, MI, serious dysrhythmias, acute respiratory episode, pneumothorax, hemorrhage, or other situations occurring because of the invasive technique.

Patients who are admitted to a PACU unexpectedly after a complication of local or regional anesthesia may be very apprehensive and are often quite alert. Their anxiety may stem from many factors: justifiable fears of physical pain or complications, mental sequelae of local anesthesia toxicity, worry about their waiting family members, or reactions to, and fear of, the PACU environment, where critically ill patients are within their sight and hearing.

The PACU nurse may be called on to assist with regional blocks, both for surgical anesthesia and for therapeutic pain control, or sympathetic blockade. Chapter 14 contains a discussion of local and regional anesthesia and potential complications.

NURSING CARE AFTER EPIDURAL AND SPINAL ANESTHESIA

Patients having central regional blocks, specifically epidural and subarachnoid (spinal) anesthesia, are admitted to the PACU for care until the major effects of the anesthesia have passed and potential complications are less likely to occur. Untoward sequelae that can occur in that period include hypotension, tachycardia or bradycardia, hypothermia, pressure injury or unnoticed trauma to tissues, anxiety related to the loss of motor and sensory abilities, and, rarely, epidural hematoma. A period of close observation is necessary.

Spinal anesthesia is technically easier and often a less time-consuming approach than others. It is effective and adequate for many ambulatory procedures. Conversely, there are several benefits of an epidural anesthetic. The first is the anesthesiologist's ability to control the titration of medication through a continuous catheter, although the short nature of most ambulatory procedures does not demand that precise an approach. Also, an uncomplicated epidural approach (without dural puncture) does not carry the possibility of entry of foreign or infectious material into the cerebrospinal fluid (CSF).

Nursing care after these two approaches is essentially identical because of the similarity in anesthetic effects. One important difference is that postanesthesia headaches, although uncommon, are more likely to occur after a spinal approach. Barring the complication of an inadvertent dural puncture, an epidural injection does not involve entering the subarachnoid space; thus, there is no leakage of CSF to cause a headache. The following discussion pertains to both epidural and spinal anesthesia unless specific reference is made to one or the other approach.

The patient is often quite awake and aware of the surroundings on admission to the PACU. Encouragement of deep breathing to prevent hypoventilation and close observation for signs of airway or respiratory incompetence are important, especially if sedation was administered intraoperatively. Protective airway reflexes are not affected by regional anesthetic unless the patient has been given significant sedating drugs. Oxygen therapy may be ordered for the early phase of PACU recovery if the patient is shivering or sedated.

After initial assessment of the patient's vital systems, the level of anesthesia blockade is assessed by evaluating the patient's sensory and motor abilities. The reference is based on the dermatomes, areas innervated by particular spinal nerves, as illustrated in Figure 20–5. Major landmarks and their spinal nerve levels are as follows:

T4—sensation at nipple line
T10—sensation at umbilicus
L2 and L3—raising the knee
L4 and L5—flexion of the knee
S1 and S2—dorsiflexion of the foot

Having an ambulatory surgery patient with high or total spinal anesthesia in which the upper extremities or respiratory and cardiac functions are involved would be unusual. Still, this complication is possible at the time of injection as a result of

- Increased intrathecal pressure from coughing or straining
- Too rapid an injection or too large a volume of the anesthetic agent
- Positioning of the patient in a head-down inclination before the anesthetic agent has set at the intended spinal level

Initial treatment of this rare complication includes mechanical ventilation, oxygen therapy, IV fluids, vasopressors, and atropine or glycopyrrolate for treatment of bradycardia. Emotional support and appropriate interventions are continued until the effects of the anesthetic resolve and the patient's normal cardiorespiratory functions return.

Immobility related to central regional anesthesia predisposes the patient to tissue injury. Gentle passive movement of the lower extremities and periodic repositioning help prevent pressure on tissues and provide the patient with a change in position. The patient's proper body

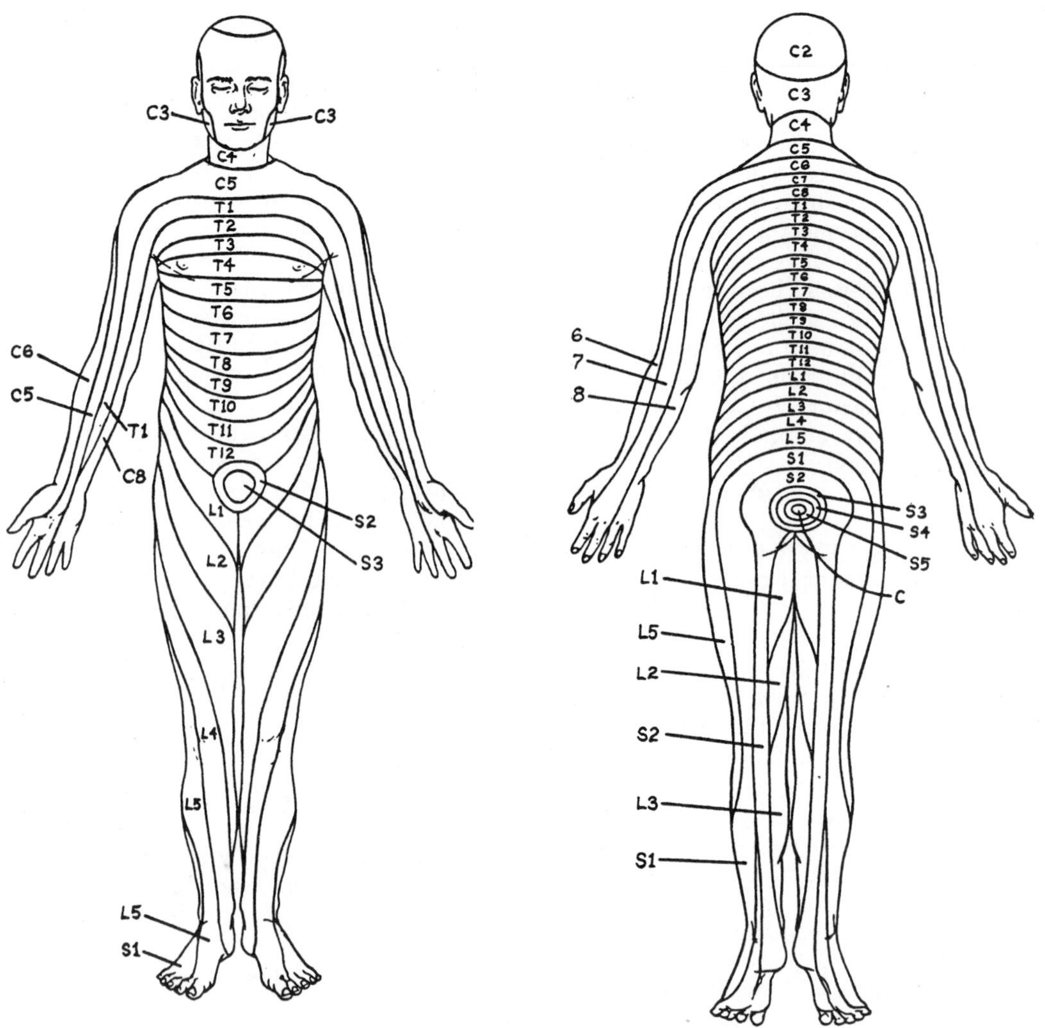

Figure 20–5. The dermatomes. (From Stewart J: Clinical Anatomy and Physiology for the Frustrated and Angry Health Professional. Miami: MedMaster, 1986, p 89.)

alignment helps prevent musculoskeletal injury and lingering muscle soreness.

The vasodilation of a large portion of the vasculature that accompanies spinal and epidural anesthesia is one of the more common untoward effects. It can lead to significant pooling of blood in the lower extremities. Arteries and arterioles in the region of the block are unable to constrict in response to lowered blood pressures; thus, the patient loses an important compensatory mechanism, and hypotension can result. Because of the patient's precarious physiologic state, the nurse should move the patient gently and slowly to avoid causing further hypotension. Elevation of the head of the stretcher should be accomplished in small increments, and blood pressure should be measured frequently during the process.

Intravenous fluids are maintained until full motor and sensory functions return. Aggressive hydration is often instituted to prevent or treat pronounced hypotension. Not only is hypotension a dangerous cardiovascular occurrence, particularly for the patient with pre-existing coronary artery disease, but it can also lead to nausea, vomiting, and faintness. The patient who has undergone spinal anesthesia may not be physically able to turn to the side to vomit without help and could aspirate vomitus, particularly if he or she is sedated. Nausea related to hypotension often responds to hydration and lowering of the head to supine. More aggressive therapy for hypotension with or without nausea is 10 to 25 mg of ephedrine, diluted and given slowly IV.

Peripheral dilation of blood vessels related to

sympathetic blockade contributes to hypothermia, and thus the patient should be kept warm. Warming should be undertaken carefully, however, because it can contribute to additional vasodilation and can promote hypotension.

Hemorrhage at the site of injection is extremely rare but particularly perilous. Internal pressure from an epidural hematoma can compromise the spinal cord, resulting in permanent neurologic damage. Patients at the greatest risk are those with coagulation defects or those who have taken anticoagulants. Rapid onset of a neurologic deficit, such as return of paralysis or paresthesia after the block has once resolved, must be reported to the anesthesiologist immediately. Another presenting symptom can be severe back pain. Quick diagnosis by myelography or computed tomography is necessary because surgical treatment is most likely to be effective if it is performed within 12 hours of the beginning of symptoms.[47]

Resolution of Anesthetic Effects

The duration of regional blocks is related to the type and the dose of anesthetic agents and to the addition of epinephrine or other vasoconstrictors, which prolong the actions of an anesthetic agent. For instance, lidocaine is a short-acting agent that generally dissipates within 90 minutes of injection. Tetracaine and bupivacaine blocks last approximately 150 minutes and are used when longer procedures are projected.[47]

After spinal or epidural anesthesia, sensation generally returns first to the areas most distal to the site of injection. The accepted progression for return of neurologic function is in reverse to the sequence in which it was lost. Some investigators have demonstrated that autonomic control returns before movement and sensation.[48] The most widely accepted sequence is that the sense of proprioception, the location of the extremity in relation to the body and stretcher, is usually the first to return.[48] After that comes the return of pressure, movement, touch, pain, sense of temperature, and finally, sympathetic functions, such as vasomotor and bladder control (Table 20–10). It follows, then, that some patients can move their legs before they can feel that they are doing so or before they sense operative pain.

Another implication has more clinical importance. Because autonomic control is the last function to return, the potential for hypotension secondary to decreased vasomotor tone can extend beyond the period that the nurse often associates with the resolution of the spinal or epidural anesthesia, that is, the return of movement and sensation. Elevation and ambulation should be cautiously approached in these patients.

Some patients may become anxious or agitated because of inability to move or feel their legs in the early period of recovery. Reassurance and diversion are usually effective in helping the patient tolerate a period of motor and sensory loss. Sedation may be necessary in the PACU if the patient is particularly anxious, but reunion with a family member or a friend who serves as support and distraction is often preferred to sedation.

Autonomic Innervation and Urinary Bladder Tone

Bladder distention may occur as a result of decreased bladder muscle tone after sympathetic blockade. The patient may exhibit restlessness, hypertension, or bradycardia and may or may not feel suprapubic pain, depending on the level

Table 20–10. **Generally Accepted Progression of the Loss and Return of Neurologic Function with Epidural or Spinal Anesthesia**

RESOLUTION OF BLOCK		INDUCTION OF BLOCK
First to return		Last to be lost
↓	Proprioception (location of the extremity in relation to the body)	↑
↓	Pressure	↑
↓	Movement	↑
↓	Touch	↑
↓	Pain	↑
↓	A sense of temperature	↑
↓	Sympathetic functions (vasomotor, bladder control)	↑
Last to return		First to be lost

of sensory blockade. Because the symptoms of bladder distention can mimic those of hypoxia, a careful differential diagnosis must be undertaken.

Thorough, periodic assessments of the bladder after major sympathetic blockade should alert the nurse to a problem. Although there is classic evidence that autonomic function (i.e., bladder tone) returns once the patient exhibits motor function of the legs, proprioception of the great toe and perianal sensory return[49]; others dispute that fact and have shown that complete return of bladder detrussor muscle tone may not occur for up to an additional 1 to 2 hours.

Treatment for bladder distention may be as simple as having the patient void, or it may require obtaining a physician's order for catheterization. Difference of opinion exists about the care of the patient with a full bladder who is unable to void in the early postanesthesia period. One choice is to insert an indwelling catheter and either hospitalize the patient or discharge the patient with the catheter in place. Another philosophy is to straight-catheterize the patient, thus ensuring that the bladder is empty before discharge, with the expectation that bladder tone will sufficiently return before subsequent bladder fullness. Either way, the patient requires specific instructions about bladder or catheter care.

Post–Dural Puncture Headache

A postspinal headache (also called post–dural puncture headache, PDPH, or post–dural puncture cephalgia) is an unpleasant side effect of spinal or epidural anesthesia. Many patients express concern or fear of central regional anesthesia primarily because of stories they have heard from family or friends regarding debilitating postanesthetic headaches. The cause is thought to be leakage of CSF through the dural puncture site. This decreases intrathecal pressure and allows traction on pain-sensitive intracranial sensors. With adequate hydration, the patient is better able to replenish CSF. Other signs of dural leakage of CSF include muscle aches in the neck, double vision, other visual disturbances, and auditory difficulties.

With the current anesthesia techniques using very small-gauge needles for subarachnoid blocks, the potential for this occurrence is small. Also, needles with rounded point bevels (Whitacre, Quincke, Sprotte) have been designed to spread or split, rather than cut, the fibers of the dura.[50] In this way, a permanent track that would allow leakage of CSF is not created. Needle gauge also closely parallels the occurrence, duration, and severity of PDPH,[50] with a higher frequency occurring in women than in men and in patients between 20 and 40 years of age.[50]

Current research indicates that requiring the patient to remain in a recumbent position for several hours after the block is of no value in preventing PDPH and is unnecessary.[1, 11] Head elevation and progressive ambulation should be gradual. However, this is more because of the propensity for hypotensive occurrences than because of a relationship to PDPH.

Although the small-gauge needles used for spinal anesthesia are not likely to promote CSF leakage, an inadvertent dural puncture with a large-bore epidural needle can predispose the patient to a significant headache. When the CSF is entered in error during an epidural technique, it is called a "wet tap." When this occurs, the practitioner may inject saline into the epidural space before removing the needle or catheter to increase epidural pressure. By reducing the difference in pressure between the intrathecal and the epidural spaces, flow of CSF into the epidural space is discouraged.[51] An epidural blood patch (which is described later) may be performed before the catheter is removed in an attempt to prevent the headache, but more often, it is a secondary intervention only after the actual diagnosis of PDPH.

A PDPH may appear within a few hours after the puncture, but one that is evident after 1 or 2 days is more typical.[1] Thus, when PDPH does occur in the ambulatory surgical patient, it is usually after discharge, even up to the 6th postoperative day. This situation can frighten the patient and complicate or delay definitive therapy. The nurse is challenged to instruct the patient appropriately before discharge to report any significant or prolonged headache to the physician without unduly frightening the patient or suggesting that a spinal headache will occur.

Pain associated with PDPH is usually occipital, but it may occur in the frontal or vertex areas or may be described as behind the eyes. It is more intense when the patient sits up, stands, moves the head, flexes the neck, or coughs.[1, 50] PDPH is relieved when pressure is placed on the abdomen. In fact, relief of pain with firm abdominal pressure while the patient is sitting or standing is considered diagnostic.[3, 51] For a persistent headache, treatment includes the use of analgesics, subdued lighting and noise, aggressive IV and oral hydration, recumbency, and use of an abdominal binder to increase pressure in the epidural venous plexus. IV caffeine may be a highly effective treatment for PDPH.[51]

Severe and unrelenting headaches may require more aggressive intervention. The injection of the patient's own blood into the epidural space surrounding the original dural puncture obliterates the puncture site with a clot and effectively stops a slow leak of CSF. This technique, called an epidural blood patch, is sometimes performed in the PACU. First, an IV line is established under aseptic technique. Once the anesthesiologist has made an epidural puncture at the level of the dual leakage, the nurse aseptically withdraws approximately 10 ml of venous blood that the anesthesiologist injects into the patient's epidural space. The needle is removed and the patient is instructed to sit up. Immediate relief of the headache usually occurs as a result of increased intrathecal pressure. Vital signs are assessed, and the epidural site is observed for signs of bleeding. The patient is then maintained supine in bed for approximately 1 hour to allow the clot to adhere firmly to the dura. During this time, the patient is observed for complications. The patient's activity at home is generally not restricted, and improvement is usually dramatic.

DOCUMENTATION OF CARE

The initial concept of ambulatory surgery called for brief documentation that would streamline nursing time, thereby cutting costs. However, the ever-increasing age and acuity of patients combined with the progressive invasiveness of ambulatory surgical procedures have altered that original approach. The current litigious climate also plays a role because defensive charting is critical to the nurse's protection in court. Therefore, the goal is to provide a method that allows comprehensive documentation of patient events, assessments, and treatments using the least amount of time and effort.

Charting formats should provide ease of documentation to accommodate the typically short ambulatory procedure times, frequent admissions, and rapid turnovers. The PACU form should allow for checklist documentation for routine care rather than narrative format. The narrative notes should focus on deviations from expected outcomes and individual patient responses to treatment and interventions. Specific descriptions of the operative site and associated information are also included in the narrative section.

DISCHARGE FROM A POSTANESTHESIA CARE UNIT

Discharge Criteria

In most facilities, the anesthesiologist is responsible for the discharge of patients from the PACU. Internal policy may require the physician's attendance for discharge at the time of readiness or may allow the postanesthesia nurse to discharge patients who meet predetermined criteria approved by the medical staff.

Before the patient leaves the PACU, certain criteria for safe discharge must be met. Written criteria should address many parameters of physical and cognitive recovery and must be appropriate to the unit or location to which the patient is transferred. For instance, the phase II area of a particular ambulatory surgery center may have only recliners in the unit and may be geared toward receiving only those patients who are ready to get out of bed. In other facilities, the phase II area may be prepared to care for patients who require continued bedrest for a time, up to 23 hours. Obviously, the patient who is being discharged directly to home from the PACU must meet more stringent criteria. In that situation, the addition of the criteria described for home readiness in a later chapter must be added to those appropriate for PACU discharge.

Numeric scoring systems provide objective methods with which the patient's condition can be evaluated and described in a variety of parameters. This scoring, which is used on admission, throughout the PACU stay, and on discharge, provides a concise way to document certain aspects of the patient's condition. Several scoring systems are in use, the most popular of which is the classic but outdated Aldrete/Kroulik Score.[52] This measures five parameters in which the patient may be given a score ranging from zero to 2. The five parameters evaluated are activity, respiration, circulation, consciousness, and color. An Aldrete score of 9 or 10 is generally required for PACU phase I discharge unless a specific physician's order preempts that policy. Certain patients may never reach an ideal score of 10 because of preexisting situations. For instance, the paraplegic or hemiplegic patient may have permanent paralysis of one or more extremities, or the person with Raynaud's disease may have persistent peripheral cyanosis. Another system, devised in the mid-1980s, includes temperature and eliminates the often subjective assessment of color. The name of this scoring system is REACT,[53] an acronym for its components, including *r*espiration, *e*nergy (movement), *a*lertness, *c*irculation, and *t*emperature.

Criticism of the Aldrete scoring system is based on the inclusion of color and blood pressure. Color is a subjective finding in patients. The surrounding wall or curtain color and the type of lighting in the PACU affect the patient's skin tone. The use of mucous membrane color to determine oxygenation level was, and is, an imprecise measurement. Table 20–11 shows an updated (modified) version of the Aldrete score that reflects the use of pulse oximetry for a more precise monitor of oxygenation status.[54, 55] Forty percent or more of the ambulatory surgery patients scheduled for surgery have only one documented preoperative blood pressure that may be artificially high as a result of anxiety about the anticipated surgery.[3]

These scoring systems do provide a method of evaluating certain factors, but they are limited and do not address many important aspects of the patient's condition, for instance, presence of nausea, vomiting, or pain; emotional status; chills or shivering; condition of the operative site or bleeding; fluid and urinary status; cognitive abilities; peripheral circulation; and in the Aldrete score, temperature. These parameters must be evaluated and considered in the decision for PACU discharge in addition to the patient's score computed in any numeric system.

After spinal or epidural anesthesia, return of strength and sympathetic innervation must be assured before ambulation. Depending on the facility policy, the patient may be discharged to a phase II unit with continued orders for bedrest or may be kept in the PACU until the spinal effects are gone and the patient is ready for ambulation. Most PACUs require that the patient have a return of movement and sensation before discharge.

Another point of view regarding the PACU discharge of the post–spinal anesthesia patient is held by some who believe that a prolonged PACU stay while return of movement or sensation is awaited is unnecessary. The absence of orthostatic hypotension must be tested for and ensured to allow for PACU discharge after spinal or epidural anesthesia. Patients can be safely discharged from the PACU if they demonstrate less than a 10% drop in mean arterial pressure in response to two tests.[54] The test consists of checking the blood pressure in both the sitting and the supine position.

For patients who are discharged to a second phase of care before return of full movement, sensation, and strength, the staff, patient, and family must be properly educated. Communication about the individual patient's status must be provided. The accepting nurse should understand the implications for care to provide a safe environment for continued progression of care.

Transfer and Report

Immediately before the patient's transfer from the PACU, the nurse completes a comprehensive assessment, noting the condition of the

Table 20–11. Aldrete's Modified Phase I Postanesthesia Recovery Score

PATIENT SIGN	CRITERION	SCORE
Activity	Able to move 4 extremities*	2
	Able to move 2 extremities*	1
	Able to move 0 extremities*	0
Respiration	Able to deep breathe and cough	2
	Dyspnea or limited breathing	1
	Apneic, obstructed airway	0
Circulation	BP ± 20% of preanesthesia value	2
	BP ± 20–49% of preanesthesia value	1
	BP ± 50% of preanesthesia value	0
Consciousness	Fully awake	2
	Arousable (by name)	1
	Nonresponsive	0
Oxygen saturation	Spo_2 > 92% on room air	2
	Requires supplemental O_2 to maintain Spo_2 > 90%	1
	Spo_2 < 90% even with O_2 supplement	0

*Voluntarily or on command.

BP, blood pressure; Spo_2, oxygen saturation as measured by pulse oximetry.

Modified from Aldrete JA: Discharge criteria. In Thomson D, Frost E (eds): Baillière's Clinical Anaesthesiology: Postanaesthesia Care. London: Baillière Tindall, 1994, pp 763–773.

operative site, the vital signs, and the patient's level of consciousness, comfort, and other appropriate parameters. The patient's skin should be cleaned to remove any antiseptic solutions that could stain clothing or irritate the skin with prolonged contact. Blood or surgical drainage should be removed from the skin for aesthetic, safety, and emotional reasons. The nurse ensures that the dressing is dry and intact and that the IV line is patent and empties all drainage containers, such as wound drainage systems and urinary drainage bags. Whenever possible, the patient's sensory aide, eyeglasses, dentures, and other personal items should be returned in order to encourage a sense of normalcy and dignity.

Transfer of patients from the PACU to the phase II unit requires the interaction and cooperation of staff members in the two units. Although the specific transfer procedure differs from one facility to another, the underlying goal is the timely and safe transport of patients so that they are able to reunite with family or friends and continue the process of recovery. The timing of the transfer is dependent on the patient's readiness and nursing care needs coupled with consideration for the availability of staff and the current patient load in the two areas.

Although conflicts can occur when two busy nursing units must depend on each other for services like transportation, transfers, and acceptance of patients, it is important that no adversarial relationship exists between the PACU and the ambulatory surgery unit. All team members should interact in a professional and mutually respectful manner. When transferring the patient to the care of nurses in the phase II recovery area, the PACU nurse should supply the accepting nurse with comprehensive information, including any medications the patient has been given, physician's orders that affect the immediate period, the patient's response to PACU interventions, any complications experienced, and any known information about the patient's waiting family and home support plans.

The transporting and accepting nurses should cooperate in settling the patient safely, and the PACU nurse should await the patient's current vital signs, as determined by the phase II nurse, before relinquishing responsibility for the patient's nursing care. Such a team effort not only promotes a safe environment for the patient but also encourages the patient's confidence in the competency and professionalism of the staff.

FOCUSING ON "SUCCESS"

Measuring the "success" of nursing care in a PACU is difficult, both in concept and in reality. What is success in postanesthesia care for the ambulatory patient? Surely, the definition is as broad as the number of people attempting to define it. One measurement might be expressed as a fourfold focus for postanesthesia nurses:

1. Being a catalyst who helps the patients to return as closely and rapidly as possible to their preoperative condition and to their families
2. Being totally attentive for potential complications and helping to avoid them whenever possible
3. Discharging each patient to the phase II unit as awake, pain free, and nausea free as possible
4. Ensuring that each patient is treated with dignity and as a person who is important and special

Anesthesia or surgical complications, excessive sleepiness, pain, and GI upset are unpleasant for any surgical patient. For the ambulatory surgery patient, these events have an extensive impact because they directly affect the time of discharge to home, plans for transportation, home care, and other family members' schedules. PACU nurses and physicians must be aware of the criteria for ultimate patient discharge for the facility and must base medical and nursing decisions on the patient's projected discharge plans, even in the early minutes of the PACU stay. The result is the perfect combination of safe, attentive physical care along with a pleasant and caring 1-day experience for ambulatory patients.

SPECIAL CONSIDERATIONS IN POSTANESTHESIA CARE UNIT CARE

Medical Support

Of particular importance to nurses practicing in an ambulatory surgery setting is the medical support that is available while patients are in the unit. Nurses often receive direction for the patient's care from both the physician who performs the procedure and the anesthesiologist involved with that patient. Individual facilities differ in the line of medical responsibility imposed during the postoperative stay, but there are some very definite statements in that regard made by the American Society of Anesthesiologists. The American Society of Anesthesiologists Standards for Postanesthesia Care approved in 1988 and amended in 1994 are presented in Table 20–12. Although these are

Table 20–12. American Society of Anesthesiologists' Standards for Postanesthesia Care

(Approved by House of Delegates on October 12, 1988 and last amended on October 19, 1994)

These Standards apply to postanesthesia care in all locations. These Standards may be exceeded based on the judgment of the responsible anesthesiologist. They are intended to encourage high-quality patient care, but cannot guarantee any specific patient outcome. They are subject to revision from time to time as warranted by the evolution of technology and practice. *Under extenuating circumstances, the responsible anesthesiologist may waive the requirements marked with an asterisk (*); it is recommended that when this is done, it should be so stated (including the reasons) in a note in the patient's medical record.*

Standard I

ALL PATIENTS WHO HAVE RECEIVED GENERAL ANESTHESIA, REGIONAL ANESTHESIA, OR MONITORED ANESTHESIA CARE SHALL RECEIVE APPROPRIATE POSTANESTHESIA MANAGEMENT

1. A Postanesthesia Care Unit (PACU) or an area which provides equivalent postanesthesia care shall be available to receive patients after anesthesia care. All patients who receive anesthesia shall be admitted to the PACU or its equivalent except by specific order of the anesthesiologist responsible for the patient's care.
2. The medical aspects of care in the PACU shall be governed by policies and procedures which have been reviewed and approved by the Department of Anesthesiology.
3. The design, equipment and staffing of the PACU shall meet requirements of the facility's accrediting and licensing bodies.

Standard II

A PATIENT TRANSPORTED TO THE PACU SHALL BE ACCOMPANIED BY A MEMBER OF THE ANESTHESIA CARE TEAM WHO IS KNOWLEDGEABLE ABOUT THE PATIENT'S CONDITION. THE PATIENT SHALL BE CONTINUALLY EVALUATED AND TREATED DURING TRANSPORT WITH MONITORING AND SUPPORT APPROPRIATE TO THE PATIENT'S CONDITION.

Standard III

UPON ARRIVAL IN THE PACU, THE PATIENT SHALL BE RE-EVALUATED AND A VERBAL REPORT PROVIDED TO THE RESPONSIBLE PACU NURSE BY THE MEMBER OF THE ANESTHESIA CARE TEAM WHO ACCOMPANIES THE PATIENT.

1. The patient's status on arrival in the PACU shall be documented.
2. Information concerning the preoperative condition and the surgical/anesthetic course shall be transmitted to the PACU nurse.
3. The member of the Anesthesia Care Team shall remain in the PACU until the PACU nurse accepts responsibility for the nursing care of the patient.

Standard IV

THE PATIENT'S CONDITION SHALL BE EVALUATED CONTINUALLY IN THE PACU.

1. The patient shall be observed and monitored by methods appropriate to the patients' medical condition. Particular attention should be given to monitoring oxygenation, ventilation, and circulation. During recovery from all anesthetics, a quantitative method of assessing oxygenation such as pulse oximetry shall be employed in the initial phase of recovery.* This is not intended for application during the recovery of the obstetrical patient in whom regional anesthesia was used for labor and vaginal delivery.
2. An accurate written report of the PACU period shall be maintained. Use of an appropriate PACU scoring system is encouraged for each patient on admission, at appropriate intervals prior to discharge, and at the time of discharge.
3. General medical supervision and coordination of patient care in the PACU should be the responsibility of an anesthesiologist.
4. There shall be a policy to assure the availability in the facility of a physician capable of managing complications and providing cardiopulmonary resuscitation for patients in the PACU.

Standard V

A PHYSICIAN IS RESPONSIBLE FOR THE DISCHARGE OF THE PATIENT FROM THE POSTANESTHESIA CARE UNIT.

1. When discharge criteria are used, they must be approved by the Department of Anesthesiology and the medical staff. They may vary depending upon whether the patient is discharged to a hospital room, to the ICU, to a short stay unit, or home.
2. In the absence of the physician responsible for the discharge, the PACU nurse shall determine that the patient meets the discharge criteria. The name of the physician accepting responsibility for discharge shall be noted on the record.

*Refer to *Standards of Post Anesthesia Nursing Practice 1992* published by the ASPAN, for issues of nursing care.

From American Society of Anesthesiologists. Standards for Post Anesthesia Care. Park Ridge, IL: Published by Author, 1994.

medical guidelines, they are included in this text because of their implications for PACU nurses.

Quality Improvement Practices

Addressing quality-of-care issues in their daily work setting is important for all PACU nursing staff members. Involvement in ongoing clinical studies and audits can identify valuable trends and information that affect current and future patient care. The postanesthesia period is ripe with topics for investigation (Table 20–13).

An important issue to consider in any quality improvement study is its actual usefulness. Will the results tell the staff something that is helpful in determining future change in nursing care plans or in nursing or medical management? Will the study provide valuable statistical data that will influence staffing or productivity? Is the study in question a paper shuffle to pacify a certifying or licensing agency? The latter is the least desirable motivating factor. Other members of the anesthesia and surgical team can and should be involved in multidisciplinary studies.

Table 20–13. **Topics for Quality Improvement Study in the Postanesthesia Care Unit**

Topics
Administration of antihypertensives
Administration of antidysrhythmics
Untoward drug reactions
Code situations and outcomes
Arrival of intubated ambulatory surgical patients
Incomplete report to PACU nurse
Unexpected admission to PACU nurse
Unexpected admission to PACU after local or regional anesthesia
Unanticipated intraoperative change to general anesthesia
Incidence of shivering and response to therapeutic interventions
Radiologic exposure in PACU
Incidence and treatment of nausea/vomiting
Incidence and treatment of pain
Return to surgery for second procedure
Antibiotic therapy—cost studies, allergic reactions, proper dilution, and labeling
Postoperative sequelae related to intraoperative tourniquet
Infiltrations/phlebitis of veins
Length of PACU stay related to anesthetic approach
Time studies in relation to transfer to phase II
Response of physicians to requests/needs of postanesthesia staff
Response of patients having family members allowed in PACU

PACU, postanesthesia care unit.

The staff nurse should look at the overall quality improvement process as a challenge to improve the care rendered on a day-to-day basis. Rather than perceive a quality improvement program as a nuisance, the nurse is called on to think of the provision of quality as a professional duty to all patients. Quality-of-care issues then become a continuous state of mind rather than a periodic task. A more comprehensive discussion is provided in Chapter 8.

The Postanesthesia Care Unit as a Treatment and Anesthesia Site

Depending on the policies and the physical setup of the ambulatory surgery center, the patient may be taken to the PACU for the administration of local or regional anesthesia before surgery, particularly if sedation will be required during the local anesthetic injection. The PACU is an excellent location because it is fully equipped with ECG and blood pressure monitors, oximetry, oxygen, suction, and emergency equipment. The patient who will be unconscious during local anesthesia injection must be afforded both a monitored environment and the attention of anesthesia and nursing personnel.

Often, the PACU in the ambulatory unit is also used as the site for therapeutic procedures. Pain clinic procedures are prime examples and might include epidural steroid injections, stellate ganglion blocks, and other sympathetic blocks. Electroconvulsive shock therapy, blood transfusions, and chemotherapy are other examples. Litwack,[3] in fact, identified the PACU acronym as sometimes being "*p*ut *a*ll you *c*an in the *u*nit." The diverse nature of such procedures stretches the nurses' versatility and accommodation. Care must be taken to provide staff for vigilant attention to postanesthesia patients and for those undergoing special procedures within the PACU. Separation of these two patient populations is desirable.

"Be prepared" must be the motto for the postanesthesia nurse. The nurse must be prepared and attentive when assisting with any regional anesthesia or invasive treatment and must be alert to the potential complications of local anesthesia, including toxic and allergic reactions, and should be prepared to institute appropriate emergency procedures if they occur. The basic principles of ABCD (*a*irway, *b*reathing, *c*irculation, and *d*rugs) apply. All necessary items and supplies should be prepared or gathered before any procedure or anesthetic administration. The PACU nurse who is assisting assesses the patient's vital signs and physical and emotional status; reviews the patient's history (particularly allergies and previous anesthetic experiences); and explains to the patient what to expect and what will be expected during the procedure. Positioning may be difficult or uncomfortable for the patient to maintain during the procedure, so the nurse is often called on to help the patient assume and sustain the correct position. This may require physical support or verbal encouragement and instructions.

The nurse plays a variety of roles during invasive procedures. First, the nurse is the physician's assistant, who may be required to secure further supplies, hold drapes or solutions, move equipment, lights, or the patient, and perform other duties. Another role is that of a patient supporter. Whenever possible, the nurse should be within the patient's line of vision to provide emotional support. The nurse is primarily a provider who monitors vital signs and assesses the patient's overall responses. Sometimes, the nurse is the only person who is able to visualize the patient as a whole because the physician is concentrating on the procedure and may not be in a position to see the patient's face. In this role, the nurse may identify early signs of untoward reactions to the procedure or drugs being administered. Finally, the nurse documents the procedure and the patient's responses.

The Physician's Office as a Postanesthesia Setting

Despite the physical setting, the patient recovering from any anesthesia method deserves and requires a fully staffed and equipped postanesthesia recovery site. Whether it is general, regional, topical, or local, when anesthesia is administered in the physician's office, there is no less chance of complications than in the hospital setting. Administration of anesthesia to inherently poor-risk patients is avoided in an office setting. This careful selection process may help to decrease the occurrence of serious complications in a physician's office. However, unexpected complications, such as toxicity, allergic reaction, laryngospasm, respiratory depression, cardiopulmonary sequelae, and hemorrhage, are always possible with any patient, in any setting.

The office-based nurse should consider three separate issues before assuming postanesthesia responsibility for patients. First, does the nurse possess the knowledge, experience, and skills to identify and intercede in complications associated with anesthesia? Second, is the office fully stocked with the drugs, supplies, and equipment needed to address serious complications promptly? Finally, are knowledgeable and adequate staff available for assisting if such an untoward occurrence happens? Every nurse should be concerned with these issues and should seriously consider the danger and liability of practicing in a setting that has not provided for an adequate emergency response.

Staffing considerations and policies of the physician's office may find a single nurse responsible for preparing the patient, assisting with surgery, and settling the patient in another area after surgery. When other surgical cases are to follow, that nurse may be required to leave the postanesthesia patient in the care of a nonprofessional peer or the patient's family member. Obviously, the patient who has been given a general anesthetic cannot be placed in nonprofessional care until he or she has sufficiently recovered, but even a local injection or a regional block can cause untoward symptoms that require immediate intervention. Staffing should be provided to allow sufficient attention to each patient before, during, and after the procedure.

If the office-based nurse does not have experience with, or sufficient knowledge of, postanesthesia nursing care, educational courses and texts that can provide that information are available. Another way to gain confidence and experience is to spend time in a nearby PACU as an observer or an intern.[56] Physician-office–based nurses should be certified in basic life support. Advanced cardiac life support or its equivalent is considered essential nursing preparation[5] in all phase I PACU settings.

Emergency equipment, a plan for obtaining blood products, and a predetermined system for securing outside help are essential. It is recommended that a local ambulance company be contacted to discuss the office location and the types of emergencies that might necessitate an ambulance response. The physician should also have an agreement with a nearby hospital for acceptance of emergency admissions.

Preparedness is the key work for the office-based nurse. Serious complications may seem remote and, as such, may not be consciously considered in day-to-day operations. The unfortunate truth was clearly brought to light in one office setting when a healthy woman of 36, the mother of two small children, underwent a breast augmentation. She suffered a toxic reaction from a local anesthetic agent injected at the incisional site and experienced a cardiac arrest. Resuscitation attempts were unsuccessful. Such a devastating occurrence may not be avoidable because no one has future vision, but the nurse can surely increase the chance of a successful outcome through vigilance and preparedness of the setting and the adequacy of emergency skills.

References

1. Drain C: The Post Anesthesia Care Unit: A Critical Care Approach to Post Anesthesia Nursing. Philadelphia: WB Saunders, 1994.
2. Aker J: Immediate care in the postoperative period. Curr Rev Postanesth Nurses 16:146–156, 1994.
3. Litwack K: Post Anesthesia Care Nursing. St. Louis: Mosby, 1991.
4. Perry K: Increasing patient satisfaction: Simple ways to increase the effectiveness of interpersonal communication in the PACU. J Postanesth Nurs 9:153–156, 1996.
5. American Society of Perianesthesia Nurses: ASPAN Standards of Perianesthesia Nursing Practice. Thorofare, NJ: ASPAN, 1998.
6. Feeley T: The design and staffing of a modern post anesthesia care unit. Curr Rev Postanesth Nurses 15:129–136, 1993.
7. Joint Commission on Accreditation of Healthcare Organizations: 2000–2001 Comprehensive Accreditation Manual for Ambulatory Care. Oakbrook Terrace, IL: Published by Author, 1999.
8. Ignatavicius D, Workman M, Mishler M: Medical Surgical Nursing: A nursing process approach, 2nd ed. Philadelphia, WB Saunders, 1995.
9. Kahn R: Approaching common problems in the PACU. Curr Reviews for Postanesth Nurses 19:161–168, 1996.
10. Omoigui S: The Anesthesia Drug Handbook, 2nd ed. St. Louis, Mosby, 1995.
11. Jacobsen W: Manual of Post Anesthesia Care. Philadelphia: WB Saunders, 1992.
12. Grove T. Management of problems in the PACU: Part II. Curr Rev Postanesth Nurses 18:9–16, 1996.
13. Nachman J: Pulse oximetry: History, technical aspects and clinical considerations. Curr Rev Postanesth Nurses 16:73–80, 1994.
14. Domino K: Anesthetic management in the patient with chronic obstructive pulmonary disease. Curr Rev Postanesth Nurses 18:25–36, 1996.
15. Maree S: Aspiration prophylaxis: An update. Curr Rev Postanesth Nurses 16:61–72, 1994.
16. Reed C: Care of postoperative patients with pulmonary edema. J Perianesth Nurses 11:164–169, 1996.
17. Aker J: Neuromuscular relaxants: A primer. Curr Rev Postanesth Nurses 17:113–124, 1995.
18. Einhorn G, Chant P: Postanesthesia care unit dilemmas: Prompt assessment and treatment. J Postanesth Nurs 9:28–33, 1994.
19. Callahan L: The effect of surgical stress on postoperative care of the patient. Curr Rev Postanesth Nurses 15:129–136, 1994.
20. Wetchler BV (ed): Anesthesia for Ambulatory Surgery, 2nd ed. Philadelphia: JB Lippincott, 1991.
21. NDH: Nursing 97 Drug Handbook. Springhouse, PA: Springhouse Corporation, 1997.
22. Callahan L: Anesthesia for electroconvulsive therapy. Curr Rev Postanesth Nurses 15:9–16, 1993.
23. Dubin D: Rapid Interpretation of ECG. St. Louis, Mosby-Year Book. 1996.
24. Biddle C: Should we really be "banking" on autologous blood? Curr Rev Postanesth Nurses 17:149–156, 1996.
25. Heres E, Gravlee G: Approaches and techniques to minimize blood transfusions. Curr Rev Postanesth Nurses 17:45–76, 1996.
26. Krenzischek DA, Frank SM, Kelly S: Forced-air warming versus routine thermal care and core temperature measurement sites. J Postanesth Nurs 10:69–78, 1995.
27. Ciufo D, Dice S, Coles C: Rewarming hypothermic postanesthesia patients: A comparison between a water coil warming blanket and a forced-air warming blanket. J Postanesth Nurs 10:155–158, 1995.
28. Vogelsang J, Hayes S: Stadol attenuates postanesthesia shivering. J Postanesth Nurs 4:222–227, 1989.
29. Grove TM: Management of problems in the post anesthesia care unit: Part I. Curr Rev Postanesthesia Nurses 18:1–8, 1996.
30. Knowles R: Standardization of pain management in the postanesthesia care unit. J Perianesth Nurs 11:390–398, 1996.
31. Dixon CL: Pain management in the recovery room. Curr Rev Postanesth Nurses 15:153–160, 1993.
32. Sullivan LM: Factors influencing pain management: A nursing perspective. J Postanesth Nurs 9:83–90, 1994.
33. Salerno E: Race, culture, and medications: Pharmacolgenetic variations. J Emerg Nurs 21:560–562, 1995.
34. Mendelson L: Pain management for ambulatory surgery. J Postanesth Nurs 3:109–113, 1988.
35. Alexander C, Wetchler B, Thompson R: Infiltration of the mesosalpinx with bupivacaine 0.5% effectively relieves pain following laparoscopic tubal sterilization. Third Annual Symposium on Anesthesia for Ambulatory Surgery, Williamsburg, VA, 1985.
36. Bosek V: The role of non-steroidal anti-inflammatory agents in perioperative pain therapy. Curr Rev Postanesth Nurses 17:133–140, 1995.
37. Wetchler BV: Anesthesia for Ambulatory Surgery. Philadelphia: JB Lippincott, 1991.
38. Kovac AL: The difficult postoperative patient with nausea and/or vomiting. Curr Rev Perianesth Nurses 19:25–36, 1997.
39. Watcha MF, White PF: Postoperative nausea and vomiting: Its etiology, treatment, and prevention. Anesthesiology 77:162–284, 1992.
40. Nachman JA: Postoperative nausea and vomiting. Curr Rev Postanesth Nurses 15:37–44, 1993.
41. Anderson R, Crohg K: Pain as a major cause of postoperative nausea. Can Anaesth Soc J 23:336, 1976.
42. Bodner M, White P: Antiemetic efficacy of ondansetron after outpatient laparoscopy. Anesth Analg 73:250–254, 1991.
43. Saga-Rumley SA: Intravenous Regional Anesthesia (IRA). Current Rev Perianesth Nurses 19:65–76, 1997.
44. Fiorentini SE: Evaluation of a new program: Pediatric parental visitation in the postanesthesia care unit. J Postanesth Nurs 8:249–256, 1993.
45. Poole EL: The effects of postanesthesia care unit visits on anxiety in surgical patients. J Postanesth Nurs 8:386–394, 1993.
46. Frost EAM: Post Anesthesia Care Unit: Current Practices, 2nd ed. St. Louis, CV Mosby, 1990.
47. Kang SB, Rudrud L, Nelson W, Baier D: Postanesthesia nursing care for ambulatory surgery patients post-spinal anesthesia. J Postanesth Nurs 9:101–106, 1994.
48. Pflug A, Aasheim G, Foster C: Sequence of return of neurological function and criteria for safe ambulation

following subarachnoid block (spinal anesthetic). Can Anesth Soc J 25:133, 1978.
49. Axelsson K, Mollefors K, Olsson J, et al: Bladder function and spinal anesthesia. Acta Anaesth Scand 29:315, 1985.
50. Mulroy M: Local and regional anesthesia. In White P (ed): Ambulatory Anesthesia and Surgery. London: WB Saunders, 1997.
51. Aldrete J, Kroulik D: A postanesthetic recovery score. Anesth Analg 49:924–933, 1970.
52. Reiser LS: Regional anesthesia: PACU considerations. Curr Rev Postanesth Nurses 20:177–176, 1993.
53. Fraulini K, Murphy P: REACT: A new system for measuring postanesthesia recovery. Nursing 84, April: 101–102, 1984.
54. Marley RA, Moline BM: Patient discharge from the ambulatory setting. J Perianesth Nurs 11:39–49, 1996.
55. Aldrete JA: Discharge criteria. In Thomson D, Frost E (eds): Baillieres Clinical Anaesthesiology—Postanaesthesia Care. London: Bailliere Tindall, 1994, pp 763–773.
56. Bauer J: Who is that new nurse? J Perianesth Nurs 11:374, 1996.
57. Brown E: Heart drug still used for wrong—and potentially dangerous—reasons. Med Update 20:2, 1997.

Chapter 21

Progressive Postanesthesia Care: Phase II Recovery

Shauna Smith

Things which matter most must never be at the mercy of things which matter least.

—Johann Wolfgang von Goethe

As the patient progresses and no longer requires the intensive nursing care provided in a postanesthesia care unit (PACU), an operating room (OR), or another procedure room, a second phase of recovery is appropriate in which a different focus of care is emphasized. In many facilities, the area is called the "discharge unit," although it serves many other functions. There are many names given to such units, for instance, *step down*, *sit up*, and *progressive care*. In this chapter, *Phase II* is used to describe the area.

The Phase II area of an ambulatory surgery center (ASC) may be a separate unit used solely for the care of awake patients nearing discharge. Most freestanding centers are designed with dedicated Phase II units that function in this manner. In many hospital-based units, the Phase II area is often synonymous with the ASC as a whole because patients are admitted there preoperatively, then cared for after surgery by the same nurses in a multipurpose setting. Patients may undergo certain special procedures or treatments on an ASC unit or go to an operating room or other special departments for procedures. Thus, it is often difficult to isolate Phase II as a separate function or area in many ASCs.

This chapter deals with the use of Phase II as a setting for the aftercare of ambulatory surgery patients. Readers are encouraged to apply the ideas and information presented to their individual work settings and to apply information in the previous chapter (Chapter 20) regarding PACU care.

A major characteristic of the department lies in its versatility as a nursing unit. Patients arrive in a Phase II area from a variety of places: from the PACU, from the OR, and from specialty departments such as radiology, endoscopy, and the cardiovascular laboratory. Preoperative patients arrive from home for preparations before surgery and from other hospital departments when the ASC is used for special procedures. This varied activity and patient population involves a constant turnover of short-term patients with a variety of nursing care needs.

In addition to postoperative care of patients, many ASCs use this multifunctional department as a primary care setting for procedures such as diagnostic or therapeutic lumbar puncture, pain clinic treatments, laser therapy, liver biopsy, chemotherapy, antibiotic and blood administration, electroconvulsive shock therapy (ECT), bronchoscopy, and endoscopy. These special procedures are discussed in Chapter 38.

Nurses who function well in this demanding

environment characteristically are organized, energetic, versatile, and independent thinkers. They must possess common sense and work efficiently and independently. A nurse with a positive attitude that can be combined with physical and emotional support gives the patient confidence, comfort, and understanding of his or her recovery needs. The Phase II nurse should have previous medical–surgical nursing experience, strong teaching skills, a basic understanding of anesthetic agents and their side-effects, and a caring attitude. Because most of the patients in this area will be going home to continue their recuperation without the advantage of nursing or medical supervision, Phase II nurses must have strong clinical assessment skills and expertise in teaching and can be relied on to heed details that may affect patient recovery at home.

Although a Phase II area cannot be termed a critical care area in the strict sense, patients there are often in a delicate physiologic state after anesthesia and invasive procedures. They can have complications and deteriorate without warning. A critical care background in a PACU, a surgical intensive care unit (SICU), or a cardiac care unit (CCU) is a definite advantage for the nurse in this department.

Educational requirements for the ASC nurse include a basic arrhythmia interpretation and treatment course and ongoing certification in cardiopulmonary resuscitation (basic life support [BLS]). The nurse must have a knowledge of the policies and procedures of the ASC and should be expected to attend general nursing in-service programs; infection control lectures; meetings and presentations pertinent to the practice of ambulatory surgery; and presentations on fire, electrical, and disaster safety. Because of the diversity and responsibility of primary patient care and assessment for discharge, the care for each patient should be provided by or directly supervised by a registered nurse (RN). Licensed practical nurses (LPNs) and nursing assistants can be used as assistants to RNs.

All staff members must have a thorough orientation to procedures and policies of the unit to allow them to respond independently to most situations without the need to seek advice or direction from other busy staff members. This does not mean that collaboration should not occur, only that nurses in the unit should be able to work independently. Consistency in documentation practices allows staff members to identify current patient needs and to share responsibilities in patient care.

EQUIPMENT AND ENVIRONMENTAL CONCERNS

An ASC should be efficient and functional as well as visually appealing to patients and their families. Patient needs in a Phase II area require the availability of recliners, beds or stretchers, bathrooms, dressing areas, nourishment and medication stations, storage for surgical supplies and equipment, an emergency equipment area, and a clerical area for charting and other paperwork. There should be a means of summoning help in all patient locations. These and other functions often are addressed in decorative and camouflaged ways to allow the ASC to remain visually appealing, for example, with wallpaper and paneled cabinets, hidden electronic controls and oxygen and suction panels, and privacy screens instead of ceiling-hung cloth curtains.

"Noise can be a most noxious stressor"[1] to recovering patients and should be controlled. This can be accomplished by design during construction of new buildings. In existing units, installing carpeting and wall fabrics, lowering ceilings, placement of live or silk plants, or a continuous running water fountain for "white" noise can prove beneficial to patients.

Progressive facilities are pleasing to the eye, comfortable settings for the patients and visitors using them. Sufficient space to allow visitors to rejoin the patient is important in planning ASCs. This supports the family-oriented philosophy and allows the responsible adult caring for the patient at home to take part in the patient's care and discharge instructions. Figure 21–1 illustrates the family-oriented setting and decorative appeal of one freestanding center.

The needs of special patient groups should be considered in the planning and management of a Phase II unit. Provisions must be made for appropriate isolation of patients with communicable diseases. Other patients may require or prefer a private area for emotional, social, or aesthetic reasons. A separate area for postoperative care of children and their parents is beneficial both for them and for other recovering adult patients. This separation allows the child to cry, talk, or play without reproach from adult patients who may want a quieter environment. It also spares the children and parents from seeing unpleasant situations occurring with other patients. Recovering children often want to be held by their parents. Rocking recliners can be soothing to child and parent while conveying a homelike atmosphere as well.

The physical layouts of ASCs are widely di-

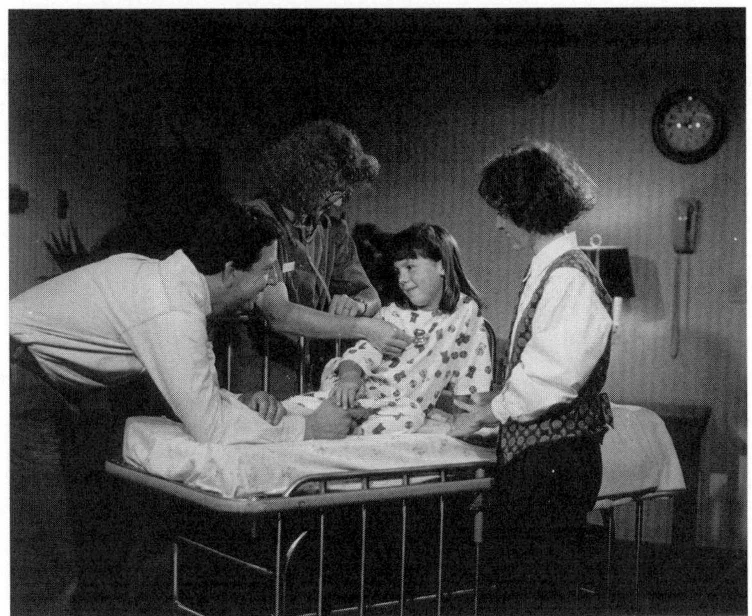

Figure 21–1. The Phase II area provides patients with both function and beauty in this unit decorated with silk and live plants, gentle colors, and overstuffed furniture. The soothing sounds of a small water fountain provide audio relief in the pediatric area. (With permission from Idaho Falls Surgical Center, Idaho Falls, Idaho.)

vergent from one facility to another. Some have private and semiprivate rooms in Phase II areas that are furnished with recliners or beds. Beds provide a more comfortable setting for patients who are expected to stay in the unit for an extended period, but they do not encourage activity or project the sense of wellness intended in an ASC and should be used with discretion.

Some ASCs have small patient rooms with stretchers, rather than beds, for recovery. This setup provides privacy and more comfort than a recliner, but still is seen by the patient as a transition to home and his or her own bed. In this more private environment, patients and family may find it easier to ask questions about postoperative care. Dressing changes and other medical activities, such as catheter care, can be demonstrated freely. Because the patients are already on stretchers, they can be moved quickly in case of emergency.

In many ASCs, a number of recliners often are arranged in one large community room. This setting enhances the sense of normalcy and encourages patients to socialize with those around them. However, privacy can be difficult or nonexistent unless curtains or screens are drawn. Even with barriers, sounds and odors may penetrate the entire room. One method of providing for patient privacy is the use of a nearby designated area for dressing, checking operative sites, and explaining personal instructions. Bathrooms should be available nearby, with a nurse call bell and a door that can be opened from the outside at all times. In a Phase II unit that is furnished solely with recliners, a stretcher should be quickly accessible for any emergency situation that requires the patient to be placed recumbent or rapidly transferred back to the PACU or the OR.

Equipment and supplies required on this unit are diverse to address the patients' medical, surgical, and nursing care needs. The American Society of PeriAnesthesia Nurses (ASPAN) Standards of Perianesthesia Nursing Practice, Resource 5, "Recommended Equipment for Preanesthesia Phase, PACU Phase I and II,"[2] is a good starting point for planning (Table 21–1). A method for replenishing and ensuring the availability of all necessary supplies should be in place. Phase II units in which invasive procedures are performed require the availability of equipment for those procedures and related emergencies.

Safekeeping and Return of Patient Valuables

In a Phase II unit, the nurse must ensure that all belongings are returned to the patient. Lockers may be used for securing patient belongings, or personal items and clothing may remain on the stretcher to accompany the patient throughout the transfer from one department to another. Religious medals or other valuables that have accompanied the patient to the OR should be reported to the Phase II nurse so that they are not discarded unintentionally with the linen.

Table 21–1. American Society of PeriAnesthesia Nurses (ASPAN) Standards of Perianesthesia Nursing Practice, 1998: From Resource 5, Recommended Equipment for Preanesthesia Phase, PACU Phase I and Phase II

RECOMMENDED EQUIPMENT FOR PHASE II PACU

1. Each patient care unit will be equipped with the following:
   a. Means to deliver oxygen
   b. Constant and intermittent suction
   c. Means to monitor blood pressure
   d. Adjustable lighting
   e. Capacity to ensure patient privacy
   f. Means of monitoring patient temperature.
2. An EKG monitor and pulse oximeter will be readily available for use in Phase II PACU.
3. A bag-valve mask, adult and pediatric, must be readily available at all times.
4. A means to monitor patient temperature will be available. Supplies to handle a malignant hyperthermia crisis must be readily accessible. These supplies should include:
   a. Means to deliver 100% oxygen
   b. Dantrolene
   c. Mannitol
   d. Bicarbonate
   e. Antidysrhythmic agents
   f. Cool IV fluids and irrigants
   g. External cooling methods.
5. A method of calling for assistance in emergency situations shall be provided.
6. An emergency cart will be in Phase II PACU at all times.
7. A defibrillator with adult and pediatric paddles must be readily available.
8. Stock medications should include the following:
   a. Antibiotics
   b. Antiemetics
   c. Anesthesia reversal agents
   d. Analgesics, opioids, and nonopioids.
9. IV supplies shall include:
   a. Various types of solutions
   b. Various types of intravenous catheters
   c. Various types of IV tubing
   d. IV dressing supplies per hospital protocol.
10. Stock supplies should include:
   a. Dressings
   b. Facial tissues
   c. Gloves
   d. Bedpans and urinals
   e. Syringes and needles
   f. Emesis basin
   g. Patient linens
   h. Alcohol swabs/wipes
   i. Ice bags
   j. Tongue blades
   k. Foley insertion supplies
   l. Personal protective equipment
   m. Access to latex-free supplies and equipment.
11. A means to safely transport patients from phase II PACU.

EKG, electrocardiogram; IV, intravenous; PACU, postanesthesia care unit.

Reprinted with permission of the American Society of PeriAnesthesia Nurses (ASPAN): Standards of Perianesthesia Nursing Practice 1998. Thorofare, NJ: ASPAN, 1998, pp 36–37.

The safekeeping of prostheses is especially important to patients. The return of hearing aids, eyeglasses, breast and leg prostheses, dentures, and wigs are often top priorities for patients, for both function and dignity. Their early return usually is appreciated. If the patient is unable to use a particular sensory aid postoperatively, the staff should ensure that the patient receives that item before discharge.

When valuables are returned postoperatively, the medical record should reflect that the patient has received them before discharge. Some facilities require the responsible adult (or patient who is not sedated) to sign a statement that all valuables have been received. Quite appropriately, the patient's physical status and concerns relating to the surgery and anesthesia are more important to the patient and family in an early postoperative period than thoughts about belongings. These concerns and the lingering sedative and amnesic effects of medications can cloud the patient's memory of receiving valuables before discharge, and thus, specific documentation identifying what was given and to whom can prove very helpful.

POLICIES AND PROCEDURES

As in all nursing departments, a Phase II area must have specific policies and procedures for guidance of nursing care. The policy manual should be available within the unit for ease of referral. It should be reviewed in its entirety by each nurse at least annually, and the review should be documented. Each facility must prepare policies and procedures that address specific patient needs within the unit and community and that complement the philosophy of the individual ASC.

The medical department policy regarding the responsibilities of surgeons and anesthesiologists should be communicated to nurses in the Phase II unit. With the advent of ambulatory surgery, anesthesiologists are playing a more active role in the aftercare of many surgical patients and often have the primary responsibility for decisions such as medicating and discharging ambulatory surgery patients. Frequently, an anesthesiologist is the medical director of the ASC.

Accrediting bodies such as the Joint Commission on Accreditation of Healthcare Organizations (JCAHO)[3] and the Accreditation Association for Ambulatory Health Care (AAAHC)[4] state that a physician or other licensed independent practitioner who is familiar with the patient should be present or immediately available until all patients operated on each day have been evaluated and discharged. National leaders in ambulatory anesthesia go one step further. Wetchler, for example, notes that it is in both the patient's and the anesthesiologist's best interest for the anesthesiologist to remain in the facility until all patients for the day have been discharged. The anesthesiologist must assess whether the patient has recovered from the anesthesia sufficiently to return home to continue to recover and be able to seek help should an unexpected complication arise.[5]

Occasionally, serious or even life-threatening situations call for immediate interventions. If the surgeon or anesthesiologist is not immediately available, an alternate plan should be in effect. Emergency protocols (standing orders) that are initiated by the nursing staff must have been approved by the governing medical body of the ASC before their enactment by nursing personnel. When these orders are used, a copy must be placed in the patient's medical record and signed by the attending physician as soon as possible. This system allows the nurse to respond immediately to the patient's emergency needs.

Staffing needs throughout the day depend on a variety of factors, such as patients' ages, medical conditions, and educational requirements; type of procedures; the day's mix of anesthesia approaches; the number of primary procedures being done in the ASC; and the projected length of recovery periods. Staffing should address the peak periods of Phase II admissions and discharges. A suggested nurse-to-patient ratio is provided in Resource 3 of the ASPAN Standards of Perianesthesia Nursing Practice[4] (Table 21–2).

In many facilities, those patients who are not ready to be discharged at the Phase II unit's usual closing time are transferred to in-house status or temporarily are cared for on a different designated nursing unit until discharge. In other facilities, Phase II nursing staff members remain

***Table 21–2.* American Society of PeriAnesthesia Nurses (ASPAN) Standards of Perianesthesia Nursing Practice, 1998: From Resource 3, Patient Classification—Phase II**

Class 1:3	One Nurse to Three Patients a. Over 5 years within 1/2 hour of procedure/discharge from phase I b. 5 years of age and under within 1/2 hour of procedure discharge from phase I with family present
Class 1:2	One Nurse to Two Patients a. 5 years of age and under without family or support staff present b. Initial admission of patient postprocedure
Class 1:1	One Nurse to One Patient a. Unstable patient of any age requiring transfer

*Two competent personnel, one of whom is an RN, are present whenever a patient is recovering in Phase II. An RN must be present at all times in Phase II.

Reprinted with permission of the American Society of PeriAnesthesia Nurses (ASPAN): Standards of Perianesthesia Nursing Practice 1998. Thorofare, NJ: ASPAN, 1998, p 28.

until all patients have been discharged. Staffing patterns are dependent on these and other variables.

PATIENT CARE GOALS

A Phase II unit provides care for patients and families who have experienced a period of significant stress relating to surgery and anesthesia. In light of that fact and the patients' physical and emotional needs, the following unit goals often prevail:

1. To provide close assessment of and attention to the patient's physical, emotional, and educational needs in the postoperative period.
2. To provide an environment and personnel who are prepared for emergency interventions at all times.
3. To provide family-oriented care that stresses the concept of wellness and acknowledges the integral relationship of the patient and family or other supporting adult.
4. To encourage the patient toward as much self-sufficiency as possible, given the type of surgery and anesthesia performed.
5. To respect the patient's right to confidentiality, privacy, and respectful, compassionate nursing care.
6. To maintain accurate records of patient-related care and environmental preparedness.
7. To interact with physicians and other health-care providers in a professional manner that results in high-quality patient care.
8. To provide patients and families with a resource for questions, comments, and nursing information during their stay and in the immediate period after discharge.

GENERAL NURSING CARE

The patient has physical, emotional, social, and educational needs during this subacute recovery period. Careful monitoring is needed to identify and, hopefully, avoid potential emergency occurrences. Patients in this unit already have regained or have never lost their basic physiologic protective reflexes. Barring complications that affect their cardiovascular or respiratory status, they are generally ambulatory and able to take part in their own care and recovery process.

Nursing care must be planned with consideration to each patient's individuality, including their pre-existing physical and emotional needs and unique responses to surgery and anesthesia. Major areas of concern in Phase II care include:

1. Stability of vital signs, including cardiovascular and respiratory parameters
2. Progression and encouragement of ambulation
3. Nutrition and fluid status
4. Prevention or aggressive treatment of nausea and vomiting
5. Provision of adequate analgesia
6. Observation of the operative site and associated symptoms
7. Psychosocial support, including a speedy reunion with the supporting adult
8. Educational needs of patient and responsible adult escort
9. Evaluation of patient progress toward home readiness
10. Determination of abilities of responsible adult to provide adequate home support.

After local and regional anesthesia, the nurse specifically observes and protects locally anesthetized areas and provides information and encouragement to those patients regarding the return of sensation and movement.

Table 21–3 is a sample Patient Outcomes Grid identifying potential patient needs based on nursing diagnoses, goals, suggested nursing interventions, and possible resources to use in attaining the outcomes. Systems such as these have replaced the cumbersome care plans of the past, although they are nearly identical in purpose.

Nursing Report and Initial Phase II Nursing Assessment

Because of the relatively short time for preoperative assessment in many ASCs, the ambulatory surgery patient often challenges postoperative nurses to provide care with a limited database. The Phase II nurse may or may not have had an initial contact with the patient preoperatively. Often, historic information about special problems or needs must be obtained from the nursing record. Many patients arrive in Phase II as strangers to the nursing staff, so it is imperative that comprehensive written assessments and verbal reports are provided by the transporting team.

A few of the more important parameters of the admission report include the type of procedure, anesthesia, and drugs given before Phase II admission; the location and type of dressings, drains, tubings, catheters, and appliances; pre-existing diseases, sensory losses, special emotional needs, and allergies; and specific physician's orders regarding aftercare. The report to

Table 21–3. **Phase II Recovery Patient Outcomes Grid from Morton Plant Mease Trinity Outpatient Center, New Port Richey, Florida**

POTENTIAL AND ACTUAL PROBLEMS/NURSING DIAGNOSES	OUTCOME GOALS—PATIENT WILL BE ABLE TO:	NURSING INTERVENTIONS	RESOURCES
Altered thought processes and/or memory loss R/T sedation/anesthesia	Display/verbalize appropriate orientation to surroundings and situations Respond lucidly to questions Avoid self-injury R/T altered thought patterns Assume self-care activities within parameters of surgical restrictions Rely on RA who understands nature of patient's temporarily altered thought patterns and responsibility for patient care	Provide frequent affirmations of orientation to time, place, and events Assess patient's orientation Monitor and oversee patient care while patient is vulnerable to environment Provide adequate time for drug clearance before patient discharge Administer medications with caution to avoid further sedation that would greatly alter patient's mental status	Comprehensive report from prior caregivers regarding sedative medications, prior mental status Predetermined discharge criteria that include assessment of mental status and availability of RA to drive and provide home support ASPAN Standards of Perianesthesia Nursing Practice
Ineffective airway clearance Potential for aspiration Ineffective breathing patterns, respiratory depression R/T sedation, anesthesia, positioning, pain, increased respiratory secretions, vomiting, or untoward reactions to medications or local anesthetics	Maintain normal respiratory parameters (rate, depth, ease, clarity of breath sounds) Maintain clear airway Avoid aspiration Maintain adequate oxygenation of tissues Avoid symptoms of hypoxia Perform effective cough and deep breath exercises	Knowledge of effects of anesthetics, analgesics, sedatives, and muscle relaxants and associated drug interactions Airway maintenance techniques, including suctioning and bag-valve-mask resuscitative techniques as needed Apply stir-up regimen Administer oxygen per protocols Continuous assessment of respiratory status Timely report of untoward symptoms to anesthesiologist/surgeon Provide adequate hydration and safe positioning Identify pre-existing respiratory disease and individualize care appropriately	Physiologic monitoring equipment, oxygen, suction and emergency equipment available in unit Crash cart, resuscitator bag, ventilator, airway maintenance supplies, drugs Adequate staffing patterns to ensure proper nurse:patient ratio Immediate access to anesthesia provider Comprehensive anesthesia and/or nursing report before transfer of patient care ASPAN Standards of Perianesthesia Nursing Practice Facility policies regarding interventions for cardiovascular/respiratory problems Intravenous fluids and venipuncture supplies Spirits of ammonia available, especially in bathrooms Emergency call bell system functional
Potential alteration in tissue perfusion Cardiovascular instability	Maintain normal cardiovascular parameters, avoiding hypertension and hypotension Demonstrate expected postoperative arousal and mental status Demonstrate normal parameters of peripheral circulation Ambulate without faintness or hypotension	Assess all parameters of vital signs in ongoing fashion, including heart rate and rhythm, BP Assess mental status and progression Assist patient in progressive ambulation within individual patient's abilities Check peripheral pulses, color, and sensory adequacy in ongoing fashion Timely report of untoward symptoms to anesthesiologist/surgeon Maintain adequate fluid balance and hydration	

Table continued on following page

Table 21–3. **Phase II Recovery Patient Outcomes Grid from Morton Plant Mease Trinity Outpatient Center, New Port Richey, Florida** *Continued*

POTENTIAL AND ACTUAL PROBLEMS/NURSING DIAGNOSES	OUTCOME GOALS—PATIENT WILL BE ABLE TO:	NURSING INTERVENTIONS	RESOURCES
Altered skin integrity R/T surgical wound Potential for infection at surgical site	Experience appropriate and uncomplicated wound healing Avoid fever	Use aseptic technique and teach to family and patient Enhance circulation of surgical wound site Avoid constricting bandages at surgical site Assess surgical site throughout Phase II stay	Universal precautions PPE and sterile dressing supplies Intravenous fluids Antibiotics, if ordered
Alterations in comfort—pain	Express acceptable comfort level Maintain normal CV, R parameters	Administer appropriate analgesics, cold therapy Position patient for comfort Provide positive reinforcements and encourage philosophy of wellness throughout process Encourage appropriate pace for increased activities	Physician's orders for analgesics Analgesic medications Knowledge of nursing interventions for comfort—positioning and support of body areas, breathing exercises, positive reinforcement of comfort
Alterations in comfort—nausea and vomiting	Express acceptable comfort level Avoid vomiting and retching	Encourage appropriate pace for oral intake of fluids Administer antiemetics as needed Administer intravenous solutions for hydration as ordered Provide positive reinforcements and encourage philosophy of wellness throughout process	Physician's orders/prescriptions for antiemetics Intravenous fluids Literature R/T reducing GI symptoms Appropriate food and beverages—avoid acid producing juices, spicy or difficult-to-digest foods
Self-care deficit	Display sufficient level of alertness and self-care for safe discharge to home with RA	Provide comprehensive nursing care modified to patient's abilities Assess patient for ability to ambulate and call for assistance before discharge Assure availability of RA before discharge	Discharge criteria

Actual or perceived loss of privacy or dignity	Express content at level of privacy provided Maintain dignity and sense of self-esteem	Support patient's right to privacy and dignity Promote unit philosophy that demands support of patient's right to privacy Explain and demonstrate to patient before surgery that privacy and dignity will not be invaded while patient is asleep or sedated Provide privacy—curtains, blankets, clothing that covers patient Allow patient as much decision-making as is possible and encourage RA to do same	Surroundings that are friendly, family focused, private, and apart from view of other patients or staff Patient Bill of Rights Patient linens that provide adequate cover Cubicle curtains
Risk of hemorrhage	Maintain blood volume at normal level Maintain blood pressure at normal levels—avoid hypertension	Assure availability of intravenous solutions Observe surgical site for signs of bleeding and report to physician Administer anxiolytic and/or antihypertensive medications as ordered Instruct patient on appropriate support of surgical site	Blood bank contract and policies for rapid availability of blood products Antihypertensives Anxiolytic medications Intravenous fluids and supplies
Anxiety R/T fear of home care without nursing support, separation from family, potential diagnosis, etc.	Express lingering fears, questions about home care or other topics Display calm demeanor Verbalize reduced anxiety Rely on RA for support in the home setting	Provide written and verbal information and ongoing explanations regarding care issues within limits of nursing Assure home support before discharge Encourage questions from patient and RA	Verbal and written discharge instructions that include emergency contact information Responsible adult willing and able to provide home support
Potential for injury R/T faintness, weakness, fatigue, prolonged regional block, altered sensory perception	Remains free from injury Ambulates without faintness or injury	Encourage appropriate pace for progression of ambulation Monitor vital signs in relationship to ambulation Reduce obstacles to safe ambulation—wet floors, slippery shoes, improper fit of slings, braces, surgical shoes, crutches, etc. Provide ongoing assessments for potential complications R/T ambulation	Safe environment Nursing attendance during ambulation attempts and while patient in bathroom Evaluation of patient's home setting during preadmission assessment Responsible adult in home setting

ASPAN, American Society of PeriAnesthesia Nurses; BP, blood pressure; CV, cardiovascular; GI, gastrointestinal; PACU, postanesthesia care unit; PPE, personal protective equipment; PRN, as needed; R, respiratory; RA, responsible adult; R/T, related to.

the Phase II nurse also should include the extent of ambulation or head elevation that the patient has tolerated and the amount and type of oral intake and medications that have been given.

The postoperative patient may arrive in Phase II on a stretcher or wheelchair or may walk there, depending on facility policies and the geographic limitations of the unit. The initial nursing assessment focuses first on critical areas of concern: the airway, respiratory adequacy, and cardiovascular status. Subsequent evaluation includes:

1. A check of all vital signs, including blood pressure, heart rate, temperature, and respiratory effort
2. General appearance and level of consciousness
3. Neurovascular and muscle strength assessments, as appropriate
4. Inspection of the operative site and associated areas or drainage devices
5. Level of comfort
6. Gastrointestinal (GI) status
7. Urinary bladder status
8. Intravenous (IV) fluids and site
9. Skin condition and position; and
10. Assignment of a numeric score if in use by the facility.

Aldrete recently offered a criteria-based scoring system designed specifically for the Phase II recovery area (Table 21–4).[6] This numeric system offers consistency of patient evaluation and could be tailored to meet the specific needs of different types of ASCs. It should, however, be integrated into the comprehensive nursing assessment and not be used as the sole source of patient evaluation.

After nursing assessment is complete, initial interventions in Phase II usually include helping a patient to redress. The nurse should remove any remaining disinfectant preparatory solutions that could stain the patient's clothing, irri-

Table 21–4. **Aldrete's Phase II Postanesthetic Recovery Score**

PATIENT SIGN	CRITERION	SCORE*
Activity	Able to move 4 extremities†	2
	Able to move 2 extremities†	1
	Able to move 0 extremities†	0
Respiration	Able to breathe deeply and cough	2
	Dyspnea, limited breathing, or tachypnea	1
	Apneic or on mechanical ventilator	0
Circulation	BP +/− 20% of preanesthesia level	2
	BP +/−20–49% of preanesthesia level	1
	BP +/−50% of preanesthesia level	0
Consciousness	Fully awake	2
	Arousable on calling	1
	Not responding	0
Oxygen saturation	$SpO_2 > 92\%$ on room air	2
	Requires supplemental O_2 to maintain $SpO_2 > 90\%$	1
	$SpO_2 < 90\%$ even with O_2 supplement	0
Dressing	Dry and clean	2
	Wet but stationary or marked	1
	Growing area of wetness	0
Pain	Pain free	2
	Mild pain handled by oral medication	1
	Severe pain requiring IV or IM medication	0
Ambulation	Can stand up and walk straight	2
	Vertigo when erect	1
	Dizziness when supine	0
Fasting–feeding	Able to drink fluids	2
	Nauseated	1
	Nauseated and vomiting	0
Urine output	Has voided	2
	Unable to void but comfortable	1
	Unable to void and uncomfortable	0

IV, intravenous; IM, intramuscular.
*Note: The total possible score is 20. A score of ≥ 18 is considered appropriate for patient discharge.
†Voluntary or on command.
Reprinted with permission from Aldrete JA: Discharge criteria. In Thomson D, Frost E (eds): Baillieres Clinical Anaesthesiology-Postanaesthesia Care. London: Bailliere Tindall, 1994, pp 763–773.

tate the skin, or limit accurate postoperative skin assessments. An early return to normal attire helps to reinforce the patient's sense of normalcy and wellness promoted in the ASC.

In addition to the obvious benefits of maintaining the patient's dignity and avoiding embarrassment, having the patient dress before ambulating to a recliner can be a time-saver when the nurse combines helping the patient to dress with the initial physical assessment. If young children are frightened or agitated, putting on their own clothes may provide a sense of normalcy and comfort.

There are times, of course, when it is more appropriate for the patient to remain in a hospital gown for a period of time, for instance:

1. When there is a significant chance of bleeding or drainage from the procedure site;
2. When the patient's personal clothing is tight, constrictive, difficult to get on, or significantly restricts observation of the operative site;
3. When the stability of the patient's cardiovascular status is in question;
4. When a temporary urinary catheter is present;
5. When the patient is in obvious discomfort or is nauseated; or
6. When dressings or drains need attention before discharge.

After an initial assessment, ongoing nursing care reflects a balance between actual physical assistance and encouragement of patient and family involvement in the patient's care. Ongoing patient assessment parameters are listed in Resource 4 of the ASPAN Standards of Perianesthesia Nursing Practice[4] (Table 21–5).

Table 21–5. American Society of PeriAnesthesia Nurses (ASPAN) Standards of Perianesthesia Nursing Practice, 1998: From Resource 4, Preanesthesia, Postanesthesia—Data Required for Initial, Ongoing, and Discharge Assessment

Ongoing Assessment: Phase II

Ongoing patient care and assessment should include but not be limited to the following:

1. Identification of patient and name family normally uses
2. Monitor, maintain, and/or improve respiratory function
3. Monitor, maintain, and/or improve circulatory function
4. Promote and maintain physical and emotional comfort
5. Monitor surgical/procedural site
6. Interpret and document data obtained during assessment
7. Administer analgesics as necessary, record results
8. Administer other medication as ordered, record results
9. Provide maximum degree of privacy
10. Provide for safety
11. Provide for confidentiality of information and records
12. Encourage fluids by mouth as indicated
13. Ambulate with assistance
14. Position patient gradually from supine to Fowler's position
15. Ask patient to urinate prior to discharge if indicated
16. Review discharge planning with patient, family/ accompanying responsible adult as appropriate; provide written home care instructions
17. Provide follow-up for extended care as indicated: follow-up phone call to evaluate status

Reprinted with permission of the American Society of PeriAnesthesia Nurses: ASPAN Standards of Perianesthesia Nursing Practice 1998. Thorofare, NJ: ASPAN, 1998, pp 31–32.

Cardiovascular and Respiratory Concerns

The patient should have passed any period of cardiovascular or respiratory instability before transfer to Phase II, but sometimes that judgment is elusive. The patient may or may not have progressed in activity level in the previous department. Assessment of the patient's tolerance of the sitting position is impossible until it is tried, and thus, initial ambulation to a chair should be combined with frequent observation of the blood pressure, pulse, sensorium, and general condition. Some facilities require blood pressure and pulse readings every 5 to 10 minutes, two to three times after initial ambulation. At least one set of vital signs should be obtained soon after ambulation, even for the patient who received a local anesthetic without adjunctive sedation. A series of vital signs is necessary to ascertain stability or trends. The frequency of those assessments is dictated by facility policies and patient condition.

Changes in the patient's position may cause fluctuations in blood pressure. The resultant hypotension may be related to anesthesia-induced loss of compensatory mechanisms, such as reflex sympathetic constriction, changes in extravascular pressure, loss of venous tone, and lack of skeletal muscle contraction.[7] Fainting is always a possibility, particularly with initial ambulation attempts. Postural hypotension must be treated promptly by lowering the patient to a supine position, elevating the legs if the patient is in a chair, and often with increasing the rate of IV fluid administration.[8] Occasionally, more aggressive therapy is necessary, and the patient may require the administration of oxygen and pharmacologic interventions. Effective therapy often includes ephedrine 0.5 mg/kg intramuscular (IM) 10 to 25 mg IV given slowly,[8] or 0.2 to 0.5 mg of atropine IV when bradycardia coexists with hypotension. After an episode of postural hypotension, ambulation should be undertaken gradually with close observation for a second occurrence.

A vagal reaction is always a potential complication in the postanesthesia period. It can be in response to anesthetic agents, breath-holding, gagging, vomiting, straining, or the effects of sympathetic blockade from major regional anesthesia.[9] It results in bradycardia and, when accompanied by hypotension over a prolonged period, can be dangerous, particularly to a patient with primary heart disease. Treatment is generally IV atropine.

Hypertension is also a potential complication in Phase II. Once the anxiety of awaiting surgery has passed, the patient who has exhibited perioperative hypertension often will return to a more normal range of blood pressure. When significant hypertension does occur during or after surgery, the physician often chooses to observe or treat the patient in the monitored setting of the PACU before the transfer to Phase II. When the patient is transferred, the Phase II nurse should be informed of the time and dosages of any antihypertensive agents or sedatives that have been given. Vital signs should be observed closely. In this situation, ambulation should be gradual because the combination of drug therapy and reduced anxiety can result in a significant reduction in blood pressure.

The hypertensive patient may be asked to bring prescribed oral antihypertensive agents to take after surgery. The nurse should assess the patient's GI status before oral therapy. Again, close observation for signs of hypotension or fainting is essential when the patient first ambulates.

Patients usually are not admitted to Phase II with observable respiratory distress or when oxygen therapy still is indicated. Rather, PACU care for stabilization is preferred. One exception is a chronically oxygen-dependent patient. Use of the facility's oxygen while the patient is in the ASC helps to prevent depletion of the patient's personal tank so that adequate oxygen is available for transit to home.

Oxygen must be readily available in a Phase II unit. The appropriate physician, most often an anesthesiologist, should be contacted immediately to examine any patient experiencing respiratory compromise. Appropriate therapy must be instituted vigorously and can be as varied as bronchodilators for asthmatic attacks, antihistamines for allergic reactions, diuretics for cardiac-related complications, or chest tube insertion for pneumothorax related to surgery or to a regional anesthesia technique. Although the patient may be transferred back to PACU for these interventions, the Phase II nursing staff must remain prepared to handle respiratory emergencies.

Progression of Ambulation

The postoperative patient should ambulate slowly, with gradual progression from one activity to the next. This includes dangling on the side of the stretcher or bed before standing, sitting, and walking. The stretcher should be positioned close to the recliner or chair for the initial transfer. Other safety measures include

1. Locking the wheels and lowering the stretcher before transfer;
2. Eliminating environmental dangers such as wet floors or obstacles;
3. Having a sufficient number of assistants to help, based on the patient's size and mobility; and
4. Using nonslip shoes or slippers while the patient is walking.

The patient with dizziness, faintness, or significant hypotension or bradycardia should postpone ambulation until the sensorium clears and vital signs are more reflective of the patient's preoperative normal range.

Several factors, including the procedure, the type of anesthesia, and pre-existing physical problems, affect the patient's ability and desire to ambulate. The surgical procedure may preclude weight-bearing on an extremity or limit ambulation for several days. Crutches, walkers, wheelchairs, walking casts, and surgical boots all are aids that the patient can use to support walking and to protect the operative site from trauma.

Unless the patient has used crutches extensively within a reasonable time before surgery, the nurse should assess the patient's crutch-walking ability during the Phase II stay. Initial instructions and demonstrations should be given before surgery and anesthesia, but a return demonstration by the patient is appropriate postoperatively. A pair of adjustable crutches kept in the Phase II unit for such demonstrations is helpful when the patient has not brought his or her own to the ASC. Family members should be instructed about the need for any physical support until the patient is proficient in ambulating.[10] Hospital-based facilities may have access to a physical therapy department to teach and assess crutch-walking demonstrations, but the nurse is primarily responsible in many ASCs.

The patient's preoperative abilities must be considered when encouraging postoperative ambulation. Those with significantly impaired mobility are likely to require special assistance. Special preparations may be required for the patient whose preoperative status will significantly alter the usual postoperative course. Examples include patients who are severely obese or arthritic or a person with hemiparesis who is having a procedure that usually requires the use of crutches postoperatively. If that patient's inherent inability to use crutches is identified before surgery, an alternate plan can be initiated without the stress or embarrassment of failed attempts or accidents in trying to use crutches. A walker or wheelchair might be suggested, or the physician may provide extra support in the form of a walking cast or brace that allows the patient to place weight on the operative extremity without causing injury.

The type of anesthesia given also affects the extent of postoperative ambulation. After general anesthesia, the patient is observed for a period of time to ascertain cardiovascular stability before ambulation. Symptoms such as faintness, hypotension, and diaphoresis may be signs of hypovolemia and vasodilatation, which delay ambulation. Appropriate therapy may be required before the patient's attempts to sit or stand.

Ambulation attempts after regional anesthesia depend on the type and site of anesthetic block. Regional anesthesia of an upper extremity rarely affects the patient's ability to ambulate in the early postoperative period. Local infiltration of anesthetics to the foot or ankle usually does not delay ambulation unless no weight-bearing has been ordered or extensive sedation has been given. Conversely, patients who have had major regional anesthesia such as spinal and epidural techniques require close observation and physical support for their first attempts to walk. In addition to primary weakness of the legs, lingering sympathetic blockade can result in hypotension, nausea, vomiting, and lightheadedness with initial attempts to ambulate. Sedative medications given during the procedure can complicate further the patient's attempts to ambulate.

Significant changes have occurred in the theories surrounding postspinal anesthesia care, specifically in relation to head elevation and ambulation. Current thinking allows and encourages both activities. Sudden head movements and abruptness in sitting or standing are discouraged on the day of surgery, but moderate activity is not limited unless the patient has a strong contributing history that increases the likelihood of complications.

Traditional postspinal anesthesia protocol requiring lengthy bedrest reflected the main goal of decreasing potential leakage of cerebral spinal fluid (CSF) from the subarachnoid space, thus reducing the possibility of postspinal anesthesia headache. With the current use of specially designed small-gauge needles, leakage of CSF is considered negligible or insignificant. Also, current practitioners aggressively hydrate patients intravenously to support volume in the vasculature and to provide fluids for the ongoing production of CSF, particularly in young women who are more likely to develop postspinal anesthesia headache than other patients. These measures have resulted in most practitioners allowing early ambulation after the patient demonstrates vasomotor stability and a return of strength and movement in the legs.

Vasomotor stability can be determined by postural blood pressure assessments performed while the patient is recumbent. Blood pressures are measured with the patient flat and again when he or she is sitting at least twice at 30-minute intervals. The mean arterial blood pressure (MABP) should not decrease more than 10% when the patient assumes a sitting position.[11]

Patients who have had an inguinal infiltration anesthetic may experience significant leg weakness for a period of time if there has been an inadvertent block of the femoral nerve. The nurse who assists the patient in ambulating for the first time after an inguinal block should assess carefully the patient's leg strength and motor abilities and should provide physical support. It is wise to have two attendants for the patient's first attempt to stand and to warn the patient about the potential for temporary leg weakness.

Fluids and Nutrition

Certain safety practices should be observed when providing postanesthesia nourishment. First, the patient's ability to swallow and gag must be established as a primary determinant of readiness. This is evidence that the protective airway reflex is present. It is best for the patient to be sitting up when taking nourishment to avoid choking or difficulty in swallowing. Water (or ice) is usually the first fluid allowed because it is the least likely to cause lung damage if it is aspirated. The patient then can progress to noncaffeinated soda, tea, or juices. Hot beverages must be used with caution to prevent burns. They must be easily accessible, and the patient should be assisted if there is a chance of spillage, for example, in the case of the patient with severely arthritic hands or Parkinson's disease, the patient with impaired depth perception because one eye is patched, the very old or very young patient, or the sedated patient. Straws intensify the temperature of hot beverages, so they should be used with caution. The nurse should use professional judgment in limiting or suggesting moderation in the amount and type of nourishment taken.

If oral analgesics have been ordered for postoperative comfort, tolerance of oral intake must be evaluated before discharge.[10] Phase II patients are often ready for oral fluids and nourishment on admission and usually may drink unless it is contraindicated by anesthesia, procedure restrictions, or GI upset. Although some practitioners believe that room-temperature beverages cause less nausea than iced or cold ones,[5] others have not identified a difference in patient tolerance of cold or warm beverages.

After general anesthesia, nausea is relatively more likely to occur, and it is best to provide clear liquids and bland foods such as crackers or toast in limited amounts. In particular, coffee, citrus juices, and dairy products tend to promote GI upset and vomiting, especially when combined with the subsequent automobile ride home. Regional and local anesthetics, unless they affect the patient's ability to swallow or gag, often do not affect the patient's ability or desire to drink and eat, and the patient is allowed a choice of nourishments. Anxiety and the psychological stress of surgery can promote GI upset in any patient, so moderation is advised for all.

The patient's appetite often is considered the best indicator of readiness to eat and drink[12] and should be used as the main guide for giving nourishment. To insist that a reluctant patient drink usually results in poor tolerance of the beverage. The decision to allow a patient to go home without having tolerated oral fluids is one that is based on the individual physician's and nurse's experience, practice standards, and the facility's discharge criteria. The attending physician may require that the patient remain at the surgery center until oral intake is tolerated, whereas other physicians may feel comfortable allowing the patient who is not interested in eating or drinking to go home. In most instances, healthy adult patients who are not hungry or thirsty and are not having significant nausea do very well when allowed to go home and proceed with nourishment and fluids at their own pace. Many ASCs have changed discharge criteria to reflect this less restrictive philosophy.

For patients who are observed in Phase II for extended periods, a meal tray or snack often is provided. Because appetite usually is diminished and digestion already is slowed during times of physiologic stress, food choices should be light, nonspicy, and low fat. By addressing the patient's primary need for nourishment, the nurse actually is helping to heighten the patient's ability to concentrate on other needs, particularly educational ones.

Nausea and Vomiting

Nausea and vomiting can significantly prolong the patient's postoperative stay.[8] Three issues stand out as the main determinants of nausea and vomiting: patient predisposition to nausea and vomiting (history), appropriate prophylaxis and therapy, and psychological expectations. First, patients' previous experiences with anesthesia and personal predisposition to motion sickness influence their responses. Second is the attention given to appropriate and aggressive antiemetic therapy and prophylaxis perioperatively. The preoperative use of histamine- or serotonin-blocking agents, antisalients, and antiemetics can help reduce postoperative nausea, as can the choice of anesthetic agents and analgesics with low potential for producing nausea. After surgery, bland foods such as a cracker or piece of unbuttered toast may be an excellent deterrent to nausea and vomiting when the patient expresses great hunger. Providing some food in the stomach is particularly helpful before any oral analgesics are given.

The third issue is one that often is overlooked but has tremendous impact. Preoperatively and throughout the ambulatory stay, the nursing staff and anesthesiologists are able to influence the patient's psychological and emotional expectations. The concept of self-fulfilling prophecy is very much at work when the patient is encouraged continually to expect a nausea-free recovery. By expressing confidence in the staff's ability to prevent nausea and vomiting, the nurse helps the patient to form those same expectations. When the patient successfully undergoes the day of surgery without GI complications, the nurse can use the opportunity to extend that same expectation to potential future encounters.

Sometimes, no matter what is done to prevent it, nausea and vomiting accompany the Phase II period of recovery. When the patient is nauseated, a gentle approach is the best policy. Caution in ambulation, head elevation, and oral intake usually helps to diminish the symptoms. Nausea related to hypotension or hypovolemia often responds well to IV hydration and a period of recumbency.[8] Investigators also have noted a significant relationship between postoperative pain and nausea.[12–14] Adequate analgesia is often a primary deterrent to nausea and vomiting, and thus the nurse must consider the patient's complaints of pain when planning interventions for nausea and vomiting.

Antiemetic drugs may be necessary. All possible routes of administration must be considered in Phase II, but parenteral and rectal routes are the most likely. A major side effect of some of these drugs is somnolence, which can delay or preclude discharge, and doses should be calculated individually to avoid oversedation. Agents relatively free of side effects (e.g., ondansetron) should be considered for patients in whom nausea and vomiting develop in Phase II.[10]

Depending on facility policy, patients receiving antiemetics in Phase II may be required to remain in the ASC for 1 hour or more after administration to assess both the effectiveness of the therapy and the potential sedative effects. Some physicians may discharge the patient soon after antiemetic therapy is given so that the patient can get settled in bed at home and sleep with the medication.

Emesis basins should be kept out of sight whenever possible to avoid the suggestion of nausea. When the patient is actively vomiting or retching, privacy is a great concern, both for that patient and for others in the room. Privacy screens or curtains are effective in blocking the view of others but cannot block sounds. When possible, the patient who is vomiting should be cared for in a separate, private area.

Analgesia

The basic analgesia principles discussed in Chapter 20, Phase I Recovery, continue to apply in Phase II. Refer to that chapter for medication actions as well as other general information regarding analgesia for the postoperative patient.

Once the patient has recovered from anesthesia, the mainstay of pain assessment should be the patient's self-report to assess pain perceptions (including description, location, intensity/severity, and aggravating and relieving factors) and cognitive response. Patient self-report is the single most reliable indicator of the existence and intensity of acute pain, discomfort or distress.[15] Vital signs, patient behavior, and body language may be misleading regarding actual pain level. Some patients are able to talk and make jokes even while experiencing severe pain. Humor, anger, or sleeping may be coping mechanisms used by patients to deal with pain.

Preventative preoperative and intraoperative pain control is becoming an accepted method of analgesia nationwide. Once sensitized, pain receptors become more and more irritated and the consequent pain increasingly difficult to control.[15] Patients should be taught preoperatively of the need to report pain accurately and early for optimum comfort. This teaching should begin with the surgeon's explanation of the operative procedure and then can be reinforced during the preadmission interview and the admission nursing assessment.

Many facilities use some sort of self-report "scale" or other pain assessment tool for clarity of pain descriptions. Three common self-report measurement tools useful for assessment of pain intensity and affective distress in adults and many children are: (1) a numerical rating scale (NRS); (2) a visual analog scale (VAS); and (3) an adjective rating scale (ARS).[15] Examples of each of these can be seen in Table 21–6. The NRS and ARS methods are verbal methods, whereas the VAS is a visual chart on which the patient points to his or her level of pain. An adaptation of the VAS tool has been made for children using simple smiling faces, frowning faces, and a face with tears for the worst possible pain. Children can easily point to the face that shows what they are feeling.

When the patient is in pain, it is difficult, if not impossible, to concentrate on discharge instructions or other self-care issues. Once these basic comfort needs are met, the patient can be taught dressing care and other pertinent issues necessary for a safe discharge.

Nonpharmacologic methods of analgesia are sometimes effective in reducing the patient's perception or experience of pain. Comfortable positioning, dimmed lighting, back rubs, and the presence of a family member or loved one may provide effective comfort. Other ap-

***Table 21–6.* Pain Assessment Tools**

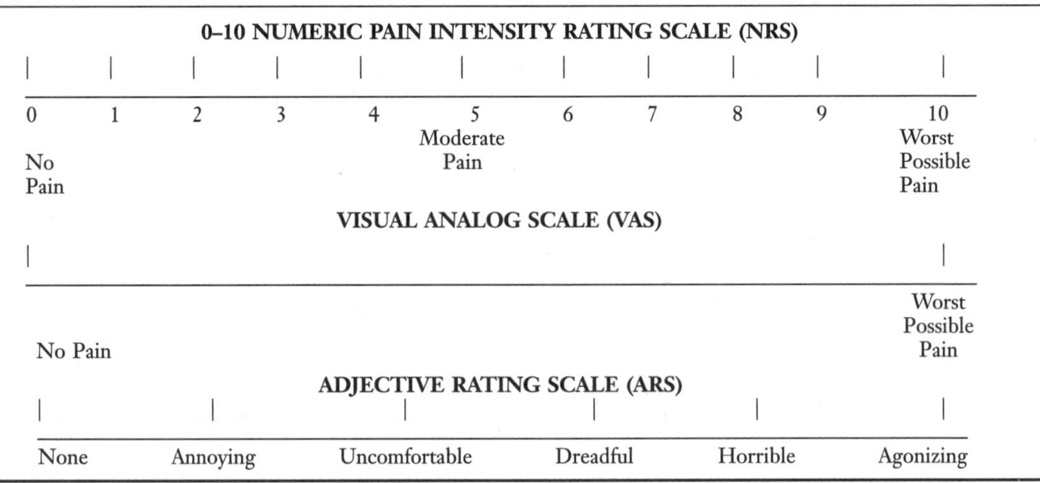

Reprinted from: Acute Pain Management Guidelines Panel: Acute Pain Management: Operative or Medical Procedures and Trauma. Clinical Practice Guideline. AHCPR Pub. No. 92-0032. Rockville, MD: Agency for Health Care Policy and Research, Public Health Service, U.S. Department of Health and Human Services, Feb 1992.

proaches to pain control include imagery, hypnosis, and even music and aroma therapy. These techniques are somewhat controversial and probably would be used only in an ambulatory setting at the patient's request. When nonpharmacologic methods are ineffective, the patient still has a basic right to adequate pain management.

Individual therapy is based on the patient's actual needs and the type of medications already administered. The patient's analgesic needs should be balanced with the appropriate type and route of medication. Many narcotic and non-narcotic analgesics are available. Of note are the nonsteroidal anti-inflammatory drugs, for example, ketorolac, which currently is available in an oral form. Patients who have had procedures that typically result in significant postoperative discomfort may require parenteral drug therapy in Phase II. Because discharge can be delayed if the patient is heavily sedated, an attempt should be made to provide medications and dosages that provide pain relief without undue somnolence. The goal is to provide comfort for the trip home and beyond without so much sedation that the patient is unable to walk without dizziness or faintness. The responsible adult who accompanies the patient who has had medication affecting sensorium must understand his or her responsibility to closely observe and attend the patient at home.

There may be patients who are given several types or doses of analgesics yet continue to express discomfort and ask for more medication. Careful assessments must be undertaken to identify any reason that might be contributing to the high level of discomfort. Some examples include bleeding with hematoma, wound dehiscence, bladder distention, obstructed circulation caused by dressing or cast, historically low tolerance for pain, and chronic analgesic use resulting in enzyme induction that increases the patient's tolerance of current therapy.

It may not be possible to relieve every pain or discomfort, and the patient may have unrealistic goals of being totally pain free. An honest explanation and dialogue between the nurse, family, and patient may help the patient to better understand and accept the reality of minor discomfort.

Operative Site and General Assessments

Observation of the operative site must continue throughout the entire postoperative stay. This ongoing assessment incorporates many clinical observations depending on the patient's procedure and anesthesia. Frank hemorrhage, hematoma formation, and dehiscence are potential wound complications in the early postoperative period. Circulatory impairment and nerve compression are occurrences that may complicate healing of the surgical area or surrounding tissues. Parameters of clinical assessment associated with the operative procedure include:

1. Size, location, and condition of dressings;
2. Direct visualization of suture lines or drainage from body cavities;
3. Status of the surrounding skin for swelling or bruising;
4. Peripheral circulation, as evidenced by color, capillary refill time, pulses, sensation, and movement of distal areas;
5. Location and correct fit of appliances such as slings, casts, and braces;
6. Girth and firmness of surrounding tissues;
7. Urinary output and hematuria;
8. Vaginal flow;
9. Neurovascular assessments of areas supplied by peripheral, cranial, or spinal nerves distal to the operative site; and
10. Abdominal or other pain that is unexpected or out of proportion for the procedure performed.

In addition to incision or surgery complications, other symptoms relating to the procedure may occur. These include anesthesia-related sequelae and complications of positioning. Patients have been known to have local reactions to electrocautery grounding pads or tape used to pull excess skin folds away from operative sites. These sites should be checked before discharge and their condition noted in the nursing notes. In addition to examining the surgical site and peripheral circulation, the injection site of any local or regional anesthetic should be examined on arrival in the ambulatory care unit and again before discharge, and the condition of the area should be documented. Although complications are rare at the injection site, hematoma formation or frank bleeding are possibilities. Should such an occurrence arise, the anesthesiologist should be notified to evaluate the patient and direct any necessary treatments.

Regional anesthetics such as spinal and epidural blocks, brachial plexus and intravenous (Bier) blocks, intercostal nerve block, and various infiltrating blocks of the ankle, hand, or wrist can affect large portions of the body and require special nursing attention in Phase II. First, anesthesia complications may occur, as discussed in Chapter 14. Although it is more common for problems to occur in the procedure room immediately after injection of the local anesthetic, they may become apparent only after the patient's transfer to the Phase II unit. Occurrences such as toxic or allergic reactions, convulsions, chest pain, myocardial infarction (MI), serious arrhythmias, pneumothorax, and hemorrhage are also possible subsequent to an invasive anesthetic technique. Nursing interventions can range from emotional support and observation of a small hematoma to emergency procedures to maintain heart and lung functions or to abate hemorrhage. Emergency preparedness is essential for unexpected complications. An IV access should be available on all patients who have had regional anesthesia until the time of discharge.

Residual motor and sensory effects from any block require that the patient be protected from injury. Appropriate support and elevation are required for involved extremities. Patients and family members must have immediate, clear instructions regarding restrictions of movement and care of any affected area as soon as they arrive in the Phase II unit. In most cases, these instructions will need to be reinforced several times before discharge. An example is the patient who, after a brachial plexus block, has limited control of the upper arm but none in the forearm and wrist. Attempting to move the affected arm while the patient is recumbent could result in injury to the surgical site or to the patient's face or nose, particularly if the extremity is in a cast. The admitting nurse should assess immediately the patient's arm control and explain the need to leave the arm undisturbed until a sling is applied for protection. Improper positioning on a stretcher or recliner predisposes the patient to involuntary slipping of the arm from pillows or padding, and thus, correct positioning must be carefully monitored and maintained. This provides the nurse an avenue to begin patient and family instruction. Family members can provide valuable assistance and at the same time begin to take responsibility for caring for the patient.

Patients with residual block of limited areas may be eager to show their control over the anesthetized area so that they can go home or to satisfy their own need to be in control of their bodies. These efforts are usually futile and tiring to the patient, both physically and emotionally. The nurse may need to encourage the patient to be tolerant of the lingering block and provide frequent, periodic reassurance that the effects are not permanent. Family members should be included in all nursing instructions and asked to reinforce them to the patient.

Patients may complain of a diversity of other symptoms, for example:

1. Sore throat or hoarseness following intubation;[16]
2. Stiff or aching muscles after an episode of shivering or after administration of succinylcholine, which may precipitate fasciculations;

3. Headache;
4. Muscle or joint soreness relating to the surgical position;
5. A sore lip or tongue from biting it or having it caught between the teeth and an airway;
6. Extremity coldness or discomfort after intraoperative tourniquet use;
7. Double or blurred vision after the use of intraocular ointments to protect the corneas during general anesthesia.

It may be impossible to ascertain the reason for every symptom, but all must be investigated carefully and appropriate corrective action taken.

The nurse may find that the patient continues to have lingering fears or concerns about unexpected or untoward symptoms. Providing an explanation about the cause of minor symptoms can be the only action necessary to alleviate the patient's concerns. To be able to provide accurate explanations, the nurse must understand or investigate the physiologic reasons for these potential sequelae. Depending on the problem identified by the patient, suggestions may be made for comfort measures that can be taken at home, for example: cool compresses, ice packs, dim lighting, quiet environment, warm soaks, heating pad, elevation of affected area, and other such actions can prove helpful. The nurse must make certain none of these actions are contraindicated before advising the patient.

Psychosocial Needs

The patient is reunited with family or friends as soon as possible based on individual recovery rate and the needs of other patients in the immediate surroundings. Some facilities do not allow visitors in a Phase II area until it is time to review discharge instructions. Others allow no visitors. This latter policy may be the result of tradition or space limitations; however, an early reunion supports the family-oriented approach to ambulatory surgery and is usually beneficial to the entire family. The nurse is able to assess the patient and also the learning needs and abilities of the adult who will assume responsibility for that patient in the home setting.

The nurse who observes the relationship that exists between the patient and adult supporter is better able to develop a plan that provides appropriate guidance. A supporting adult who is overbearing, aggressive, negative, uninterested, meek, or fearful can be more deleterious than helpful to the patient during recuperation at home. The nurse who has the opportunity to provide instructions, encouragement, and information may help to mold the supporting adult's attitude and knowledge base into a more positive mode.

There are patients with very special social and emotional needs who positively require early reunion with family or friends. An infant or child is the most obvious example. In fact, many progressive ASCs allow and encourage parents to come to the PACU as soon as the child awakens or before. Patients who are mentally challenged, either through illness or developmental delay, often respond more favorably to familiar people. Those with significant sensory deficits may be able to communicate with only a few people and should be afforded that benefit whenever possible. The inclusion of such resource people is usually a boon, rather than a hindrance, to the nurse who is attempting to assess and communicate with the patient.

There are other benefits to allowing family members into a Phase II unit. It often is comforting to the patient for several reasons. The first is the patient's need for personal attention and for the emotional comfort of a familiar person. Some patients may worry about family members who are waiting in the lobby or waiting room. They may be concerned that their loved ones are experiencing too long a wait or undue worry or concern. Also, a family member who will be providing care in the home should be allowed to participate in postoperative patient care. This provides an enhanced understanding of care to be provided at home and fosters a trust between the nursing staff, patient, and adult companion, which in turn allows for more open communication of questions and concerns.

Educational Needs

Patient education is a long-standing nursing tradition. Nursing has used patient education as a tool for providing safe, cost-effective, quality healthcare since the middle of the 19th century. Nurses are ethically and legally bound to teach.[17]

Alert patients, family members, and other supporting adults all are likely candidates to receive ongoing health information. As a healthcare professional who interacts with many people, a Phase II nurse should seize any opportunity to provide guidance, not only specific to the procedure at hand but to many issues regarding general health and wellness. The nurse should be prepared to provide information about such topics as diet, exercise, smoking, cholesterol levels, hygiene, and stress reduction. There may be opportunities to address the need for ongoing home examinations, such as breast or testicular self-examination, and for annual physicals, mammograms, rectal examinations, and so forth. Some ASCs have developed pamphlets or brochures on such topics, whereas others act as distributors for literature published by health organizations and societies such as the American Heart Association and the American Cancer Society.

A large segment of the population sees a physician only when absolutely necessary for a specific problem. Whenever health-related information can be provided to the public, it is truly a professional service. In an ASC, there is a wonderful opportunity to address such needs in a subtle yet authoritative manner because of the trust that the patient and family place in the ambulatory surgical nurse.

Many general questions relating to the surgery or the aftercare are within the realm of the Phase II nurse to answer. This requires the nurse to have a comprehensive knowledge and understanding of the procedures being performed in the facility. Questions of a specific medical nature should be referred to the physician either immediately, by the nurse contacting the physician, or later, by directing the patient to discuss special concerns and questions during the postoperative office visit. One facility has posted a sign in the conference room to remind families to ask surgeons about issues sometimes forgotten in the postoperative consultation (Table 21–7).

Information and instructions specific to the patient's individual procedure must be both verbal and written. Teaching actually is ongoing throughout the Phase II stay, but it culminates with formally presented instructions when the patient nears the time of discharge. This process, which should include the supporting adult, is discussed in Chapter 22.

Table 21–7. Reminder to Families

FAMILY!
REMEMBER TO ASK
THE DOCTOR ABOUT:

- ☐ Dressing changes
- ☐ Return to work
- ☐ Appointment
- ☐ Bathing

Used in Physician/Family Conference Room at the Idaho Falls Surgical Center, 1945 E. 17th St., Idaho Falls, ID 83404.

NURSING CARE OF THE PATIENT AFTER UNSUPPLEMENTED LOCAL ANESTHESIA

A patient whose procedure has been performed under local anesthesia without any adjunctive sedation often is allowed to walk from surgery or ambulate immediately after arrival in Phase II. Although facility-specific criteria may vary, the patient usually is allowed to leave the center after:

1. Evaluation of the surgical site;
2. One set of vital signs, including blood pressure, pulse, respirations, and temperature, is taken; and
3. Receipt of discharge instructions.

Fewer physical restrictions are placed on these patients in the immediate postoperative period, but an important anesthesia-related instruction is to avoid injury to any anesthetized area that may remain insensitive to pressure or heat. With the physician's written orders, facility protocol may allow the patient who had no sedation to leave the surgery center without adult companionship and to drive, unless the procedure performed inhibits safe driving.

Although the patient may have undergone the simple excision of a superficial skin or subcutaneous lesion or another minor procedure, the possibility of upsetting emotional sequelae may predispose cardiovascular response. The patient may fear the diagnosis, particularly when a malignancy is suspected, or may be concerned about facial scarring or disfigurement. This may not be the first time a similar procedure has been performed, and previous results may have been either favorable or not. Emotional assessment and support remain important nursing functions for the patient who has had even a minor procedure under local anesthesia.

DOCUMENTATION OF CARE

As in all areas of an ASC, there is rapid turnover of patients because of the scheduling of many short-duration cases. Accurate and comprehensive documentation of each patient's care becomes a challenge in this high-volume setting. However, that volume makes accurate documentation especially important because a later attempt to remember a patient or an incident is not likely to be accurate unless the documentation reflects actual care. Additionally, there may be several nurses caring for the same patients, and documentation of nursing actions must be clear to prevent duplication and provide for a smooth progression of care.

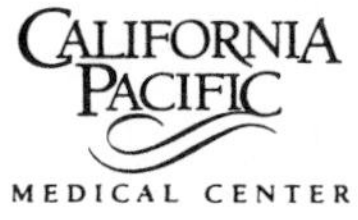

PEDIATRIC POST-OPERATIVE ASSESSMENT AMBULATORY CARE SERVICE

CALIFORNIA PACIFIC MEDICAL CENTER
P.O. BOX 7999
SAN FRANCISCO, CA 94120

		POST-OP						
	PRE-OP	Arriv.	1/2°	1°	2°	3°	4°	Discharge
TIME								
INITIALS								
TEMPERATURE								
PULSE								
RESPIRATION								
BLOOD PRESSURE								
Respirations — 2 Appropriate rate and depth for age (birth to 3 mos.: 30-40/min, 3 mos. to age 4: 20-30/min. >age 4: 14-20/min) 0 Croupy, wheezing, retractions or cyanosis; any evidence of airway obstruction								
Activity / Exercise — 2 Normal age-appropriate pre-op activity 1 Awake 0 Arouses with difficulty								
Circulation — 2 Rate appropriate for age with normal peripheral perfusion (birth to 6 mos. 120 to 150/min, 6 mos. to age 4: 90-120/min., > age 4: 70-100/min) 0 Sustained tachycardia, vasoconstriction or poor capillary refill								
Nausea and vomiting — 2 minimal 1 moderate 0 severe								
Cognitive / Perceptual — 2 Discomfort appropriate to procedure 1 Medicated for discomfort (PO) 0 Requires parenteral analgesic								
Bleeding — 2 Bleeding appropriate to procedure 1 Moderate amount of bleeding 0 Large amounts of bleeding								
Discharge Score ≥ 9 TOTAL								

POST OPERATIVE STANDARD OF CARE UTILIZED
Patient outcomes achieved Yes ☐ No ☐
If "No", document in Nurses Comments

Standard of Care utilized: ____________________

Patient outcomes achieved: Yes ☐ No ☐
If "No", document under Nurses Comments.

Anesthesia Sign Out (general, MAC, regional)
Discharge when criteria met:
Discharge Score ≥ 9
Signature of Anesthesiologist: ____________
Comments: ____________________

____

Nursing Comments:

____

____

____

____

____

____

____

____

____

____

Name of Physician notified if score 8 or less at D/C

____

Admitted to hospital/SSU/OBS Room # ________

Reason for Admission: ____________

Report given to: ____________
Patient has His/Her belongings. Yes ☐ No ☐
Written Discharge Instructions given. Yes ☐ No ☐

Mode of Discharge: ☐ Ambulatory ☐ Gurney
☐ Carried ☐ Wheel Chair
☐ Other ____________
Time of Discharge: ____________
Accompanied by: ____________

Signature: ____________ RN/LVN

CALIFORNIA CAMPUS
PACIFIC CAMPUS

Figure 21–2. A sample Phase II flowsheet. (Developed by and reprinted with permission of California Pacific Medical Center, 2351 Clay, San Francisco, CA.)

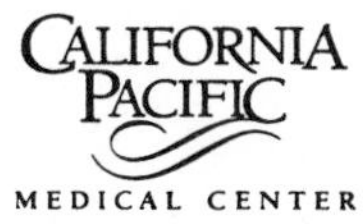

PEDIATRIC POST-OPERATIVE ASSESSMENT AMBULATORY CARE SERVICE

CALIFORNIA PACIFIC MEDICAL CENTER
P.O. BOX 7999
SAN FRANCISCO, CA 94120

TIME RETURNED:__________ DATE: __________

ACCOMPANIED BY: __________

PROCEDURE: __________

RETURNED TO UNIT VIA: Ambulatory ☐ Gurney ☐ Crib ☐ Wheel Chair ☐ Other ☐ __________

ALLERGIES: Yes ☐ No ☐ __________

IV: Yes ☐ No ☐ If Yes: Solution __________ Amount remaining upon return: __________

Site: Left Arm ☐ Right Arm ☐ Other ☐

Time Discontinued Amount infused in Unit: __________

DRESSING SITE AND TYPE: __________

Condition of drainage: Dry and Intact ☐ Stained and Intact ☐ Bloody and Intact ☐

Other: __________

Amount of Drainage: Minimal ☐ Active ☐ Other: __________

PAIN: Location #1 ☐ Surgical site **Rating (see scale)**

#2 ☐ Other __________ Initial Assessment __________

Discharge Assessment __________

0 — 5 — 10

No Pain — Moderate Pain — Severe Pain

RELIEF:

LOCATION	RATING	MEDICATION	DOSE	ROUTE	TIME	GIVEN BY	RELIEF OBTAINED

SCALE FOR RELIEF OBTAINED: 1) Resolved 2) Pain decreased and tolerable 3) Pain remains unchanged

NURSING COMMENTS:

CALIFORNIA CAMPUS
PACIFIC CAMPUS

44329 (10/95)

Figure 21–2 *Continued.*

ABINGTON MEMORIAL HOSPITAL
SAME DAY PROCEDURES RECORD

DATE ________ TIME ________ ROOM NO. ________ INFORMANT ________

AMBULATORY ________ OTHER ________

REASON FOR ADMISSION ________

TO BE DISCHARGED WITH ________

RELATIONSHIP ________ PHONE NO. ________

BASELINE DATA: HEIGHT ________ WEIGHT ________

ALLERGIES: ________

VITAL SIGNS: T ________ P ________ R ________ BP ________

CURRENT MEDICATIONS	TIME OF LAST DOSE

PREOPERATIVE CHECKLIST N/A ☐	Y	N	NA	INITIALS
Consent signed and in chart				
History and Physical in chart				
Current lab results in chart				
Type/Rh charted ________				
Chest x-ray report in chart				
ECG report in chart				
Abnormal test results reported				
Orientation to unit				
I. D. bracelet on patient				
N. P. O. since ________				
Voided at ________				
Pre-op teaching completed				
Surgical site prepped				
Prepped by ________				
Contact lenses removed				
Eyeglasses removed				
Dentures removed				
Permanent bridgework				
Hearing aid removed				
Other ________				
Valuables, jewelry removed				
Jewelry taped ________				
Ready for O. R. at ________				

Patient identified prior to transport:

Date: ________ Time: ________

Nurse ________

Escort ________

PREOPERATIVE PARENTERAL FLUIDS N/A ☐

Type/Amount ________

Site ________ Size ________ Rate ________

Signature ________

MEDICATIONS GIVEN PREOPERATIVELY N/A ☐

MED/DOSAGE/ROUTE	SITE	TIME ADM	INITIALS

INJECTION SITE KEY: RGA - 1, LGA - 2, RAT - 3, LAT - 4, RLT - 5, LLT - 6

NURSES' INITIALS, SIGNATURES AND TITLES		

Comments:

Patient's ID Label

30-97-108800 Rev (8/93)

Figure 21–3. A sample flowsheet for postoperative and discharge assessment. (Developed by and reprinted with permission of Ruth Seitter, RN, MSN, and with permission of Abington Memorial Hospital, 1200 Old York Road, Abington, PA.)

S.D.P. ADMISSION ASSESSMENT

VISION	Y	N	NA	COMMENTS
Glasses				
Contacts				
Other				
HEARING	R	L	NA	COMMENTS
Hearing deficit				
Aid				
Other				
DENTAL	U	L	NA	COMMENTS
Full dentures				
Partial dentures				
Capped teeth				
Bridgework				
Other				
RESPIRATORY	Y	N	NA	COMMENTS
Lungs - clear				Site:
Cough				
Dyspnea/SOB				
Other				
CARDIOVASCULAR	Y	N	NA	COMMENTS
Chest pain				
Edema				
Peripheral pulses				
Other				
GI/GU	Y	N	NA	COMMENTS
Bowel Sounds				
Abdomen soft				
Abdomen convex				
Urinary problems				
Other				
NEUROLOGICAL	Y	N	NA	COMMENTS
Alert				
Oriented x 3				
Sensation - Normal				
Movement - Normal				
Other				

SKIN	Y	N	NA	COMMENTS
Color - Normal				
Warm/Dry				
Rash(es)				
Bruise(s)				
Abrasion(s)				
Other				
HEALTH HABITS	Y	N	NA	COMMENTS
Tobacco use				
Sleep problems				
Other				
PSYCHO/SOCIAL	Y	N	NA	COMMENTS
Knowledge of dx.				
Other				
Date	By			R. N.

TIME	NURSES' NOTES

Figure 21–3 *Continued.*

Illustration continued on following page

Although patient care and documentation are planned for each patient individually, the nurse often finds the need to include relatively standard assessments and comments in many patients' charts. The obvious answer to this need is to have checklists and other preprinted information available on the nursing record to allow rapid, yet comprehensive documentation by checking off, filling in, or circling items. When such time-saving steps are multiplied by 8 or 10 assessment parameters and by that many patients per day, the amount of nursing hours saved is obvious. Figures 21–2 and 21–3 are examples of Phase II nursing records that incor-

S.D.P. NURSING CARE PLAN

Outcome Goal: Patient will adapt successfully to an uncomplicated surgical and recovery process ☐

Patient will respond to medical treatment without adverse complications ☐

A. NURSING DIAGNOSIS B. EXPECTED OUTCOME	NURSING INTERVENTIONS	INITIALS	EVALUATION	INITIALS
Knowledge Deficit R/T perioperative routine. ☐ E.O. Patient will verbalize an understanding of the perioperative routine and/or experience a reduction of anxiety preoperatively.	- Assess patient's ability to learn and learning needs. - Explain perioperative routine: • S.D.P. • O.R./Holding Area • PACU • Family Lounge		- Patient and/or significant other expresses an understanding of the perioperative routine. Yes ☐ No ☐ - If no, explain other interventions.	
Knowledge Deficit R/T post-discharge care. ☐ E.O. Patient and/or significant other will verbalize understanding of post-discharge care.	- Assess patient's ability to learn and learning needs. - Give printed instruction sheet. - Explain discharge instructions.		- Patient and/or significant other expresses an understanding of post-discharge care. Yes ☐ No ☐ - If no, explain other interventions.	

Other care plans added -

Yes ☐ No ☐

If yes, list plans added

INITIALS	SIGNATURE/TITLE	INITIALS	SIGNATURE/TITLE

TIME	NURSES' NOTES
	Plan of care reviewed with patient______family______.

Patient's ID Label

Figure 21–3 *Continued.*

POSTOPERATIVE/DISCHARGE ASSESSMENT

SURGICAL PROCEDURE:			ANESTHESIA: Spinal/Epidural ____ IV Block ____ Block ____ General ____ MAC ____ Local ____
TIME RETURNED	SKIN COLOR Normal ____ Other ____	SKIN TEMPERATURE Warm ____ Dry ____ Moist ____	BREATH SOUNDS - BILATERALS: Clear ____ Abnormal ____ See Notes ____
ICE BAG (site applied)		ELEVATION (site)	ABDOMEN: Soft ____ Convex ____ Other ____

NEUROVASCULAR ASSESSMENT:
Site ____ Temp ____ Color ____
Movement ____ Sensation ____ Capillary Refill ____ Pulse(s) ____

INTAKE		SOLUTION TYPE	SITE	AMOUNT REMAINING	RATE	AMOUNT ABSORBED IN SDP	TIME ABSORBED	INITIALS	OUTPUT	TIME	URINE	EMESIS	INITIALS
	IV												
	IV												

MEDS	TIME	DRUG	DOSE	ROUTE	EFFECTIVENESS	SIGNATURE

TIME	TEMP	P	R	BP	DISCHARGE CRITERIA SCORE: VITAL SIGNS	MENTAL STATUS	ACTIVITY	PAIN	INTAKE	OPERATIVE SITE	TOTAL SCORE	INITIALS
PRE-OP												

KEY FOR DISCHARGE CRITERIA SCORES:

Vital Signs	2 = BP ± 0-20 mm Hg from pre-anesthesia level 1 = BP ± 20-30 mm Hg 0 = BP ± >30 mm Hg
Mental Status	2 = fully awake and alert 1 = sleepy, responds readily 0 = sleepy, sedated
Activity	2 = OOB ab lib 1 = OOB w assistance 0 = unable to ambulate
Pain	2 = absent or mild 1 = moderate or controlled w p. o. meds 0 = severe or requires IM meds
Intake	2 = tolerates p. o. fluids w/o N/V 1 = tolerates ice chips/sips fluid/mild nausea 0 = unable to tolerate p. o. fluids
Operative Site	2 = absence of or minimal bleeding 1 = moderate bleeding 0 = large amount bleeding

TIME	NURSES' NOTES

DISCHARGE ASSESSMENT

PACKING Yes ____ No ____ Site ____ Removed at ____ Initials ____			DR. TO SEE PT. BEFORE D/C Yes ____ No ____	INITIALS
TIME	DISCHARGE VIA Ambulatory ____ Wheelchair ____ Other ____	ACCOMPANIED BY	INSTRUCTIONS Given by M. D. Printed ____ Verbal ____ Given by R. N. Printed ____ Verbal ____	

NURSES' INITIALS, SIGNATURES & TITLES				

Figure 21–3 *Continued.*

porate checklists and other mechanisms for speed and consistency in documenting nurse care. Narrative notes then can address specific issues of importance for individual patients.

IMPROVING AND MONITORING QUALITY OF CARE

A Phase II unit offers both the opportunity and the mandate to monitor nursing and medical care provided to patients. All nurses in the unit should take an active role in quality improvement activities. Concurrent audits of care can be performed by an independent observer, but more often, clinical studies and chart audits form most quality monitors. Some of the questions and topics that might be considered are included in Table 21–8. One of the many issues of quality care is preventing infections. Nurses should follow the basics of Standard Precautions and appropriate aseptic technique when providing care for a surgical site or drainage systems. In a Phase II unit, infection control also includes ongoing education of the patient and family about methods to prevent infections after discharge.

PREPARING THE PATIENT FOR DISCHARGE

The Phase II unit nurse has significant responsibilities in the care of an ambulatory surgical patient. First, the nurse must constantly monitor and assess patients who have had a wide variety of procedures and anesthetic approaches. That nurse also is balancing two divergent patient care goals: that of encouraging self-care while simultaneously providing for the patients' physical needs. Motivating or convincing the patient to take responsibility for some aspects of self-care sometimes is difficult. Even more difficult can be the job of convincing family members that it is beneficial for the patient to resume self-care.

The Phase II nurse's duties are interesting and varied. These include assessing the patient's physical and mental condition, remaining prepared for emergencies, providing education and encouragement, promoting a sense of wellness, and including family members in the plan of action. All these concerns are focused toward one end: the safe discharge of patients to their home settings. The patient does not come to that point merely by accident or luck, but rather through the direction, care, and encouragement of the nursing staff. When the nurse has accomplished these many functions, the patient is ready for more formal instructions about home care and is prepared for discharge. Chapter 22 presents a detailed discussion of discharge instructions and criteria.

***Table 21–8.* Quality Improvement Indicators Applicable to Phase II Recovery**

Admission criteria being met
Clinical complications
Adequacy of pain and nausea management
Returns to surgery or PACU
IV site complications
Medication errors
Complaints related to privacy
Timeliness of reuniting patient with family/friends
Nurse:patient ratio
Late hours required for patient care and reasons
Discharge criteria/length of stay
Unplanned admissions for overnight care
Falls, injuries
Criteria for discharge met and found in documentation
Medications and treatments all have signed physician orders
Patient complaint
Thrombophlebitis
Pain medication > 4 times
Prolonged headache after spinal anesthesia

IV, intravenous; PACU, postanesthesia care unit.

References

1. Malkin J: Health Facilities Manage 6:2, 1993.
2. ASPAN Standards of Perianesthesia Nursing Practice. Thorofare, NJ: American Society of Perianesthesia Nurses, 1995.
3. Joint Commission on Accreditation of Health Care Organizations: 1996 Accreditation Manual for Ambulatory Health Care. Chicago: JCAHO, 1996.
4. Accreditation Association for Ambulatory Health Care: Accreditation Handbook for Ambulatory Health Care. Skokie, IL: AAAHC, 1992.
5. Wetchler B: Anesthesia for Ambulatory Surgery, 2nd ed. Philadelphia: JB Lippincott, 1991.
6. Aldrete JA: Discharge criteria. In Thomson D, Frost E (eds): Baillieres Clinical Anaesthesiology-Postanaesthesia Care. London: Bailliere Tindall, 1994, pp 763–773.
7. Gruendeman B, Fernsebner B: Comprehensive Perioperative Nursing. Boston: Jones & Bartlett Publishers, 1995.
8. Marley RA: Postoperative nausea and vomiting: The outpatient enigma. J Postanesth Nurs 11:147–161, 1996.
9. Fraulini K: After Anesthesia: A Guide for PACU, ICU and Medical–Surgical Nurses. Norwalk, CT: Appleton & Lange, 1987.
10. Marley RA, Moline B: Patient discharge from the ambulatory setting. J Postanesth Nurs 11:39–49, 1996.
11. Alexander C, Teller L, Gross J, et al: New discharge criteria decrease recovery room time after subarachnoid block. Anesthesiology 70:640–643, 1989.

12. Anderson R, Crohg K: Pain as a major cause of postoperative nausea. Can Anaesth Soc J 23:366, 1976.
13. Kallar S, Everett L: Nausea and vomiting: Eitiology, prophylaxis, and therapy. In McGoldrick K (ed): Ambulatory Anesthesiology: A Problem Oriented Approach. Baltimore: Williams & Wilkins, 1995, p 626.
14. Bresson V: Postoperative nausea and vomiting. In Jacobsen W: Manual of Post Anesthesia Care. Philadelphia: WB Saunders, 1992, pp 180–186.
15. Acute Pain Management Guideline Panel: Acute Pain Management: Operative or Medical Procedures and Trauma. Clinical Practice Guideline. AHCPR Pub. No. 92-0032. Rockville, MD: Agency for Health Care Policy and Research, Public Health Service, U.S. Department of Health and Human Services, Feb 1992.
16. Stout D, Bishop M, Dwersteg J, et al: Correlation of endotracheal tube size with sore throat and hoarseness following general anesthesia. Anesthesiology 67:419–421, 1987.
17. Fox VJ: Patient teaching and discharge planning: The short stay challenge. Capsules Comments Perioperative Nurs I:98–111, 1995.

Chapter 22

Patient Discharge Issues

Rex A. Marley and Beverly M. Moline

The essence of professional nursing lies not in its environment or the use of specialized equipment, but in its decision-making on the part of the nurse.

— Helen Creighton, RN, MSN, JD.

The time necessary for recuperation after surgery and anesthesia is contingent upon several variables: (1) the type and length of the surgical procedure performed, (2) the anesthetic agents, sedatives, and analgesics administered during the perioperative phase, and (3) the manner in which the patient reacts to these influences. The ideal anesthetic agent for the continually expanding ambulatory surgical practice is one that possesses the pharmacokinetic traits of rapid onset and offset, short half-life, inert metabolites, and insignificant cardiovascular or other side effects. Pivotal strides in attaining the ideal anesthetic have been realized with the introduction of the newer anesthetic agents (e.g., propofol, desflurane, sevoflurane, alfentanil, remifentanil). However, residual anesthetic effect still dictates that the ambulatory surgical patient receive a period of postoperative observation plus an organized evaluation prior to discharge.

Operating efficiency is an important component for the business success of an ambulatory surgical facility when a major concern of healthcare delivery is bottom line cost. Safe, appropriate, and timely discharge of patients is crucial to this efficiency. Premature dismissal can lead to complications requiring unplanned hospital admission or visits to the emergency room, both of which have a negative economic impact. Conversely, delayed discharge reduces the ambulatory surgical unit's efficiency and increases cost to the consumer. A practical and systematic patient discharge plan is an essential component in the daily operation of the contemporary ambulatory surgical facility.

GOALS OF PATIENT DISCHARGE

A primary goal of discharge planning is for the patient, who has sufficiently recovered from the effects of surgery and anesthesia, to be "home ready" or "fit for discharge" and safely discharged within a minimal period of time (usually within 1 to 1.5 hours). Certain comprehensive objectives should be met to provide consistent, efficient, and cost-effective quality care to the ambulatory surgical patient (Table 22–1).[1]

STANDARDS AND POLICIES OF PATIENT DISCHARGE

Accrediting and Provider Organizations

General guidelines for discharging the patient from the ambulatory surgical facility have been established by two national accrediting organizations—the Joint Commission for Accreditation of Healthcare Organizations' Ambulatory

Table 22–1. Patient Discharge Goals Following Ambulatory Surgery and Anesthesia

To promote patient satisfaction by minimizing disruptive influences associated with the patient's perioperative care
To optimize quality patient care such that patients can be safely discharged from the facility
To educate patients regarding the anticipated recovery process, thus facilitating patient participation and compliance with postoperative care plus early recognition of problems
To proficiently manage patients to minimize costs to the patient, medical facility, and third party payers

Modified from Marley RA, Moline BM: Patient discharge from the ambulatory setting. J Post Anesth Nurs 11:40, 1996.

Care Accreditation Services[2] and the Accreditation Association of Ambulatory Health Care,[3, 4] plus anesthesia[5, 6] and postanesthesia[7] provider associations. The recommendations offered by these groups are designed to establish standards to maintain quality care for ambulatory surgical facilities (Table 22–2).[1]

Institutional Discharge Policy

Each ambulatory facility must establish a written protocol dealing specifically with patient discharge to a remote recovery location, typically the patient's home. This institutional discharge policy should specify discharge criteria for determining the "home readiness" of the patient. This process promotes quality patient care and provides a foundation for practice decisions. It is imperative that the discharge policy is well documented and uniformly employed as a standard of patient care.

Table 22–2. Guidelines for Discharging the Ambulatory Surgical Patient

Institutional guidelines are developed and approved by the anesthesia department and the medical staff for patient discharge.
Patient evaluation before discharge is the responsibility of a licensed independent practitioner.
A *responsible adult* must accompany any patient who has received other than unsupplemented local anesthesia.
Written postoperative and follow-up care instructions are provided the patient and responsible caregiver.
A written transfer agreement must exist between a freestanding facility and a nearby hospital in the event that hospitalization for more definitive or prolonged care becomes necessary.

From Marley RA, Moline BM: Patient discharge from the ambulatory setting. J Post Anesth Nurs 11:40, 1996.

Patient Evaluation

A licensed independent practitioner is responsible for making the final decision to discharge a patient from the ambulatory facility.[2] A licensed independent practitioner is any individual who is permitted by law and by the organization to provide patient care services without direction or supervision, within the scope of the individual's license and in accordance with individually granted clinical privileges.[2] Depending on state law or institutional policy, this responsibility for patient discharge lies with the surgical, dental, or anesthesia staff. If the primary licensed independent practitioner is not personally present to evaluate the patient's readiness for discharge: (1) a detailed process (i.e., protocol, policy, standing orders, collaborative practice) for patient discharge shall be followed and documented by the phase II nurse, and (2) the responsible practitioner's name will be recorded in the patient's medical record.[2]

Responsible Adult

A responsible adult can be any willing person who is intellectually and physically capable of providing care to the patient.[8] This individual may be expected to: (1) assist with activities of daily living as needed, (2) ensure patient compliance with postoperative instructions, and (3) monitor the patient's progress toward recovery.[1] Ensuring the availability of a responsible adult is best addressed in the preadmission workup of the patient, allowing adequate time for the rearrangement of schedules and anticipatory planning to meet postoperative needs. The time that the services of the caregiver is needed will be dependent on the surgical procedure, the length and type of anesthesia, and the patient's age and general health status. Generally, 24 hours is the recommended time frame for requiring postoperative assistance, but in patients with operative limitations (e.g., bilateral carpal tunnel release), young or elderly patients,[9] and patients for whom anesthesia lasted longer than 2 hours,[10] care may be required for up to 48 hours. Approximately 40% of ambulatory surgical patients report their return to normal activities the day after surgery and anesthesia.[11] Patients receiving local anesthesia without sedation may be discharged without an accompanying adult escort.

Written Instructions

A verbal review of the written discharge instructions is carried out with the patient and the responsible adult before discharge.[2] Validation and documentation of their understanding of crucial instructions is an important component of the discharge process. Ideally, general postoperative instructions should be given during the preadmission or preoperative phase because pain, anxiety, and residual drug effect can impair concentration or recall for the postoperative patient.

General instructions are those that are relevant to almost all outpatients (Table 22–3).[1] These instructions provide the patient with an understanding of limitations and expectations relative to their recovery. The instructions should be written clearly and comprehensively such that the needs of the patient are met as effectively as possible. Documentation that these instructions were conveyed to and under-

***Table 22–3.* Key Education Points for Discharge Instructions**

MEDICATIONS

Note the name, purpose, and dosage schedule for each medication; emphasize the importance of following the directions on the label.

The patient should resume medications taken before surgery per the physician's order.

If pain medication is not prescribed, nonprescription, nonaspirin analgesics (e.g., acetaminophen, ibuprofen) may be effective for mild aches and pains.

Additional pain medication may be ordered by the physician after surgery. The patient should take these medications as directed, preferably with food to prevent gastrointestinal upset.

ACTIVITY RESTRICTION

Advise the patient to take it easy for the remainder of the day after surgery. Dizziness or drowsiness is not unusual following surgery and anesthesia.

For the next 24 hours, the patient should not:

- Drive a vehicle or operate machinery or power tools
- Consume alcohol, including beer
- Make important personal or business decisions or sign important documents

Activity level: In specific behavioral terms (e.g., do not lift objects heavier than 20 lb), describe any limitation of activities.

DIET

Explain any dietary restrictions or instructions.

If no dietary restriction exists, instruct the patient to progress as tolerated to a regular diet.

SURGICAL AND ANESTHESIA SIDE EFFECTS

Anticipated sequelae of surgery (e.g., bleeding and pain) should be delineated.

Common side effects associated with anesthesia include dizziness, drowsiness, myalgia, nausea and vomiting, or sore throat.

POSSIBLE COMPLICATIONS AND SYMPTOMS

Instruct the patient and responsible adult in pertinent signs and symptoms that could be indicative of postoperative complications.

The patient should call the responsible physician if he or she develops:

- Fever > 38.3°C (101°F) orally
- Persistent, atypical pain
- Pain not relieved by medication
- Bleeding or unexpected drainage from the wound that does not stop
- Extreme redness or swelling around the incision site or drainage of pus
- Urinary retention
- Continual nausea or vomiting

TREATMENT AND TESTS

Procedures that the patient or responsible adult is expected to perform (e.g., dressing changes or the application of warm moist compresses) should be described in detail.

A complete list of necessary supplies should be included.

If any postoperative tests are to be conducted, instructions as to the date, time, test location, and any previsit preparation should be listed.

ACCESS TO POSTDISCHARGE CARE

Note the telephone number of the responsible and available physician.

Include the telephone number of the ambulatory center and the hours of operation.

Note also the name, address, and telephone number of the appropriate emergency care facility.

FOLLOW-UP CARE

Identify the date, time, and location of the patient's scheduled return visit to the clinic or surgeon.

Modified from Marley RA, Moline BM: Patient discharge from the ambulatory setting. J Post Anesth Nurs 11:41, 1996.

stood by the patient and escort is an important medicolegal consideration, because one study noted that almost 30% of patients admitted driving a vehicle or consuming alcohol within 24 hours of surgery.[12] In addition to general discharge instructions, the patient receives home care instruction specific to the surgical procedure or anesthetic technique when necessary.

Transfer to Inpatient Status Considerations

Unanticipated Hospital Admission

With contemporary standards of anesthesia care, major morbidity and mortality following ambulatory surgery is remarkably low. A review of ambulatory surgical care encompassing 45,090 patients over a 3-year period at a rural-based referral center found that the majority of postoperative morbidity (1:1455) occurred within the first 48 hours, whereas no deaths occurred during the first week after surgery.[13] Many factors account for unexpected hospitalization following ambulatory surgery; surgical-related complications (e.g., more extensive surgery, hemorrhage, wound dehiscence) are responsible for more hospital transfers or return emergency room visits than are persistent pain or unrelenting nausea and vomiting.[14–19] The unanticipated hospital admission rates have been reported to range between 0.2% and 33%.[14, 17, 19–27] This divergency in hospital admission rates is a reflection of policies and practices of the various ambulatory facilities, appropriate patient selection, and the type of surgical procedures performed. Certain procedures (e.g., laparoscopic sterilization, head and neck procedures, urologic procedures) account for the higher reported incidence of hospital admissions; when these higher at-risk-for-admission procedures are considered and averaged, the overall hospital admission rate following ambulatory surgery approaches 0.5% to 1.5%.

Admission Plan and Implementation

A written protocol is necessary to facilitate patient transport to the nearby hospital if the patient requires a higher level of care than the freestanding ambulatory center can offer. An ongoing review of this policy and process with the ambulatory staff is necessary so that proficiency is maintained in: (1) activation of the transport team (i.e., paramedics and ambulance), (2) patient stabilization, and (3) the use of emergency equipment. To guarantee patient access to the full-service hospital, either a written transfer agreement between the free-standing facility and hospital is present or the ambulatory surgical facility grants privileges only to physicians who have admission privileges at the nearby hospital.[4]

STAGES OF RECOVERY FROM ANESTHESIA

Three basic stages of recovery from anesthesia are recognized and of concern to the postoperative nurses while evaluating the patient's cognitive, psychomotor, and physiologic recovery following anesthesia (Table 22–4).[28] A fourth stage of recovery, known as the emergence from anesthesia, beginning in the operating room, has been suggested.[29] Some overlap may exist between this stage and the early stage of recovery. For the phase I postanesthesia care unit (PACU) nurse, patient care concerns (i.e., patient awakening and recovery of vital reflexes) will be the same as identified in the early stage of recovery.

Early Stage of Recovery

The early stage of recovery encompasses the time from the termination of anesthetic agent administration till such time that the patient is alert and oriented to person, place, and time. The patient will be admitted to the phase I postanesthesia care area for continuous observation and monitoring. There is a restoration of the fundamental reflexes of the cardiovascular system and upper airway during this stage. The patient remains in this environment until he or she is physiologically stable and has recovered sufficiently so that he or she may be safely transferred to the phase II area.

Tests to Evaluate Early Stage Recovery

Assessment for the early stage of recovery consists of cognitive tests (e.g., eye opening to command, orientation to person, place, and time). In addition, the return of motor activity is observed during this time. Traditional quantitative methods for evaluating recovery from the phase I setting have utilized the Aldrete and Kroulik postanesthetic recovery (PAR) score.[30] A revised version was offered by Aldrete in 1994 to reflect the clinical ability to routinely quantitate oxygenation with the pulse oximeter

Table 22–4. **Stages of Recovery**

STAGES OF RECOVERY	CLINICAL DEFINITION AND ENDPOINTS
Stage I	*Awakening:*
Early recovery (in phase I recovery)	Responds to verbal commands, progressing to being awake and alert*
	Recovery and stabilization of vital reflexes:
	Return of protective reflexes and cough and swallowing reflexes
	Can maintain a clear airway unaided
	Oxyhemoglobin saturation (Spo_2) > 94% with or without supplemental oxygen therapy
	Stable vital functions (e.g., blood pressure, respiration, heart rate)
	Absence of surgical (e.g., bleeding) or anesthetic (e.g., laryngeal edema) complications
	Aldrete score ≥ 8 or fulfills a similar scoring system
Stage II	*Immediate clinical recovery:*
Intermediate recovery (in phase II recovery)	Normal Spo_2 in room air* Stands and walks unaided to bathroom*
"Home readiness"	*Home readiness:*
	Fulfills institutional discharge criteria
	Absence of any major complications or side effects
Stage III	*Psychological recovery:*
Late recovery (phase III)	Return of memory and cognitive function*
	Return of concentration, discrimination, reasoning*
Complete recovery to "street fitness"	*Full recovery:*
	Return of psychomotor functions to preoperative baseline status
	Can perform normal daily activities (e.g., return to work)

Data from Korttila KT: Post-anaesthetic psychomotor and cognitive function. Eur J Anaesth 12:43–46, 1995; Pandit SK, Pandit UA: Phases of the recovery period. In White PF (ed): Ambulatory Anesthesia and Surgery. Philadelphia: WB Saunders, 1997, pp 457–464.

*Or return to preoperative baseline status.

(see Table 20–11).[31] Usually upon achieving a score of ≥ 8, the patient will be transferred to the phase II recovery area.

Intermediate Stage of Recovery

The period from the return of vital reflexes (e.g., hemodynamic, neurologic, pulmonary) till phase II discharge criteria are met is called the intermediate stage of recovery. The phase II postanesthesia care setting is appropriate for this stage of recovery. Upon completion of surgery with general anesthesia, the alert and stable patient who meets standard phase I discharge criteria while in the operating room and who can demonstrate the ability to move may be admitted directly to the phase II area if he or she is comfortable and free of nausea and vomiting.[32, 33] Patients having received monitored anesthesia care and select regional anesthetic techniques can be expected to return directly to the phase II area for postoperative recovery. These patients require less intensive monitoring and can be cared for in an environment with a reduced staffing ratio. In this environment, interaction with the patient's family is resumed; patient mobilization is encouraged; patient instructions are reinforced; and the patient is prepared and evaluated for dismissal.

Tests to Evaluate Intermediate Stage Recovery

Various clinical tests (e.g., sitting unaided, walking in a straight line, countdown test from 100, and reaction time), pencil-and-paper tests (e.g., Trieger, perceptual speed, 'p'-deletion, and digit symbol substitution), and psychomotor tests (e.g., Maddox Wing, Critical flicker fusion, and Choice reaction time) have been used to determine home readiness. Many of these cognitive and psychomotor ability tests require comparison with the patient's preoperative values; many tests are time-consuming, costly, and complex or require sophisticated equipment; or the tests lack standardization and thus are impractical for routine clinical use in the busy ambulatory setting. A criteria-based postanesthesia scoring system provides an objective, consistent, and efficient method of assessing a patient's readiness for discharge.

Late Stage of Recovery

The patient continues to recover from anesthetic effects once he or she is dismissed from the ambulatory facility. This late stage of recovery progresses until the patient safely resumes normal daily activities consistent with preoperative status.

CRITERIA-BASED SCORING SYSTEMS

Helpful in the decision to discharge patients from the ambulatory facility are discriminating scoring systems. Unfortunately, the most commonly used postoperative recovery evaluation method developed by Aldrete and Kroulik[30] in 1970 and recently updated[31] is not meaningful for the phase II ambulatory population with regard to comprehensive "home readiness." Newer, more discriminate models such as the Modified Postanesthesia Discharge Scoring System[34] and Aldrete's phase II postanesthetic recovery score[31] address items specific to suitability for home discharge (i.e., ambulation, bleeding, comfort level, and nausea and vomiting) following ambulatory surgery and anesthesia. A systematic approach to patient evaluation by the nursing personnel is necessary as a method of determining the patient's postoperative recovery and suitability for discharge.

Aldrete's Phase I Postanesthetic Recovery Score

The patient scoring system that has received nearly universal acceptance for discharge readiness from phase I is the Aldrete and Kroulik PAR score.[30] For numerous years we have been aware that observation of the patient's skin or mucous membranes to determine the patient's ability to oxygenate was an imprecise science.[35] Aldrete updated his original phase I PAR score in 1994 to reflect the contemporary ability to monitor oxygenation in a more precise manner with pulse oximetry (see Table 20–11).[31]

The Aldrete phase I PAR scoring system is not specific for evaluating the ambulatory patient's readiness for home discharge. Limitations of this scoring system for discharging ambulatory patients include no mention of the patient's: (1) ability to ambulate, (2) hydration status, (3) comfort level, or (4) whether persistent nausea or vomiting is present. These are important issues that require evaluation before dismissing the patient from the phase II recovery area.

Aldrete's Phase II Postanesthetic Recovery Score

A criteria-based scoring system specific to the ambulatory setting has been introduced by Aldrete.[31] In addition to the categories found in his phase I discharge criteria (activity, respiration, circulation, consciousness, and oxygen saturation), this scoring system was developed to include five additional criteria (dressing, pain, ambulation, fasting-feeding, and urine output) specific to ambulatory patients (see Table 21–4).[31]

Modified Postanesthesia Discharge Scoring System

In 1991, Chung and associates first proposed using a discriminative discharge scoring system for ambulatory surgical patients, termed the Post Anesthesia Discharge Scoring System (PADSS).[36] Refinements in the original PADSS (such as removing the criteria of whether or not the patient took oral fluids or could void) led to more clinically practical discharge criteria known as the modified PADSS (Table 22–5).[34] This revised scoring system identifies five areas of evaluation: (1) vital signs, (2) ambulation, (3) nausea and vomiting, (4) pain, and (5) surgical bleeding. When ensuring that the patient's ability to drink and void was removed as a discharge criterion, 20% of outpatients were able to be discharged earlier.[34]

These two phase II criteria-based discharge scoring systems offer easy and objective methods of assessing "home readiness"; however, they should not replace critical and individualized patient assessment. These scoring systems provide sound discharge goals that offer direction to our decision-making process of home discharge, yet these systems can still fail the patient if we blindly look at the present criteria to the exclusion of the entire picture.

Table 22–5. **Modified Postanesthesia Discharge Scoring System**

PATIENT SIGN	CRITERION	SCORE
Vital Signs	< 20% of preoperative value	2
	20–40% of preoperative value	1
	> 40% of preoperative value	0
Ambulation	Steady gait; no dizziness	2
	With assistance	1
	None; dizziness	0
Nausea/Vomiting	Minimal	2
	Moderate	1
	Severe	0
Pain	Minimal	2
	Moderate	1
	Severe	0
Surgical Bleeding	Minimal	2
	Moderate	1
	Severe	0

Note: The total possible score is 10. Patients scoring ≥ 9 are considered fit for outpatient discharge.

Modified from Theodorou-Michaloliakou C, Chung FF, Chua JG: Does a modified postanaesthetic discharge scoring system determine home-readiness sooner? Can J Anaesth 40:A32, 1993.

For example, we might consider the patient presenting in phase II: (1) who has a blood pressure of 114/62 (preoperative baseline was 148/74; Aldrete phase II PAR score = 1), (2) who expresses moderate nausea (Aldrete phase II PAR score = 1), (3) who has some discomfort (oral medication is adequate for pain control; Aldrete phase II PAR score = 1), and (4) who has not voided but denies bladder discomfort (Aldrete phase II PAR score = 1). This patient's Aldrete's phase II PAR score would not meet discharge criteria.

A critical and individualized patient assessment reveals a history of: (1) mild nausea following all previous surgeries, which generally resolves later that day or the next, (2) nothing by mouth 7 hours before surgery, (3) adequate hydration, and (4) no pre-existing health problems. The surgical procedure did not involve the pelvic region or genitourinary system. The patient denies any urge to void, and the bladder region is not distended. Pain control is reported by the patient to be satisfactory, and the patient is enjoying conversation with a friend. The current blood pressure is compatible with intraoperative and postoperative values. This patient appears to be a viable candidate for discharge even though the patient failed to meet the required score of 18 or higher. Retaining the patient in the phase II recovery area until an adequate score of 18 is reached may not be the most efficient approach.

The cost of prolonging phase II recovery until the patient has voided or nausea has resolved is a relevant concern in the changing healthcare arena. Nausea and voiding are problems that can be managed at home with clear directions on when to contact appropriate resources should symptoms persist. Pain is not expected to decrease in the immediate future, and the blood pressure may not return to preoperative levels considering the patient's recent surgical experience. Although significant progress has been made in attempts to develop a meaningful discharge scoring system for the ambulatory surgical population, a definitive tool that is sensitive to the patient, surgical procedure, and anesthetic technique, as well as compatible with today's economic concerns, has yet to be finalized.[1]

CLINICAL READINESS CRITERIA FOR DISCHARGE

For discharge to occur, the patient must be clinically stable and able to continue the recovery process at a remote recovery location. The decision to discharge is best made on objective criteria outlined in the policies of each ambulatory surgical facility. Noncriteria-based systems have been offered, e.g. Wetchler (Table 22–6)[37, 38] and Korttila (Table 22–7),[39] which look for specific clinical parameters as indicators for successful dismissal from the ambulatory center. Distinct objective discharge criteria must be addressed when assessing home readiness of the patient. Individually, the following clinical markers should be evaluated in an organized, concise manner.

Prior to discharge from phase I, the patient's vital signs will be stable; there will be no respiratory impairment; protective reflexes of swallow and cough will be present; and the patient will be oriented to person, place, and time. It is assumed that the status of these parameters will not deteriorate during the patient's stay in Phase II.

Vital Signs

When only one set of preoperative vital signs is available as a baseline, it is important to con-

Table 22–6. Wetchler's Guidelines for Safe Patient Discharge After Ambulatory Surgery and Anesthesia

Stable vital signs: these include temperature, pulse, respiration, and blood pressure when appropriate. Vital signs should remain stable for a period of not less than 30 minutes and be consistent with the patient's age and preanesthesia levels.

Ability to swallow and cough: the patient must demonstrate ability to swallow fluids and be able to cough.

Ability to walk: the patient demonstrates ability to perform movement consistent with age and development level (e.g., sit, stand, walk).

Minimal nausea, vomiting, and dizziness:

Minimal nausea: absence of nausea, or, if nausea is present, the patient can still swallow and retain some fluids.

Minimal vomiting: vomiting is either absent or, if present, does not require treatment. Following vomiting that requires treatment, the patient should be able to swallow and retain fluids.

Minimal dizziness: dizziness is either absent or present only upon sitting and the patient is still able to perform movement consistent with age.

Absence of respiratory distress: the patient exhibits no signs of snoring, obstructed respiration, stridor, retractions, or croupy cough.

Alert and oriented: the patient is aware of his or her surroundings and what has taken place and is also interested in returning home.

From Wetchler BV: Problem solving in the postanesthesia care unit. In Wetchler BV (ed): Anesthesia for Ambulatory Surgery, 2nd ed. Philadelphia: JB Lippincott, 1991, p 421.

Table 22–7. Korttila's Guidelines for Safe Patient Discharge After Ambulatory Surgery and Anesthesia

Vital signs stable for 1 hour
The patient must be:
 Oriented to person, place, and time
 Able to tolerate orally administered fluids*
 Able to void†
 Able to dress
 Able to walk without assistance
The patient must not have:
 More than minimal nausea or vomiting
 Excessive pain
 Bleeding
The patient must be discharged by both the person who gave anaesthesia and the person who performed surgery, or their designees‡
Written instructions for the postoperative period at home, including a contact place and person, need to be reinforced
Patients must have a responsible "vested" adult to escort them home and to stay with them at home

From Korttila K: Recovery from outpatient anesthesia: Factors affecting outcome. Anaesthesia 50(Suppl):24, 1995.

* Drinking is recommended before discharge but is not mandatory.

† Voiding is recommended as a criterion for discharge but is not mandatory. It should be required after spinal or epidural blocks and after pelvic-related surgery.

‡ It is not mandatory that these persons are physically present upon discharge if a discharge note has been signed and discharge is carried out following strict policy.

sider the circumstances by which the data were obtained. An anxious patient presenting to the ambulatory center in discomfort or one who is hurried in preparation for surgery may not present with vital signs reflective of his or her normal baseline values. Discharge evaluation of vital signs should consider age-appropriateness, the patient's general health status, anesthetic technique, a comparison with not only preoperative values but also intraoperative and postoperative values, and the patient's position when blood pressure and heart rate were monitored. Vital signs should be stable for at least 30 minutes prior to patient discharge.[40]

The blood pressure and pulse rate should fall ideally within ±20% of their preoperative value. Occasionally, the licensed independent practitioner must depend on the entire clinical picture to make an informed, realistic decision to discharge in cases in which the established criteria have not been satisfied. Clinical signs of orthostatic hypotension (e.g., dizziness, nausea, syncope, tachycardia) should be assessed, especially when the patient is sitting and then standing.

The patient's body temperature may drop 2°C to 3°C following ambulatory surgery. This is typically well tolerated and of no clinical consequence.[41] A patient temperature of less than 35°C should be treated aggressively with active skin-surface warming devices (e.g., forced air warmer). The usefulness of establishing a minimum temperature criterion prior to patient discharge has yet to be demonstrated.[42]

Respiratory Status

The patient with significant respiratory impairment is not a candidate for home discharge. Adequate oxyhemoglobin saturations via pulse oximetry on room air, respiratory rates consistent with age and preoperative health status, and an uncompromised airway permit further evaluation of the patient to meet other discharge criteria. The patient should be free of respiratory distress (e.g., croupy [barky] cough, dyspnea, nasal flaring, retractions, snoring, stridor, or wheezing). With appropriate respiratory care and extended observation, patients experiencing adverse respiratory events (e.g., pulmonary aspiration of gastric contents[43]; postextubation laryngeal edema[44]) who no longer display symptoms may be considered for home discharge.

Reflexes

The swallowing and coughing protective airway reflexes must be present before discharge. Particularly careful evaluation of these reflexes should occur after procedures that involve airway manipulation or administration of topical anesthesia to the upper airway. Usually, the patient must demonstrate adequate swallowing before discharge. If the physician orders the patient to remain nil per os (NPO) for several hours after discharge, instructions to the patient should include time-specific parameters prior to drinking at home. Water is suggested as the initial liquid until adequate swallowing is ensured, and the patient should be instructed to pay attention to swallowing the beverage and avoid drinking while talking, walking, or turning the head.

Another protective reflex—that of blinking—may be absent at the time of discharge after eye surgery; however, bandaging of the eye with the upper lid closed prevents drying of or injury to the cornea. Rarely, a special instance may occur when the patient has had regional anesthesia of the eye but the surgery is canceled.

If the blink reflex is absent the upper eyelid should be taped closed or a bandage placed over the closed eye until return of the protective reflex.[45]

Orientation

The patient should be oriented to person, place, and time or at a level appropriate for the patient's developmental and preoperative status. Additional patient observation and evaluation may become necessary for the patient not returning to the normal preoperative mental state. The patient who is confused in Phase I will likely remain in that setting while evaluation as to the etiology of the confusion is initiated.

Surgical Considerations

Bleeding

Bleeding from the surgical site needs to be minimal or appropriate for the surgical procedure. The expertise of the phase II recovery nurse is crucial when evaluating appropriate surgical bleeding. With some procedures no bleeding is anticipated, whereas with others it is expected that dressing changes will be required. Communication with the surgeon is important to establish permissible levels of drainage (e.g., blood, urine, or other fluids) from the surgical site. Discharge evaluation of the condition of dressings, casts, and drains must be documented. It is important for the patient to be informed of the expected wound drainage and to be skilled in managing dressing changes and drain care, if relevant.[1]

Extremity Circulation

If an intraoperative limb tourniquet was utilized, admission assessment of the extremity may reveal skin that is pale, flushed, or mottled. The patient should not be dismissed until skin color and capillary refill have returned to normal limits.

Plaster or fiberglass casts or encircling dressings can compromise circulation, and their presence demands frequent extremity assessment. Neurovascular integrity, skin color and temperature, pulses, capillary refill, sensation (sharp and tactile), and movement of the affected extremity are regularly assessed throughout recovery and on discharge. Skin temperature can be an unreliable indicator of circulatory status, because cool room temperature in the operating room or PACU may produce vasoconstriction of the surgical extremity. Comparing the operative with the nonoperative extremity is helpful in identifying surgically induced compromise.[45]

Pain

In addition to protracted emesis, postoperative discomfort secondary to the surgical intervention is a common management issue which leads to unanticipated hospital admissions.[46, 47] The goal of acute pain management in the ambulatory setting is to have a patient free of unreasonable surgical discomfort, recover, and be discharged free of side effects in the most expedient manner possible. Inadequate postoperative pain management continues to be a problem for adult and pediatric populations. Severe pain (defined as moaning or writhing in pain at any time, initial nursing care dominated by pain control, or requiring more analgesics than ordered) was noted in 5.3% of ambulatory patients in the PACU and again at 24 hours postoperatively.[48] This deficiency in care is typically attributed to an inadequate prescribed dosage regimen by the physician, underutilization of postoperative analgesics by nursing personnel, and lack of communication on the patient's part in requesting medication.

Etiology

Postoperative pain resulting from direct tissue or nerve injury is a physiologic process consisting of an inflammatory response, hyperalgesia, and nociceptor activation. The physiologic response of the nervous system involves two modifications—peripheral and central sensitization. Peripheral sensitization consisting of nociceptor activation involves the release of endogenous pain-producing substances or ions from the cell that either directly or indirectly sensitize nociceptors, thus lowering the stimulus threshold. Identified mediators that lower the painful stimulus threshold include bradykinin, histamine, leukotrienes, prostaglandins, serotonin, and substance P. Central sensitization describes the excitable reaction of the spinal neurons in response to noxious stimuli produced as a result of the surgical trauma. Local anesthetic agents and the opioid analgesics are effective in preventing the establishment and suppression of central sensitization.

Pain Prophylaxis

An effective and organized approach to the management of postoperative pain begins with its anticipation. Preemptive analgesia has been shown to be a more effective method of pain control than to reactively address the issue. Anticipation of the occurrence of pain before it occurs should be a goal in the postoperative care of the patient. Considerations relating to preemptive analgesia follow.

Open Communication. Encourage the patient to communicate discomfort and request measures to relieve pain. The patient's self-report of pain offers a consistent, reliable means of quantifying pain.[49] Several Lickert type numeric pain intensity scales (see Table 21–6 for pain assessment tools) are available for use in adults and the older pediatric patient. For the younger pediatric patient, the Wong-Baker FACES Pain Rating Scale (see Table 26–13) should prove useful.[50]

Consider Analgesics. Give pre- and intraoperative analgesic medications in those surgical procedures associated with significant discomfort following emergence from anesthesia. Administration of analgesics before the pain becomes intense makes pain management easier. A multimodal analgesic treatment regimen is directed at altering the central and peripheral sensitization responses to the surgically induced trauma. Pharmacologic therapy with analgesic medications attempts to inhibit the nociceptor response either centrally (within the central nervous system) or peripherally (at the site of insult). Opioid analgesics are effective in modulating afferent nociceptive impulses at several anatomic sites (e.g., the brain and the dorsal horn of the spinal cord). Peripheral anti-inflammatory and analgesic effects are instituted by the prototypical nonsteroidal anti-inflammatory drugs (NSAIDs). This combination therapy offers the best approach for preemptive analgesia in the ambulatory setting.

Administration of a longer-lasting opioid analgesic (i.e., fentanyl), along with non-narcotic analgesics, should be considered so that a sustained effect carries over into the immediate recovery phase. An additional benefit seen with the administration of these potent analgesics is a reduction in the intraoperative anesthetic requirement. Unless contraindicated, consideration should be given for including a non-narcotic analgesic during this time. Single doses of these analgesics (e.g., acetaminophen, ibuprofen, ketorolac) are effective in reducing postoperative pain when dispensed before or during surgery. These drugs may also be administered via the rectal (e.g., acetaminophen) or parenteral routes (e.g., ketorolac) once the patient is anesthetized. One advantage of employing these agents is their opioid dose-sparing analgesic effect, which should reduce the need for narcotic supplementation and help minimize narcotic-induced side effects (i.e., nausea and vomiting, sedation).

Wound Infiltration with Local Anesthetic Agents. Intraoperatively infiltrating the wound with long-acting local anesthetic agents should be used whenever possible. Effective application of local anesthetics to the operative site may reduce or eliminate the need for parenteral analgesics in the immediate postoperative phase.

Peripheral or Regional Nerve Blocks. Peripheral or regional nerve blocks are an effective and underutilized method of sheltering the patient from pain. This concept is becoming more popular especially in the pediatric population (e.g., caudal block). Nerve blocks will complement a general anesthetic by:

- Contributing to a smoother, more pleasant emergence from general anesthesia.
- Reducing the need for narcotic and non-narcotic analgesics postoperatively.
- Promoting earlier ambulation.
- Allowing early resumption of normal appetite.
- Reducing phase I and II recovery times.

Pain Management

Any pain experienced by the patient should be consistent with the surgical event and controllable by the prescribed postoperative analgesics. In most situations, the preferred route of analgesic administration is oral. Once the patient is tolerating oral fluids, pain should be manageable with standard oral analgesics.

Before discharge from the facility, the patient may be started on his or her prescribed oral analgesic to evaluate analgesic efficacy. For mild to moderate postoperative pain, short-term oral NSAIDs may be all that is required. When prescribed, the NSAIDs should be administered continuously for the first 24 to 48 hours. For severe or breakthrough pain, a combination of narcotic and NSAIDs will provide more effective relief than each of the drugs individually. Patient controlled analgesia (PCA) may be utilized if the patient is being discharged to a skilled care facility or to a homecare agency.

The patient's perception of pain dictates the level of pain therapy instituted. The location, type, and intensity of pain should be consistent with anticipated postoperative discomfort. Atypical pain (e.g., abdominal pain [as opposed to expected cramping] following a diagnostic dilatation and curettage) would require further patient evaluation.[40]

Nonpharmacologic Pain Management Strategies. Nonpharmacologic techniques of modifying the response to pain have been advocated and employed in recent years. Included in such measures are reassurance, relaxation techniques (e.g., visualization, music therapy), massage, thermal packs, acupuncture, and use of transcutaneous electrical nerve stimulation (TENS).

Nausea and Vomiting

One of the more common and disturbing adverse effects of surgery and anesthesia is postoperative nausea and vomiting (PONV). Approximately one fourth to one third of all patients having surgery will experience PONV.[51–55] Protracted nausea and vomiting is: (1) the main reason for delayed discharge from the ambulatory center[56]; (2) a leading reason for unanticipated hospital admission[14, 27, 57]; and (3) responsible for increases in patient cost.[58] Postoperative nausea and vomiting has been reported to be more incapacitating than the consequences of the surgery in almost 40% of outpatients.[59]

Generally, this annoying side effect is self-limiting and improves with time. The causes of PONV are multiple and may be attributable to anesthetic or nonanesthetic factors.[60] However, for the patient able to be discharged with minimal nausea and vomiting, patient evaluation and management options should be known and utilized.

Patient Evaluation

When faced with problematic postoperative nausea and vomiting, several factors need to be assessed when evaluating whether the patient should be discharged home.

1. The patient's general health status preoperatively and the consequences of not tolerating oral intake once the patient is discharged must be considered. It may be acceptable for a healthy adult to continue his or her recovery at home and abstain from eating or drinking until he or she is free of nausea and vomiting. However, this plan of patient management would not be acceptable for certain populations (e.g., the diabetic patient).
2. The patient's age is important, because the geriatric and pediatric populations present greater risks than does the otherwise healthy adult patient if he or she is unable to resume caloric intake.
3. The patient's hydration status is an important component that must be evaluated. Certain variables to observe include: (1) the time of fasting before surgery, (2) the amount of perioperative intravenous fluids infused plus oral fluids retained, (3) the amount of fluid loss during surgery and through emesis, and (4) the amount of urinary output and the color and odor of the urine.
4. The probability of the nausea and vomiting resolving, continuing, or progressing must be evaluated. Several variables that are part of this assessment include the type of surgery, the intensity and pattern of the nausea and vomiting, the patient's historical experience with nausea and vomiting, and the patient's response to interventions directed at alleviating the nausea and vomiting. The patient should exhibit only minimal nausea or vomiting, and this pattern should be stable or improving before the patient is discharged.

Postoperative Management of Nausea and Vomiting

Nausea and vomiting affects the patient's overall perception of the ambulatory surgical experience.[61, 62] This often-associated "bad reaction" to anesthesia as expressed by the patient confirms that nausea and vomiting is not an acceptable sequela of ambulatory surgery. Patient management problems designed to minimize PONV would include the following issues.

Antiemetic Prophylaxis. Antiemetic drug therapy is aimed at alleviating the multiple trigger mechanisms by which the vomiting reflex may be initiated. This helps to explain why particular antiemetics are effective in a given situation whereas others are not. Combination multimechanism drug therapy may be more effective in managing nausea and vomiting, yet the likelihood of side effects is increased. Pharmacologic antiemetic therapy for all patients is not recommended secondary to the increased potential for adverse drug effect (e.g., cardiovascular changes, dysphoria, extrapyramidal symptoms). Preemptive antiemetic prophylaxis should be considered pre- or intraoperatively in the high-risk patient. Indications for prophylactic antiemetic therapy would include[63]:

- A history of protracted postoperative emesis.
- Operations associated with a high incidence of nausea and vomiting.
- Mandibular surgery when the jaws are wired shut.

- Circumstances in which retching could jeopardize the surgical result (e.g., plastic or eye procedures).

Appropriate Hydration. Maintaining appropriate hydration in the surgical patient is important for minimizing the incidence of dizziness and postural hypotension. Reducing the NPO interval decreases the time that patients must fast and curtails problems associated with prolonged fasting.[64] Providing sufficient intravenous fluid hydration, such as perioperatively administering at least 20 ml/kg of isotonic electrolyte solution, will improve the postoperative course of the healthy patient (e.g., less dizziness, drowsiness, or faintness; shorter hospital stay; earlier return to work).[65, 66]

Postural hypotension may become apparent when the patient attempts to sit or stand up in the phase II recovery area. Ensuring adequate hydration before mobilizing the patient and avoiding rapid postural changes are important in preventing postural hypotension. In otherwise healthy individuals, ephedrine, a sympathomimetic agent, in a dose of 0.5 mg/kg intramuscularly, has been effective in preventing postoperative nausea and vomiting possibly by preventing postural hypotension and by improving medullary blood flow.[67]

Minimize Motion. Minimizing unnecessary movement may be helpful. Sensitization of the vestibular system, secondary to agents such as nitrous oxide or narcotics, may produce nausea and vomiting when the patient moves.

Minimize Narcotic Analgesics. Narcotic agents administered intraoperatively[68–70] or postoperatively[71] will: (1) increase the incidence of PONV, (2) contribute to a greater need for rescue antiemetic therapy, and (3) delay patient discharge from the ambulatory facility. The use of narcotic analgesics can be reduced by employing non-narcotic analgesics (e.g., NSAIDS, acetaminophen), peripheral or regional nerve blocks, and operative site infiltration with long-lasting local anesthetic agents.

Oral Intake

A protective airway reflex should be confirmed prior to the patient's discharge from phase I. The patient should demonstrate the ability to swallow and cough. Unless crucial to his or her continued convalescence at home (e.g., diabetic patient; patients requiring oral analgesics), the otherwise healthy outpatient who is sufficiently hydrated should not be forced to take oral fluids.[72] Requiring the patient to consume fluids before he or she is ready will increase the incidence of vomiting.[73] Schreiner and associates[73] found an approximately 60% higher incidence of nausea and vomiting in patients who were forced to drink than in those patients who drank only when they requested liquids.

Just because a patient is able to take and retain oral fluids prior to discharge from the ambulatory center does not ensure that the patient will avoid dehydration once he or she returns home. Recent evaluations have documented a 35% to 50% incidence of vomiting once patients were discharged from the ambulatory facility.[74, 75]

Voiding

Patient evaluation relative to postoperative voiding should consider the patient's age, hydration status, psychomotor state of arousal, type of surgery, and anesthetic technique. Patients may not exhibit a need to void who:

1. Have voided just before surgery
2. Have fasted extensively (e.g., NPO since the evening before surgery)
3. Are not afforded an understanding, relaxed, private environment (particularly with children)[76]
4. Have received minimal intravenous hydration in the perioperative setting

Certain surgical procedures (e.g., gynecologic, inguinal herniorrhaphy, urologic) are associated with a higher incidence of postoperative urinary retention. These patients should demonstrate the ability to void before discharge. Following cystoscopic procedures, the urine should be observed to ensure that hematuria, if present, is within clinically acceptable limits. Patients who receive a central neuraxial block should demonstrate the ability to void prior to dismissal, because intact functioning of the autonomic nerve supply to the bladder and urethra is essential for micturition. In select patients who cannot urinate, bladder catheterization along with explicit instructions (e.g., signs of urinary retention and when to contact the responsible physician if unable to urinate) may permit patient discharge.

Anesthesia Considerations

Malignant Hyperthermia–Susceptible Patient

The malignant hyperthermia (MH)–susceptible patient is one who has had: (1) a previous episode of MH, (2) masseter muscle rigidity with previous anesthesia, or (3) a first-degree relative with history of an MH episode or a positive muscle biopsy.[77] The patient susceptible to MH who has undergone a routine trigger-free anesthetic will not require hospital admission based exclusively on being MH susceptible.[78] The surgery should be scheduled as early in the day as possible to permit extended patient monitoring of 4 to 6 hours.[79] The lack of symptoms of malignant hyperthermia should be ensured before patient discharge is considered. Extended patient observation would include monitoring for the signs and symptoms of malignant hyperthermia (Table 22–8).[80, 81]

The extended observation unit is appropriate for the MH-susceptible patient in which reservations about discharge exist. For the MH-susceptible patient to be considered for discharge home, it is important to have a strong support network (i.e., responsible and informed escort, telephone access, and transportation if return to medical care is necessary). The responsible adult should be knowledgeable as to the signs and symptoms of MH and the required action to take if any symptoms are present.

The increase in body temperature associated with MH typically develops late in the course of the disease. Exhaled carbon dioxide level determination on a continual basis is not a commonly employed PACU monitoring tool and is subject to limitations, especially in the nonintubated patient. The patient emerging from general anesthesia is subject to factors that may predispose the patient to hypercarbia other than secondary to malignant hyperthermia (e.g., hypoventilation). It is important to differentiate between a primary hypercarbia secondary to alveolar hypoventilation and hypercarbia secondary to a metabolic crisis. If the patient exhibits signs and symptoms consistent with malignant hyperthermia, arterial blood gas analysis should be performed to evaluate oxygenation, ventilation, and acid-base status.

***Table 22–8.* Signs and Symptoms of Malignant Hyperthermia**

Increased carbon dioxide production: the most sensitive indicator of potential MH in the operating room; doubling or tripling of end-tidal carbon dioxide may occur acutely or gradually over 10 to 20 minutes.
Total body rigidity: the most specific sign of MH; watch for subjective patient complaints of muscle aches
Unexpected signs and symptoms that are common with MH: tachycardia, tachypnea, and jaw muscle rigidity
Acidosis occurring early in MH: respiratory, metabolic
Elevated body temperature: often a late sign of MH
Occurrence of dark urine

MH, malignant hyperthermia.

Regional Anesthesia

Central Neuraxial Techniques. Central neuraxial techniques (e.g., spinal or epidural anesthesia) require total recovery from motor, sensory, and sympathetic blockade prior to discharge. Patients receiving this form of anesthesia will be required to meet the same discharge criteria as patients receiving general anesthesia. Appropriate central neuraxial recovery may be assessed as follows:

- Recovery of sensory function can be assessed by return of skin prick sensation to the perianal region, which requires residual central neuraxial block to have receded to at least dermatome S4-5.[82]
- Recovery of sympathetic tone can be evaluated once sensory function has returned. Permit the patient to sit up while monitoring for signs of hypotension and syncope, which are indicators of inadequate recovery.
- Recovery of motor function can be assessed by the patient being able to take each heel and move it contralaterally from the big toe to the knee and back.[83]

If the patient tolerates sitting well and demonstrates motor strength recovery, he or she can best confirm complete recovery by walking to the bathroom and urinating.[39]

Peripheral Nerve Blocks. With proper patient selection and instructions, individuals receiving peripheral nerve blocks, such as brachial plexus or foot blocks, can be expected to be discharged with residual anesthesia.

Ambulation

It is necessary for the patient to have the ability to sit, stand, and walk prior to discharge. These tasks should be on a par with the patient's preoperative abilities, giving consideration to the surgical event. Such activity will identify potential problems, including orthostatic hypotension. If the surgical event requires utilization of assistive devices (e.g., crutches, walkers, slings), verify the patient's understanding and ability to use these items before discharge.

DISCHARGE INSTRUCTIONS

Comprehensive and individualized patient instructions are an essential component of successful ambulatory surgery. The importance of discharge instruction is underscored by several regulatory and professional associations (see Accrediting and Provider Organizations).[2–7] *A Patient's Bill of Rights*, a pamphlet prepared by the American Hospital Association, emphasizes the importance of educating patients regarding ongoing health care requirements following discharge.[84] From a medicolegal perspective, effective patient education cannot be overstated as a method of minimizing risk of lawsuit.[85]

The ASPAN standards state that the patient is to be provided with written discharge instruction.[7] These printed or written instructions offer the advantage of being available to the patient following discharge from the surgical facility and can stimulate recall of information discussed by the nurse. Medical terminology should be avoided or defined in common terms that can be understood by the patient.

The final phase of ambulatory anesthesia recovery, phase III (see Table 22–4), typically occurs in the patient's home, while under the supervision of a responsible adult. Concurrent with this recovery phase, the surgical healing process is beginning. Both of these events require the patient and caregiver to be knowledgeable of normal expectations, physician directed limitations, and potential complications. Failure to provide sufficient, easily understood information can have a negative impact on patient outcomes.

Format

The surgeon and anesthesia provider offer relevant discharge instructions and assume responsibility for the necessary discharge information to be conveyed to the patient. This can be achieved through handwritten orders but is commonly accomplished with standing orders, protocols, collaborative practice guidelines, or preprinted instructions. Preprinted discharge instructions addressing the common surgical procedures and anesthesia techniques may be available for each surgeon or anesthesia provider. An alternative to personalized orders would be a generic postoperative discharge instruction form with check boxes or blanks in which to individualize postoperative patient care. A defined method of periodic evaluation and updating of these materials must be established for each ambulatory surgical facility.

Other preprinted materials that provide discharge instructions include handouts covering specific topics such as: (1) prescribed therapies (e.g., thermal applications, exercises, extremity elevation), (2) care of surgical dressings, wound drains, casts or splints, or (3) proper self-medication (e.g., ophthalmic, otic, or nose drops). These forms offer the advantage of providing complete and consistent information and also serve as a home resource for the patient. A possible disadvantage of this educational technique lies in overwhelming the patient when he or she leaves the facility with a handful of instruction papers.

When preprinted materials are to be used, several factors must be considered during the development: (1) *Make them reader friendly.* Readability is affected by headings, line width, type font and size, and drawings. Utilize headings to draw attention to specific topics of importance. In general, print layout should be of sufficient size to be easily read by the target audience. (2) *Make them understandable.* Address the educational level of the target audience. Comprehension is decreased when the reading level of the material exceeds the cognitive skills of the patient. Various formulas (e.g., SMOG, FOG, or Fry) can be used to assess appropriate reading levels for discharge instructions.[86]

The populations commonly served by the ambulatory facility need to be considered. The geriatric population, for example, will benefit from block print on nonglossy warm colors. The information may also need to be produced in several languages to accommodate frequently represented groups.

Regardless of the format for discharge orders, the nurse must be sure the patient and caregiver are able to comply with the instructions. The nurse must review the orders with the patient and caregiver and provide explanation and clarification of instructions or referral to the physician as appropriate. Additionally, the patient's knowledge and understanding of instructions must be validated and, if necessary, appropriate resources should be activated to assist the patient in complying with the instructions (e.g., family resources, community assistance programs, or state and federal social services).

The physician will sometimes privately give the patient or caregiver verbal instructions. When this occurs, the nurse should ask the patient if there are any questions regarding the physician's instructions or concerns about being able to follow the instructions. The nurse should then document that verbal instructions were provided by the physician and the patient and caregiver stated that they understood the instructions and had no questions or concerns regarding the information.

Process

Providing the patient and caregiver postoperative instructions is a process that utilizes the professional judgment and skills of the nurse. Assessment of the patient's learning needs, learning style, readiness to learn, and barriers to learning are critical components of appropriate patient education. Information from this assessment provides a guide for the delivery of the instructions. After providing the information, there must be validation that the patient and caregiver understand and are able to comply with the instructions. Nursing documentation in the patient's medical record must accurately reflect details of the process.

Assessment

Assessment of learning needs is initiated in the preoperative interview or admission phase and is ongoing. An effective evaluation of the patient's understanding of the procedure and expected postprocedural recovery process is fundamental in mutually determining the patient's learning needs. An assessment is made of the patient's preferred method of learning new material (i.e., observing, performing, reading, or listening). Providing instructions in the desired format will increase the information learned and retained. Various teaching tools should be available and selected to best meet the needs of the patient. Anatomic models, charts, diagrams, illustrations, and videos are useful teaching resources. Employing teaching strategies, such as rephrasing and repeating important information, will help with retention of critical details.

Establishing the patient's readiness to learn is part of the teaching-learning process.[86] Some questions to consider when determining the patient's learning readiness include:

- Does the patient perceive a need for postdischarge information?
- What is the current level of patient understanding?
- Is there motivation for the patient to follow the instructions?

The likelihood of the patient following postoperative instructions is directly related to his or her appreciation of the benefits of such a plan of postoperative care.

Throughout the patient's stay, barriers to learning, whether real or potential, are assessed and minimized to the extent possible. These barriers are multidimensional and may be functional, cultural, socioeconomic, physical, or environmental. Impaired vision, hearing, and intellectual ability are examples of a functional barrier. Cultural barriers to learning might be language or ethnicity related. Impaired functional vocabulary and educational levels are types of socioeconomic barriers in the healthcare environment. Physical barriers are an especially important aspect of patient education in the perioperative setting. Pain, anxiety, nausea and vomiting, and drug influence will impair motivation, learning, and recall. Environmental barriers are created by entities such as visual and auditory distractions, poor room lighting, and lack of privacy. Information gleaned from the assessment of learning needs is used to individualize and continuously modify the patient's plan of care.

Plan

The goals of patient education are typically categorized into three domains: (1) cognitive, (2) affective, and (3) psychomotor. The cognitive domain relates to knowledge and understanding, affective domain reflects attitudes, and the psychomotor domain refers to motor skills. When providing postoperative instructions to patients and caregivers, these domains provide a framework for structuring the educational process. For example, the physician's postoperative instruction may be to "keep ice on an elevated extremity." Explaining to the patient that this action will reduce surgical swelling provides the cognitive information (knowledge) that is needed to understand the reason for the order. The affective domain is addressed by getting a buy-in by the patient on the importance of following the instruction by adding that excessive swelling will increase discomfort and can impair circulation, which will delay wound healing and may lead to postoperative complications. The psychomotor skills associated with this learning need include proper elevation of the extremity and the ability to empty, fill, and secure ice bags.

Implementation

Ideally, postoperative instructions are provided during the preadmission interview when the patient is more likely to be free of drug influence, which can impair attention and recall. In addition, this time frame facilitates advanced preparation for limitations and expectations following surgery, such as obtaining needed supplies (e.g., crutches, additional dressings), arranging transportation, adjusting schedules of others in the household, and modifying living environments. If a preadmission interview has not been done, postoperative instructions should be addressed during the admission process, because it has been demonstrated that even a brief period of general anesthesia can hinder retention of new information for as long as 24 hours.[87] However, it must be realized that this environment is less than ideal for patient education because many barriers exist. Patient anxiety, a noisy or distractive environment, or short preoperative phase packed with numerous activities and tasks are all barriers to effective learning.

Ideally in the phase II setting, the nurse reviews and updates instructions, which may be new or have changed because of operative events. Before this review, it is crucial to assess the barriers to learning, especially physical and environmental. The patient in uncontrolled pain, plagued by nausea and vomiting, or distracted by the unfamiliar medical environment is not a proper candidate for education. Such barriers to learning must be minimized as much as possible before the education process is undertaken.

Environmental barriers to learning are common in many phase II facilities, which consist of large open environments. Although the open area is helpful for visualizing patients at all times, it presents a less than ideal learning environment. Attempts should be made to reduce visual and auditory distractions when providing discharge instructions. The patient's privacy is also a consideration; when possible, select a private area or provide privacy by using a curtain or screen. It may be appropriate to move the patient to another location such as the far end of the room or to an enclosed dressing area. If these options are not reasonable, consider turning the patient to face a wall or away from the visual distractions.

Sit or stand in close proximity to the patient and speak in a low and slow speech pattern. Maintain good eye contact, and observe for nonverbal reactions to instructions (e.g., explore why the patient grimaces when told to change a dressing in 24 hours). Provide ample opportunities for the patient and caregiver to ask questions. Include the rationale for a specific instruction to the patient and caregiver. Explain the purpose and care of equipment such as drains. Clarify whether crutches are ordered for the patient's comfort only or is the intent of the crutches to avoid weight-bearing on the operative leg. Demonstrate dressing changes, how to empty drains, or other psychomotor skills. It is imperative that the nurse review with the patient possible signs and symptoms that require immediate notification of the physician. An understanding of what is "normal" and what is "abnormal" during the recovery process is essential if complications are to be identified early by the patient or caregiver.

Barriers to communication should be proactively addressed by each facility. Methods of accessing available resources, either commercial or volunteer, must be defined by protocols or guidelines. Both commercial and volunteer services are available in many communities; the American Red Cross and university or college services often provide interpreters. Organizations for the visual or hearing impaired can assist in locating both human and technologic resources. Often a family member or friend can assist in communicating with the patient; however, the ideal facilitator is a disinterested third party.

Evaluation

Validate a patient's understanding of instructions by asking open-ended questions, for example, "Can you tell me when you need to call the doctor?" Ask the patient or caregiver to explain the purpose of or reason for an instruction (e.g., care of a surgical drain). Request a return demonstration on how to empty the surgical drain or change a sterile dressing. Verify that there is an understanding of what actions are to be taken if the patient encounters an unexpected problem after discharge.

Documentation

The patient care record must reflect what instructions were provided, to whom the instructions were provided, the recipient's response, and the nurse's assessment of the patient and caregiver's understanding of the postoperative instructions. The caregiver who will be overseeing the patient's progress at home should be included in the discharge teaching. Generally, space is provided on the instruction form where the nurse providing the information and the patient or caregiver provide written acknowledgment that the instructions were thoroughly conveyed. A copy of this signed instruction form is retained in the patient's medical record. If the escort with the patient is only providing transportation, discharge instructions can be conveyed to the caregiver by telephone to reinforce the written instructions sent with the patient.

A competent patient's request for confidentiality must be respected. With the patient's permission, it may be possible to provide instructions related to the signs and symptoms of potential complications without disclosing the procedure or its outcome. Each confidentiality situation must be carefully evaluated and concerns for safe outcomes discussed with the patient. A mentally competent patient is the final decision-maker regarding what if any information may or may not be disclosed. Accurate and comprehensive documentation of the discussion regarding confidentiality must follow. Meticulous documentation is essential to protect the patient and the nurse (Welsh RS: Personal Communication, 1997).

Content

Discharge instructions provide the patient and caregiver with a plan of postoperative care that extends into the home environment. General expectations, procedural specific information, and anesthetic precautions are included in this comprehensive educational plan.

General Expectations

The patient and caregiver should leave the healthcare facility with a reasonable understanding of the recovery process and their role and responsibilities in this process. This requires information regarding activity, diet, hygiene, and medications.

Activity. The patient and caregiver should be informed of minor discomforts that may be experienced in the recovery process. Muscle aches, headache, and sore throat are common but generally not serious and can be relieved with the usual remedies, such as mild over-the-counter analgesics (if not contraindicated), throat lozenges, or warm gargles. Fatigue and low energy levels can also be expected as the body recovers. Advise the patient to plan a gradual return to normal activities and to include periods of rest into the day's activities. Excessive activity can result in increased pain, bleeding, swelling in the surgical site, and extreme physical fatigue. Performing strenuous activities or heavy lifting requires clearance by the surgeon.

While cautioning the patient against excessive physical activity, the nurse should also caution against lack of physical activity. Ambulating about the home, sitting at the table for meals, and frequent change of position offer the advantages of promoting deep breathing and increasing circulation. These activities stimulate the cardiovascular system and bring oxygen and other nutrients to the cells, facilitating healing and decreasing complications.

Instructions for specific limitations (e.g., no weight-bearing) or specific activities (e.g., extremity exercises) are generally related to the patient's procedure or dictated by the patient's preprocedural condition. When instructions are in conflict with the patient's preprocedural abilities or restrictions, clarification by the physician will be necessary before the patient is discharged.

Unless contraindicated by the procedure, sexual activity may be resumed when patient comfort permits. After genitourinary or gynecologic procedures, any restrictions must be clearly understood by the patient and partner. Sexual intercourse, as well as the use of tampons or douches, may place a female patient who has had a gynecologic procedure at risk for infection. A male patient who has had a vasectomy for sterilization needs to understand that he can still impregnate a female for a period of time. As with all instructions, an understanding of the reason will increase compliance.

Diet and Elimination. Ideally, a patient will return home and resume normal dietary and elimination patterns. However, it is more likely the patient will experience gastrointestinal effects following a surgical and anesthetic episode. As long as the patient is healthy and well hydrated, it is acceptable for the patient to avoid consuming food and fluid for the remainder of the day. When nausea resolves, a slow return to a normal diet is advised while avoiding heavy, greasy foods and excessive dairy products. The focus should be on the patient maintaining an adequate fluid intake. Frozen juices, popsicles, and ice chips are refreshing and can often be tolerated when consumed in small amounts at frequent intervals. Nausea precipitated by medication may be minimized by eating crackers, toast, or a small snack before taking the medication.

Patients who will be taking narcotics for pain control should be informed of the potential constipating side effect associated with the use of these medications secondary to decreased peristaltic motility.[88] A reduction in normal physical activities may also predispose the patient to constipation. An increase in the amount of fluids, fiber, and fresh fruits in the diet can help to offset this annoying problem. Awareness of this potential side effect and implementation of the dietary modifications may minimize the occurrence of this uncomfortable complication.

The ability of patients to urinate prior to discharge is usually not a discharge standard except for high-risk procedures (e.g., urologic, gynecologic, inguinal herniorrhaphy). When voiding is not part of the discharge criteria, the patient should be instructed in what time frame following discharge (e.g., after 6 to 8 hours) he or she should contact the physician if unable to urinate.

Strategies that may help the patient to urinate include providing a private and peaceful environment, listening to the sound of running water, and sitting in a tub of warm water. Parents of small children can be taught how to observe and palpate for a distended bladder. Patients and caregivers should be instructed on monitoring the adequacy of hydration (e.g., urinary frequency, amount, and concentration [color and odor] of the voided urine). Hematuria after a urinary procedure may be acceptable, but active bleeding or passing blood clots demands further evaluation. Based on professional knowledge and experience, "active bleeding" is a term that the nurse is comfortable with, but the patient or caregiver will need clear guidelines regarding what is acceptable and when notification of the surgeon is appropriate.

Hygiene. Depending on the procedure and type of dressings, bathing or showering may need modification. In some situations, the surgeon may permit removal of dressings in 24 to 48 hours after surgery and allow the patient to take a shower. Incisions protected by adherent plastic dressings also permit showering. Bathing in a tub is usually limited to surgical procedures where the incision will remain above the water line. Patients with soft dressings that will stay in place until the first postoperative visit or those with splints or casts may find sponge bathing more convenient and easier than waterproofing the surgical area. The upper extremities are easier to protect than the lower extremities because an arm can be held outside of the shower flow. It is essential to convey the importance of keeping a cast clean and dry. A wet cast predisposes the underlying incision to infection and may collapse in areas, causing inappropriate pressure on soft tissues.

Medications. One of the most important topics in the realm of discharge instructions is patient self-medication. Many healthcare facilities offer preprinted instruction sheets for commonly prescribed medications. Possible interactions with food and other drugs must be considered and clearly communicated to the patient. This requires a knowledge of all prescribed and over-the-counter drugs that the patient may be taking. If the patient is to continue a medication started in the facility, the time of the next dose must be clearly established verbally and in writing. Leader[89] found that when prescriptions were not explained, complications once the patient was discharged increased 9-fold. It is not sufficient that the patient and caregiver understand just the purpose and expectations of a medication, they must be knowledgeable as to the common side effects that can occur and the appropriate actions to be taken should adverse signs and symptoms present. Specific instructions regarding the timing (e.g., every 6 hours vs. qid) and consumption (e.g., empty stomach or with food) of the medication must be clarified. When medications are prescribed on an as needed basis, the patient or caregiver becomes a decision-maker; therefore, it is important that the purpose and limitations of the medication be clearly understood.

Analgesic medications are probably the most common drugs dispensed to the ambulatory surgical patient. For optimal pain relief with minimal side effects, the patient needs clear instructions on the use of this type of drug. If the patient has had the surgical incision injected with a long-acting local anesthetic, there may be no surgical pain at the time of discharge. The patient should realize that this is not a continual pain-free situation, and as the medication is absorbed there will be an awareness of increasing pain, which can become intense within a short time. Managing surgical discomfort from a prophylactic approach is more effective than trying to gain control of accelerating pain. Therefore, it is not advisable for the patient to wait until the pain is quite pronounced before taking the analgesic medication. The patient should be informed of a realistic time frame for the onset of analgesic action.

Empowering the patient to contact the physician is a very important aspect of the discharge instructions. Clarify for the patient that the physician is expecting the recovery process to go well. If situations arise that were not addressed in the discharge instructions or if the prescribed medications are not effective, the physician needs to be made aware of the problem so that adjustments in care can be made (e.g., patient evaluation for potential complications, changes in medication dosage, or trying an alternative medication).

Procedural Specific Information

Surgical discharge instructions are as varied as there are procedures but have common aspects that include incisional care, expectations, and limitations.

Incisional Care. Incisional care encompasses the changing of dressings, application of medications, and observation of the operative site for signs of infection, bleeding, and the anticipated healing. Caring for the incisional area starts and ends with good handwashing. If wound dressings are to be changed, a demonstration as to proper technique and return demonstration by the patient or caregiver are appropriate. Elements to address include use of aseptic technique in removal and replacement of the dressing, proper disposal of the dressing, and observation of the site and any drainage that may be present on the dressing.

Emphasize to the patient that keeping the wound clean and dry reduces the chance of infection. Although a slight redness adjacent to the incision or puncture site is a normal inflammatory response, patients and caregivers need a clear understanding of what is acceptable and what is cause for concern and requires notification of the physician. In addition to the redness of the inflammatory response, other signs of infection that should be listed in the discharge instructions and discussed with the patient include: (1) abnormal drainage that may be foul smelling or purulent, (2) increased tenderness, warmth, or swelling in the surgical area, (3) a fever over 38.3°C (101°F), and (4) possibly chills. Providing the patient with a time frame for these symptoms to occur is beneficial, because typically an operative site infection will demonstrate symptoms 36 hours or later postoperatively.[45] A low-grade fever the day after surgery is not unusual and reflects the body's normal healing response.[90]

Expectations. What the patient can expect postoperatively may be focused on the surgical site (e.g., drainage, bleeding, healing), his or her level of activity (e.g., limb positioning or exercises, overall activity), and follow-up care. Providing the patient and caregivers with clear expectations for the next few days promotes compliance with discharge instructions and facilitates good decision-making when concerns arise.

If bleeding or drainage is expected, the amount and character that is acceptable must be clearly understood. The amount of drainage should be clarified in terms such as: (1) the number of dressing changes per hour, or (2) size of drainage on a dressing expressed in inches, etc., and not by terms that are open to subjective interpretation (e.g., "large," "excessive"). The character of the drainage is equally important; a patient or caregiver may view any red drainage as "bleeding" when in fact it may be serosanguineous or blood-tinged. Both the amount and character of normal drainage vary greatly with the procedure and surgical technique. To provide realistic information, nurses in the ambulatory setting need to be knowledgeable of what constitutes normal postoperative drainage, such as the anticipated drainage after surgery in vascular areas (e.g., nose, oral cavity).

Providing instructions related to positioning should include not only the correct position but also details of what makes it correct or incorrect. For example, it is inadequate to provide the instruction to elevate the casted distal left arm on two pillows. Important details would be that the arm should be higher than the level of the heart with the fingers higher than the elbow to facilitate venous return, and the elbow should be flexed comfortably but not at an angle that compromises circulation. Unless contraindicated, instructions to extend and flex fingers several times an hour will help stimulate circulation. Demonstrate to the patient how to conduct a neurovascular assessment; explain what observations should be made, and when the physician should be contacted. Explain what are acceptable assessments and observations and what are unacceptable findings when checking the finger tips for color, warmth, capillary refill, sensation, and motion. Terms such as duskiness and mottling may not be understood, whereas pale, white, bluish, or spotty may be more meaningful to the patient.

All postoperative instructions should include information regarding follow-up care. Often the first postoperative checkup is already established, having been scheduled at the time of the patient's preoperative visit with the surgeon. The nurse, however, must confirm whether a follow-up appointment is already scheduled. Some ambulatory centers facilitate scheduling appointments by calling or allowing the patient to call the surgeon's office prior to discharge home.

In addition to follow-up details, the patient and caregiver must have a clear understanding of the sequence of the actions to be taken in the event that unexpected problems arise. It may be possible to delineate the appropriateness of contacting the surgeon versus the anesthesia provider when the patient has postoperative problems or concerns (e.g., the patient who develops a severe sore throat after knee surgery). There should also be an understanding of when it is more appropriate to seek emergency health services. Postoperative hemorrhage, respiratory distress, and falling with resultant injury are relevant examples.

Limitations. The surgical procedure may necessitate that limitations be imposed secondary to mobility restrictions, sensory impairment, or potential damage to the surgery itself. For example, the surgeon may impose driving restrictions beyond the 24-hour time frame normally recommended from an anesthetic perspective, for any of the aforementioned reasons. However, most discharge instructions are focused on expectations; for example, what actions are to be taken by the patient to contribute to the recovery process. Often these expectations produce limitations on activities of daily living (ADL) to varying degrees. Keeping the feet elevated, for example, has a greater impact on the ADL than keeping the distal arm elevated. Too many limitations can negatively affect patient compliance.

Once the patient has achieved good pain control, returned to a normal diet, and perceived a normal energy level, there can be a desire to resume role responsibilities. This urge may be self-imposed by the patient or directly or indirectly expressed by other members of the household. If limitations are expected, the patient and caregiver must understand the rationale supporting these instructions. Acknowledging that it would be normal to experience conflict in adhering to instructions can be helpful with effective coping measures. Reinforce with the patient and caregiver that adhering to the recommended limitations is an investment in achieving optimal surgical outcome.

Anesthesia Precautions

Discharge instructions regarding anesthesia are primarily guided by the anesthesia technique employed. However, with rare exceptions, most anesthesia techniques utilize various medications that continue to have an impact on the patient beyond discharge. Sedatives and narcotics can cause sleepiness and impair psychomotor and cognitive skills and can lead to impaired judgment and slower reaction times. General instructions to the patient related to these side effects include a caution not to sign legal documents, operate a motor vehicle, or carry out any activity that requires judgment or quick reaction for at least 24 hours. These cautions may extend beyond this time frame if potent medications will be required for pain control. The patient should also be advised not to consume alcohol (including beer and wine) or use recreational drugs for 24 hours. The explanation for this instruction should be a nonjudgmental statement that these substances can be potentially dangerous because of interactions with medications used during the procedure.

The patient who received a sensory block will have loss of protective pain sensation for an extended time. While this provides the patient with analgesia, it also prevents a normal response to a painful superficial injury such as a burn. Patients and caregivers need to be mindful of positioning and protection of the affected area until the sensory block has subsided. Next day follow-up contact with the patient is important to determine if there is persistent sensory or motor blockade.

Brachial Plexus Block. Following brachial plexus blockade, the patient will be instructed to support the arm in a sling until sensory and motor function have returned. Specifically, the patient and responsible adult will be instructed to protect the extremity from injury (e.g., smoking or cooking) until sensation and reflexes have normalized.

Foot Block. A bulky dressing is desirable to provide padding for the patient recovering from a foot block. The patient should be instructed on the proper use of crutches and should be monitored to assure proper crutch operation. If the patient experiences difficulty in mastering the crutch, the responsible adult must be physically able to assist the patient.

Central Neuraxial Techniques. Postoperative instructions for the patient who had spinal anesthesia include the signs and symptoms of a postdural puncture headache (PDPH) and who the patient should contact if the symptoms appear. The patient should also be told that the incidence of PDPH is quite low and that effective treatments are available if the symptoms occur.

Intravenous Catheter Site. Slight redness or tenderness at the intravenous site can be treated with warm moist compresses, but if the redness or tenderness persists or increases, the patient should be given a resource to contact.

Follow-up

Prior to leaving the facility, the patient should be informed that a follow-up telephone call will be made to check on his or her recovery progress. An estimated timetable should be made, and the patient should be asked if the time is convenient. If the patient does not have a telephone, explore the possibility of telephone contact for messages or having the patient contact the facility within a specific time frame.

This call offers the opportunity to confirm that recovery is occurring as expected, clarify concerns, answer questions, and receive feedback on the services provided by the facility. It also offers an opportunity to gather information for quality assurance outcomes.[91] A thoughtfully designed ambulatory process, clear discharge criteria, and comprehensive discharge information contribute to a successful outcome and customer satisfaction.

DISCHARGE OPTIONS

Transportation

A postoperative patient who has had anesthesia or sedation should not be allowed to travel home unsupervised. Another of the discharge nurse's responsibilities is to evaluate the capabilities of the caregiver who will be transporting and providing care to the patient. A person who is impaired secondary to alcohol or another drug is not a candidate to transport the patient home. Once arrangements seem appropriate, the final interaction between the ambulatory staff on the day of surgery is to accompany the patient to the transport vehicle and ensure that the seat belt is secured for the drive home. An infant or small child should be fastened in a car seat that is approved according to state and local regulations.[45]

Extended Observation

Patients who do not meet the discharge criteria outlined in the policies of the ambulatory surgical center (e.g., persistent nausea and vomiting, disabling pain not controlled with oral analgesics) will benefit from the monitoring and care of an extended observation unit. This transitional status between inpatient and outpatient care allows prolonged observation and care for select patients.

Discharge Against Medical Advice (AMA)

The patient should understand that admission to an extended care facility may be required if a responsible adult is not available. Whether due to fear, hostility, independence, or simply a person's unique personality, some patients are unwilling to comply with the policies and protocols regarding discharge standards of a facility. Patients sometimes demand to leave the ambulatory surgical facility before medical discharge and cannot be dissuaded. An adult patient has the legal right to choose a mode of treatment or refuse it. Any form of restraint could be considered battery and violation of a person's right to leave.[45] If a patient is found to be without a vested adult escort postoperatively and refuses the extended observation option, he or she must sign an AMA release. It is important to realize that there is real concern about the legality of the patient's signature on an AMA release when the patient has had any type of mind-altering medication. In fact, the nurse could be questioned later about the appropriateness of even asking for a signature in such a case when it is known that the patient has been recently medicated. As with all issues of this nature, each facility's legal counsel should be consulted for direction and suggestions regarding the policy.[45]

References

1. Marley RA, Moline BM: Patient discharge from the ambulatory setting. J Post Anesth Nurs 11:39–49, 1996.
2. Joint Commission on Accreditation of Healthcare Organizations: Surgical and anesthesia services. In 1994 Accreditation Manual for Ambulatory Health Care. I: Standards. Oakbrook Terrace, IL, 1993, pp 37–41.
3. Accreditation Association for Ambulatory Health Care: Anesthesia services. In 1994/1995 Accreditation Handbook for Ambulatory Health Care. Skokie, IL, 1993, p 37.
4. Accreditation Association for Ambulatory Health Care: Overnight care and services. In 1994/1995 Accreditation Handbook for Ambulatory Health Care. Skokie, IL: 1993, p 40.
5. American Association of Nurse Anesthetists: Postanesthesia Care Standards for the Certified Registered Nurse Anesthetist. In Professional Practice Manual for the Certified Registered Nurse Anesthetist. Park Ridge, IL: 1992, p 2.
6. American Society of Anesthesiologists: Guidelines for ambulatory surgical facilities. In ASA Standards, Guidelines and Statements. Park Ridge, IL: 1994, p 9.
7. American Society of Post Anesthesia Nurses: Preanesthesia, postanesthesia data required for initial, ongoing and discharge assessment. In Standards of Perianesthesia Nursing Practice. Thorofare, NJ: 1995, pp 42–45.
8. Griffith JL, McLaughlin SH: Legal implications. In Wetchler BV (ed): Anesthesia for Ambulatory Surgery, 2nd ed. Philadelphia: JB Lippincott, 1991, pp 61–62.
9. Weintraub HD: Anesthetic management of the geriatric outpatient. In Barash PG (ed): ASA Refresher Courses in Anesthesiology. Philadelphia: JB Lippincott, 1986, pp 237–246.
10. Korttila KT: Practical discharge criteria for the 1990s: Assessing home readiness. Anesthesiol Rev 18 (Suppl 1): 23–27, 1991.
11. Philip BK: Patient's assessment of ambulatory anesthesia and surgery. J Clin Anesth 4:355–358, 1992.
12. Lichtor JL, Sah J, Apfelbaum J, et al: Some patients may drink or drive after ambulatory surgery. Anesthesiology 73:A1083, 1990.
13. Warner MA, Shields SE, Chute CG: Major morbidity

and mortality within 1 month of ambulatory surgery and anesthesia. JAMA 270:1437–1441, 1993.
14. Biswas TK, Cleary C: Postoperative hospital admission from a day surgery unit: A seven-year retrospective survey. Anaesth Intensive Care 20:147–150, 1992.
15. Fancourt-Smith PF, Hornstein J, Jenkins JC: Hospital admissions from the Surgical Day Care Centre of Vancouver General Hospital 1977–1987. Can J Anaesth 37:699–704, 1990.
16. Duncan PG, Cohen MM, Tweed WA, et al: The Canadian four-centre study of anaesthetic outcomes. III: Are anaesthetic complications predictable in day surgical practice? Can J Anaesth 39:440–448, 1992.
17. Rudkin GE, Osborne GA, Doyle CE: Assessment and selection of patients for day surgery in a public hospital. Med J Aust 158:308–312, 1993.
18. Meeks GR, Meydrech EF, Bradford TH, et al: Comparison of unscheduled hospital admission following ambulatory operative laparoscopy at a teaching hospital and a community hospital. J Laparoendosc Surg 5:7–13, 1995.
19. Twersky R, Fishman D, Homel P: What happens after discharge? Return hospital visits after ambulatory surgery. Anesth Analg 84:319–324, 1997.
20. Osborne GA, Rudkin GE: Outcome after day-care surgery in a major teaching hospital. Anaesth Intensive Care 21:822–827, 1993.
21. Chung F: Recovery pattern and home-readiness after ambulatory surgery. Anesth Analg 80:896–902, 1995.
22. Chung F, Ritchie E, Su J: Postoperative pain in ambulatory surgery. Anesth Analg 85:808–816, 1997.
23. Cardosa M, Rudkin GE, Osborne GA: Outcome from day-care knee arthroscopy in a major teaching hospital. Arthroscopy 10:624–629, 1994.
24. Cade L, Kakulas P: Ketorolac or pethidine for analgesia after elective laparoscopic sterilization. Anaesth Intensive Care 23:158–161, 1995.
25. Brooks DC: A prospective comparison of laparoscopic and tension-free open herniorrhaphy. Arch Surg 129:361–366, 1994.
26. Helmus C, Grin M, Westfall R: Same-day-stay head and neck surgery. Laryngoscope, 102:1331–1334, 1992.
27. Meeks GR, Waller GA, Meydrech EF, et al: Unscheduled hospital admission following ambulatory gynecologic surgery. Obstet Gynecol 80:446–450, 1992.
28. Korttila KT: Post-anaesthetic psychomotor and cognitive function. Eur J Anaesth 12:43–46, 1995.
29. Pandit SK, Pandit UA: Phases of the recovery period. In White PF (ed): Ambulatory Anesthesia and Surgery. Philadelphia: WB Saunders, 1997, pp 457–464.
30. Aldrete JA, Kroulik D: A postanesthetic recovery score. Anesth Analg 49:924–933, 1970.
31. Aldrete JA: Discharge criteria. In Thomson D, Frost E (eds): Baillière's Clinical Anaesthesiology: Postanaesthesia Care. London: Baillière Tindall, 1994, pp 763–773.
32. Apfelbaum JL, Grasela TH, Walawander CA, et al: Bypassing the PACU—a new paradigm in ambulatory surgery. Anesthesiology 87:A32, 1997.
33. Bell S, Hill N: Factors facilitating PACU bypass in ambulatory surgery. Anesthesiology 87:A34, 1997.
34. Theodorou-Michaloliakou C, Chung FF, Chua JG: Does a modified postanaesthetic discharge scoring system determine home-readiness sooner? Can J Anaesth 40:A32, 1993.
35. Comroe JH Jr, Botelho S: The unreliability of cyanosis in the recognition of arterial anoxemia. Am J Med Sci 214:1–6, 1947.
36. Chung F, Ong D, Seyone C, et al: PADS—A discriminative discharge index for ambulatory surgery. Anesthesiology 75:A1105, 1991.
37. Wetchler BV: Postanesthesia scoring system. AORN J 41:382–384, 1985.
38. Wetchler BV: Problem solving in the postanesthesia care unit. In Wetchler BV (ed): Anesthesia for Ambulatory Surgery, 2nd ed. Philadelphia: JB Lippincott, 1991, pp 375–434.
39. Korttila K: Recovery from outpatient anaesthesia: Factors affecting outcome. Anaesthesia 50 (Suppl): 22–28, 1995.
40. Reed WA: Recovery from anesthesia and discharge. In Shultz R (ed): Outpatient Surgery. Philadelphia: Lea & Febiger, 1979, p 45.
41. Mecca RS, Sharnick SV: Common postanesthesia care unit problems. In McGoldrick KE (ed): Ambulatory Anesthesiology: A Problem-Oriented Approach. Baltimore: Williams & Wilkins, 1995, pp 582–618.
42. Fetzer-Fowler SJ, Huot S: The use of temperature as a discharge criterion for ambulatory surgery patients. J Post Anesth Nurs 7:398–403, 1992.
43. Warner ME: Risks and outcomes of perioperative pulmonary aspiration. J PeriAnesth Nurs 12:352–357, 1997.
44. Marley RA: Postextubation laryngeal edema: A review with consideration for home discharge. J PeriAnesth Nurs 13:39–53, 1998.
45. Burden N: Discharge. In Ambulatory Surgical Nursing. Philadelphia: WB Saunders, 1993, pp 340–371.
46. Fortier J, Chung F, Su J: Predictive factors of unanticipated admission in ambulatory surgery: A prospective study. Anesthesiology 85:A27, 1996.
47. Gold BS, Kitz DS, Lecky JH, et al: Unanticipated admission to the hospital following ambulatory surgery. JAMA 262:3008–3010, 1989.
48. Reference deleted.
49. Rittenmeyer H, Dolezal D, Vogel E: Pain management: A quality improvement project. J PeriAnesth Nurs 12:329–335, 1997.
50. Wong D: Whaley and Wong's Nursing Care of Infants and Children, 5th ed. St. Louis: Mosby-Year Book, 1995, p 1085.
51. Forrest JB, Cahalan MK, Rehder K, et al: Multicenter study of general anesthesia. II: Results. Anesthesiology 72:262–268, 1990.
52. Larsson S, Lundberg D: A prospective survey of postoperative nausea and vomiting with special regard to incidence and relations to patient characteristics, anesthetic routines and surgical procedures. Acta Anaesthesiol Scand 39:539–545, 1995.
53. Karlsson E, Larsson LE, Nilsson K: Postanesthetic nausea in children. Acta Anaesthesiol Scand 34:515–518, 1990.
54. Patel RI, Hannallah RS: Anesthetic complications following pediatric ambulatory surgery: A 3-year study. Anesthesiology 69:1009–1012, 1988.
55. Cohen MM, Cameron CB, Duncan PG: Pediatric anesthesia morbidity and mortality in the perioperative period. Anesth Analg 70:160–167, 1990.
56. Green G, Jonsson L: Nausea: The most important factor determining length of stay after ambulatory anaesthesia: A comparative study of isoflurane and/or propofol techniques. Acta Anaesthesiol Scand 37:742–746, 1993.
57. Patel RI, Hannallah RS: Complications following pediatric ambulatory surgery—less of the same? Anesthesiology 79:A223, 1993.
58. Metter SE, Kitz DS, Young ML, et al: Nausea and vomiting after outpatient laparoscopy: Incidence, impact on recovery room stay and cost. Anesth Analg 66:S116, 1987.

59. Kovac AL, Pearman MH, Khalil SN, et al: Ondansetron prevents postoperative emesis in male outpatients: S3A-379 study group. J Clin Anesth 8:644–651, 1996.
60. Marley RA: Postoperative nausea and vomiting: The outpatient enigma. J PeriAnesth Nurs 11:147–161, 1996.
61. Watcha MF, Bras PJ, Cieslak GD, et al: The dose-response relationship of ondansetron in preventing postoperative emesis in pediatric patients undergoing ambulatory surgery. Anesthesiology 82:47–52, 1995.
62. Sikich N, Carr AS, Lerman J: Parental perceptions, expectations and preferences for the postanaesthetic recovery of children. Paediatr Anaesth 7:139–142, 1997.
63. Marley R: Outpatient anesthesia. In Nagelhout JJ, Zaglaniczny KL (eds): Nurse Anesthesia. Philadelphia: WB Saunders, 1997, pp 1018–1037.
64. Pandit UA, Pandit SK: Fasting before and after ambulatory surgery. J PeriAnesth Nurs 12:181–187, 1997.
65. Keane PW, Murray PF: Intravenous fluids in minor surgery: Their effect on recovery from anaesthesia. Anaesthesia 41:635–637, 1986.
66. Cook R, Anderson S, Riseborough M, et al: Intravenous fluid load and recovery: A double-blind comparison in gynaecological patients who had day-case laparoscopy. Anaesthesia 45:826–830, 1990.
67. Rothenberg DM, Parnass SM, Litwack K, et al: Efficacy of ephedrine in the prevention of postoperative nausea and vomiting. Anesth Analg 72:58–61, 1991.
68. Gaskey NJ, Ferriero L, Pournaras L, et al: Use of fentanyl markedly increases nausea and vomiting in gynecological short stay patients. AANA J 54:309–311, 1986.
69. Vasquez J, Sukhani R, Pappas A, et al: Propofol for ambulatory gynecological laparoscopy: Does omission of intraoperative opioid alter postoperative emetic sequela and recovery. Anesthesiology 83:A29, 1995.
70. Zuurmond WWA, van Leeuwen L: Recovery from sufentanil anaesthesia for outpatient arthroscopy: A comparison with isoflurane. Acta Anaesthesiol Scand 31:154–156, 1987.
71. Rose DK, Cohen MM, Yee DA: Reducing postoperative nausea and vomiting: What works and what doesn't. Anesth Analg 80:S403, 1995.
72. Schreiner MS, Nicolson SC: Pediatric ambulatory anesthesia: NPO—before or after surgery? J Clin Anesth 7:589–596, 1995.
73. Schreiner MS, Nicolson SC, Martin T, et al: Should children drink before discharge from day surgery? Anesthesiology 76:528–533, 1992.
74. Davis PJ, McGowan FX Jr, Landsman I, et al: Effect of antiemetic therapy on recovery and hospital discharge time: A double-blind assessment of ondansetron, droperidol, and placebo in pediatric patients undergoing ambulatory surgery. Anesthesiology 83:956–960, 1995.
75. Carroll NV, Miederhoff P, Cox FM, et al: Postoperative nausea and vomiting after discharge from outpatient surgery centers. Anesth Analg 80:903–909, 1995.
76. Hjalmas K: Urodynamics in normal infants and children. Scand J Urol Nephrol 114 (Suppl):20–27, 1988.
77. McGoldrick K: Is malignant hyperthermia a contraindication for outpatient surgery? Soc Ambulatory Anesth Newslett 7:11, 1992.
78. Spieker M: Patients susceptible to malignant hyperthermia. In McGoldrick KE (ed): Ambulatory Anesthesiology: A Problem-Oriented Approach. Baltimore: Williams & Wilkins, 1995, pp 318–331.
79. Yentis SM, Levine MF, Hartley EJ: Should all children with suspected or confirmed malignant hyperthermia susceptibility be admitted after surgery? A 10-year review. Anesth Analg 75:345–350, 1992.
80. Malignant Hyperthermia Association of the United States: Clinical Update 1997/98, Managing Malignant Hyperthermia. Sherburne, NY: MHAUS, 1997.
81. Snyder DS, Pasternak LR: Facility design and procedural safety. In White PF (ed): Ambulatory Anesthesia and Surgery. Philadelphia: WB Saunders, 1997, pp 61–76.
82. Pflug AE, Aasheim GM, Foster C: Sequence of return of neurological function and criteria for safe ambulation following subarachnoid block (spinal anaesthetic). Can Anaesth Soc J 25:133–139, 1978.
83. Chung FF: Discharge requirements. In White PF (ed): Ambulatory Anesthesia and Surgery. Philadelphia: WB Saunders, 1997, pp 518–525.
84. American Hospital Association: A Patient's Bill of Rights. Catalog No. 157759, Chicago, IL: AHA, 1992.
85. Kinnaird LS: Managing risk through patient education. In Giloth BE (ed): Managing Hospital-Based Patient Education. Chicago: American Hospital Publishing, 1993, pp 115–128.
86. Redman BK: The Process of Patient Education, 7th ed. St. Louis: Mosby-Year Book, 1993, pp 140–156.
87. Health PJ, Ogg TW, Gilks WR: Recovery after daycare anaesthesia: A 24-hour comparison of recovery after thiopentone or propofol anaesthesia. Anaesthesia 45:911–915, 1990.
88. DeLuca A, Coupar IM: Insights into opioid action in the intestinal tract. Pharmacol Ther 69:103–115, 1996.
89. Leader S: The outpatient surgical experiences of aged Medicare enrollees. Am Assoc Retired Persons August pub no. H-11, 1990.
90. Tortora GJ, Anagnostakos NP: Principles of Anatomy and Physiology 6th ed. New York: Harper & Row, 1990, p 817.
91. Kleinpell RM: Improving telephone follow-up after ambulatory surgery. J PeriAnesth Nurs 12:336–340, 1997.

Chapter 23

Extensions of Care: Phase III Recovery

Mary C. Redmond

THE QUESTIONS

Surgery and anesthesia may have been simple and uneventful or perhaps somewhat more complicated with a few harrowing moments. Nevertheless, the patient proceeded successfully through phases I and II recovery, benefiting from high-quality nursing care every step along the way. Now that patient is finally ready for discharge to phase III recovery. But what is phase III recovery? What happens to the patient during this time? Who is responsible for the patient's care during this time? Does the perianesthesia nurse have any responsibility to the patient or other concerned parties during phase III recovery? If so, what is that responsibility? What is the role of the perianesthesia nurse during phase III recovery? How long does phase III recovery last? Why should perianesthesia nurses be concerned with and involved in phase III recovery once the patient is discharged from the ambulatory surgery unit?

THE ANSWERS

Phase III Recovery: An Overview

Phase III recovery is the period of extended postoperative recuperation after discharge from the hospital-based or free-standing ambulatory surgery center (ASC).[1, 2] Usually, patients and families believe that this period begins when the patient leaves phase II recovery. However, nurses actually start preparing for phase III when the patient is scheduled for surgery and continue the process on the day of surgery and beyond. Customarily, ASC nurses have assumed some degree of responsibility for their patients in phase III recovery for an arbitrary period of 24 hours postoperatively or until they completed the follow-up phone call, but when their responsibility actually ends is not exactly clear.

Phase III recovery seems to be a rather gray area of concern and responsibility for ASC perianesthesia nurses. Although they cannot be all things to all patients at all times, ASC nurses nevertheless have a responsibility to provide for the needs of their patients. Those needs vary with the individual patient's surgical procedure, physiologic, and psychosocial status, support system, course of recovery, and the involvement of external case managers. The perianesthesia nurse must be flexible, adaptable, and well prepared to work with available resources to meet the ever-changing and challenging needs of our patients. Table 23–1 presents a number of desired patient outcomes for the home, or phase III recovery time period.

Discharge to a Responsible Adult

Traditionally, discharge of a patient to phase III recovery meant release of the patient to a responsible adult caregiver. Because of some dilemmas, nurses have raised legal and ethical questions about "responsible adults." For example, what constitutes a responsible adult? The legal definition is age 18, 19, or 21 years, de-

Table 23–1. Patient Outcomes Grid—Home Care Needs

POTENTIAL AND ACTUAL PROBLEMS/ NURSING DIAGNOSES	OUTCOME GOALS—THE PATIENT WILL BE ABLE TO	NURSING INTERVENTIONS/EVAL (THROUGHOUT PROCESS AND PER PHONE DURING HOME RECOVERY PROCESS)	RESOURCES
Knowledge deficit R/T appropriate actions for medical emergencies (bleeding, impaired circulation, etc.)	Identify untoward/unexpected symptoms that should be reported Appropriately report symptoms of complications to surgeon, other physician, or nurse Appropriately seek emergency medical help	Provide information regarding access to physician after discharge (written and verbal) Provide information regarding access to emergency medical care on written discharge instructions Provide telephone number and name at surgery facility in case patient has further questions	ASPAN Standards of PeriAnesthesia Nursing Discharge instructions that include details on access to emergency medical care, physician's telephone number, and untoward symptoms to report Postdischarge telephone call
Alterations in health that can complicate home recovery course	Express understanding of how medical factors relate to surgery, anesthesia, and recovery process Comply with instructions for preoperative activities to optimize medical status before DOS Comply with instructions for postoperative activities and self-care to minimize chance of complications R/T health status	Encourage patient to provide accurate and complete historical health information Provide information regarding health practices and relationship to surgery within scope of nursing Provide comprehensive, individualized written and verbal discharge instructions in language that the patient and family can understand Involve primary care physician for home support	Primary care physician for care of ongoing health conditions Literature/brochures outlining patient expectations/responsibilities to provide information and home healthcare needs Books and references on patient assessment and relationship of health status to surgery and anesthesia Written and verbal discharge instructions R/T health status Postdischarge telephone call
Alterations in comfort—pain	Express acceptable comfort level during home recuperation Enact appropriate physical and pharmacologic interventions to reduce pain (i.e., positioning of surgical site, applying cold therapy) Take prescription drugs appropriately Provide self-care within activities limitations R/T surgery	Encourage proper and early use of prescription analgesics to reduce pain Ensure patient has obtained prescriptions for and physician instructions regarding home interventions to reduce pain Explain positioning of surgical site, application of cold therapy as ordered Provide positive reinforcements and encourage philosophy of wellness throughout process Encourage appropriate pace for activities	Analgesic medications at the facility and prescriptions for home Literature/patient instructions about pain management Philosophy of wellness Postdischarge telephone call Home health nurse

Alterations in comfort—nausea and vomiting	Express acceptable comfort level during home recuperation Identify foods and beverages that will help reduce or prevent PONV Eat, drink, and retain nourishment Avoid vomiting and retching	Encourage appropriate pace for oral intake of food and fluids at home (written and verbal) Encourage proper and early use of prescription drugs to prevent/reduce PONV Encourage taking analgesics with food	Antiemetic medications at the facility and prescriptions for home Literature/patient instructions about reducing GI symptoms Appropriate food and beverages at home
Self-care deficit	Perform self-care in relation to abilities and imposed activity restrictions R/T procedure and anesthetic interventions Rely on RA for needed assistance Display sufficient level of self-care for safety in home setting with RA before discharge	Demonstrate alternative methods of self-care modified to patient's abilities Assess patient and RA abilities to provide needed care	Preadmission instructions—(written and verbal) outlining home care needs and need for driver and RA in home setting Admitting form that prompts admitting nurse to identify availability of RA support
Constipation R/T physical inactivity and/or use of opioid medications	Maintain normal bowel habits Verbalize the fact that increased oral fluids and increased physical activity are deterrents to constipation Increase physical activity and oral fluids within surgical limits	Encourage activity at home within surgical limits Suggest increased oral fluids, bulk while taking narcotic analgesics Encourage patient to consult with physician should constipation occur	Listing of foods and beverages that promote regular bowel habits
Altered thought processes and/or memory loss R/T effects of sedation, anesthesia or analgesics	Display/verbalize appropriate orientation to surroundings and situations Avoid self-injury R/T altered thought patterns Rely on RA who understands nature of patient's temporarily altered thought patterns and responsibility for patient care	Provide frequent affirmations of orientation to time, place, and events Assess orientation Provide written and verbal information for family/RA regarding discharge instructions	Pharmaceutical literature outlining effects of anesthesia, sedative, analgesic medications Predetermined discharge criteria that include assessment of mental status and standards for identification of home support before discharge Postdischarge telephone call
Increased potential for injury or falls R/T weakness, altered comfort, faintness, orthostatic hypotension and impaired physical mobility	Demonstrate safe ambulation within parameters of surgical restrictions before discharge and at home Demonstrate proper use of assistive devices where appropriate Maintain normal cardiovascular parameters with activity before discharge and at home	Assess/document stable physiologic parameters before discharge Provide information and demonstration of proper ambulation techniques to patient and responsible adult Provide information on interventions for faintness, weakness (i.e., supine position, increasing fluid intake)	Policy supporting proper application of discharge criteria Written instructions for use of assistive devices Intravenous fluids, vasopressor medications HHN agencies Facility resources for transportation and overnight care ASPAN Standards of PeriAnesthesia Nursing Practice Postdischarge telephone call

Table continued on following page

***Table 23–1.* Patient Outcomes Grid—Home Care Needs** *Continued*

POTENTIAL AND ACTUAL PROBLEMS/ NURSING DIAGNOSES	OUTCOME GOALS—THE PATIENT WILL BE ABLE TO	NURSING INTERVENTIONS/EVAL (THROUGHOUT PROCESS AND PER PHONE DURING HOME RECOVERY PROCESS)	RESOURCES
Knowledge deficit R/T home care needs	Verbalize appropriate understanding of and preparation for home care needs Verbalize lingering questions R/T home care Ask appropriate questions Demonstrate procedures that will be needed at home for self-care activities	Provide preadmission information about home care needs Verify patient's home care plans before procedure being done Assess patient's knowledge, instruct patient and RA on home care needs	Patient-focused literature detailing home care needs and expectations of patient and family/RA Equipment, teaching tools (charts, models, etc.) for demonstration/redemonstration Postdischarge telephone call
Inadequate social support	Rely on RA to provide transportation and home care Accept assistance from outside sources for transportation and home support Accept overnight care or home nursing care if RA not available	Provide written and verbal information for family/RA regarding discharge instructions Query patient about availability of home care before the start of any procedure or anesthetic Coordinate home health nurse or companion services	Family/RA or friends of patient HHN services Hospital or other facility overnight services Facility transportation service Facility policy regarding discharge criteria
Noncompliance with discharge instructions (medications, diet, activity, wound care, RA care, driving, follow-up)	Verbalize appropriate understanding of consequences of actions/choices Verbalize responsibility for actions/choices	Provide information to patient/RA on consequences of noncompliance Provide information re: access to physician after discharge, emergency medical care and number and name at surgical facility and/or emergency room	Facility policy Facility legal counsel Patient education materials

ASPAN = American Society of PeriAnesthesia Nurses; DOS = day of surgery; GI = gastrointestinal; HHN = home health nurse; PAT = preadmission testing; PONV = postoperative nausea and vomiting; RA = responsible adult; R/T = related to.

pending on the state in which you live, but does age alone determine responsibility? At what age is a person too young or too old to be responsible? Many teenagers at 16 or 17 years of age are able to responsibly care for a parent after a minor surgical procedure. Many married couples in their 90s are active, in reasonably good health, and have successfully cared for each other for many years.

What if the caregiver is old enough and responsible but is suspected of being unable to care adequately for the patient? For example, the caregiver may appear physically debilitated, or complicated postoperative instructions may seem beyond his or her comprehension. Must a responsible adult be present for 24 hours? What if no one is available to stay overnight or the patient is reluctant to ask or refuses to have someone stay overnight? After 24 hours, if the patient experiences persistent nausea and vomiting, if pain is severe and uncontrolled with existing medications, or if the patient experiences prolonged vertigo or amnesia from anesthesia and the responsible adult caregiver no longer can remain with the patient, what can and should be done? All these questions are typical, but none have easy answers. Each one must be addressed in view of the individual patient, problem, and available resources, and in compliance with the ASC's policies, procedures, and standards of care.

Responsible Adult Role

The role of the responsible adult in phase III recovery is that of caregiver, troubleshooter, and cheerleader. Although nurses tend to take many care activities for granted because they do these tasks regularly and routinely, the responsible adult needs to be taught to meet the basic needs of the patient.

Caregiver

The caregiver first needs to learn how and why it is important to provide for the overall comfort of the patient. This includes providing a quiet, therapeutic environment, free of stress to the extent possible; properly positioning the patient; applying ice or heat to the operative site according to discharge instructions; checking extremities regularly, if appropriate, for good circulation and sensation; giving back rubs and massages to relieve sore, tense muscles; helping splint an abdominal incision; and encouraging coughing and deep breathing. These simple but effective measures enhance the patient's well-being.

Analgesics also play an important role in maintaining comfort. The perianesthesia nurses must teach the caregiver and patient that they can successfully achieve and maintain pain relief by taking analgesics regularly and when pain is mild so that it never becomes severe, especially in the early stages of phase III recovery. Patients then may gradually wean off prescription analgesics and substitute over-the-counter analgesics, if appropriate, as healing progresses to wellness. Many patients find it especially helpful to use a pain scale, which helps them visualize and express the intensity of their pain, as well as appreciate the degree of pain relief achieved.[3, 4] Remind patients that it is helpful to take analgesics with food, rather than on an empty stomach, to prevent nausea. "With food" can mean with soda crackers and a carbonated beverage and need not be a full meal.

As caregiver, the responsible adult also needs to see that the patient receives the other medications ordered, including medications that the patient was taking before surgery. The ASC nurse must consult with the patient's physicians regarding which medications should be resumed and when, and which ones should be discontinued.

Providing proper nutrition and hydration for the patient is yet another caregiver responsibility. The responsible adult must be instructed to make sure that patients who have local anesthesia for nasopharyngeal/laryngeal procedures have a swallowing reflex before giving them water or ice chips to avoid choking. Carbonated drinks and citrus juice should be avoided to reduce local irritation until these areas are healed. Avoid hot liquids for patients who have a local anesthesia in place for oral procedures to prevent burns. Unless otherwise ordered, offer a light first meal of clear juice, soda, soup, gelatin or fruit, and progress to the patient's normal diet as tolerated.

It is especially important to provide adequate liquid intake to children and the elderly, who can dehydrate rapidly. If necessary, almost anything the patient enjoys and is not contraindicated can be put in near-liquid or soft form with the aid of a food processor or blender to encourage intake. Once the patient is taking fluids, the caregiver then needs to monitor for adequate urinary output or inability to urinate resulting in bladder distention. After several days of altered food intake, reduced physical activity, and opioid use, constipation is another potential problem that should be anticipated and prevented.

Another duty of the responsible adult is to

provide for the basic safety of the patient. It can take many forms. For example, one way is by making the home environment barrier free, with chairs and tables moved out of the patient's way and throw rugs and extension cords removed. The patient will need an area of comfortable rest, easily accessible to a bathroom, where the patient can avoid climbing stairs unnecessarily. A night light or flashlight may be helpful. Appropriate phone numbers should be placed beside a conveniently located phone, and large, easy-to-read print should be used for names and numbers. Regarding physiologic safety, the caregiver should observe for a fever, dehydration, edema of an area, or unusually large amounts of unexpected or foul-smelling drainage. The patient should be observed for vertigo, somnolence, disorientation, nausea, vomiting, diarrhea, rash, or hives, which may indicate an untoward reaction to medications.

The responsible adult also needs to provide basic assistive care to the patient. Such care can include dressing changes, active and passive range-of-motion exercises to extremities, application of braces or splints, and transfer to and from a bed, wheelchair, car, and the bathroom. Finally, ASC nurses need to send the patient home with a sufficient amount of basic supplies, for example, dressings and tape, ice bags, and slings, and help the responsible adult locate and make arrangements for other equipment as necessary.

Troubleshooter and Cheerleader

In addition to the role of caregiver, the responsible adult needs to be a "troubleshooter" for the patient. The nurse can help build caregiver confidence by reviewing the potentially problematic signs and symptoms that need to be identified and reported to the physician. The staff also needs to provide a contact telephone number for the ASC and to reassure the caregiver that no questions are too simple or too trivial. The caregiver is there to obtain help for the patient in time of need, and the ASC staff is available as a resource for the patient and caregiver.

Finally, the responsible adult also must act as "cheerleader." Because it is easy to become discouraged because of frustration or perceived slow progress during recovery, the patient may need positive reinforcement and encouragement. The responsible adult needs to understand discharge instructions and to reinforce them to the patient who often accepts such instructions better knowing that they come from the physician or nurses rather than from the caregiver.

Support Mechanisms

Responsible adults are more likely to leave the ASC confident of their ability to care for the patient if they know that there is an adequate support system available to them in time of need. The support system begins with careful and complete teaching that includes both the patient and the responsible adult. Information needs to be very basic, practical, and relevant to the needs of the individual patient. To facilitate learning, all instructions should be in writing and should be reviewed with the involved parties using the adult principles of learning[5] (Table 23–2). Include information on where to call in case of further questions and how to obtain help in case of need during regular working hours, after hours, and in case of emergency. Finally, the patient and responsible adult should be reassured that the ASC nurse will contact them in a routine telephone call, according to facility policy or patient need, to check on their status and to answer any questions that they may have. Table 23–3 provides an overview of important educational points related to home recovery.

However, sometimes no amount of careful planning and preparation can overcome the single-minded determination of some patients. The following case study indicates a typical example of a patient's noncompliance with discharge instructions.

Case Study

Mr. R was a 62-year-old, take charge, no nonsense, burly man who had a knee arthroscopy with lateral release under general anesthe-

***Table 23–2.* Adult Learning Principles**

Treat each learner as an individual.
Build on the learner's basic knowledge—discover, reinforce, correct, elaborate.
Use language appropriate to the learner—clear, simple, concise, sixth-grade level.
Be patient—repeat, reinforce, answer questions.
Use various teaching modes—reading, touching, demonstrations, analogies, comparisons.
Sequence from simple to complex, known to unknown—repeat, summarize, question.
Give positive encouragement—reinforce, reassure.

Data from Redmond MC: The importance of good communication in effective patient–family teaching. J PostAnesth Nurs 8:109–112, 1993.

Table 23–3. Key Educational Points: Home Care Issues

SUPERVISION

By responsible adult
For length of time appropriate to patient needs, surgical procedure/anesthesia

GENERAL COMFORT/SAFETY

Safe, quiet environment
Activity permitted/restrictions
Positioning, support of extremity
Coughing, turning, deep breathing, splinting incision

MEDICATIONS

Analgesics as ordered, according to pain scale
Other prescriptions to be started and when, duration
Preoperative prescriptions to be resumed and when
Preoperative prescriptions to be discontinued

HYDRATION/NUTRITION/ELIMINATION

Provide adequate liquids
Prevent nausea, dehydration
Monitor adequate urine output, check distention
Type of diet with any restrictions
Prevent constipation

WOUND CARE

If/when to change dressings, frequency
Observation of operative site: drainage, odor, temperature, color, edema, altered sensation or circulation, impaired movement
If/how to redress wound, type of dressing, sterile technique
If/when to remove dressing

SPECIAL INSTRUCTIONS

Use of restrictive devices (e.g., braces, splints, slings)
Use of assistive devices (e.g., crutches, walker, wheelchair)
Use of special equipment (e.g., PCA pumps, CPM devices, catheters, drains)
Cold/heat application, length of time, duration
Elevation of extremity
Weight-bearing status
Bathing/shampoo restrictions
Therapy (e.g., physical, occupational, respiratory, speech); when to begin and location
Arrangements with outside agencies (e.g., home health care)

FOLLOW-UP APPOINTMENT WITH PHYSICIAN

Call to arrange date, time, and location
Purpose of visit

FOLLOW-UP CONTACT BY ASC NURSE

Notify patient/caregiver of date, approximate time of call
Obtain phone number where patient can be reached

HELP AFTER LEAVING ASC

Facility phone number, name of nurse
Physician's office and answering service phone numbers

WHEN/IF TO CALL THE PHYSICIAN

Allergic reaction or compromised condition related to medications/anesthetics: respiratory distress, shock, confusion, pruritus, hives, nausea, vomiting, diarrhea
Persistent, unrelieved nausea/vomiting beyond 24 hours in adults
Unrelieved pain after use of analgesics as ordered
Compromised circulation: changes in color, sensation, temperature, movement
Edema at operative site greater than expected
Drainage from operative site in greater amounts than expected
Fever greater than 100°F in adults
Urinary retention, bladder distention
Alteration in concurrent medical condition
Persistent altered thought process inconsistent with preoperative status
Whenever questions arise

ASC = ambulatory surgery center; CPM = continuous passive motion; PCA = patient-controlled analgesia.

sia. Preoperatively, he impatiently tolerated nurses' questions, explanations, and preparations, and he asked no questions. At the scheduled surgery time, he marched into the operating room, dismissing his passive wife to the waiting room.

Surgery and phases I and II recovery were uneventful. Because of intraoperative infiltration of local anesthesia, he required no analgesics. After he and his wife hurriedly read the discharge instructions, he insisted on leaving, and his wife readily agreed. Because he was stable and met discharge criteria, he was released home with the knowledge and approval of both his surgeon and the anesthesiologist.

By early evening, Mr. R's wife telephoned the ASC nurses in tears. She explained that he had driven home, had been up walking with full weight-bearing all day, and refused to elevate his leg or apply ice to the knee. At the time of her call, the local anesthetic had worn off, and he had significant knee edema. The oral analgesics he had taken were not yet effective, and he could be heard screaming and swearing in the background.

Mr. R was referred to the facility's emergency room. After treatment for pain and edema, he was kept overnight in 23-hour observation for further pain management and monitoring of his circulatory status. His wife went home to rest.

Telephone contact with his wife 2 days later revealed that Mr. R's perianesthesia behavior was typical. "I never could tell him what to do." Except for significant discomfort, Mr. R had an otherwise uneventful recovery.

Later discussion with the staff and surgeon concluded that the potential for noncompliance with discharge instructions might have been better identified preoperatively. However, it was doubtful that the situation could have been avoided because Mr. R was strong willed, insistent on having surgery, and had a history of doing what he wanted to do.

Common Reasons for Assisted Care

For various reasons, not all patients are able to be discharged home postoperatively to the care of a responsible adult without some additional form of assisted care. Patients may lack a social support system because they live alone and have no family or friends to look after them, or the spouse or other responsible adult is unwilling or physically unable to care for them. Because of many stairs or a difficult transfer, the patient's home environment may not support ease of care. Postoperative care may be quite complex, including wound care, a complicated medication regimen, or complex equipment or devices. Another challenge can be that the patient may exhibit personal coping deficits, for example, depression, anxiety, denial of medical problems, or orientation or memory problems, necessitating additional help.[6] Age alone should not be included in screening criteria because the young may be as much in need of assisted care as are the elderly.[7, 8] Whatever the situation, the goal of assisted care is to meet the needs of the patient and responsible adult while avoiding an unplanned, unnecessary, and costly inpatient hospital stay whenever possible.[2]

There are several problems that frequently occur in phases I and II recovery and may extend into phase III recovery. Two of the most common are pain and postoperative nausea and vomiting (PONV). Both these problems can be treated before discharge, but either one may require assisted care after discharge to avoid an otherwise unnecessary admission. Other considerations that frequently need to be addressed in phase III recovery are the management of concurrent medical conditions and the management of various medical devices as a result of surgery.

Pain

There are several important factors influencing the occurrence, intensity, quality, and duration of postoperative pain. They include the site, nature, and duration of the surgery; the patient's physiologic and psychological makeup; the preoperative pharmacologic and psychological preparation of the patient; the presence of postoperative complications; and the anesthetic management before, during, and after surgery.[4, 9, 10]

Common methods of pain management after ambulatory surgery include the administration of analgesics intravenously (IV), orally, intramuscularly, and via local infiltration or nerve blocks. One of the newer routes of administration gaining popularity in selected patients and procedures is the subcutaneous (SC) route with a patient-controlled analgesia (PCA) pump. Use of PCA morphine, for example, provides for intermittent on-demand or continuous plus intermittent on-demand pain control.[3, 4] The advantages are that the patient can enjoy more stable serum levels of analgesia without the fear or inconvenience of an IV line. Achieving consistently better pain management promotes early ambulation with fewer side effects, generally resulting in a more rapid recovery. After approximately 24 hours, when there usually is less incidence of PONV, the patient can convert easily to equianalgesic doses of oral medications.[3]

Patient selection for the use of PCA depends on several factors: operative procedure, the perceptions and cooperation of the patient and responsible adult, insurance coverage, and home healthcare availability in the community. Once selection criteria have been met, teaching must include selecting the SC site that can be kept clean, dry, and free of restrictive clothing and observing the site at least twice daily for edema, redness, or leakage of fluid; properly using the equipment with return demonstrations; effectively using the analgesic, stressing prevention or control of pain, titration or adjustment of doses for prevention or control of side effects, and safety; and observing for side effects including respiratory depression, excessive sedation, dry mouth, nausea and vomiting, confusion, vertigo, restlessness, or muscle spasms. As with any narcotic use, patients should be cautioned against simultaneously engaging in potentially dangerous activities and alcohol ingestion.[3]

Nausea and Vomiting

When patients have had a bad past experience with PONV, they often fear repeating that experience more than they fear the surgical procedure or postoperative pain. Risk factors generally associated with PONV include anesthetic techniques, anesthetic agents, narcotics, age, gender, weight, type of surgical procedure, pain, and a history of prior nausea and vomiting or motion sickness.[4]

It is usually easier to prevent than to treat PONV, and for that reason, it is vitally important that patients at risk of becoming nauseated be identified by a thorough history as early as possible. Ideally, prophylactic antiemetics can be given preoperatively or intraoperatively. Prevention or early treatment results in increased patient comfort, reduced nursing care time, and increased patient satisfaction. In extreme cases of persistent PONV, patients may need to be sent home with a prescription for antiemetic suppositories or may require hospital admission.

Most patients are able to be discharged home once PONV is under control. To help reduce the chance of vomiting during transit, patients should be taught to remain upright, look straight ahead, and take slow deep breaths during the ride home to maintain equilibrium. In anticipation of potential vomiting en route, send an emesis basin and tissues home with the patient. Once home, the patient should take sips of water and a light diet before advancing to a regular diet and should take medications with food. ASC nurses should offer the needed positive reinforcement, provide phone numbers for contacting help in case of need, and follow up with the patient on the next day.

Concurrent Medical Conditions

Another reason for assisted care in phase III recovery may be instability of concurrent medical conditions. Once home, patients may require continued observation, monitoring, or intervention for chronic cardiovascular, respiratory, endocrine, or other systemic conditions that may or may not have been well controlled preoperatively or postoperatively.

Needs for assisted care may include observation and assessment to evaluate treatment modifications or need for additional procedures; planning, management, and evaluation of a patient care plan for complex conditions and potential complications; or reinforcement of teaching and training activities taught in the institutional setting. Postoperative management of pre-existing, changing medical conditions may necessitate performing laboratory tests or adjusting and administering complicated medication regimens or medical gases.[11] Further information about these services is discussed in the section on Home Health Care later in this chapter.

Management of Equipment and Devices

As technology and new surgical techniques are perfected, associated equipment and devices seem to increase proportionately. When equipment or devices appear in conjunction with patient care, several pieces of information need to be determined before the patient's discharge to phase III recovery. Is the equipment or device going to be sent home with the patient? Was the use of the equipment or device preplanned or unplanned? Will the patient or caregiver be responsible in any manner for the equipment or device? If so, does the patient or responsible adult know its purpose and how to operate it? Does the patient or responsible adult demonstrate capability and confidence in managing the equipment or device, or do they express fear, reluctance or doubt about it?

Some items used for patient care may be in place postoperatively, with their operation explained to the patient and responsible adult before discharge from the ASC. Examples include catheters, drains, infusion ports, and braces. Other items may have been delivered to the home and demonstrated to the patient and responsible adult before the day of surgery, such as continuous passive motion (CPM) devices. Assisted care may be necessary postoperatively to actually apply and adjust the equipment properly. Still other equipment may be explained preoperatively but delivered and attached only after the patient has returned home postoperatively. PCA pumps or IV infusion devices for antibiotics are examples. In any case, staff providing assisted care after discharge from the ASC can provide technical expertise and education, answer questions and allay fears, and serve as a resource to patients and responsible adult caregivers alike.

Assisted Care Decision Process

Many parties can and should have input regarding whether a patient needs some type of assisted care after discharge from phase II recovery. When scheduling the patient for the procedure, the surgeon should take into account the nature of the surgical procedure, time of day for which it is scheduled, length of the procedure, type of anesthesia, and general medical condition of the patient. The medical doctor may be able to provide additional significant information about the patient's medical and psychosocial history, available support system, and anticipated postoperative needs.

During the preoperative phone call(s), the patient or family may be able to identify justifiable medical or psychosocial needs for assisted care. However, staff members must clarify that approval for assisted care and payment likely will be denied if the request is due to a matter of convenience or patient/responsible adult preference.

Undoubtedly, the nurse is in a key position to identify a patient's or responsible adult's need for assisted care during phase III recovery. Using the nursing process, the nurse assesses the needs based on scheduling information, demographic information, insurance coverage, interview information including the medical and surgical history, the preoperative assessment, and the anticipated status of the patient postoperatively. In planning and goal setting, the nurse must determine actual patient needs, available options within the community, and the patient's qualifying factors; then obtain appropriate orders. During implementation, the nurse needs to discuss patient and responsible adult needs with the involved physicians, social services representatives, if available, home health agency, and the business office/insurance company to set in motion the process of arranging assisted care. Finally, on the day of surgery, the nurse must re-evaluate those needs before discharge and adjust plans according to postoperative orders, patient condition, and patient/responsible adult needs.

Another determinant is the managed-care system. Internal and external case managers can be a valuable source of information about a particular patient's needs and history. The case manager is also familiar with the services available within a given system and community and knows how to qualify the patient and access the system.

Lastly, third party payers, for example, Medicare, Medicaid, health maintenance organizations (HMOs), preferred provider organizations (PPOs), and private insurance carriers, have significant input regarding whether a patient actually receives assisted care during phase III recovery, even if others already have determined that the need may exist. Business office personnel must determine requisite qualifications and obtain necessary approvals in advance of care arrangements.

Assisted Care Alternatives

As the nature of society, healthcare reform, and surgical procedures have become more complex, so too have the variety of assisted care options available during phase III recovery. In response to varying needs of the parties concerned, many creative programs have been developed, some more successful than others. These programs range from the very simple short stay arrangements in self-care rooms or hotels with custodial services to more long-term arrangements with home healthcare agencies. These options continue to evolve rapidly to meet the ever-changing needs of the people we serve. Alternatives currently available include those services offered within a hospital, those offered outside but in conjunction with a hospital or ambulatory center, and those services offered in the home.

Twenty-Three Hour Observation

After ambulatory surgery in an ASC, some patients receive phase III extended care in a 23-hour observation unit. This option is perhaps the simplest, most familiar, most convenient, and most readily available for patients. Whether preplanned or not, the patient transfers from phase I or II recovery to a hospital room on a separate unit or on a regular medical–surgical unit. During the stay, the patient receives the full complement of nursing care, treatments, and medications, as well as any other services necessary and available from the ancillary departments.[8]

Insurance carriers and Medicare reimburse a hospital for these services at reduced outpatient rates only if certain conditions are met. The first condition is a limited time factor. As the name implies, "currently the maximum time allowed for Medicare reimbursement at most facilities under state and local regulations is 23 hours and 59 minutes."[12] Most insurance carriers impose the same limitation. Patients whose medical condition warrants a longer stay then must be admitted as hospital inpatients. In such instances, any necessary approval must be obtained from Medicare or insurance carriers according to specified requirements.

The other major condition is that the patient's stay must be medically warranted. For example, the patient must have a surgical complication, intractable pain or PONV, or a preexisting medical condition that needs to be monitored postoperatively for actual or potential complications, for example, cardiac arrhythmias. Documentation in the medical record must reflect appropriate observations, interventions, and outcomes concerning the reasons for the patient's stay, or ultimately reimbursement may be denied. No longer may patients stay in 23-hour observation as a matter of preference, convenience, or for a social need unless they are willing to pay expenses out of pocket, generally prohibitive for most people. Fortunately, many other care alternatives are available for those in need.

Short Stay Units

Sometimes what a patient needs more than anything else during early phase III recovery is "tincture of time." Alegent Health Bergan Mercy Medical Center in Omaha, Nebraska, has a brief stay unit, known as short-term care, which offers time and nursing care to patients before discharge home. Registered nurses staff this hospital unit 12 hours a day, Monday through Friday.

The unit serves a variety of medical and surgical patients who need to be observed for a few hours after simple procedures. For example, a patient who has had ambulatory surgery can go to that unit for a stay of several hours, eat as tolerated, void, relax in privacy with family, or wait for a responsible adult to get off work to provide home care. Nurses in the unit provide observation, general nursing care, and comfort measures, including medications. Patients are required to be healthy adults having elective procedures and expected to be discharged by 7:30 PM. If any patient experiences problems or is unable to leave by the designated time, the nurse notifies the patient's physician and the patient is transferred to an appropriate nursing unit for observation or inpatient status.

Patients qualify for these services in the same way as 23-hour observation patients. Room rates are hourly up to 6 hours, then convert to 23-hour observation room rates. Insurance carriers and Medicare reimburse at reduced rates for these ambulatory services.

A similar type of unit popular in both the United States and Canada is a somewhat longer short stay or interim stay unit. This hospital unit is open from midmorning on Monday to early evening on Friday for the postoperative care of ambulatory surgery patients. Those patients who are not able to be discharged home by Friday at closing time are transferred to another surgical ward that can meet their needs.[13, 14]

These cost-effective units usually have specific admission criteria. For example, the length of stay is limited to 72 hours; patients must have the ability to meet basic self-care needs, as well as the cognitive and psychomotor capabilities for learning self-care; and there must be a likelihood of reasonable pain control within the 72-hour limit.[13] Insurance coverage depends on the carrier and must be investigated in advance of need.

Hospital Self-Care

Burden[8] cites yet another short stay alternative called "Rest Assured." In this example, a hospital converted otherwise unused rooms on a medical–surgical unit into self-care rooms. Patients undergoing minor procedures can stay overnight for a prepaid, out-of-pocket, nominal fee that includes a meal and medications. Although routine nursing care is not provided, nurses respond in case of emergency. Because patients are not counted in the census, they cannot figure into the staffing needs of the unit. This unit is helpful for those patients who do not meet criteria for insurance coverage of care but are in need of a low-cost alternative, that is, people with no home support for the first 24 hours.

Hospital Hotels/Motels

Some hospitals make arrangements with nearby, freestanding hotels or motels owned by nonhospital developers. These facilities often provide rooms at reduced rates to out-of-town patients who are undergoing procedures at the local hospital. Special services they provide may include transportation and special diets.[13, 14] The patient is responsible for self-payment of these short-term expenses.

Certain programs require that another person reside in the hotel with the patient. In any case, the ASC staff must provide proper postoperative instructions to patients and families, if present, including observations and how to seek help if necessary. Before discharge from the ASC, nurses also must obtain the patient's hotel phone number and room number to make a follow-up telephone call. Hotel/motel personnel assume no other responsibility for patients but will call 911 for patients in need of emergency assistance.

Package Plans

For the patient who is able to go directly home from the ASC but briefly needs minimal assistance, one health system in west central Florida offers a "Coming Home" package through its home health agency. For an out-of-pocket nominal fee, an employee of the home health agency transports the patient postoperatively from the ASC, picks up prescriptions and groceries that the patient pays for, and stays with the patient for 4 hours to make sure he or she is doing well.[15]

Yet a different type of package plan is available for the patient who is able to go home directly from the ASC after more complex procedures and needs a longer period of assisted care postoperatively. Burden[8] cites Texas Outpatient Surgicare (TOPS) in Houston, Texas, as an example. This ASC worked with a home health agency to arrive at a package price for surgery and home nursing care, medications, and surgical supplies for home use. A home health agency nurse accompanied the patient home via ambulance and provided care for 24 to 48 hours after discharge.

To qualify for the package plan, the patient had to meet the criteria determined by the physician, facility, and home health agency. The billed insurance carrier also had to pre-approve the billed services. Finally, the patient and responsible adult also had to approve the plans. Such an arrangement remained below the cost of a traditional inpatient day.

Since then, this ASC has developed into a licensed hospital facility that provides short-term overnight care for surgical patients. Such specialty surgical hospitals, combined with overnight beds, provide yet another type of assisted care alternative.

Recovery Centers

Recovery centers are short stay units that house essentially healthy patients recovering from uncomplicated, elective orthopedic and podiatric, gynecologic, urologic, plastic, ear/nose/throat (ENT), or general surgery. These centers offer around-the-clock care provided by an RN-led staff with emphasis on pain management, treatments, and teaching. Services emphasize wellness and preparation for discharge. The setting is a comfortable, hotel-like atmosphere of private rooms with safety backups of oxygen and suction, amenities such as big screen cable television and VCR, and dinner provided by room service. Many centers also provide guest accommodations for one other accompanying person.

These centers were introduced in California in the 1980s to complement the growth of physician-owned freestanding surgery centers. At that time, the length of stay was limited to 72 hours but averaged 48 hours. Many states currently limit stays at these recovery centers to 23 hours. New federal restrictions apply to doctors sending patients to physician-owned surgery centers, and managed care has transferred patient control from physicians to insurance companies.[16] Medicare and Medicaid do not pay for most types of recovery centers that charge an average of 40% less than hospitals.[16, 17] As a result, some freestanding surgery centers, such as Fresno Surgery Center, have chosen instead to operate as Medicare-approved hospitals. Many hospitals looking to establish a solid outpatient services division have added surgery centers with recovery care facilities. Large healthcare chains like Columbia/HCA Healthcare Corporation operate freestanding surgery centers with recovery care centers.[17]

Home Health Care

For the patient in need of assisted care beyond these options, home healthcare agencies offer yet another alternative. This service allows patients with functional disabilities to recuperate safely and independently at home with the help of a responsible adult under nursing supervision.

Care Providers

A number of sources provide home healthcare services. Historically, the largest and best known provider has been the Visiting Nurses Association (VNA). However, in recent years, other service providers include nationally owned and operated agencies, often patterned after the VNA. Although some of these agencies provide a full range of services, others specialize in limited services, such as parenteral therapy. In view of the growth of partnerships and managed care, many medical centers either have their own division of home healthcare services or work in agreement with centers that have such services. The trend is to work not only locally, but more likely within a certain radius in outlying communities to meet the needs of growing numbers of patients and families who need extended care.

Financing

The means of payment depends on the patient's insurance coverage. For example, there are important differences among private insurance carrier policies, Medicare, and Medicaid[19] (Table 23–4). The healthcare team needs input from the business office and sometimes the social services department to determine whether

Table 23–4. **Private Insurance, Medicare, and Medicaid Differences**

	PRIVATE INSURANCE	MEDICARE	MEDICAID
Eligibility*	Meet policy requirements	Age ≥ 65 years or < 65 years and disabled	People with low income and few financial resources Patients may have to impoverish themselves by paying for medical treatment, home health, or nursing homes before applying for Medicaid
Financed by	Individual	Federal government; administered by Health Care Financing Administration	Federal, state, and local funding; state determines eligibility Covered services vary by state and are broader than Medicare coverage
Criteria for covered services	Depends on specific policy coverage; most do not cover long-term care	Services must be ordered by a physician Services must be reasonable and medically necessary to the treatment of the illness or injury Patient must be homebound; care is provided in lieu of hospitalization Patient must need a skilled primary service, i.e., skilled nursing care; speech, physical, or occupational therapy; home health aide service; medical social services; or medical supplies and equipment Services must be provided on an intermittent or part-time basis Patient must have restorative potential if ongoing therapy visits are planned There is no provision for long-term maintenance services	Patient need not be homebound Patient need not meet skilled nursing criteria Covers home care services for the chronically ill; pays more extensive home health aide and home attendant services Covers skilled nursing facility (nursing home) costs

*Patients may have both Medicare and Medicaid if the eligibility requirements for each are met.
Data from Corkery E: Discharge planning and home health care: What every staff nurse should know. Orthop Nurs 8:18–27, 1989.

and how the patient qualifies. Most older postoperative patients needing assisted care through a home health agency are covered by Medicare within certain guidelines. There are nine regional Medicare Fiscal Intermediaries for processing home healthcare claims throughout the country. Because interpretation of the billing guidelines may differ slightly from one intermediary to another, information must be verified with the intermediary in the patient's specific region.[19]

Medicare-Covered Services

Patients who qualify can receive several different types of services. These services include skilled nursing care; other therapeutic services such as physical, speech, or occupational therapy; medical social services; and home health aide services.

There are 16 categories of skilled nursing services covered by Medicare, including assessment, instruction, treatments in such areas as wound and skin care, care of the urinary and respiratory systems, nutrition, including enteral and parenteral feedings, ostomy care, rehabilitation, monitoring of vital signs, and medication administration[11, 19] (Table 23–5). Services are intermittent rather than continuous and are meant to supplement care provided by the patient's own responsible adult caregiver. The number of nursing visits, types of services per day and per week, as well as over what period of time, depends on the patient's needs, physician's orders, and availability of resources within a particular community.[2, 19]

Home health aides perform a different level of care under the supervision of nurses. Tasks include applying or reinforcing dressings, taking and recording vital signs, assisting patients with the care of urinary drainage bags or ostomy bags, assembling supplies for tracheostomy care, preparing special diets, and assisting with active and passive range-of-motion exercises. These functions may vary from state to state according to the state department of health.[2]

When unskilled care is sufficient to meet the needs of patients, home attendants provide basic personal and chore services including assistance

Table 23–5. Skilled Nursing Services Covered by Medicare

1. Observation and assessment to evaluate treatment modification or need for additional procedures
2. Planning, management, and evaluation of a patient care plan for complex conditions and potential complications
3. Reinforcement of teaching and training activities taught in the institutional setting
4. Administration of medications IV, IM, SC, infusions, hypodermoclysis or IV feedings, and frequently adjusted oral medications
5. Nasogastric and percutaneous tube feedings, as well as replacement, adjustment, stabilization, and suctioning to treat the illness or injury
6. Aspiration of nasopharyngeal and tracheostomy tubes PRN
7. Insertion, sterile irrigation, and replacement of catheters cyclically or PRN
8. Wound care for direct treatment, teaching, and/or skilled observation and assessment
9. Ostomy care for teaching purposes, postoperatively, or if associated with complications
10. Heat treatments in conjunction with skilled observation and evaluation of the patient's progress
11. Medical gases for skilled observation and evaluation of the patient's response and for patient and family teaching
12. Rehabilitation nursing including bowel and bladder training
13. Venipuncture when necessary to the patient's diagnosis and treatment and the specimen cannot be collected via routine visits to a physician
14. Cataract care and eye drops when aides help patients to administer eye medications. Skilled nursing care is covered for observation, assessment, and teaching if actual or potential complications exist
15. Diabetic care in unstable patient conditions, or if the patient is mentally or physically incapable of self-care
16. Foot and nail care for patients with diabetes or circulatory problems

IM = intramuscular; IV = intravenous; PRN = as occasion requires; SC = subcutaneous.
Data from Redmond MC: Using home health agencies to meet patient needs in phase III recovery. J PostAnesth Nurs, 10:23–25, 1995. Reprinted with permission.

with activities of daily living, meal preparation, shopping, and housekeeping. Other resources, such as Meals-on-Wheels and local self-help groups, also may be available in the community.[2]

Phase III Recovery: The Nurses' Follow-up Role

For all the rewards of working with ambulatory surgery patients and families, there also are disadvantages. Perhaps the most notable are the limited contact and general inability of ASC nurses to observe patients for an extended period of time to determine their general progress. However, there exists a professional, moral, and ethical nursing responsibility to patients separate from but in conjunction with that of physicians to provide a continuum of care beyond phase II and into recuperation during phase III recovery.

Burden[8] emphasizes that the responsibility for follow-up extends to everyone who has been a patient in the ASC, regardless of his or her discharge status or destination. Thus, whether a patient is discharged home to the care of a responsible adult, receives assisted care from a home healthcare provider, or stays overnight in 23-hour observation or a recovery center, he or she is entitled to the same standard of care, that is, follow-up by ASC nurses after phase II recovery discharge, even though it may seem redundant in some cases.

There are several ways in which ASC nurses follow patients during phase III recovery. In some medical centers, these nurses may be cross-trained in home healthcare services and visit the patient at home. "With the increase in managed care and efforts to decrease costs we likely will see more practices where one nurse becomes the patient's primary nurse, providing preadmission assessment, tests, and teaching in the home or at a facility, care on the day of the procedure, and follow-up in the home during the recovery time."[20] More common methods of follow-up are telephone calls, surveys, or a combination of the two.

Telephone Calls

Telephone calls usually focus on the general physical well-being of patients. However, they also may cover some issues of satisfaction or dissatisfaction, questions about care, or actual or potential problems and complications.

Before discharge, all patients or responsible adults should be told that they will be contacted postoperatively for routine follow-up. In preparation for the call, certain information should be verified before discharging the patient from the ASC, including accurate telephone number and the patient's anticipated location (at home, relative's home, hotel, etc.), special requests or constraints (do not call at work, do not give information to family members, etc.) and preferred contact time.

Although the staff may be very busy, follow-up telephone calls should be made by registered nurses rather than by clerical or technical personnel. Professional judgment is necessary to evaluate the health information described by the patient or responsible adult and to formulate appropriate action steps when necessary.[8]

When the nurses actually make the follow-up telephone calls varies according to the patients' needs and circumstances as well as staff convenience. In some cases, it is appropriate to telephone the patient on the day of the procedure after questionable transportation home, for example, when you suspect that the patient drove him- or herself home instead of leaving with family. If the patient insists on leaving against medical advice, it is prudent to check on the patient to make sure he or she has arrived home safely with no untoward effects because of his or her decision. In most cases, the nurse makes the routine follow-up call within 24 hours of discharge. However, depending on the individual patient, it may be appropriate to call a second time up to several days postoperatively.

Mechanism

To facilitate efficient phone calls, it is helpful to have a preprinted form or standard computer screen on which to record the information. There should be room to record unsuccessful attempts to contact the patient, as well as room for information obtained during the first and any subsequent telephone calls. This information then should become a permanent part of the patient's record.

Beginning at a reasonable hour or the specific time arranged with the patient, make the postoperative telephone call to the agreed-on location. This may be at the patient's home or other alternative care site, at work, at school, or at some other location. The patient's privacy should be protected because others may not be aware that the patient has had surgery. Therefore, when contacting the patient, identify yourself and ask the patient if he or she is able to talk conveniently at that time before proceeding. Conversely, if the patient is not in or is not able to talk at that time, leave a message to return your call. For example, at one facility, nurses leave a message for the patient to call Ruth Reynolds, a fictitious "code name," indicating to whomever answers at the ASC that the caller is a patient returning a postoperative call.

Nurses at most facilities make initial follow-up telephone calls within 24 hours of the patient's discharge from the ASC or on the next work day. In some cases, nurses take follow-up sheets home to complete these calls on weekends or holidays, when the ASC is closed, thus providing the same quality of care to Friday's patients as is given to patients having procedures Monday through Thursday.[20]

The number of days and attempts made to contact patients postoperatively depends on the patient's condition and circumstances and varies with different facilities. If a patient cannot be reached within 1 or 2 days postoperatively and there is actual or potential reason for concern, the ASC nurse may contact the physician's office to determine the patient's condition or to check on the patient's circumstances. Nurses at some facilities send letters or postcards to patients stating that attempts to reach them have been unsuccessful. They then request that if there are any questions or problems, the patient or responsible adult contact the facility, thereby placing shared responsibility with the patient.

Content

The purpose of the follow-up telephone call is twofold: to obtain information about the patient and to give information to the patient. During the call, the nurse can best elicit information about the patient's general condition by using open-ended questions rather than those requiring a simple "yes" or "no" response. Conversation also enables the nurse to evaluate the patient's comprehension of discharge instructions, check compliance, reinforce information and instructions, and give encouragement and positive reinforcement to the patient as well as to the responsible adult caregiver. This is also a time to answer questions and to clarify any information or correct any misconceptions that may have arisen. Information obtained and instructions given should be documented concisely and completely in the patient's record.

During follow-up telephone calls, the patient may discuss specific concerns with the ASC nurse. These concerns may range from minor to significant problems. To properly assess the situation, the nurse must listen carefully and obtain all relevant information from the patient or responsible adult. If they describe symptoms or situations with a potential for serious complications, the nurse needs to take appropriate action. Such action can include directing the patient to contact the physician, then calling the patient again later to see that those instructions were followed. At other times, it means personally notifying the patient's physician or anesthesiologist to intercede for the patient.

In such situations, additional appropriate follow-up depends on the nature of the problem, needs of the individual patient, and institutional policy. Contact with the physician's office may prove sufficient. Conversely, the patient may need additional telephone calls in a few days or further intervention, such as referral to home healthcare services. In the end, it must be demonstrated that the patient's needs were identified, a plan of action was developed and implemented, and the plan met the needs of the patient.

Again, any information obtained, instructions given, and action taken must be documented in the patient's record. Some facilities keep a log book for patient problems and complications, separate from the medical record, containing the same information. This log, kept in the ASC, provides easy and quick reference in case a question arises about the patient after the chart is sent to medical records for coding and storage.[21]

Satisfaction Surveys

Printed satisfaction surveys usually focus on broad issues of overall facility acceptability and satisfaction. Surveys can be specific to the ASC or a section of a larger survey for the entire institution. Used as a marketing tool, they are useful in identifying problems and making changes for improvement.

Although patients and families may not be able to identify the technical aspects of quality nursing care, they generally know what they want and expect. Forbes and Brown[22] suggest that satisfaction with nursing care can be divided into four domains:

- Caring—focuses on respect, concern, and compassion
- Continuity of care—focuses on services, treatments, and outcomes of care
- Competency—focuses on the patient's perception of the behavior and manner in which services, information, and care are administered
- Education—focuses on clear, effective communication techniques

The extent to which these needs are met determines, from the patient's perspective, whether nursing care was good and met expectations.

To add greater meaning, additional questions on the survey should be tailored to provide specific information useful to the ASC. For example, Burden[8] suggests questions such as "Was waiting time minimal?" "Were financial arrangements explained to your satisfaction?" "Were pain management measures explained adequately?" "Was your privacy maintained?" Staff members then can use feedback to modify systems involving arrival and waiting times, better explain charges, and other factors. Questions relating to issues that are not easily changed are of little value, for example, questions about the structure of the building or the distance from the parking lot.

Patients should be told that they will receive the surveys and that you would appreciate their completion because their response is important and useful to the staff. Surveys may be simple checklists or computer-personalized forms with clear instructions. They also should allow for any additional comments that patients wish to make privately and anonymously. To encourage return of surveys, they should be preaddressed with postage prepaid. At some facilities, patients receive the survey before discharge. In other cases, surveys are mailed to the patient's home several weeks after surgery.

Finally, there needs to be a mechanism for ensuring that comments requiring a response are addressed. This is especially important if a patient or family makes a complaint. Such situations need to be followed up in a timely manner with personal communication from the nurse involved in the patient's care or, if necessary, from the manager. Regardless of who responds to the patient's complaint, the manager should be made aware of the situation.[8]

Other Follow-up

Like many service-oriented businesses, healthcare facilities realize the importance of offering their customers a cathartic opportunity to comment on likes or dislikes, discuss problems, or register complaints or compliments. When appropriate, a personal follow-up in the form of a telephone call or written note to the patient can serve as an additional marketing tool. In some instances, according to Burden,[8] it may be as simple as expressing appreciation for someone's patience during an unavoidable delay. At other times, the situation may be of a more serious nature. For example, there may be a need to apologize for a problem that occurred, a personal item that was misplaced, or perceived rude treatment. Such intervention may not only help to diffuse anger but also may prevent potential litigation in the future. Any response should be prompt and sincere, especially when a complaint is involved. As a result, the patient and family should feel the goodwill and positive concern of the facility's employees and administration for their general well-being.

Sometimes patient and family comments and actions are of a more positive nature. They, too, deserve feedback from the staff. Just a simple comment to thank the person for notable kindness and to express appreciation for the opportunity to be of service is not only thoughtful but also serves as a powerful marketing tool.

There may be other occasions when it is necessary or prudent to follow up with a telephone call to a physician's office. For example, if nurses have been unsuccessful in trying to contact a patient postoperatively, a call to the office may provide helpful information about the patient. In this case, the patient may have decided to stay at a relative's home without telling the ASC staff. Nurses also can use a follow-up call to report problems experienced by the patient who "doesn't want to bother the doctor," for example, abnormal bleeding, prolonged nausea and vomiting, or unrelieved pain. On other occasions, the nurse may call a physician to report problems that could lead to an otherwise unexpected hospitalization, or to learn about an unexpected hospitalization resulting from a postoperative problem. Finally, it is especially helpful to work with physicians' offices when identifying and tracking postoperative infections for ASC infection control purposes.

Such follow-up with physicians' offices can have several positive effects. Through prudent follow-up, the ASC staff demonstrates excellence in practice and genuine concern for their patients. Physicians make note of where their patients receive competent care and do not hesitate to voice their concerns and complaints when and where quality is lacking. Thus, well-cared-for and satisfied patients ultimately contribute to physician satisfaction. In this era of managed care, a continuum of efficiency and effectiveness is important to the very economic survival of practices and facilities.

Phase III Recovery: The Nurses' Need for Involvement

During preoperative preparation, surgery, and phase I and II recovery, patients receive high-quality care appropriate to their needs before being discharged to phase III recovery. Once patients leave the ASC, why do nurses need to be involved in phase III recovery follow-up, especially if responsible adult caregivers have been given instructions, or the patient is receiving home health–assisted care?

There are a number of reasons that nurses need to pursue patient follow-up in phase III recovery:

1. The nurse may identify areas of health-related problems and help the patient to address or solve problems. Information obtained, advice given, and actions taken by the nurse are a reflection of the quality of care provided by the ASC staff.
2. Follow-up contacts indicate compliance with accrediting bodies, professional associations, community standards, and institutional policies and procedures.
3. Within the realm of risk management, nurses need to be aware of how legal considerations, bioethical considerations, and quality improvement considerations affect care to address actual or potential problems at the earliest opportunity.
4. Changing economic situations necessitate that nurses be able to function effectively within the managed-care environment, contributing relevant information to case managers during the multiple phases of the patient's surgical experience.
5. Follow-up affords the patient one more example of the caring attitude that was established during the surgical experience.
6. The staff gains a sense of job completion and satisfaction.

Quality of Care and Caring

The nurse and the ASC have a responsibility to patients to provide high-quality care and to facilitate their safety and well-being. This responsibility extends into phase III recovery and applies to all patients whether they go home to the care of a responsible adult, are referred to another facility for assisted care, or qualify for home health care.

One way to extend quality care is by means of the postoperative phone call. During the call, the nurse can evaluate several factors. What is the patient's present condition? The nurse can elicit general information such as the presence or absence of nausea, amount and type of fluid and food intake and tolerance, presence or absence of fever, adequate output; color, consistency, odor, and amount of drainage; circulation, sensation, and edema of extremities; and adequate pain management.

Do the patient and responsible adult understand the discharge instructions? Nurses can evaluate general information, such as overall compliance with instructions, comprehension and adherence to the medication regimen, making a follow-up appointment with the physician, and observance for signs and symptoms specific to the procedure that should be reported to the physician as potential complications.

Does the patient or responsible adult have questions about anything that he or she was told? Does he or she have questions about anything that was not discussed previously? Ideally, all information should have been discussed completely with questions answered before discharge, but realistically, sometimes that does not happen. Thus, the follow-up call is the ideal time to discover information that is altogether absent, inaccurate, or unclear; to provide correct information; and to elaborate on information as necessary.

This is also a time to bolster sagging spirits and to give positive reinforcement to patients. It is not uncommon for patients to wonder whether their course of recuperation is proceeding normally, especially if they have not had previous surgery or know of no one who has had similar surgery. This is a time to empathize, to offer any necessary simple explanations, and to reinforce the wellness concept within the context of the patient's prognosis.

During the postoperative call, the nurse may discover that the responsible adult caregiver, too, needs some positive reinforcement. Even after a brief period of time, it is not uncommon for the caregiver to experience "role strain." The diagnosis, prognosis, outcome of caregiving activities, length of time that caregiving is required, nature of the caregiving tasks, and relationship between the caregiver and patient affect caregiving strain.[23] Caregivers might need and appreciate a word of encouragement, reassurance about the appropriateness and adequacy of their performance, or suggestions on how to resolve problems or improve situations.

Are the patient and responsible adult satisfied with the type and quality of care provided? Could nurses have done things differently, resulting in a better outcome? Encourage the patient and family to express their feelings during the follow-up telephone call and to complete the satisfaction survey. Accurate or not, to them perception is reality. Because nothing fosters more goodwill among the patients and their families than to know that they are important as human beings, reinforce that the staff and administration truly value their feelings, opinions, concerns, and suggestions for improvement.

Based on information obtained during the postoperative telephone call, the nurse also should evaluate whether any referrals were appropriate. For example, did a patient really need 23-hour observation, or could arrangements have been made for a responsible adult to care for that patient at home? Should the nurse have anticipated a patient's postoperative need for a recovery center or 23-hour observation based on the preoperative physiologic and psychosocial assessments? Does new information about a patient's postoperative status warrant an otherwise unanticipated referral to home health care for additional services? Certainly what is learned from one patient's situation can be applied to future patients' needs.

Compliance with Standards

Another reason for ASC nurses to be involved in phase III recovery is to comply with standards. According to the American Society of PeriAnesthesia Nurses (ASPAN), "Professions have a responsibility to identify and regulate their practice in order to protect consumers by assuring the delivery of quality service. One means to meet this professional charge is to develop standards of practice."[24]

There are several different accrediting bodies, professional organizations, and standards with which ASCs comply, such as the Joint Commission on Accreditation of Healthcare Organizations (JCAHO), the Accreditation Association for Ambulatory Health Care, Inc. (AAAHC), ASPAN, community standards, and institutional policies and procedures.

Accrediting Bodies

A JCAHO continuum of care standard states, "The discharge process provides for continuing care based upon the patient's assessed needs at the time of discharge." The intent is to identify the needs that the patient may have after discharge and to make arrangements to meet those needs. As an example of implementation of the standard, JCAHO further states, "For postdischarge follow-up care, primary nurses provide telephone follow-up assessment to surgical patients between 48 and 72 hours after discharge. Additional teaching, counseling, and referral are provided based on the assessment." Additionally, JCAHO also recommends that an evaluation of patient satisfaction be monitored.[25]

The AAAHC, in describing the quality of care provided, makes reference to characteristics of an accredited organization. Among those characteristics is continuity of care.[26] Although there is no specific recommendation for follow-up phone calls or satisfaction surveys, the facility likely would be held to the same standard as other facilities within the community or region.

Professional Organizations

ASPAN outlines data required for initial, ongoing, and discharge assessment of surgical patients. The organization recommends that ongoing patient care and assessment should include follow-up for extended care as indicated with a follow-up telephone call the next day to evaluate the patient's status.[24] This type of follow-up assessment applies in phase III recovery to all patients, whether hospitalized for observation or discharged home or to another type of setting, with or without assisted care.

Community Standards

Likewise, an ASC is held to the generally accepted standards established within the local community and the regional area. Patients and families tend to develop their expectations based on several factors, including the reputation of the facility and its staff within the community, prior personal experience, experiences of family and friends, and recommendations of family, friends, and physicians. As a result, patients and families expect care, attention, and service that are the same or better than that of another community facility. "This expectation then becomes an issue of compliance with standards that have been set by others in the community."[8] The follow-up telephone call and satisfaction survey thus enable the ASC staff to meet community standards while reinforcing the caring concern of the staff for the patient's well-being and to solicit personal comments and suggestions from patients and families.

Institutional Policies and Procedures

Finally, there are institutional policies and procedures to which the ASC staff must adhere. These policies and procedures more specifically address issues such as discharge criteria, discharge to a responsible adult, measures to be taken when a patient has no ride home or no responsible adult caregiver at home, and responsibility for discharge instructions to a non-English speaking patient without an interpreter. When actual or potential problems arise, ASC nurses must be involved actively with problem solving. Likewise, it is prudent to follow up with postoperative telephone calls at times appropriate to the patient's condition and situation after discharge from phase II recovery.

Risk Management

The ASC nurse also needs to be involved in phase III follow-up for risk management purposes. According to Keen,[27] "Risk management integrates a program of loss prevention into the medical, surgical, anesthesia, and nursing management of ambulatory surgery patients . . . The goals of a comprehensive program are consistent: to protect the financial resources of the ambulatory surgery nurse and the facility and to ensure quality patient care." Risk management encompasses legal, bioethical, and quality improvement considerations.

Legal Considerations

According to Murphy,[28] "Ambulatory surgery settings and the circumstances of ambulatory care create additional liability exposure for nurses. Ambulatory surgery nurses have less ability than inpatient nurses to control patient behavior preoperatively and postoperatively." In the ASC, she describes patients as "more partners in their care rather than recipients of the nurses' care."[28]

For patients and their responsible adult caregivers to be able to act in partnership postoperatively, they must be taught what they need to know. For example, minimal information must include: how to take care of themselves at home; what signs and symptoms can be expected; which symptoms need to be brought to the healthcare professional's attention and when; how to reach a professional who can answer other concerns that may arise; and a time, place, and date for a follow-up contact. During the postoperative follow-up telephone call, the nurse has an ideal opportunity to discover information that may be absent, inaccurate, or unclear; provide correct information; and elaborate on information as necessary.

Duration of Responsibility

Furthermore, Murphy[28] states that contrary to nurses' belief that they are responsible for whatever may happen to patients for only 24 hours after discharge, "This is not true. Ambulatory surgery nurses are responsible for assessing patients' abilities to safely care for themselves (or caregivers' abilities to care for patients) until the patients' next contact with healthcare professionals (usually the follow-up visit to the physician)." Perhaps the ASC nurse's responsibility actually lies somewhere between these two extremes. Thus, the follow-up telephone call takes on added importance.

Documentation

Likewise, documentation is important to risk management efforts. Documentation of information in the patient's medical record is a "primary means by which various care providers communicate pertinent facts, observations, and assessments related to the patient's diagnosis, condition and response to therapy."[29] The content should reflect care in the ASC as well as information pertinent to phase III recovery obtained in the follow-up phone call. As outlined by Eng,[30] documentation should be accurate (factual and timely); brief (avoid duplication); complete (document signs and symptoms, refusal of care or noncompliance with instructions, reasons for omission of treatments or medications); objective (use supportive, subjective patient statements; avoid judgmental, derogatory remarks); comprehensive; and legible. Although computerized documentation may significantly simplify and enhance comprehensive documentation, input ultimately depends on the professional nurse. "What is documented reflects the character, the competency, and the caring of the nurse."[31]

Incident Reports

Incident reports can be useful in both the risk management program and the quality improvement program, and it may not be until the patient is recovering at home that symptoms or issues arise.

When the nurse discovers information during the follow-up telephone call of a nature that indicates potential patient injury, complications, or poor outcome, an incident report should be completed according to the facility's policies. Chapter 9 provides useful guidelines.

Litigation Prevention Through Diffusion

Follow-up during phase III recovery can serve another very important function in the area of risk control. During a follow-up telephone call or in response to the satisfaction survey, the ASC nurse or manager must address issues of patients and families who believe that they have been treated poorly or wronged. For example, the patient or family may have a complaint about physical care; a lost personal belonging; lack of privacy, respect or courtesy; breach of confidentiality; or the attitude of the staff or physicians.[8, 32] Whether the situation or complaint is actual or perceived, to the patient and family it is reality. By appropriately responding to the patient and family in a timely manner, the nurse may be able to diffuse anger and possibly avoid further action such as litigation.

Bioethical Considerations

Legal and ethical issues may be linked throughout the perioperative experience. Ethics concerns human behavior and makes value judgments about what is good or bad and right or wrong. More specifically, bioethics is the study of ethics as applied to health care.[33] Many of the ethical issues that concern ASC nurses in phase III recovery actually begin in the preoperative, intraoperative, or immediate postoperative periods. However, the impact of the ethical concerns may begin to surface in phase III recovery.

There are many ethical issues involved, including patient's rights, confidentiality, and privacy. Among the most significant in ambulatory surgery are the allocation and distribution of limited resources. These resources include nursing time, skill, knowledge, expertise, and availability of appropriate follow-up care of the type needed postoperatively. When any of these is lacking, the patient's safety and well-being may be at risk.[34] For example, are resources as readily available to both the "haves" and the "have nots"? Are patients at both ends of this spectrum respected and treated equally? With respect to the elderly and mentally or physically impaired, has surgery improved their quality of life or merely added revenue to the physician and the ASC? Could the resources have been better allocated to the young or unimpaired?[35] In noncompliant patients, are resources wasted and costs more expensive in the long run?[33] Do patients with cultural differences have a right to refuse recommended services when their beliefs differ from those of the community, especially if such refusal likely will result in more expensive future treatment?[36]

There are no simple answers, and the ASC nurse cannot resolve many of these ethical concerns. However, nurses need to be aware of these ethical problems, which they may identify in follow-up with patients during phase III recovery. Ultimately, trends need to be identified, and problems and input must be given to administration or the ethics committee.

Quality/Performance Improvement

Whether the term used is quality improvement (QI), continuous quality improvement (CQI), total quality management (TQM), or continuous performance improvement (CPI), the goal is to prevent problems by improving the process of care delivery across the organization. One way that nurses become involved is through making follow-up telephone calls to patients to assess their condition, offer appropriate advice as necessary, and complete the nursing process. Together, telephone calls and satisfaction surveys provide information that management needs to compile, summarize, evaluate, and share with the nursing, anesthesia, and medical staff, as appropriate. The results enable the staff at all levels to examine the adequacy of the facility's system as a whole.[8]

Maintaining quality control programs continues to be a JCAHO standard that applies across departments and disciplines.[25] Survey results may identify systems' problems, such as the continuum of care, information sharing, or staff or departmental deficiencies. Such feedback can prompt the formation of multidisciplinary groups to resolve problems more efficiently and effectively and provide the opportunity to implement suggestions from patients and staff for improvement.

Infection Control

Another area closely related to quality improvement and risk management is infection control monitoring. One of the advantages of surgery in the ASC is that patients spend minimal time in the facility, thus limiting their potential for exposure to infections. Thorough preoperative assessment for contributory risk factors, strict adherence to aseptic technique and standard precautions, and meticulous discharge instructions on proper wound care help limit postoperative infections. Nevertheless, a simple but effective monitoring system needs to be in effect to identify and report postoperative infections because symptoms may not be apparent at the time of the postoperative follow-up telephone call. Results of the monitoring then need to be compiled and shared with the appropriate staff members. If problems are identified, then policies, procedures, and practice need to be examined, with necessary changes implemented to improve patient care.[37]

Because these areas are so closely related, Pfaff[38] states, "There is a growing movement toward integrating infection prevention and control, quality improvement and risk management programs. Such an approach may be especially cost-effective [for ASCs]."

Economics

Nurses also need to be involved in phase III recovery because of ongoing economic changes, namely the healthcare reform strategy of managed competition.

Managed Competition

The goal of managed competition is to make healthcare services more efficient through controlled costs and improved quality of care. Health care currently is viewed as a continuum with emphasis on promotion of wellness rather than on care for isolated episodes of illness, enhanced continuity and coordination of care, increased patient and family education and involvement, and cross-training of staff for patient care.[39, 40]

There are several elements necessary for facilities to succeed in the healthcare reform environment. These include development of and involvement in integrated delivery systems, which Rothrock[41] refers to as "womb to tomb" continuity of care. Other elements include continued attention to clinical quality and customer service satisfaction, state-of-the-art information systems, and flexibility and innovation in new program development. Eventually, ongoing innovations will be "more evolutionary rather than revolutionary."[42]

By being involved in phase III recovery, nurses can contribute important information as new systems continue to evolve in the managed-care environment. Follow-up telephone calls reinforce continuity of care and caring after patient discharge, thus enhancing patient satisfaction. As families receive more detailed instructions and assume more responsibility for providing sometimes complicated care after discharge, they need and appreciate a readily available resource of information and encouragement when questions or problems arise. Problems averted or identified and treated in a timely manner generally save more costly future treatment and losses. Follow-up in the form of telephone calls and surveys also provides significant information for quality improvement efforts.

Case Management

An integral component in managed care is case management of the individual patient. Case management focuses on coordination and integration in the delivery of services to those in need, places controls on all the resources used for care, increases involvement of nurses and other healthcare providers in decisions regarding practice, and promotes continuity and consistency of care. These positive outcomes counteract some of the negative aspects of changes in health care, including fragmentation of patient care resulting from changes in the physical setting, caregiver, and plan of care; increased patient acuity; and increased workloads.[43]

Case management consists of two components: internal components, which span the acute episode of hospitalization, and external components, which span the continuum of care before and after discharge.[43] Care paths, pathways, or care maps structure the internal component of case management, providing general multidisciplinary guidelines for patient care in a cost-effective manner. Nurses in ASCs can expect to develop and work with internal care paths that apply to the perianesthesia and perioperative care of patients, then make adjustments based on variance tracking and analysis that is communicated to the organization as a whole. External care paths involve ASC nurses working with physicians' offices and patients and families on preoperative and postoperative education and with home health care and other community services, arranging and coordinating care during phase III recovery.

Satisfaction

For years, business and industry have understood the importance of consumer service and satisfaction. More recently, health care, influenced by fierce competition, not only has emphasized providing quality care and containing costs, but also has focused on consumer satisfaction. Although our customers include many parties, follow-up in phase III recovery enhances satisfaction particularly for patients and families, and for nurses as well.

Patients and Families

Telephone calls and satisfaction surveys in phase III recovery reinforce the caring concept of the staff toward the patient and family. These tools also give the patient and family important opportunities to vent positive as well as negative feelings. The survey should encompass the cycle-of-care concept, including the patient's entire experience from scheduling to follow-up telephone call or beyond.[44]

Feedback from patients about their ASC experience is important because of the potentially far-reaching effects. One study found that satisfied consumers tell four or five other customers about their experience. However, dissatisfied customers tell an average of 9 to 10 people, with 13% of dissatisfied customers telling more than 20 people.[45] Thus, follow-up telephone calls and satisfaction surveys are important marketing tools for an ASC. It is always the intent that patients and families have a positive experience in the ASC. But should anyone express a negative comment about their experience, it is especially important to follow-up further with them to determine the exact nature and extent of the problem and to take appropriate action when warranted. For, to the patient and family, perception is reality.

Staff

Likewise, follow-up via telephone calls and surveys is important for several reasons to the staff. Nurses need to feel a sense of job completion by bringing a conclusion to the nursing process.[8] Having followed a patient through the ambulatory surgical experience, the nurse, during the follow-up telephone call, has a final opportunity to evaluate the patient's condition, answer questions, reinforce teaching, give appropriate nursing advice and emotional support, and generally tie up any loose ends. In addition, calls can prove to be a learning experience in which nurses can evaluate their personal performance in light of patients' needs.

The nurse also can use the follow-up call as a means of evaluating the patient's experience as a whole. For example, nurses at one facility ask patients whether anything could have been done differently that would have made the surgical experience any better. Information from telephone calls and satisfaction surveys then should be compiled and shared with the nursing staff and with other members of the healthcare team in an appropriate manner. Positive comments help to reinforce the satisfaction of a job well done. Negative comments can be a catalyst for evaluating current performance and redesigning systems that provide optimal care that results in patient, family, and staff satisfaction.

Summary

As the walls of our once physically constraining facilities open up in the ambulatory setting, so do our practices and responsibilities expand to meet the growing needs of our consumers. Perianesthesia and perioperative boundaries blur as we better realize the opportunities and the needs of those we serve. Currently, we are challenged more than ever to anticipate those needs and to meet them as our responsibilities stretch beyond phase II and into phase III recovery.

References

1. Kromminga S, Ostwald S: The public health nurse as a discharge planner: Patients' perceptions of the discharge process. Publ Health Nurs 4:224–229, 1987.
2. Redmond MC: Phase III recovery: Referral options in postoperative discharge planning. J Post Anesth Nurs 9:353–356, 1994.
3. McCaffrey M, Beebe A: Pain: Clinical Manual for Nursing Practice. St. Louis: Mosby–Year Book, 1989, pp 48–110.
4. Litwack K: Post Anesthesia Care Nursing, 2nd ed. St. Louis: Mosby–Year Book, 1995, pp 496–499, 525–529.
5. Redmond MC: The importance of good communication in effective patient–family teaching. J Post Anesth Nurs 8:109–112, 1993.
6. Corkery E: Discharge planning and home health care: What every staff nurse should know. Orthop Nurs, 8:18–27, 1989.
7. Cramer C: Ambulatory surgery: Nursing considerations. Curr Rev Nurse Anesth 10:146–151, 1988.
8. Burden N: Ambulatory Surgical Nursing. Philadelphia: WB Saunders, 1993.
9. Chadwick H, Ross B: Analgesia for post cesarean delivery pain. Anesth Clin North Am 7:133–153, 1989.
10. Rawal N: Postoperative pain and its management. In Raj P (ed): Practical Management of Pain, 2nd ed. St. Louis: Mosby–Year Book, 1992, pp 367–387.
11. Blue Cross/Blue Shield of Iowa: A Medicare Guide to Billing for HHAs. Federal Medicare Intermediary and Carriers. Des Moines: IASD Health Services Corp, 1991, pp 1–12, 18–34.
12. Davis JE: Ambulatory surgery . . . how far can we go? Med Clin North Am 77:365–375, 1993.
13. Llewellyn JG: Short stay surgery: Present practices, future trends. AORN J 53:1179–1191, 1991.
14. Stuttard D: The effects of minimally invasive surgery on the future of perioperative nursing. Can Operating Room Nurs J 12:5–12, 1994.
15. Even the best discharge planning can go bust: What do you do? Same Day Surg 19:41–45, 1995.
16. Burns J: Hospitals could save floundering industry of recovery care. Mod Healthcare 25:36, 1995.
17. Graves JM: Postop chocolates on your pillow. Fortune 131:34, 1995.
18. Detmer DE, Gelijns AC: Ambulatory surgery: A more cost-effective treatment strategy? Arch Surg 129:123–127, 1994.
19. Redmond MC: Using home health agencies to meet patient needs in phase III recovery. J Post Anesth Nurs 10:21–26, 1995.
20. Burden N: Personal communication, Feb 1997.
21. Mamaril M: Clinical practice: Response to question on follow-up phone calls. Breathline ASPAN Newsletter 15:15, 1995.
22. Forbes ML, Brown HN: Measuring patient satisfaction. AORN J 61:737–742, 1995.
23. Burns C, Archbold P, Stewart B, et al: New diagnosis: Caregiver role strain. Nurs Diagn 4:70–76, 1993.
24. American Society of Post Anesthesia Nurses: Standards of Perianesthesia Nursing Practice 1998. Thorofare, NJ: ASPAN, 1998, pp 31–32.
25. Joint Commission on Accreditation of Healthcare Organizations: 1996 Comprehensive Accreditation Manual for Hospitals. Oakbrook Terrace, IL: JCAHO, 1996, CC.4, CC.5, CC. 6.1, pp 231–232.
26. Accreditation Association for Ambulatory Health Care, Inc: Accreditation Handbook for Ambulatory Health Care, 1996–97 ed. Skokie, IL: AAAHC, 1996, CC.6.1, p 180.
27. Keen LH: Risk management in the ambulatory surgery setting. In Burden N (ed): Ambulatory Surgical Nursing. Philadelphia: WB Saunders, 1993, pp 601, 607–608.
28. Murphy EK: OR nursing law—liability exposure in ambulatory surgery settings. AORN J 54:1287–1289, 1991.
29. Allen A: Does your documentation defend or discredit? J Post Anesth Nurs 9:172–173, 1994.
30. Eng M: If it isn't charted, it isn't done. Presentation to the Nebraska Association of Post Anesthesia Nurses, Omaha, NE, Feb 22, 1992.
31. Feutz-Harter S: Documentation principles and pitfalls. J Nurs Admin 19:7, 1989.
32. Silver I: Liberate yourself from the liability trap: 10+ risk management tips for PACU nurses. 12th National ASPAN Conference Abstracts. J Post Anesth Nurs 8:225, 1993.
33. Haddad AM: Ethical and Legal Issues in Home Health Care. Norwalk, CT: Appleton & Lange, 1991, p 8.
34. Edwards BJ: Ethics. In Gruendemann BJ, Fernsebner B (eds): Comprehensive Perioperative Nursing, Vol. 1 Principles. Boston: Jones & Bartlett Publishers, 1995, p 111.
35. Curtin LL: How much is enough? Nurs Man 25:30–31, 1994.
36. Beiser EN: Medical ethics in an outpatient setting: Conflicting cultural values. Rhode Island Med 75:413–416, 1992.
37. Redmond MC: Infection control monitoring in the ambulatory surgery unit. J Post Anesth Nurs 8:28–34, 1993.
38. Pfaff SJ: Infection prevention and control. In Burden N (ed): Ambulatory Surgical Nursing. Philadelphia: WB Saunders, 1993, p 643.
39. Spitzer-Lehmann R: Managed care: What's ahead? Surg Serv Manage 1:18–21, 1995.
40. Kaiser Foundation Health Plan, Inc., Northern California Region: Public Relations Materials. Oakland, CA: Kaiser Foundation, Aug 1993.
41. Rothrock JC: Editorial comment. Capsules Comments Periop Nurs 1:29, 1995.
42. Clark CS, Schuster TB: Managed care innovation and new product development. J Ambulatory Care Man 17:18–28, 1994.
43. Gibbs B, Lonowski L, Meyer PJ, et al: The role of the clinical nurse specialist and the nurse manager in case management. J Nurs Admin 25:28–34, 1995.
44. Cohen L, Delaney P, Boston P: Listening to the customer: Implementing a patient satisfaction measurement system. Gastroenterol Nurs 17:110–115, 1994.
45. Press I, Ganey RF, Malone MP: Satisfied patients can spell financial well-being. Healthcare Financial Man 45:34, 1991.

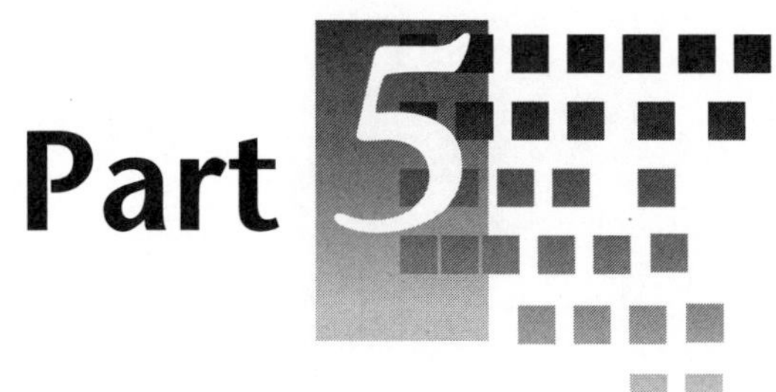

Patients with Special Needs

Chapter 24

Special Emotional, Social, and Cultural Needs

Nancy M. Saufl

The ambulatory surgery patient population is amazingly varied. Many patients are healthy, but those who have special needs relating to health, sensory, and developmental limitations and those from varied socioeconomic and cultural backgrounds must be prepared for surgery with the greatest care. Most ambulatory surgical, endoscopic, and other procedures are elective rather than urgent, so time usually is available to ensure that patients are prepared effectively before their procedures. The needs of these patients require that a structured program be available for ensuring their adequate assessment and education.

Underneath all the concerns and plans and challenges of caring for a diverse population stands the blanket fact that even as healthcare providers we are different one from another as much as from our patients and their families. The world continues to become a more and more homogenous place, with the continued increase in population; travel; availability of information; and vast technical, social, and economic pressures. The nurse and other providers are exposed to the rich tapestry of our ever-changing culture each day. If we are to provide the best possible care to all our customers—patients, families, physicians, and others—we must be able to do so without limitations of prejudice or of class, abilities, or social distinctions. When such concerns are considered and successfully addressed individually and collectively by healthcare providers, the best possible setting can be provided for each customer.

Even the most "normal" people have challenges that set them apart as individuals, things as simple as fears, dietary preferences, family problems, and predetermined ideas about their procedures or goals. Others have specific challenges related to a variety of issues. For example, people with mental or emotional challenges may have difficulty concentrating or understanding the surgical experience. These patients need careful teaching, reassurance, and reinforcement. Bolstering the patient's sense of self-worth and providing an accepting environment are important elements of emotional care.

Physical and sensory deficits also can add many challenges for the patient and family who will face surgical interventions. Some examples include negotiating the physical environment of the outpatient center, providing self-care with surgical limitations, receiving and sharing personal and procedure-related information, and communicating with the facility and medical staff members. Cultural, religious, and sexual differences add yet other facets to the challenge of ensuring that our care is appropriate and unbiased.

For specially challenged families, the nurse can provide further encouragement by validating the patient's current knowledge and abilities and by providing necessary information that the patient and family can use to formulate plans for home care after surgery.[1] The patient and family who have difficulty coping with the added demands of surgery may benefit from referral to an appropriate agency for assistance.

For these more complex patients, the ambulatory surgical nurse must manage nursing care in a manner that reduces the occurrence of complications related to both the anesthesia and the surgical intervention. This level of care is reflected in care planning, symptom assessment, and discharge instructions tailored to each patient's specific social, emotional, and cultural needs. Nurses play an important role in the identification and avoidance of complications in all patients; but nursing vigilance, knowledge, and interventions are especially important when caring for those patients with special needs.

MENTAL DISABILITIES

Patients who have mental disabilities can benefit from ambulatory surgery because this approach causes less disruption in their usual daily routines than does hospitalization. Specific advantages include minimal separation from family or familiar caretakers, a personal setting geared toward family involvement, and a limited number of healthcare providers involved with each patient.

Developmentally disabled patients need simple and direct instructions and continual affirmation of their abilities to follow directions. Praise is often the best motivator to encourage self-care. The nurse, however, must be cautious that expectations are not set too high for the patient's abilities but are based on knowledge of the patient's actual developmental level.

The nurse should look for signs of coexisting, associated physical or neurologic abnormalities in the developmentally disabled patient. For instance, 50% of patients with Down syndrome may have congenital heart disease. Many also have epilepsy, skeletal abnormalities, such as scoliosis, a small mandible and maxilla, a smaller than usual larynx for age, abnormal dental structures, and immunologic deficiency. Weakness of the pharyngeal muscles and a large tongue also complicate airway management.

Of special note to the anesthesia provider is the tendency in a small percentage of patients with Down syndrome toward instability of the atlantoaxial joint at the base of the skull. This defect can result in the rare occurrence of subluxation (overriding of bones) during neck extension for laryngoscopy or airway management.[2] Hyperextension of the neck should be avoided and cautious airway management employed because the development of quadriplegia is a serious, although rare, consequence of this complication.

The mentally disabled patient requires a calm and supportive environment. Patients may present with a number of psychiatric conditions, for example, depression, mania, delusions, neuroses, schizophrenia, and hallucinations. It is imperative that the staff is aware of the patient's psychological needs to adequately plan nursing care. A primary nursing approach that limits the number of people who interact with the patient can be helpful. Care should be planned efficiently so that the patient has minimal stimulation.

Unless an adversarial relationship exists, the family or responsible adult should remain with the patient as long as possible and should be reunited as soon as possible after surgery. Personal belongings left with the patient may provide special comfort. A family member or other responsible family member should remain at the surgery center throughout the day because his or her support and intervention may be needed if the patient becomes agitated or frightened. In rare cases, the caregiver even may accompany the patient into the operating room.

The nurse enlists aid from the family or other knowledgeable adult to supply information about the medical and social history, special likes and dislikes, and any other important idiosyncrasies. The patient should be included in questions and discussions to the extent of his or her ability. The necessary consent for surgery and anesthesia must be obtained from the legal guardian. This is best accomplished before the day of surgery. If the legal guardian lives out of state, consent can be obtained using certified mail.

The patient's underlying psychological or emotional pathology, along with the effects of psychoactive mediations, can result in unusual or inappropriate verbal and physical behaviors; thus, constant nursing observation and intervention are essential. Many mentally disabled patients have gentle, quiet personalities, but the antisocial behavior of some can be disturbing to other patients or visitors. The nurse must react with great sensitivity to avoid embarrassing situations for all parties. Providing a private area for care supports a patient's privacy and dignity.

Violent behavior can result in injury to the patient or to others. Indications of such an impending event should alert nursing personnel to intercede as necessary. The patient with a known history for self-abuse or violence requires constant attention by an experienced attendant.

The suicidal patient must be attended constantly to prevent self-inflicted injury. It is often the responsibility of the original facility or unit to provide an attendant who is trained in mental health nursing interventions. Otherwise, the ambulatory surgery center (ASC) staff should obtain specific information about the patient's previous actions and methods being used to prevent self-injury.

Gentle physical restraint may be necessary to provide patient safety and should be undertaken only after other measures have been ineffective. Restraint use is generally a last resort, and less restrictive measures should be considered first.[3] The nurse should know and follow the facility's policy on the use of restraints. The policy should include the need for a physician's order, proper application and frequent monitoring, periodic removal for exercise and movement, and the provision of clear explanations to the patient and family indicating that safety, not punishment, of the patient is the reason for the use of restraints.

Perioperative medication protocols must be determined individually, considering the patient's usual psychoactive drug therapy. Some mentally fragile patients may require aggressive sedation to reduce anxiety and to ensure their compliance with the plan of care.

General anesthesia is most often the choice for this group of patients, who may be unable to cooperate with local or regional anesthesia techniques. The patient who is uncooperative may receive sedation with intramuscular ketamine or midazolam (Versed) to encourage calmness and cooperation before general anesthesia induction with a mask or intravenous agent.[4]

Potential interactions are possible between perioperative medications and psychoactive drugs. Tranquilizers, antianxiolytics, and antidepressants may be synergistic with anesthetics and sedatives, resulting in prolonged somnolence, reduced airway reflexes, passive regurgitation, orthostatic hypotension, and respiratory depression. Delayed recovery from anesthesia is not unusual for patients who are taking such medications.[5]

Usual medication protocols should be disrupted as little as possible, although two groups of antidepressants present special concerns regarding the potential for untoward interactions with perioperative drugs. Tricyclic antidepressants, such as amitriptyline (Elavil), desipramine (Norpramin, Pertofrane), doxepin (Sinequan), and imipramine (Tofranil) inhibit the uptake of previously released norepinephrine, causing an overabundance of it in the circulation. Ephedrine is an indirect-acting sympathomimetic that often is used as a vasopressor. When given to a patient with high levels of norepinephrine, it can precipitate a hypertensive crisis; thus, it should be avoided in patients taking these drugs. Combining halothane and pancuronium with tricyclics can increase catecholamine levels, potentially causing cardiac arrhythmias. Cardiac conduction defects can be associated with tricyclic antidepressants as well.

Monoamine oxidase inhibitors (MAOIs), which include isocarboxazid (Marplan), phenelzine (Nardil), and tranylcypromine (Parnate), also cause an increase in the available circulating norepinephrine but do so by inhibiting its breakdown. Again, hypertensive crisis is a potential occurrence with the administration of ephedrine to these patients. Concurrent use of opioid drugs can cause respiratory depression, high fever, seizures, and cardiovascular collapse. Also, the effects of barbiturates, benzodiazepines, and central nervous system (CNS) depressants are potentiated by MAOIs. Many practitioners suggest that nonurgent surgery be deferred until the patient has discontinued MAOIs for 14 to 21 days before surgery,[6] whereas others proceed, using a carefully planned anesthetic approach.

The adult patient with Alzheimer's disease needs special consideration. This form of senile dementia is a complex degenerative disorder typified by memory loss and inability to concentrate, which complicate the patient's ability to provide self-care. Besides having difficulty in providing an accurate and reliable medical history, the patient is likely to forget pre- and postoperative instructions and may become agitated when pressured to comply with directives.

Care should be provided by one nurse as much as possible to increase familiarity and continuity of care. Repeated verbal and simple written instructions should be given. A small amount of information should be given at one time. In addition, the caretaker must ensure that the patient complies with preoperative instructions, such as NPO (nothing by mouth) requirements. Postoperatively, repeated orientation to surroundings by the nurse and quick reunification with a familiar caretaker are helpful interventions for the patient who is confused.

Patients with advanced Alzheimer's disease may pose airway management problems. Some cannot swallow, and some forget to swallow saliva; thus, aspiration is a constant risk. Also, Alzheimer's disease can be associated with impairment of the cholinergic system, and anticholinergic mediations such as atropine and scopolamine should be avoided because they can precipitate untoward behavioral activity.[7]

The patient may have difficulty verbalizing thoughts accurately, so the nurse must observe for nonverbal clues to the patient's needs. Social behavior may be aberrant, and both the patient and family may require special support during periods of patient agitation, combativeness, and confusion. Restraints should be avoided unless absolutely necessary for the patient's own protection.

Developmental disability (formerly termed mental retardation) is a problem with many etiologies, including chromosomal abnormalities, genetic defects intrauterine, and perinatal, neonatal, and postnatal causes. Developmental disability refers to substantial limitations in present functioning and is characterized by significantly subaverage intellectual function, existing concurrently with related limitations in two or more of the following skill areas: communication, self-care, home living, social skills, community use, self-direction, health and safety functional academics, leisure, and work. Mental manifestations become evident before 18 years of age.[8]

Developmental disabilities range from mild or moderate to severe and profound. Patients with mild disability have social and communication skills and functional literacy. Moderately disabled patients may have speech deficits but are able to manage personal care skills, such as dressing, eating, and washing. Patients with severe developmental problems have limited speech and language and poor motor development and need supervision. Profoundly disabled patients have neurologic defects, poor cognitive social ability, and absent speech, and may cause self-harm. Care should be individualized according to each patient's needs. The family or responsible caregiver should be allowed to stay with the patient as much as possible to help provide a supportive and calm environment.

The perianesthesia nurse should assess each patient's level of understanding and plan patient education accordingly. Patients with poor verbal or cognitive skills may be unable to express their needs in the usual manner. Pain management must be addressed by careful objective nursing assessments, for instance, restlessness not related to hypoxia, pulling or rubbing a body part, grimacing, aggressiveness, or withdrawal and crying. Local anesthesia infiltration or regional blockade is an excellent method to reduce postoperative pain, especially for those who may have difficulty understanding why they are having pain or verbalizing it.

A responsible adult is essential to provide aftercare at home. Discharge instructions must reflect the patients' psychosocial needs. Unusual dressings may be necessary to protect the surgical site; for example, casting may be needed over a dressing to prevent the patient from removing the dressing or injuring the incision. Straight-arm splints may be needed to prevent the patient from disturbing an operative site near the head and neck.

COMMUNICATION CHALLENGES

Low Literacy

Literacy levels should also be considered when caring for the ambulatory surgical patient. Two of every 10 Americans are functionally illiterate and may have difficulty with the simplest of handouts, audiotapes, or even videotapes.[9] Patients may have learning deficits that involve reading, writing, listening, and even speaking skills. Patient education materials may be written at fifth- or sixth-grade level, but low-literacy patients may still be unable to learn from them. Illiteracy is found in all walks of life and socioeconomic levels. The person may have an average or above-average intelligence quotient (IQ) or may have limited comprehension skills. Perianesthesia nurses should assess the patient's abilities to read and identify those at risk of not understanding information. The nurse should observe for signs, such as those presented in Table 24–1, that may suggest illiteracy.

When teaching patients with low literacy the following strategies may be of help:

- Focus on the most significant and necessary knowledge.
- Teach the smallest amount of information possible.
- Have the patient demonstrate understanding when appropriate.
- Repeat and summarize information.
- Ask patients to put their understanding of the information into their own words.
- Review, clarify, and reteach as necessary.[9]

Learning styles should be individualized. Having several types of teaching aids available is beneficial for the teaching process (Table 24–2).

Table 24–1. Cues That Suggest Illiteracy

Lack of interest in materials	Inability to answer questions about text
Expressions of frustration	Limited vocabulary
Lack of reading speed	Requests to let someone else read the text

From Revell L: Understanding, identifying, and teaching the low-literacy patient. Semin Periop Nurs 3:168, 1994.

Table 24–2. **Learning Styles and Teaching Methodologies**

AUDITORY LECTURE	VISUAL DEMONSTRATION	TACTILE SIMULATION
Audiotapes	Videotapes	Practice
Videotapes	Charts	Models
	Graphs	
	Chalkboards	
	Flipcharts	
	Photographs	
	Slides	

From Revell L: Understanding, identifying, and teaching the low-literacy patient. Semin Periop Nurs 3:171, 1994.

Low-literacy patients may need more than one type of teaching method or style.

Surgical consent, anesthesia consent, discharge instructions, and other paperwork involved in the care of the ambulatory surgical patient should be reviewed for reading levels and revised as necessary to promote patient understanding. The perianesthesia nurse should be aware of the needs of the low-literacy patient and ensure that educational tools are appropriate.

Non-English Speaking

The non-English speaking patient is at a disadvantage in sending and receiving messages. Nonverbal communication using gestures and facial expressions is limited in its scope, and every effort should be made to ensure that appropriate translation of information occurs. Usually, the non-English speaking patient is urged or required to bring a translator to the surgery center with them. It is ultimately the responsibility of the facility to ensure availability of a translator. Resources exist for commercial translator services by telephone. Although most people seem to prefer the translation services of a family member or friend, others may prefer the privacy of a third party who does not know the patient or family. Consideration should be given to providing a translator of the same gender, particularly when relaying personal and sensitive information.

If a third party is used to translate information to the patient or family, the nurse should attempt to ensure that the interpreter does, in fact, understand the information he or she is being asked to translate. The risk of faulty translation or misunderstanding is real, particularly if complex material or medical jargon is used that does not translate easily into other languages. The nurse should include the patient and family in the conversation, using facial expressions, eye contact, gestures, and touch. The name and relationship, if any, of the interpreter should be documented in the patient's record, along with a notation of what information was translated. In areas with large populations of non-English speaking residents, informational literature should be provided in the primary languages spoken in the area.

Speech Impairment

A variety of conditions can result in the patient having difficulty communication verbally. Rarely, a patient may be mute or totally unable to speak. Others may suffer from any degree of aphasia. Speech impairment can be associated with neurologic diseases. Parkinsonism, Alzheimer's disease, stroke, and brain tumors are conditions in which patients may have difficulty with verbal expression of ideas.

Aphasic patients should be given small amounts of information, slowly and clearly. Distractions in the environment should be kept at a minimum, and the patient should be given enough time to respond. Frustration on the part of both the patient and the nurse is not uncommon in a busy setting such as an ASC. Aphasic patients may benefit from receiving written instructions to review at their leisure before the day of surgery.

Family members may have more success in communicating with the patient because they may better understand the patient's gestures and attempts at formulating sentences or words. The patients should not be omitted from conversations simply because he or she has difficulty responding verbally. The tendency to speak louder than usual should be avoided unless the patient has a hearing deficit as well.

The patient with a language barrier may find other means of communication to be helpful. Pictures or models may provide a medium for demonstration and for assessment of the patient's understanding of instructions. A note pad and pencil may be helpful means of expression for the patient.

Hearing Impairment

Hearing loss is another barrier to effective communication that can affect comprehension of instructions before, during, and after surgery. The hearing-impaired patient may feel isolated from the environment and may be excessively anxious. Deafness denies the patient not only the spoken word but also other environmental sounds that can be soothing.[10] Other reassurances, such as the presence of the nurse or family, a smile, or a touch are alternative measures to decrease anxiety. The nurse can avoid startling a hearing-impaired patient by approaching within the patient's line of vision to avoid the surprise of an unexpected touch.

Misconceptions persist regarding hearing impairment. First, a hearing deficit is not reflective of low intelligence. Second, not all hearing-impaired people can lip-read or understand sign language. Most people whose hearing impairment was acquired rather than congenital can speak, although their speech may be unusual because of their inability to hear their own voices. The ability to read and write is partially dependent on verbal and hearing skills[10]; thus, complicated written instructions may be as overwhelming as complex verbal messages.

People who communicate primarily through lip-reading rely on certain cardinal rules: face the person, speak slowly and clearly, and use the smallest number of words necessary to communicate the message. Yelling is counterproductive and can cause the person embarrassment. Eye contact should be maintained. Good lighting is helpful so that the patient can see the speaker's lips. The speaker should avoid chewing gum or food, covering his or her mouth, or turning away during the conversation.[11] Only 30% of what is spoken in the English language is visible on the lips, so gestures and facial expressions are important adjuncts to verbal communication. One of the best methods to verify that the patient has understood a message is to ask directly. Other forms of communication that may be used include written messages, sign language, demonstrations, and gestures.

Hearing-impaired patients who rely on hearing aids should be allowed to wear the hearing aid throughout the ambulatory surgery experience if possible. Another device that can aid in communication is a battery-powered microphone into which the nurse or others speak. Attached to the microphone is a wire and earpiece that amplifies the sound, similar to that of a transistor radio. The earpiece must be disinfected between patient uses.

Almost 2 million Americans have some degree of hearing loss.[12] Therefore, it is almost a certainty that all perianesthesia nurses will provide nursing care for hearing impaired or deaf patients at some point. As with all patients, education should be tailored to the individual patient needs. Some do's and don'ts for teaching the hearing-impaired patient are described in Table 24–3.

Vision Impairment

The sightless or visually impaired person uses many other means with which to sense the environment, particularly sound and touch. The staff should provide the patient with a description of the new surroundings and allow time and opportunity for the patient to explore that environment within safe parameters. Before providing physical direction, it is advisable to ask patients how much assistance they need or want so as not to impose on their sense of independence. The nurse assumes a grave responsibility in ensuring that environmental hazards do not threaten the patient's well-being, particularly one who is sedated. Safety devices such as siderails and straps for stretchers are important, but more so is frequent verbal contact. A nurse call system should be within the patient's reach at all times.

Sightlessness does not preclude all self-care postoperatively, although more direction and supervision may be necessary. The time delegated for patient and family education must be adequate to allow for demonstration and redemonstration of needed self-skills. The adult companion must provide assessments for bleeding, ecchymosis, and other signs of complications.

One special consideration is the patient who has temporary loss of vision due to the surgery performed, for example, a patient who is blind in one eye and has the other eye bandaged after surgery. This can be particularly difficult for a person who is not accustomed to being totally sightless. One intercession may be the use of a perforated eye shield to protect the surgical eye without using an eye pad directly over the eyelid. This protects the surgical eye while allowing some vision through the perforated shield. Before surgery, the patient should be informed of the amount and duration of visual compromise that is projected for the operative eye.

SOCIOECONOMIC ISSUES

Patients cared for in ASCs include people from various types of socioeconomic backgrounds. Millions of Americans do not have health insurance, and this phenomenon is not limited to the unemployed or those in lower socioeconomic levels. While health insurance

Table 24–3. Tips for Talking with Hard-of-Hearing Persons

According to *Healthy People 2000: National Health Promotion and Disease Prevention Objectives*, impaired hearing becomes increasingly common after 50 years of age, affecting 23% of people aged 65 through 74 years; 33% of those 75 through 84 years; and 48% of those who are 85 years of age and older. These figures are considered to be underestimates.

Healthy People 2000 emphasizes that: ". . . patient and family communication training and environmental structuring can help to enhance the . . . quality of life for the hearing-impaired . . ." Greater awareness of the adverse effects on a person because of hearing impairment and using easy tips such as the following, will facilitate communication between the hard-of-hearing and "normal-hearing" persons.

- Whenever possible, face the hard-of-hearing person directly and on the same level.
- Your speech will be more easily understood when you are not eating, chewing, smoking, etc.
- Reduce background noises when carrying on conversations—turn off the radio or television.
- Keep your hands away from your face while talking.
- If it is difficult for a person to understand, find another way of saying the same thing rather than repeating the original words. Move to a quieter location.
- Recognize that hard-of-hearing people hear and understand less well when they are tired or ill.
- Do not talk to a hard-of-hearing person from another room. Be sure to get the attention of the person to whom you will speak before you start talking.
- Speak in a normal fashion without shouting or showing impatience. See that the light is not shining into the eyes of the hard-of-hearing person.
- A woman's voice is often harder to hear than a man's because of its pitch. A woman might try to lower the pitch of her voice when talking to the hard-of-hearing to see if that helps.
- Speak slowly and clearly.
- If the hard-of-hearing person wears a hearing aid, make sure that it has batteries installed, that the batteries work, that the hearing aid is turned on, and that the hearing aid is clean and free from ear wax.
- If you know (or if it becomes evident) from which side the person hears best, talk to that side.
- It is better to speak directly face to face in situations in which relatively diffuse lighting is adequate and lights the speaker's face. This allows the hard-of-hearing listener to observe the speaker's facial expressions and lip movements.
- Persons with hearing impairment also can benefit from seating themselves at a table where they can best see all parties (e.g., from the "end" of a rectangular table).
- Announce beforehand when you are going to change the subject of conversation. Doing so might avoid an unfortunate faux pas by a hard-of-hearing listener.
- Sometimes hard-of-hearing persons have "good" or "better" sides—right or left—ask them if they do. If they indicate a preference, direct your remarks to the "good" side or face to face, as they wish.
- Check to see that a light is not shining in the eyes of the hard-of-hearing person. Change position so that you are not standing in front of a light source, such as a window, which puts your face in shadow or silhouette and makes it hard for the hard-of-hearing person to "speech read."
- Avoid abrupt changes of subject or interjecting small talk into your conversation because hard-of-hearing listeners often use context to understand what you are saying.
- If the hard-of-hearing person wears an aid, try raising the pitch of your voice just slightly. If the hard-of-hearing listener is not wearing an aid, try lowering the pitch of your voice.
- If all else fails, rephrase your remarks or have someone whose voice is familiar to the hard-of-hearing person repeat your words.
- Do not talk too fast.
- Pronounce words clearly. If the hearing-impaired person has difficulty with letters and numbers say: "M as in Mary," "2 as in twins," "B as in boy," and say each number separately, like "five six" instead of "fifty-six." The reason for doing so is that m, n and 2, 3, 56, 66 and b, c, d, e, t and v sound alike.
- If you are around a corner, or turn away, you become much harder to understand.
- Keep a note pad handy, and write your words out and show them to the hard-of-hearing person if you have to—do not just walk away, leaving the hearing-impaired listener puzzling over what you said and thinking you do not care.
- Be patient.

Note: These tips originally appeared on the Gerinet listserv list. The author encouraged further dissemination without additional permission. From the government site http://www.aoa.gov/elderpage/hohtips.html, November 1998.

premiums continue to rise, so do the number of uninsured or underinsured Americans.[13] According to the Agency for Health Care Policy and Research (AHCPR) 27% of uninsured families had difficulty obtaining health care, primarily because of cost.[13] Although the unemployment rate has decreased in the United States in recent years, the number of uninsured continues to climb. Many employers are finding it difficult or impossible to continue providing the same level of health insurance benefits to their employees.

Some uninsured people may obtain health care by paying full charges for services. Others, however, may get reduced or waived fees, visit emergency departments, or use community health systems. Persons of low socioeconomic status often use emergency departments because they have no other choice for health care. State, federal, and community programs offer coverage for some citizens. The Children's Health Insurance Plan (CHIP) and the Health Insurance Portability and Accountability Act (HIPAA) have been created to help make health care more available to children, working families, and those who are between jobs, have preexisting medical conditions, or are self-employed.[13]

Access to health insurance varies widely among the different states. For example, in Tennessee, uninsured families with income up to 40% of the poverty level may buy into Medicaid on a sliding-scale level. Other states, however, allow only families living substantially below the poverty level to be eligible for welfare.[14] Therefore, depending on the state, poor adults may be two to three times more likely to be uninsured in Florida or Texas as they would be in Minnesota or Oregon.

ASCs associated with public, tax-supported healthcare systems may see a higher percentage of patients from varied socioeconomic backgrounds than those centers that are private, for-profit centers. The quality of care provided to this group of patients should be no different than that provided to those patients with insurance payers. Some studies have documented the adverse affects of lack of health insurance on patient outcomes. A 1991 study reported by Hadley and associates compared privately insured and uninsured hospital patients according to admission, use of resources, and discharge outcome. They found, with few exceptions, that people without insurance had a greater chance of dying in the hospital.[15]

Homelessness is a social, economic, and public health problem of increased magnitude in the United States. The approaches to the delivery of health care to those without homes have been inadequate because of many complex problems facing the homeless population.[16] Homelessness exists in virtually every community, and a community-based service delivery system to meet the needs of the homeless is needed. This problem poses significant challenges for aftercare arrangements, and the nurse must call on a variety of agencies and community services to ensure a safe haven for the homeless person facing ambulatory surgery.

Patients without access to health care and therefore, no primary care physician, may present to the ASC with various medical problems, such as uncontrolled hypertension, that can be linked with adverse outcomes. Clearly, these patients can provide challenges for the healthcare providers in the ASC. Medical "clearance" for surgery may be difficult to obtain, and collaboration among the physicians, nurses, and social workers is needed, along with public health departments and community health centers.

Significant others are an important part of the care provided for ambulatory surgery patients. Ideally, the individuals who are responsible for the patient's immediate aftercare are identified during the pre-admission testing visit. The nurse should have an understanding of the patient's home support before planning care and providing individual instructions. When the patient does not have an adequate support system at home, the ASC nurse may need to seek the direction of the physician or administrator.

Home health agencies are one source of assistance but may not be financially feasible. Specific insurance guidelines and Medicare/Medicaid guidelines determine whether the home visits meet their criteria for home visits. A 23-hour hospital admission may be the answer to some of the postsurgical nursing care needs for many patients. Many hospital-based centers provide this type of care for observation after complex procedures or if the patient experiences postoperative complications. Unfortunately, the practice of using 23-hour programs for patients strictly with social needs is becoming obsolete. Creative alternatives need to be established to help meet the needs of these patients.

Financial concerns also can be a problem area for this group of patients. They may be unable to purchase prescription drugs and nutritious food. Transportation to and from pre- and postoperative medical appointments may also be a problem. If a social services department is available, that resource should be consulted to help meet these needs. In a freestanding surgery center without such resources, the physician should be informed and asked to intercede appropriately. The physician may be able to assist the patient by supplementing their medication supply with pharmaceutical company samples or by writing for low-cost or generic drugs. The Council on Aging and other community resources may be able to help with the provision of meals and transportation needs. Shelters may be available for patients with no homes. It is important not to pass judgment on these patients and to try to meet their individual needs in a caring, compassionate, and respectful manner.

CULTURAL DIVERSITY

Cultural competence requires sensitivity, understanding, and acceptance of uniqueness, worth, and value of each individual. Cultural diversity is who we are and how we relate to each other, regardless of the setting. As healthcare providers, we have a professional responsibility to enhance and value the worth of those entrusted in our care.[17]

Cultural and ethical beliefs influence patients' attitudes and responses regarding medical intervention as well as that of each staff member. Bille points out that modern medicine often ignores sociocultural forces that are not in agreement with current scientifically based health care.[18] Many cultures have beliefs based on spiritual control over the body, on faith healing, on being one with the environment; and various other beliefs that many people would consider superstitious.

It may be very difficult for people from other cultures to look to modern surgical interventions without a sense that they have abandoned a part of their upbringing. They may accept only a portion of the explanations or instructions that a nurse or physician offers and may have different perspectives about life and health than the nurse. Healthcare workers must respect each patient's beliefs, regardless of whether they agree with them. How the patient's beliefs affect understanding and compliance with the surgical and nursing plans of action is an issue that must be assessed and addressed on an individual basis.

Demographers report that the largest population increase in the United States (all ages) is among minority groups of racial and ethnic origin.[19] Two thirds of all global migration is into the United States.[20] Cultural diversity is addressed in the JCAHO standards relating to patient assessment, education, and rights.[21] A social assessment of patients is required and should include social and cultural influences, such as beliefs, values, and spiritual orientation. What the patient believes is the cause of the illness may affect how he or she accepts the recommended treatment or his or her adherence to the treatment plan. The American Nurses Association has published a position statement on cultural diversity in the workplace (Table 24–4).[22] This position states that knowledge of cultural diversity is vital at all levels of nursing practice. Cultural diversity will have a profound impact on health care in hospitals and community settings and will pose a tremendous challenge for nurses practicing in the 21st century.

Patients cared for in ambulatory surgical programs include people from many ethnic, racial, and religious groups. Although people from a particular background may not necessarily have healthcare needs identical to others of their race or group, similarities sometimes exist. Generalizations can be made about various ethnic practices and beliefs, but the nurse should recognize that generalizations are just that, and the individuality of each patient must be addressed when planning care.

Social and health beliefs as well as the importance generally ascribed to the family unit are passed on through generations. Dietary patterns in a particular culture tend to be similar as well. Health beliefs may differ from the nurse's, and an understanding of and sensitivity to the patient's value system is important when planning care. Although large ethnic groups share many similarities, such as history, ancestry, language, and traditions, each has many subgroups with unique and distinguishing social and cultural practices. For example, Mexicans, Puerto Ricans, and Cubans all are considered Hispanic Americans, but they vary widely in their cultural beliefs and practices, so generalizations would be faulty.[23] Another example is that some Hispanic women may avoid discussing family planning and do not use birth control, and thus detailed personal instructions after gynecologic procedures may be embarrassing for them, particularly in the presence of another person, even a family member. In traditional Chinese families, respect for elders is imperative, and women are often given a lower status in the family than men. The Chinese-American woman in a relationship based on traditional Chinese norms

Table 24–4. Cultural Diversity in Nursing Practice

Summary: This ANA Position Statement describes the features of an operational definition of cultural diversity as it is expressed in nursing practice, education, administration, and research.

Knowledge of cultural diversity is vital at all levels of nursing practice. Ethnocentric approaches to nursing practice are ineffective in meeting health and nursing needs of diverse cultural groups of clients. Knowledge about cultures and their impact on interactions with health care is essential for nurses, whether they are practicing in a clinical setting, education, research, or administration. Cultural diversity addresses racial and ethnic differences; however, these concepts or features of the human experience are not synonymous. The changing demographics of the nation as reflected in the 1990 census will increase the cultural diversity of the U.S. population by the year 2000, and what have heretofore been called minority groups will, on the whole, constitute a national majority (American Nurses Association, 1990).

Knowledge and skills related to cultural diversity can strengthen and broaden healthcare delivery systems. Other cultures can provide examples of a range of alternatives in services, delivery systems, conceptualization of illness, and treatment modalities. Cultural groups often utilize traditional healthcare providers, identified by and respected within the group. Concepts of illness, wellness, and treatment modalities evolve from a cultural perspective or worldview. Concepts of illness, health, and wellness are part of the total cultural belief system. Culture is one of the organizing concepts upon which nursing is based and defined. Nurses need to understand:

- How cultural groups understand life processes
- How cultural groups define health and illness
- What cultural groups do to maintain wellness
- What cultural groups believe to be the causes of illness
- How healers cure and care for members of cultural groups
- How the cultural background of the nurse influences the way in which care is delivered

It is important that the nurse consider specific cultural factors impacting on individual clients and recognize that intracultural variation means that each client must be assessed for individual cultural differences.

Nurses bring their personal cultural heritage as well as the cultural and philosophical views of their education into the professional setting. Therefore, it is important for the nurse to understand that nurse–patient encounters include the interaction of three cultural systems: the culture of the nurse, the culture of the client, and the culture of the setting. Access to care can be improved by providing culturally relevant, responsive services. Individuals need choices of delivery systems in seeking health care. Nurses in clinical practice must use their knowledge of cultural diversity to develop and implement culturally sensitive nursing care. Nurses take pride in their role as client advocates.

Recognizing cultural diversity, integrating cultural knowledge, and acting, when possible, in a culturally appropriate manner enables nurses to be more effective in initiating nursing assessments and serving as client advocates. All nursing curricula should include pertinent information about diverse healthcare beliefs, values, and practices. Such educational programs would demonstrate to nursing students that cultural beliefs and practices are as integral to the nursing process as are physical and psychosocial factors. Nurse administrators need to foster policies and procedures that help ensure access to care that accommodates varying cultural beliefs. Nurse administrators need to be knowledgeable about and sensitive to the cultural diversity among providers and consumers. Nurse researchers need to utilize the cross-cultural body of knowledge in order to ask pertinent research questions. Through exploration of other cultures, nurse researchers and practitioners find that while cultures differ, there are also many similarities among groups. Nurses are in a position to influence professional policies and practice in response to cultural diversity.

Definitions

Cultural diversity in nursing practice derives its conceptual base from nursing, other cross-cultural health disciplines, and the social sciences such as anthropology, sociology, and psychology. Culture is conceptualized broadly to encompass the belief systems of a variety of groups. Cultural diversity refers to the differences between people based on a shared ideology and valued set of beliefs, norms, customs, and meanings evidenced in a way of life. Culture consists of patterns of behavior acquired and transmitted symbols, constituting the distinctive achievement of human groups, including their embodiment in artifacts; the essential core of culture consists of historically derived and selected ideas and especially their attached values (Kroeber and Kluckhohn, 1952).

The impact of culture as a causative influence on the perceptions, interpretations, and behaviors of persons in specific cultural groups is important. Issues such as cultural differences in defining health and in designing treatments are also important. As knowledge of specific cultures is gained, cross-cultural comparison can lead to recognition of possible universal aspects as well. Ideology is comprised of the ideas of a group, their nature and source, and the doctrines, opinions, or ways of thinking of a group. These are attached to an agreed-upon set of beliefs or a creed. Values refer to the especially favorable way of regarding the ideas, behaviors, customs, and institutions of a group as desirable, useful, estimable, important, or truthful. Ethnocentrism is the belief that one's own culture is superior to all others. This belief is common to all cultural groups; all groups regard their own culture as not only the best but also the correct, moral, and only way of life. This belief is pervasive, often unconscious, and is imposed on every aspect of day-to-day interaction and practices, including health care. It is this attitude which creates problems between nurses and clients of diverse cultural groups.

References

American Nurses Association: Code with Interpretive Statements. Kansas City: ANA, 1985.

American Nurses Association: Cultural Diversity in Nursing, ANA House of Delegates, 1986. U.S. Census Bureau, The 1990 Census, 1990.

Kroeber AL, Kluckhohn C: Culture: A Critical Review of Concepts and Definitions. New York: Random House, 1952.

may have little support from her husband in regard to household chores, but the extended family unit is strong. Other females family members often are available to help after surgery.

When patients present to the ASC, the nurse should interview the patient and learn about the patient's living situation and location, religious beliefs that may affect patient care, socioeconomic status, family structure, current health status, and view of health and illness. A Native American living on a reservation is likely to have more strongly held ethnic beliefs than one living in a more heterogeneous community.[23] Table 24–5 provides suggestions on how to enhance cultural communications.[20] Patient assessment also should include areas to help determine the patient's cultural needs.[20] These are described in Table 24–6.

Posing questions of cultural and religious matters must be done tactfully and respectfully. Some questions presented in this table may not be appropriate to the ASC setting, and the nurse must make individual judgments about which questions are pertinent. One way of posing a question regarding religious or cultural needs might be, "Is there anything in your cultural or religious beliefs that you want to tell me that is important for your care today?"

Illnesses may be prevalent in a particular ethnic group for a number of reasons. Genetic predisposition, or heredity, cannot be eliminated as a source of disease. Sickle cell anemia and essential hypertension in African Americans are examples. A family tendency toward malignant hyperthermia (MH) is particularly noteworthy in a setting in which anesthetics will be administered. MH often can be tracked to geographic patterns, where many descendants of predisposed people settle in one area of the country.

Dietary patterns can predispose patients to diseases such as obesity, hypertension, and malnutrition. Environmental factors can result in widespread acquired illnesses in a group of people. Lead poisoning and parasitic diseases due to environmental exposure can affect people living in similar settings. Social pressures in the environment can be causative as well; an example is the high incidence of alcoholism seen in some Native American cultures. Table 24–7 lists a number of illnesses and conditions frequently associated with different ethnic groups. The ambulatory surgical nurse should consider these when planning care for people from various cultural backgrounds.

Ambulatory surgery nurses often are required to obtain the patient's signature on the surgical consent form. Ideally, the consent confirms that the physician has provided the patient with adequate information with which to make an informed decision about treatment and care. The nurse is the witness to the signature. Cultural as well as language differences may make it challenging to obtain the surgical consent. Cultural differences between the patient and the healthcare system may impair true understand-

Table 24–5. Enhancing Cultural Communication

- Determine the level of fluency in English and arrange for an interpreter, if needed.
- Speak directly to the patient, whether the interpreter is present or not.
- Ask how the patient prefers to be addressed.
- Allow the patient to choose seating for comfortable personal space and eye contact.
- Avoid body language that may be offensive or misunderstood.
- Choose a speech rate and style that promotes understanding and shows respect for the patient.
- Avoid slang, technical jargon, and complex sentences.
- Give the patient time to formulate an answer.
- Use open-ended questions or questions phrased in several ways to obtain information.
- Determine the patient's reading ability before using written materials in the teaching process.

From Stewart B: The culturally diverse patient. Semin Perioperative Nurs 3:163, 1994.

Table 24–6. Cultural Assessment

AREA OF CONCERN	HELPFUL QUESTIONS
Religion	Inquire about religious practices. What is allowed/what is forbidden (relating to care)? What influences does God have on health?
Alternative medicine	What home remedies, if any, are used? What is the choice of practitioner? When do you see other practitioners?
Are specific rituals followed re:	Birth, infancy, marriage, old age, death?
Pain	How is pain expressed?
Illness	Identify specific illness behaviors.
Family communication patterns	Identify patterns of authority and family responsibility.

From Stewart B: The culturally diverse patient. Semin Perioperative Nurs 3:165, 1994.

Table 24–7. Illnesses Related to Various Ethnic Groups

ETHNIC GROUP	ASSOCIATED ILLNESSES
African Americans	Sickle cell anemia, hypertension, keloid formation
Latin Americans/Hispanics	Anemia in females, diabetes mellitus, parasites, obesity, lactose intolerance, lead poisoning, tuberculosis, malnutrition with associated infant mortality
Native Americans	Alcoholism, trachoma, tuberculosis, diabetes mellitus, high infant mortality, liver and heart disease
Filipino Americans	Diabetes mellitus, tuberculosis, cancer of the liver, hyperuricemia, cardiovascular–renal disease
Chinese Americans	Lactose and alcohol intolerance, tuberculosis, dermatitis
Japanese Americans	Alcohol intolerance, lactose deficiency, CVA, cancer of esophagus, stomach, liver, and biliary system, ulcers, colitis, psoriasis
South Vietnamese Americans	Tuberculosis, intestinal parasites, anemia, malnutrition, skin diseases, malaria, hepatitis, dental problems
Gypsies	Hypertension, diabetes mellitus, coronary artery disease, peripheral vascular disease, obesity, elevated triglycerides or cholesterol

CVA = cerebrovascular accident.
From Groah L: Operating Room Nursing—Perioperative Practice, 2nd ed. Norwalk, CT: Appleton & Lange, 1990, pp 99–104. Adapted with permission.

Table 24–8. Using Continuous Quality Improvement (CQI) to Achieve Cultural Diversity

Achieving a culturally diverse workforce at South Miami Hospital in Miami, Florida, was accomplished by use of the continuous quality improvement (CQI) process. To enhance the ability to care for their patients and to promote understanding and harmony, a team was developed that drew on the strength of a culturally diverse staff and community. The first step was to collect patient mix data. The data showed a patient mix of 48% Caucasian, 7% African American, 41% Hispanic, and 4% other. The employee mix was 42% Caucasian, 27% African American, 29% Hispanic, and 2% Asian. The team then began to brainstorm and developed an affinity diagram to look at the sources of variations to develop a better cultural understanding. The different culture variables were patients, families, physicians, and staff. The team then took steps to prioritize and work on one opportunity at a time by using the cycle of improvement (Plan, Do, Check, Act—PDCA).

Language and bilingual information was the first issue to be addressed. All brochures and patient forms were translated from English into Spanish. In addition, Spanish classes were offered to the hospital switchboard operators. The goal was to have the operators communicate using common phrases used in telephone conversations with Spanish-speaking customers. Also, a list of all the employees at the hospital who speak 24 different languages was distributed to all departments. All Spanish-speaking employees were given identification buttons with the symbol Ñ, which is a letter used only in the Spanish alphabet. This identification button would inform the patients that the employee was able to speak Spanish. Finally, in an effort to assist the non-Spanish speaking staff, common phrases were printed in Spanish in the hospital newsletter, *FYI*.

To help the staff learn about cultural diversity, the hospital began to provide "Cultural Special Events." For example, a Black History Month Celebration was planned and included fashion shows, art displays, guest speakers, and other similar activities. Other successful events included the development of a Cultural Choir, Ethnic Foods Specialty Days, and the Maria Paradox Program.

The next step of the program was to facilitate hospital visits for international patients. The staff began to identify international patients by placing green armbands on them upon admission to the hospital. This allowed for recognition of their special needs. These patients also were provided with a packet of information that included area maps, local shopping plazas, nearby area restaurants, discount coupons, telephone calling cards, and other pertinent information.

A patient satisfaction survey was developed to help the team determine whether the program was meeting its goals. Questions on the survey included: "Is the staff considerate of your needs?" and "Was information provided in your primary language?" During the third quarter, the team noted that there was a decrease in patient satisfaction. Through the CQI process, the team learned that there was a need to work further on staff education and this was incorporated into the *culture tool* to help us meet the needs of our culturally diverse patient population in South Florida.

Printed with permission of Carmen Rodriguez, RN, South Miami Hospital. Personal contact, November 1998.

ing of the procedure and consequences.[24] Translators can be of paramount importance when obtaining consent from patients. An interpreter of the same gender is best because many patients do not feel comfortable revealing personal concerns to those of the opposite sex. Chaplains also may provide assistance with cultural support. Perianesthesia nurses need to be aware of cultural factors when witnessing the patient's signature on surgical consent forms.

The ASC nurse must collaborate with peers, physicians, and other community resources to meet the varied needs of their patients from many backgrounds and ethnic groups. Table 24–8 illustrates the efforts of a Miami, Florida, hospital to address multicultural issues using a continuous quality improvement model. This same staff created a Culture Tool to assist them in identifying and understanding some of the cultural needs of their multicultural patient population (Table 24–9).

All nurses must recognize the importance of understanding the values, beliefs, attitudes, and health practices of the multicultural American society and thus be able to provide appropriate care to these patients. Additionally, nurses must recognize their own cultural biases. That is sometimes a more difficult obstacle. By becoming aware of culturally relevant issues, nurses can better assess, plan, implement, and evaluate patient care.

CULTURE IN THE WORKPLACE

The character of the current workforce is changing rapidly. Only approximately 15% of new workers are white men. Of new entrants into the workforce, 29% are minorities; a large percentage of new entrants into the workforce are immigrants, and two thirds of those entering the workforce are women.[25] These trends present challenges and opportunities in nursing. Fostering diversity in the workplace is about building an organizational culture that embraces personal differences and encourages heterogeneous persons to work together toward a common end.[26] Managing diversity allows healthcare leaders to develop the potential of all employees while improving performance and productivity.

Managers need to effectively prepare for an increasingly diverse workforce. Education is needed to increase awareness and sensitivity of the managers' own cultural beliefs and values, as well as those of the staff. Managers need to build human resource skills to help deal with individuals who have different attitudes and beliefs regarding life and work. Sensitivity and understanding will help with problem solving and conflict resolution. Poor intercultural communication can result in low morale, lack of teamwork, charges of discrimination, and other negative behaviors that can affect productivity.[27]

Working relationships in multicultural environments will be enhanced if there is commitment, empathy, and sensitivity from everyone, including administrators, educators, managers, and staff.[28] Points to remember include:

- Respect your differences—respect your colleagues' values, beliefs, customs, just as you would those of your individual patients.
- Get out of the comfort zone—clustering with one's own group prevents the staff from getting to know people and learning about their cultures.
- Resist judgmental reactions until you obtain sufficient information—do not use your own standards as a frame of reference; "different" does not mean "inferior."
- Learn to communicate effectively—listen closely and also pay attention to nonverbal cues; give feedback.
- Accentuate the positive—share positive aspects of your culture; organize potluck meals where everyone brings typical ethnic dishes.
- Gain cultural knowledge—read, observe, ask questions.
- Confront prejudices—denying prejudices keeps you from moving toward multiculturalism.[27, 28]

Managers must respond to the needs of diverse staff members to promote teamwork and productivity in the workplace.

SUMMARY

Patients with special emotional, social, and cultural needs require careful preoperative assessment and planning of care. The ASC nurses need to anticipate each individual patient's specific needs and provide discharge instructions and education that will facilitate the patient's recovery phase.

Addressing the widely diverse needs of patients seeking care in the ASC setting is not a one-time event. Nurses are challenged everyday with yet another never-before-presented issue or patient need. The nurse must continually develop critical-thinking and problem-solving skills to provide individualized care for the special needs of patients and their families.

Text continued on page 571

Table 24–9. **The Culture Tool**

CULTURE GROUP AND LANGUAGE	BELIEF PRACTICES	NUTRITIONAL PREFERENCES	COMMUNICATION AWARENESS	PATIENT CARE/HANDLING OF DEATH
American English	Christian and Jewish beliefs are prominent; many others exist in smaller numbers. Family-oriented.	Beef, chicken, potatoes, vegetables, fast food, ethnic foods.	Talkative, shake hands, not much touching during conversation. Prefer to gather information for decision-making. Some hugging and kissing, mainly between women.	Family members and friends visit in small groups. Expect high-quality care.
Argentinian Spanish	90% Catholic, some Protestant and Jewish. Strong belief in saints, purgatory, and heaven. People from rural areas may be more superstitious.	Emphasis on meat, especially beef with homemade pastas, pastries, and local wines. Maté: national beverage that is stimulating and "addictive" like coffee.	Talkative, very expressive, direct, and to the point; extroverted; good eye contact; like personal and physical contact such as holding hands, hugging, and kissing.	Educated, yet reluctant to get medical attention or accept new medical advancements. Independent; often deny disability. Believe in natural and holistic remedies: herbal teas, pure aloe, natural oils, poultices. Family gets involved with caring for the ill family member.
Brazilian Portuguese Diverse cultural backgrounds including: European, African, Indian.	Mostly Catholic; some Spiritism. Growing Evangelical representation. Candomble and Macumba—similar to Santeria.	Beans and rice are staples. Feijoada—black beans, beef, pork. Churrasco (charcoal-broiled meats). Manioc (vegetable). Tropical fruits.	Very sociable. Will stand close to each other. Social kissing, hugging, touching. Good eye contact.	Emphasis on family unity—will want to be actively involved. Tend to trust medical personnel; place great faith in doctors and nurses. Some believe in herbal treatments, teas, and balsams.
Canadian English; French and Innuit (Eskimo)	Protestant, Catholic, and Jewish.	Comparable to the American diet. French influence in Montreal and Quebec.	May prefer no touching or kissing. Take things at face value.	Follow nurses' instructions. Accustomed to socialized medicine, less litigation. Take physicians at their word. Willing to wait for treatment.
Cayman English with some changes in accent and verbs.	People are very religious. The majority of the island is Baptist or "Church of God." *Voodoo and psychics are outlawed.*	Fish, turtle, beef, goat, and conch. Rice, beans, and plantains. Fried food very rich in fat: cooked or fried in coconut oil or milk.	Like to be acknowledged. Good eye contact. Prefer no touching or kissing. Very talkative and known for their friendliness. Everyone on the island knows each other.	Like to be told what is going on by the doctor. Would rather talk to doctors than to nurses. Prefer one-to-one care.

Chinese Many dialects spoken; one written language.	Religions: Taoism, Buddhism, Islam, Christianity. Harmonious relationship with nature and others; loyalty to family, friends, and government. Public debate of conflicting views is unacceptable. Accommodating, not confrontational. Modesty, self-control, self-reliance, self-restraint. Hierarchical structure for interpersonal and family interactions.	Diet consisting of vegetables and rice. Tofu (bean curd) can be prepared in various ways. Soy sauce, MSG, and preserved foods. Belief in theory of "yin" (cold) and "yang" (hot) when they are sick. No food with "yin" after surgery (e.g., cold desserts, salad). Often lactose intolerant.	Quiet, polite, unassertive. Suppress feelings of anxiety, fear, depression, and pain. Eye contact and touching sometimes seen as offensive or impolite. Emphasize loyalty and tradition. Self-expression and individualism discouraged.	Women uncomfortable with exams by male physicians. May not adhere to fixed schedule. May fear medical institutions. Use a combination of herbal and Western medicine. Traditional: acupuncture, herbal medicine, massage, skin scraping, and cupping. Alcohol may cause flushing.
Cuban Spanish	Catholic with Protestant minority. Santeria, which can include animal sacrifice.	Cuban bread, café con leche, Cuban coffee. Roast pork, black beans, and rice. Plaintains, yuca, chicken, and rice.	Some may have a tendency to be loud when having a discussion. Use their hands for emphasis and credibility, and prefer strong eye contact.	Culture requires visiting the sick. The extended family supports the immediate family. It is an insult to the patient if there is not a large family/friend presence.
Ecuadorian Spanish Quechua-Indian	Primarily Catholic. Increase in Protestant, Baptist, and Jehovah Witness. Very respectful toward religious leaders. Small percentage of population is wealthy with much political control. Family size is usually large.	Diet high in fruits and proteins, starches: rice, potatoes, corn. Food is prepared fresh daily, usually with salsa. Coastal diet: rice, fish (ceviche). Drink beer, soda.	Extremely polite; reserved; respectful; especially helpful.	Prefer pampering ill family members; stay overnight with the patient. Not stoic when it comes to pain. Very private, modest. Embarrassed if they do not look their best. Extremely protective of family; often elderly parents live with grown children.
Filipino English; Spanish; Tagalog (80 dialects)	Catholic. Seek both faith healer and Western physician when ill. Belief that many diseases are the will of God.	Theory of hot and cold food. Certain foods in the Philippines are traditionally eaten hot *or* cold (e.g., milk is only taken HOT). Fish, rice, vegetables, fruit. Meals have to be HOT.	Value and respect elders. Loving, family-oriented. Set aside time just for family.	Family decision important. Ignore health-related issues; often noncompliant. In spite of Western medicine, they often leave things in the hands of God, with occasional folk medicine. Home remedies: herbal tea, massage, sleep. May subscribe to supernatural cause of diseases.
Guatemalan Spanish; Mayan heritage; European influence.	Primarily Catholic. Increase in Protestants. Very respectful toward elders. European heritage; strong family ties.	Diet high in fruits, vegetables, rice, beans, and tortillas (corn flour bread).	Quiet, reserved, and respectful. Will not question for fear of insulting the professional.	Modest, private, and stoic. Believe in alternative methods of healing.

Table continued on following page

***Table 24–9.* The Culture Tool** *Continued*

CULTURE GROUP AND LANGUAGE	BELIEF PRACTICES	NUTRITIONAL PREFERENCES	COMMUNICATION AWARENESS	PATIENT CARE/HANDLING OF DEATH
Haitian Creole; French is taught in schools.	Catholic and Protestant. Voodoo is practiced. Large social gap exists between wealthy and poor citizens.	Large breakfast and lunch. Light dinner. Rice, fried pork grillot, and red beans. Herbs and cloves.	Quiet, polite. Value touch and eye contact.	Obedient to doctor and nurse but hesitant to ask questions. View use of oxygen as indication of severe illness. Occasionally share prescriptions and home remedies.
Hindu Hindi	The belief of cyclic birth and reincarnation lies at the center of Hinduism. The status, condition, and caste of each life is determined by behavior in the last life.	Cow is sacred. No beef. Some are strictly vegetarian.	Limit eye contact. Do not touch while talking.	Do not try to force foods when religiously forbidden. Death—the priest may tie a thread around the neck or wrist to signify a blessing. This thread should not be removed. The priest will pour water into the mouth of the body. Family will request to wash the body. The eldest son is responsible for the funeral rites.
Jamaican English; Patois (broken English)	Christian beliefs dominate (Catholic, Baptist, Anglican). Some Rastafari influence.	Beef, goat, rice and peas, chicken, vegetables, fish, lots of spices. Some avoid eating pork and pork products because of religious beliefs.	Respect for elders is encouraged. Reserved; avoid hugging and showing affection in public. Curious and tend to ask a lot of questions.	Will try some home remedies before seeking medical help. Like to be completely informed before procedures. Respectful of doctor's opinion. May be reluctant to admit that they are in pain. May not adhere to a fixed schedule.
Japanese Japanese	Self-praise or the acceptance of praise is considered poor manners. Family is extremely important. Behavior and communication are defined by role and status. Religion includes a combination of Buddhism and Shinto.	Food presentation is important. Fish and soybean are main sources of protein, as well as meats and vegetables (some pickled). Rice and noodles, tea, soy sauce. Often lactose intolerant.	Use attitude, actions, and feelings to communicate. Talkative people are considered show-offs or insincere. Openness considered a sign of immaturity, lack of self-control. Implicit nonverbal messages are of central importance. Use concept of hierarchy and status. Avoid conflict. Avoid eye contact and touch.	Family role for support is important. Insulted when addressed by first name. Confidentiality is very important for honor. Information about illness is kept in immediate family. Prone to keloid formation. Cleft lip or palate not uncommon. Alcohol may cause flushing. Tendency to control anger. May be reluctant to admit that they are in pain.

Jewish Many from E. European countries. English; Hebrew; Yiddish. Three basic groups: Orthodox (most strict), Conservative, Reform (least strict).	Israel is the holy land. Sabbath is from sundown on Friday to sundown on Saturday. It is customary to invite other families in for Friday evening Sabbath dinner.	Orthodox and some conservatives maintain a Kosher diet. Kosher food is prepared according to Jewish law under Rabbinical supervision. Eating of unclean animals is forbidden. Blood and animal fats are taboo (blood is synonymous with life). Do not mix meat with dairy products.	Orthodox men do not touch women, except their wives. Touch only for hands-on care. Very talkative and known for their friendliness.	Stoic and authoritative. Appreciate family accommodation. Jewish law demands that they seek complete medical care. Donor transplants are not acceptable to Orthodox Jews but are to Conservative and Reform. Death—cremation is discouraged. Autopsy is permitted in less strict groups. Orthodox believe that entire body, tissues, organs, amputated limbs, and blood sponges need to be available to the family for burial. Do not cross hands in postmortem care.
Korean Hangul	Family-oriented. Believe in reincarnation. Religions include: Shammanism, Taoism, Buddhism, Confucianism, Christianity. Belief in balance of two forces: hot and cold.	High fiber; spicy seasoning; rice; Kim Chee (fermented cabbage). Often lactose and alcohol intolerant. Speak little during meal.	Reserved with strangers. Will use eye contact with familiar individuals. Etiquette is important. First names used only for family members. Proud, independent. Children should not be used as translators due to reversal of parent/child relationship.	Family needs to be included in plan of care. Prefer non-contact. Respond to sincerity.
Mexican Spanish; people of Indian heritage may speak one of more than 50 dialects.	Predominantly Roman Catholic. Pray, say rosary, have priest in time of crisis. Limited belief in "brujeria" as a magical, supernatural, or emotional illness precipitated by evil forces.	Corn, beans, avocado, chilies, yellow rice. Heavy use of spices.	Tend to describe emotions by using dramatic body language. Very dramatic with grief but otherwise diplomatic and tactful. Direct confrontation is rude.	May believe that the outcome of circumstances is controlled by an external force; this can influence the patient's compliance with health care. Women do not expose their bodies to men or other women.
Muslim Language of the country and some English.	Believe in one God, "Allah," and Mohammed, his prophet. Five daily prayers. Zakat, a compulsory giving of alms to the poor. Fasting during the month of Ramadan. Pilgrimage to Mecca is the goal of the faithful.	No pork or alcohol. Eat only Halal meat (type of Kosher).	Limit eye contact. Do not touch while talking. Women may cover entire body except the face and hands.	Do not force foods when it is religiously forbidden. Abortion before 130 days—fetus is treated as discarded tissue; after 130 days, as a human. Before death, confession of sins with family present. After death, only relatives or priest may touch the body. Koran, the holy book, is recited near the dying person. The body is bathed and clothed in white and buried within 24 hours.

Table continued on following page

Table 24–9. The Culture Tool *Continued*

CULTURE GROUP AND LANGUAGE	BELIEF PRACTICES	NUTRITIONAL PREFERENCES	COMMUNICATION AWARENESS	PATIENT CARE/HANDLING OF DEATH
Northern European Language of the country and some English.	Similar to American customs. Protestant, Catholic, and Jewish. Multiethnic groups.	Comparable to American diet: meat, vegetables, and starches. Coffee, hot tea, and beer.	Courtesy is of utmost importance. Address by surname and maintain personal space and good eye contact.	Maintain modesty at all times. Stoic regarding pain tolerance. Death is often taken quietly with little emotional expression. Patients/family tend not to question medical authority.
Southern European Language of the country and some English.	Roman Catholic, Protestant, Greek Orthodox, and some Jewish.	Main meal at midday: pasta, meat, and fish with cheeses and wine. Fresh fruit. Espresso coffee.	Talkative, very expressive. Direct and to the point. Extroverted. Good eye contact. Like personal and physical contact: holding hands, patting on the back, kissing.	Educated, yet reluctant to get medical attention. Very independent. Birth control and abortion are accepted in some countries and not in others. Family gets involved with caring for ill family member.
Vietnamese Vietnamese language has several dialects—also French, English, Chinese.	Family loyalty is very important. Religions include Buddhism, Confucianism, Taoism, Cao Di, Hoa Hoa, Catholicism, occasional ancestral worship. General respect and harmony. Supernatural is sometimes used as an explanation for disease.	Rice often with green leafy vegetable, fish sauce added for flavor. Meat used sparingly and cut into small pieces. Tea is main beverage. Often lactose and alcohol intolerant.	Communication—formal, polite manner; limit use of touch. Respect conveyed by nonverbal communication. Use both hands to give something to an adult. To beckon someone, place the palm downward and wave. Don't snap your fingers to gain attention. Person's name used with title, i.e., "Mr. Bill," "Director James." "Ya" indicates respect (not agreement).	Negative emotions conveyed by silence and reluctant smile; will smile even if angry. Head is sacred—avoid touching. Back rub—uneasy experience. Common folk practices—skin rubbing, pinching, herbs in hot water, balms, string tying. Misunderstanding about illness—drawing blood seen as loss of body tissue; organ donation causes suffering in next life. Hospitalization is a last resort. Flowers only for the dead.

The Culture Tool has been assembled from anecdotal information and sharing by the Culture Connection CQI Team at South Miami Hospital, and Transcultural Nursing by Joyce Newman Giger and Ruth Elaine, Mosby 1995.

References

1. Gull H: The chronically ill patient's adaptation to hospitalization. Nurs Clin North Am 22:593–601, 1987.
2. Miller W: Other hereditary disorders. In Katz J, Benumof J, Kadis L (eds): Anesthesia and Uncommon Diseases, 3rd ed. Philadelphia: WB Saunders, 1990, pp 144–152.
3. Johnson R, Beneda H: Reducing patient restraint use. Nurs Manage 29:32–34, 1998.
4. Bogetz M, Resnikoff E: Management of the mentally handicapped surgical outpatient SAMBA Newsletter 2:7, 1988.
5. Waugaman W: Surgery and the patient with Alzheimer's disease. Geriatr Nurs 9:227–229, 1988.
6. Stoelting R, Miller R: Basics of Anesthesia, 2nd ed. New York: Churchill Livingstone, 1989.
7. Drachman D, Leavitt J: Human memory and the cholinergic system: A relationship to aging? Arch Neurol 30:113–121, 1974.
8. Simensen R: Mental retardation. In Dambro MR, Griffith JA (eds): The 5 Minute Clinical Consult. Baltimore: Williams & Wilkins, 1995, pp 664–665.
9. Revell L: Understanding, identifying, and teaching the low-literacy patient. Semin Periop Nurs 3:168–171, 1994.
10. Bleidt B, Clouse E: Counseling techniques for the hearing-impaired. US Pharmacist 14:51–57, 1989.
11. Johnson D: Shattered silence. J Post Anesth Nurs 1:215–218, 1986.
12. Ekstrom I: Communicating with the deaf patient. Plast Surg Nurs 14:31–32, 1994.
13. Gunderson L: Number of uninsured continues to rise. Ann Intern Med 129:513–515, 1998.
14. Gesensway D: Limited reforms revive insurance debate. From ACP Observer, American College of Surgeons, Dec 1997.
15. Hadley J, Steinberf E, Feder J: Comparison of uninsured and privately insured hospital patients: Condition on admission, resource use, and outcome. JAMA 265:374–379, 1991.
16. Plumb J, McManus P, Carson L: A collaborative community approach to homeless care. Prim Care 23:17–30, 1996.
17. Gullatte MM: Caring for patients from diverse cultures. American Society of Post Anesthesia Nurses 14th National Conference, Atlanta, GA, 1995.
18. Bille D (ed): Practical Approaches to Patient Teaching. Boston: Little Brown, 1981.
19. Bushy A: Ethnocultural sensitivity and measurement of consumer satisfaction. J Nurs Care Qual 9:16–25, 1995.
20. Stewart B: Teaching culturally diverse populations. Semin Perioperative Nurs 3:160–167, 1994.
21. Grossman D: Cultural diversity: Meeting JCAHO requirements. Florida Nurs Spectrum 7:5, 1997.
22. American Nurses Association: Position Statement on Cultural Diversity in Nursing Practice. Oct 1991.
23. Price J, Cordell B: Cultural diversity and patient teaching. J Continuing Educ Nurs 25:163–166, 1994.
24. Mailhot CB: Culture and consent. Nurs Man 28:48P, 1997.
25. Veninga RL: Valuing our differences. Health Progress 75:30–33, 54, 1994.
26. Lappetito J: Workplace diversity: A leadership challenge. Health Progress 75:22–27, 33, 1994.
27. Taylor R: Check your cultural competence. Nurs Man 29:30–32, 1998.
28. Grossman D, Taylor R: Cultural diversity on the unit. Am J Nurs 95:64–67, 1995.

Chapter 25

Patients with Special Medical Needs

Nancy Burden and Jan Odom

Young, active, healthy people do not make up the majority of the patients in most ambulatory surgery facilities. On the contrary, chronic and acute disease processes are prevalent in this population, so healthcare providers must maintain a well-disciplined approach to managing patients during the perianesthesia period. In the past 10 to 20 years, research has identified many new concepts, treatment protocols, and disease etiologies that affect the ASC patient population.

For understanding and application of effective patient management in the light of disease processes, it is essential that healthcare providers continue to learn throughout their careers. A current knowledge base requires ongoing reading and attendance at educational workshops. Another important tool is the existence of unit-based resources, for instance, a library specific to the needs of the ASC. Current textbooks, Internet sites, and journals and newsletters pertinent to the specialty provide quick and useful references when questions arise.

This chapter touches upon some of the major chronic diseases and conditions that nurses will encounter but is not intended as a comprehensive and singular source. The reader is referred to the mass of literature available.

SUBSTANCE ABUSE

Addiction can be defined as a pathologic relationship to a mood-altering experience or substance that has life-damaging consequences. Another definition is that it is a behavioral pattern of substance use characterized by overwhelming involvement in the use of a drug, the securing of its supply, and a high tendency to relapse into its use after its withdrawal. Addictions of all kinds are evident in all levels of society and are a major concern in the United States and throughout most of the world. The psychosocial and biogenetic nature of addiction means that a person is influenced by social, psychological, and biogenetic factors toward abuse.

By far the most common substance abused today is food. Tobacco, alcohol, and recreational drugs are also frequently abused. Nursing care of patients with a history of current or past abuse must integrate physiologic, social, emotional, and psychological aspects of care in a planned approach to making the perianesthesia period as safe as possible. Moral judgment or condemnation is not appropriate, particularly if one is to gain trust of the patient and obtain an essential and accurate history. Rather, the nurse must provide adequate information for the patient to make appropriate choices and must incorporate knowledge of the physiologic effects of addicting substances into the plan of care.

Obesity

Obesity is the most common nutritional disorder in the United States. The Centers for Disease Control and Prevention report that in

1997, 54% of adults in the United States were overweight[1] and that 5% were morbidly obese, a risk factor that increases the mortality rate of this group 3.9 times that of a nonobese person. One half of adults in the United States have blood cholesterol levels of greater than the desired 200 mg/dl level. Given the fact that 30% to 40% of coronary heart disease deaths are attributed to obesity and high blood cholesterol and that over 300,000 deaths each year are associated with poor dietary and activity patterns, it would seem that a trend toward healthier weight levels would be evident. However, the opposite is true, with obesity affecting adults, children, and adolescents at an alarming rate. Obesity can have a profound effect on anesthesia outcome. Airway management becomes a challenge, along with ventilatory concerns and altered pharmacokinetic and physiologic responses.

Obesity has been defined in a number of ways. The most common is that of being 20% over ideal body weight. Morbid obesity can be defined as being twice ideal body weight,[2] or 70% to 100% over ideal body weight, or 100 lb over ideal weight. The ambulatory setting may not be the most appropriate setting for the morbidly obese patient because of increased perioperative morbidity and mortality rates in this group.

Obesity is considered a disease with many causes—social, metabolic, physiologic, and psychological. Although increased caloric intake ultimately leads to increased size of adipose tissue cells, the underlying metabolic cause has not been identified. The cerebral cortex controls behaviors such as eating and the hypothalamus controls appetite, but genetic predisposition, physiologic alterations, and psychological factors such as stress, depression, anxiety, fatigue, and loneliness must also be considered.

The increased risks that the obese patient faces with anesthesia and surgery present unique challenges to the nursing staff. Nursing interventions must address a variety of physiologic and emotional needs as well as the mechanical issues of access to the large patient for blood pressure measurements, turning or other care. Medical complications are more likely to be encountered in the obese patient, including hypertension, obstructive sleep apnea, hiatal hernia, certain cancers, osteoarthritis, cholelithiasis, cardiac disease, joint disorders, varicose veins, and cerebral vascular disease. The obese person is twice as likely to have diabetes as a normal weight counterpart.

These and other factors can pose increased risk during anesthesia and surgery. Wound complications, airway challenges including loss of airway control, pulmonary and cardiac dysfunction, and thromboembolism are a few areas at higher risk. In fact, thromboembolism is the leading cause of perioperative death in the morbidly obese population.[3]

Psychological support is important, and nursing interventions should maintain every patient's dignity and sense of self-worth. Examples of caring interventions for the obese patient include ensuring privacy for dressing and for procedures, avoiding asking the obese patient to sit in chairs that are too narrow, providing appropriately sized nightshirts, and allowing the patient to move at his or her own speed.

The literature is full of references to negative attitudes on the part of healthcare providers toward obese patients. In a 1983 study, body weight was surpassed only by skin color as the most stigmatizing physical feature.[4] Schwartz suggests that cultural bias against obese women plays a major role in the origin of their low self-esteem, depression, weight loss and gain, and binge eating.[5] A more recent study of RN students found that a stigma still exists toward thinking about and caring for obese adult patients.[6] Focused discussions at staff meetings may be a way for nurses and other providers to confront personal biases and develop healthy attitudes toward caring for obese patients. The obvious goals are to maintain respectful conversations and a professional, caring relationship with the obese patient and to avoid derogatory comments among staff members.

Physiologic challenges are great, affecting all organ systems. The cardiopulmonary effects can be profound; thus, the nursing plan must address not only the effects of outpatient anesthesia and surgery, but also those effects in the habitus of obesity. Important physiologic changes are listed in Table 25–1. Because cardiovascular changes can be significant, preoperative assessment generally includes an electrocardiogram to identify conduction, ischemic, and ventricular changes that can complicate care.

Respiratory challenges are especially problematic. Metabolic needs relating to the large body mass lead to increased oxygen consumption and carbon dioxide production, which can approach twice the normal values. Concurrent pulmonary and cardiac changes make it difficult for the person to meet those needs. Respiratory rate and effort increase as weight increases, but eventually the patient is not able to keep up

Table 25–1. Physiologic Changes Related to Obesity

CARDIOPULMONARY CHANGES

Large body mass → increased metabolic demand → increased cardiac output
Increased blood volume (although lower percentage of total body weight); blood volume can be as low as 45 ml/kg
Left ventricular hypertrophy/dilatation due to increased stroke volume and work
Hypoxia/hypercapnia → pulmonary vasoconstriction → chronic pulmonary hypertension and right-sided heart failure
Increased risk of arrhythmias due to hypertrophy, hypoxemia, fatty infiltration of cardiac conduction system, use of diuretics, increased incidence of coronary artery disease, increased catecholamines, and sleep apnea
Excess metabolically active adipose tissue with increased workload on supportive muscles → increased oxygen consumption and increased carbon dioxide production
Decreased myocardial compliance (as low as 35% of normal), increased work of breathing and decreased efficiency
Decreased resting functional residual capacity will decrease further with induction

GASTROINTESTINAL CHANGES

Increased incidence of gastroesophageal reflux, hiatal hernias and abdominal pressure → severe risk of aspiration
Fatty liver changes may be present but may not be reflected in liver function tests

Data from Langer R: Anesthesia and the morbidly obese. Accessed via http://www.gasnet.org on Oct. 31, 1999.

with the demand, and hypoventilation and decreased oxygenation result from the following:

- Decreased pulmonary volumes, particularly functional residual capacity
- Elevation of the diaphragm due to large abdominal size
- Chest wall stiffness due to the thick layer of adipose tissue

Increased abdominal mass reduces thoracic cavity expansion, limiting full expansion of the lungs. This reduced capacity means that obese patients have less oxygen reserve to sustain them through periods of apnea, such as during intubation or laryngospasm. The risk of aspiration is also increased because of obesity, and aggressive antiemetic prophylaxis may be indicated (Table 25–2). Additionally, to avoid further respiratory compromise, particularly in the obese patient who may concurrently suffer from sleep apnea, the anesthesia provider often avoids any type of preoperative sedation, although histamine blockers or metaclopromide may be indicated as antiemetics. Intramuscular injections are avoided because of inconsistent absorption. Obstructive sleep apnea syndrome (OSAS) challenges the perioperative nurse not only with potential airway maintenance problems but also with related arrhythmias and possible depressed central control of breathing.[7]

Problems associated with difficult intubation include a short, thick neck, large tongue, and reduced cervical mobility due to adipose tissue. Thus, awake nasotracheal intubation may be chosen to reduce the chance of aspiration. Attentive emotional support by the nurse is important because of the patient's heightened anxiety and discomfort with this procedure. Regional anesthesia may be chosen in an attempt to avoid general anesthesia and airway management challenges, but the potential for airway disaster can still be present. Caregivers must always be prepared to respond to loss of airway and other related emergency interventions in the severely obese patient.

Postoperatively, the most important intervention to prevent aspiration and improve ventilatory capacity is to raise the patient's head. Sitting or standing is the preferred position to enhance cardiopulmonary function. Supine and prone positioning severely compromise the patient's chest expansion. Cautious airway management is also essential in the early postoperative period. Oxygen administration, vigilant nursing observation and lateral positioning are key elements of airway protection. Elevation of the head of the bed is also advised, even when the patient is in a lateral position.

Many anesthetic agents, particularly intravenous agents, are lipophilic. This affinity for fat can prolong the effects such drugs as barbiturates, fentanyl, meperidine, sufentanil, and diazepam, all of which are stored in adipose tissue and metabolized slowly over hours or days.

Table 25–2. Factors Predisposing the Obese Patient to Aspiration

Difficult airway maintenance due to increased neck and chest bulk
Increased gastric volumes and higher acidity of stomach juices*
Increased intra-abdominal pressure
Increased occurrence of hiatal hernias
Inability to rapidly turn or move the unconscious, obese patient
Difficult or impossible intubation leading to mask ventilation

*Data from Vaughn R, Bauer S, Wise L: Volume and pH of gastric juices in obese patients. Anesthesiology 43:686, 1975.

Long-acting agents such as pancuronium and morphine are generally avoided. Prolonged somnolence can increase initial recovery time and discourage activity and exercise in the immediate postoperative period. Early ambulation, deep breathing, and exercise are encouraged in this population that has a predisposition to thrombotic events.

Cardiovascular factors related to obesity include increased cardiac output, increased arterial blood pressure, pulmonary hypertension, increased risk of coronary artery disease, and increased blood volume. These risk factors make it important for nursing care to be planned in a manner that reduces the patient's physical exertion, reduces stress on the heart and lungs, avoids overhydration, and ensures appropriate medication administration that limits excessive sedation. It is important to use the correct size blood pressure cuff to ensure accurate readings. The cuff should be 20% longer than the circumference of the patient's arm and the width should be more than one third the circumference of the arm. A cuff that is too small will overestimate blood pressure readings. The conical shape of the upper arm in some patients may necessitate using the forearm for cuff application.

Other logistic challenges that could be encountered may be difficult intravenous access, securing of adequately sized procedural instrumentation and equipment, and issues of positioning and ambulation. The scheduling physician or the preanesthesia nurse should alert the procedural team as early as possible about unusually large (or small) patients so that appropriate plans can be made and equipment prepared to avoid cancellation or delay of the procedure. A turning sheet or other assistive device should be used to protect the staff from injury when moving the unconscious patient and to assist in rapid repositioning for airway safety should the need arise. Extra personnel and adequate mechanical aids such as blankets, pillows, and other padding are essential. The awake patient should be encouraged to actively move and is usually more comfortable, both physically and emotionally, when able to do so.

Ambulation can be another problem for the obese patient who is required to maintain little or no weight bearing on one lower extremity. A walker may be easier to manage than crutches. Despite the difficulties the patient may face in ambulating, it is essential that the patient do so to reduce the occurrence of pulmonary and venous complications, such as deep vein thrombosis and pulmonary congestion or embolus, that are related to prolonged inactivity. This instruction, along with the others noted in Table 25–3, is a key element of patient education. Aggressive pain management is essential so that the obese patient will be able to adequately move and breathe, and rest periods should be encouraged between strenuous activities.

Table 25–3. Key Education Points for the Obese Patient

Perioperative nutrition to support wound healing
Pulmonary toilet to ensure that respiratory function is optimum prior to elective procedures and to prevent postoperative complications
Measures to prevent thrombosis—hydration, activity, positioning to avoid groin and popliteal pressure
Ambulation—importance and assistive aids
Wound care and reportable symptoms
Maintenance of medication protocols for comorbid conditions
Expectations and rights regarding dignity and privacy

Wound healing is another area of special concern for the obese patient. Subcutaneous fat is relatively avascular, with resulting decreased oxygen delivered to the tissues of the operative site. This predisposes the individual to infection and delayed healing and can lead to wound dehiscence. Meticulous wound care should be stressed, along with proper perioperative nutrition that includes adequate protein, fluids, vitamins, and minerals. Symptoms of infection such as fever, redness, or drainage at the site should be reported to the physician immediately. Patients should be encouraged to take all doses of prescribed antibiotics. The extremely obese patient with severe respiratory limitations has further reduction in oxygenation of tissues and is best monitored in the hospital setting in the early recovery period.

Smoking

Despite the efforts of the medical community and organizations such as the American Heart Association and the American Cancer Society, cigarette smoking remains a significant health threat and is the leading preventable cause of death in the United States. Consider these staggering statistics:

- More than 400,000 annual deaths are attributed to tobacco use.

- Each year smoking kills more people than AIDS, alcohol, drug abuse, automobile accidents, murders, suicides, and fires combined.
- Tobacco use causes about one in every five deaths annually.
- One of every two lifelong smokers will die from smoking.
- Every day, almost 3,000 young people under the age of 18 become regular smokers.
- More than 5 million children living today will die prematurely because of a decision to smoke cigarettes.
- Since the Surgeon General's 1964 report linking smoking to increased death rates, 10 million people in the United States have died from smoking-related causes.
- In 1993 the direct medical costs associated with smoking were estimated at $50 billion, or 7% of the total health care costs in the USA.[8]

Cigarette smoking has been the most popular method of taking nicotine since the beginning of the 20th century. In 1989, the U.S. Surgeon General issued a report that concluded that cigarettes and other forms of tobacco, such as cigars, pipe tobacco, and chewing tobacco, are addictive and that nicotine is the drug in tobacco that causes addiction. In addition, the report determined that smoking was a major cause of stroke and the third leading cause of death in the United States. Despite this warning, about 62 million Americans age 12 and older (29%) are current cigarette smokers, making nicotine one of the most heavily used addictive drugs in the United States.

Respiratory changes associated with smoking include early closure of small airways, paralysis of cilia, chronic increase of secretions, and eventual consolidation or destruction of lung tissue with ensuing chronic obstructive pulmonary disease and cancer. Vital capacity and functional reserve are reduced and eventually oxygenation of body tissues is compromised.

Chronic smoking results in 10% to 15% reduction in functional hemoglobin concentration.[9] The carbon monoxide in cigarette smoke attaches to hemoglobin, producing carboxyhemoglobin, which is ineffective in carrying oxygen to the tissues. Unfortunately, carboxyhemoglobin can produce falsely high oxygen saturation readings by pulse oximetry, so alternative methods of clinical assessment must be considered in conjunction with oxygen saturation levels.

Discontinuation of smoking for 12 to 18 hours preoperatively can result in significant reduction in carboxyhemoglobin, freeing up hemoglobin for the essential task of tissue oxygenation. Cessation of smoking for that short a period does not reverse other negative effects of smoking such as increased sputum production, chronic irritation of the tracheobronchial tree, and ciliary paralysis in the airways. Bronchospasm can be extreme and, in rare patients, intractable, leading to death.

The cardiovascular effects of smoking are equally dangerous. Nicotine is a potent vasoconstrictor that leads to increased heart rate, arterial hypertension, and reduced peripheral and coronary blood flow. Smoking has recently joined hypercholesterolemia and hypertension as the three major risk factors for coronary artery disease. The risk of myocardial infarction is twice as high in smokers as nonsmokers, and those who smoke have two to four times the chance of sudden cardiac death.

Other potential effects of smoking include many types of cancer, diffuse peripheral vascular disease, aortic aneurysm, cerebral vascular accident, liver enzyme induction, and gastrointestinal disease such as peptic ulcer and esophageal reflux. Cutaneous blood flow is reduced, contributing to poor tissue oxygenation and delayed wound healing.

Important preoperative education includes encouraging the patient to avoid smoking for 12 to 18 hours before surgery. Owing to the addictive nature of cigarette smoking, this instruction may or may not be followed, especially during this time of heightened stress related to the upcoming procedure. Encouraging the patient to do the best he or she can to reduce smoking is probably a more reasonable expectation and may result in better compliance. Preoperative assessment should include auscultation of the chest, careful history taking, and sometimes chest radiography or pulmonary function testing. The anesthesia provider and the nurse plan care based on current pulmonary status and the projected potential for complications.

Stormy emergence from general anesthesia, a higher than usual likelihood of pulmonary complications such as laryngospasm and bronchospasm, and prolonged PACU (postanesthesia care unit) stay are frequent postoperative outcomes for smokers. Spasmodic coughing can be detrimental to the patient's respiratory function as well as to the integrity and comfort of the surgical site. To reduce the chance of serious pulmonary complications, breathing exercises and adequate activity should be encouraged after the procedure.

The nursing contact with all patients in the

ambulatory surgery setting is an opportunity to provide general health education, and this one should not be missed in providing information to the patient about the health value of stopping smoking altogether. Table 17–3 provides some useful Internet sites with information to help patients who want to stop smoking. Because smoking contributes to both respiratory sequelae and delayed wound healing, the patient should be instructed to delay resumption of smoking for as long as possible during the early recovery stage. Special wound care attention should be encouraged to prevent infection and to encourage healing.

In light of the vast body of information about the negative effects of smoking, both from primary and secondary smoke, coupled with the increased cost of providing health care to employees who smoke, many health care facilities and campuses are designated as nonsmoking areas. This policy contributes to a more aesthetically pleasing environment, addresses the health of employees, and sends a positive health message to visitors, patients, and staff. The nurse is a very visible healthcare professional who is looked upon as a role model regarding health practices.

Drug and Alcohol Abuse

The use of alcohol and recreational and prescription drugs is widespread in our society and crosses all socioeconomic, age, and other demographic lines. Concerns related to the effects of anesthesia and surgery on the addict or abuser center on the following:

1. How the long-term metabolic effects of the substance have altered the body's normal reaction to anesthetic drugs
2. Whether acute intoxication exists at the time of surgery
3. The patient's level of compliance with pre- and postoperative instructions and restrictions[10]
4. The patient's general state of health

Although chronic substance abuse does not necessarily preclude anesthesia and surgery, healthcare professionals should be aware of the patient's substance history so that care can be planned in relation to the potential associated complications. A private, nonjudgmental interview may help to elicit honest answers from the abuser during the preoperative assessment. Information gleaned should be shared confidentially with only those health professionals who will take care of the patient in order to protect the person's privacy. A healthy skepticism is warranted during this information-gathering period because total honesty about current and recent drug use is not likely to be forthcoming from the patient.

Acute intoxication or recent substance ingestion demands cancellation or delay of elective or nonurgent procedures due to the abnormal and potentially harmful responses to anesthesia administration, for instance untoward cardiovascular and autonomic effects.[11] Any suspicion of current intoxication should be relayed to the anesthesiologist prior to the patient being transferred to surgery. Signs include, but are not limited to, slurred speech, disorientation, dysphoria, agitation, combativeness, inappropriate verbal responses, grogginess, pupillary constriction, and the smell of alcohol on the breath. Recent ingestion of hallucinogens such as LSD and mescaline can result in pupillary dilatation, nausea, anxiety, and reflex activity. Amphetamines can produce sweating, tachycardia, hypertension, hyperactive bowel sounds and increased motor activity.[12]

Depression, fatigue, and altered self-concept often plagues the addicted person, and noncompliance with instructions is common. Great tact and diplomacy are needed to secure cooperation with appropriate behavior such as refraining from substance ingestion and driving in the early recovery period. Family relationships may be strained, and the nurse may have to negotiate issues regarding care that would otherwise fall to the family support system. Furthermore, withdrawal symptoms are possible in as little as 8 hours after cessation of alcohol intake, and thus the potential for associated symptoms is considerable, even in an ambulatory surgery setting.

Pain management becomes a challenge for patients who have a variety of concurrent chemical dependencies. Chronic use of alcohol, narcotics, and other drugs results in a permanent induction of liver enzymes used in the metabolism of these substances. Even a former alcoholic who has not consumed alcohol for many years will have residual enzyme induction. As a result, larger-than-usual doses of sedatives and analgesics are needed to produce effective results.

The right to adequate pain relief is not relinquished by the person who has a substance abuse problem, and the provision of that comfort rests in the hands and creativity of the healthcare providers. Limiting or withholding pain medication results in needless suffering.

This quandary over the prescription of powerful pain relievers continues while investigators search for new ways to control pain. Researchers funded by the National Institute on Drug Abuse are spearheading the exploration for new pain killers that are effective but nonaddicting.

In recent years research has shown that doctors' fears that patients will become addicted to pain medication are largely unfounded. Studies indicate that most patients who receive opioids for pain, even those undergoing long-term therapy, do not become addicted to these drugs. The very few patients who develop rapid and marked tolerance and addiction to opioids are usually those who have a history of psychological problems or prior substance abuse.

One study found that only 4 out of over 12,000 patients who were given opioids for acute pain actually became addicted to the drugs. Even long-term therapy has limited potential for addiction. In a study of 38 chronic pain patients, most of whom received opioids for 4 to 7 years, only 2 patients actually became addicted, and both had a history of drug abuse.[13]

Organic changes associated with chronic substance abuse complicate medical management. Table 25–4 lists a number of systemic complications associated with chronic alcohol and drug abuse. Postoperative instructions should emphasize the potential danger of combining drugs or alcohol with the lingering sedative and depressant effects of anesthetic and adjunctive agents. Good nutrition should be encouraged to assist in the healing process including the prevention of wound infection.

The healthcare worker should consider the personal risks associated with caring for patients who have a high potential for illicit intravenous drug use and whose associated social behaviors may place them at increased risk for infectious disease. Standard precautions are designed to protect personnel and others from personal exposure to blood and body fluids that may pose a threat to health.

Alcohol

According to the National Council on Alcoholism and Drug Dependence, more than 13 million Americans abuse alcohol. The widespread use of alcohol is the result of many factors, most notably its availability and social acceptance. Many factors contribute to alcohol dependence and include personality characteristics, stress, family environment, heredity, and the addictive nature of alcohol. Drinking among U.S. workers can threaten public safety, impair job performance, and result in costly medical, social, and other problems. Productivity losses attributable to alcohol were estimated at $119 billion in 1995 alone.

As the elderly population increases in size, it

***Table 25–4.* Complications Associated with Chronic Substance Abuse**

DEFICIENCY/DEFECT	PHYSIOLOGIC EFFECT
Alcohol	
Malnutrition/vitamin deficiency	Delayed wound healing, peripheral neuropathy, electrolyte disturbances
Blood dyscrasias: Anemia, Prolonged prothrombin time, Altered platelet function, Bone marrow depression	Bleeding, delayed wound healing, respiratory challenge to provide adequate tissue oxygenation
Hepatic dysfunction: Cirrhosis/hepatitis, Vitamin K deficiency	Bleeding, altered drug metabolism, diminished reserve against infection
Cardiac changes: Conduction defects, Cardiomyopathy	Arrhythmias, conduction defects, diminished cardiac reserve, heart failure
Organic brain syndrome	Seizures, psychoses, personality disorders
Illicit/Recreational Drugs	
Cardiorespiratory dysfunction	Arrhythmias, respiratory depression, chronic aspiration pneumonia, pulmonary emboli, pulmonary edema
Exposure to blood-borne infections	Septic emboli, septicemia, AIDS, hepatitis, osteomyelitis, endocarditis
Alternative social behavior	Sexually transmitted diseases, noncompliant personality, lethargy, sedative effects

will be increasingly important to adequately assess for alcohol consumption and its related health implications. Many surveys of the general public suggest that people over 65 ingest less alcohol than younger counterparts. However, surveys in healthcare settings find increasing prevalence of alcoholism in the elderly. From 6% to 11% of elderly people admitted to hospitals exhibit signs of alcoholism, as do 20% of those admitted to psychiatric hospitals and 14% presenting in emergency rooms. Social drinking in adult retirement communities may result in late onset alcohol problems. Healthcare providers are significantly less likely to recognize alcoholism in an older patient than in younger ones.[14]

Alcohol has the most far-reaching and direct physiologic effects on organ systems of all substances discussed in this chapter. Although research has shown an association between moderate alcohol consumption and lowered risk for coronary heart disease, many other negative effects outweigh that potentially positive effect. Many organs are adversely and permanently affected by alcohol. Destruction of cortical brain tissue leads to dementia and personally changes. Cardiomyopathy is the most common cardiac occurrence, and anemia, malnutrition, and ulcerative gastrointestinal disease also occur. Esophageal reflux predisposes the alcoholic patient to aspiration. Liver cells are destroyed with each ingestion. Although liver cells regenerate, eventually they become sclerosed. Cirrhosis and ascites follow, with loss of hepatic functions, such as coagulation and drug metabolism. In advanced cases, esophageal varies may occur, predisposing the patient to acute hemorrhage during intubation and placement of airways or gastric tubes.

Many alcoholic patients tend to underreport or deny the amount of alcohol they consume. Some physical manifestations that might indicate chronic alcohol use include spider veins on the face, hand tremors, and a reddened, bulbous nose. A number of serum enzymes can be ordered to assess hepatic function, but simple and reliable indicators are the prothrombin time (PT) and partial thromboplastin time (PTT) because coagulation is one of the first functions to be affected by cirrhotic changes when production of the proteins needed for clotting is diminished.

Illicit Drug Use

A plethora of drugs exist that continue to exert their effects on the health and welfare of Americans. Cocaine, heroin, narcotics, anabolic steroids, hallucinogens, marijuana, stimulants, Ecstasy, methamphetamines, phencyclidine (PCP), lysergic acid diethylamide (LSD), and inhalants all extract a huge financial, social, physical, and psychological toll. ASC nurses will very likely continue to have increased encounters with drug-using patients. Unfortunately, the drug use behaviors of many of these patients will be unspoken and can remain unknown to the healthcare team, creating an environment of even higher risk to those patients. Great vigilance and conscious attention to potential signs and symptoms are essential. The challenge to provide nonjudgmental, professional care is omnipresent. The following discussion includes some of the more prevalent substances that will be encountered in the ASC population.

Narcotics

Illicit use of narcotics such as heroin, morphine, and codeine is prevalent throughout all parts of the country; however, substances such as crack cocaine may be easier to secure and less expensive. A 1996 study[66] (National Household Survey on Drug Abuse) showed a significant increase from 1993 in the estimated number of current heroin users, with the term "current" being defined as use in the past month of the survey. The estimates have risen from 68,000 in 1993 to 216,000 in 1996. The abuse problem crosses all socioeconomic lines, and the ASC nurse must consider not only the recreational drug user, but also the many patients regularly taking prescribed narcotics for chronic pain and cancer pain.

Heroin abuse is associated with acute overdose, spontaneous abortion, collapsed veins, and infectious diseases. Postinjection euphoria is accompanied by warm flushing of the skin, dry mouth, and heavy extremities. After this initial euphoria, the user goes "on the nod," into an alternately wakeful and drowsy state. Mental function becomes clouded owing to CNS depression. Withdrawal symptoms include drug craving, restlessness, muscle and bone pain, insomnia, diarrhea and vomiting, cold flashes, and other symptoms. Even though sudden withdrawal can prove fatal, heroin withdrawal is still considered much less dangerous than alcohol or barbiturate withdrawal. Chapter 38 includes a discussion of a new procedure for controlled medical withdrawal from opiates with anesthesia oversight.

Chronic narcotic use does not cause primary organ damage like alcohol. Rather, complications result from the techniques of administration. An example is pulmonary embolism due to drug impurities or injection of air intravenously. Infections such as phlebitis, subacute bacterial endocarditis, pulmonary abscess, hepatitis, AIDS, and septicemia occur from use of contaminated needles and inappropriate social activities that sometimes surround the use and acquisition of these drugs. Overdose is another related complication.

Opiates are drugs that come from the opium poppy plant, and opioids are drugs that affect the opiate receptors in the brain. Opioids can be synthetic drugs such as fentanyl and meperidine, and may be agonists or antagonists to these receptors. Effects of these drugs include respiratory depression, analgesia, sedation, and pupillary constriction. Such effects can be additive with anesthetics and other perioperative drugs.

The perioperative period is not an appropriate time to withhold narcotics from the habitual user because a serious or even fatal withdrawal episode can occur. Larger-than-usual doses of pain medications are needed to provide adequate pain relief. Agonist/antagonist drugs such as nalbuphine and butorphanol should be avoided in this population because they can precipitate acute withdrawal symptoms. Regional anesthetics, wound infiltration, and nonsteroidal anti-inflammatory drugs may be helpful supplements to pain management.

One of the more common perioperative complications associated with chronic narcotic use is noncardiogenic pulmonary edema. A definitive cause has not yet been determined, but theories suggest that it may occur as a result of anaphylaxis or heart failure from an overdose of quinine, which is used to mix heroin. Pulmonary endothelial damage, hypoxemia, hypotension, and neurogenic causes also must be considered.[15] Treatment is discussed in Chapter 11.

Cocaine

Cocaine is a physiologically dangerous drug and its abuse is widespread in the United States. Cocaine continues to dominate the nation's illicit drug problems. In 1996, about 1.7 million Americans were current (at least once per month) cocaine users. This number accounts for about 0.8% of the population age 12 and older. About 668,000 of these used crack. The rate of current cocaine use in 1996 was highest among Americans ages 18 to 25 (2%). The rate of use for this age group was significantly higher in 1996 than in 1995, when it was 1.3%. These staggering statistics from the National Institute on Drug Abuse make it very clear that cocaine is abundantly available throughout the USA. ASC nurses are caring for many known and unknown cocaine users, and that care must center on scrupulous assessment and attention to symptoms that may herald significant risk in the perioperative period.

Not a narcotic, cocaine is a local anesthetic that exerts a significant effect on the pleasure center of the brain. Cocaine is a strong central nervous system stimulant that interferes with the reabsorption process of dopamine, a chemical messenger associated with pleasure and movement. Dopamine is released as part of the brain's reward system and is involved in the high that characterizes cocaine consumption. Physical effects of cocaine use include constricted peripheral blood vessels, dilated pupils, and increased temperature, heart rate, and blood pressure. Euphoria, hyperstimulation, reduced fatigue, and mental clarity are the effects that the abuser experiences. Some users of cocaine report feelings of restlessness, irritability, and anxiety. In rare cases, sudden death can occur on the first use of cocaine or unexpectedly with subsequent use. However, there is no way to determine who is prone to sudden death.

High doses of cocaine or prolonged use can trigger paranoia. Smoking crack cocaine can produce a particularly aggressive paranoid behavior in users. When addicted individuals stop using cocaine, they often become depressed. This also may lead to further cocaine use to alleviate depression. Prolonged cocaine snorting can result in ulceration of the mucous membrane of the nose and can damage the nasal septum enough to cause it to collapse. Thus, intubation, extubation, suctioning, and insertion of gastric tubes can pose the threat of hemorrhage.

Cardiovascular complications of cocaine abuse include tachycardia, aortic vasoconstriction, myocardial ischemia, and acute myocardial infarction. Cocaine-related deaths are often a result of cardiac arrest or seizures followed by respiratory arrest. Sudden death secondary to ventricular fibrillation can occur in young, otherwise healthy people from the sudden adrenalin rush from cocaine use. Cocaine can cause coronary artery spasm or thrombosis even in people with normal coronary arteries. Ventricular fibrillation and asystole can result from cocaine's direct action on the myocardium or from alterations in catecholamine production. Toxic depressant effects on the cardiac conduction system can result in cardiac arrest that is extremely difficult, if not impossible, to reverse.

Cerebral vasoconstriction or subarachnoid bleeding can result in a cardiovascular accident (CVA). Severe hypertension occurring from stimulation of α- and β-adrenergic receptors is treated with esmolol, nitroprusside, or a combination of phentolamine and a β-blocking agent to reduce blood pressure and slow heart rate. Cardiovascular side effects can be potentiated in the perianesthesia period by the concurrent administration of epinephrine or aminophylline.

A lowered seizure threshold with resulting muscle twitching and convulsions is treated with diazepam, phenobarbital, and phenytoin. Cocaine-induced pulmonary complications include reduced pulmonary function, bronchospasm, and pulmonary edema. Hepatotoxicity, muscle tissue damage resulting in renal damage, and memory and judgment challenges are all potential side effects. Table 25–5 provides key points in anesthetic management of cocaine users.

Anabolic Steroids

Anabolic steroids are synthetic derivatives of the male hormone testosterone that promote the growth of skeletal muscle and increase lean body mass. Athletes and others abuse anabolic steroids to enhance performance and also to improve physical appearance. In recent years there has been a significant increase in use by females.

Anabolic steroids are taken orally or injected, and athletes and other abusers take them typically in cycles of weeks or months, rather than continuously. Reports indicate that use of anabolic steroids increases lean muscle mass, strength, and ability to train longer and harder. Long-term, high-dose effects of steroid use are largely unknown. Many health hazards of short-term effects are reversible. In addition, people who inject anabolic steroids run the additional risk of contracting or transmitting hepatitis or HIV, which leads to AIDS.

The major side effects of anabolic steroid use include liver tumors, jaundice, fluid retention, high blood pressure, and unhealthy cholesterol changes. Severe acne and trembling can occur. Additional side effects include the following:

- For men: shrinking of the testicles, reduced sperm count, infertility, baldness, development of breasts
- For women: growth of facial hair, changes in or cessation of the menstrual cycle, enlargement of the clitoris, deepened voice
- For adolescents: growth halted prematurely through premature skeletal maturation and accelerated puberty changes

Aggression and other psychiatric side effects may result from anabolic steroid abuse, including wild mood swings and manic symptoms leading to violent, even homicidal, episodes.[16]

The ASC nurse has good reason to identify patients taking steroids. The chronic use of steroids suppresses the natural cortisone production in the adrenal cortex, leading to the inability to demonstrate an adequate response to the stress of surgery and anesthesia. Body builders and well-developed athletic individuals should be questioned directly about the use of steroids in a nonjudgmental manner that focuses on the safety of the patient in the perioperative period. The anesthesia provider may choose to provide intravenous steroid coverage for this individual during the perioperative period.

Table 25–5. Anesthetic Management of Cocaine User

System review, including an electrocardiogram
Sympathetic nervous system stimulation:
  hypertension and tachycardia
  Avoid use of phenylephrine and ephedrine
  Selective β_1-antagonist: esmolol
  Direct vasodilator: nitroprusside
  Nitroglycerine for coronary vasoconstriction
Cautious use of halogenated agents
Barbiturates, nitrous oxide, opioids

From Culver J, Walker J: Anesthetic implications of illicit drug use. JOPAN 14:86, 1999.

THE PATIENT USING HERBAL SUPPLEMENTS

The use of alternative medicine practices has risen sharply in the past few years. Believing that the body is naturally inclined toward health and has the capacity to heal itself when given the proper natural therapies like exercise and herbal supplements, many people incorporate the use of herbs, homeopathic medicines, massage, meditation, and acupuncture into their daily routines. Herbalism is the therapeutic use of plants containing various chemicals as pain relievers, hormone balancers, calmers, energizers, sleep aids, stomach soothers, and general tonics.[17] Comparing the data from 1990 to 1997, one study identified a 380% increase in the use herbal remedies among several thousand respondents.[18] In fact, Americans spent an estimated $1 billion on herbal products in 1993,[19] and estimates of up to $5 billion were projected for herbal sales in 1999.

Although herbs are natural, they often act like other medications and may potentiate or otherwise interact with prescription and other medications being used. It is estimated that up to 70% of herbal medicine users do not tell their physicians about the products that they are taking. Consumers should be made aware that natural does not necessarily mean safe, and that a physician should supervise the use of herbal remedies just like prescription medications. As dietary supplements, many herbal products are not scrutinized or regulated by any government agencies in regard to their effectiveness, potency, ingredients, or safety. In fact, products may contain little or none of the ingredient claimed. Although some have been scientifically researched and found to have some benefits, many herbs have no proven positive effects and some have been shown to be harmful.[20] Some effects are thought to be placebo in origin.

In addition to their ability to affect the body's metabolic and chemical mechanisms, herbs can also interact with anesthetics and other drugs given during the perioperative time, thus it is important for the perianesthesia nurse to carefully elicit a thorough history of herbal use during the preoperative assessment. Although the American Society of Anesthesiologists does not take a formal position on herbal remedies, it does warn patients to stop taking any herbal products several weeks prior to having surgery. If time does not allow this discontinuation, patients should bring the original containers of herbs to the facility to show the anesthesiologist.[21] Educating staff members at the referring physicians' offices can help them understand and convey to patients the need to refrain from taking herbal supplements prior to surgery, thus providing a larger window of opportunity to clear the herbs out of their system.

Patients should be specifically queried about the use of vitamins, minerals, and herbal supplements. Similarly, postoperative instructions from the physician should include information on when medications, including herbal supplements, can be resumed safely. If the patient indicates the use of a potentially harmful herb, the perianesthesia nurse has an opportunity for patient education that may prove very important in the patient's overall future health. Table 25–6 lists a number of herbal supplements along with their intended uses and potential side effects.

***Table 25–6.* Common Herbal Remedies and Potential Effects**

HERB AND ACTIVE INGREDIENT	PROMOTED USES AND CLAIMED BENEFITS (UNPROVED)	CLINICAL TRIALS AND OUTCOMES	POTENTIAL SIDE EFFECTS/ CONTRAINDICATIONS
Comfrey	Treat pulmonary disorders, sprains, boils, and skin ulcers		Harmful to liver; in fact, roots contain world's richest source of hepatotoxin
Ginkgo biloba (flavonoids, terpenoids, organic acids)	Treat vascular disease, memory improvement, increase blood circulation, reduce peripheral claudication, potent antioxidant	Modest improvement in cognition and social functioning in Alzheimer's patients; reduced pain of claudication and increased ability to walk	Generally safe and well tolerated; may reduce platelets and affect clotting—do not use concurrent with antithrombotic agents; minor gastrointestinal distress, rare headache or dizziness, asthma
St. John's wort (hypericin)	Treat anxiety, mild depression, and sleep disorders (widely prescribed in Germany), MAO-like effect	One study found the herb to be 2.7 times more effective for mild depression than placebo	Reasonably safe, but may cause dry mouth, dizziness, fatigue, constipation, nausea, and photosensitivity; avoid use with selective serotonin reuptake inhibitors and MAOIs—synergistic effects; may intensify sedation effects of narcotics and anesthetic agents

Table 25–6. Common Herbal Remedies and Potential Effects *Continued*

HERB AND ACTIVE INGREDIENT	PROMOTED USES AND CLAIMED BENEFITS (UNPROVED)	CLINICAL TRIALS AND OUTCOMES	POTENTIAL SIDE EFFECTS/ CONTRAINDICATIONS
Echinacea (daisy family)	Boost immune system response, prevention and treatment of upper respiratory viral infections, supportive measure for urinary tract infection and superficial wound application	None proved; clinical trials for upper respiratory tract infections showed no significant effect compared to placebo	Little is known of toxicity and effects; possible anaphylaxis, may exacerbate immune system dysfunction
Garlic (allicin)	Potential to lower serum lipids and control hypertension	Reduction of total cholesterol in one study by 12% compared to placebo; little effect on high blood pressure found during studies	Basically benign except for halitosis, unproved reports of predisposition to postoperative bleeding
Ginger (zingiber officinale)	Treat nausea, vomiting, vertigo, and motion sickness; reduced risk of gastric cancer	One trial showed decreased postoperative nausea after major gynecologic surgery; another study showed some improvement in vertigo as compared to placebo	Minimal; can increase bleeding, so avoid with oral anticoagulant therapy
Ephedra (ma huang)	Contains ephedrine; used as bronchodilator, sympathetic nervous system stimulant, and weight loss product; combined with other products it is marketed as "herbal fen-phen"; also compounded with other products to form "herbal ecstasy" to provide a "natural high"		Considered dangerous; excessive doses often present in products; linked to hundreds of adverse effects and at least 38 deaths; adrenergic effects on heart and blood vessels lead to hypertension and tachycardia
Ginseng	Improve body's resistance to stress, increase vitality, energy, lower cholesterol, treat impotence, elevate mood	Some studies confirm benefits to reduce cholesterol and fasting blood glucose levels None proved regarding vitality	Sleeplessness, hypertension, tachycardia Wide variation in product concentrations of active ingredients; associated with estrogenic effects and vaginal bleeding and painful breasts
Saw palmetto	Diuretic properties, treatment of benign prostatic hyperplasia (BPH)	Antiandrogenic—reduces BPH; may have some benefit in prostatic cancer, but more studies needed	Deep venous thrombosis, gastrointestinal disturbances, male breast enlargement, arrhythmias

Note: Of the vast body of information about herbal preparations, little has been scientifically proved; thus, it is important to weigh the potential, unproved benefits against the potential risks.

Data taken from the following sources:

American Society of Anesthesiologists: Anesthesiologists' warning: If you're taking herbal products, tell your doctor before surgery. Public Education as accessed via www.asahq.org on Nov. 7, 1999.

Glisson J, Crawford R, Street S: The clinical applications of gingko biloba, St. John's Wort, saw palmetto, and soy. Nurse Practitioner 24(6):28, 31, 35, 36, 38, 43–49, 1999.

Lerner J: Herbal therapy: There are risks. RN 60(8):53–54, 1997.

Maclay P: Herbal medicine—what you don't know can hurt you. Presentation to the 30th annual Seminar for Perianesthesia Personnel, Florida Society of Perianesthesia Nurses, Orlando, Oct. 26, 1999.

Murphy J: Preoperative considerations with herbal medicines. AORN J 69:73–83, 1999.

Ness J, Sherman F, Pan C: Alternative medicine: What the data say about common herbal therapies. Geriatrics 54:33–43, 1999.

THE PREGNANT PATIENT

During pregnancy women may undergo surgery for delivery or termination of the pregnancy or for any number of nonobstetric causes. The anatomic and physiologic changes that occur throughout pregnancy contribute to the complex decision to perform elective or emergency surgery on a pregnant woman and the decision as to what type of anesthesia and medications to administer. Nursing care throughout the perianesthesia period must consider both the mother and fetus in all care decisions. Forming collaborative relationships with obstetric nurses can help perianesthesia nurses to increase their knowledge and understanding of and their responses to the unique needs of this patient population.[22]

Abdominal surgery during early pregnancy has been associated with spontaneous abortion,[23] but in later months preterm labor is likely, probably due to manipulation of the uterus. One study of 5405 women showed the incidence of premature birth to be 46% higher in women who underwent surgery during pregnancy when compared with those who did not.[24] In general, whenever possible, elective surgical intervention should be postponed until the postpartum period, when maternal anatomy and physiology has returned to normal.

Surgical intervention during pregnancy is sometimes necessary. The most common problem reported for pregnant woman is the "acute abdomen," generally associated with acute appendicitis. Gallbladder and biliary tract diseases are also common.[25] Other reasons for surgical intervention include blunt trauma to the abdomen, torsion or rupture of ovarian cysts, breast tumors, ectopic pregnancy, placenta previa, abruptio placentae, and uterine rupture. Ectopic pregnancy is a life-threatening condition encountered during the first trimester that requires surgical intervention.

Anatomic changes affect all aspects of the pregnant woman's physiology: the cardiovascular, respiratory, gastrointestinal, renal, and other systems. Table 25–7 provides a synopsis of those changes. The perianesthesia nurse must incorporate this knowledge into the care of the pregnant patient.

Whatever the reason for surgical intervention, there are legal and ethical considerations prior to surgery. Pregnancy should be ruled out for any woman of childbearing age who is scheduled to undergo an elective procedure. Preoperative diagnostic testing for pregnancy should be considered for all women of childbearing age according to facility policies

***Table 25–7.* Physiologic Changes in the Pregnant Patient**

INTEGUMENTARY SYSTEM
Reddish streaks on abdomen and thighs
Palmar erythema
Vascular spiders on face and upper chest
CENTRAL NERVOUS SYSTEM
40% decrease in inhalation anesthetic requirements
40% decrease in spinal/epidural anesthetic requirements
Increased neurosensitivity to local anesthetics
BLOOD
Increased coagulation factors except XI and XIII
ENDOCRINE
Increased thyroid activity
REPRODUCTIVE TRACT
Increased uterine blood flow
Increased size and weight
RESPIRATORY SYSTEM
40% increase in tidal volume
15% increase in respiratory rate
20% increase in oxygen consumption
Increased Pa_{O_2} by 5–10 mm Hg
Decreased Pa_{CO_2} to about 32 mm Hg
30% decrease in compliance
35% decrease in resistance
Nasal and respiratory tract mucosa becomes edematous and hyperemic
CARDIOVASCULAR SYSTEM
35–40% increase in blood volume in single fetus pregnancy
Increased plasma volume from 40 to 70 ml/kg
Increased RBC volume from 25 to 30 ml/kg (lesser rate than plasma—explains anemia of pregnancy)
30–50% increase in cardiac output
15% increase in heart rate
15% decrease in peripheral vascular resistance
RENAL SYSTEM
50–60% increase in glomerular filtration rate
50–60% increase in renal blood flow
Increased creatinine clearance
40% decrease in BUN and creatinine
Increased incidence of urinary tract infections due to pressure on ureters, thus urinary stasis
GASTROINTESTINAL SYSTEM
Decreased gastric emptying
Decreased gastric pH
Increased gastric reflux due to incompetence gastric reflex
HEPATIC SYSTEM
Hepatic blood flow shows little or no change
Liver function tests abnormal, but no evidence of altered liver function
Anesthetic agents metabolized in liver over same duration

Data taken from the following:

Fullerton J: Surgery during pregnancy. Semin Periop Nurs 8(3):101–108, 1999.

Litwack K: Practical points in the care of the obstetric surgical patient. JOPAN 5(3):183, 1990.

Odom J: Pre, intra, and post-operative special needs patient. Specialty Learning Labs Learningbook. Pittsburgh: RTN HealthCareGroup, 1997, 28.

and the clinical judgment of the attending physicians. The most common test is a qualitative hCG (human chorionic gonadatropin) level. β-hCG is detectable in the mother's blood and urine within 8 to 9 days after conception. When a pregnant woman is scheduled to undergo a surgical procedure, informed consent must include consideration of fetal risks, many of which are unknown or, at best, speculative.

The administration of anesthesia and analgesic agents is also of concern, and consideration should be given to the possibility that certain agents are teratogenic. A diverse and varied menu of inhalation agents, muscle relaxants, maintenance agents, antiemetics, and narcotic antagonists have been used. During the first trimester, thiopental, muscle relaxants, and narcotics are considered safe, although regional or local anesthesia remains the first choice of anesthesiologists for the patient in her first trimester. The safety of nitrous oxide, benzodiazepines, and inhalation agents is more controversial.[26] When administering medications, the lowest effective dose is preferred.

Nursing considerations must be clearly defined and implemented for the safety of the patient and fetus. Table 25–8 lists important goals of nursing care. Intraoperatively and during the immediate postoperative period, auscultation of the fetal heart is recommended after the 16th week of gestation,[27] using either a hand-held fetal stethoscope or Doppler device or continuous electronic monitoring. The normal fetal heart rate averages between 120 and 160 beats/min. A rate over 180 or under 100 beats per minute is considered markedly abnormal and demands immediate attention.[28]

In the PACU, pregnant or immediate postpartum patients must be critically observed for embolic events and other potential complications, including signs of premature labor. The following symptoms should be reported to the physician immediately: significant changes in fetal heart rate, contractions, and unexpected vaginal drainage. Oxygen administration is indicated when abrupt changes in fetal heart are present. Interventions to halt premature labor include intravenous hydration, oxygenation, and the administration of tocolytic agents to halt contractions.[21]

Although anesthetic recovery is similar to that for any patient, several additional issues should be addressed. Positioning the patient in a left lateral tilt position reduces the pressure of the uterus on the mother's vena cava. Such pressure, left unaddressed, can lead to reduced maternal afterload, resulting in maternal hypotension and a decrease in uterine blood flow leading to decreased placental perfusion and decreased fetal oxygenation.[29] Fetal monitoring as appropriate and constant emotional support are other specific postanesthesia interventions for this group of patients. Pain management requires judicious use of medications after diversion and general comfort measures are employed.

The emotional and social aspects of the pregnant patient's care cannot be overstated. Not only is the pregnant woman often fearful for the safety of her unborn child, but she may also be dealing with guilt relating to the need for surgery. However illogical that guilt may be to the nurse, it may be very real to the mother. Physiologic discomfort and pain may accompany psychological and emotional trauma, complicating the woman's normal coping strategies. Emotional support, privacy and caring attention are particularly important for the woman whose pregnancy is terminated either purposefully or due to unexpected complications. The presence of a supporting adult, particularly the baby's father, is paramount and should be encouraged during all possible phases of care.

Table 25–8. Goals for the Pregnant Patient Undergoing Surgery and Anesthesia

1. Protect the mother
   - Maintain maternal oxygenation and perfusion
   - Protect the mother's airway during intubation
   - Maintain normotension
2. Maintain uterine blood flow
   - Maintain adequate maternal perfusion
   - Avoid placing patient supine (left lying removes uterine pressure on mother's vena cava)
3. Maintain fetal oxygenation
   - Fetal monitoring to detect fetal distress secondary to hypoxemia
4. Avoid teratogenic drugs
   - Ideal is to avoid any anesthetic exposure during pregnancy, especially during first trimester
   - Most data are anecdotal concerning anesthetic exposure during pregnancy
5. Prevent preterm labor
   - Risk of preterm labor greater than fetal anomalies
   - Preterm labor due to surgical disease rather than either surgery or anesthesia technique
   - 8.8% of women who have surgery while pregnant develop preterm labor

Adapted from Litwack K: Post Anesthesia Care Nursing. St. Louis, MO: Mosby, 1995, p 379.

The assessment and management of the pregnant patient requires a complete understanding of the anatomic and physiologic variations that accompany pregnancy. Ambulatory surgical nurses play a key role in providing care to this segment of the population. Nurses who are skilled and knowledgeable in the care of the pregnant patient will help to assure positive outcomes.

CARDIOVASCULAR DISEASE

Cardiovascular disease (CVD) claimed 953,110 lives in the United States in 1997, a staggering 41.2% of all deaths, or 1 of every 2.4 deaths. CVD was about 60% of the total mention mortality rate in 1997, which means that of the more than 2 million deaths from all causes, CVD was listed as a primary or contributing cause in about 1.4 million death certificates. Coronary artery disease remains the leading cause of death in the United States for those 40 years and over (Table 25–9).

- Since 1900, CVD has been the number 1 killer in the United States in every year but one (1918).
- More than 2,600 Americans die each day of CVD, for an average of 1 death every 33 seconds.
- CVD claims more lives each year than the next seven leading causes of death combined.
- About one-sixth of people killed by CVD are under age 65.

The ASC sees many patients with various levels of cardiovascular compromise. The most common CV diseases encountered in the ASC setting include coronary artery disease, hypertension, congestive heart failure, artificial pacemakers, and arrhythmias. To be considered an appropriate candidate for the ambulatory approach, these patients should be under adequate medical control, because perioperative cardiac mortality is the number one cause of death following general anesthesia and surgery.[31] The challenge for the staff is to identify the people at increased perianesthesia risk so as to maintain or improve their status and avoid related complications in the perioperative period. Complications of hypertensive disease include aortic aneurysm, aortic dissection, central hemorrhage, congestive heart failure, cardiomegaly, left ventricular hypertrophy, renal failure, and retinopathy. Atherosclerosis with its associated coronary artery disease predisposes the patient to ischemic changes, which include angina, myocardial infarction, and sudden death.[32]

Table 25–9. Prevalence of Cardiovascular Disease*

High blood pressure†—50,000,000
Coronary heart disease—12,000,000
  Myocardial infarction—7,000,000
  Angina pectoris—6,200,000
Stroke—4,400,000
Rheumatic fever/rheumatic heart disease—1,800,000
Congenital cardiovascular defects—1,000,000
Congestive heart failure—4,600,000
1 in 5 males and females have some form of CVD
1 in 3 men can expect to develop some major cardiovascular disease before age 60; the odds for women are 1 in 10

*58,800,000 Americans have one or more types of cardiovascular disease (CVD) according to current estimates

†A person is considered to have high blood pressure when he or she has a systolic pressure of 140 mm Hg or greater and/or a diastolic pressure of 90 mm Hg or greater, or is taking antihypertensive medication.

Data taken from the following sources:

Phase I, National Health and Nutrition Examination Survey III (NHANES III), 1988–1991, CDC/NCHS and the American Heart Association.

National Health and Nutrition Examination Survey III (NHANES III), 1988–1994, CDC/NCHS and the American Heart Association.

National Health and Nutrition Examination Survey II (NHANES II), 1976–1980, CDC/NCHS and the American Heart Association.

Hurst, The Heart, Arteries and Veins, 9th ed. New York: McGraw-Hill, 1998, pp 3–17.

Nursing care of the patient with CVD includes careful ongoing assessment of vital signs and respiratory function, careful administration of vasoactive medications, adequate oxygenation, and cautious fluid replacement. An important goal of nursing care is to limit patient exertion, anxiety, pain, and stress to reduce oxygen consumption. Adequate pain and nausea management and maintenance of normotension and normal heart rate are important adjuncts to achieve this goal. Treatment protocols for perioperative hypertension, myocardial infarction, and arrhythmias are discussed in Chapter 11.

Coronary Artery Disease

About 7 million people suffer from coronary artery disease (CAD), which is caused by the accumulation of lipids, fibrous tissue, and calcium deposits that narrow or obstruct the arterial lumens, decreasing and sometimes completely cutting off the supply of oxygen and nutrients to the myocardium. Coronary artery spasm, although relatively rare, is another process that can result in decreased coronary blood flow. Through either mechanism, decreased blood supply to the myocardium can result in acute and permanent damage due to myocardial ischemia or infarction, angina, and serious arrhythmias including cardiac arrest.

The right coronary artery originates from the right aortic sinus and supplies nourishment to the right atrium and ventricle, the sinus node, and the atrioventricular node. The left coronary artery originates from the posterior aortic sinus and branches into two divisions, the left descending coronary artery, which supplies the anterolateral aspects of the left ventricle, and the circumflex coronary artery, which supplies the lateral left ventricle. ECG leads that correspond to these areas of the heart are listed in Table 11–6.

Preoperative evaluation should include questions to identify the patient at risk for or with existing CAD. High blood cholesterol, hypertension, hereditary predisposition, increasing age, and smoking all contribute to CHD. Obesity and physical inactivity are other factors that can lead to CHD, as is the postmenopausal period and use of birth control pills in females. Also, left coronary artery disease is five times more prevalent in a person with diabetes mellitus than in the nondiabetic patient. In addition to considering risk factors, the assessment should elicit historical information about chest pain, angina, exercise intolerance, and previous myocardial infarction (MI). Prior MI is one of the most important factors to consider when predicting perioperative cardiac morbidity.[33]

Diagnostic tests may be ordered in clinically questionable patients and include electrocardiogram, stress testing, Holter monitoring, and chest radiography. Asymptomatic, undiagnosed CAD greatly increases perioperative risk for the patient, particularly left main with significant stenosis, which is life-threatening. The second and third postoperative days are the most common time for MI in the noncardiac surgery patient with CAD; thus, careful patient selection for the ambulatory surgery setting is important. Aspirin or other medications may be considered to reduce the chance of coronary thrombosis.[34]

Appropriate perioperative care necessitates the proper management of the patient's cardioactive medications, maintaining myocardial oxygenation, reducing myocardial oxygen consumption, and identifying and reversing early ischemic changes. Concurrent treatment for hypertension may be necessary, because elevated blood pressure often coexists with CAD. Table 25–10 summarizes occurrences to avoid in the patient with CAD.

Classic ischemic changes appear on the ECG as depression of the ST segment and T wave inversion. Tissue damage related to infarction can manifest itself with ST segment elevation, and eventual appearance of a Q wave greater than 0.03 second when tissue necrosis has occurred. These ECG changes alone are not necessarily diagnostic of damage or ischemia, but are used in conjunction with other symptoms such as anginal or atypical chest pain, shortness

Table 25–10. Occurrences to Avoid in the Patient with Coronary Artery Disease

OCCURRENCES	POSSIBLE CAUSES	UNTOWARD RESULTS
Hypoxemia	Inadequate airway maintenance Inadequate oxygen therapy Pain, anxiety Respiratory depression Fever	Decreased myocardial oxygenation
Hypotension	Hypovolemia Hemorrhage Anesthetics, sedatives, narcotics	Decreased coronary artery perfusion Decreased myocardial oxygen supply
Hypertension	Pain, anxiety (↑ catecholamines) Fluid overload Omission of antihypertensive medications Intubation Presence of artificial airway Shivering	Increased work of heart to pump Increased myocardial oxygen consumption
Tachycardia	Pain, stress Hypotension, bleeding Light anesthesia level Shivering, fever	Increased myocardial oxygen consumption Decreased diastole time Decreased coronary artery perfusion

of breath, nausea, vomiting, and pallor in making a diagnosis.

Nitrates, β-blockers, calcium channel blockers, aspirin, and anticoagulants may be prescribed to treat CAD. Except for aspirin and anticoagulants, these drugs are usually continued up until the time of surgery and resumed shortly after. The nurse should ensure that the patient understands and follows the physician's directions.

Nitrates, such as nitroglycerin products and isosorbide, work by dilating the coronary arteries, thus increasing myocardial oxygen supply and reducing demand. Concurrent peripheral vasodilation reduces vascular resistance (both preload and afterload), reducing the work of the heart. Total coronary blood flow in patients with existing myocardial ischemia from coronary occlusion is not increased, but nitrates appear to cause redistribution of coronary blood flow, which reduces ischemia.[35] Nitrates are administered orally and transdermally for long-term effects, and the patient is generally instructed to maintain his or her usual scheduled doses on the day of surgery. Intravenous nitrates are available for emergency use.

β-Adrenergic blocking agents inhibit circulating catecholamines from stimulating β-receptor sites. Nonselective β-blockers such as propranolol, nadolol, timolol, and pindolol affect both β_1- and β_2-receptors. The cardiac selective agents, atenolol and metoprolol, affect only the β_1 sites, resulting in decreased heart rate and contractility, thus reducing myocardial oxygen demand. Side effects of a β_1-block include heart block, bradycardia, heart failure, and hypotension.

β_2-Receptor blockade causes bronchoconstriction, coronary artery vasoconstriction, and peripheral vascular vasoconstriction, which are the undesirable side effects of the nonspecific β-blocking drugs. As expected, nonspecific β-blockers are contraindicated in people with asthma, significant bradycardia, or greater than first-degree heart block.

Calcium channel blockers such as diltiazem, nicardipine, nifedipine, and verapamil also reduce myocardial oxygen demand and increase coronary blood flow. They are also used for primary antihypertensive therapy. By inhibiting the flow of calcium across cell membranes they reduce natural pacemaker activity, heart rate, blood pressure, and myocardial contractility. They also cause dilation of coronary and peripheral arteries. Their dilating effect on coronary arteries reduces vasospasm and helps to prevent anginal pain. Side effects include dizziness, headache, flushing, bradycardia, and hypotension.

Aspirin and anticoagulants may be used in conjunction with other medications to reduce the chance of clot formation within small coronary vessels. They may be discontinued appropriately before surgery, but an increased potential for bleeding should still be considered in the nursing care plan. Before discharge the nurse should ensure that the patient is instructed about the physician's directions for resumption of cardioactive and other medications.

Congestive Heart Failure

Congestive heart failure (CHF) is a widespread problem with 4.7 million Americans afflicted. Over 250,000 die each year of CHF.[36] The patient with symptoms of significant CHF is not a candidate for outpatient surgery. In fact, the presence of heart failure is a significant perioperative risk factor. The many etiologies of CHF include primary heart disease, the effects of medication protocols, pulmonary embolism, and the aging process in general.

Symptoms reflect the heart's attempt to compensate for altered pumping ability. Left ventricular failure is often the result of an acute myocardial infarction or hypertension. Associated increased left ventricular pressure causes increased pressure in the pulmonary vasculature with resulting pulmonary symptoms of dyspnea and orthopnea. As the pressure increases, the lungs become fluid-filled, leading to pulmonary edema and eventually to right ventricular failure with the classic occurrence of peripheral edema.

Both general and regional anesthesia have associated cardiovascular effects, so the anesthesia provider and nursing staff must be continually alert to any progression of symptoms. Volatile anesthetic gases and intravenous agents must be given judiciously because they invariably cause some level of respiratory depression. Regional anesthesia is another consideration; however, profound vasodilatation with resulting hypotension is also undesirable and should be avoided.

Perianesthesia care and assessment is similar to that described for coronary artery disease, but the importance of pulmonary auscultation cannot be overstated. Identifying pulmonary congestion before it compromises the patient's condition is a primary goal of nursing care. Changes in sensorium, air hunger, dyspnea, pallor, diaphoresis, tachycardia, and hypotension are all signs of decompensation and impending acute pulmonary involvement. Fluid management must be cautious, and the patient's usual medication protocols should be carefully managed. Typically medications are continued until the time of surgery except for diuretics that may cause intraoperative urinary urge or incontinence. Chapter 11 includes a discussion of treatment for acute pulmonary edema.

Heart Valve Disease

Valve disease creates the problem of impeding forward flow of blood through the heart and major vessels. The type of disease is identified by the pathophysiology (for instance, stenosis or incompetence of the valve) and the valve involved. A stenotic, or obstructed, valve results in pressure overload in the chamber from which the blood is being pumped. Regurgitation, or incompetence, occurs when the valve does not close properly, allowing the backflow of blood into the chamber from which it was pumped. Although all valves can be affected, those on the left side of the heart create the most far-reaching symptoms.

The mitral valve controls the flow of blood from the left atrium to the left ventricle, while the aortic valve connects the left ventricle to the aorta. Disease in either of these valves can seriously compromise the heart's ability to pump oxygenated blood into the peripheral and cerebral circulation. These patients have little reserve to increase cardiac output to respond to increased circulatory demand, so a major focus of perioperative care is to maintain homeostasis and reduce any increased cardiac demand. Tachycardia and hypovolemia should be avoided. Preoperative antibiotics that may be indicated prior to some procedures as prophylaxis against endocarditis are listed in Tables 38–8 and 38–9. Patients who have had prior valve surgery may be on long-term anticoagulant therapy, and nursing assessment should focus on the potential effects relating to perioperative bleeding.

Mitral valve stenosis is almost always a result of an episode of childhood rheumatic carditis. Symptoms usually do not appear until about 20 years later, often when added demands are placed on the heart during illness or pregnancy. Postoperatively, the patient with mitral stenosis is at high risk for pulmonary edema, paroxysmal atrial fibrillation or flutter, and right-sided heart failure. These patients have little reserve to increase cardiac output to meet increased metabolic demands. Nursing considerations include maintaining adequate fluid status and analgesia, providing a calming influence, monitoring heart rhythm, and ensuring that ordered antibiotic coverage is given appropriately.

Calcification and stiffening of the aortic (bicuspid) valve creates a fixed resistance to blood flow from the left ventricle to the aorta. Stenosis, which can be in or near the valve, results in chronically increased left ventricular pressure and ultimately left ventricular hypertrophy as the heart attempts to pump blood through a narrowed aorta. Loss of compliance and decreased stroke volume follow.

Aortic valve disease increases the risk of myocardial infarction surrounding noncardiac surgery. Myocardial oxygen demand can exceed supply by two mechanisms. First, angina unrelated to coronary artery disease may appear due to the oxygen needs of the increased left ventricular muscle mass. Also, increased left ventricular pressure that causes compression of subendocardial coronary vessels can mechanically decrease myocardial oxygenation.

Valve disease can remain undiagnosed for many years and be quite advanced by the time it is diagnosed. Symptoms include a systolic ejection murmur at the second right intercostal space, dyspnea, angina, syncope, and exercise intolerance.[10] The combination of aortic stenosis with tachycardia or hypotension poses a serious threat to the patient, and all efforts should be made to maintain heart rate and blood pressure in a normal range. The patient with aortic stenosis is at risk for sudden death when increased cardiovascular demands occur. Resuscitation from associated cardiac arrest is difficult, if not impossible.

Artificial Pacemakers

The ASC nurse should attempt to secure information when a patient presents with an artificial pacemaker. For instance, is the type of pacing on demand or continuous and is it AV sequential or atrial? Besides this information, the nurse should ask about the rate at which the pacer is set, the name of the patient's cardiologist, the brand of pacer, the date of implantation, and the most recent battery change or check. One way to assess the battery function is to compare the rate of fire with the rate at which the pacer is set. If the current rate is 10% or more below the present rate, the battery function is questionable. Many patients are, however, unable to provide detailed information about their pacemaker.

Cardiographic monitoring to identify adequate capture and response is important, along with physical assessment of pulse rate and character, blood pressure, normal sensorium, and adequacy of peripheral circulation. Subjective symptoms that can indicate pacemaker malfunction include fatigue, weakness, and dizziness.

Anesthesia and nursing care are not significantly affected by the presence of a pacemaker as long as it is functioning properly. Atropine and isoproterenol should be available to temporarily support heart rate in the event of pacemaker failure. The availability of a noninvasive, external pacemaker is also suggested. No special anesthesia plan is necessary, although all perioperative healthcare providers should note that any physiologic demand for increased heart rate may not be answered in the patient with a pacemaker, so hypovolemia should be avoided. Electrical equipment must be used according to manufacturer's directions to avoid interference with pacemaker function.

Automatic Implantable Cardiac Defibrillator

Automatic implantable cardiac (or cardioverter) defibrillators (AICDs) are becoming more common in the patients seen in the ASC. Approximately 10,000 people undergo AICD implantation each year as a defense against sudden cardiac death. Seventy-six percent of AICD patients are male. Although the device is not a risk in itself, the underlying disease must be considered. Implantation is for spontaneous, life-threatening ventricular dysrhythmias that can occur perioperatively. These patients are frequently (80%) taking concurrent antidysrhythmic medications.

An AICD has both sensing and defibrillation components; some also have a pacing component. Electromagnetic interference can cause the AICD to malfunction. An AICD should be turned off preoperatively using an external magnet. This renders the resuscitative mechanism of the device inactive, and transthoracic therapy must be employed during the time period. The presence of an experienced representative from the AICD manufacturer as well as the patient's cardiologist is often sought for support and response to perioperative emergencies.

Depending on the type of facility, whether freestanding or hospital-based, these patients may or may not be appropriate candidates for ambulatory surgery. Not only is the support of emergency backup lacking in the freestanding facility, but also the existing nursing and other personnel may have had little or no prior experience with an ACID, limiting their response effectiveness should complications occur.[37]

PULMONARY DISEASE

Pulmonary complications are the most frequent and often the most devastating complications associated with anesthesia and surgery. The patient with pre-existing disease already has some extent of respiratory compromise and requires skillful and attentive care to reduce the potential for complications such as aspiration, bronchospasm, airway obstruction, and traumatic intubation or extubation. Care must consider both perioperative processes and the patient's underlying disease. Figure 25–1 provides a visual overview of pulmonary anatomy.

Pulmonary health must be a major assessment parameter throughout the perianesthesia period. Lung disease, the fourth leading cause of death in the United States, is pervasive throughout the population, particularly among current or past tobacco smokers. A plethora of information about all types of lung disease is available for the public and for health professionals from the National Heart, Lung, and Blood Institute (NHLBI), a division of the National Institutes of Health (NIH). The NHLBI Information Center can be accessed by Internet site http://www.nhibi.nih.gov/health/infoctr/index.htm or by telephone (301-592-8573) or fax (301-592-8563). The postal address is National Heart, Lung, and Blood Institute, Division of Lung Diseases, Two Rockledge Center, 6701 Rockledge Drive, MSC 7952, Suite 10018, Bethesda, MD 20892-7952. This source can be of great assistance to the nurse in preparing patient education material both for content and as a reference site for patients and families. For example, *The Lungs in Health and Disease* is a 39-page booklet available singly or in bulk by ordering NIH Publication #97-3279 or by downloading it from the NIH Web site.[38] There is also a method to download this information into a format that can be accessed by audible synthesized speech readers for the visually impaired or blind user.

Patients with chronic pulmonary disease may present with a range of problems with minor to marked restrictions. Careful medical assessment is essential to identify those who are appropriate candidates for the ASC. Oxygen-dependent patients are not necessarily precluded from ambulatory care, but the invasiveness of the intended procedure must be appropriate, and nursing care must be tailored to their special needs. In fact, avoiding hospitalization for minor surgery may be beneficial to patients with pulmonary challenges by avoiding exposure to hospital-acquired complications and by limiting the dis-

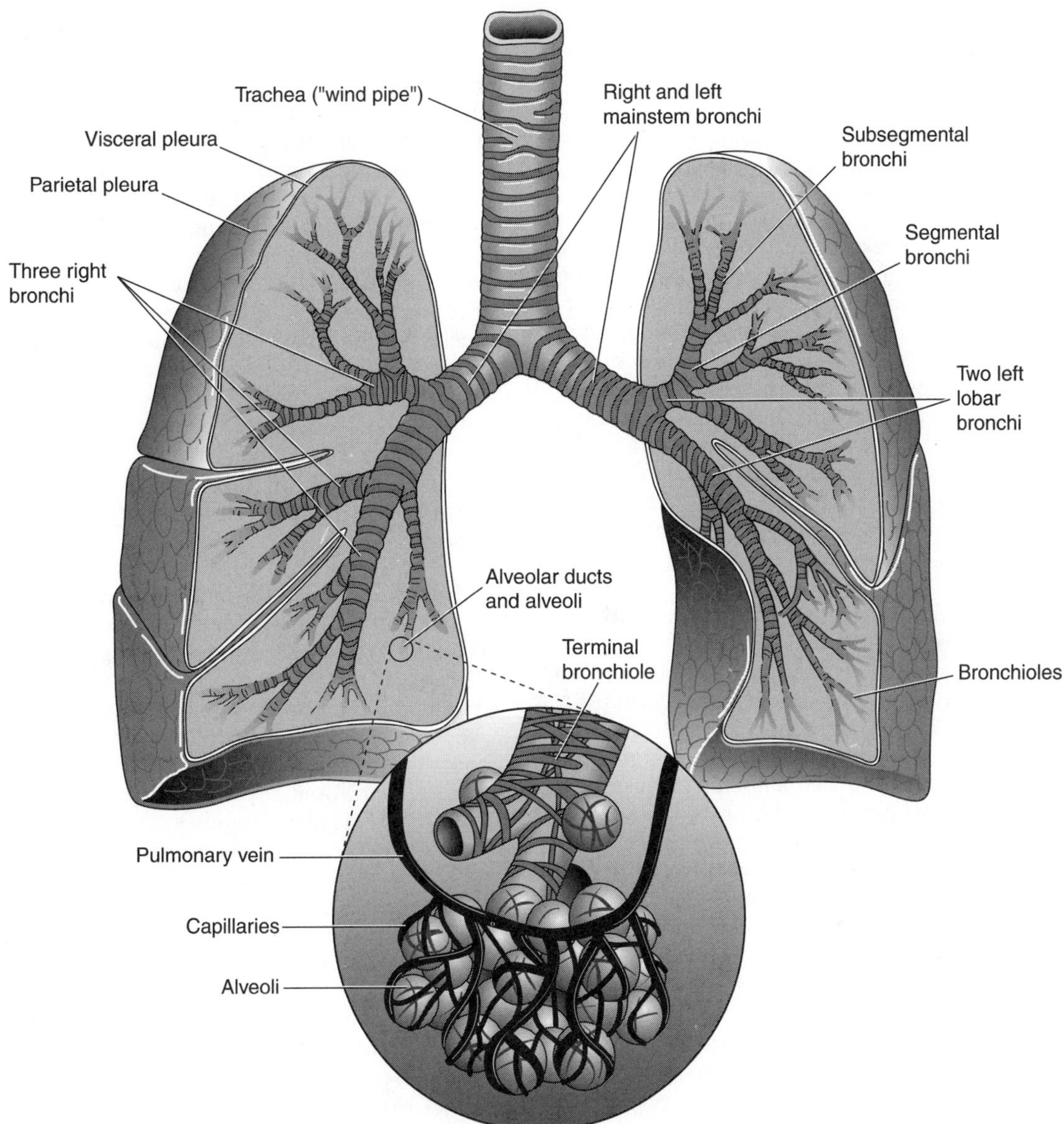

Figure 25–1. Structures of the respiratory tract.

ruption in their daily routines and medication protocols.

Pulmonary complications in the postoperative period can affect recovery and result in unplanned hospitalization and major medical complications. Risk factors increasing the chance of pulmonary complications include preexisting pulmonary disease, smoking, advancing age, and poor general health. Obesity, often assumed to be a major risk factor, does not have a major impact according to a number of clinical studies.[39] Preoperative assessment should include questions about smoking habits because this risk factor can have significant effects on patient outcomes.

Meticulous respiratory assessment must be ongoing to ensure rapid identification of any deterioration so that aggressive interventions can be initiated. Patient needs center on the following goals.

1. Ensuring that the patient's respiratory status is as optimal as possible prior to surgery
2. Identifying the patient with an active acute respiratory process and avoiding surgery

3. Decreasing the patient's oxygen needs and increasing oxygen supply whenever possible
4. Avoiding complications that would further tax the patient's respiratory status—for instance, aspiration, pneumothorax, laryngospasm, bronchospasm, oversedation, and airway obstruction

To limit or prevent acute pulmonary events, nursing interventions should focus on reducing workload, anxiety, pain, nausea, vomiting, restlessness, and shivering. Care should be planned to help the patient conserve energy and movements. For instance, extra time devoted to admission procedures will help to avoid rushing the patient. Gentle airway manipulations, judicious use of sedating medications, and avoidance of coughing and retching are also important. Prior to any pharmacologic interventions for restlessness, hypoxia must be ruled out as a cause.

Medication protocols for the patient with existing pulmonary disease generally include maintaining the usual medication schedule up to the time of the procedure and resuming it soon afterward. Patients should be instructed to bring their usual medications, including inhalants, to the ASC so that subsequent doses can be taken postoperatively. A physician's order should be secured for administration of the patient's own medications. Having the patient's own inhalant medications available not only provides for rapid administration, but also provides some measure of psychological comfort to the patient who may feel anxious without this resource close by.

Patients with symptomatic obstructive disease are often treated with inhaled ipratropium, with inhaled β-adrenergic receptor agonists added as needed up to four times a day. These agents have an additive effect.[40]

Preoperative assessment may include a chest radiograph and pulmonary function testing, depending on the clinical examination and the physician's judgment. Recent studies show that spirometry results have a variable predictive value, and are generally not as reliable as clinical findings in predicting pulmonary complications.[38] Test results should be on the medical record and should be reviewed by the physician before the patient is transferred to the procedure room. Although cautious respiratory evaluation is primarily the responsibility of the anesthesia provider, that responsibility is shared by the perianesthesia nurse, who should assess and document baseline examination results for comparison during the postoperative course. Assessment includes, but is not limited to, general well-being, skin color and temperature, and bilateral breath sounds, along with the ease, rate, and depth of respirations. Oximetry is an essential tool throughout the patient's experience.

Chest auscultation should be performed before and periodically after sedation and surgery. Rhonchi (low-pitched snoring sounds that are coarse in nature) occur when air flows through passages narrowed by secretions, for instance, in the patient with pulmonary involvement subsequent to congestive heart failure. A higher pitched wheezing sound is indicative of bronchospasm, such as that which occurs in asthma, bronchitis, and allergic reactions.

Chronic Obstructive Pulmonary Disease

Advanced chronic obstructive pulmonary disease (COPD), or emphysema, involves alveolar destruction with loss of gas exchange surface area, loss of elastic recoil, and distention of remaining lung tissues. Loss of elasticity promotes airway obstruction and reduces air movement. Air becomes trapped in the lungs, increasing functional residual capacity (FRC). Increased dead space requires the patient to breathe more rapidly to maintain a normal Pa_{CO_2}. The characteristic puffing respirations, pursed lip breathing, a barrel chest, abdominal breathing, and elevated shoulders are all mechanisms the patient uses to enhance respirations in permanently damaged lungs. Bronchospastic disease or bronchitis often coexist and complicate management.

Techniques previously discussed to reduce physical workload and effort for cardiovascular or obese patients also apply to those with pulmonary challenges. The preoperative history should include ascertaining the patient's tolerance for activity, oxygen dependency, smoking habits, level of dyspnea, and medications. Diagnostic testing is based on the clinical status.

A specific consideration for patients with a chronically compromised respiratory system is the possibility of a change in their primary mechanism of ventilatory drive. In the healthy person, respirations increase when chemoreceptors in the brain sense a rise in carbon dioxide levels. The patient with COPD with chronic elevation of CO_2 levels becomes insensitive to that stimulus to breathe, and hypoxia becomes the primary driving force for ventilatory effort.

The administration of high-flow oxygen for a prolonged period can be detrimental to the

COPD patient who depends on this hypoxic drive; thus, a low flow of 2 to 3 L/min is preferred along with careful monitoring of the patient's respiratory effort, especially after discontinuation of the oxygen. Pulse oximetry monitoring should continue after discontinuation of oxygen administration to evaluate the patient's response to breathing room air.

Emotional support has special meaning in the care of a person with compromised breathing. Many COPD patients become anxious, demanding, and agitated as it becomes more difficult to get enough air with each breath. Aggressive and demanding patient behavior may challenge the nurse's patience in providing compassionate attention. The patient may fear being alone, having further respiratory deterioration, and not having medications and oxygen available.

Home instructions focus on avoiding further respiratory compromise in the early recovery period after discharge. This goal is primarily in the patient's own hands through proper deep breathing exercises and coughing as demonstrated by the nurse, avoidance of smoking, and resumption of usual medication protocols. The patient should avoid people with respiratory infections and should take all doses of any prescribed antibiotics. Proper hydration and nutrition are important for overall health and energy maintenance and for surgical healing.

Reactive Airway Disease

Reactive airway disease comprises a number of conditions that can occur from childhood through old age, including asthma and chronic bronchitis. Given the widespread occurrence of these conditions, it is logical to expect that a vast number of patients seen in ambulatory surgical settings will be affected.

Asthma, a reactive airway disease, occurs in about 12 million people in the United States. Perioperative risk associated with asthma may be related to the degree of preoperative control attained. The tendency to develop asthma is often inherited. Although the exact etiology is unknown, three physiologic processes are involved: (1) adreneric activity of the sympathetic nervous system (α- and β-adrenergic receptors), (2) cholinergic responses and vagal activity of the parasympathetic nervous system, and (3) the antigen-antibody response.

In the third case, inhalation of an irritant (antigen) in a predisposed person can cause the production of antibodies with subsequent release of histamine and other substances from the mast cells of the lungs. This reaction is responsible for the asthmatic symptoms, which are due to reversible obstruction and irritability of the airways. Symptoms include dyspnea, bronchoconstriction, bronchial edema, cough, and increased mucus production that further narrows air passages. As airflow diminishes, symptoms include dyspnea, tachypnea, and anxiety. Expiratory time is increased and wheezing is common. The pitch of sound produced by wheezing becomes higher as the bronchial lumen narrows.

Atopic individuals are at increased risk for asthma and should be regarded with suspicion and close monitoring, particularly when they have a history of prior asthmatic events. Besides environmental allergens such as dust, cigarette smoke, feathers, sprays, and fragrances, excessive dryness or moisture in the air can precipitate an attack. Childhood exposure to tobacco smoke, allergens, and bronchial wall infections may predispose that person to develop asthma later in life. Occupational exposures to grain, dust, latex, and other allergens may predispose an event, but the most common trigger of asthma attacks is a respiratory tract infection.[41] Other triggers are listed in Table 25–11. Prodromal symptoms such as tightness in the chest, wheezing, and coughing can precede an acute event and should be aggressively treated in the predisposed patient.

Table 25–11. Potential Triggers of Bronchoconstrictive Reactions

ENVIRONMENTAL
Fragrances
Dust
Feathers
Sprays
Perfumes
Cigarette smoke
Excessive humidity or dryness
Cold air
Respiratory infection
PERIOPERATIVE
Medications
Environmental latex
Aspiration of gastric contents
Intubation or extubation during light plane of anesthesia
EMOTIONAL
Stress
Fear
Anger
Crying
Overexertion

The best treatment for an acute attack is surely prevention. Besides limiting the triggers previously mentioned, it is important to avoid or to be cautious about administering medications that are known to cause bronchoconstriction, for instance, barbiturates, morphine, cholinesterase inhibitors such as neostigmine and pyridostigmine, and histamine-releasing drugs like tubocurarine and succinylcholine. Regional anesthesia is often preferred to reduce respiratory insult. When general anesthesia is used, isoflurane, enflurane, or halothane may be the agent of choice because of their bronchodilating effects. Another agent with bronchodilating characteristics is ketamine. Avoidance of overinflation of the lungs is important during mechanical ventilation. To avoid tracheal stimulation during the lighter planes of general anesthesia, which is often employed for ambulatory procedures, a facemask or laryngeal mask may be used rather than intubation.[42]

Acute, rapidly occurring symptoms can be mild or severe, requiring interventions such as the administration of bronchodilators, oxygen, mucolytic agents, and inhalation treatments. Maintaining a calm and supportive environment is important in helping the patient gain confidence in the healthcare providers. This, in turn, helps to reduce anxiety that could exacerbate symptoms. Coughing and deep breathing can help the patient raise secretions and clear airways. Oxygen therapy helps avoid or reverse hypoxia, and airway management should be gentle to avoid trauma. Adequate intravenous hydration helps to decrease viscosity of the bronchial secretions.

Pharmacologic treatment is directed at relaxing bronchial smooth muscles. First-line management includes oxygen, inhaled albuterol, and systemic corticosteroids. Subcutaneous epinephrine or terbutaline may be required if the patient is unable to take or does not respond to inhalation therapy. Terbutaline is preferred in the pregnant patient. For those patients who do not respond to initial therapy, a second-line drug is the anticholinergic agent ipratropium bromide, which blocks muscarinic receptors in the airway, thus inhibiting vagally induced bronchoconstriction.[41] Although methylxanthines such as theophylline and aminophylline are well established as effective agents used in chronic reactive airway disease, their usefulness in acute situations has been questioned.

After a patient has suffered an acute asthma attack, discharge should be delayed until all symptoms have abated and the physician has examined the patient. Oximetry and bedside spirometry are simple, useful tools for ascertaining if the patient has recovered to baseline status. The physician's instructions for continuing maintenance doses of bronchodilating medications should be reviewed, and the patient most assuredly should be in the care of an adult for the first 24 hours after discharge. Hospitalization may be indicated.

Throughout the perioperative care of the patient with pre-existing pulmonary disease, it is helpful for the nurse to realize that the patient and family have personal experience with the patient's stamina and responses related to the disease. Their opinions and ideas should be respected and carefully considered by all healthcare providers during care decisions. A questioning attitude along with active listening, astute observation, and intelligent choices in therapy, medications, and activity demands all play a role in successfully managing the person with respiratory compromise.

RENAL FAILURE

Almost 12 million people in the United States suffer from some degree of renal, or kidney, disease. Chronic renal disease comprises a number of conditions such as chronic nephrotic syndrome, glomerulonephritis, and renovascular hypertension. Depending on the extent of illness, the patient may require hospitalization after even minor surgery, for instance, when complicating multisystem diseases develop secondary to the renal failure. However, avoiding hospitalization and associated disruption of hemodialysis appointments is usually a significant benefit of ambulatory care for these patients, who may present for unrelated procedures or for primary care of an arteriovenous shunt, such as establishing a new shunt or declotting an existing shunt.

Renal failure leads to untoward changes in many body systems. Failure of the kidneys to perform excretory functions leads to volume overload, accumulation of products of catabolism (e.g., potassium and hydrogen ions), and platelet dysfunction.[43] Hypertension, left ventricular failure, coronary artery disease, hyperkalemia with associated dysrhythmias, pulmonary edema, peripheral and autonomic neuropathy, and chronic anemia are a few outcomes of this dysfunction. The frequent coexistence of diabetes mellitus is another consideration.

The person in end-stage kidney failure is readily identifiable and is most likely on renal dialysis. The patient with less obvious renal disease may be difficult to identify because up to 50% of kidney function can be lost prior to definitive laboratory changes.[10] Symptoms suggestive of renal disease include fever, fatigue, weight loss, dyspnea, chest pain, edema, anorexia, nausea and vomiting, polyuria, dysuria, flank pain, hematuria, and passage of renal stones.[44]

Laboratory findings include elevated blood urea nitrogen (BUN), serum creatinine level, and creatinine clearance rate. These readings may not always be elevated, nor do their values always reflect the severity of disease present. Also seen are hyperkalemia, hypermagnesemia, hypocalcemia, and coagulopathies.

Anemia is often severe. Hemoglobin and hematocrit levels may drop as low as 5 to 8 g/dl and 15% to 25%, respectively. Because the drop is gradual, the patient becomes accustomed to low hemoglobin and hematocrit levels over a period of time. This reduced oxygen-carrying capacity makes administration of supplemental oxygen to support tissue oxygenation essential. The nursing plan should address the patient's general lack of energy and stamina.

The patient in renal failure poorly tolerates stress, both physical and emotional. Extremes of blood pressure should be avoided, and fluid balance should be monitored carefully. Hypotension can further reduce the patient's already compromised renal blood flow and glomerular filtration rate. Hypertension can lead to congestive heart failure and cardiomegaly. Extreme hypertension due to fluid overload may require dialysis to adjust the patient's fluid volume. Until that can be accomplished, a direct-acting vasodilator such as sodium nitroprusside, hydralazine, or labetalol may be used to reduce blood pressure. Accompanying liver disease is not uncommon because of hepatic venous congestion. Nausea with vomiting or delayed gastric emptying predispose the patient to aspiration. Primary concerns in the perioperative course include hyperkalemia, balance fluid volumes, and avoiding exaggerated and prolonged drug effects.

Hemodialysis brings special concerns. To avoid unnecessary jeopardy to the patient the scheduling of an elective procedure should take the patient's dialysis schedule into consideration. Electrolyte imbalances occur as a result of the disease as well as secondary to dialysis treatments. Securing laboratory values close to the time of surgery and after the most recent dialysis treatment is important. Anticoagulation related to dialysis techniques is assessed by laboratory measurements just prior to surgery.

The patient with an arteriovenous shunt for dialysis requires special care. The nurse must avoid using the shunted arm for blood pressure readings. Hypotension should be avoided to reduce the chance of thrombus formation in the shunt. Hepatitis is always a possibility in patients who have had multiple dialysis exposures, thus staff protection is a concern.

Medications must be given judiciously, reducing the usual doses of certain perioperative medications such as thiopental, benzodiazepines, phenothiazines, and narcotics. Avoiding renally excreted drugs and neuromuscular blockers such as pancuronium and vecuronium is wise. Anticholinergics such as atropine, scopolamine, and glycopyrrolate can be given in usual dosages. Monitoring for prolonged effects of all drugs is important, and patient discharge should not be hurried. Perioperative fluid and dietary protein intake may be limited, and such restrictions should be taken into consideration in the nursing plan.

Discharge instructions stress the prevention of infection and a return to usual medication, dietary, and hemodialysis schedules. The patient should be instructed to immediately report untoward symptoms such as persistent nausea and vomiting, increased anorexia, or cardiovascular symptoms such as chest pain. Patients are referred back to the care of their nephrologists for medical management.

HEPATIC DYSFUNCTION

The liver has myriad functions such as fat metabolism, glucose homeostasis, protein synthesis, drug and hormone metabolism, production of coagulation factors, and bilirubin formation and excretion. Like renal disease, liver dysfunction results in diverse systemic effects including coagulopathies, reduced drug metabolism, drug toxicity, cardiovascular compromise, and hypoglycemia. Typical laboratory abnormalities include elevated prothrombin time, reduced plasma albumin levels, and increased globulin and bilirubin levels.

Acute hepatitis is most likely a result of viral infection. It can follow drug toxicity, sepsis, congestive heart failure, and pregnancy. Elective surgery is avoided in the person with acute hepatitis.

Chronic hepatitis disease (cirrhosis) may be the result of hepatitis, acute or chronic. More often it is a result of chronic alcohol consumption. Cirrhosis is typified by an interference of bile production resulting in aberrations in gastrointestinal absorption of fat and fat-soluble vitamins such as vitamin K. Not only is digestion affected, but prothrombin production and clotting ability are altered as well. Bleeding abnormalities may dictate the avoidance of invasive regional anesthetics. Fluid and sodium retention are also common, and fluid replacement should be carefully monitored. Eventually, obstruction of blood flow in the liver with portal hypertension can result in esophageal and gastrointestinal varices.

Altered drug metabolism occurs for several reasons. First, reduced blood flow through the consolidated liver slows the metabolic process. Reduced protein (albumin) synthesis leads to inadequate protein-binding sites for drugs, so much of the drug that was administered remains active in the circulation, unbound, while the slow metabolic process occurs. Thus, patients require smaller doses to reach desired effects, and the possibility of toxicity is increased. Also the production of hepatic microsomal enzymes is reduced in the cirrhotic liver, further diminishing the body's ability to metabolize and detoxify drugs.

The liver has a tremendous reserve capacity, and only when there is severe liver damage is there significant alteration in drug metabolism.[45] Still, it is wise to avoid or reduce dosages of drugs that are primarily metabolized in the liver. Some of those drugs include diazepam, meperidine, morphine, halothane, lidocaine, vecuronium, and other benzodiazepines. Isoflurane is considered the favored inhalation agent, and there are no contraindications to nitrous oxide.[46]

Other nursing considerations include maintaining suspicion regarding the patient's predisposition to bleeding and using care with airway manipulations to avoid bleeding from nasotracheal or esophageal trauma. These patients may be taking steroids as part of long-term therapy, so parenteral replacement may be needed perioperatively to supplement the patient's diminished stress response. The patient may be a carrier of hepatitis B virus, so careful self-protection measures are important.

NEUROMUSCULAR, SKELETAL, CONNECTIVE TISSUE, AND IMMUNE SYSTEM DISEASES

The many forms of arthritis and diseases of the musculoskeletal system, bones, and skin afflict millions of Americans, causing tremendous human suffering and disability and complicating the perioperative period and home recovery. Economic costs of arthritis, musculoskeletal and bone diseases, and skin diseases exceed $100 billion a year. These diseases represent some of the most common causes of chronic illness in the United States and are the leading reasons for time lost from work. Many of these diseases disproportionately affect women (lupus, scleroderma, fibromyalgia, osteoporosis), minority populations, the elderly (osteoarthritis, osteoporosis), and children (juvenile rheumatoid arthritis, epidermolysis bullosa).

Almost every household in the United States is affected in some way by one or more of these diseases. Forty million Americans have some type of arthritis. Ten million Americans have osteoporosis, and 18 million more have low bone mass, placing them at risk for the disease. Eight of ten Americans have had a low back pain problem at some time. Skin problems are responsible for 63 million visits to the doctor annually.

Information useful for professional learning and for patient education material is available from the National Institute of Arthritis and Musculoskeletal and Skin Diseases (NIAMS), which is a component of the National Institutes of Health (NIH), within the federal government. This site can be accessed at www.nih.gov/niams, or information can be obtained from the NIAMS Clearinghouse at 1 AMS Circle, Bethesda, MD 20892-3675, telephone 301-495-4484. Chapter 17 includes discussion of several conditions including patients with spinal cord injury, multiple sclerosis, and Alzheimer's disease.

Arthritis

Many types of arthritis exist, including the common forms of osteoarthritis and rheumatoid arthritis. Although etiology varies, the effects and nursing needs are similar for these patients. Osteoarthritis, also called degenerative joint disease or DJD, typified by degenerative changes in the articulating cartilage in a few or in many joints, often accompanies aging. Rheumatoid arthritis is a progressive systemic inflammatory process that affects the synovium of the joints, eventually leading to joint destruction. In both disease processes, the symptoms include pain, stiffness, inflammation, heat, muscle spasm, and joint deformity.

Additional systemic symptoms that may accompany rheumatoid arthritis include fever, anorexia, paresthesia, weakness, and fatigue. Later symptoms include osteoporosis, anemia, subcutaneous nodules, endocarditis, fibrotic lung disease, and vasculitis.[47]

A wide variety of medications may be prescribed for the palliation of arthritic symptoms and include nonsteroidal anti-inflammatory drugs (NSAIDs), steroids, immunosuppressants, calcium, analgesics, vitamins, and gastric acid suppressants. Proper identification of and instructions about medications that can have untoward effects during the perioperative period are essential to reduce the opportunity for related complications such as gastric irritation, bleeding, decreased stress response, and infection. Preoperative coagulation studies may be indicated.

Pain management must address both acute surgical pain and chronic arthritis pain. NSAIDs may be useful; however, the patient's chronic use of many drugs may necessitate that larger-than-normal doses are prescribed postoperatively. Adjunctive treatments may also help alleviate pain, for instance, topical application of cold.

Two other challenges facing the arthritic patient are emotional/psychological and mobility concerns. These individuals often require more time for basic admission tasks such as undressing and moving from one surface to another. Careful and gentle positioning is essential and should take into consideration specific information about limitations and range of motion provided to the nurse by the patient during the assessment phase of care. In particular, the sedated or unconscious patient must rely on the nurse to oversee positioning in a conscientious manner when the patient is unable to verbalize comfort level. Careful, documentation should indicate specific positioning and aids used.

Postoperative activity should be encouraged within the patient's ability to maintain joint mobility and muscle strength and avoid problems related to inactivity. Aids such as wheelchairs and walkers to assist with ambulation should be available. Again, sufficient time should be provided for activities relating to preparation for discharge.

The chronicity of arthritis can result in depression, lowered self-esteem, dependence, altered body image, and a feeling of hopelessness. Empathic encouragement can help the patient assume perioperative responsibilities within the patient's ability. The added stress of surgery and anesthesia can be particularly difficult for those who deal with chronic pain, and nursing compassion is an important adjunct to any analgesic protocol.

Neuromuscular Diseases

Neuromuscular disorders originate from and affect both nerve and muscle function. Muscle diseases are those in which an intrinsic disorder of skeletal muscle cells exists, generally at or distal to the neuromuscular junction. Muscular dystrophy, myasthenia gravis, and myotonic dystrophies are examples. Specific planning of nursing care is essential and should be based on the patient's specific disorder rather than on generalities. Perioperative hospitalization may be indicated for the patient with extensive disease. For patients who return home on the day of surgery, caution and patience should be applied to avoid premature discharge prior to return of preoperative muscle function. Of particular concern is respiratory function.

Decreased muscle strength and little or no reserve to sustain even that level of strength during times of stress can lead to ventilatory and mobility complications. Anesthesia management is essentially the same for these patients as for others, although decreased doses of sedatives, anesthetic agents and muscle relaxants are often in order to avoid profound, sustained muscle weakness, and respiratory depression. The effects of local anesthetics can be unpredictable.

In addition to having weakness in the primary muscles of respiration, these patients can experience oropharyngeal weakness, reduced cough effort, and inadequate swallowing, making it difficult for them to handle secretions. Central nervous system and cardiac involvement can further complicate cardiorespiratory function in some.

Nursing care focuses on aggressive assessment, oximetry monitoring, supplemental oxygen administration, reduced doses of sedating medications, extra time for patient activities, adequate time for resting, and environmental controls to reduce stress. Passive exercises may be indicated to prevent stasis of blood flow during times of immobility. The patient with long-standing myotonic disease may have contractures and require special positioning and support of extremities or the head.

Myasthenia Gravis

Myasthenia gravis (MG) is a progressive autoimmune disease affecting the skeletal muscles. MG affects about 10,000 to 15,000 people of all races in the United States and is twice as likely to affect women as men.[48] MG is characterized by fluctuating muscle weakness that usually progresses during the day as the patient becomes tired. The pathophysiologic abnormality is a defect in the transmission of impulses from the nerve to the muscle cells, specifically a decrease in the number and effectiveness of acetylcholine receptors at the neuromuscular junction or a decreased amount of acetylcholine produced in the presynaptic membrane of the junction.[49] Either option results in reduced innervation of skeletal muscle.

Frequently ocular muscles are affected with resultant ptosis and diplopia. Facial and throat weakness can result in loss of facial expression, drooling, choking, swallowing difficulty, and weakness of the voice. Inability to adequately clear the throat of secretions and aspiration are potential problems. Respiratory muscle weakness is not common but is most often encountered during a myasthenic crisis. Likewise, muscle atrophy is not common. The potential for postoperative ventilatory failure or pneumonia due to weak cough effort and clearance of secretions must be considered in the medical and nursing plans for these patient.

Edrophonium (Tensilon) is a very short-acting anticholinesterase drug used to diagnose MG. Edrophonium blocks the destruction of acetylcholine, resulting in an immediate increase in neural transmission and muscle strength.[50] When given intravenously, edrophonium temporarily reverses muscle weakness that typifies the condition. Dramatic improvement of ptosis and diplopia is considered diagnostic.[51]

Oral anticholinergic medications used for treatment include pyridostigmine (Mestinon) or neostigmine (Prostigmin) to increase the response of muscles to nerve stimulation. Many perioperative medications can reverse these anticholinergic drugs that are essential for ensuring the patient's adequate muscle strength. These include nondepolarizing muscle relaxants, mycin-type antibiotics, and aminogycosides, morphine, and procainamide. The astute nurse or anesthesia provider must be able to recognize and respond to such unwanted effects. Steroids, immunosuppressants, azathioprine, and intravenous immunoglobulin are other drugs that may be used to treat myasthenia, along with plasmapheresis to lower acetylcholine receptor antibodies and thymectomy.[48] Regional anesthesia with an amide-type of agent is a preferred anesthetic approach when possible.

Nursing care must address respiratory and swallowing challenges as well as the patient's ability to provide for personal care. It should be noted that stress can cause increased symptoms, so the nursing plan should strive to provide as calm an environment as possible. Key points of education for the patient and family include resumption of normal medication protocols, pulmonary toilet as appropriate, resuming preprocedural levels of activity as soon as possible, avoiding sources of infection, and reporting complicating symptoms to the physician immediately.

Parkinson's Disease

This progressive neurologic disease affects about 1% of the population over 50 years old, with the highest prevalence in 40- to 60-year-old men. Onset is gradual, but the disease is progressive to a point of dementia (in 50% of those affected), inability to swallow, violent tremors, and respiratory compromise. About 90% of cases are considered idiopathic because the cause is unknown. A discussion of symptoms and assessment parameters is presented in Chapter 17.

Perioperative concerns include the patient's increased sensitivity to anesthetic agents, poor respiratory effort, inability to handle oral secretions, and tremors that can mimic ventricular fibrillation on an ECG monitor. The patient's usual medications should be continued up until the time of surgery and resumed as soon as possible postoperatively, so preoperative instructions should encourage patients to bring their usual medications with them to the facility. Drugs that treat Parkinson's disease act in one of two ways: to increase the functional ability of the underactive dopaminergic system or to reduce excessive influence of excitatory cholinergic neurons on the extrapyramidal tract.[52] Typical pharmacologic treatment includes levodopa combined with alpha-methylhydrazine (Sinemet), bromocriptine, and lergotrile to stimulate dopamine receptors, and others.[53] Muscle rigidity that can occur when the patient omits medication can make ventilation of the patient difficult and can predispose to venous thrombosis and increased psychological sequelae. Drugs that exacerbate extrapyramidal symptoms should be avoided perioperatively. These drugs include metoclopramide (Reglan), droperidol (Inapsine), and phenothiazines such as promethazine (Phenergan), and chlorpromazine (Thorazine).

Difficult mobility and self-care problems should be addressed by the nurse and a responsible caregiver who will assist at home. Seborrhea is common and is related to neuroendocrine dysfunction. Excessive hormones released by the anterior pituitary gland produce excessive secretion of sebum along the hairline and in chin and nasal creases.

Hypotension and cardiac arrhythmias are not uncommon and are complicated by hypovolemia and the patient's inadequate physiologic response to hypotension. Increased potential for orthostatic hypotension implies the need to ambulate these patients gradually and with assistance. Vital signs should be evaluated along the continuum of ambulation. Choking and aspiration are real threats given diminished muscle control, so drinking and eating should be observed closely and attempted only when the patient is sitting up and attentive to the task.

Parkinson's disease does not rob the patient of intelligence. Often they are struggling to control their own muscles and body responses and may be experiencing great frustration and depression, as may their caregivers. Respect of the patient's dignity, independence, and intelligence should be part of the plan of care.

Systemic Lupus Erythematous

This systemic disease affects mostly women of childbearing age and is typified by periods of exacerbations and remissions. It is thought to have an autoimmune etiology with genetic predisposition. Diagnosis is not simple. The characteristic erythematous butterfly mask occurs in only about 50% of patients. Multiple body systems are affected with complications including kidney disease with glomerular nephritis, cardiac abnormalities of the endocardium and pericardium, clotting abnormalities, neurologic changes relating to personality and cognition, and peripheral neuropathy. Usual treatment includes rest, steroids, salicylates, azathioprine, cyclosporine, and plasmapheresis.[54]

Perioperative concerns include reduction or avoidance of stress and maintenance of kidney function. Hypotension that results in reduced renal blood flow and nephrotoxic drugs should be avoided. Regional anesthesia is acceptable unless the patient exhibits signs of bleeding, such as petechiae. Patients on long-term corticosteroid therapy should have parenteral steroids perioperatively to support their response to surgical stress. Perioperative relapse is a possibility for those in remission.

Acquired Immunodeficiency Syndrome

Acquired immunodeficiency syndrome (AIDS) and human immunodeficiency virus (HIV) infection are rampant worldwide. Statistics are always out of date by the time they are published because of the explosive spread of this devastating disease. AIDS was first reported in the United States in 1981 and has since become a major worldwide epidemic. AIDS is caused by the HIV. By killing or impairing cells of the immune system, HIV progressively destroys the body's ability to fight infections and certain cancers. Individuals diagnosed with AIDS are susceptible to life-threatening diseases called opportunistic infections (OI), which are caused by microbes that usually do not cause illness in healthy people.

More than 600,000 cases of AIDS have been reported in the United States since 1981, and as many as 900,000 Americans may be infected with HIV. The epidemic is growing most rapidly among minority populations and is a leading killer of African-American males. In fact, the prevalence of AIDS is six times higher in African-Americans and three times higher among Hispanics than among whites.[55] Although it is still more prevalent in homosexual males and intravenous drug abusers, heterosexual spread has increased significantly, and it is believed that undiagnosed cases continue to proliferate on a massive scale.

In recent years, medical science has made great progress in successful treatment protocols for HIV infection and associated opportunistic infections. Wider use of medications for preventing tuberculosis, *Pneumocystis carinii* pneumonia (PCP), toxoplasmosis, and *Mycobacterium avium* complex (MAC), for example, has helped reduce the number of people with HIV who develop serious illness and die from AIDS. Also, several new compounds in a new class of drugs, called protease inhibitors, have been federally approved to treat HIV infection. These drugs, when taken in combination with previously approved drugs such as zidovudine (ZDV, also called AZT), lamivudine (3TC) and dideoxyinosine (ddl), reduce the level of HIV particles circulating in the blood (viral load) to very low levels in many individuals. Treatment results using these drugs have been extremely encouraging, because these drug combinations are more effective than any previously available therapies. Researchers are hopeful that this type of combination therapy, with further study, will prove effective over the long term and increase the healthy life span of more HIV-infected individuals.[56] These new combination therapies reduce the serum concentration of HIV, but there is no evidence that HIV is eradicated from the body. Also, the drugs do not work for some people, nor do they eliminate the chance of transmission of HIV to others.

Work continues to develop an effective vaccine against HIV. It is estimated that over 30 million individuals worldwide are infected with HIV, the vast majority of whom live in the developing world. One country in particular, Thailand, has experienced a rapidly escalating and severe HIV epidemic since 1988. Among the 60 million inhabitants of Thailand, as many as 800,000 people are currently believed to be living with HIV. Despite innovative and persistent preventions efforts, HIV continues to spread rapidly, particularly among Thailand's population of injection drug users (IDUs). Thailand has emerged as one of the nations most committed to ending its toll. To address the urgent need for an HIV vaccine, Thai officials have been working with many international agencies, including the Centers for Disease Control and Prevention (CDC), since 1991 to prepare for HIV vaccine efficacy trials. In February 1999, Thailand became the first developing nation to announce a phase III vaccine field trial.

A phase III trial is done to determine if a vaccine is effective in protecting against infection or disease and is an important step in the evaluation process leading to licensure. A 3-year collaborative research trial is under way to evaluate the ability of AIDSVAX to prevent HIV infection among uninfected IDUs in Bangkok, Thailand. AIDSVAX was developed by VaxGen, a US vaccine developer. Early reports from several smaller trials of AIDSVAX in Thailand and the United States, involving about 2000 persons, have shown the vaccine to be safe and capable of inducing antibodies against these strains of HIV. Still, caution is advised in considering this a magic answer to stopping the spread of HIV.

After initial exposure, antibodies to HIV appear within weeks to months or for up to 1 year. During this early time period the virus replicates rapidly, primarily in the T_4 lymphocyte cells. Often macrophages are infected, including those in the central nervous system, contributing to the dementia complex that accompanies the disease in some people. The patient is most infectious to others during this early period and again when the immune system begins to fail.[57]

Symptoms during the early acute infectious stage resemble those of mononucleosis or flu, for instance, sore throat, general malaise, myalgia, lymphedema, and rash. Later symptoms are body wasting, weight loss, diarrhea, fatigue, neurologic impairment, and the appearance of opportunistic infections and cancers.

Kaposi's sarcoma (KS) is the most frequent cancer associated with AIDS. Small purplish-brown skin lesions are only surface evidence of greater sites in the GI tract, lymph nodes, and lungs. PCP is a common infection plaguing people with AIDS, along with innumerable other types of infections from fungal, viral, protozoan bacterial, and other sources.

Complex medical and nursing needs attend these patients whose body systems are fragile. In particular, the patient must be shielded from sources of nosocomial infection. They need emotional support, careful attention to their tenuous physiologic balance, and nursing care that focuses on their immediate needs as well as on their support system in the home setting.

Maintaining the Patient's Physiologic Balance

Affected patients will present in the ASC in all phases of the disease, from seemingly healthy to severely compromised. Regardless of the current state of health, their disease can become acute at any time. These patients need a gentle approach that includes immaculate general nursing care related to nutrition, positioning, fluid replacement, and hygiene. Patients in advanced stages may be dyspneic and require supplemental oxygen and other methods to improve their respiratory status.

Although the ASC stay is generally short, nursing needs may be intense. Typical reasons for care may include endoscopic examination or parenteral therapies. Their surgical and anesthetic needs must be met, but in addition, they may have ongoing needs for mouth care, decubitus care, attention to hygiene related to body wastes, and other needs that are not typical of the ambulatory surgical patient population.

Neurologic symptoms may require simplified instructions, but care must be taken to avoid talking down to the adult patient as though he or she is a child. Thought processes and physical movement may be diminished, so self-care may be difficult or impossible. Seizure precautions may be necessary, and the patient may need frequent reorientation to the surroundings.

Preventing Nosocomial Infection

The HIV infected patient must be protected from threats in the environment. Infections can be acquired very easily when the immune system is weakened, so the nurse must monitor and control the personnel and equipment coming into contact with the patient to avoid infectious exposures. Antiseptics and disinfectants used for equipment and surfaces must be proved effective against pathogens. People with obvious or suspected infections such as upper respiratory infections or influenza, should not be near patients with compromised immune systems. Avoiding the potential infectious exposures of the inpatient world is one benefit of using an ambulatory surgical approach for these susceptible people.

Emotional and Home Support

These often young patients have emotional needs that far surpass most other patients. They are or may have been dealing with grief, depression, anger, isolation, financial ruin, loss of self-esteem and sexuality, rejection, loss of body functions, generally failing health, inability to provide self-care, and the fear or dread of death. Many are alone and may be estranged from their families.

Nurses in the ASC can offer these patients an environment of honesty, acceptance, and privacy. They can make the short time spent in the ASC a period in which the patient feels safe in expressing opinions and feelings and is encouraged to provide self-care within his or her limits. Some patients have said that the most important things a nurse can do are to act normal, to touch them, and to care.[58]

Healthcare workers should explore their personal feelings about caring for patients with HIV infection. Outside support and guidance may be available within the facility to help the nurse who is dealing with fears, feelings of powerlessness, or other emotions related to HIV and AIDS patient care. State and federal laws should be consulted to understand and ensure compliance with statutes regarding testing for HIV, confidentiality, health reporting, nondiscriminatory policies, and disclosure of infections of healthcare workers.

Social isolation may or may not pose a problem for the patient with HIV. Those in early stages and with few, if any, presenting symptoms may have no concerns for home support, while patients with advanced disease may require extensive home support and care. Avoidance of hospital admission is important whenever possible to avoid hospital-acquired infection. Financial struggles may force the patient into one setting or another, depending on the status of healthcare insurance and benefits already used.

The patient with advanced disease may be unable to recall or understand home instructions if confused, distracted, or even more restricted mentally. A responsible adult is an essential support system for such patients, and the companion should be included in all instructions. The need for good nutrition and wound care to avoid infection should be addressed in the discharge instructions.

Preventing Spread in the Healthcare Setting

HIV infection is known to spread through blood, semen, vaginal secretions, other body fluids containing visible blood, and possibly through breast milk, particularly in the first few months post partum. HIV is also spread through contact with infected blood. Prior to the screening of blood for evidence of HIV infection and before the introduction in 1985 of heat-treating techniques to destroy HIV in blood products, HIV was transmitted through transfusions of contaminated blood or blood components. Today, because of blood screening and heat treatment, the risk of acquiring HIV from such transfusions is extremely small.

Accidental exposure by needlestick or contact of broken skin or mucosa with infected blood is a risk that continually threatens healthcare workers. Table 25–12 provides insights regarding behaviors and responsibilities of both employers and healthcare workers to reduce exposures related to needles and sharps.

It should go without saying that a major concern is the prevention of spread of infection to the healthcare workers. All people encountered in the ASC setting should be managed under the assumption that they pose an infectious threat to the healthcare worker either from HIV or from another pathogen such as hepatitis B or other devastating infection. This potential mandates the continuous, impeccable application of standard precautions in all phases of each patient's care. Standard precautions apply to the handling of all bodily fluids, even though they have an unknown risk factor, these fluids include cerebrospinal, synovial, pleural, peritoneal, pericardial, and amniotic fluids (Table 25–13).

ENDOCRINE DISORDERS

Adrenocortical Insufficiency

Organic disease such as Addison's disease or previous adrenalectomy may be the cause of

Table 25–12. Reducing Needlesticks and Sharps Injuries

RESPONSIBILITIES SHARED BY EMPLOYERS AND HEALTHCARE WORKERS

In preventing needlestick/sharps injuries, both employers and employees have specific responsibilities.

Employer	*Employee*
Ensure a safe environment	Maintain current knowledge base on blood-borne disease and safety measures
Inform employees of workplace hazards	Recognize own high-risk behavior
Provide educational programs	Attend educational programs
Establish guidelines for sharps safety	Know hospital policies and procedures
Provide employees with health infection control programs	Change high-risk behavior
Enforce adherence to policies/procedures	Comply with safety policies
Provide equipment and supplies	Use resources consistently
Monitor or follow up all injuries	Report all injuries

SHARPS PRECAUTIONS

1. Dispose of needles and sharps immediately
2. Do not recap, bend, or break needles
3. Do not remove needles from syringes
4. Use puncture-resistant disposal containers
5. Containers should be in the immediate area of disposal
6. Containers should not be above eye level
7. Containers should be confined to an area that is for disposal purposes only
8. Wear gloves when handling blood specimens or body fluids, and when handling contaminated sharps, needles, IV insertion apparatus, or other blood-access equipment
9. Wash hands thoroughly and immediately if contamination occurs, after removing gloves and/or gown, and before leaving the area
10. Needlestick or sharps injuries should be followed with appropriate testing and treatment

RISK MANAGEMENT ACTIVITIES

Encourage reporting of all sharps injuries
Review all employee and patient sharps injuries
Identify units with high rates of sharps injuries
Identify individuals with high-risk behavior
Conduct audits and other monitoring activities to determine causes of incidents
Evaluate sharps disposal policies
Stay current on new sharps safety technology
Evaluate sharps safety program on a regular basis
Explore alternate methods of sharps disposal

Reprinted with permission from Slack, Inc. De Laune S: Risk reduction through testing, screening, and infection control measures—with special emphasis on needlestick injuries. Infect Control 11 (suppl)(10):563–565, Oct. 1990.

adrenocortical insufficiency, but suppression of cortisone production in the adrenal cortex due to long-term steroid therapy is a more common cause. Patients may be taking steroids for arthritis, inflammatory or allergic conditions, renal disease, organ transplant, or chronic obstructive lung disease. Because of their inability or reduced ability to produce endogenous adrenocorticosteroids, such patients may demonstrate a limited response to the stresses of surgery and anesthesia. For example, they may not have the ability to increase blood pressure and heart rate appropriately.

Also important is the identification of patients who use anabolic steroids for building muscle mass. Male and female body builders should be directly questioned about the use of steroids in a nonjudgmental manner and provided with information that focuses on their perioperative safety. Their positive answer should be a matter of record but held in confidence, as should all portions of the medical record.

The adrenal cortex requires 2 weeks or more to recover and begin production of cortisone after replacement steroid therapy is discontinued. The anesthesiologist should be informed of the patient's medication history including the dose, duration, and discontinuation of therapy, if any. Abrupt discontinuation of steroids prior to surgery is dangerous.

It remains controversial as to whether the patient who has minor surgery requires steroid replacement therapy. Some experts believe that coverage should be considered for the patient who has taken corticosteroids within the immediate preoperative period or for more than

Table 25–13. Standard Precautions

HOSPITAL INFECTION CONTROL PRACTICES ADVISORY COMMITTEE (HICPAC) ISOLATION PRECAUTIONS

There are two tiers of HICPAC isolation precautions. In the first, and most important, tier are those precautions designed for the care of all patients in hospitals, regardless of their diagnosis or presumed infection status. Implementation of these standard precautions is the primary strategy for successful nosocomial infection control. In the second tier are precautions designed only for the care of specified patients. These additional transmission-based precautions are for patients known or suspected to be infected by epidemiologically important pathogens spread by airborne or droplet transmission or by contact with dry skin or contaminated surfaces.

STANDARD PRECAUTIONS

Standard precautions synthesize the major features of universal (blood and body fluid) precautions (designed to reduce the risk of transmission of blood-borne pathogens) and body substance isolation (designed to reduce the risk of transmission of pathogens from moist body substances). Standard precautions apply to: (1) blood; (2) all body fluids, secretions, and excretions except sweat, regardless of whether or not they contain visible blood; (3) nonintact skin; and (4) mucous membranes. Standard precautions are designed to reduce the risk of transmission of microorganisms from both recognized and unrecognized sources of infection in hospitals. Use standard precautions, or the equivalent, for the care of all patients.

1. Handwashing
   Wash hands after touching blood, body fluids, secretions, excretions, and contaminated items, whether or not gloves are worn. Wash hands immediately after gloves are removed, between patient contacts, and when otherwise indicated to avoid transfer of microorganisms to other patients or environments. It may be necessary to wash hands between tasks and procedures on the same patient to prevent cross-contamination of different body sites.
   Use a plain (nonantimicrobial) soap for routine handwashing.
   Use an antimicrobial agent or a waterless antiseptic agent for specific circumstances (e.g., control of outbreaks or hyperendemic infections), as defined by the infection control program.
2. Gloves
   Wear gloves (clean, nonsterile gloves are adequate) when touching blood, body fluids, secretions, excretions, and contaminated items. Put on clean gloves just before touching mucous membranes and nonintact skin. Change gloves between tasks and procedures on the same patient after contact with material that may contain a high concentration of microorganisms. Remove gloves promptly after use, before touching noncontaminated items and environmental surfaces, and before going to another patient, and wash hands immediately to avoid transfer of microorganisms to other patients or environments.
3. Mask, Eye Protection, Face Shield
   Wear a mask and eye protection or a face shield to protect mucous membranes of the eyes, nose, and mouth during procedures and patient care activities that are likely to generate splashes or sprays of blood, body fluids, secretions, and excretions
4. Gown
   Wear a gown (a clean, nonsterile gown is adequate) to protect skin and to prevent soiling of clothing during procedures and patient care activities that are likely to generate splashes or sprays of blood, body fluids, secretions, or excretions. Select a gown that is appropriate for the activity and amount of fluid likely to be encountered. Remove a soiled gown as promptly as possible, and wash hands to avoid transfer of microorganisms to other patients or environments.
5. Patient Care Equipment
   Handle used patient care equipment soiled with blood, body fluids, secretions, and excretions in a manner that prevents skin and mucous membrane exposures, contamination of clothing, and transfer of microorganisms to other patients and environments. Ensure that reusable equipment is not used for the care of another patient until it has been cleaned and reprocessed appropriately. Ensure that single-use items are discarded properly.
6. Environmental Control
   Ensure that the hospital has adequate procedures for the routine care, cleaning, and disinfection of environmental surfaces, beds, bed rails, bedside equipment, and other frequently touched surfaces and ensure that these procedures are being followed.
7. Linen
   Handle, transport, and process used linen soiled with blood, body fluids, secretions, and excretions in a manner that prevents skin and mucous membrane exposures and contamination of clothing, and that avoids transfer of microorganisms to other patients and environments.
8. Occupational Health and Blood-borne Pathogens
   Take care to prevent injuries when using needles, scalpels, and other sharp instruments or devices; when handling sharp instruments after procedures; when cleaning used instruments; and when disposing of used needles. Never recap used needles, or otherwise manipulate them using both hands, or use any other technique that involves directing the point of a needle toward any part of the body; rather, use either a one-handed "scoop" technique or a mechanical device designed for holding the needle sheath. Do not remove used needles from disposable syringes by hand, and do not bend, break, or otherwise manipulate used needles by hand. Place used disposable syringes and needles, scalpel blades, and other sharp items in appropriate puncture-resistant containers, which are located as close as practical to the area in which the items were used, and place reusable syringes and needles in a puncture-resistant container for transport to the reprocessing area.
   Use mouthpieces, resuscitation bags, or other ventilation devices as an alternative to mouth-to-mouth resuscitation methods in areas where the need for resuscitation is predictable.
9. Patient Placement
   Place a patient who contaminates the environment or who does not (or cannot be expected to) assist in maintaining appropriate hygiene or environmental control in a private room. If a private room is not available, consult with infection control professionals regarding patient placement or other alternatives.

Reprinted from Hospital Infection Control Practices Advisory Committee. Guidelines for Isolation Precautions in Hospitals. Atlanta: Centers for Disease Control and Prevention. Jan. 1, 1996. Accessed at www.epo.cdc.gov/wonder/prevguid on Nov. 27, 1999.

1 month within the prior 6 months. Dosage is calculated individually for each patient, but typically a 70-kg person would receive a 100-mg intravenous dose of hydrocortisone phosphate before minor surgeries. It may be sufficient for patients currently on long-term steroid therapy to increase or double the usual oral dosage on the night prior to surgery. In that case, intravenous hydrocortisone should be on hand in the operating room and PACU to respond to symptoms of acute adrenal insufficiency.[67] Dexamethasone is an incomplete corticosteroid and is not adequate for replacement.

Rare complications associated with perioperative administration include aggravated hypertension, hyperglycemia, fluid retention, stress ulcers, and psychiatric disturbances.[59] Discharge instructions should include specific information from the physician about when to resume usual steroid replacement therapy.

Delayed wound-healing and masking of signs of infection are possible complications related to long-term steroid use because of suppression of the body's inflammatory response. Discharge instructions should be very precise relating to good nutrition, aseptic wound care, and reporting of any untoward symptoms to the physician. All prescribed antibiotics should be taken.

*Diabetes Mellitus**

An estimated 16 million people in the United States have diabetes mellitus, a serious, lifelong condition. About half of these people do not know they have diabetes and are not under care for the disorder. Each year, about 798,000 people are diagnosed with diabetes. Although diabetes occurs most often in older adults, it is one of the most common chronic disorders in children in the United States. About 123,000 children and teenagers age 19 and younger have diabetes.

Diabetes is widely recognized as one of the leading causes of death and disability in the United States. According to death certificate data, diabetes contributed to the deaths of more than 193,140 persons in 1996. Diabetes is associated with long-term complications that affect almost every major part of the body. It contributes to blindness, heart disease, strokes, kidney failure, amputations, and nerve damage. Uncontrolled diabetes can complicate pregnancy, and birth defects are more common in babies born to women with diabetes. Diabetes cost the United States $98 billion in 1997. Indirect costs, including disability payments, time lost from work, and premature death, totaled $54 billion; medical costs for diabetes care, including hospitalizations, medical care, and treatment supplies, totaled $44 billion.

Diabetes is a disorder of metabolism. Most of the food that we eat is broken down by the digestive juices into a simple sugar called glucose. For glucose to get into the cells, insulin must be present. In people with diabetes, however, the islets of Langerhans in the pancreas either produces little or no insulin, or the body cells do not respond to the insulin that is produced. As a result, glucose builds up in the blood, overflows into the urine, and passes out of the body. Thus, the body loses its main source of fuel even though hyperglycemia occurs.

The three main types of diabetes are type 1 diabetes, type 2 diabetes, and gestational diabetes which occurs during pregnancy. Type 1 diabetes (insulin-dependent diabetes mellitus or juvenile diabetes) is considered an autoimmune disease. The immune system attacks the insulin-producing beta cells in the pancreas and destroys them; the pancreas then produces little or no insulin. At present, scientists do not know exactly what causes the body's immune system to attack the beta cells, but they believe that both genetic factors and viruses are involved. Type 1 diabetes accounts for about 5% to 10% of diagnosed diabetes in the United States.

Type 1 diabetes develops most often in children and young adults, but the disorder can appear at any age. Symptoms of type 1 diabetes usually develop over a short period, although beta cell destruction can begin years earlier. Symptoms include increased thirst and urination, constant hunger, weight loss, blurred vision, and extreme tiredness. If not diagnosed and treated with insulin, a person can lapse into a life-threatening coma.

Daily injections of insulin are the basic therapy for type 1 diabetes. Insulin injections must be balanced with meals and daily activities, and glucose levels must be closely monitored through frequent blood sugar testing. Table 25–14 provides an overview of various types of insulin.

The most common form of diabetes is type 2 diabetes (non–insulin-dependent diabetes mellitus, or NIDDM). About 90% to 95% of people with diabetes have type 2 diabetes. This form usually develops in adults over 40 years of age and is most common among adults over age 55.

*This introductory information is taken substantially from National Institutes of Health, National Institute of Diabetes and Digestive and Kidney Diseases.[60]

Table 25–14. **Onset, Peak, and Duration of Action of Various Insulins**

TYPE	ONSET	PEAK	DURATION
Short-acting			
Regular Iletin	15–30 min	2–4 hr	5–7 hr
Humulin R	30 min	2–4 hr	6–8 hr
Intermediate-acting			
Lente	1–2 hr	6–12 hr	18–24 hr
NPH	1–2 hr	6–12 hr	18–24 hr
Humulin N	1–3 hr	6–12 hr	14–24 hr
Long-acting			
Ultralente	4–6 hr	14–24 hr	28–36 hr
Humulin U	4–6 hr	8–20 hr	24–28 hr

About 80% of people with type 2 diabetes are overweight.

In type 2 diabetes, the pancreas usually produces insulin, but for some reason, the body cannot use the insulin effectively. The end result is the same as for type 1 diabetes, hyperglycemia and an inability of the body to make efficient use of its main source of fuel. The symptoms of type 2 diabetes develop gradually and are not as noticeable as in type 1 diabetes. Symptoms include fatigue, malaise, frequent urination (especially at night), unusual thirst, weight loss, blurred vision, frequent infections, and slow healing of sores. Diet, exercise, and blood testing for glucose are also the basis for management of type 2 diabetes, and some people with type 2 diabetes take oral drugs or insulin to lower their blood glucose levels. Table 25–15 lists a number of oral hypoglycemic medications in use.

The goal of diabetes management is to keep blood glucose levels as close to the normal, nondiabetic range as safely possible. In addition to the current medications available today, recent advances in diabetes research have led to better ways to manage diabetes and treat its complications. Major advances include:

- New forms of purified insulin, such as human insulin produced through genetic engineering
- Better ways for doctors to monitor blood glucose levels and for people with diabetes to test their own blood glucose levels at home
- Development of external and implantable insulin pumps that deliver appropriate amounts of insulin, replacing daily injections
- Laser treatment for diabetic eye disease, reducing the risk of blindness
- Successful transplantation of kidneys in people whose own kidneys fail because of diabetes
- Better ways of managing diabetic pregnancies, improving chances of successful outcomes
- New drugs to treat type 2 diabetes and better ways to manage this form of diabetes through weight control
- Evidence that intensive management of blood glucose reduces and may prevent development of microvascular complications of diabetes
- Demonstration that antihypertensive drugs called angiotensin converting enzyme (ACE) inhibitors prevent or delay kidney failure in people with diabetes[60]

Perioperative implications for diabetic patients include monitoring and reporting of blood glucose levels and precise instructions to patients regarding their usual hypoglycemic protocols. Many ambulatory surgical procedures performed on older adults do not substantially affect dietary intake, and those patients are often encouraged to take their usual medication after nourishment has been resumed postoperatively. Instructions prior to the day of surgery should tell patients to bring usual medications with them to the ASC and inform patients of the types of food available in the ASC.

The patient on insulin requires especially close monitoring. Urine glucose is an inaccurate measure of blood glucose levels and is not suggested. Bedside monitoring using impregnated strips or glucose monitoring devices provides rapid determination but depends on the accuracy of the equipment and the personnel. Calibration of equipment, periodic skill checks of personnel, checking of equipment, and other precautions are dictated by the Clinical Laboratory Improvement Act. See Chapter 3 for further information.

Insulin shock due to hypoglycemia or diabetic ketoacidosis is more likely in the type I patient who requires close control of diet, IV replacement fluids, and insulin therapy. Predisposing factors include noncompliance with diet and medication protocols, exercise, drugs, and

Table 25–15. **Oral Hypoglycemic Medications**

DRUG	TRADE NAMES	CLASSIFICATION	ACTION	HOW SUPPLIED	ONSET OF ACTION	PEAK OF SERUM LEVEL	DURATION OF ACTION	SIDE EFFECTS/ ADVERSE REACTIONS
Acetohexamide	Dymelor	Antidiabetic agent, sulfonylurea	Probably stimulates insulin release from the beta cells and reduces glucose output by the liver	250 mg, 500 mg	1 hr	1.5–2 hr	8–24 h	Nausea, heartburn, vomiting; skin rash, pruritus, facial flushing; hypersensitivity reactions, sodium loss
Chlorpropamide	Diabenese, Glucamide	Antidiabetic agent, sulfonylurea	Probably stimulates insulin release from the beta cells and reduces glucose output by the liver	100 mg, 250 mg	1 hr	2–4 hr	24–72 hr	Nausea, heartburn, vomiting; skin rash, pruritus, facial flushing; hypersensitivity reactions, sodium loss
Gliclazide	Diamicron (not available in US)	Antidiabetic agent, second generation sulfonylurea	Probably stimulates insulin release from the beta cells and reduces glucose output by the liver	80 mg	—	4–6 hr	24 hr	Nausea, heartburn, vomiting; skin rash, pruritus, facial flushing; hypersensitivity reactions, sodium loss
Glipizide	Glucotrol, Glucotrol XL	Antidiabetic agent, second generation sulfonylurea	Probably stimulates insulin release from the beta cells and reduces glucose output by the liver	5 mg, 10 mg, and extended release	15–30 min	2–4 hr	12–24 hr	Dizziness; nausea, vomiting, constipation; cholestatic jaundice; skin rash, pruritus, facial flushing

Glyburide	DiaBeta, Glynase PresTab, Micronase	Antidiabetic agent, second generation sulfonylurea	Probably stimulates insulin release from the beta cells and reduces glucose output by the liver	1.25 mg, 2.5 mg, and micronized 1.5 mg, 3 mg, 5 mg	1 hr (micronized form); 2 to 4 hr (nonmicronized form)	Nonmicronized 3.4 to 4.5 hr; micronized 2.3 to 3.5 hr	24 hr	Nausea, epigastric fullness, heartburn; cholestatic jaundice; skin rash, pruritus, facial flushing
Metformin hydrochloride	Glucophage	Antihyperglycemic agent, biguanide	Decreases hepatic glucose production and intestinal absorption of glucose and improves insulin sensitivity	500 mg, 850 mg	Not known	Unknown	Unknown	Diarrhea, nausea, vomiting, abdominal bloating, flatulence, anorexia; megaloblastic anemia, rash, dermatitis, lactic acidosis, metallic taste
Tolazamide	Tolamide, Tolinase	Sulfonylurea	Unknown, probably stimulates insulin release from the beta cells and reduces glucose output by the liver	100 mg, 250 mg, 500 mg	4–6 hr	3–4 hr	10–20 hr	Nausea, vomiting; skin rash, urticaria, facial flushing; hypersensitivity reactions
Tolbutamide	Apo-Tolbutamide, Oramide, Orinase	Sulfonylurea	Unknown, probably stimulates insulin release from the beta cells and reduces glucose output by the liver	250 mg, 500 mg	1 hr	3–4 hr	6–12 hr	Nausea, heartburn; rash, pruritus, facial flushing, hypersensitivity reactions, decreased blood sodium levels

Reprinted with permission from Gray M: Historical developments in the drug therapy of diabetes. Orthopaedic Nurs 16(2):86, 1997.

stress. Anxiolytic medication and emotional support are important nursing interventions to reduce stress.

The occurrence of hypoglycemic symptoms in the type 1 diabetic patient should alert the nurse to escalating potential problems, and an immediate bedside glucose determination should be performed. Hypoglycemic symptoms include confusion, changes in level of consciousness, lethargy, fatigue, visual disturbances, tachycardia, seizures, anxiety, extreme hunger, and circumoral numbness. The awake patient can be urged to take oral sugar such as honey, milk, hard candy, juice, or a regular soda. Intravenous administration of 50% dextrose is rapidly effective for the patient with altered consciousness. Intravenous glucagon can be given in a dose of 0.5 mg to 1 mg and repeated one or two more times at 20-minute intervals.[61] If a vein is not available, 1 mg of glucagon can be given intramuscularly to stimulate glycogenesis in the liver. When the crisis has passed, the patient will need further dietary or parenteral glucose intake to prevent another episode.

All possible measures should be taken to reduce perioperative nausea and vomiting because serious problems may result if the diabetic patient is unable to eat for an extended period of time. Changes in drug therapy or even hospitalization may be necessary.

Other complications of diabetes may surface in the ASC. Difficult voiding as a result of autonomic neuropathy of the bladder may add to surgical or anesthesia-related voiding issues. Spontaneous voiding is much preferred to avoid the possibility of urinary tract infection. If catheterization is necessary, strict aseptic technique must be followed. Diabetes also affects the gastrointestinal system with reduced esophageal and gastric motility, termed gastroparesis, which makes the patient prone to pooling of gastric contents and possible esophageal reflux. Thus, aspiration becomes another concern.

Predisposition to cardiac, vascular, and renal disease, as well as diverse neuropathy and atherosclerosis make the diabetic patient prone to other perioperative complications. Microvascular changes can affect the retina, coronary and cerebral arteries, and peripheral vessels. Peripheral neuropathy reduces sensation and awareness of pressure or pain in the extremities, and silent myocardial infarction or angina is not uncommon, so a preoperative ECG is a frequent assessment parameter for the complex diabetic patient. Smoking compounds the risk of myocardial infarction or cardiovascular accident (CVA) for these patients.

Wound-healing is negatively affected for several reasons, including the following:

1. Predisposition to infection
2. Reduced nutrition due to altered fat, protein, and glucose metabolism
3. Peripheral vascular disease and neuropathy, decreasing blood supply
4. Inadvertent injury and unawareness of complications as a result of reduced sensation

For these reasons, the patient should be carefully instructed on the importance of aseptic wound and dressing care; frequent wound examinations; maintaining a nutritious diet, good hydration, and normal blood glucose levels; and reporting signs of infection immediately.

Prior to discharge, the patient also needs specific instructions from the physician about drug and dietary management. Diabetic retinopathy can impede the patient's vision, making it difficult to read medicine bottles and postoperative instructions. Peripheral neuropathy can rob the patient of motor and sensory innervation in the hands, complicating self-care. A reliable home companion to assist with care is an important support for these complicated patients. Although the patient with diabetes is at higher risk than unaffected patients, when careful preoperative assessment is performed and their diabetes is under control, they are considered appropriate candidates for ambulatory surgery. A list of Internet sites providing information on diabetes is found in Table 25–16. Also, the American Diabetes Association can be reached by calling 1 (800) DIABETES, or 1 (800) 342-2383.

HEMATOLOGIC DISEASES

A variety of genetic and acquired blood disorders can affect the patient's tolerance for anesthesia and surgery. The blood is integral in the uptake, distribution, metabolism, and elimination of anesthetic drugs and adjuvants. It also functions in tissue oxygen delivery, carbon dioxide elimination, transport of nutrients in the body, hemostasis, and immunity to disease.

Serious blood dyscrasias should be identified during the preadmission assessment so that necessary maintenance or corrective actions can be initiated to reduce or eliminate related perioperative complications. For instance, a person with significant anemia may require preoperative transfusion or drug therapy prior to surgery or may need prolonged perioperative oxygen administration. Patients on anticoagulant ther-

Table 25–16. **Internet Resource Sites for Diabetes**

NAME	INTERNET ADDRESS
National Institute of Diabetes and Digestive and Kidney Diseases at the National Institutes of Health	www.niddk.nih.gov/health/diabetes/pubs
Joslin's Online Diabetes Library	www.joslin.harvard.edu/wlist.html
American Diabetes Association	www.diabetes.org
Doctor's Guide	www.pslgroup.com/dg/5ffe.htm
On Health Guide	www.onhealth.com/ch1/resource/index.asp

apy may need to modify or stop drug therapy prior to surgery so that clotting will be adequate for hemostasis. In the case of someone with sickle cell disease or thalassemia, the physician is concerned that perioperative stress or certain anesthetic agents will precipitate an acute episode. Medical and nursing planning must take the patient's specific condition into account during all phases of the procedure.

Anemia

Anemia is a symptom rather than a disease, and it has many causes. It can be defined as a hemoglobin concentration less than normal for the patient's age and gender. Normal ranges are 14 to 18 g/dl for males and 12 to 16 g/dl for females. The usual range for children is 12 to 14 g/dl.

Hemoglobin is the primary oxygen and carbon dioxide transporter to and from tissues, respectively. Traditional thinking was to avoid nonurgent surgery on anyone with a hemoglobin level lower than 10 g/dl, but it is more common now to consider the patient individually and to assess the cardiovascular and respiratory systems, the chronicity of the anemia, and the extent to which the body has compensated. Myocardial ischemia with or without infarction is a possibility when oxygenation is not sufficient. Thus, anesthetic goals aim at avoiding hypovolemia, maintaining a high PaO_2, keeping the patient warm, avoiding shivering, and maintaining the hemoglobin level above critical level. In patients with concurrent coronary artery disease, extubation is the time of greatest risk.[62]

Nursing implications include monitoring oxygen saturation during the perioperative period, providing supplemental oxygen as appropriate, and reducing stress and workload to reduce oxygen demand. The latter is addressed by keeping the patient warm to avoid shivering, providing aggressive pain and nausea management, and maintaining normotension. Restlessness should be investigated carefully to rule out hypoxia as a cause.

Sickle Cell Disease

Sickle cell disease (SCD) is the term for a group of genetic disorders characterized by the predominance of hemoglobin S. The name comes from the diagnostic sickle shape of the affected red blood cells. It is an inherited disorder that can be mild to severe, including fatal. There are two cardinal pathophysiologic features of sickle cell disorders: chronic hemolytic anemia and vaso-occlusion, which results in ischemic tissue injury. Sickle cell trait, on the other hand, is not a disease but a disorder that rarely results in the crises seen in the disease state. Sickle cell disorders are found in people of African, Mediterranean, Indian, and Middle Eastern heritage.

The definitive diagnosis of sickle cell disease is not simple and requires a variety of laboratory tests. Approximately 1000 babies affected by sickle cell disease are born in the United States each year. Estimates are that about 2.5 million Americans have the sickle cell trait, and about 700,000 suffer from sickle cell disease. Careful preoperative assessment should include questioning about family and personal history and symptoms that could indicate SCD.

Erythrocyte sickling occurs more readily in the presence of low oxygen partial pressures and acidosis; thus, if hemoglobin oxygen saturation levels drop, the chance of sickling increases. The abnormally shaped cells rupture and chronic hemolytic anemia results. Sickle cells also become trapped in small vessels, reducing blood flow to distal tissues. Peripheral and organ damage results from thrombosis and infarction of tissues. The brain and kidneys are most affected from these periodic crises because of their constant need for oxygen. Vessel occlusion causes ischemic pain that can be severe, particularly in the hands and feet.[63]

The most acute manifestation of SCD is called a sequestration crisis, during which large amounts of blood pool in the spleen and liver. Liver function is seriously affected, and multiple areas of infarction occur throughout body systems. Anemia increases as abnormal cells break down, and cardiovascular collapse can occur.

Perioperatively the goals are to identify patients with potential for SCD and, in known patients, to provide comfort and reduce the risk of a sickling crisis. Preoperatively the patient should be well hydrated and assessed for signs of vaso-occlusion, fever, infection, and dehydration. More extensive preoperative diagnostic tests may be performed based on the individual patient's needs. The ECG, along with oxygen saturation levels, is monitored closely. The operating room should be warm, and oxygen is often administered in higher than usual concentrations, at least 50%. Postoperatively oxygen should be administered until the effects of anesthesia have worn off and oxygen saturation monitoring should be continued. Intravenous hydration is often maintained for a period of time, and pulmonary care is aggressive to minimize pulmonary complications.[64]

Other nursing care goals include avoidance of environmental and positional causes of circulatory compromise and venous stasis, maintenance of proper body alignment, avoidance of pressure points, cautious use and monitoring of pneumatic tourniquets, judicious use of blood pressure cuffs, maintenance of normothermia, support of adequate hydration, and prevention of acidosis.[65] Careful assessment for peripheral ischemia is essential.

Bleeding Disorders

The process of clot formation is complex and requires the interaction of platelets, enzymes, and many other factors, many of which are manufactured by the liver. Dysfunction at any step in this process can result in inadequate hemostasis and the chance of significant perioperative bleeding.

Three elements are necessary for adequate hemostasis: vascular constriction, adequate platelets, and coagulation factors. When damaged, a blood vessel constricts to help divert blood away from the point of injury. Normally platelets adhere to the exposed subendothelial portion of the damaged vessel, triggering adherence of more platelets (platelet aggregation) and the formation of a plug that is reinforced by fibrin strands formed from the proteins of coagulation.

It is important to identify patients with compromised hemostatic ability before surgery. The major causes of coagulopathy besides inadequate surgical hemostasis include disorders of the platelets of coagulation factors, excessive fibrinolysis, and the presence of an anticoagulant. Hepatic disease, alcoholism, vitamin K deficiency, and excessive use of aspirin or other medications that affect platelet production are all potential causes of bleeding disorders. Other risk factors include the following:

- Prior history of perioperative or dental bleeding
- Family history of bleeding
- Significant epistaxis or menorrhagia
- Medication history
- Alcohol abuse
- History of hepatitis or other liver disease
- History of biliary tract disease.

Preoperative assessment includes physical examination for bruising, petechiae, or signs of liver disease such as jaundice, ascites, spider angiomas, or Dupuytren's contracture. Patients with prior history will require laboratory screening to evaluate different steps of the coagulation process. Prothrombin time (PT) evaluates the extrinsic pathway and the partial thromboplastin time (PTT) measures the intrinsic pathway in the formation of activated factor X, which is one of the factors needed to transform prothrombin into thrombin.

The normal range for platelets is 150,000 to 400,000 per mm^3. A minimal level of 50,000 per mm^3 is necessary to prevent surgical bleeding. Platelet production can be altered by bone marrow depression, medications such as aspirin and NSAIDs, thrombocytopenic purpura, and massive transfusions. Platelets have a lifespan of 1 to 2 weeks, after which they are gradually consumed and new platelets form. For this reason, medications that affect platelets should be stopped 1 to 2 weeks before surgery to allow proper regeneration of normal platelets. The availability of proper blood or blood components to treat the patient's specific coagulopathy should be ascertained prior to surgery.

Postoperative bleeding can be insidious. Some covert signs include increased girth, ecchymosis, frequent swallowing, and pain that is difficult to control. Simple procedures such as venipuncture and phlebotomy for blood sampling can result in prolonged bleeding, particularly in people who are taking anticoagulants, so careful hemostasis must be ensured. Patients with known or suspected coagulation deficiencies should have 3 to 5 minutes or more of pressure applied to venipuncture sites. Patients should avoid exertion during the early recovery phase after surgery and should know the insidious signs of bleeding to report. Patients with significant blood dyscrasias may require hospitalization for perioperative management.

CONCLUSION

All patients undergoing surgery and anesthesia have individual physical, emotional, social, and educational needs. Those who have significant pre-existing diseases or risk factors have an even greater need for careful attention that addresses their special challenges. Nurses in the ASC setting must evaluate each patient's medical, surgical, social, and emotional history and collaborate with the anesthesia and surgical team members to communicate special needs and risks. Patients whose conditions are compromised by pre-existing illness require care planning that depends on a multidisciplinary approach to ensure that comprehensive care is provided.

References

1. Fastats, Centers for Disease Control and Prevention. Available at www.cdc.gov/nchs/fastats.overwt.htm. Accessed Oct. 31, 1999.
2. Langer L: Anesthesia and the morbidity obese. Available at http://www.gasnet.med.yale.edu/gta/obese.html. Oct. 31, 1999.
3. Polk S: Anesthesia for the morbidity obese patient—proceed with care. Wellcome Trends Anesthesiol 6(6):3–9, 1988.
4. Wooley S, Wooley O: Should obesity be treated at all? Psychiatric Ann 13:884–888, 1983.
5. Schwartz F: The relationship among personality characteristics of dieting and weight. AAOHN J 41(10):504–509, 1993.
6. Culbertson M, Smolen D: Attitudes of RN students toward obese adult patients. J Nurs Educ 38:84–87, 1999.
7. Jarrell L: Preoperative diagnosis and postoperative management of adult patients with obstructive sleep apnea: A review of the literature. JOPAN 14:193–200, 1999.
8. Centers for Disease Control and Prevention: Accessed at Internet site www.cdc.gov/tobacco/issue.htm on Oct. 31, 1999.
9. Groah L: Operating Room Nursing Perioperative Practice, 2nd ed. Norwalk, CT: Appleton & Lange, 1990.
10. Mason R: Anaesthesia Datebook: A Clinical Practice Compendium. Edinburgh: Churchill Livingstone, 1990.
11. Feeley T, Botz G: Factors influencing choice of anesthetic technique. In White P: Ambulatory Anesthesia and Surgery. Philadelphia: WB Saunders, 1997, pp 190–197.
12. Caldwell T: Anesthesia for patients with behavioral and environmental disorders. In Katz J, Benumof J, Kadis L: Anesthesia and Uncommon Diseases, 3rd ed. Philadelphia: WB Saunders, 1990, pp. 792–922.
13. National Institute on Drug Abuse at National Institutes of Health: Pain Medications. No. 13553. Accessed via the Internet at www.nidda.nih.gov/Infofax/PainMed.html on Nov. 4, 1999.
14. National Institute on Alcohol Abuse and Alcoholism at National Institutes of Health: Alcohol Alert No. 40-1998. Accessed via the Internet at www.silk/nih.gov/silk/niaaa1/publication/aa40.htm on Nov. 4, 1999.
15. Huckabee M: Perioperative care of the active substance abuser. JOPAN 3:254–259, 1988.
16. National Institute on Drug Abuse at National Institutes of Health: Steroids. No. 13557. Accessed via the Internet at www.nidda.nih.gov/Infofax/steroids.html on Nov. 4, 1999.
17. American Herbalist Guild: Accessed at www.healthy.net/herbalists on Nov. 5, 1999.
18. Eisenberg D, Davis R, Ettner S, et al: Trends in alternative medicine use in the United States, 1990–1997. JAMA 280:1569–1575, 1998.
19. Malik T: The safety of herbal medicine. Alternative Ther Health Med 1:27–28, Sept. 1995.
20. Murphy J: Preoperative considerations with herbal medicines. AORN J 69:73–83, 1999.
21. American Society of Anesthesiologists: Public education document. Accessed at www.asaho.org on Nov. 6, 1999.
22. Gabrielse L, Boosamra S: Obstetrical patient postanesthesia management protocol. JOPAN 12(4):245–251, 1997.
23. Duncan P, Pope W, Cohen M, et al: Fetal risk of anesthesia and surgery during pregnancy. Anesthesiology 64:790–794, 1986.
24. Kendrick J, Woodard C, Cross S: Surveyed use of fetal and uterine monitoring during maternal surgery. AORN J 62:386–391, 1995.
25. Fullerton JT: Surgery during pregnancy. Semin Perioperative Nurs 8:101–108, 1999.
26. Twersky R, Phillips R: Pregnancy testing. In Roizen M, Fleisher L: Essence of Anesthesia Practice. Philadelphia: WB Saunders, 1997, p 572.
27. Odom J: Pre, intra, and post-operative special needs patient. Specialty Learning Labs Learningbook. Pittsburgh: RTN HealthCareGroup, 1997.
28. Drain C: The Post Anesthesia Care Unit. Philadelphia: WB Saunders, 1994, p 554.
29. Scott J, Disaia P, Hammond C, et al: Danforth's Obstetrics and Gynecology, 7th ed. Philadelphia: JB Lippincott, 1994, pp 119–299.
30. American Heart Association: Accessed via www.americanheart.org/statistics/index.html on Feb. 19, 2000.
31. Walton J: Nursing interventions to reduce perioperative cardiac morbidity and mortality. Dimen Crit Care 17(6):282–293, 1998.
32. Thomas R: Cardiovascular disease in blacks: Planning a successful treatment strategy. US Phamacist Cardiovascular Supplement, March 1991, p 35–41.
33. Brown S: Coronary artery disease—Considerations in postanesthesia care. JOPAN 3:240–246, 1988.
34. Reves J: Coronary artery disease. In Roizen M, Fleisher L: Essence of Anesthesia Practice. Philadelphia: WB Saunders, 1997, p 91.
35. Abrams J: Hemodynamic effects of nitroglycerin and long acting nitrates. Am Heart J 110:216–224, 1985.
36. D'Altellis N, Baron J: Congestive heart failure. In Roizen M, Fleisher L: Essence of Anesthesia Practice. Philadelphia: WB Saunders, 1997, p 86.
37. Echenbrecht P: Implantable cardioverter-defibrillators (ICDs): Management. In Roizen M, Fleisher L: Essence of Anesthesia Practice. Philadelphia: WB Saunders, 1997, p 189.

38. National Institutes of Health, National Heart, Lung, and Blood Institute: The Lungs in Health and Disease. Washington, DC: US Department of Health & Human Services. NIH Publication No. 97-3279, Aug. 1997.
39. Smetana G: Preoperative pulmonary evaluation. N Engl J Med 340(12):937–943, 1999.
40. The COMBIVENT Inhalation Aerosol Group Study: In chronic obstructive pulmonary disease, a combination of ipratropium and albuterol is more effective than either agent alone: An 85 day multicenter trial. Chest 105:1411–1419, 1994.
41. Corbridge T, Hall J: Asthma, acute. In Roizen M, Fleisher L: Essence of Anesthesia Practice. Philadelphia: WB Saunders, 1997, p 34.
42. Gold B, Fleisher L: Management of patients with associated pre-existing diseases. In White P: Ambulatory Anesthesia and Surgery. Philadelphia: WB Saunders, 1997, p, 138–154.
43. Prough D: Renal failure, chronic. In Roizen M, Fleisher L: Essence of Anesthesia Practice. Philadelphia: WB Saunders, 1997, p 273.
44. Maree S: Advanced scientific concepts: Update for nurse anesthetists: Part II—The renal system: Physiology, pathophysiology and anesthesia management. Am Assoc Nurs Anesth J 55:269–282, June 1987.
45. Strunin L, Eagle C: Liver diseases. In Katz J, Benumof J, Kadis L: Anesthesia and Uncommon Diseases, 3rd ed. Philadelphia: WB Saunders, 1990, p 512–536.
46. Pregler J: Hepatitis—alcoholic. In Roizen M, Fleisher L. Essence of Anesthesia Practice. Philadelphia: WB Saunders, 1997, p 155.
47. Ignatavicius D: Meeting the psychosocial needs of the patient with rheumatoid arthritis. Orthop Nurs 6:16–21, 1987.
48. Borel C: Myasthenia gravis. In Roizen M, Fleisher L: Essence of Anesthesia Practice. Philadelphia: WB Saunders, 1997, p 224.
49. Ignatavicius D, Bayne M: Medical-Surgical Nursing: A Nursing Diagnosis Approach. Philadelphia: WB Saunders, 1991.
50. Hardy E, Rittenberry K: Myasthenia gravis: An overview. Orthop Nurs 13:37–42, 1994.
51. Goldblum K: Nursing care of the patient with myasthenia gravis. Insight. Newsletter Am Soc Ophthalmic Reg Nurses 16:7, 1991.
52. Porth C: Pathophysiology: Concepts of altered health states, 3rd ed. Philadelphia: JB Lippincott, 1990, pp 1036–1038.
53. Sharpe M, Zimmerman W: Parkinson's disease. In Roizen M, Fleisher L: Essence of Anesthesia Practice. Philadelphia: WB Saunders, 1997, p 242.
54. Robinson D: Systemic lupus erythematosus. In Roizen M, Fleisher L: Essence of Anesthesia Practice. Philadelphia: WB Saunders, 1997, p 305.
55. National Institutes of Health, National Institute of Asthma and Infectious Diseases: Basic information about AIDS and HIV. Accessed at www.niaid.nih.oov/daids/vaccine/basicinfo.htm on Nov. 27, 1999.
56. Centers of Disease Control and Prevention: Recent HIV/AIDS treatment advances and the implications for prevention. Accessed at www.cdc.gov/nchstp/hivaids/pubs/facts/treatment.htm on Nov. 27, 1999.
57. Merigan T: Recent advances in antiretroviral therapy. Part 1: HIV. In Richman D (series ed): Continuing Medical Education Program for the Specialist in Virology. San Diego School of Medicine, University of California, 1(2):1990.
58. Ignatavicius D, Bayne M: Medical-Surgical Nursing: A Nursing Diagnosis Approach. Philadelphia: WB Saunders, 1991.
59. Roizen M: Diseases of the endocrine system. In Katz J, Benumof J, Kadis L: Anesthesia and Uncommon Diseases, 3rd ed. Philadelphia: WB Saunders, 1990, p 245–292.
60. National Diabetes Information Clearinghouse: Diabetes overview. National Institutes of Health, National Institute of Diabetes and Digestive and Kidney Diseases. Accessed at www.nih.gov/health/diabetes/pubs on Nov. 27, 1999.
61. Nurse's PDR Resource Center: Accessed at www.nursespdr.com on Feb. 19, 2000.
62. Spahn D: Anemia—chronic disease. In Roizen M, Fleisher L: Essence of Anesthesia Practice. Philadelphia: WB Saunders, 1997, p 17.
63. Martinelli A: Sickle cell disease: Etiology, symptoms, patient care. AORN J 53:716–724, 1991.
64. National Heart, Lung and Blood Institute: Management and Therapy of Sickle Cell Disease, 3rd ed. Bethesda, MD: National Institutes of Health. NIH Publication No. 96-2117, pp 109–110, 1995.
65. Dewhirst W, Glass D: hematologic diseases. In Katz J, Benumof J, Kadis L: Anesthesia and Uncommon Diseases, 3rd ed. Philadelphia: WB Saunders, 1990, pp 378–436.
66. U.S. Dept. of Justice Drug Enforcement Administration. Accessed at http://www.usdoj.gov/dea/stats/overview.htm on November 28, 1999.
67. Green C, Pandit S: Preoperative preparation. In Twersky R: The Ambulatory Anesthesia Handbook. St. Louis: CV Mosby, 1995, pp 171–202.

Chapter 26

Pediatric Patients and Their Families

Delores Ireland

Children are the hands by which we take hold of Heaven.
— Henry Ward Beecher

Children are excellent candidates for ambulatory surgery. Most children are healthy, and most surgeries performed on children are simple procedures associated with prompt recovery. It is not surprising, therefore, that up to 60% of pediatric surgeries in this country are performed as ambulatory procedures.[1]

Pediatric patients are not "miniature adults," although the goals and standards of care remain the same as for adults. Effective and developmentally appropriate preparation, thorough assessment of preoperative and postoperative needs, and implementation and delivery of care provide the pediatric patient with a safe return to the preanesthesia state.

The perianesthesia nurse deals not only with the child as a patient but also with the parents during the child's care. The integrity of the family unit must be maintained, allowing parents to be active partners in the caregiving process. The nurse can assist parents through this educational process by providing them with the necessary information to make informed decisions and provide emotional support for their children.

Children should be seen from a wellness viewpoint. Individual strengths and weaknesses should be assessed according to developmental levels. Children should be encouraged to function at their level throughout the perianesthesia experience and return home to a state of wellness within the family.

The focus in this chapter is on the special needs of the pediatric patient. The importance of meeting these needs as they relate to the family and the adequate preparation of the family as an integrated unit are stressed. The statement that "children have the right to be treated with dignity and respect,"[2] taken from older standards of the American Nurses' Association (ANA), remains a valid challenge to nurses caring for pediatric patients.

FAMILY-CENTERED CONCEPTS

Bill of Rights

Facilities providing services to children should have a policy on the rights and responsibilities of these patients and of their parents and/or guardians.[3] Many facilities have developed a "bill of rights" (see example in Table 26–1), which is presented to families at the time of admission and displayed in highly visible locations. Legal and ethical considerations are also important, especially when caring for the pediatric patient. Nurses should be aware of these legal requirements (Table 26–2) when caring for children.

Table 26–1. Bill of Rights for Children and Teens

In this hospital you and your family have the right to:
- Respect and personal dignity
- Care that supports you and your family
- Information you can understand
- Quality health care
- Emotional support
- Care that respects your need to grow, play, and learn
- Make choices and decisions

From Association for the Care of Children's Health: *A pediatric bill of rights,* Mt. Royal, NJ, 1998. A detailed explanation of each right is available for a fee from the Association for the Care of Children's Health, 19 Mantua Road, Mt. Royal, NJ 08061, (609) 224-1742.

Family Support

Parents remain the greatest source of support for children undergoing surgery. We cannot assume that parents automatically come equipped with the knowledge necessary to prepare their children for this experience. Parents need to be given the proper educational tools and information to make informed decisions in the best interests of their child.

Children and their parents will feel more in control when they know what to expect. Numerous articles support the theory that stress is reduced within the family when everyone knows and understands what is expected.[4]

Healing Triangle

There is a delicate balance that exists among the child, the family, and the nurse. All three interact to aid in the healing process. The nurse assesses the patient's physical condition, developmental levels, behavioral reactions, and learning readiness and interprets verbal and nonverbal clues. The parents participate by learning the disease process and surgical and discharge preparation and aid in interpretation of the child's emotional responses. The child learns independently out of interest and curiosity with a desire to maintain some degree of control.

Table 26–2. Legal and Ethical Considerations

The nurse or physician must obtain informed consent before any procedure or treatment that is potentially harmful to the child. These include immunizations and participation in research. A parent, an adolescent older than 18 years, or an emancipated minor (a minor child who is no longer dependent upon parents for either emotional or financial support) may give consent.

Children able to understand the procedure and its implications should be included in the decision making.

In certain cultures, the primary caregiver is not the child's legal guardian and cannot give consent. To give culturally sensitive care, include all the child's significant caregivers in the decision-making process.

From Luckmann J (ed): Saunders Manual of Nursing Care. Philadelphia: WB Saunders, 1997, p 475.

PHYSICAL ENVIRONMENT

Environment and Safety

Cost-effective and safe ambulatory surgery can be achieved in both hospital-based and free-standing centers. Regardless of where the surgery is performed or the site chosen there are certain safety factors that must be employed:

- Available resuscitation equipment specific to meet pediatric requirements
- Stretchers with appropriate side-rail padding
- Cribs with side rails in tallest position and fastened securely
- Supplies and equipment kept out of children's reach
- Age-appropriate toys without small pieces that are nonallergenic and washable

In addition, if children are allowed to move about in a preoperative "play" area there should be child-size furniture available and nonslippery floor surfaces, and care should be taken to have rounded edges on all counters and furniture. Electrical outlets should be covered with plastic protectors or be placed out of reach. If children change into hospital pajamas in such an area, feet should be covered with slippers that have nonskid bottoms. Preoperative and postoperative areas should be separated so those children who are NPO (nothing by mouth) do not come in contact with food or drinks.

Hospital-Based Programs

Hospital-based programs offer a more extensive back-up support system if an emergency situation occurs. If a procedure becomes more extensive than originally planned or the child cannot meet discharge criteria, a hospital-based program prevents the need for a transfer to another hospital for overnight care. Many hospital-based centers also require their ambulatory staff to assume the preoperative teaching and preparation of pediatric patients who are scheduled to go to an inpatient hospital bed after discharge from the postanesthesia care unit (PACU).

Freestanding Programs

Freestanding facilities are safe, cost-effective alternatives to hospital-based programs. Overall, the procedures performed tend to be less complex and the pediatric patients have potentially fewer underlying health problems. Freestanding facilities should be located in close proximity to a hospital with prearranged guidelines for transfer in the case of an emergency or if a child is unable to meet the necessary discharge criteria.

DEVELOPMENTAL CONSIDERATIONS

Erickson presented the most widely used theory of personality development.[5] It is built on freudian theory but stresses a healthy personality instead of a pathologic approach. Erickson shows specific age-related stages and defines the changes that take place within these stages (Table 26–3).

Infant (Birth–1 Year)

The infant has two major stressors to hospitalization and surgery: separation and pain. The infant reacts to these stressors through protest, despair, and detachment. Key interventions in caring for the infant are

- Meet needs promptly
- Allow unrestricted visiting by parents
- Use comfort measures, such as blanket, pacifier, special toy, stroking skin

Toddler (1–3 Years)

The toddler has three major stressors to hospitalization and surgery: separation, loss of control, and bodily injury and pain. The toddler's loss of control centers around physical restriction, loss of daily routine, loss of everyday rituals, and dependency on others. The toddler's prime reactions are identical to those of the infant's but, in addition, the toddler reacts with resistance, physical aggression, verbal uncooperativeness, regression, negativism, and temper tantrums. Key interventions in caring for toddlers are

- Allow them to express feelings of protest within safety limits
- Accept regressive behavior without comment
- Incorporate home routine and comfort measures
- Allow early parental visits

Preschool (3–6 Years)

The preschool child's stressors are also separation, loss of control, and bodily injury and pain, but their reactions differ from those of the toddler. Protests are less direct and aggressive. Despair and detachment are directed to loss of control. Aggression and regression are reactions the preschooler has to bodily injury and pain. Key interventions for this age group are

- Accept and acknowledge fears and anxieties
- Demonstrate equipment with hands-on application by child
- Encourage verbalization of feelings
- Allow early parental visits

School Age (6–12 Years)

The school-age child continues to react to the same major stressors. However, the children in this age-group have wide differences in their reactions. They have an increased ability to express feelings verbally. Reactions will vary from isolation and withdrawal, inquisitiveness, and detailed questioning to displaced anger and total frustration. Occasionally, the school-age child will show passive acceptance of procedures and pain, "trying to act brave." Key interventions for the child of school age are

- Allow expression and acknowledge fears
- Encourage questions and use more detailed explanations
- Include child in simple decisions concerning care
- Increase hands-on demonstrations of equipment

Adolescent (12–18 Years)

The unique world of the teenager can be a challenge for both healthcare providers and parents. The adolescent focuses on two stressors: loss of control and bodily injury and pain. Stress from separation can be experienced, but it is from their peer group and friends when hospitalization is prolonged. The behavioral reactions displayed by teens are often as wide and diverse as their mood swings. Key interventions include

Table 26–3. Growth and Development

DEVELOPMENTAL LEVEL	COGNITIVE (PIAGET)	PSYCHOSOCIAL		MORAL (KOHLBERG)
		Erikson	*Freud*	
Infant (Birth to 1 year)	*Sensorimotor stage:* initial reflex actions become more repetitive and intentional as the infant learns to elicit a response from self or objects in the environment; beginning "object permanence," the ability to understand that an object or person exists even if not seen	*Trust vs. mistrust:* learns to trust the environment through having basic needs met in an adequate and consistent manner	*Oral stage:* increases understanding of the environment through activities associated with the mouth (e.g., sucking, mouthing, chewing)	
Toddler (1–3 yr)	*Sensorimotor stage (until age 2 years):* learns cause-and-effect relationships and begins to actively use memory to solve problems; beginning of imitation, speech, and use of symbols; increasing understanding of space and time; advanced concept of object permanence *Preoperational stage (Preconceptual, 2–4 years):* increasing use of symbols in the form of language and imaginative play; egocentric, unable to view situations from another's perspective	*Autonomy vs. shame and doubt:* begins to develop independence and control of physical skills and mental processes with the positive encouragement and support of caregivers	*Anal stage:* develops control over the environment as sphincter control develops	*Preconventional:* determines right and wrong by making decisions according to rules imposed by others or by gratifying impulses; behavior is guided by the expectation of reward or punishment
Preschool (3–6 yr)	*Preoperational stage (intuitive, 4–7 years):* improves language development, which allows the child to gather information through questioning; less egocentric; unable yet to fully understand the changing or reversible properties of objects	*Initiative vs. guilt:* initiates goal-directed exploration and manipulation of the self and the environment, with increasing self-confidence and sense of responsibility for actions	*Phallic stage:* gender identity emerges as a result of unconscious conflict and subsequent identification with the parent of the same sex	
School age (6–12 yr)	*Concrete operational stage (7–11 years):* refines logical thought processes by dealing with objects and actions that can be seen and manipulated; develops ability to sort, classify, and order objects, and solve problems systematically and concurrently; understands that certain properties of objects remain the same even though their action or appearance changes (conservation); views a situation from another's perspective	*Industry vs. inferiority:* develops the ability to achieve and the necessary skills to complete activities and projects successfully, with positive feedback from peers and family	*Latency:* resolves previous conflicts and develops greater interest in others	*Conventional:* bases moral behavior on values and expectations of others (e.g., family, peers, teachers) and on respect for authority and established rules
Adolescence	*Formal operational stage (11 years and older):* develops abstract reasoning, hypothetical thinking, deduction, and synthesis of information	*Identity vs. identity diffusion:* develops a positive sense of self, allegiance to a set of values, and mastery of social skills by experimenting with different roles	*Genital stage:* constructs appropriate relationships with members of the opposite sex	*Postconventional (autonomous):* makes moral, rational decisions based on an understanding of law and social order beyond the immediate environment, and considers right and wrong within the context of what is best for the individual as well as society as a whole

From Luckmann J (ed): Saunders Manual of Nursing Care. Philadelphia: WB Saunders, 1997, p 472.

- Provide detailed explanations, often including benefits of procedures and reasons why
- Encourage adjustment to and acceptance of new authority figures
- Encourage questioning and allow expression of feelings
- Respect privacy and concern over appearance
- Include in decision making

Knowing the expected reactions that are seen with different developmental levels allows the nurse to adjust preparation accordingly. Considering children's developmental needs and cognitive abilities is helpful in preparing children for procedures. The healthcare professional should always consider the individual child's personality, what coping skills are being used, and previous experiences when developing an individualized plan of preparation.

PREADMISSION TEACHING

Teaching Programs

Many facilities have developed some type of preoperative teaching program for children and their families awaiting surgery. Programs are developed to standardize information and reduce perioperative anxiety of the child and parents. Key education points to keep in mind when developing teaching programs can be found in Table 26–4.

Preoperative teaching programs come in a

Table 26–4. **Key Education Points**

1. Develop a relationship (rapport) with the child and parents.
2. Determine the developmental level of the child.
3. Determine the domain of learning needed: cognitive, affective, psychomotor.
4. Assess the learning style of family and adjust teaching style accordingly.
5. Use a variety of teaching materials based on assessment findings.
6. Stress important information first and keep instructions short and simple.
7. Repeat information until feedback received ensures understanding.
8. Allow time for questions and answers.
9. Be specific; avoid hospital terms; and clarify unfamiliar terms.
10. Use hospitalization to incorporate teaching on other health issues: e.g., hygiene, disease process, immunizations (see box below)
11. Regular evaluation of education program and teaching effectiveness.

	MONTHS								YEARS		
	Birth	*1*	*2*	*4*	*6*	*12*	*15*	*18*	*4–8*	*11–12*	*14–18*
Hepatitis B Hepatitis B	■	■	■	■	■	■	■	■		(■)	
DTap or DTP Diphtheria, Tetanus, Pertussis (Whooping Cough)			■	■	■	■	■	■	■		
Tetanus-Diphtheria Tetanus-Diphtheria										■	■
Hib *Haemophilus influenzae* type B			■	■	■	■	■				
Polio (OPV or IPV)			■	■	■	■	■	■	■		
MMR Measles, Mumps, Rubella						■	■		■		
Varicella Chickenpox						■	■	■		(■)*	

Shaded bars indicate range of acceptable ages for vaccination. These recommended ages should not be thought of as absolute. Vaccine schedules are changed as new vaccines, combinations of current vaccines, and indications are licensed. (■) Previously unimmunized preadolescent/adolescents should be immunized. (■)* Those who have not had a documented case of chickenpox or have not been immunized should receive the vaccine. For more specific information, parents are encouraged to contact their pediatrician, health department, or another healthcare provider.

variety of shapes and sizes. Some programs are very informal, offering an open invitation for a question and answer session. Other programs, such as the Surgical Safari program, at William Beaumont Hospital in Troy, Michigan, incorporate tours, videos, dressing up, and demonstrations as part of their program. Whatever teaching methods are chosen, the underlying philosophy behind these programs is to:

- Provide information to children and parents about the surgical experience
- Minimize postoperative complications
- Reduce preoperative stress levels of children and parents
- Create a positive attitude toward the hospital visit

The choice between a simple or more involved program will often be based on the resources each institution has available. Teaching is more effective when more than one methodology is included in the program. There is, however, no single method that will be effective at every facility, or even for every child in the same institution. Teaching programs should include the following objectives:

- Identify routines, procedures, and equipment related to the perioperative experience
- Explain methods used by staff and describe roles of hospital personnel
- Explain medical terminology that may be used
- Participate in a hospital tour that closely simulates the day of surgery
- Allow children and parents to express concerns and anxieties
- Verbalize understanding of sample discharge instructions
- Provide ample question and answer time
- Discuss effective coping methods
- Evaluate programs' effectiveness for child and parents

Programs should be designed to provide a fun atmosphere where learning takes place. Teaching methods can include any of the following options:

1. *Audiovisual.* Show slides or a video of the actual program. When shown at the beginning of the program this provides a preview of what to expect, and it can serve as reinforcement if shown at the end of the program.
2. *Role playing.* Allow children to dress up in surgical hats, booties, and masks. This reinforces the changing of clothes the day of surgery, and what child doesn't like to play "dress up?"
3. *Play therapy.* Allow children to act out, draw, or describe events as they see them. Puppet shows and dolls can also be used for demonstration.
4. *Handouts.* Coloring books depicting events of the surgical day are effective reinforcement tools for children. Information for parents on do's and don'ts is particularly helpful as the surgical date draws closer.
5. *Tours.* Taking children on a tour through the operating room, the PACU, and the phase II or discharge area takes away the fear of the unknown. Children get to see what the bright lights look like and sit on the operating room table. They can smell the oxygen as it comes through the tubing or watch as they are connected to an electrocardiographic monitor. Allowing children to touch, feel, and smell reduces fantasies they may imagine.
6. *Models.* Allow children to touch and manipulate as much of the equipment as is feasible.
7. *Question and Answer Time.* Allow ample time for parents and children to ask questions of the day's events. Parents sometimes fear asking what they think is a silly question; thus, they should be made to feel comfortable asking questions.
8. *Evaluation.* It is important to have an evaluation tool that will monitor the effectiveness of the program. Parents should be encouraged to comment on how they feel the program helped their child. There may also be activities that parents and children do not like, and this allows the teaching program to be adjusted.

The timing of the visit may positively influence the outcome. Children aged 7 to 12 years benefit most from preparatory information given about 1 week before the experience, whereas children aged 4 to 7 years benefit from information given closer to the date of the procedure.[6] The nurse must be sure to give the family guidelines about how to reinforce and review the information at home before the surgical visit.

Telephone Screening

Preoperative telephone calls are used by some facilities in place of a formal teaching program. They can also be helpful to the family that has attended a teaching program. Preoperative routines, time schedules, and feeding instructions can be reviewed and reinforced by the nurse. The family is given an opportunity to ask last-minute questions or to report a change in the child's condition. Changes in health status should be reported to the anesthesiologist and surgeon. Specific preoperative instructions, such as antibiotics, can also be reinforced at this time.

Same-Day Preparation

There may be instances when children are unable to attend a teaching program. Procedures that are scheduled quickly may miss the scheduled program date, or it may be impractical for families traveling a long distance from the facility. Children with chronic health problems or repeated surgeries may already be familiar with the facility and routine and find such a program unnecessary. Assessment of these children can be made on the day of surgery with staff reinforcing teaching according to the needs of the child.

PREOPERATIVE CARE

Nursing Process

Nurses assist the family to maintain optimal health by providing anticipatory guidance, assisting with problem solving, identifying actual or potential problems, and making necessary referrals. The nursing process serves as a systematic approach for the nurse to use to care for the child and family.

The assessment phase is crucial to the entire process, establishing a baseline on which other subsequent phases are built. Assessment includes an evaluation of the child's physical, emotional, developmental, and psychological health status. In addition to assessing child and parent readiness to learn, information is gathered concerning past, present, and projected needs. The nurse will consider the ability of the caretakers, the potential for language problems, previous surgical experiences, and fears or inaccurate information, which are being communicated. Questions and observations allow the nurse to classify the learning needs of the child and family into one or more of the following learning domains[7]:

Cognitive—needing further knowledge
Affective—needing a change in attitude
Psychomotor—needing to learn a skill

Documentation of assessment findings is an important part of the process. All caregivers should have easy access to the tool chosen for communication; information should be documented in writing, the tool easy to use, and the information recorded in one place.

The planning phase allows information obtained to be organized into learning priorities. Participation by the child and family in setting these priorities should be encouraged. Allowing the child to participate, when age appropriate, gives the child a feeling of control over the hospitalization. Coordination among all health-care providers establishes who is responsible for which priority.

Interventions are based on the findings obtained. Abnormal assessment results may require additional information. Finding a previously undiagnosed health problem may result in the need for a more detailed health workup and a revised anesthesia plan or delay of surgery. Individualized interventions will be based on each patient's assessment data and plan of care.

Evaluation, the final step in the nursing process, is often overlooked. Accurate assessments, effective plans, and interventions may be determined by evaluating preoperative and postoperative patient care outcomes.

Preparation

The essential preoperative requirements for safe conduct of anesthesia in pediatric outpatients are the same as those for inpatients. A complete history and physical examination performed by a member of the medical staff, appropriate laboratory tests, consultations when indicated, an appropriate fasting period, and a chance to personally evaluate and establish rapport with the child and the parents are the standard preanesthetic requirements.[1]

History and Physical Examination

Children undergoing ambulatory surgery are generally in good health. If a child has a systemic disease it should be under good control. A review of physical systems the day of surgery allows for discovery of any new symptoms. A baseline set of vital signs is also obtained at this time, including an accurate weight. Further information includes an accurate feeding history, medications the child is presently taking, and allergies the child may have to medications, food, or latex products. Latex allergies are being seen in children who have repeated procedures involving latex products such as urology procedures. Latex sensitivity is discussed in detail in Chapter 10. An additional listing of suggested assessments important to the pediatric patient can be found in Table 26–5.

Table 26–5. Preoperative Assessments Important to the Pediatric Patient

Physical
Head circumference
Loose teeth
Skin: rashes, possible signs of communicable disease
Recent exposure to communicable disease
Currency of vaccinations
Recent illness of child or siblings

Social
Parental validation of NPO status
Preferred name to be called
Specific fears
Typical behavior patterns when in pain

Developmental
Pet names for objects or functions
Use of pacifier, bottle, cup
Loved objects
Communication skills and level
Potty training status

Parental
Understanding of preoperative instructions, especially NPO ramifications
Availability of child care assistance for travel
Availability of child car seat/appropriate restraint device
Resources for postoperative care of child
Understanding of potential complications: signs and symptoms, when to call for help

Preoperative Fasting

The need for pediatric ambulatory patients to undergo prolonged fasting before elective surgery has recently been challenged.[8] Studies have shown that children who are allowed to drink clear liquids until 2 to 3 hours before anesthesia induction do not have higher gastric volume or acidity than children who fast overnight.[8] Recent literature suggests that pediatric anesthesiologists have now liberalized their NPO orders. Solid food, milk, formula, and milk products are still withheld, usually for 8 to 12 hours before the scheduled surgery.[9] Children may drink clear liquids (Table 26–6) until 2 to 3 hours before the scheduled surgical time and breast-feed until 3 hours before surgery. Preoperative fasting requirements continue to vary among institutions and individual practice, but the literature suggests that studies conducted at this point open the door for modification of previously established fasting guidelines. Whichever fasting orders are observed, clear, concise instructions need to be given to the parents. Emphasis must be placed on the importance of following these instructions before anesthesia.

Preoperative Laboratory Testing

Laboratory testing is another parameter that is in the process of change. Until recently, the minimum laboratory requirements were a complete blood cell count and urinalysis. Often, if the procedure was prone to bleeding, such as a tonsillectomy, additional coagulation studies were performed. Many anesthesiologists no longer require routine urinalysis unless there is evidence of genitourinary disease. Controversy still surrounds the issue of hemoglobin and hematocrit studies.

The incidence of anemia in healthy children is extremely low and does not usually require therapeutic intervention or modification of the anesthetic.[10] Anesthesiologists are now comfortable requesting preoperative hemoglobin and hematocrit testing only when the medical history suggests that significant anemia may be present. This applies to infants, adolescent females, and children with chronic disease. There are some states that still mandate routine laboratory testing regardless of private practice.[11]

Preoperative Medication

There is no one consensus that exists on the optimal method of preanesthesia medication for children. The American Academy of Pediatrics states that drugs should achieve five goals: (1) to guard the patient's safety and welfare; (2) to minimize physical discomfort or pain; (3) to minimize negative psychologic responses to

Table 26–6. Guidelines for Preoperative Feeding

At midnight the evening before surgery, stop all food, including:
- Solid food, candy,* and chewing gum*
- Milk, milk products, and formulas†
- Orange juice and juice containing pulp

Breast-feeding may continue until 3 hours before surgery.
Clear fluids may be continued until 2 hours before surgery.
Clear fluids include water, apple juice, clear juice drinks, plain gelatin, clear broth, Pedialyte, and ice pops.

*Sucking hard candy is probably of little concern, and a variety of opinions exist regarding the significance of gum chewing.
†The duration for fasting after formulas is uncertain, and shorter intervals may be appropriate.
From Wong DL: Whaley & Wong's Nursing Care of Infants & Children, 6th ed. St. Louis: Mosby–Year Book, 1995, p 1222.

treatment by providing analgesia and to maximize the potential for amnesia; (4) to control behavior; and (5) to return the patient to a state in which safe discharge, as determined by recognized criteria, is possible.[12]

The decision to administer preoperative medication to children will be directed by the facility's department of anesthesia. Other factors that affect the decision to premedicate are the physical layout of the facility, the length of the procedure, the period of time between sedation and induction of anesthesia, and the cooperation of the child. Several drug options are available (Table 26–7). The medication chosen should be atraumatic, with preferable choices being oral, existing intravenous, rectal, or transmucosal routes. For most children intramuscular injections cause more anxiety than the surgical procedure and should be avoided unless specific conditions warrant their use.

The oral use of midazolam (Versed), as noted in Table 26–7, is not specifically approved by the manufacturer for pediatric use, but it is the most popular pediatric premedication in the outpatient setting. Midazolam dosage is controlled by the anesthesiologist following recommended guidelines. Its taste must be masked by an equal amount of strongly flavored liquid such as cherry syrup or grape Kool-Aid or followed with a small amount of water.

The oral medication of meperidine (Demerol), diazepam (Valium), and atropine (see Table 26–7) is administered under a variety of names at many institutions across the country. The mixture is prepared by the pharmacist using the following formula guidelines[13]:

1. Add to a clean, empty container of suitable size and mix:
   a. 45 ml Demerol syrup 10 mg/ml
   b. 9 ml Diazepam oral solution 5 mg/ml
   c. 15 ml Atropine injection 0.4 mg/ml
   d. 6 ml Simple syrup
2. Obtain 15 unit dose containers for oral liquids and prepackage immediately
3. Lot numbers begin with #1 and run consecutively
4. Expiration date is 1 month from date of preparation
5. Label mixture exactly as follows:
   Pediatric pre-op (PAM) mix 5 ml Lot # ____
   Demerol 6.0 mg/ml
   Valium 0.6 mg/ml
   Atropine 0.08 mg/ml
   Usual dose = 0.25 mg/kg
   Exp. ______ Initials ______
6. Record transaction involving controlled substances in appropriate manner

Fluid restriction before induction and maximum dose allowances preclude this mixture being used in higher-weight children, and alternative choices should be made.

The child's response to any form of medication must be carefully monitored. Children should not be allowed to walk around play areas unattended after being medicated. Stretchers should have side rails up and be padded for extra protection. Parents should be instructed on the effects of the medication and how their child's sensorium may change. Normal reactions such as facial flushing and warm skin should be pointed out to avoid alarming the parents. Supplemental oxygen, pulse oximetry, and resuscitation equipment should always be immediately available in the event of respiratory depression, although incidence at these dosages is almost nonexistent.

Family Support

The presence of parents with children during induction of anesthesia is an approach that is gaining support, is being requested by parents, and is becoming accepted by many anesthesiologists. Hannallah and Epstein[1] state that the presence of an intelligent, supportive parent during induction of anesthesia may be the best available substitute for premedication.

Institutions differ in their approach to this method of induction. Some facilities have special induction rooms adjacent to the operating room where surgical attire is not needed. Others allow selected parents (with cover gown or scrubs) to accompany the child into the operating room.[14] Parent selection and education are of extreme importance in carrying out this approach. The parent must be told precisely what to expect and is escorted back to a waiting area by assigned personnel as soon as the child is asleep. Most literature advises against allowing overly anxious parents to participate in this method and cautions parents that if asked to leave by the anesthesiologist they must do so immediately.[1]

Parents remain the most significant support system for the child undergoing surgery. Children need reinforced assurance that they will be reunited with their parents after surgery. Parents should be allowed to be with their children for as long as possible and should be reunited after surgery as soon as the child awakens. Many institutions, depending on their size and policies, now allow parents into the PACU as soon as the child's condition has stabilized, airway

Table 26–7. Dosages of Drugs Commonly Used for Effective Premedication

DRUG		ROUTE	USUAL DOSE (mg/kg)
Opioids			
Morphine sulfate		Intravenous	0.1–0.3
		Intramuscular	0.1–0.3
		Rectal	Not recommended
Fentanyl		Oral transmucosal	0.015–0.020
		Sublingual	0.010–0.015
		Intravenous	0.001–0.005
Meperidine		Intravenous	1.0–3.0
		Intramuscular	1.0–3.0
		Rectal	Not recommended
Sedatives			
Diazepam		Oral	0.1–0.3
		Intravenous	0.1–0.3
		Intramuscular	Not recommended
		Rectal	0.2–0.3
Midazolam		Oral	0.5–0.75
		Intravenous	0.05–0.15
		Intramuscular	0.05–0.15
		Rectal	0.5–0.75
		Nasal	0.2–0.5
		Sublingual	0.2–0.5
Pentobarbital		Intravenous	1.0–3.0 (max. 100 mg)
		Intramuscular	5.0–7.0
Chloral hydrate		Orally/rectally	20–75 (max. 100 mg or 2.0 g)
Ketamine		Oral	3.0–10.0
		Intravenous	1.0–3.0
		Intramuscular	2.0–10.0
		Rectal	5.0–10.0
		Nasal	3.0–5.0
		Sublingual	3.0–5.0
Barbiturates			
Methohexital		Intramuscular	7.0–10.0
		Rectal (10% solution)	20.0–30.0
Thiopental		Intramuscular	7.0–10.0
		Rectal	20.0–30.0
Combinations			
DPT "lytic cocktail" "pedicocktail"			
Meperidine (Demerol)	25 mg/ml	Intramuscular	0.02–0.2 ml/kg
Promethazine (Phenergan)	6.5 mg/ml	Intravenous	Contraindicated
Chlorpromazine (Thorazine)	6.5 mg/ml		
"DAD's" solution*	"PAM" solution†		
Meperidine (Demerol)	6.0 mg/ml	Oral	0.25 ml/kg
Diazepam (Valium)	0.6 mg/ml		
Atropine Sulfate	0.08 mg/ml		
Midazolam		Oral	0.5–0.75
Children's Tylenol			10.0–15.0
Other			
EMLA Cream		Topical	Apply ½ of 5-g tube to site. Cover with occlusive transparent dressing.
Lidocaine 2.5%			Minor procedures: application 60 min.
Prilocaine 2.5%			Major procedures: application 120–180 min.

*Children's Hospital of Philadelphia.

†William Beaumont Hospital—Troy, Michigan.

Data compiled from Wong DL: Whaley & Wong's Nursing Care of Infants & Children, 5th ed. St. Louis: Mosby, 1995, pp 1144–1145; Cote CJ: Sedation for the pediatric patient. Pediatr Clin North Am 41:34–35, 1994; and Twersky RS: The Ambulatory Anesthesia Handbook. St. Louis: Mosby, 1995, pp 148–151.

obstruction is no longer a threat, and the child is awakening.

Special Considerations

As the popularity of pediatric outpatient surgery continues to increase and programs expand, concern is raised for the child who presents with significant medical disease. A bigger dilemma is the child whose disease, such as a heart murmur, is first discovered in the outpatient surgical unit. These patients can benefit from ambulatory surgery by shorter parental separation and reduced exposure to hospital pathogens. Successful management depends on coordination of their medical situation by pediatricians, surgeons, and the anesthesia team. Consultations and appropriate laboratory testing should be obtained before the surgical visit.

Some of the most common management problems that can confront clinicians in the ambulatory setting are

- The premature infant
- Runny nose
- Sickle cell disease
- Heart disease or heart murmur
- Malignant hyperthermia susceptibility
- Down's syndrome
- Cancer
- Child abuse and neglect

DeSoto's[15] suggested management of these situations could be summarized as follows: No conclusive data exist on the appropriate age for term children to undergo outpatient procedures; the former premature child should be evaluated for risk of apnea and bradycardia. Infants younger than 50 weeks postconceptual age should be admitted overnight. Older, former premature, infants without cardiopulmonary dysfunction may be managed as outpatients.

The child with a respiratory infection is at risk for perioperative respiratory problems. The history and physical examination should help the clinician differentiate an infectious from a noninfectious process. A child who has a fever and a purulent nasal discharge will most probably have an infectious process.

With an adequate facility and proper patient preparation, patients with sickle cell disease may undergo ambulatory surgery. Adequate hydration, pain management, and oxygenation should be maintained during the hospitalization.

Children with heart murmurs and/or a disease process can undergo an outpatient procedure as long as the pathophysiology is recognized, evaluated, and compensated. A cardiology consult may be necessary to differentiate an innocent murmur from a pathologic murmur. Careful evaluation of vital signs, oxygen saturation, growth and development, exercise tolerance, and other associated medical conditions will determine if this child is a candidate for ambulatory surgery.

Pediatric patients susceptible to malignant hyperthermia may be considered as outpatients. Prophylactic dantrolene is unnecessary. Triggering anesthetic agents are avoided, and the patient should be evaluated for discharge after observation for at least 4 hours. Parents should be given specific instructions about signs and symptoms to watch for after discharge.

The child with Down's syndrome should be evaluated for associated cardiac, renal, and airway problems before proceeding with outpatient surgery.

Children with cancer often undergo frequent outpatient procedures; therefore, the anesthetic approach should be aggressive toward pain management and anesthetics with minimal side effects.[15]

Child abuse and neglect come in all forms, shapes, and sizes and occur in all types of families. In most states any nurse or healthcare provider suspecting abuse or neglect is required by law to report their findings. Nurses are responsible to intervene with vulnerable clients and families; they may be the first person to see the child and parent. Nurses must be alert to bruises, welts, cigarette burns, unexplained lacerations or abrasions, and behavioral reactions such as fear of parents, withdrawal, and an overall lack of reaction to the environment.

ANATOMIC AND PHYSIOLOGIC DIFFERENCES

Pediatric Airway

When compared with adults, children have definite anatomic and physiologic differences, some of which are illustrated in Figure 26–1. The infant's head is proportionately larger in comparison to the body. The infant and child's nares are narrow, and the tongue is large. Infants are obligate nasal breathers. The larynx is high and funnel shaped, causing a natural narrowing at the cricoid ring. This rigid circular framework of cartilage contains the epiglottis and the glottis (vocal cords). The epiglottis is very high, almost to the soft palate; it is omega shaped and protrudes over the larynx about 45 degrees; vocal cords are slanted, and in infancy

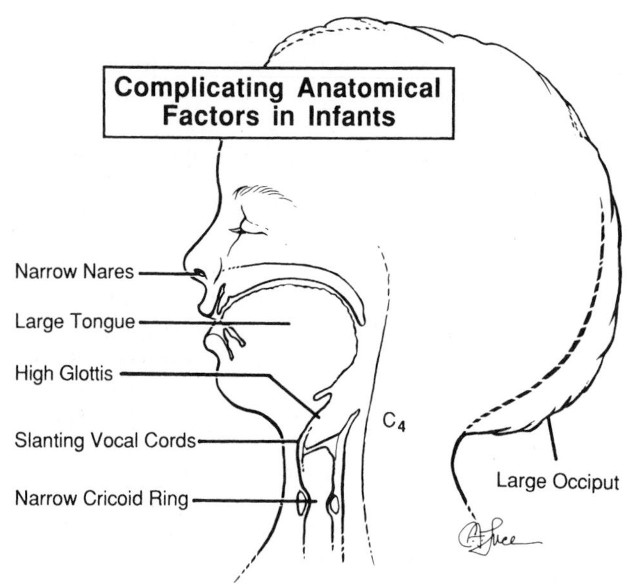

Figure 26–1. Complicating anatomic factors in infants. (From Barash PG, et al: Handbook of Clinical Anesthesia. Philadelphia: Lippincott-Raven, 1996, p 390.)

the glottis is located more cephalad than in later childhood. Laryngeal reflexes are very active. The tracheal diameter is relatively small and is located downward and posterior; this diameter triples in size by 12 years of age.

Respiratory System

Pediatric patients are predisposed to upper airway obstruction because of these anatomical differences. In addition, they have small mandibles and short necks. They have large amounts of upper airway lymphoid tissue, which add to the tendency for obstruction. Upper airway obstruction is characterized by stridor and hoarseness, whereas lower airway problems are associated with wheezing.

The amount of dead space where air passes but gases are not exchanged is large during neonatal life and infancy. Proportionately more air must be moved in and out than with the older child, which accounts for the increased respiratory rates in infants and small children; as the volume of the lungs increases with growth the respiratory rate gradually decreases.

Cardiovascular System

The circulation pathway allows for oxygenation of venous blood by the lungs and delivery of saturated blood to the systemic circulation. In attempting to meet oxygen requirements, the cardiac output of the infant is 30% to 50% greater than that of adults. The resting heart rate is two times greater than that in an adult and decreases progressively until the child reaches 12 years of age.

The systolic blood pressure is at its lowest immediately after birth. In the first 4 weeks of life the left ventricle gains strength and the systolic pressure rises. The diastolic pressure also rises with increasing age. Blood pressure readings vary more frequently in infancy owing to sleep and activity patterns. Systolic and diastolic readings continue to increase from the newborn period until the child reaches adolescence, when pressure readings assume adult levels.

Although it is challenging to obtain vital signs, especially blood pressures, on newborns or struggling toddlers, it is recommended that full parameters be assessed on all children regardless of their age. Table 26–8 shows normal ranges for vital signs in infants and children. In addition to blood pressure, pulse, and respiratory rates, temperature and pulse oximetry readings should also be taken. Infants and children experience an even greater heat loss during surgery than adults. Infants can lose up to 75% of their body heat through exposure of their heads to room air. Increased heat loss, infection, and a higher incidence of malignant hyperthermia in children make preoperative assessment values essential.

One of the most common errors in obtaining pediatric vital signs is the use of improper equipment. Proper blood pressure cuff size is necessary for accurate values. The cuff should cover approximately three fourths of the length

Table 26–8. Normal Ranges for Vital Signs in Infants and Children

AGE-SPECIFIC HEART RATES

Age	*Rate (Mean, per min)*	*Rate (Range, per min)*
0–24 hours	119	100–150
1–7 days	133	100–175
7–30 days	163	115–190
1–3 months	154	124–190
3–6 months	140	111–179
6–12 months	140	112–177
1–3 years	126	98–163
3–5 years	98	65–132
5–8 years	96	70–115
8–12 years	79	55–107
12–16 years	75	55–102

AGE-SPECIFIC RESPIRATORY RATES

Age	*Rate (per min)*
Premature infant	50–65
Newborn	30–50
2 years	24–32
6 years	22–28
10 years	20–26
12 years	18–24
Adult	16–22

AGE-SPECIFIC BLOOD PRESSURE READINGS

Age	*Reading**
Newborn—4 years	85/60
5 years	87/60
6 years	90/60
7 years	92/62
8 years	95/62
9 years	98/64
10 years	100/65
11 years	110/60
12 years	114/60
13 years	116/60
14 years	118/64

*May be + or − 10 to 15 points.

From Roberts C: The pediatric patient. In Allen A (ed): ASPAN's Core Curriculum for Post Anesthesia Nursing Practice. Philadelphia: WB Saunders, 1991, pp 46–47.

of the upper arm. A blood pressure may also be taken on the upper calf of the leg. It is important to have a variety of pediatric cuff sizes available. Electronic blood pressure devices aid in obtaining accurate preoperative and postoperative vital signs. Tympanic thermometers allow rapid and accurate evaluation of the child's temperature in a noninvasive manner. Oximetry readings are a vital part of the vital sign assessment, and children are often fascinated by the light on the end of their finger.

Central Nervous System

The nervous system comprises the central nervous system (CNS), the peripheral nervous system (PNS), and the autonomic nervous system (ANS). In proportion to other body systems the nervous system grows more rapidly before birth. Myelinization of various nerve tracts in the CNS allows progressive neuromotor function. Acquisition of motor skills depends on the maturation and myelination of the nervous system.

The CNS consists of the spinal cord and brain. The PNS encompasses the spinal nerves, cranial nerves and associated ganglia, and peripheral portions of the ANS. Cardiac muscle, smooth muscle of the viscera, arterioles, and glands are governed by the ANS, which has two components: the sympathetic and parasympathetic systems. The sympathetic system functions to maintain stability during stress, activating the "fight or flight" response. The parasympathetic system's primary function is regulating the digestive processes, acting to conserve and restore energy surpluses.

Renal System

Maturity of the kidneys is not completed until the end of the first year; glomerular filtration and absorption are low, and adult levels are not met until 1 to 2 years of age. As a result, newborns are unable to dispose of excess water and solutes as rapidly or efficiently as older children and adults. The loop of Henle, where urine is concentrated, is shorter in the newborn, causing less concentrated urine and varying specific gravities.

Postoperatively, the risks of dehydration are just as great as the risks of overhydration. Two formulas are shown (Table 26–9*A* and *B*) for replacement of fluid deficits. Normal urinary output should be 1 to 2 ml/kg/hr postoperatively. When measuring wet diapers the equation to use is 1 g = 1 ml of urine. The renal system converts up to 20% of volatile anesthetic gases into metabolites for excretion through the urinary system.

Liver

The liver is the most immature of all the gastrointestinal organs during infancy. It remains functionally immature until after the first year of life. The liver plays a vital role in metabolizing and excreting many pharmacologic

Table 26–9A. Intravenous Fluid Maintenance Formula for Infants and Children

To correct the pediatric patient's 24-hour fluid loss, the following formula for intravenous fluid replacement is applied.
For the first 10 kg of the child's weight—give 100 ml/kg/24 hr
For the second 10 kg of the child's weight—give 50 ml/kg/24 hr
For each kg of weight over 20 kg—give 20 ml/kg/24 hr
The hourly rate is obtained by dividing the total replacement needs by 24

Examples:

1. A child who weighs 21 kg (46.2 lb) requires the following fluid replacement
   First 10 kg @ 100 ml/kg = 1000 ml/24 hr
   Second 10 kg @ 50 ml/kg = 500 ml/24 hr
   Next 1 kg @ 20 ml/kg = 20 ml/24 hr
   Total 1520 ml/24 hr
   1520 ml ÷ 24 = 63 ml/hr maintenance
2. A child who weighs 14 kg (30.8 lb) requires the following fluid replacement
   First 10 kg @ 100 ml/kg = 1000 ml/24 hr
   Next 4 kg @ 50 ml/kg = 200 ml/24 hr
   Total: 1200 ml/24 hr
   1200 ml ÷ 24 = 50 ml/hr maintenance
3. A newborn who weighs 3 kg (6.6 lb) requires the following fluid replacement
   First 3 kg @ 100 ml/kg = 300 ml/24 hr
   300 ÷ 24 = 12.5 ml/hr maintenance

   Approximate blood volumes:
   Infants 80–90 ml/kg
   Children 70–80 ml/kg

Maximum allowable blood loss should not exceed 20% of total blood volume (depending on preoperative hematocrit).

Data from Frochtman D: Principles of Nursing Care for the Pediatric Surgical Patient. Boston: Little, Brown, 1976; and Cohen M: Administering IV fluids to children. In Hayman L, Sporing E (eds): Handbook of Pediatric Nursing. New York: Fleschner, John Wiley, 1985.

agents used with anesthesia. This functional immaturity may result in prolonged effects of muscle relaxants and narcotics in neonates and infants.

Table 26–9B. Fluid Replacement as Determined by Site and Duration of Surgery

Short Surgical Procedure with Minimal to Moderate Third-Space Loss

5% Dextrose in lactated Ringer's solution for maintenance and third-space loss (limit to 15–20 $ml \cdot kg^{-1}$ to avoid hyperglycemia)

Long Surgical Procedure with Moderate to Extensive Third-Space Loss

5% Dextrose in 0.25 normal saline for maintenance and lactated Ringer's solution for third-space loss

Massive Third-Space Loss

5% albumin to restore one third to one quarter of the loss

Daily Fluid Maintenance Requirements

First 10 kg	$4\ ml \cdot kg^{-1} \cdot h^{-1}$
Second 10 kg	$2\ ml \cdot kg^{-1} \cdot h^{-1}$
>20 kg	$1\ ml \cdot kg^{-1} \cdot h^{-1}$

From Barash PG, et al: Handbook of Clinical Anesthesia. Philadelphia: Lippincott-Raven, 1996, p 405.

Endocrine System

The endocrine system of the newborn is developed but functions immaturely. The posterior lobe of the pituitary gland produces limited quantities of antidiuretic hormone, which inhibits diuresis, causing the newborn to be more susceptible to dehydration.

COMMON PEDIATRIC AMBULATORY SURGICAL PROCEDURES

The pediatric patient adapts well to many procedures that can be accomplished in a safe, cost-effective ambulatory setting. Table 26–10 presents some of the most common ambulatory surgical procedures. As ambulatory services continue to expand, additional types of surgeries will be done in the ambulatory setting. Diagnostic tests such as esophagoscopy, colonoscopy, gastroscopy, sigmoidoscopy, magnetic resonance imaging, computed tomography, and bone marrow aspirations are also performed as outpatient procedures with mild sedation or general anesthesia.

POST ANESTHESIA, PHASE I

Children emerge from anesthesia differently than adults. It is vitally important for the PACU nurse to meet the emotional, as well as physical, needs of the pediatric patient. Comfort measures such as pacifiers, blankets, and special toys are encouraged. Individual policies vary, but many facilities now allow parents to join their children in the PACU.[16] The most effective approach to care is a calm atmosphere, soothing voice, and constant reassurance at the child's developmental level.

Safety

All children who have been given anesthesia are classified as a 1:1 nurse-patient acuity until reflexes and consciousness return. Nurse-patient ratios are addressed in Resource 3 of the Standards of PeriAnesthesia Nursing Practice published by the American Society of PeriAnesthesia Nurses (ASPAN).[17] See Table 20–2.

Safety devices must be implemented to protect children from injury. Side rails should be maintained in the upright position at all times, and bumper pads or blankets should be used to protect children from injury due to thrashing or kicking. Safety vests, seat belts, arm restraints, and stretcher security straps are sometimes necessary to protect children from additional movement and injury. If age appropriate, explanations should be given to the children about these safety devices so that they know they are not being punished.

Transport

Pediatric patients should be transported from the operating room to the PACU by the anesthesia team and the operating room nurse. When transferring the patient from phase I to phase II the postanesthesia care nurse should accompany the child during this transfer and give a full report to the next caregiver. Assessment of the airway is crucial during these transfers, and emergency equipment such as oxygen, bag and mask system, and portable suction may be necessary depending on the child's condition.

Length of Stay

Length of stay in the phase I PACU varies from one institution to another. The anesthesia department generally establishes the guidelines for duration of stay.

Pediatric patients should not be released from phase I until they are awake and have returned to their baseline status. Many facilities no longer have minimum observation times but choose to base the length of stay on specific criteria such as consciousness, vital signs, postoperative bleeding, nausea and vomiting, and pain control.

Fluid Replacement

The anesthesiologist is responsible for determining preoperative and postoperative fluid deficits. Fluid replacement is determined by a variety of factors: (1) number of hours the child was NPO before surgery, (2) hours of surgery, and (3) blood loss. It is important to correct and maintain proper fluid balance because energy is used on maintaining ventilation, cardiac output, regulating temperature, and muscle activity. Caution must be taken with neonates and infants to avoid overhydration; correction of fluid loss over a longer period of time is suggested.

Equipment

Appropriate respiratory equipment must be available when caring for the pediatric patient. Ideally this equipment is located at each cubicle in the PACU. Necessary equipment includes infant and child size masks; face tents; bag and mask system; infant, pediatric, and adult size nasal cannulas; and suction catheters. Pulse oximetry should be maintained throughout the operating room and initial postanesthesia period to assess oxygen needs. Fingers, toes, and earlobes are the most common sites used for oximetry readings. Humidifiers and nebulizers should both be available.

As previously discussed, accurate blood pressures depend on proper cuff size. A variety of cuff sizes should be available to accommodate all children's sizes. Cardiac monitoring is at the discretion of the anesthesiologist. Initially, all pediatric patients should be placed on the bedside monitor. Additional monitoring guidelines are appropriate for the infant whose conceptual age is 50 weeks or less; for infants with a history of apnea, bradycardia, or breathing abnormality; for infants with a documented incidence of apnea or bradycardia during surgery and/or the immediate postanesthesia period; and for any other pediatric patient for whom the attending anesthesiologist specifically orders monitoring. The anesthesia department of each individual hospital or freestanding center establishes these guidelines.

***Table 26–10.* Common Pediatric Ambulatory Surgical Procedures**

SURGERY	DEFINITION	INDICATIONS FOR SURGERY	NURSING CONSIDERATIONS	DISCHARGE INSTRUCTIONS
Strabismus repair	Surgery to correct misalignment of one or both eyes	Unresponsive to medical regimen of patching; avoid permanent impairment of vision; improve cosmetic appearance	Restrain if necessary to avoid pulling at eyes and dressings. Provide comfort by medicating for pain/nausea. Decrease stimulation and dim lights. Reunite with parents ASAP.	Stress importance of not rubbing eyes. Observe for signs of infection: redness, matting, discolored drainage. Reassure parents that tears may be blood tinged initially. Decrease stimulation and light. Call physician if eyes become malaligned or signs of infection occur.
Myringotomy with/without tympanostomy tube	Facilitate drainage of fluid and allow continued ventilation of middle ear	Treatment for chronic otitis media	Provide comfort by medicating for pain. Pulling/tugging may indicate pain. Observe color and amount of drainage.	Keep water out of ears during bath/shower. Earplugs may be recommended. Swimming, diving, jumping, and submerging are usually discouraged. Parents should be instructed that tube may fall out naturally.
Adenoidectomy	Removal of the adenoids	Recurrent otitis media, hearing loss, nasal airway obstruction: snoring, heavy respirations, and nasal speech	Observe for signs of increased bleeding: Increased bleeding from nose, tachycardia, pallor, frequent clearing of throat, restlessness, vomiting bright red blood. Position for drainage. Medicate for pain. Encourage fluids when reactive and bleeding and emesis are under control.	Avoid irritating tender tissue. Give soft foods that are cool and bland. Use analgesics as ordered. Observe for signs of infection: increased temperature, severe earache, cough. Quiet housebound activities, increase per physician's instructions. Instruct parents that tonsil scab falls off 5–10 days postoperatively.
Tonsillectomy	Removal of palatine tonsils	Massive hypertrophy, obstruction of airway, difficulty eating, malignancy, and chronic tonsillitis	Same as above	Same as above

Hemiorrhaphy	Prolapse of a portion of the intestine into the inguinal ring; most common infant procedure	Persistent painless inguinal swelling, partial obstruction of bowel, and incarcerated hernia	Comfort measures: pain medication or injection of local at site. Position with pillows under knees. Change diapers often.	Observe for signs of infection: redness, tenderness, increased temperature. Frequent diaper changes. Sponge baths first 2–5 days. Older children should be cautioned against lifting, pushing, wrestling, and athletics for 2–3 wk.
Hydrocelectomy	Presence of fluid in the persistent processus vaginalis	Communicating hydrocele that does not resolve in 1 year; potential for herniation	Same as with hernia. Advise parents that temporary swelling and discoloration of scrotum resolves spontaneously.	Same as above
Hypospadias	Urethral opening is located below the glans penis or anywhere along the ventral surface of the penile shaft	Enable child to void in standing position with voluntary direction of urine in normal manner; improved physical appearance for psychological reasons; produce sexually adequate organ	Prepare parents and child for type of procedure and what results to expect. Urinary diversion sometimes necessary for optimum healing. May have indwelling catheter or stent. Restrain as necessary. Medicate for pain.	Teach parents catheter care: avoid kinking, twisting, or blocking catheter/stent. Show how to empty urine bag. Encourage fluid intake. Bathe twice daily. Wear loose clothing. Avoid sandboxes, straddle-type toys, swimming, and rough activity until physician permits.
Orchiopexy	Undescended testes brought down into the scrotum and secured in position	If undescended spontaneously. Surgery performed between age 1–2 yr to prevent: damage to testicle by exposure to higher body heat, tumor formation, trauma and torsion, cosmetic and psychological handicap	Comfort measures: Medicate for pain/nausea. Position with pillows under knees. Injection with local at site is helpful. Usually done as outpatient.	Instruct parents on prevention of infection: show proper cleaning of site. Frequent cleaning after urination and bowel movements. Restrict activity. Provide counseling referral to family for questions on fertility.
Closed reduction of fracture	Bone fragments realigned and immobilized by traction or by closed manipulation and casting	To regain alignment and length of bony fragments (reduction): to retain alignment and length (immobilization); to restore function to injured parts	Observe neurovascular status; check regularly for edema, allow cast to dry uncovered. Medicate for pain.	Instruct parents on cast care and proper positioning. Show how to check for adequate circulation. Avoid small items that can be put inside cast by small children.

Data compiled from Wong DL: Whaley & Wong's Nursing Care of Infants and Children, 5th ed. St. Louis: CV Mosby, 1995; Luckmann J: Saunders Manual of Nursing Care. Philadelphia: WB Saunders, 1997; Litwack K: Core Curriculum for Post Anesthesia Nursing Practice, 3rd ed. Philadelphia: WB Saunders, 1995; and Suddarth DS: The Lippincott Manual of Nursing Practice, 5th ed. Philadelphia: JB Lippincott, 1991.

Thermometers are available in a variety of modes: oral, tympanic, axillary, and rectal probes should all be available in the PACU setting. Oral temperatures are difficult to obtain with accuracy owing to humidified oxygen use, oral secretions, and the inability to hold a thermometer sublingually after anesthesia. Rectal temperatures are the least favored because of their invasiveness and distress to the child.

Warming blankets and overhead radiant warmers should be available for hypothermia but are not commonly used for children.

Emergency equipment must be readily available. PACUs caring for the pediatric population must be equipped with a wide range of pediatric specific supplies and medications. The ASPAN Standards of PeriAnesthesia Nursing Practice gives a list of suggested emergency equipment and drugs in Resource 7. Advanced cardiac life support is addressed in Resource 6.[17] Pediatric cardiopulmonary resuscitation guidelines are shown in Figure 26–2.

It is helpful to have a pediatric drug dosage chart available with the emergency supplies. Charts that give dosages corresponding to weight in kilograms are recommended for proper dosages. An example is the Broselow Pediatric Emergency Tape (800-323-4220).[18] The child's weight in kilograms corresponds to a coded color on the tape. Each color code lists emergency drugs with appropriate dosages, emergency supplies needed, and correct sizes for

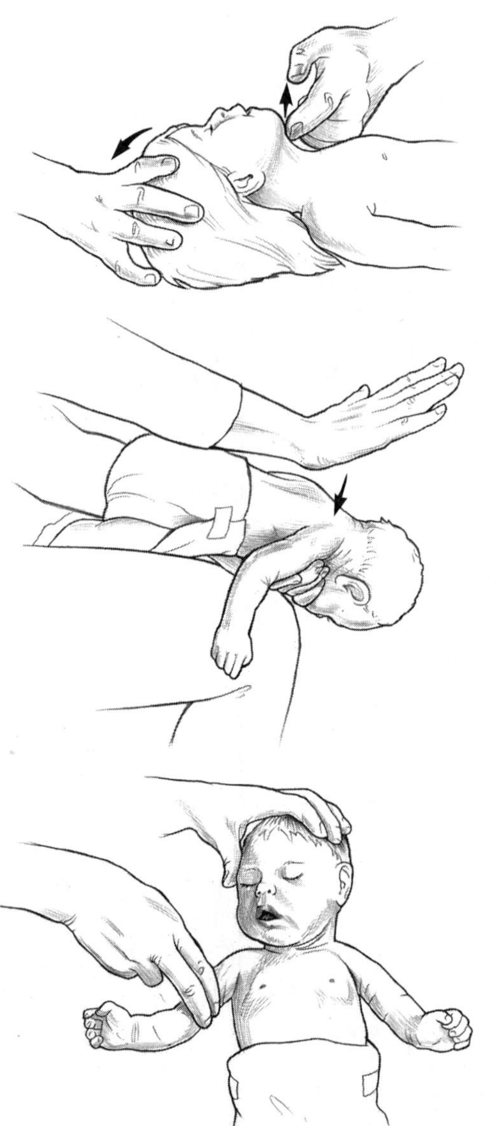

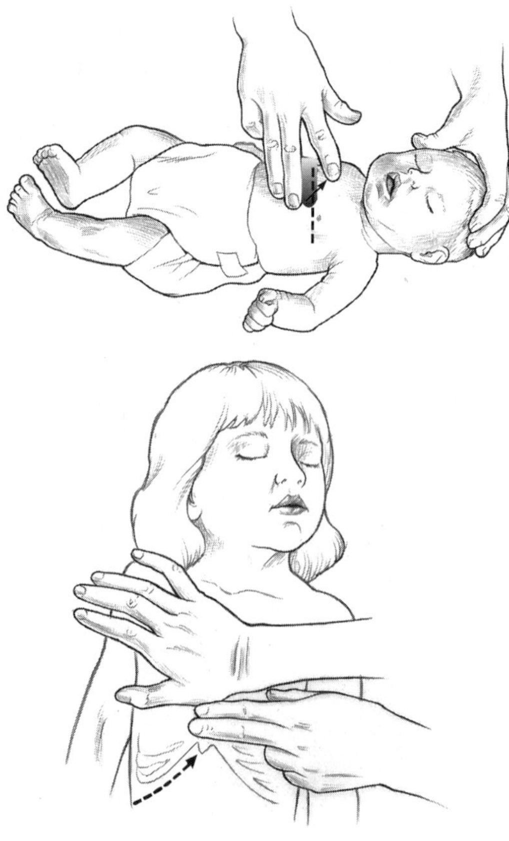

Figure 26–2. Cardiopulmonary resuscitation for infants and children. (From Luckmann J [ed]: Saunders Manual of Nursing Care. Philadelphia: WB Saunders, 1997, pp 547–548.)

emergency equipment. Nurses using the Broselow tape recommend taping a copy of the appropriate color-coded box directly to the chart in the preadmission phase so that emergency information is immediately available. The algorithm decision trees for pediatric bradycardia, asystole, and pulseless arrest are shown in Figures 26–3 and 26–4. Emergency drug dosages used in pediatric advanced life support (Table 26–11) serve as a guideline. Physicians' specific dosage and administration recommendations should be followed.

COMPLICATIONS AND TREATMENT

Preventing complications in the PACU begins when the pediatric patient is transported into the unit. Assessment at frequent and regular intervals is essential to prevent complications. Vital signs should be assessed every 15 minutes, more frequently if the condition warrants, for the duration of the initial postoperative period. Temperatures are taken on admission and should be monitored continuously if the patient is hypothermic or hyperthermic. The child should be positioned according to the procedure performed. Prone and semi-prone positions facilitate drainage and help to prevent aspiration if the child should vomit.

In general, the major respiratory complications seen in the postanesthesia care unit include the following:

- Airway obstruction
- Secretions/suctioning
- Stridor

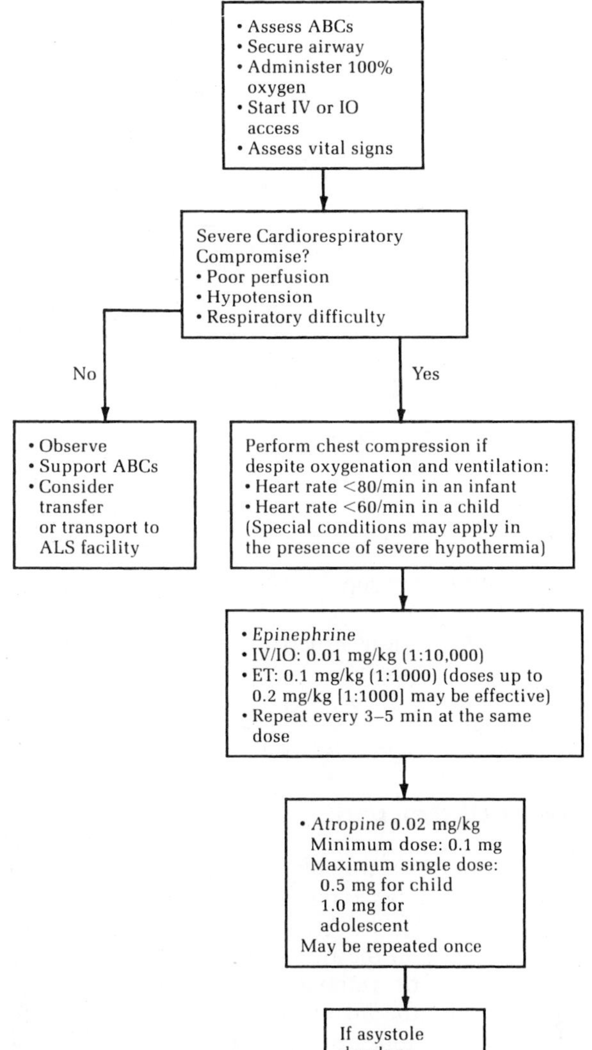

Figure 26–3. Pediatric bradycardia decision tree. American Heart Association guidelines for cardiopulmonary resuscitation and emergency cardiac care. (From Barash PG, et al: Handbook of Clinical Anesthesia. Philadelphia: Lippincott-Raven, 1996, p 600.)

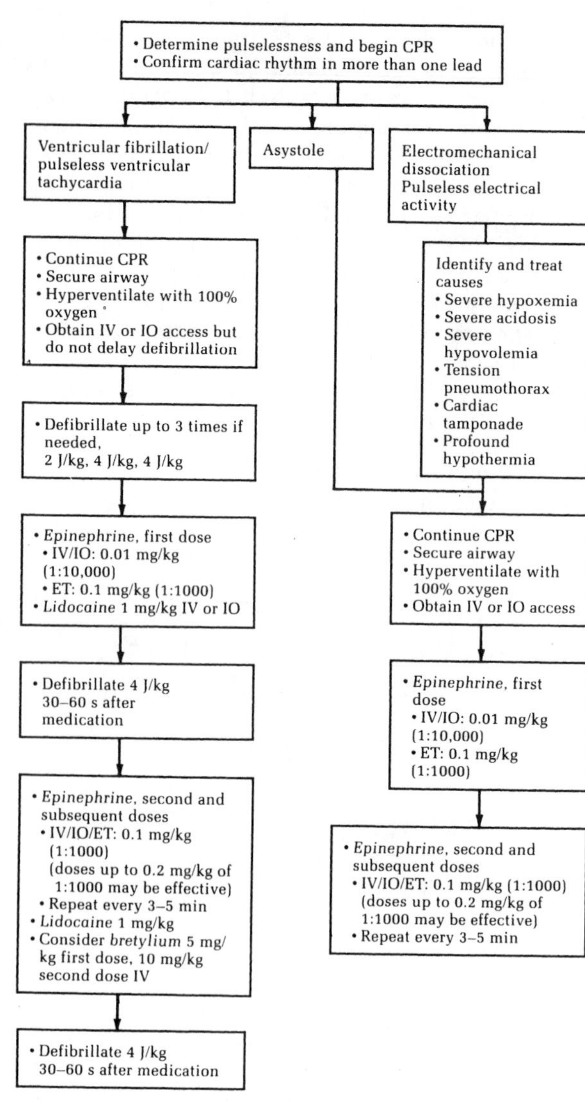

Figure 26–4. Pediatric asystole and pulseless arrest decision tree. American Heart Association guidelines for cardiopulmonary resuscitation and emergency cardiac care. (From Barash PG, et al: Handbook of Clinical Anesthesia. Philadelphia: Lippincott-Raven, 1996, p 601.)

- Postextubation croup
- Laryngospasm
- Laryngeal edema/obstruction
- Respiratory depression
- Bronchospasm
- Aspiration

Airway Obstruction

Although infants are obligatory nasal breathers, the large tongue tends to fall back and produce pharyngeal obstruction. The tongue may also adhere to the roof of the mouth. Obstruction may be relieved by pinching the cheeks, holding the infant in a sitting position, pulling the chin forward, and using a pacifier.[17] If these manipulations are ineffective, oral or nasal airways may be used. Hyperextension of the jaws in the infant generally results in obstruction rather than clearing.

Secretions/Suctioning

Excessive secretions can rapidly obstruct the airway causing respiratory problems. Proper positioning can eliminate many risks associated with increased secretions. When secretions cannot be controlled with positioning the nurse must use suctioning techniques to control the excessive secretions. Suctioning must be done carefully and with the correct-size suction catheter. Table 26–12 shows correct catheter sizes for suctioning endotracheal tubes; sterile technique should always be used. Careful suctioning of the nonintubated child is also necessary. The

Table 26–11. Drugs Used in Pediatric Advanced Life Support

DRUG	DOSE	REMARKS
Adenosine	0.1 to 0.2 mg/kg Maximum single dose: 12 mg	Rapid IV bolus
Atropine sulfate	0.02 mg/kg per dose	Minimum dose: 0.1 mg Maximum single dose: 0.5 mg in child, 1 mg in adolescent
Bretylium	5 mg/kg; may be increased to 10 mg/kg	Rapid IV
Calcium chloride 10%	20 mg/kg per dose	Give slowly
Dopamine hydrochloride	2–20 μg/kg/min	α-Adrenergic action dominates at ≥15–20 μg/kg/min
Dobutamine hydrochloride	2–20 μg/kg/min	Titrate to desired effect
Epinephrine For bradycardia	IV/IO: 0.01 mg/kg (1:10,000) ET: 0.1 mg/kg (1:1000)	Be aware of effective dose of preservatives administered (if preservatives are present in epinephrine preparation) when high doses are used
For asystolic or pulseless arrest	First dose: IV/IO: 0.01 mg/kg (1:10,000) ET: 0.1 mg/kg (1:1000) Doses as high as 0.2 mg/kg may be effective Subsequent doses: IV/IO/ET: 0.1 mg/kg (1:1000) Doses as high as 0.2 mg/kg may be effective	Be aware of effective dose of preservative administered (if preservatives present in epinephrine preparation) when high doses are used
Epinephrine infusion	Initial at 0.1 μg/kg/min Higher infusion dose used if asystole present	Titrate to desired effect (0.1–1 μg/kg/min)
Lidocaine	1 mg/kg per dose	
Lidocaine infusion	20–50 μg/kg/min	
Sodium bicarbonate	1 mEq/kg per dose or 0.3 × kg × base deficit	Infuse slowly and only if ventilation is adequate

IV, intravenous route; IO, intraosseous route; ET, endotracheal route.
From Barash PG, et al: Handbook of Clinical Anesthesia. Philadelphia: Lippincott-Raven, 1996, pp 602–603.

infant's nares should be suctioned first because of the obligate nasal breathing. Excessive suctioning or suctioning too deeply are actions that may trigger a laryngospasm.

Table 26–12. Endotracheal Tube/Catheter Size for Suctioning

TUBE SIZE (mm)	CATHETER SIZE (FRENCH)
2–2.5	No. 5
3–3.5	No. 6.5
4–4.5	No. 8
5–6.5	No. 10
7 and up	No. 14

From Roberts C, Okula N: The pediatric patient. In Litwack K (ed): ASPAN's Core Curriculum for Post Anesthesia Nursing. Philadelphia: WB Saunders, 1995, p 67.

Stridor

The "crowing" sound of stridor is an unmistakable sound; it is most often seen in children who have been intubated during surgery. The irritation and edema resulting from intubation are the common causes of stridor. Treatment of stridor involves

- Oxygen mist
- Racemic epinephrine via nebulizer with oxygen

Racemic epinephrine is used for its vasoconstrictive properties and has a well-known rebound phenomena. Within 2 hours, the clinical effects dissipate and obstruction can be worse than before.[15] If used, the child must be closely monitored for 2 to 3 hours afterward to detect possible rebound edema and symptoms.[14]

Tachycardia can also be a side effect of this treatment.

Postintubation Croup

Postintubation croup can be a frequent complication after traumatic intubation, prolonged intubation, improper endotracheal tube size, excessive coughing on the endotracheal tube, and surgical trauma. There is an increased incidence in the 1- to 4-year-old age group. It can be accompanied by stridor and is characterized by a "barklike" cough. Treatment is similar to the care for stridor:

- Calm reassurance
- Oxygen mist. Depending on severity this may be recommended overnight. If a tent is used it can be referred to as "raindrops" or a "rain forest" to reduce fear.
- Racemic epinephrine via nebulizer and/or dexamethasone
  - Racemic epinephrine (RE) by nebulization: 0.5 ml of 2.25% RE in 2.5 ml of saline
  - Dexamethasone: 4 to 8 mg intravenously[19]
- Reintubation may be necessary if condition is severe or worsens after initial treatment.

Laryngospasm

Laryngospasm may occur on emergence from anesthesia. Children with irritable airways are especially prone to this complication. Laryngospasm occurs at the site of the vocal cords and can be self-limiting or proceed to total obstruction. Irritation from the endotracheal tube and/or oral airway, excessive suctioning, and excessive secretions can trigger a laryngospasm. Characteristics of a laryngospasm in order of appearance are dyspnea, "crowing" sound on inspiration, rocking motion of chest wall indicating accessory muscle use, and aphonia. Aphonia (no sound) indicates total blockage has occurred. Treatment of laryngospasm is as follows:

- Remain calm; assemble help during the early warning signs
- Positioning
- Positive pressure with 100% oxygen ventilation
- Succinylcholine administration if spasm unrelieved by positive pressure
- Airway and ventilation support if muscle relaxants are required
- Continued observation after spasm is resolved

Laryngeal Edema/Obstruction

Edema can occur due to irritation from the endotracheal tube and from the mechanical irritation of suctioning. The small diameter of children's airways increases the potential risk of any condition that reduces airway size.[5] A mere 1 mm of circumferential edema in the infant's trachea, at the cricoid level, can decrease the diameter of the airway by 75%.[20] The most common cause of laryngeal edema/obstruction is the use of inappropriate-sized endotracheal tubes for intubation. Cuffed endotracheal tubes are never used in children younger than 7 to 8 years, because they reduce lumen size, increase airway resistance, and put pressure on the tracheal mucosa. Characteristics include croupy cough, hoarseness, inspiratory stridor, and aphonia. Early signs of impending airway obstruction include increased pulse and respiratory rate; substernal, suprasternal, and intercostal retractions; flaring nares; and increased restlessness.[5] Treatment includes the following:

- High, humidified oxygen therapy
- Body hydration
- Antibiotics (if contributing factor is an infection)
- Corticosteroids (decrease laryngeal inflammation)

Respiratory Depression

Respiratory depression is seen in children for many reasons. The most common reasons producing depression are

- Inadequate reversal of muscle relaxants, causing residual neuromuscular blockade
- Residual effects of inhalation agents, barbiturates, and narcotics
- Pre-existing pulmonary disease

Treatment of respiratory depression involves evaluating the cause, determining the proper treatment, and then assessing the child's response to the treatment selected. Treatment can include any or all of the following:

- Verbal and tactile stimulation by the PACU nurse. This stimulation, sometimes called the "stir-up regimen," may be all that is needed to stimulate spontaneous respirations.
- Naloxone may be used to reverse narcotic-induced depression. Renarcotization may occur, thus children should be observed closely after the 30- to 60-minute duration of action of naloxone.

- Additional reversal agents may be used to reverse the effects of nondepolarizing relaxants.
- Close observation of vital signs, color, oxygen saturation, and respiratory effort and characteristics are necessary throughout the course of the respiratory depression.
- Additional ventilation may be necessary.

Bronchospasm

Bronchospasm is another problem resulting in diminished ventilation. It is more common in the child with a pre-existing bronchospastic disease, such as asthma. High-pitched wheezing is an indication of this spasm and can be heard on auscultation along with coarse rales. Characteristics include skin color changes, flaring nostrils, increased respiratory rate, coughing, and restlessness. Treatment centers on the following:

- Positioning
- Calm environment
- Coughing deeply and/or suctioning if needed
- Oxygen therapy
- Parenteral and inhaled bronchodilating drugs such as intravenous aminophylline and isoetharine (Bronkosol)/metaproterenol (Alupent) inhalers

Aspiration

Aspiration after emesis produces complications in pediatric patients that are similar to adult patients. Aspiration of gastric secretions may cause irritation of the trachea and bronchi. The diagnosis is made on the basis of tachypnea, dyspnea, bronchospasm, cyanosis, shock, and pulmonary edema.[21] Treatment should include the following:

- Positioning with the child's head down and turned to one side to aid in drainage
- Suctioning of the mouth and oropharynx to remove residual secretions
- Oxygen (100%) by face mask
- Diagnostic tests such as arterial blood gas analysis and chest radiography
- Support of the respiratory and cardiovascular systems

Nonrespiratory Complications

Emergence Delirium

Children emerge from anesthesia much differently than adults. They can open their eyes gently and awaken quietly or emerge in a state of complete delirium. The delirious state can last from 30 seconds to 5 minutes. Protection from injury is the primary responsibility during these episodes. Children will fall back to sleep (normally or through the administration of medication) and reawaken calmly without recollection of the event. Characteristics of emergence delirium, which can differentiate this phenomenon from an ordinary excitable emergence or a temper tantrum, are:

- Dissociative state
- Unresponsive to verbal commands
- Appearance of being confused, disoriented
- Generalized purposeless movements
- Amnesic during entire episode

No treatment is necessary, although intravenous medications are often given to hasten the return to sleep and alleviate postoperative pain, which may be a factor in the occurrence. Additional caregivers may be necessary to assist the primary nurse in protecting the child from injury during an episode of delirium, although excessive restriction of movement and forceful restraint should be avoided.

Malignant Hyperthermia

Malignant hyperthermia (MH) is discussed in detail in Chapter 11, but a discussion of the condition is included because the incidence of MH is increased for children to approximately 1 in 14,000. This genetically determined condition is triggered by the depolarizing muscle relaxant succinylcholine and by inhalation anesthetic agents such as halothane. The pathophysiology of MH centers on the enhanced release and diminished reuptake of calcium in the skeletal muscle. This causes sustained skeletal muscle contraction and, ultimately, profound hyperthermia.[20] The presenting symptoms are likely to be end-tidal CO_2 levels and/or rigidity of the jaw (masseter muscle rigidity) after the initial dose of succinylcholine. Anesthesia and surgery are immediately stopped to help avoid a full-blown crisis. Masseter muscle rigidity sometimes does not occur, and the anesthesiologist is then presented with an unexplained tachycardia. Other signs that occur with MH are dark blood in the operative field, ventricular arrhythmias, skin color changes, skeletal muscle rigidity, and, very late in the crisis, the high temperatures for which the condition is named.

In most cases MH occurs in the operating room; however, it can occur in the PACU or a relapse can occur after it has initially been treated successfully. The anesthesia/surgical team must respond immediately to the early signs exhibited and stop all anesthesia, hyperventilate with 100% oxygen, and terminate surgery as quickly as possible. Dantrolene is the only specific treatment for MH. Administration should begin immediately. Recommended dosage is 2 to 3 mg/kg as an initial bolus repeated every 5 to 10 minutes until symptoms are controlled. Occasionally, a total dose of 10 mg/kg or more may be required.[22]

DeSoto recommends that two criteria be met before accepting a child susceptible to MH for outpatient surgery. Dantrolene must be available, and the facility must have monitoring capabilities, including a laboratory, which can perform quantitative acid-base determinations.[15] The minimum observation period for an MH-susceptible child is not known. Recent literature has reported that if a child is asymptomatic after a postoperative observation period of at least 4 hours, the patient may be safely discharged.[23] There have been no deaths from MH in previously diagnosed MH-susceptible patients when the anesthesiologist was aware of the problem and proper management was followed. This information can alleviate patients' preoperative anxiety.[24] The routine use of succinylcholine has decreased owing to its implication in increased potassium levels and cardiac arrest, as well as MH with undiagnosed myopathies.

POSTOPERATIVE PAIN MANAGEMENT

Children deserve and should receive adequate pain management. Unfortunately, their pain is often managed less well than pain in adults. The Agency for Health Care Policy and Research (AHCPR) produced a clinical practice guideline that describes in detail acute pain management for infants, children, and adolescents.[25] AHCPR bases their guidelines on the following principles: (1) unrelieved pain has negative consequences and aggressive pain prevention yields short- and long-term benefits; (2) prevention is better than treatment; (3) successful assessment and control depends, in part, on a positive relationship between healthcare professionals and children and their families; (4) children and their families should be actively involved in the assessment and management; and (5) it may not be practical to eliminate all pain but techniques are now available to reduce pain to acceptable levels.

The aim in postoperative pain management is to have children be cooperative, recover quickly, and have minimal side effects. The difficulty in treating children for pain has multiple reasons. Some healthcare professionals still question the existence of pain in children, assessment of pain can be very difficult, especially with the infant and nonverbal child, and there remains a lack of research on pain management for children.

Assessment of pain should involve the parents so that the nurse is familiar with words and actions the child uses when hurting. Assessment methods (pain rating scales, or tools) provide a subjective measurement of pain. Many pain scales exist (Table 26–13) and should be selected based on the child's age, abilities, and preference. Scales with facial expressions are well liked by children and are suitable for the very young child. Observation remains the most important tool available, especially with the preverbal and nonverbal child. Children should be observed for facial expressions, motor responses, body positioning and activity, and words or sounds they make, understanding that individual children will react to pain in a variety of ways. The World Health Organization has adopted the definition of pain as being "whatever the experiencing person says it is, existing whenever the person says it does."[5]

There are two levels to the management of pain: non-pharmacologic strategies and pharmacologic agents. Optimal application of pain control methods depends on cooperation among different members of the healthcare team throughout the child's course of treatment.[25] Nonpharmacologic strategies consist of music therapy, play therapy, distraction techniques, physical therapy, and comfort measures such as pacifiers, blankets, and special toys. Pharmacologic agents used in the treatment of pain are nonopioids, nonsteroidal anti-inflammatory drugs, opioids, and regional analgesia. Commonly used analgesic drugs and dosage recommendations can be found in Tables 26–14 and 26–15. The optimum dosage controls pain without causing undesirable side effects.

AHCPR made the following statement regarding addiction from opioid use in pain management for children: "There is no known aspect of childhood development or physiology that indicates any increased risk of physiologic or psychologic dependence from the brief use of opioids for acute pain management."[25]

Other pharmacologic approaches available are patient-controlled analgesia and epidural and intrathecal analgesia. New products on the market include oral transmucosal fentanyl (Fen-

Table 26–13. Pain Rating Scales

SCALE/DESCRIPTION	INSTRUCTIONS	RECOMMENDED AGE
FACES Pain Rating Scale* (Nix, Clutter, and Wong, 1994; Wong and Baker, 1988): Consists of six cartoon faces ranging from smiling face for "no pain" to tearful face for "worst pain"	Explain to child that each face is for a person who feels happy because there is no pain (hurt) or sad because there is some or a lot of pain. Face 0 is very happy because there is no hurt. Face 1 hurts just a little bit. Face 2 hurts a little more. Face 3 hurts even more. Face 4 hurts a whole lot, but Face 5 hurts as much as you can imagine, although you don't have to be crying to feel this bad. Ask child to choose face that best describes own pain. Record the number under chosen face on pain assessment record.	Children as young as 3 years
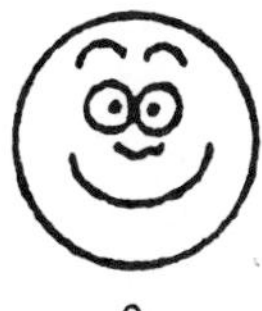 0 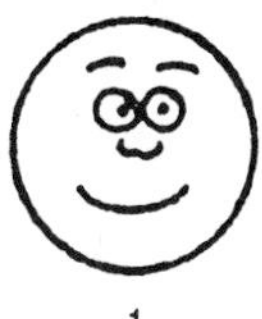 1 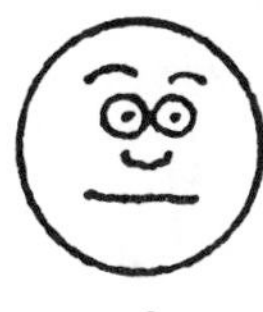 2 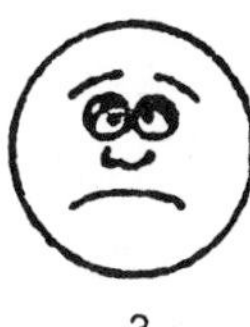 3 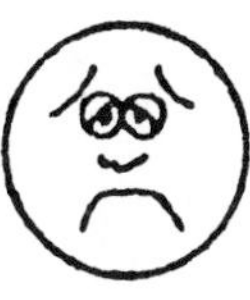 4 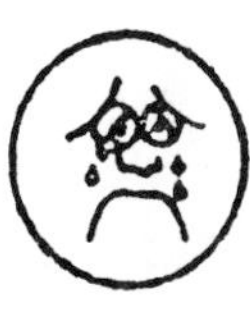 5		
Oucher (Beyer, 1989): Consists of six photographs of child's face representing "no hurt" to "biggest hurt you could ever have"; also includes a vertical scale with numbers from 0 to 100; scales for African-American and Hispanic children have been developed (Villarruel and Denyes, 1991) and validated (Beyer, Denyes, and Villarruel, 1992)	*Photographs:* Explain to child that face at bottom has "no hurt"; second picture, "just a little bit of hurt"; third picture, a "little bit more"; fourth picture, "even more hurt"; fifth picture, "*pretty* much hurt"; and last picture, "biggest hurt you could ever have." Ask child to choose face that best describes own pain. *Numbers:* Explain to child that 0 means you have "no hurt"; 0 to 29, "little hurts"; 30 to 69, "middle hurts"; 70 to 99, "big hurts"; and 100, "biggest hurt you could ever have." Ask child to choose any number between 0 and 100, not just numbers pictured on Oucher, that best describes own pain.	Children 3–13 years; use numeric scale if child can count to 100 by 1s and identify larger of any two numbers (as in original instructions), or by 10s (Jordan-Marsh and others, 1994); otherwise use photographic scale
Numeric Scale: Uses straight line with end points identified as "no pain" and "worst pain"; divisions along line are marked in units from 0 to 10 (high number may vary)	Explain to child that at one end of the line is a 0, which means that a person feels no pain (hurt). At the other end is a 10, which means the person feels the worst pain imaginable. The numbers 1 to 9 are for a very little pain to a whole lot of pain. Ask child to choose number that best describes own pain.	Children as young as 5 years, provided they can count and have some concept of numbers and their values of more or less
No pain 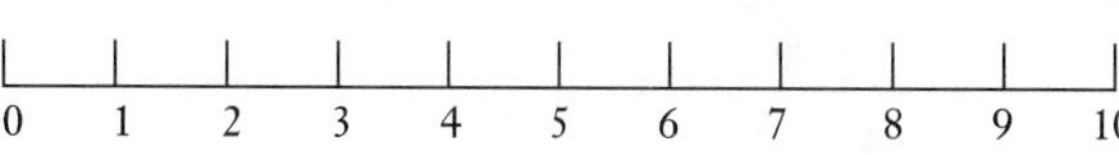 Worst pain		

Table continued on following page

Table 26–13. Pain Rating Scales *Continued*

SCALE/DESCRIPTION	INSTRUCTIONS	RECOMMENDED AGE
Poker chip tool: Uses four red poker chips placed horizontally in front of child	Tell child, "These are pieces of hurt." Beginning at the chip nearest child's left side and ending at the one nearest child's right side, point to chips and say, "This [the first chip] is a little bit of hurt and this [the fourth chip] is the most hurt you could ever have." For a young child or for any child who does not comprehend the instructions, clarify by saying, "That means this [the first chip] is just a little hurt; this [the second chip] is a little more hurt; this [the third chip] is more hurt; and this [the fourth chip] is the most hurt you could ever have." Ask child, "How many pieces of hurt do you have right now?" Children without pain will say they don't have any. Clarify child's answer by words such as "Oh, you have a little hurt? Tell me about the hurt." Elicit descriptors, location, and cause. Ask the child, "What would you like me to do for you?" Record number of chips selected. *Spanish Instructions:* Follow English instructions, substituting the following words. Tell parent, if present: "Estas fichas son una manera de medir dolor. Usamos cuatro fichas." Say to child: "Estas son pedazos de dolor: una es un poquito de dolor y cuatro son el dolor maximo que tu puedes sentir. Cuantos pedazos de dolor tienes?"	Children as young as 4 to 4½ years, provided they can count and have some concept of numbers
Word Graphic Rating Scale (Tesler and others, 1991): Uses descriptive words (may vary in other scales) to denote varying intensities of pain	Explain to child, "This is a line with words to describe how much pain you may have. This side of the line means no pain and over here the line means worst possible pain." (Point with your finger where "no pain" is, and run your finger along the line to "worst possible pain," as you say it.) "If you have no pain, you would mark like this." (Show example.) "If you have some pain, you would mark somewhere along the line, depending on how much pain you have." (Show example.) "The more pain you have, the closer to worst pain you would mark. The worst pain possible is marked like this." (Show example.) "Show me how much pain you have right now by marking with a straight, up-and-down line anywhere along the line to show how much pain you have right now." With a millimeter ruler, measure from the "no pain" end to the mark and record this measurement as the pain score.	Children as young as 5 years, although words may need explanation; words shown below were used with children ages 8 to 17 years

No pain — Little pain — Medium pain — Large pain — Worst possible pain

Table 26–13. Pain Rating Scales *Continued*

SCALE/DESCRIPTION	INSTRUCTIONS	RECOMMENDED AGE
Visual Analogue Scale: Uses 10 cm horizontal line with end points marked "no pain" and "worst pain"	Ask child to place a mark on line that best describes amount of own pain. With a centimeter ruler, measure from the "no pain" end to the mark and record this measurement as the pain score.	Children as young as 4½ years; vertical or horizontal scale may be used (Walco and Ilowite, 1991)
Color Tool (Eland, 1993): Uses markers for child to construct own scale that is used with body outline	Present eight markers to child in a random order. Ask child, "Of these colors, which color is like . . .?" (the event identified by the child as having hurt the most). Place the marker away from the other markers. (Represents severe pain.) Ask child, "Which color is like a hurt, but not quite as much as . . .?" (the event identified by the child as having hurt the most). Place the marker with the marker chosen to represent severe pain. Ask child, "Which color is like something that hurts just a little?" Place the marker with the other colors. Ask child, "Which color is like no hurt at all?" Show the four marker choices to child in order from the worst to the no-hurt color. Ask child to show on the body outlines where they hurt, using the markers they have chosen. After child has colored the hurts, ask if they are current hurts or hurts from the past. Ask if child knows why the area hurts if it is not clear to you why it does.	Children as young as 4 years provided they know their colors, are not color blind, and are able to construct the scale if in pain

*Wong-Baker FACES Pain Rating Scale.
Reprinted with permission from Wong DL: Whaley & Wong's Nursing Care of Infants & Children. St. Louis: Mosby-Year Book, 1995, pp 1085–1086.

Table 26–14. Commonly Used Analgesic Drugs and Dosages

DRUG	ROUTE	DOSE	DURATION OF ACTION (hr)
Acetaminophen	PR/PO	10–15 mg/kg*	4–6
Ketorolac	IM/?IV	1 mg/kg (max. of 30 mg)	6–8
	PO	1 mg/kg (max. of 10 mg)	4–6
Ibuprofen	PO	5 mg/kg	6–8
Codeine	PO	0.5–1 mg/kg	4–6
Naproxen	PO	10 mg/kg	6–8
Fentanyl	IV	1–2 μg/kg	0.5–1
Meperidine	IV/IM	0.5–1 mg/kg	2–4
Morphine	IV/IM	0.05–0.1 mg/kg	2–4

*Acetaminophen suppositories are available in 120-mg, 325-mg, and 650-mg sizes. Usually the calculated dose is rounded up or down to the nearest whole or half size suppository.
From Hannallah RS, Patel RI: Pediatric considerations. In Twersky RS (ed): The Ambulatory Anesthesia Handbook. St. Louis: Mosby-Year Book, 1995, p 163.

Table 26–15. Regional Techniques for Pediatric Ambulatory Surgery

SURGICAL PROCEDURE	BLOCK	DRUG	DOSE
Inguinal hernia, hydrocelectomy, orchiopexy	Caudal	Bupivacaine 0.25%–0.125%	0.75–1.0 ml/kg
	Ilioinguinal/iliohypogastric	Bupivacaine 0.25%	0.3–0.5 ml/kg
	Instillation	Bupivacaine 0.25%	0.5 ml/kg
		Bupivacaine 0.25%	0.5 ml/kg
Umbilical hernia	Infiltration	Bupivacaine 0.25%	0.3–0.5 ml/kg
	Caudal	Bupivacaine 0.125%	1.25 ml/kg
Circumcision, hypospadias	Caudal	Bupivacaine 0.25%	0.5 ml/kg
	Dorsal nerve	Bupivacaine 0.25%	4–6 ml
	Ring block	Bupivacaine 0.25%	4–6 ml
	Topical (end of surgery)	Lidocaine jelly or ointment (2%)	
Tonsillectomy and adenoidectomy	Infiltration	Bupivacaine 0.25% with epinephrine 1:200,000	0.5 ml/kg
	Topical	Lidocaine 10% spray	4 mg/kg
Extremities	Peripheral nerve blocks (e.g., axillary)	Bupivacaine	2.5 mg/kg
		Lidocaine	5 mg/kg
Airway endoscopy	Topical	Lidocaine	2 mg/kg

From Hannallah RS, Patel RI: Pediatric considerations. In Twersky RS (ed): The Ambulatory Anesthesia Handbook. St. Louis: Mosby–Year Book, 1995, p 164.

tanyl Oralet) and the fentanyl transdermal patch (Duragesic). Controversy surrounds the use of fentanyl lollipops because dosage is difficult to determine if the entire lollipop is not eaten and objection has been made to the message of candy and drugs. The transdermal patch has a potential for respiratory depression, and care must be taken to remove the patch before discharge. An anesthetic cream called EMLA provides localized atraumatic treatment for a variety of procedures such as intravenous access, lumbar punctures, implanted port access, bone marrow examinations, and superficial biopsies. EMLA is a eutectic mixture of local anesthetics (lidocaine 2.5% and prilocaine 2.5%). A thick layer of cream is applied and covered with an occlusive transparent dressing for 1 hour or more depending on the duration of the procedure to be performed. In some facilities where use is anticipated parents are given instructions for application at home.

Regardless of the pain intervention used it is necessary to evaluate the results. Careful monitoring and assessment is necessary to document the effectiveness of pain intervention methods. Research on pediatric pain management continues to grow, and it will soon be unacceptable, socially and medically, to ignore the pain children experience.

PHASE II DISCHARGE CRITERIA AND INSTRUCTIONS

Discharge Criteria

It is important that the child return to his or her baseline level of functioning. Individual facilities have predetermined guidelines for the criteria that must be met before the child is discharged. Some decisions are based entirely on the physician's clinical judgment; other factors that influence discharge time are administration of medications, extubation time, ability to urinate and ambulate, fluid intake, and control of postoperative nausea and vomiting. There is controversy over demanding that children drink and/or urinate before discharge. Many facilities now discharge children without these requirements, provided they are addressed in the discharge instructions.

Written Instructions

During the postoperative discharge period (phase II) family members are included in the care of their child. The nurse should demonstrate and receive a return-demonstration, of any techniques that the family will need to continue at home. This is an excellent time to reinforce teaching, which was started preoperatively.

Written discharge instructions should complement the verbal instructions and teaching given by the PACU nurse. These instructions serve as a reference for the parents as they care for their child at home. Telephone numbers of the physician, emergency department, and PACU are included in the discharge instructions and given to families in case of an emergency after returning home.

Safe transportation home is a matter of concern for all who discharge children. Safety concerns are difficult to dictate and enforce. Recommendations include that two adults accompany the child home—one to drive and one to care for the child's needs—and that the child is adequately secured in an approved restraint device. These recommendations should be included in the preoperative teaching along with community resources for obtaining help if needed.

Call Back System

Many facilities have some form of system in place to initiate calls within 24 hours after surgery. This allows the nurse to evaluate the effectiveness of interventions and postoperative teaching. Call backs also provide an additional opportunity for parents to ask or clarify a particular question they may have on returning home. The return call, comments, and any action taken should remain a permanent part of the patient's record.

QUALITY IMPROVEMENT

Evaluation of patient care outcomes, preoperatively and postoperatively, is necessary to serve as a quality improvement mechanism. Good indicators for measuring effectiveness with preoperative instructions are the assessment of compliance with feeding and medication schedules, and if a preoperative teaching program has been successful. Postoperatively, evaluating parental performance related to skills taught as well as validating understanding of home care can be accomplished through the follow-up phone call.

Quality improvement processes should be used to obtain feedback from children and parents to ensure that pain management practices are being followed. Outcomes of the procedure or surgical process can be tabulated and can monitor care standards developed by the professional nursing staff. By reviewing the audit outcomes, issues relating to infection, responses to teaching, or readmission to the hospital within a 24-hour period can be evaluated. From the information collected, alterations in the program can be made to achieve the desired patient goals and outcomes of each ambulatory surgical unit.

RESEARCH

Nursing care is expanding rapidly as different models of care are developed and the types of ambulatory procedures continue to increase. Nursing practice succeeds as technical and educational issues are systematically evaluated through research.

Research does not have to be complex or overwhelming, but nursing routines, procedures, and teaching must be continually validated and altered by documented research. The large volumes of patients and the variety of ages and diagnoses make the pediatric ambulatory population a valuable resource for systematic investigation that will ultimately improve care for all patients.

SUMMARY

Surgery for pediatric patients in an ambulatory setting continues to be developed. This chapter has attempted to address the special needs of the pediatric population. Integrating psychosocial, developmental, and cognitive domains are principles stressed throughout the entire chapter. The family (parents and child) must be cared for as an integral unit because to care for only one part of the unit fails both.

The framework for delivery of nursing care is built on the ANA Standards of Maternal and Child Health Nursing and Pediatric Clinical Nursing Practice, ASPAN Standards of Peri-Anesthesia Nursing Practice, and AORN Standards and Recommended Practices. The nursing process serves as the practice model.

Effective preparation, delivery of care, and the prevention of physiological and behavioral problems for the pediatric patient and family are complex, but rewarding goals. When nurses, the family, and the child all work together, goals are met, desired patient outcomes are accomplished, and satisfaction will be achieved.

References

1. Hannallah RS, Epstein BS: The pediatric patient. In Wetchler BV (ed): Anesthesia for Ambulatory Surgery, 2nd ed. Philadelphia: JB Lippincott, 1991, pp 131–195.
2. American Nurses' Association: Standards of Maternal and Child Health Nursing Practice. Kansas City: ANA, 1983.
3. Joint Commission on Accreditation of Healthcare Organizations: Comprehensive Accreditation Manual for Hospitals: The Official Handbook (CAMH). Chicago: JCAHO, 1997.
4. Mansson ME, et al: Comparison of preparation and narcotic-sedative premedication in children undergoing surgery. Pediatr Nurs 18:337–342, 1992.
5. Wong DL: Whaley & Wong's Nursing Care of Infants and Children. St. Louis: Mosby–Year Book, 1995.
6. Bates T, Broome M: Preparation of children for hospitalization and surgery: A review of the literature. J Pediatr Nurs 1:230–239, 1986.

7. Rankin SH, Stallings KD: Patient Education: Issues, Principles, Practices, 3rd ed. Philadelphia: Lippincott-Raven, 1996.
8. Pandit UA, Pandit SK: Fasting before and after ambulatory surgery. J Perianesth Nurs 12:181–187, 1997.
9. Schreiner MS: Preoperative and postoperative fasting in children. Pediatr Clin North Am 41:111–120, 1994.
10. Steward DJ: Screening tests before surgery in children. Can J Anesth 38:693–695, 1994.
11. Roy WL, et al: Is preoperative haemoglobin testing justified in children undergoing minor elective surgery. Can J Anesth 38:700–703, 1991.
12. American Academy of Pediatrics: Committee on drugs: Guidelines for monitoring and management of pediatric patients during and after sedation for diagnostic and therapeutic procedures. Pediatrics 86:1110–1115, 1992.
13. William Beaumont Hospital, Troy, Michigan. Pharmacy Services, 1997.
14. Hannallah RS, Patel RI: Pediatric considerations. In Twersky RS (ed): The Ambulatory Anesthesia Handbook. St. Louis: Mosby–Year Book, 1995, pp 145–167.
15. DeSoto H: Management dilemmas of pediatric patients. In Twersky RS (ed): The Ambulatory Anesthesia Handbook. St. Louis: Mosby–Year Book, 1995, pp 123–141.
16. Fina DK, et al: Parent participation in the postanesthesia care unit: Fourteen years of progress at one hospital. J Perianesth Nurs 12:152–162, 1997.
17. American Society of PeriAnesthesia Nurses: Standards of Perianesthesia Nursing Practice. Thorofare, NJ: ASPAN, 1998.
18. Broselow J, Luten R: Broselow Pediatric Emergency Tape: Scientific and Technical Assistance. Lincolnshire, UK: Armstrong Medical Industries, Inc.
19. Roberts CC, Okula NS: The pediatric patient. In Litwack K (ed): Core Curriculum for Post Anesthesia Nursing Practice. Philadelphia: WB Saunders, 1995, pp 62–77.
20. Drain CB. The Post Anesthesia Care Unit. Philadelphia: WB Saunders, 1994.
21. Balan N, Hollinger I: Children in the PACU. In Frost EAM (ed): Post Anesthesia Care Unit. St. Louis: CV Mosby, 1990, pp 75–92.
22. Malignant Hyperthermia Association of the United States: Emergency Therapy for Malignant Hyperthermia. Sherburne, NY: MHAUS, 1995.
23. Yentis SM, et al: Should all children with suspected or confirmed malignant hyperthermia susceptibility be admitted after surgery? A ten year review. Anesth Analg 75:345–350, 1992.
24. Barash PG, et al: Handbook of Clinical Anesthesia. Philadelphia: Lippincott–Raven, 1996.
25. Agency for Health Care Policy and Research: Acute Pain Management in Infants, Children, and Adolescents: Operative and Medical Procedures. Clinical Practice Guidelines. Publication No. 92–0020. Rockville, MD, AHCPR, 1992.

Chapter 27

Special Needs of the Older Adult

Melissa Marshall Koehle

For age is opportunity no less
Than youth, though in another dress
And as the evening twilight fades away
The sky is filled with stars, invisible by day
— Morituri Salutamus, Longfellow

Aging is a normal and expected process in which changes occur that may decrease a person's ability to adapt physically, emotionally, and psychologically. Surgery, particularly ambulatory surgery, burdens the older adult with stresses that may be particularly difficult to manage.

Many older adults are physically healthy, self-sufficient, and mentally astute well into their 90s, with active lifestyles, close families, and large social circles. Others, however, may be less well off, being chronically ill, debilitated, or cognitively impaired or requiring around the clock care. With the trend being toward a more mobile society, the result has been that many seniors are living far apart from their extended families. The provision of care for these disenfranchised adults can be challenging.

Clearly, healthcare providers must be aware of continuum of care requirements between these two extremes. Increasingly, the myth connecting age and functional ability is being shattered, as evidenced by 80-year-old marathon runners, 84-year-old weightlifters, and increasing enrollments of older people in both job retraining programs and academic programs in institutions of higher learning.

This chapter deals with the nursing needs of elderly patients who require ambulatory surgery. These needs vary enormously from patient to patient, depending on the functional status of each person. The challenge to the ambulatory surgical nurse is to appropriately apply the issues discussed, particularly when considering the generally greater needs of the frail elderly patient.

The approach to providing care to the geriatric patient must be multifaceted and multidimensional. First, these patients require care that is appropriate for the anesthetic and surgical interventions. The normal aging process, perhaps unrelated to the surgery, may dictate what additional nursing needs are required. Furthermore, it may be difficult to distinguish between the effects of normal aging and the disease processes that are common, but by no means inevitable, in the older population. We discuss these differences later in the chapter.

A substantial proportion of older people report having at least one chronic condition or disease, including arthritis, osteoporosis, hypertension, anemia, heart disease, hearing impairments, visual impairments (especially cataracts), orthopedic problems, and diabetes.[1] Anesthesia, surgery, aging and pre-existing disease: one need is not greater than any other; they are interwoven and inter-dependent.

Healthy and lucid seniors and those with moderately or well-controlled disease processes make up a large number of the patients encountered in an outpatient or ambulatory surgical setting. However, as the proportion of frail elders increases, increasing numbers of chronically ill, debilitated, or mildly demented patients will be seen in these settings. Appropriate resources must be available to deal with their special needs, including adequate staffing for their more time-consuming care. Equipment, supplies, and medications for the short-term nursing needs of chronically ill patients must be available. Both assessment and instruction techniques must be altered if the patient has psychological, cognitive, or physical limitations. It is essential that the support people caring for these patients at home or in nursing homes are included in the patient's plan of care.

The term *elderly*, generally defined as "anyone aged 65 years or older," is a useful measure for making financial and job- or retirement-related decisions. Medically, however, people must be assessed to determine their functional or physiologic age with respect to their chronologic age. Many 70-year-olds are vigorous and healthy and maintain a physiologic age years younger than indicated by their birth certificates. Conversely, a chronically ill man of 55 years with end-stage emphysema and diabetes functions at a significantly older age than 55 years. Still, caution is advised that the obvious health of any older adult does not lull the healthcare team into overconfidence in administering drugs or anesthetic agents. One generally agreed on result of the aging process is the body's decreased ability to respond or adapt to stress.[2] The apparently well-controlled elderly diabetic who attends the ambulatory surgery center (ASC) for cataract surgery and interrupts his or her normal dietary schedule may have a higher likelihood of hypoglycemic or hyperglycemic reaction than the young teenager whose ability to adapt to interruptions or stressors is much greater.

In approaching the care of elderly patients, health professionals must consider one or two common pitfalls. First, inadequate evaluation and treatment of older patients can occur if symptoms that might be pathologic or reversible are attributed to the normal process of aging. Second, the use of heroic and excessively invasive efforts may not be appropriate in all circumstances. Somewhere in the continuum lies the best approach.

DEMOGRAPHICS AND SOCIAL TRENDS

The popular phrase "the graying of America" (and Canada) is no more frequently observed than in the healthcare settings, where increased numbers of older and sicker patients are undergoing ambulatory surgical procedures than ever before. In 1940, there were 9 million people aged 65 years and older in the United States. Projections place 39.4 million people aged 65 years and older by the year 2010 and 69 million older than 65 years by the year 2030. Even more significant is the proportion of those who will be 85 years and older, often referred as the "old-old." From 1995 through 2010, this group is expected to grow by 56%, compared with the 13% growth of people aged 65 to 84.[3–5]

Extensive information regarding demographic trends can be found in the Internet Web site for the Administration on Aging at www.aoa.dhhs.gov or at the National Aging Information Center at 330 Independence Avenue, SW, Washington, DC 20201; (202) 619-0724; TDD: (202) 401-7575; FAX: (202) 260-1012.

Another resource for information on aging and its effects is the National Institute on Aging Information Center at P.O. Box 8057, Gaithersburg, MD 20898-8057; (800) 222-2225; TTY: (800)222-4225; or Web site: www.nih.gov/nia.

Many ambulatory surgical settings, especially those in retirement communities, see 70% or more of their patients in the 65 years and older age range. Those older than 75 years require more surgeries, and predictably, more focused and intense nursing care than any other age group.

Several factors have contributed to this trend toward an aging population. Modern advances in technology, with the ability to continually decrease mortality rates, have prolonged the average life expectancy dramatically since the turn of the century. Immigration of young people, such as was seen in the earlier pioneer days, helped to maintain a young working population, but this has decreased in recent years. The generation of baby boomers has not been as fertile as past generations, with the consequence that as they age, the proportion of elders will grow disproportionately higher. At the same time, pressures are on governments and other insurers to encourage fiscal responsibility and appropriate use of scarce resources. This means a reduction in the use of resources and in the lengths of stay in hospitals and clinics.

While recognizing the need for conserving these scarce resources and controlling costs, nurses must also recognize their role as patient advocates within this system. Patient safety and care must always be forefront in the nurse's mind if ever there is question as to, for example, the readiness of a patient for discharge. It is frequently a difficult decision and must be thoroughly and carefully thought out with the patient's best interests in mind.

Since the turn of the century, the educational level of the senior population has gradually risen. In Canada in 1991, 60.4% of seniors reported 9 or more years of schooling, up considerably over previous years.[3] More and more seniors will be college or university educated in the near future. The level of education and comprehension of those in our care affect both the methods and the effectiveness of patient teaching. Nurses must be aware of the changing educational needs of the elderly population over time.

Socially, the older generation in North America was held in great esteem in generations past. With urbanization and industrialization of the mid-19th century came a shift toward a more youth-oriented culture. The social status afforded to the elderly dropped to its lowest point by the mid-20th century, but social programs instituted after World War II have gradually reversed this trend. Due in part to their greater visibility, increased political activism, and increased financial status, the elderly are once again enjoying the status they so richly deserve within our society. Despite this increased awareness of the social status of the elderly in today's society, or perhaps because of it, there has been an alarming increase in cases of elder abuse and neglect. Far from being a problem experienced only by children in our society, abuse of the elderly is a very real concern.

ELDER ABUSE

Definition

Elder abuse is generally defined as the mistreatment of older people by those in a position of trust, power, or responsibility for their care. Four common kinds of elder abuse exist:

1. Physical abuse—the infliction of physical pain or injury, e.g., slapping, bruising, sexual molesting, and restraining
2. Psychological abuse—the infliction of mental anguish, e.g., humiliating, intimidating, and threatening
3. Financial abuse—the improper or illegal use of the resources of an older person without his or her consent for someone else's benefit
4. Neglect—the failure to fulfill a care-taking obligation to provide goods or services, e.g., abandonment, denial of food, water, medicine, or health-related services[6]

Neglect may also include such other behaviors as denial of therapy, nursing services, clothing, therapeutic and equipment aids, and even visits from people who are important to the elderly individual. Elder neglect may be either intentional or unintentional on the part of the caregiver; it is by no means always a consciously malicious act.

Elder abuse or neglect has become an increasing problem in our society. According to the Sudbury Elder Abuse Committee, it is estimated that 1.5 million individuals are victims of elder abuse or mistreatment every year,[7] with only one in five cases being reported. The ambulatory surgery patient is likely to be much more affected by lack of social or family support than the hospitalized patient who is cared for around the clock in an acute care facility. Nurses working in the ambulatory setting are ideally situated to recognize the signs of neglect or abuse of an elderly patient, and then to take action on these findings, according to their agency policy.

Risk Profile

Although not restricted to any one economic, social, or cultural group, there are characteristics of both abused and abusers that may be observed. These include, for the abused, being Caucasian, widowed, female, isolated, 75 years of age or older, physically or cognitively impaired, not financially self-sufficient, and living with relatives. The abuser, on the other hand, is generally a close relative or spouse of the abused, middle aged or older, living with the abused elder, and often experiencing stress such as financial problems, medical problems, marital conflict, substance abuse, and unemployment. This individual may have been an abused child or may harbor some other form of lowered self-esteem or ineffective coping mechanisms.

Recognizing Elder Abuse

Elder abuse is difficult to identify unless outright battery is visible. Elders frequently do not

Table 27–1. Potential Signs of Elder Abuse

- Patterns of "health hopping," i.e., relying on walk-in clinics, with no regular physician follow-up
- Previous unexplained injuries, e.g., hemorrhage beneath the scalp, which may indicate repeated hair pulling
- Burns in unusual locations
- Presence of old and new bruises, forming recognizable patterns or shapes
- Multiple unexplained fractures of ribs or long bones
- Sprains or dislocations
- Genital/anal bruises or bleeding
- Poor personal hygiene
- Signs of sexually transmitted diseases
- Extreme mood changes
- Depression or oversedation
- Lack of glasses, hearing aids, or dentures
- Fearfulness
- Complaints of sleep disorders
- Feelings of guilt, hopelessness, or helplessness

report being abused; this may jeopardize their already tenuous relationship with their caregiver. Some signs and symptoms, or indicators that may be used for the detection of abuse in the elderly in an ambulatory surgical setting, are listed in Table 27–1. The assessor must not fall into the trap of assuming abuse based on these observations, because many of the signs and symptoms listed may be due to the aging process. Accurate and comprehensive documentation must be maintained, and information should be shared with the other members of the staff at the clinic or facility in order to arrive at a plan of care for each individual patient.

Assessing Patients for Elder Abuse or Neglect

If the patient being interviewed attends the clinic with his or her caregiver, they should be interviewed together and then alone. A nonjudgmental, nonthreatening approach is essential for interviewing these patients; the interviewer must be seen as a helper and supporter of the elder. Behavioral observation of the two together may provide clues to emotional abuse. Careful observation of the patient may reveal a state of generalized fear and anxiety. The caregiver may appear to be obsessed with control, show excessive concern, and display hostility toward the patient or interviewer. The caregiver may also provide improbable explanations for symptoms and dwell on the day-to-day burdens of care giving.

Interventions for Suspected Elder Abuse

Every case of suspected abuse or neglect is unique and requires an individualized approach. Nonetheless, the first step must always be to establish whether the patient is in any immediate danger, whether hospitalization is required, or whether it is safe for the patient to remain with the current caregiver. The patient's surgeon and primary physician should be notified as soon as possible. If overt physical abuse is evident, reporting the case to adult protective services and assisting in removing the patient from his or her current home situation may be necessary. The ASC nurse must be aware of the ethical, moral, and legal implications of elder abuse and must be knowledgeable of his or her state or provincial regulations regarding reporting and intervening in cases of suspected abuse.

Under normal circumstances, it can be assumed that a patient who attends an ambulatory surgical facility is competent to make decisions for himself or herself. If, however, the ASC nurse assesses that a patient may not be mentally competent and may be at risk for abuse by the accompanying caregiver, steps must be taken to establish a substitute decision maker or temporary guardian for the at-risk senior. Once again, the nurse should be aware of the resources available in the community. Table 27–2 provides two such resources.

There may be other times when the nurse suspects abuse or neglect, but the patient involved is assessed to be legally competent and capable of making rational decisions regarding care. The patient's autonomy must be maintained under these circumstances, and the temptation to provide unsolicited help should be avoided. Reassurance may be given, however,

Table 27–2. Resources on Elder Abuse

National Center on Elder Abuse (NCEA)
1225 I Street, NW Suite 725
Washington, DC 20005
(202) 898-2586
E-mail: NCEA@NASUA.org
Web site:
http://www.gwjapan.com/NCEA

For information about state elder abuse contacts, call NCEA. The NCEA web site also includes a state-by-state listing of statewide toll-free telephone numbers for reporting/receiving domestic and institutional elder abuse that help is available at any time it is requested. Should the competent patient choose not to accept the services or interventions offered, this decision must be accepted, while assurance is provided that help is available if needed.

Intervention strategies are directed toward the patient, the care provider, and the family of the patient. Primary prevention addresses the issue of elder abuse and neglect through education. Referrals to appropriate community resources, including the patient's family physician, caregiver associations, social services, and so on, may be helpful. The nurse should be aware of the other available resources to assist the elderly and their caregivers, such as homemakers services, alternative housing services, respite care, adult day care services, "Meals on Wheels," financial counseling services, and legal assistance.

Interventions for abusers include legal proceedings (for intentional abuse), immediate relief from stress for the caregiver through assistance in care of the elder, counseling, education, and linking up with appropriate resources in the community. The pressure placed on all members of the healthcare team to reduce hospital admissions and hospital stays is making it increasingly difficult to justify hospitalization for social reasons. Nurses, then, must continually act as the patient's advocate and be watchful for suspected social or housing circumstances that may place their elder patients at risk for abuse or neglect.

THE CARING ENVIRONMENT

Most older adults have been productive and vital members of their families, the workforce, and society. As such, they deserve respectful and considerate treatment. Ideally, those working with the elderly ought to incorporate what the person used to do and be into "who they are now." The psychological and emotional pressures of growing older may be softened slightly by this kind and respectful, nonpatronizing care offered by nurses and all other healthcare providers.

Besides offering expert physical care, the nurse should provide an atmosphere that encourages elderly patients to maintain their self-esteem through retaining as much control over their environment as possible. Older adults should participate as fully as they are able in their care and in setting goals for that care. Competent patients must be permitted to make their own decisions, including the right to refuse care, a situation that the family and nurses may occasionally find difficult to accept. If it is determined that a patient is incompetent to make his or her own decisions, it is important to follow the guidelines provided in each particular institution. Issues of individual rights and autonomy have been the subjects of much discussion and scrutiny in both the United States and Canada. As the population ages, these issues are likely to become more and more contentious, as increasing numbers of seniors choose to question, rather than passively accept, decisions made about their health.

Aging does not mean loss of intelligence. Older people should not be treated as children or as though they are incapable of understanding. Although measures of abstract intelligence such as mathematics, puzzle solving, or object assembly may show a decline in the elderly, intelligence related to vocabulary, comprehension, and acquired information remains essentially unchanged. It is more likely that any intellectual changes noted may be attributed to declining sensory function, lessened ability to assimilate new information, and increased time requirements for processing that information. The nurse must allow sufficient time for the patient to respond to questions and to process the information being required. It must also be remembered that the motivation to learn to follow directions may be related to depression, a very common and very treatable condition in the elderly population.[8, 9]

Time is a precious commodity in a busy ambulatory surgical unit. Nurses must be particularly creative and resourceful to provide as much time as possible for interactions with their older patients. The elderly can become confused or disoriented by hasty instructions or rapid activity. Presenting an unhurried demeanor in the face of constant pressures to perform numerous functions is a real talent. Sitting down, even briefly, for an interchange with the patient may neutralize the appearance of haste and impatience. Further, it enhances mutual responsibility for care rather than an authoritarian relationship.

The issue of time provides an excellent opportunity for the nurse to act as a patient advocate. As pressures increase to "do more with less," the operating slates become longer and longer on any given day. This is appropriate if the patient population consists of a homogenous group of young, able-bodied people. However, how does one manage a group of 30 to 40 elderly patients, many of whom may require that little extra time and or assistance? By discussing these patient-focused concerns about the speed at which the elderly can be appropriately expected to move and think with those in charge, nurses may be able to effectively lobby for improved patient conditions and, serendipitously, improved nurses' work lives.

There is evidence to suggest that memory for recent events declines with advancing years, whereas long-term memory remains essentially intact. This is an issue of particular importance to the nurse providing preoperative or discharge instructions to the elderly patient. Elders appear to learn more efficiently when they are allowed to set their own pace. Sensory losses (especially hearing), distractions, and a decrease in motivation to learn, perhaps related to depression, can also reduce the ability and the desire to remember instructions.[10, 11]

Many people who have outlived family and friends are chronically deprived of the warmth of human touch, a gift that can readily be given in any nursing setting. Sometimes, the nurse is the only person, or one of a few, who may show genuine concern for an elderly person who is living alone. Simple, but genuine, compliments are appreciated by, for example, the woman who painstakingly applies her makeup and lipstick every day or by the 82-year-old gentleman who proudly wears Bermuda sox with his short pants. Arguably, the most effective show of concern the nurse can offer is a patient manner, a gentle touch, and the ability to listen, not just hear.

Some elderly people complain about a multitude of minor or perceived problems. The compassionate and astute nurse considers the patient's history and possible loneliness as one of several bases for such complaints. From that perspective, a caring approach, rather than one tinged with impatience or curtness, is more likely. Because each patient is seen for only a short time in an ambulatory surgery setting, compared with weeks and months in long-term care units, the nurse should be less apt to respond negatively to the patient who is perceived to be chronically complaining.

Still, it is vitally important not to ignore or avoid the patient who is complaining. A real medical problem may be overlooked or missed when the behavior is seen out of context to the individual's ordinary daily behavior. It is a challenge to detect a subtle change in behavior and then try to determine whether it is related to a true medical problem. The nurse must understand the many effects of aging as well as the symptoms of chronic diseases and be able to differentiate between them. After careful assessment, a nursing plan of care can be formulated to assist each older adult through a safe surgical and recovery course.

ENVIRONMENTAL CONCERNS

Providing a safe and comfortable setting for older patients requires meticulous attention to numerous environmental issues. Floors must be free of obstruction and not slippery. The elderly are generally more sensitive to extremes in room temperatures, particularly cold air conditioning or nearby fans, so a moderate room temperature should be maintained. Rooms should be well lit with nonglare lights. Choice of wall and door colorings is important. A darker contrasting color around the door frame helps the older people identify exits. Colors brighter than pastels are detected better by the aging eye. Handrails provided in bathrooms and hallways help patients ambulate more safely. Nearby wheelchair-accessible bathrooms are appreciated.

Furniture should be selected for comfort, including appropriate height for older people, who may have limited motion or strength. Ease of cleaning is an important consideration in furniture selection. Stretchers that lower for easy access without the use of a stepstool are ideal. When stepstools are used for access to higher surfaces, nontipping stools with attached handrails provide steadier assistance. Covered entrances and exits should be available to protect patients from weather. This is particularly important for older adults, who could easily fall in the rain or ice.

AMBULATORY SURGERY VERSUS HOSPITALIZATION FOR THE OLDER ADULT

Governments and other insurers drive increased use of ambulatory surgical services. Although technology and improved anesthesia techniques have facilitated this change in care delivery, some older patients may be concerned or frightened at the rapidity at which they are expected to recover from their procedure and go home. Ambulatory surgical nurses play an important role in explaining the medical rationale behind the current practice of same-day surgery in order to dispel any doubts the patient may have about the safety or the quality of care.

Advantages of Ambulatory Surgery for the Elderly

The ambulatory approach offers the elderly person certain advantages over traditional overnight stays. The decreased risk of nosocomial infection, particularly wound and respiratory infections, is one of the greatest advantages because the ability to combat infection may be altered in the aging immune system. There is less likelihood of mental confusion related to environmental changes and less disruption and loss of control over the older person's personal habits, eating schedules, and medication routines. Reduction in the time spent away from home, family, and friends is also an advantage that most elderly patients appreciate. This maintenance of control over their lives may or may not be overshadowed by more challenging factors related to early discharge.

The reaction of family members to the same-day approach usually depends on the physical and mental ability of each patient and the amount of responsibility the family has assumed for that elder's care. If the patient is able to provide self-care after the initial 24 hours after surgery, the family may well consider the process advantageous. The family should, nonetheless, be particularly attentive for a period of time, regardless of the patient's physical and mental status.

Ambulatory surgery is usually more cost-effective than hospital admission, so there is a financial advantage for third party payers and patients. Medicare regulations require each patient to pay a co-payment, a percentage of the allowable fee for surgery. Thus, patients can reap savings on their personal portion of the payment in the most cost-effective setting.

In contrast, the Canadian healthcare system provides universal healthcare that does not levy a user fee, other than for surgeries that may be considered "nonmedical," such as some plastic surgery procedures. What is important, however, is the savings to the taxpayer when overnight hospital stays are reduced. It is hoped that future studies will demonstrate whether this hypothesis is, indeed, true. There may be a risk involved in returning elderly patients back to their home, with insufficient home care support. Without appropriate home care nursing or community follow-up, the increasing trend toward more and more procedures being performed on an outpatient basis may backfire.

Disadvantages of Ambulatory Surgery for the Elderly

Disadvantages of same-day surgery are often related to, and increased by, the presence of diminishing mental abilities. Forgetful patients may drink or eat before surgery and may not remember or be able to tell the clinic staff. After surgery, they may not follow directions or take medications as prescribed. At home alone, they may fall, contaminate the wound site by handling the dressing, or suffer from an exacerbation of a chronic systemic illness—all without the knowledge of their families or physicians, and without assistance (see Patient and Family Key Education Point 1). Being alone after surgery, fearing complications, and coping with changes in daily routines necessitated by new medication protocols or care related to the surgery can be unsettling.

Transportation issues can be a financial and logistical burden, particularly when numerous trips to various care sites are required before and after surgery. Nurses can assist in coordinating the necessary tests, such as laboratory and radiologic studies, so that they are integrated into a single visit, while at the same time not tiring to the patient.

The lack of appropriate home support creates another difficult situation for many older adults. Some patients may actually be the support or caregiver for a spouse or family member who requires daily care. If the patient is the only automobile driver in the home, this may create additional hardships regarding transportation needs. The older adult may refuse to have friends or neighbors help for various reasons, ranging from privacy to pride. Regardless of the reason given, the nurse must persist until a mutually agreed on plan has been reached to ensure the appropriate home support.

Financial concerns can also be a problem for the elderly, particularly for those with a fixed income. One reason for financial hardship might be the inability to purchase prescription drugs and nutritious food. Another problem might be the cost of transportation to and from medical appointments. A social services representative can be consulted to consider appropriate alternatives. In a freestanding surgery center or another facility without such a resource, the physician should be asked to intercede appropriately. Supplementing the patient's medication supply with pharmaceutical company samples and writing prescriptions for lower-cost drugs are ways the physician can assist.

Patient and Family Key Education Point 1

In view of the increased risk of sepsis in the elderly, providing appropriate information for avoiding infection to these individuals at discharge becomes a critically important nursing responsibility. Using thorough handwashing techniques, properly caring for dressings, practicing good nutrition, not touching surgical areas, and avoiding people with infectious diseases are all important methods of sepsis prevention that should be discussed or reviewed. Symptoms of infection specific to the procedure should be provided in writing, with an emphasis on reporting suspicions to the physician, surgeon, or primary healthcare worker, who in some cases may be the nurse.

PHYSIOLOGIC EFFECTS OF AGING

Many changes occur in virtually every system of the body as part of the normal aging process. These changes may vary from patient to patient. They are not universal in the sense that they occur in every individual at exactly the same time, or in the same order, as illustrated by the story of the 94-year-old man who visits his doctor complaining of a sore right knee. The doctor looks at him, and says in a mildly patronizing way, "Ralph, you're 94 years old, you should expect a few aches and pains, it's part of the territory." Ralph thinks about this for a minute and replies, "But doc, my left knee is 94 years old too, and it doesn't hurt!" Simplistic yes, but it does serve to illustrate the danger of assuming age-related pathology.

It is also critical to differentiate the normal changes related to aging from the pathologic changes of disease. Despite these warnings, there are still some relatively common physiologic and psychological characteristics that the perianesthesia nurse should be aware of when working with the elderly (see Table 27–3).

Anesthesia-Related Changes

Perianesthesia nurses must be attuned to all the immediate effects of anesthesia and surgery in relation to the physiology of aging. Ambulatory surgery nurses must also anticipate potential and actual long-range effects that can extend into the home environment and instruct patients and families accordingly. For instance, the frail 84-year-old patient who has received a benzodiazepine, such as diazepam or midazolam, may have prolonged sedative and amnesic effects after discharge, so the companionship of a supporting and responsible adult must be ensured for an appropriate time period. Another example is the elderly patient with particularly fragile veins and tissues, who should be instructed to protect the venipuncture site after removal of an intravenous catheter and to remove the tape (preferably paper tape or another nontraumatic type) from the skin carefully. Skin damage or discomfort related to the venipuncture site or other taped area can be bothersome and dangerous to the older patient with a compromised immune system.

Generalized Physiologic Changes

Certain changes affect the body as a whole. There is an overall reduction in the body's ability to respond to stress of any type, such as changes in blood pressure, decreased oxygen levels, and decreased airway secretions. Tissues become less elastic and resilient, and reflexes become slower. There is a general decrease in neuromuscular response and in the efficiency of the immune system.

An overall decrease in the number of cells in the body diminishes the effectiveness of virtually all organs and affects functions such as drug elimination via the liver and kidneys and cognitive skills such as remembering instructions. Elasticity of tissues is reduced, resulting in decreased lung compliance, arterial rigidity, and wrinkling of the skin. Wound healing is slowed because of diminished response to inflammatory stimuli, slowed rate of wound contraction, cellular aging, and inadequate amounts of protein and vitamins as a result of poor nutrition.[12] Aging also leads to a decrease in fibroblasts, the cells that are responsible for synthesis of protein and collagen.[13] Other factors that can lead to delayed wound healing include circulatory changes, poor nutrition, and decreased resistance to infection.[14]

Circulatory Changes

Because of a decreased blood volume, the elderly patient is at higher risk for hypovolemia. Oxygenation of tissues can be affected owing to the decreased ability of the blood to transport oxygen and possibly to a degree of anemia, which is a frequent finding among the elderly. The situation is further complicated by sclerosis of the vessels, which mechanically limits the blood flow to the periphery.

Physical Changes

Physical appearance changes as well. At approximately 50 years, people may begin to lose height. The loss of connective tissue results in a further changing of body contour. Hair becomes thin and gray, and freckles or lentigines appear. Lentigines are flat, brown macular areas often referred to as "age" or "liver spots."[8]

The percentage of various tissues changes with the aging process. Despite an overall increase in body fat content, the amount of subcutaneous fat actually decreases with age. This relative decrease in subcutaneous fat promotes loss of body heat and provides less padding for bony prominences. The overall increase in body fat promotes absorption of, and provides increased storage depots for fat-soluble anesthetic drugs and agents. Both the tissues that store water and the total amount of intracellular water decrease proportionately. Given this smaller fluid volume, the older adult is at increased risk for both dehydration and fluid overload. Typically drier mucous membranes and wrinkled skin may complicate the assessment of dehydration in the elderly.

Nutritional and Pharmacokinetic Changes

Chronic malnutrition leading to dietary deficiencies may be a problem for some older adults. A normal decrease in appetite is one reason, along with a loss of interest in food, particularly for the person who must eat alone. If the eating alone is a result of recent widowhood or loss of a partner, this disinterest in food may be exacerbated by reactive depression or grieving.[15] Economic factors cannot be dismissed, because the cost of food is increasing disproportionately to the fixed incomes of many people. Also, many elderly people are unable, physically or intellectually, to prepare wholesome meals, and others are unable to eat properly because of dental, orthodontic, and digestive changes.

Several physiologic changes may combine to affect the way in which medications are absorbed, metabolized, and excreted. Protein-binding capacity is affected as the body ages. The effectiveness of many drugs and anesthetic agents is dependent on the amount of drug that remains unbound to serum proteins in the bloodstream. The unbound drugs are those that are pharmacologically active. The older adult who has less serum protein is thus at greater risk for developing toxic levels of drugs that are circulating unbound to protein molecules. This is particularly true of a drug such as digoxin that, with an already narrow therapeutic window, has the ability to produce toxicity in an older person very quickly. Decreased cardiac output in the elderly results in a decrease in renal and hepatic blood flow, an overall decrease in the number of neurons and neuromuscular connections, and a slower circulating time. These factors and many others may contribute to the clinical consequence of medications' producing stronger and more lasting effects than would the same amount given to a younger patient with higher serum protein levels.

Table 27–4 outlines some of these many physiologic changes that affect various body systems and offers related nursing implications. Their inter-relationships can complicate assessment and can affect the progress of the older surgical patient who has been given an anesthetic and other drugs. The reader must always remember that these physiologic changes are oversimplified here for the purposes of presenting an overall picture of the aging adult body. They are by no means linear, and they may not occur in every older patient. Assumptions about physiologic function based on age that are not supported by the clinical data can lead to problems. "Decades of study of normal and abnormal aging have shown, perhaps more clearly than anything else, that the older people become, the less like each other they become."[16]

Table 27–3. Potential Characteristics of Old Age

Increased pain threshold
Reduced requirement for anesthetic agents
Frequency of co-existing diseases, e.g., diabetes, hypertension, arteriosclerosis, anemia
Delayed drug clearance
Reduced renal and hepatic function
Diminished autonomic tone
Altered response to stress and environmental changes
Reduced thermoregulation
Edentia
Diminished protective airway reflexes
Reduced blood volume
Osteoporosis and arthritis
Decreased muscle mass
Malnutrition and anemia

Data from Nagelhout JJ, Zaglaniczny KL: Nurse Anesthesia. Philadelphia: WB Saunders, 1997.

CHALLENGES OF PATHOLOGIC AND PHARMACOLOGIC INTERVENTIONS

The elderly population experiences a variety of chronic illnesses. The disease processes and

Table 27–4. Physiology, the Aging Process, and Nursing Implications

PHYSIOLOGIC CHANGES	EFFECTS	NURSING IMPLICATIONS
Central Nervous System		
↓ Weight of brain, ↓ number of neurons ↓ Cerebral blood flow and CNS activity	↑ Potential for CNS side effects of drugs May exhibit signs of Alzheimer's disease or other organic dementias	Observe for prolonged or toxic effects Encourage reduced drug doses Enforce safety measures, siderails, observation Increase family involvement in home care Involve social services, home support services, caregiver support group for spouse or other caregiver
↓ Cognition and learning speed	↓ Understanding and memory	Allow adequate time for instructions, no distractions, ↓ noise Provide verbal and written instructions, include family
↓ Minimum alveolar concentration requirements	Prolonged emergence from general anesthesia	Provide supportive postanesthesia care for longer period Prepare for possible ↑ in length of stay in ASC
No change in intelligence		Provide respectful, adult treatment
Peripheral Nervous System		
↓ Number of neuromuscular connections ↓ Number of axons supplying peripheral muscles	↓ Dosage needs for regional anesthesia	Observe for prolonged or toxic effects of regional anesthetics
↓ Autonomic reflexes	↓ Response to stress and BP changes	Implement slower position changes Monitor fluid maintenance
Normal or lowered pain perception	Requires same or less analgesia, depending on assessment of pain	Provide appropriate analgesia based on pt assessment data. Support multimodality approach to pain management and supplemental therapies (e.g., positioning, relaxation)
Cardiovascular System		
↓ Contractility and ↓ cardiac reserve ↓ Cardiac output, atrophy of myocardial fibers	↓ Response to stress and BP changes	Ascertain cardioactive medications taken preoperatively Use caution with fluid replacement Expect slower metabolism of drugs (↓ blood to organs) Assess heart and lung sounds for signs of overload or heart failure
↑ Circulating time	Prolonged onset for drug action	Allow adequate time for response to medications before redosing
Sclerosis of coronary arteries	Potential for myocardial ischemia	Be aware of possible ↓ workload of heart Provide adequate oxygenation, monitor
Sclerosis of cardiac conduction system	Conduction delays ↑ susceptibility to dysrythmias	Use cardiac monitor in early recovery period Have medications and oxygen available Encourage deep breathing
Peripheral sclerosis and diffuse arterial disease	Potential for CVA, thrombosis, and embolism ↑ Peripheral vascular resistance	Avoid fluid overload Assess cardiovascular status Early ambulation Avoid extremes of BP Provide oxygen support for adequate tissue oxygenation
↓ Elasticity of vessels and heart valves	↓ Response to stress and BP changes Potential for orthostatic hypotension	Use slow position changes and instruct for same at home
Fragility of vessels	Bruising, difficult venipunctures	Be gentle with venipunctures; may need to avoid tourniquets and vacuum-style equipment Apply adequate pressure to site after venipuncture or catheter removed Provide care instructions to patient

Table 27–4. Physiology, the Aging Process, and Nursing Implications *Continued*

PHYSIOLOGIC CHANGES	EFFECTS	NURSING IMPLICATIONS
Respiratory System		
Edentia and ↓ bone mass of jaw	Difficult intubation and airway maintenance	Provide appropriate airways, masks, laryngeal masks, and so on Provide dentures as applicable
Depressed reflexes in upper respiratory tract and ↑ secretions	Increased potential for aspiration, regurgitation	Ascertain NPO status preoperatively Ensure reflexes before PO fluids given Position with head elevated after awake Protect unconscious airway
↓ Elasticity and recoil of lungs Calcification of costal cartilages Arthritic changes of ribs, sternum, and vertebrae Muscle strength of diaphragm and intercostal muscles	↓ Vital capacity, ↓ forced expiratory volume, ↓ residual capacity ↓ Functional residual capacity ↓ Chest expansion, stiffened chest wall ↓ Total lung capacity	Position for ease of chest expansion Elevate head when possible Provide oxygen support as needed Teach deep breathing and coughing Reduce anxiety, stress, pain
Musculoskeletal System		
Atrophy of muscle mass	Decreased strength, less regional anesthesia required	Support for walking or exercise Observe for prolonged or toxic effects of regional anesthetic
Joint stiffness, arthritis	↓ Flexibility, pain, difficult ambulation Potential for accidental falls	Provide skid-resistant slippers, handrails, other safety measures Encourage gentle exercise Administer analgesics Position for comfort
Osteoporosis	Potential for pathologic fractures	Provide careful positioning, home safety instructions
Degenerative vertebral changes, ossification of spinal ligaments	Kyphoscoliosis, ↓ body height Difficulty for spinal, epidural injections	Use special positioning for procedure, support for back
Sensory		
↓ Visual acuity, cataracts, glaucoma	Potential for confusion related to decreased sensory input	Provide large-print instructions, make magnifying glass available Provide constant reassurance and discussion about what you are doing Ascertain home support for care
↓ Hearing acuity, difficulty hearing high tones		Allow patient to wear hearing aid when possible Provide microphone-style device Increase voice volume but not pitch, speak slowly, face patient Provide written instructions Allow adequate time for feedback to verify understanding
Vestibular changes	Dizziness, loss of balance Vertigo	Use safety precautions, especially after general anesthesia; handrails; stools; help with ambulation
↓ Perception in smell and taste		
Integumentary		
Thinner layer of subcutaneous fat	Potential for hypothermia Potential for pressure sores	Provide warm blankets, ↑ room temperature when possible, cover head to prevent heat loss Pad and protect bony prominences, change position frequently
↓ Elasticity and turgor and thinner skin	Potential for injury	Pad bony prominences, use paper tape or similar, avoid pressure to or abrasion of skin
↓ Sebum secretion ↓ Collagen	Dryness of skin ↓ Subcutaneous support of blood vessels	Be aware that it may mimic dehydration Be prepared for difficult venipuncture with "rolling veins"

Table continued on following page

***Table 27–4.* Physiology, the Aging Process, and Nursing Implications** *Continued*

PHYSIOLOGIC CHANGES	EFFECTS	NURSING IMPLICATIONS
Renal/Genitourinary		
↓ Renal blood flow	↑ Excretion time for drugs ↓ Metabolism of drugs dependent on kidneys for excretion	Observe for prolonged drug effects Encourage drug doses Encourage oral fluids postoperatively
↓ GFR	Potential for fluid overload Potential for altered drug doses related to ↓ excretion, reabsorption	Monitor IV infusions and urinary output
↓ Ability to adapt to electrolyte and fluid changes	↓ Ability to conserve sodium	Consider hyponatremia (Na^+ < 135 mmol/L) as one cause of confusion
	↓ Ability to excrete potassium	Observe for cardiac dysrhythmias, ECG changes (K^+ level > 4.5 mEq/L)
Prostate enlargement in males ↓ Bladder capacity	Obstruction of urethra, dribbling	Offer urinal frequently, assist to bathroom, monitor output
Relaxation of pelvic musculature in females ↓ Bladder capacity	Stress incontinence	Provide protection for bedding and clothing Reassure and support emotionally to decrease embarrassment
Gastrointestinal		
↓ Hepatic blood flow ↓ Function of hepatic microsomal enzymes	↓ Metabolism of drugs dependent on liver for excretion	Observe for toxic or prolonged drug effects Encourage lowered drug doses dependent on assessment data
↓ Esophageal musculature	Changes in swallowing patterns May lead to reflux, spasms	Use caution with oral fluids, food Position head up if appropriate

CNS, central nervous system; BP, blood pressure; pt, patient; CVA, cerebrovascular accident; GFR, glomerular filtration rate; ASC, ambulatory surgery center; NPO, nothing by mouth; IV, intravenous; ECG, electrocardiographic.

From Eliopolis C: A Guide to Nursing the Aging. Clinical Nursing Diagnosis Series. Baltimore: Williams & Wilkins, 1987, pp 42–43.

the long-term use of medications taken for their treatment may complicate the patient's surgical course. The body systems compromised by illnesses must be considered, along with those changes related primarily to the aging process. In addition, the elderly may present with disease in a nonspecific way. If, in taking an admission history, the nurse notes any of the following, additional assessment steps should be taken:

1. Refusal to eat or drink or change in appetite
2. A history of falling
3. New incontinence
4. Dizziness
5. Acute confusion
6. New-onset or abrupt worsening of dementia
7. Weight loss
8. Failure to thrive

The appearance of any of these findings in an elderly person heralds the onset or worsening of disease and should never be attributed to old age alone.[17]

Heart disease, hypertension, respiratory disease, arthritis, senile dementia of the Alzheimer's type and other dementias, diabetes mellitus, and sensory losses are frequently present in older patients. Related systemic changes and complications significantly affect the patient's nursing needs. For instance, a calm environment should be maintained for a patient with cardiovascular disease or dementia—a challenge in any ASC. The patient with moderate-to-severe arthritis or respiratory disease requires extra time for any activity and often special positioning. Some may need help with dressing and ambulation. Very often, either the patient or the patient's caregiver can be a valuable source of information related to the specific needs or methods of meeting those needs. Taking the time to ask and listen is beneficial.

Chronic illness or disease complicates patient care, but every attempt should be made to keep the patient as close to his or her normal physiologic state as possible. Prolonged recumbency in one position can be difficult. Also, many elderly patients who have less physiologic reserve than younger people poorly tolerate long periods without food, medicine, or fluids.

Medication use generally appears to increase with age, suggesting that the frail elderly may experience the double jeopardy of diminished ability to absorb, metabolize, distribute, and excrete drugs and yet also have increased need for their benefit because of, for example, decreasing cardiovascular function. Maintaining the patient's usual medication protocol is important. Departments of anesthesia generally have policies regarding the use of antihypertensives, antiarrhythmics, mood elevators, aspirin, and anticoagulants before surgery and anesthesia. Diuretics are commonly omitted until after surgery to avoid a full bladder intraoperatively. Instructions are usually given to the patient to take specific medicines with a small amount of water on the morning of surgery. The nurse should reinforce these instructions and, on the day of surgery, verify and document that the instructions were followed.

Obtaining a complete medication history from the older adult can be a challenge. Some patients may have no idea as to the name of the medications that they take, so it may be prudent to instruct elderly patients to bring the medications with them if they seem unsure. The ASC nurse is well advised to learn to recognize some of the more common medications by color and markings. Many elderly patients forget to mention certain medications or do not consider them important enough to list on medication histories. Eye drops, inhalants, topicals, supplemental oxygen, alcohol, cough medicine, antacids, laxatives, or over-the-counter medications, such as analgesics and antihistamines, are some common examples.

The nurse must consider potential untoward interactions between the patient's usual medications and those being given in the perianesthesia period. In addition, the nurse must consider physiologic changes that occur with the aging process and adapt the medication protocol accordingly.

Anti-Inflammatory Agents

Aspirin and other anti-inflammatory agents that can interfere with blood coagulation are often taken for arthritis, bursitis, and other types of inflammatory processes. Most physicians recommend that patients discontinue such medications before the day of surgery. Although 7 to 10 days of abstinence from aspirin is suggested for effective platelet regeneration, many physicians do not recommend discontinuation of the drug long before surgery because exacerbation of the patient's chronic inflammatory disease may be more debilitating than the adverse consequences of continuation of the therapy.

Anticoagulant Agents

Many elderly patients take dipyridamole, warfarin (Coumadin), heparin, or other medications to prevent thrombosis or thromboembolism, particularly in the pulmonary and cerebral circulation. The surgeon or anesthesiologist often directs the patient to discontinue these types of drugs before surgery. For high-risk patients with complex medical histories, the patient's primary physician may be consulted about preoperative discontinuation of these medications. Bleeding and clotting studies are often required just before surgery after the drug has been stopped to ensure adequacy of the clotting mechanism. Patients should be observed for bleeding and must receive adequate physician instructions about when to resume those medications at home. They need to know about the possible symptoms of bleeding that could occur after discharge and to report these to the physician (or nurse) who is in charge of their care.

Insulin

One of the great advantages of the ambulatory approach to surgical care for the elderly is the maintenance of a more "normal" life routine, including the taking of medication and meal scheduling. This can be particularly relevant to the elderly patient with diabetes mellitus. Diabetes is a common ailment affecting the elderly population. Insulin-dependent diabetic patients need to be able to rely on a consistent and planned approach to their day to effectively manage their insulin requirements. All members of the healthcare team who communicate with the patient must be clear and consistent about the instructions regarding drug and food regimens on the day of surgery. Patients may be asked to bring their own insulin to take after they have eaten after surgery. This method is often preferred to using insulin supplied by the facility because most patients are used to a particular brand.

Maintaining both dietary and insulin schedules as close to normal as possible is beneficial to the patient both physically and emotionally. Before the day of surgery, it is helpful to tell diabetic patients of the foods and beverages that will be available at the surgery unit. They have the option of bringing their own food if they are on a particularly strict dietary regimen. A more complete discussion of diabetes mellitus and its management can be found in Chapter 25.

β-Blocking Agents

Many elderly patients take β-blocking agents. Used routinely to treat conditions associated with "old age," these agents are prescribed for everything ranging from hypertension to glaucoma. Researchers are urging caution, however, in their use with the elderly; the side effects tend to be more pronounced and potentially harmful in the older adult.[18] The primary effects of β-blockade include reduced myocardial contractility, conductivity, automaticity, and excitability, resulting in less workload for the heart—good news after, for example, a heart attack. Other effects of β-blockers, both desirable and undesirable, are listed in Table 27–5.

The postural hypotension associated with β-blockers may be more common in older people, resulting in dizziness, fainting, gait difficulties, and impaired vision, problems easily dismissed as the normal consequences of aging. By depressing the contractility of the myocardium, β-blockers place patients at risk for experiencing or exacerbating pre-existing heart failure. The lethargy and dyspnea associated with congestive heart failure are perhaps accepted as an inevitable consequence of advanced years. Hypoglycemia, which can be exacerbated by β-blockers, may be poorly detected because the β-blocker also masks the onset of tachycardia that is a frequent danger signal of impending hypoglycemia. These are just a few examples of the complex manifestations of β-blockers; they literally affect every organ system in the body. The astute ambulatory surgery nurse may be able to assess difficulties with β-blockers through an accurate history taking and thoughtful, probing questioning.

***Table 27–5.* Effects of β-Blocking Drugs**

ORGAN	EFFECT
Eye	Constriction of the ciliary muscle, causing a decline in visual acuity
Salivary glands	Depressed secretion of saliva, leaving mouth dry
Lungs	Constriction of the bronchial muscle, aggravating asthma and COPD
Pancreas	Stimulation of secretion of B cells, which enhances the hypoglycemic effects of insulin in an insulin-dependent diabetic
Heart	Slowing of heart rate or prevention of rates rising in response to exercise, illness, or other stimulation; cardiac output falls
Stomach/ Intestines	Increased motility and heightened tone, leading to such GI problems as diarrhea, nausea, and vomiting
Liver	Slowed liver perfusion; less drug available to target organs
Urinary bladder	Detrusor muscle constriction, leading to urinary retention
Arterioles	Relaxation of arterioles, causing lowered perfusion, slowing the onset of action of some drugs
Male sex organs	Potentiation of impotency in men

COPD, chronic obstructive pulmonary disease; GI, gastrointestinal.

Some practitioners feel that the long-term or intermittent use of β-blocking agents can place the patient at risk if epinephrine is administered concurrently, although controversy exists about the extent of interaction and the degree of associated risk.[19] Normally, cardiovascular response to epinephrine results from stimulation of both α- and β-receptors in the autonomic nervous system. β-Stimulation, which produces vasodilation and increased heart rate, is balanced by α-stimulation, which promotes vasoconstriction and increased arterial resistance.

In the patient taking propranolol or another β-blocking agent, the administration of epinephrine can initiate a marked hypertensive episode, followed quickly by reflex bradycardia. Hypertension occurs when the β-blocking drug blocks the peripheral β-effects of the epinephrine, which usually would be vasodilation and increased heart rate. Vasoconstriction and increased arterial resistance, the α-effects of epinephrine, are accentuated. This can be followed by a reflex bradycardia or other type of arrhythmia, during which time propranolol can prevent the cardiovascular system from responding appropriately to the α-induced peripheral resistance. The myocardium, β-blocked, is unable to respond to those increased demands, and further reflex bradycardia ensues.

Treatment is initiated with direct-acting drugs. Intravenous nitroglycerin and nitroprusside are used to decrease blood pressure. Atropine may be effective in treating associated bradycardia. Ultimately, cardiac arrest or hypertensive stroke can occur if symptoms are left untreated.

Although this occurrence is rare, it cannot be dismissed in the ASC for many reasons. These include the frequent use of local anesthetics that may contain epinephrine, the tendency to use local and regional anesthesia for elderly patients whenever possible, and the number of elderly patients who are taking long-term β-blocking agents. Some facility or anesthesia department policies discourage the use of epinephrine in patients taking β-blockers. Others are less adamant and prefer instead to monitor patients closely when epinephrine is administered.

Antidepressant Agents

Depression is a common and highly treatable illness in the elderly population. It is estimated[1] that 1% to 25% of older people experience symptoms of depression, such as low mood, sadness, pessimism, self-criticism, and difficulty sleeping, concentrating, or eating. What is generally not known is that older people have the highest rate of suicide of all age groups—two to three times higher than that of the general population. Those at greatest risk usually meet the following criteria: male; white; aged 75 years or older; low income; association with alcohol or drug abuse; single (e.g., widowed, divorced); suffering from chronic disease, especially chronic pain; and prior suicide attempt.[20]

The treatment for depression can include medications, psychotherapy, or a combination of both. Less commonly employed, but equally effective in some instances, is the use of electroconvulsive therapy, usually reserved for depression that is unresponsive to medication or for cases in which the use of antidepressant medications are contraindicated. There are many antidepressant medications on the market. They appear to work by altering how specific neurotransmitters, such as dopamine, serotonin, and norepinephrine, act on receptors in the brain. The main categories of antidepressants include

1. Tricyclic antidepressants (eg. amitriptyline)
2. Serotonin reuptake inhibitors (e.g., fluoxetine, paroxetine)
3. Monoamine oxidase inhibitors
4. Atypical antidepressants (lithium, trazodone)

All of these medications carry a wide range of side effects that can be particularly serious in elderly patients (Table 27–6). The general rule of thumb in prescribing an antidepressant to a senior is to "start low and go slow." This may help to minimize side effects, such as hypotension, anticholinergic effects, sedation, and gastrointestinal symptoms.

Orthostatic hypotension may be a problem associated with the antidepressants that have a moderate-to-strong ability to decrease blood pressure. Treatment with these drugs has been associated with an increased number of falls and fractures in the elderly patient. Those at greatest risk for developing orthostatic hypotension while taking antidepressants include the frail elderly, patients with cardiovascular disease, patients with diabetes, and those taking other medications that affect blood pressure. Symptoms that should alert the ASC nurse to a problem include dizziness on standing, lighthead-

***Table 27–6.* Antidepressants and Their Potential to Produce Side Effects**

GENERIC NAME	BP	ANTICHOLINERGIC	SEDATION	GI UPSET	OTHER
Desirable Antidepressants					
Tricyclics					
Desipramine	Mild–mod	Mild	Mild	—	—
Nortriptyline	Mild	Mod	Mild	—	—
Atypical					
Trazodone	Mod	Very mild	Mod	—	Priapism
Serotonin reuptake inhibitors					
Fluvoxamine	Mild	Mild	Mild–mod	Mod	Insomnia/agitation
Paroxetine	Mild	Mild	Mild	Mod	Insomnia/agitation
Sertraline	Mild	Mild	Mild	Mod	Insomnia/agitation
Reversible MAO inhibitors					
Meclobamide	Mod	Mild–mod	Mild	—	Agitation
Undesirable Antidepressants					
Tricyclic					
Amitriptyline	Mod	Very strong	Strong	—	—
Doxepine	Mod	Strong	Strong	—	—
Imipramine	Mod	Mod–strong	Mod	—	—
Trimipramine	Strong	Mod	Strong	—	—
Atypical					
Maprotiline	Mod	Mod	Mod–strong	—	Seizures
Serotonin reuptake inhibitors					
Fluoxetine	Mild	Mild	Mild	Mod	Long half-life Agitation Akathisia

BP, blood pressure; GI, gastrointestinal; mod, moderate.

edness, vertigo, increased number of falls, and complaints of palpitations or racing or pounding heart. Standing and lying blood pressure monitoring should be performed on patients known to be taking any of these medications.

Anticholinergic effects are similar to the effects of atropine administration, occurring because of the antidepressant drug's ability to block specific receptors in the brain and elsewhere in the body. Common symptoms may include dry mouth, dry eyes, blurred vision, constipation, and urinary retention. Less common are fatigue, memory loss, confusion, hallucinations, and delirium. Patient and Family Key Education Point 2 identifies some of the important points that the patient and family must know regarding potential anticholinergic side effects.

As with the other side effects, sedation can occur early in treatment or at each dosage increase and may be compounded by the addition of new medications or new illness. Combinations of drugs such as antianxiety medications, sleeping pills, antihistamines, and antipsychotic drugs with antidepressants can increase the sedative side effects. The mild sedative effects may actually be helpful in relieving the sleep disturbances that occur in some depressed patients. Mild daytime sedation may also help the agitated patient. However, sedation that significantly interferes with the patient's ability to eat and participate in activities is not desirable; dosage adjustments may be necessary. Patients taking antidepressants who present to the ASC with fatigue, difficulty in rousing early in the morning, late morning wakening, slurred speech, confusion, daytime sleepiness, or nighttime incontinence should be referred for further investigation of their antidepressant therapy. Once again, the difficulty in determining the difference between some of the normal patterns of aging and the dangerous side effects of drug therapy is illustrated.

The serotonin reuptake inhibitors have been reported to cause gastrointestinal upset, including nausea, vomiting, stomach pain, or a bloated feeling, in 20% to 40% of patients receiving them.[23] The severity can range from self-limited to severe. These side effects are particularly significant in an environment such as the ASC, where it is likely that procedures and medications causing further gastrointestinal upset will be administered or performed.

Patients receiving antidepressants of the monoamine oxidase inhibitor family must be evaluated particularly carefully with respect to general anesthesia. Meperidine (Demerol) especially is contraindicated in any patient receiving monoamine oxidase inhibitors. Therapeutic doses of meperidine have precipitated unpredictable, severe, and occasionally fatal reactions in patients who have received such agents within 14 days of general anesthesia. The mechanism of these reactions is unclear but may be related to a pre-existing hyperphenylalanemia. Some have been characterized by coma, severe respiratory depression, cyanosis, and hypotension and have resembled the syndrome of acute narcotic overdose. In other reactions, the predominant manifestations have been hyperexcitability, convulsions, tachycardia, hyperpyrexia, and hypertension.

Although it is not known whether other narcotics are free of the risk of such reactions, meperidine is the one most commonly cited. If a narcotic is needed for these patients, a sensitivity test should be performed in which small incremental doses of morphine are administered over the course of several hours while the patient's condition and vital signs are observed carefully. Intravenous hydrocortisone or prednisolone has been used to treat severe reactions, with the addition of intravenous chlorpromazine in those cases exhibiting hypertension and hyperpyrexia. The usefulness and the safety of narcotic antagonists in the treatment of these reactions is unknown.

In summary, the perianesthesia nurse should have a working knowledge of the various types of antidepressant medications commonly prescribed for the elderly population. The ability to recognize that one of these medications may influence the patient's ability to receive an anesthetic agent (as in the case of monoamine oxidase inhibitors and meperidine) or may be causing a dangerous side effect, such as postural hypotension, will assist the ASC nurse in providing optimum patient care.

Patient and Family Key Education Point 2

The anticholinergic effects of antidepressants may occur immediately, in fact, often before the therapeutic effects begin, or they may take some time to occur after a patient has begun taking the medication. It is possible that the ambulatory surgery nurse may be the first healthcare professional to recognize a patient who is experiencing these anticholinergic effects. The side effects vary with each drug and can be significantly worsened if a drug is used in combination with other drugs having similar effects. Commonly used agents that also have anticholinergic effects include

Antihistamines found in many allergy and cold remedies (diphenhydramine, chlorpheniramine)
Antipsychotics (chlorpromazine, thioridazine)
Antinauseants (dimenhydrinate, scopolamine)
Anti-Parkinson agents (benztropine, procyclidine)
Anti-vertigo agents (meclizine [Antivert])
Anticholinergic drugs (oxybutynin [Ditropan])

Once again, the importance of the medication history is demonstrated. Patients who are taking one or a series of "anti" drugs may be at significant risk for developing the anticholinergic syndrome. They should be warned to watch for these anticholinergic side effects. These effects are often difficult to pinpoint because in some ways they are rather vague. Once again, it is possible for patients to assume that fatigue, memory loss, and confusion are simply signs of "old age." It is important for health professionals to identify this potential cause of these worrisome side effects and intervene appropriately, by informing the patient's physician or instructing the patient to stop taking the drug immediately.

Alcohol and Substance Abuse

It is estimated that anywhere from 1% to 15% (even higher for the institutionalized elderly) of the elderly population has an undiagnosed alcohol problem.[8, 22] Physicians and others are often unwilling to recognize alcohol abuse and dependence in the elderly, perhaps believing that the elderly deserve the "last great pleasure" of alcohol (abuse). The fact remains that proper treatment can lead to productive years as a senior citizen compared with an early alcohol-related death.

Diagnostic problems constitute one of the greatest barriers to treatment of the elderly alcoholic. Where the nurse or physician perceives frailty, unsteadiness of gait, or dementia as the result of old age, such signs may herald a substance abuse problem. Table 27–7 illustrates the difficulty encountered in differentiating the various signs of aging, problem drinking, and adverse drug reactions.

Patients must be asked about their substance use in a clear, nonthreatening, nonjudgmental manner. The most widely evaluated instrument to assist in data collection is the Michigan Alcoholism Screening Test, consisting of 25 true or false items, which is reasonably valid in distinguishing alcoholic from nonalcoholic persons.[23] The CAGE (for **c**ut down, **a**nnoyed, **g**uilty, and **e**ye-opener) questionnaire, now commonly incorporated into the admission assessments of patients in both inpatient and outpatient settings, is a very simple screening tool or reference.[21] The four questions are

C: Have you ever felt a need to **c**ut down on your drinking?
A: Do you ever get **a**nnoyed by criticism of your drinking?
G: Do you ever feel **g**uilty about your alcohol consumption?
E: Do you ever feel the need for an **e**ye-opener to get started in the morning?

Generally, two of four answers in the positive indicate a problem with drinking, particularly if combined with any evidence of symptoms, such as anxiety, depression, mood swings, fragmented sleep, and personal relationship problems.

Psychoactive substance abuse and dependence often involve more than one substance and are more prevalent in women. In a practical sense, this points to the need for very thorough history taking from the elderly patient, including an inquiry as to their use of, for example, sleeping pills or antianxiety agents. These agents are often members of the benzodiazepine or hypnotic families and can potentiate the effects of alcohol. Depression, as was mentioned, may be treated with tricyclic antidepressants or selective serotonin reuptake inhibitors, again, medications that may potentiate an alcohol abuse or dependence problem. Coexisting substance abuse in the elderly person is generally of legally prescribed medications (as opposed to recreational drugs), such as antidepressants, hypnotics, and antianxiety agents.

The long-term use of benzodiazepines, such as temazepam, for the treatment of sleep disorders is important to elicit from the elderly patient in the ASC. Frequently, older patients do not consider sleeping pills "medication" or may be embarrassed to admit that they need something to help them sleep. Gentle questioning, perhaps prefaced by a reminder that the information is important to providing them with the best care possible, may help to lessen their concerns. With the addition of flumazenil to anesthesia practice, the administration of this drug to a patient who takes benzodiazepines on a regular basis could have unpleasant consequences.

Alcoholism and other drug use occurs in the elderly and may go undetected because of the

Table 27–7. **Differentiating Alcoholism, Aging, and Adverse Drug Effects**

ALCOHOLISM	AGING	ADVERSE DRUG REACTIONS
Confusion	Confusion	Confusion
Clouded sensorium	Clouded sensorium	Clouded sensorium
Disorientation	Disorientation	Disorientation
Recent memory loss	Recent memory loss	Recent memory loss
Slowed thought process	Slowed thought process	Slowed thought process
Muscle incoordination	Muscle incoordination	Muscle incoordination
Tremors	Tremors	Tremors
Inflammation of joints	Inflammation of joints	—
Gastritis	Gastritis	Gastritis
Hypertension	Hypertension	Hypertension
Depression	Depression	Depression
CHF	CHF	—
Cardiac dysrhythmias	Cardiac dysrhythmias	Cardiac dysrhythmias
Anorexia	Anorexia	Anorexia
Diminished stress response	Diminished stress response	Diminished stress response
Malnutrition	Malnutrition	—
Excess excretion of Mg^{2+} and K^+		Excess excretion of Mg^{2+} and K^+
Edema		Edema

CHF, congestive heart failure.

difficulty in differentiating the symptoms from those of other illnesses, their treatments, or simply aging itself. Early recognition and referral can significantly improve the quality of life and reduce the incidence of serious illness. Ambulatory surgical nurses, who see a large number of elderly patients in their practice, should be aware of this problem and should be prepared to recognize and refer, when appropriate. Accurate assessment of current substance use and abuse is critical to providing the most appropriate anesthetic and surgical experience for the patient. The National Institute on Alcohol Abuse and Alcoholism provides helpful information. Contact information is NIAAA, 6000 Executive Blvd., Bethesda, MD 20892-7003; telephone: (301) 443-3860. Their Web site address is www.nih.gov/nia/health/pubpub/alcohol.htm.

NURSING IMPLICATIONS: PREANESTHESIA CARE

Key nursing interventions for the care of the elderly are outlined in Table 27–8. The special needs of the older population in the surgical environment must be addressed with as much

Table 27–8. **Key Points for Nursing Interventions with Geriatric Patients**

THROUGHOUT ALL CONTACTS

Allow added time for care, instructions, and response
Avoid confusion, loud conversations, and distractions near patient
Provide warmth—room temperature, clothing as allowed, blankets, slippers, limited exposure, warm solutions
Communicate slowly, clearly, in low tones; face the patient when speaking
Use gentleness in care
Address the patient respectfully and use proper name
Observe for untoward or exaggerated effects of medications
Encourage and allow patient's independence
Include support person in care and instructions whenever appropriate

Nurse in Physician's Office

Provide written and verbal directions or map to surgery facility
Provide clear instructions for parking and for locating ambulatory surgery department
Provide brief explanation of reason for
  Preadmission interview (if one is scheduled)
  Diagnostics
  Importance of NPO and adherence to preadmission instructions

Table 27–8. Key Points for Nursing Interventions with Geriatric Patients *Continued*

Preadmission

Provide adequate time for interview and assessment*
Solicit thorough health history; include past surgeries, chronic diseases, medications taken, allergies, name of personal physician, recent diagnostics
Assess physical status; include baseline vital signs, sensory losses, limitations in mobility, prosthetic devices
Assess mental status
Secure appropriate diagnostic tests and results
Verify transportation and home support system and document
Provide verbal and written instructions in large print; include time of arrival, appropriate clothing, medications to be taken or omitted, NPO instructions

Preoperative—On Admission

Verify transportation, home support, and contact information on admission
Give instructions a few at a time; speak slowly and clearly
Ascertain adherence to NPO and requested medication protocol
Assess physical status; include lung sounds, vital signs, and AM blood glucose level as appropriate
Assist with ambulation, positioning, and belongings
Allow patient to keep sensory aids and dentures if possible
Reassure patient on location of belongings
Use gentleness in care, protect fragile skin and tissues
Use alternatives to reduce medication needs—relaxation, touch, family presence, comfort measures
Observe closely for untoward effects of preoperative medications, respiratory and cardiovascular status
Communicate special needs to OR and anesthesia team

Intraoperative

Avoid disturbing noises—instruments, loud music, inappropriate laughter and talking
Remain in visual, tactile, or voice contact with awake patient
Maintain warmth
Allow patient to keep sensory aids and dentures if possible
Positioning—change positions slowly and gently; avoid extremes (e.g., lithotomy)
Protect from skin and tissue injury
Nurse-monitored local anesthesia—provide special attention to vital signs, cardiac rhythm, sedative effects of medications

Postoperative—Phase I

Provide extra time as necessary for arousal—oxygen support, slower ambulation
Monitor vital signs, respiratory and cardiovascular status closely
Observe closely for untoward effects of medications and anesthetic agents
Avoid fluid overload
Avoid sedation when possible
Provide analgesia as appropriate
Reorient patient to surroundings frequently
Protect from skin and tissue injury

Postoperative—Phase II

Ambulate carefully—edge of stretcher first, physical support for walking, eyeglasses first, stepstool
As soon as possible
- Dress in clothes—wellness concept, warmth, familiarity
- Return belongings and sensory aids
- Reunite with support person

Include support person in instructions
Verify plans for home support
Avoid sedating drugs
Provide clear verbal and large-print written instructions
Instruct on resumption of usual medication routine
Ascertain patient's understanding of instructions and ability for self-care through demonstration of skills and repeat of instructions

After Discharge

Contact after 24 hours
Identify caller clearly and slowly
Telephone call:
- Express concern and interest
- Obtain data on physical condition, complications
- Affirm patient's understanding of and compliance with special instructions

Initiate quality improvement monitors, second telephone follow-up, physician involvement as necessary based on data collected

* If a personal visit is not possible, telephone contact should be made to confirm time of arrival, transportation and home support arrangements, patient's understanding of NPO and medication instructions, allergies, and a basic health history.
NPO, nothing by mouth; OR, operating room.

concern as exists for the pediatric patient's special needs. Are there programs that encourage spouses or friends of an elderly person to visit in the postanesthesia care unit, one way of potentially reducing the incidence of postoperative delirium? Has optimum pain management been achieved in the elderly population? Is the older adult warm enough and given enough time for activities?

A comprehensive preanesthesia workup of the patient, including nursing assessment and history taking, diagnostic testing, and patient and family instructions, is essential for the elderly patient who may present with multiple physical, sensory, and social changes. Eloquently stated by Frances Crawford of Mt. Sinai Medical Center, Miami, Florida,

> The preoperative evaluation and interview (of elderly patients) are probably the most important parts of the entire outpatient surgery process. No financial saving or administrative efficiency is worth compromising a patient's safety; proper evaluation of the geriatric patient is the key to success. Any complication is undesirable, but one resulting from poor evaluation is a tragedy because it is easily prevented.[24]

Ideally, this preparation occurs before the day of surgery. With a preadmission interview, there is a built-in period to review and compile data, identify and act on problems, and, it is hoped, avoid cancellation on the day of surgery as a result of inadequate patient preparation or selection. Most older adults are not opposed to the preadmission visit, particularly if the purposes and benefits of such a program are explained to them. While at the facility for the interview, the patient can become familiar with the layout of the building and the nearest parking areas. Meeting members of the nursing and anesthesia departments before the day of surgery often helps allay anxieties by reducing the number of unknowns.

For the patients who do not wish to make an extra trip to the hospital before the day of surgery, a structured telephone call can achieve many of the goals of the preanesthesia visit. The nurse can reaffirm what the attending surgeon and his or her staff have explained about the patient's responsibilities with respect to preoperative preparation. The nurse can also obtain the medical and social history and verify transportation and home support plans. The physician's office should provide the patient with a brochure containing clear directions, a map for locating the surgery facility, easily readable instructions, and a contact telephone number for the ASC staff.

Nursing Assessment and History

The preoperative nursing assessment helps identify potential problems so that a plan to prevent those problems can be formulated and communicated to the other members of the ambulatory surgical team. The atmosphere in an interview area should be comfortable for elderly patients. This includes a comfortable temperature, seating that is easy to get in and out of, and adequate lighting. The room should be located close to the ASC entrance to ensure as short a walk as possible for arriving patients. The interviewer must be careful not to position himself or herself in front of a brightly lit window, because the glare from the window can easily compromise the older adult's already diminishing visual acuity. A magnifying glass is helpful to some people for reading instructions or consent forms. Large-print instructions should be available, and any handwritten information should be written legibly.

Sufficient time must be allowed for assessment because, as was suggested earlier, older people may have multiple physical or social handicaps, or they may simply talk and move slower than younger patients. Attempts to speed them up because of increased workload often result in even more time being required because the patient may misunderstand something said in a hurry or may neglect to inform the interviewer of important information. Distractions should be kept to a minimum. The interviewer should face the patient and speak in a strong, low-pitched voice. Hearing deficits are common in the elderly, particularly for the high-pitched sounds that are so often those used in times of haste.

Although the nursing history and the physical assessment focus on nursing issues, this interview often precedes the anesthesiologist's examination. In some facilities, the nurse initiates referral to the anesthesiologist only if the information on the history points to the need for further evaluation. Otherwise, the anesthesiologist sees the patient on the day of surgery. The patient should have completed a health history before the interview. It is the nurse's responsibility to identify and further investigate little details that can escalate into larger problems later.

The physical assessment includes all the parameters essential to any person's care, but for the elderly person, it should focus specifically on respiratory and cardiovascular status, functional mobility, skin integrity, and sensory losses. Special attention can then be assigned to address any special needs that are identified. Where appropriate, cognitive function can be assessed with the Folstein Mini-Mental Status examination, a tool that helps recognize cognitive impairment.[25, 26] Tools such as these may become even more important in the future, when more and more patients with mild-to-moderate dementias are seen in ambulatory clinics.

The older adult's health history requires special attention. Ascertaining the extent of chronic disease allows for necessary adjustments in the planning of care. Sometimes, contact with the patient's personal physician is needed regarding specific health questions, particularly if the patient is a poor historian. If older patients do not know the names of the medications they are taking, they should be asked to provide that information before the day of surgery, so that the physician can instruct the patient about continuing or stopping the drugs before the surgical procedure.

Diagnostics

The older adult generally needs a more extensive diagnostic workup than a younger counterpart because of increased incidence of chronic disease and medication use; however, testing should be determined on the basis of clinical need rather than age alone. A complete blood count, blood glucose and potassium levels, electrocardiogram, and possibly a chest film and/or pulmonary function test may be indicated, with more or less testing required for specific situations.

Patient and Family Instructions

All patients should have adequate information regarding their responsibilities to and their expectations of the surgical facility (see Patient and Family Key Education Point 3). Special educational needs result from the sensory and cognitive losses that many older adults experience. By no means should older adults be treated as though they are incapable of hearing or understanding. If the nurse identifies such losses, however, adjustments in teaching methods should be made. Some patients may pretend to understand out of embarrassment over sensory or memory losses.

For the patient with severe physical limitations, sending pajamas or a patient gown (from the surgery center or hospital) home to wear on the morning of surgery (covered with a robe or coat) eliminates the need for the patient to dress twice that morning. It saves the patient's and family's energy as well as the nurse's time on admission. This practice, of course, must be in compliance with the facility's infection control policies and should be the exception rather than the rule.

Patient and Family Key Education Point 3

It is helpful to include a support person or caregiver during the interview. Instructions may have to be repeated more than once. They should also be provided in writing for later reference, in particular, fasting (NPO) requirements, medications protocol, appropriate clothing, time of arrival, and special home preparations (e.g., obtain a walker, hire a home health aide or nurse, or arrange for home care nursing if the community provides it). Many facilities are now insisting that the patients and/or their responsible adult sign these instructions sheets, one copy of which is then added to the patient's chart. This may help to support the claim that the patient teaching was reviewed with the patient in instances when the patient may be denying that he or she received any information. This can happen quite innocently when an older person is bombarded with information either in the preanesthetic clinic or on the day of surgery.

A warning must be issued, however, to the ambulatory surgery center nurse to be aware of the possibility of illiteracy among the aging population. If the elderly patient is unsure of the written instructions or demonstrates a reluctance to, for example, sign the instructions, the nurse should suspect this possibility. A nonjudgmental approach to the illiterate patient is important to the maintenance of the therapeutic relationship. Together, the nurse, patient, and family member can determine the best way to ensure that the patient goes home with the appropriate information that he or she will need in order to facilitate recovery. If appropriate, the nurse may wish to use the opportunity to refer the patient to community services that could assist the individual in learning to read and write.

Obtaining Consent for the Procedure

An elderly person who presents to an ambulatory surgical facility for surgical intervention is assumed by most staff to be legally competent and therefore able to complete the appropriate consent forms required by the facility in order for the surgery to proceed. Although physicians are legally obligated to obtain consent, they often enlist the assistance of the nurse in the task of documentation completion.

An individual is considered competent if and only if he or she can understand the nature, consequences, and alternatives to treatment, as explained by the physician.[27] The test of competency is the ability to repeat the diagnosis and proposed treatment in one's own words or manner. If the interviewing nurse believes that a patient is not legally competent in terms of understanding the surgery and its alternatives, it is important that the nurse follows the established institutional protocol for follow-up in these circumstances. Surgery should not go ahead without valid consents being provided. Several outcomes are possible if it is determined that the patient is incompetent, but these decisions must be made in collaboration with other key players, including physicians, social workers, other family members, or those appointed to act on behalf of the incompetent adult. Once again, it is incumbent on the nurse to have a thorough understanding of the state or provincial laws governing informed consent in acute care facilities.

Nursing Implications: The Day of Surgery and Follow-Up

Before the patient is medicated and while the family or significant other is in attendance, the person who will be responsible for postoperative transportation and home support should be identified. The telephone number of the contact person should be verified. Special calling instructions for the postoperative nurses should be documented on the medical record.

Preoperative physical assessment includes, but may not be limited to, auscultation of breath sounds, evaluation of respiratory effort, presence of peripheral edema, and apical pulse for cardiac regularity and rate. Fasting status should be confirmed and any medications taken that morning verified and documented. Preoperative medications should be used judiciously in the elderly, particularly in patients with pre-existing cardiorespiratory illness. If preoperative medications are given, the patient must be monitored carefully for any untoward effects.

Some older people are very possessive of their belongings and may need to be reassured occasionally of their whereabouts. Promoting the concepts of autonomy and normalcy can be achieved by permitting the patients to retain their wigs, false teeth, hearing aids, eyeglasses, and so on, as long as possible. In many instances, there is no need for the patient to sacrifice these items.

Of note, an interesting preoperative order was written for a person undergoing a total knee replacement under regional anesthesia. This intellectually alert 73-year-old gentleman religiously completed the New York Times crossword puzzle every day. The physician's order read, "To OR with glasses, hearing aid, Walkman and tapes, New York Times crossword puzzle, and pencil." Care must be taken, obviously, not to endanger the patients' or staffs' safety by having items in the perioperative environment that may be harmful or could interfere with the operating room equipment.

Communication of the elderly patient's special needs to the operating room and anesthesia staff is important. A consistent location for documentation should be established for special information, such as "do not place the blood pressure cuff on right (or left) arm," or "hearing aids out," "patient is deaf in both ears," "cane/walker in phase II," and "nitroglycerin tablets at foot of stretcher."

The elderly patient requires gentleness in care, both physical and emotional. The following are suggestions for addressing the elder patient's special needs in the operating room:

- Remain within the patient's sight as much as possible.
- Keep loud or disquieting noises to a minimum.
- Position carefully, avoiding extremes wherever possible.
- Place extra padding on beds and stretchers to protect fragile tissues.
- Keep perioperative environment as warm as possible. Warm blankets, slippers, or socks and a covering for the head help prevent hypothermia and may also help the older patient feel less chilled.
- During local anesthesia with or without intravenous conscious sedation, monitor the older person's cardiovascular status, cardiac monitor rhythm, and respiratory function carefully.
- Titrate drug doses to produce intended effects while avoiding somnolence or other side effects.
- Allow sufficient time to evaluate the effects of intravenous medications before a second dose is given as a result of the reduced cardiac index and circulation time of some elderly individuals.
- Provide instructions slowly and clearly.

The postanesthesia care unit staff must take into account all of the factors related to the normal physiologic changes of aging, especially cardiovascular and respiratory parameters. Anesthetic drugs may linger, producing magnified effects and slower arousal from general anesthesia. More time may be required before progress to a phase II (discharge) unit.

Because hypothermia is common in older adults, a temperature should be obtained on arrival in the postanesthesia care unit and periodically as appropriate. Rewarming may be necessary to promote recovery from general anesthesia and to provide comfort to the patient. Constant reassurance as to the completion of the procedure, and that the patient is in the postanesthesia care unit/ambulatory surgical unit helps not only to reduce anxiety but also to prevent postoperative delirium or confusion.

Acute confusion, also known as delirium and transient cognitive impairment, is a prevalent syndrome occurring in 16% to 38% of elderly patients undergoing surgery.[26] Generally, reports of acute confusion following operative procedures are higher in older than in younger patients. Acute confusion is associated with an increased risk of morbidity and mortality among the elderly and may unmask or exacerbate a chronic pre-existing cognitive impairment. Common perioperative causes of acute confusion in the older patient include hemorrhage, hypothermia, hypotension, hypoxia, and use of anticholinergic drugs, such as atropine. Uncontrolled postoperative pain, urine elimination problems, sensory disturbances, systemic infections (especially urinary tract infections), and limited physical mobility before surgery all contribute significantly to the development of postoperative delirium. Table 27–9 summarizes these causes.

The ambulatory surgical unit nurse should be aware of the constellation of risk factors that constitute patients at highest risk for developing postoperative confusion. These include

- Being 80 years of age or older
- Having a history of dementia-like symptoms
- Having multiple diseases or illnesses
- Polypharmacy
- Sensory impairments, especially sight and hearing
- Orthopedic injury
- Low mobility
- Uncontrolled pain
- Urinary elimination problems
- Pre-existing infection, especially urinary tract and respiratory
- Institutionalization before surgery
- High stress or anxiety levels[26]

It is easy to see that effective preanesthetic preparation can forestall many of these risk fac-

Table 27–9. Potential Causes of Postoperative Delirium

Physiologic

Hypoxia/hypercarbia
Cardiovascular disturbances
  Hypotension
  Blood loss
  Embolus/CVA
Drug intoxications
  Neuroleptics
  Narcotics
  Anesthetic agents
Systemic infections
  Urinary
  Respiratory
Fluid imbalances
  Dehydration
  Fluid overload
Electrolyte disturbances
  Elevated sodium (hypernatremia)
  Low serum sodium (hyponatremia)
  Decreased potassium (hypokalemia)
Metabolic disturbances
  Renal failure
  Hepatic failure
  Blood sugar alterations
Altered body temperature
  Pyrexia
  Hypothermia
Neoplasm metastasis
Type of surgery, e.g., greater with eye surgery and extensive procedures lasting a long time

Psychosocial

Severe emotional stress
  Pain
  Anxiety
  Disorientation to surroundings
  Loss of control
  Bereavement
Sensory losses, e.g., hearing and sight
Impaired ability to communicate
Sleep deprivation
Addiction
  Alcohol/thiamine deficiency
  Other substances
Increased age and history of psychiatric illness

Environmental

Unfamiliar environment
Immobility
Sleep deprivation
Sensory deprivation or overload
Social isolation

CVA, cerebrovascular accident.

Adapted from Matthiesen V, Sivertsen L, Foreman M, and Cronin-Stubbs D: Acute confusion: Nursing intervention in older patients. *Orthop Nurs* 13(2):24, 1994. Reprinted wtih permission of the publisher, the National Association of Orthopaedic Nurses.

tors. Education in a supportive and caring manner and recognition of at-risk patients may help decrease the risk of postoperative confusion. Nursing interventions for acute confusion should attempt to re-establish normal physiologic status or assist the patient in interpreting his or her environment. In other words, the cause should be treated. Sedation or restraint for the hyperkinetic patient who is confused is a last resort reserved only for the patient who is at risk for harming himself or others.

The health community generally believes that the practice of pain management ought to somehow differ for the elderly than for younger adults. Elderly patients are often given smaller amounts of analgesics than younger patients with the same magnitude of reported pain. Studies have shown, however, that older patients do not self-administer fewer analgesics than younger patients do.[28] There appears to be a lack of compelling evidence that older adults experience less pain than others. Clinical trials that have assessed the relationship between age and intensity of pain have failed to prove a significant link. According to the Agency for Health Care Policy and Research guidelines,[29] "aging does not alter pain thresholds or tolerance. The similarities of pain experience between elderly and younger patients are far more common than are the differences."

Nonetheless, there are difficulties inherent in managing the acute postoperative pain of an elderly person. Many healthcare providers and patients alike mistakenly consider pain to be a normal part of aging, something to simply be tolerated. Some elderly patients are reluctant to report their pain and stoically bear it. The Agency for Health Care Policy and Research guidelines suggest that the "old-old" (those > 85 years of age) are at particular risk for undertreatment of pain. The pain assessment process can be particularly difficult because of the patient's exhibiting concurrent physiologic, psychological, and cultural changes associated with aging, to say nothing of the compounding factor of the general or regional anesthetic. The nurse must also be aware of the potential risk for drug-drug interaction or drug-disease interaction posed by the patient with multiple chronic illnesses who may be taking numerous medications.

The problem of overmedicating an older adult can be particularly worrisome when discharge home is the goal. Choosing the appropriate analgesic dose can be a challenge. The literature does support early aggressive intravenous analgesia with narcotics, such as morphine and fentanyl or the fentanyl analogues, tapering off to the oral medications before discharge. Some hospitals and clinics are developing 23-hour surgery units, which allow patients to remain as a "day patient" as long as they are officially discharged before they have been in the facility for 24 hours. This can be an especially helpful system for the elderly patient whose pain would not be effectively controlled within the 8-hour time frame of most same day surgery units. Many of these patients are offered the use of patient-controlled analgesia pumps for the first 23 hours to get their pain under control and can be ready for home by the next day.

Additional adjuncts to pharmacologic remedies for pain should not be forgotten. Comfortable positioning, backrubs, soft music, transcutaneous electrical nerve stimulation devices, use of therapeutic touch if appropriate, and even a little "tender loving care" can be effective measures of easing pain and anxiety with minimal sedative or respiratory side effects.

Fluid administration should be closely monitored to avoid circulatory overload. Sensory aids and dentures that may have been removed for surgery should be returned as soon as is feasible—before the patient's reunion with family or friends is preferable.

Movement and positioning should be accomplished slowly to avoid injury, dizziness, or faintness related to changes in blood pressure. Ambulation to a chair should be attempted in stages, with the attendance of a nurse. Stepstools, canes, and walkers are helpful for many older adults.

Reunion with family or friends is often comforting for the older adult, who may be unsettled by the disruption in the daily schedule. The support person should be included in the home care instructions because the patient may have trouble remembering because of the anesthesia effects or declining cognitive abilities. Large-print instructions are helpful for home reference. It is important that the patient understand instructions about resuming customary medications on return to home. It is often helpful to ask the patient to perform a "return demonstration" of the discharge instructions to the nurse to help identify any misunderstandings or difficulties the patient may be having with regard to the instructions.

Slowness in thought processes, movements, activity, and responses should be expected and accommodated. It may take a longer time for the older person to recover sufficiently for discharge to home. Clearly, the elderly patient must be allowed sufficient time not only to be physically recovered before discharge from the facility but also to feel emotionally ready for discharge.

CONCLUSION

The older patient poses a real challenge to ambulatory surgical nurses to provide comprehensive care that not only encompasses their anesthetic and surgical needs but also takes their complex health and social needs into consideration. The challenge does not generally go unrewarded. Older people often exhibit an attitude of patience and true appreciation. They frequently express genuine gratitude to the nurses who care for them and by doing so, give nurses a real sense of job and personal satisfaction.

References

1. Matteson MA, McConnell ES, Linton AD: Gerontological Nursing Concepts and Practice, 2nd ed. Philadelphia: WB Saunders, 1997.
2. Humphrey JH: Stress Among Older Adults: Understanding and Coping. Springfield, IL: Charles C Thomas, 1992, p 35.
3. Gutman GM, Wister AV, Campbell H: Fact Book on Aging, 2nd ed. Vancouver: Gerontology Research Centre, Simon Fraser University at Harbour Center, 1995.
4. Administration on Aging: Growth of the Elderly Population. Based on the United States Bureau of the Census. Available at www.aoa.dhhs.gov. May 2, 1999.
5. Stone LO, Fletcher S: Population aging and the educational system in Canada. In Thornton JE, Harold SA (eds): Educational in the Third Age, Canadian and Japanese Perspectives. Vancouver: Pacific Educational Press, 1992.
6. Administration on Aging: Fact Sheet on Aging: Elder Abuse Prevention. Available at www.aoa.dhhs.gov. May 2, 1999.
7. Bourget B: Social Planning Council Sudbury Region. As reported by the Sudbury Elder Abuse Committee. Available at www.cyberbeach.net/~seac/eldabuse.htm. May 2, 1999.
8. Hazzard WR, Bierman EL, Blass JP, et al: Principles of Geriatric Medicine and Gerontology, 3rd ed. Toronto: McGraw-Hill, 1994.
9. Sanders S: Depression in the elderly. Presented at Medical Rounds, Courtenay, British Columbia, June, 1995.
10. Merriam SB: Adult Learning: Where Have We Come From? Where Are We Headed? In Merriam SB (ed): An Update on Adult Learning Theory, no. 57, Spring. San Francisco: Jossey-Bass Publishers, 1993.
11. Cross P: Patterns of adult learning and development. In Adults as Learners. San Francisco: Jossey-Bass Publishers, 1983.
12. Vowles K: Surgical Problems in the Aged. Bristol: John Wright & Sons, 1994.
13. Lapiere CM: The aging dermis: The main cause for the appearance of "old" skin. Br J of Dermatology 122 (suppl 35):5–11, 1990.
14. Lober CW, Fenske NA: Cutaneous aging: Effect of intrinsic changes on surgical considerations. South Med J 84:1444–14446, 1991.
15. Blazer D, Hughes DC, George LK: The epidemiology of depression in an elderly community population. Gerontologist 27:281, 1987.
16. Rowe JW: Interaction of aging and disease. In Gaitz CM, Samorajski T (eds): Aging 2000: Our Health Care Destiny, Vol 1: Biomedical Issues. New York: Springer-Verlag, 1985.
17. Herr KA, Mobily PR: Complexities of pain assessment in the elderly. J Gerontol Nurs, 17:12–18, 1991.
18. Newbern VB: Cautionary tales on using beta-blockers. Geriatr Nurs, May/June: 12:119–122, 1991.
19. Hansbrough J, Near A: Propranolol-epinephrine antagonism with hypertension and stroke. Ann Intern Med 92:717, 1980.
20. Kane RI, Ouslander JG, Abrass IB: Essentials of Clinical Geriatrics, 3rd ed. New York: McGraw-Hill, 1994.
21. Buchsbaum DG, Buchanan RG, Welsh J, et al: Screening for drinking disorders in the elderly using the CAGE questionnaire. J Am Geriatr Soc 40:662–665, 1992.
22. Marcus M: Alcohol and other drug abuse in elders. J ET Nurs 20:106–110, 1993.
23. Lichtenberg PA: A Guide to Psychological Practice in Geriatric Long Term Care. New York: Haworth Press, 1994.
24. Crawford F: The elderly patient. AORN J 41:356–359, 1985.
25. Ministry of Health, Province of British Columbia, Continuing Care Division: The Folstein Mini-Mental State Examination. Victoria, British Columbia, Published by Author.
26. Mattehiesen V, Sivertson L, Foreman MD: Acute confusion: Nursing intervention in older patients. Orthop Nurs. 13:21–29, 1994.
27. Ministry of Health, Province of British Columbia: Hospital Consent Guidelines. Victoria, Published by Author, 1992.
28. Duggleby W, Lander J: Cognitive status and postoperative pain: Older adults. J Pain Symptom Manage 9: 19–27, 1994.
29. Agency of Health Care Policy and Research: Clinical Practice Guidelines for Acute Pain Management: Operative or Medical Procedures and Trauma. Silver Spring, MD: AHCPR Publications Clearinghouse, 1992, p. 11.

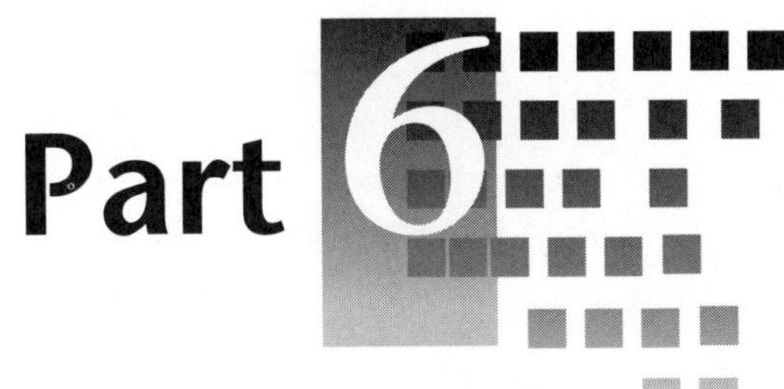

Part 6

The Surgical Specialties

Chapter 28

Minimally Invasive Surgery, Laser, and Other Technologies

Gayle Miller

As nurses working in the ambulatory surgery centers know, the trend has been toward more operative procedures being performed on an outpatient basis. Several factors have influenced this trend: new or improved short-acting pharmaceutical agents and anesthesia techniques that allow rapid recovery; technologic advances, such as laparoscopic equipment and techniques, lasers, and other modalities; the push by third party payers for healthcare dollar efficiencies; and the desire of the healthcare consumer for procedures that decrease postoperative pain or recuperation time, thereby hastening return to their routine activities. This chapter focuses on the technologies that have affected surgical care, tracing the history of minimally invasive procedures, reviewing the technologies that are currently used, and examining new technologies.

TRENDS IN TECHNOLOGY: HISTORICAL OVERVIEW OF LAPAROSCOPY

Minimally invasive techniques began as early as the 10th century, when an Arabian physician used reflected light to examine the cervix. The bladder and the nasal passages were also examined by use of reflected light.[1] Early problems included inadequate illumination and burns from light sources. An Italian physician, Philip Bozzini, in 1806 developed a "light guide," a device that used a candle for illumination. In 1853, the Frenchman Desormeaux presented to the Academy of Paris a device that used an alcohol lamp and a wick. In the 1860s, a German dentist developed a means of illumination that used a platinum wire heated by electrical current. A method of using water for cooling was still not enough to avoid the danger of burns. Edison's invention of the incandescent bulb in 1880 eliminated the need for the water cooling apparatus. Early procedures were diagnostic in nature.[2]

Pioneers in the 20th century include Kelling, who in 1901 introduced a cystoscope into the abdomen of a dog to insufflate and inspect the internal organs. This procedure was performed in humans in 1910 by Jacobaeus.[1] A simple syringe was used to instill air into the abdomen for insufflation. The air was a concern because of the risk of air embolus. In 1918, Goetz and, in 1938, Veress introduced needles for safely introducing gas into the abdomen. They initially used oxygen, but that was discontinued because introduction of electrocautery presented an increased fire hazard in an oxygen-rich environment.[3] In 1944, Palmer employed the Trendelenburg positioning to get air into the abdominal cavity after the introduction of a needle in the cul-de-sac. Palmer was early in stressing the importance of monitoring intra-abdominal pressure.

A device for automatically insufflating was

introduced by Semm in 1964. In 1966, a physicist named Hopkins, who along with Kapany developed fiberoptics in 1952, introduced a rod-lens system that greatly improved image brightness and clarity. Fiberoptic light sources also were introduced in the 1960s; these eliminated the problem of bowel burns from incandescent light. The problem of bowel burns from unipolar coagulation was decreased, but not eliminated, with the introduction of bipolar devices. Visualization was initially limited to one person and was possible only through a cumbersome system of articulated mirrors. In 1986, computer microprocessor chips and a television camera attached to a laparoscope revolutionized minimally invasive surgery. By 1994, the robotic arm was designed to hold the camera and instruments, improving the safety of the procedure and enhancing the surgeon's efficiency and ability.

Laparoscopic techniques in gynecology became widespread in the 1960s and 1970s, with 500,000 procedures performed by 1973, when the First International Congress of Gynecological Laparoscopy was held. Mouret, of France, accomplished the first laparoscopic removal of a gallbladder in 1987, and in 1988 and 1989 in the United States, McKernan and associates started the revolution in laparoscopic cholecystectomy. Within 3 years, the procedure nearly replaced the traditional open cholecystectomy.[2] The laparoscopic cholecystectomy has been described as a catalyst in the amazing growth of minimally invasive general surgery.[4]

MINIMALLY INVASIVE SURGERY

Endoscopic Applications

Arthroscopy

The introduction of arthroscopic techniques has eliminated the need for arthrotomy in many orthopedic procedures, although diagnostic arthroscopy may precede an arthrotomy, helping the surgeon to determine any needed modifications to the surgical plan. Advantages of arthroscopy to the patient include decreased infection, shortened rehabilitation time, minimal hospital stay, smaller incisions, no disruption of extensor mechanisms, and decreased postoperative pain.[2] Before surgery, it is important to have the patient abstain from aspirin products or other drugs that can affect clotting. If the surgeon plans to inject a local anesthetic agent into the joint, the patient is advised that the lack of discomfort is temporary and does not necessitate activity restrictions.

Arthroscopies are common outpatient surgical procedures and include procedures involving the knee, shoulder, elbow, and ankle.

Intraoperative Procedure. For a knee arthroscopy, the leg may be placed in a limb holder about 4 inches above the patella. After prepping, the portal sites are identified and marked before the insertion of a Veress needle or another type of irrigation cannula into the suprapatellar pouch. The joint is distended with fluid, such as lactated Ringer's solution. A sharp trocar with a scope sheath is inserted through a stab wound, and then the joint is entered with a blunt trocar. The arthroscope is inserted through the sheath, and a drainage tube, light source cord, and video camera are attached. A second stab incision is made, through which instruments can be inserted. An arthroscopy pump may be used to regulate the flow of fluid in and out of the joint and control the pressure within. When the procedure is completed, the joint is thoroughly irrigated, and the portal sites are closed by suture. Local anesthetic with epinephrine may be instilled into the joint to decrease postoperative pain and bleeding, and finally, a dressing and, if required, a splint are applied.[2]

Equipment Issues. Arthroscopic equipment may now be sterilized in a steam autoclave. The equipment can also be sterilized in an ethylene oxide sterilizer or disinfected by soaking in glutaraldehyde. If soaking is chosen, a minimum of 20 minutes is the current recommendation for disinfection. For sterilization, items must be soaked for 12 hours. Items must be thoroughly rinsed with sterile water before they are used to remove the disinfectant. The fiberoptic cables should never be kinked or twisted, because that can cause damage to the fibers, preventing the transmission of light. Use of the STERIS system or other sterilization techniques may also be appropriate, depending on manufacturer recommendations (see Chapter 36).

Cystoscopy

Examination of the urinary bladder was one of the earliest of the minimally invasive procedures in history. Modern urologic practice encompasses many commonly performed outpatient procedures, including bladder fulguration, bladder biopsy, cystoscopy, fulguration of bladder neck, ureteroscopy, stent insertion or removal, ureteral catheterization and pyelography, and transurethral ureteropyeloscopy.

Cystoscopy can be performed with either a rigid or a flexible cystoscope. The flexible scope is useful for patients with obstructive disease due to prostatic hyperplasia or for patients with limited mobility that cannot be placed in lithotomy position. The procedure can be performed under local, intravenous sedation, or general anesthesia. Diagnostic and therapeutic modalities that can be utilized in conjunction with cystourethroscopy include ultrasonography, fluoroscopy, laser, and lithotripsy (see Chapter 35).[4]

Laparoscopy

The expanding development of laparoscopic procedures has been a major reason for the growth in outpatient surgery. Gynecologists used early laparoscopic techniques initially for diagnosis and then for tubal sterilization and ovarian biopsy. General surgeons are continuing to find more applications for laparoscopic procedures to replace or supplement traditional open techniques.

Equipment and Instrumentation

Laparoscopy requires specialized equipment. The staff needs to be familiar with the use and care of all equipment and instrumentation. Improper handling can cause damage, resulting in inadequate support for the surgeon, potential injury to the patient, and considerable expense for the institution. The Association of Operating Room Nurses has published recommended practices related to the use and care of endoscopic equipment, including inspection, handling, cleaning, decontamination, sterilization, documentation, and education.[5] Equipment should not be sterilized in a steam autoclave unless this practice is approved by the manufacturer, because it can damage the scopes and the lens cement. The equipment can be sterilized in an ethylene oxide sterilizer or soaked in a liquid disinfectant. Newer sterilization modalities that use chemical processes are being adapted for use with endoscopic equipment.

The basic items needed for laparoscopy, either disposable or reusable, include[6]

Veress needle—the Veress needle is used to penetrate and insufflate the abdomen. It has a spring-loaded inner blunt tip and a sharp outer tip. When penetrating the abdomen, the blunt tip retracts, exposing the sharp beveled sheath. The blunt tip advances again to protect the underlying tissues. Insufflation tubing is attached at the hub of the needle.

Insufflator—the insufflator device delivers gas through filtered sterile tubing at a controlled rate. It also monitors the intra-abdominal pressure. The gas, CO_2, is provided in tanks.

Trocar and cannula—there are two components, an outer sheath and a sharp inner obturator. The sharp obturator penetrates the abdomen after insufflation, or the cannula is inserted by use of the open laparoscopy technique. The surgical procedure is performed through several cannulas. The trocar has a valve to attach the insufflation tubing in order to maintain pneumoperitoneum and a second valve to prevent loss of pneumoperitoneum when no instruments are in place. Cannulas come in different sizes to adapt to the laparoscope and instruments.

Laparoscope—the laparoscope consists of lenses and channels for fiberoptics and viewing. A video camera may be used with variously sized laparoscopes. Laparoscopes are available in zero-, 5-, 30-, and 45-degree angle styles. The zero-degree laparoscope views straight out, and the others provide angled views that are helpful in looking over and around intra-abdominal tissue. The laparoscope can be maintained in position by either an assistant or a mechanical scope holder attached to the operating room (OR) table. Because the surgeon is working in only two dimensions, the position of the scope must be maintained so that the orientation of the surgeon is not affected.

Light source—high-intensity light sources that use xenon, mercury, or halogen vapor bulbs provide the illumination channeled through fiberoptic cables to the laparoscope. The amount of light must be controlled so that the image is not washed out.

Camera and video—microprocessor technology has enabled the surgical team to have real-time video imaging. Earlier technology offered only the surgeon direct visualization of the operative field, unless there was a teaching port on the scope. The camera is attached to the laparoscope and transmits an image via cable through a camera box, where it is changed into a video image and displayed on a monitor. A videocassette recorder can be used to document the procedure.[7]

Instruments—both disposable and reusable instruments are available. Instruments are classified as grasping, retracting, or cutting. The instruments are insulated for use with electrosurgical devices.[6]

Laparoscopic Techniques

Insufflation

Before insufflation and attachment of the Veress needle, the pressure/flow shutoff mechanism should be tested. The insufflator is turned on to a flow of greater than 6 L/min; the pressure should register zero. The rate is then lowered to 1 L/min, and the tubing is kinked. This should cause the pressure to rise to 30 mm Hg, and flow of CO_2 should stop. The Veress needle's blunt retractable tip should also be tested before use.[5]

Procedure. The patient may be placed in the Trendelenburg position before the puncture or immediately after the pneumoperitoneum is established. The site for puncture depends on whether the patient has had previous surgery. If the patient has not had abdominal surgery, the puncture site is at the superior or inferior border of the umbilical ring or directly through the umbilicus for abdominal, gynecologic, or obese patients, respectively. After the umbilicus is stabilized, a small stab incision is made, and the needle is passed by the shaft. The surgeon should feel a change in resistance as the needle passes through the fascia and again through the peritoneum. Before proceeding, a 10-ml syringe filled with 5 ml of normal saline is used first to aspirate and check for blood or bowel contents and then to instill the saline and ascertain that there is easy flow.

The insufflator tubing is attached, and flow of CO_2 is initiated while the Veress needle is stabilized. The pressure in the abdomen should be less than 10 mm Hg at the start of the insufflation. A maximum of 15 mm Hg should not be exceeded. If the pressure is high or reached quickly, the needle may not be positioned correctly. It could be resting on omentum, adhesions, bowel, and so on. Rotating the needle may correct this, but if not, it may be withdrawn and another attempt made. The surgeon must verify needle placement before insufflation is continued. The surgeon observes the abdomen for symmetrical expansion and should note a loss of dullness with percussion over the liver. Insufflation continues until a maximum of 15 mm Hg has been reached or 3 to 6 L of CO_2 has been instilled. At this point, Veress percussion is reminiscent of a ripe watermelon. An alternate method of insufflation is to insert the Veress needle through the posterior fornix or via the transuterine route in female patients.

Alternatively, the surgeon may choose to insert a trocar before insufflation. This is accomplished by making a 1-cm incision through the skin and down to the fascia, then grasping and raising the abdominal wall manually before inserting the trocar. The same loss of resistance is noted as in the previously described technique.[8] Another option is the open cannula, or Hasson, technique. A 2- to 3-cm incision is made through the skin, the subcutaneous tissues are dissected with scissors, and the fascia is identified and incised. After the peritoneum is grasped with hemostats and incised, the surgeon manually inspects to confirm entry into the abdominal cavity and to determine the presence of adhesions. The cannula, which has a conical sleeve, is passed through the opening and secured in place by sutures that have been placed at the fascial incision. The abdominal cavity is then insufflated. The pneumoperitoneum can be achieved as rapidly if not more so than the Veress needle technique. This method is considered safer for patients who have had previous surgeries.[8]

Gasless methods of performing laparoscopies by use of mechanical lift devices are under study.[9] Although they eliminate the adverse effects associated with CO_2 absorption and pneumoperitoneum-caused increases in abdominal pressure, methods currently available offer the surgeon limited exposure of the peritoneal cavity. Refinements in abdominal lifting technology may allow these methods to gain wider acceptance.

Electrocautery

More correctly called the *electrosurgical unit*, and commonly called the *Bovie*, this device has been adapted for use in laparoscopic procedures. The electrosurgical unit generates high-frequency current that can coagulate or cut. It must be inspected carefully before each use to determine any breaks or defects in insulation, and a ground pad must be placed on the patient to prevent electrical injury to the skin if monopolar cautery is used. The pad should be on the same side and as close to the surgical site as possible and over a muscle mass, if possible. Bony prominences and hairy areas should be avoided, as should pooling of preparation solution in the area of the pad.[4]

Electrosurgery is not risk free in minimally invasive laparoscopic procedures. Leakage current can pass through a break in insulation, or by a phenomenon known as *capacitance*, to instruments or tissues. Using all-metal or all-plastic cannulas and skin anchors can decrease the risk of capacitive coupling. Creating hybrid systems with metal cannulas and plastic anchors should be avoided. Because of the limited view of the surgeon as compared with that afforded by open procedures, injuries can go undetected and have disastrous effects, such as bowel perforation, burns, and peritonitis.[10–12]

Laser

Laser, like the electrosurgical unit, can also be used to cut and coagulate. Laser is discussed later in this chapter.

Staples and Clips

Surgical clips and staples have long been used in open procedures and have been adapted for use in laparoscopy. Made of titanium, they are used to ligate vessels; to close abdominal structures with lumens, such as bowel, bladder, and ureter; and to reapproximate tissue. Two forms of clips exist: (1) occlusive and (2) tacking. They come in single or multiload appliers. Staples come in sizes varying from 2.5 to 4.8 mm and in lengths of 3 or 6 cm. When the staples are pushed into the tissue and closed, the tissue between is cut. These devices save time in surgery and are less difficult than laparoscopic knot tying, which requires considerable dexterity.[13] Disposable and reusable varieties are available.

Preoperative Issues

Patient Selection

Criteria for patient selection have broadened over the past few years. What were once considered contraindications are now conditions that demand careful consideration before proceeding.[9] Those conditions include prior abdominal/pelvic surgery, previous peritonitis or pelvic fibrosis, obesity, umbilical abnormality, abdominal/iliac artery aneurysm, severe pulmonary disease, bowel obstruction, uncontrolled coagulopathy, acute and chronic inflammation, and pregnancy. Few if any absolute contraindications to laparoscopy exist today.[13a] Those contraindications may include hypovolemic shock, large pelvic or abdominal mass, severe cardiac decompensation, congestive heart failure, increased intracranial pressure, and ventricular or peritoneal shunts.[9, 15, 15a]

Education

The patient must be educated before surgery about the usual preparatory activities that must take place. Methods of education vary and are based on the patient's ability and readiness to learn, as assessed by the nurse. Patients undergoing laparoscopic surgery tend to minimize the seriousness of the procedure. They need to be prepared for the procedure, the potential complications, and the aftercare required.

Intraoperative Issues

Room Layout

Laparoscopic procedures require a significant amount of high-technology equipment. To help ensure a smooth procedure, the equipment must be organized in the most efficient and accessible arrangement for the surgical team. To provide visualization for both the primary surgeon and the assistant, video monitors may be positioned on either side of the patient or at the foot of OR bed (table). Insufflation equipment and the electrosurgical unit or laser must be easily accessible and observable by the surgical team.

Anesthetic Considerations

Patients undergoing laparoscopic surgery are at greater risk for regurgitation and aspiration of stomach contents.[16] Precautionary measures might include strict NPO (nothing by mouth) status for at least 8 hours before surgery or a water bolus 2 to 3 hours before surgery (the bolus may stimulate gastric peristalsis and emptying), or administration of metoclopramide or an H_2 blocker, such as cimetidine and ranitidine.

Various anesthetic techniques are utilized for laparoscopic procedures. For brief, simple procedures, such as gynecologic cases, local anesthesia has been used. The technique involves injecting local anesthetic with epinephrine at each trocar site. Abdominal organs are sprayed with an anesthetic solution before being manipulated. Monitored anesthesia care may be used in conjunction with a local anesthetic technique. The advantages of these techniques are that they avoid general anesthesia risks, cause less postoperative nausea and vomiting, and have rapid postoperative recovery. The disadvantages include intraoperative anxiety, respiratory compromise, and shoulder and abdominal pain from the insufflation. Epidural anesthesia is rarely used but is a viable alternative in selected cases to avoid the risks of a general anesthetic.

General anesthesia is the most common technique for laparoscopy. Endotracheal intubation decreases the risk of regurgitation and aspiration and allows control of ventilation to compensate for compromised intraoperative pulmonary status. It is critical for the anesthesia care provider to monitor the patient closely with pulse oximetry and capnography. The goal during the anesthetic is to keep the end-tidal CO_2 at less than 40 mm Hg and the pulse oximeter oxygen saturation at least 93%.[16] Studies have compared various inhalational agents and inhalational general anesthesia versus total intravenous anesthesia. The patients receiving intravenous agents had faster recovery and less postoperative nausea and vomiting.[15]

Laparoscopy performed with pneumoperitoneum can cause profound physiologic effects on the respiratory, cardiovascular, and gastrointestinal systems.[9, 17] The cardiovascular effects are primarily related to the pneumoperitoneum created by the insufflation with CO_2. Increased pressure in the abdominal cavity can cause circulatory impairment by decreasing venous return. The resulting decreased central venous pressure can be managed with fluids. This fluid administration can lead to acute pulmonary edema in patients with cardiac compromise. The CO_2 is absorbed from the abdomen into the circulation and leads to hypercarbia and dysrhythmias. The anesthesia care provider must increase tidal volume in order to compensate. Increased tidal volume results in increased wedge pressures and decreased stroke volume and cardiac output. Cardiovascular collapse can occur from a CO_2 embolus or from vagal effects of the manipulation of abdominal organs. The pulmonary system effects include atelectasis, decreased functional residual capacity, and high peak airway pressures. Gastrointestinal effects have already been discussed, and in addition to preoperative measures noted, the anesthesia care provider decompresses the stomach with a nasogastric or an orogastric tube. This also decreases the risk of injury to organs during trocar placement.

In addition to the systemic effects noted, studies have shown that pneumoperitoneum can have a profound effect on the kidneys. Renal cortical perfusion is diminished with a pressure of 15 mm Hg, resulting in oliguria. The perfusion is rapidly restored when the pressure is released, but the urinary output may not return promptly. This may be the result of abdominal compartment syndrome, which has been studied in patients with ascites, in which there is an effect on antidiuretic hormone and aldosterone.[18, 19]

Complications

Abdominal trauma is most likely to occur during insertion of the Veress needle or placement of the trocar.[17] Vascular injury can be either minor, controllable with pressure, or major, requiring clips, suturing, or open vascular repair. Techniques and equipment have greatly reduced the incidence of vascular injury, but the surgical team must be prepared to respond to such emergencies.

The Veress needle, the trocar, various instruments, the electrosurgical unit, or the laser can cause injury to the bowel. Although puncture injuries are usually seen at the time of occurrence, thermal injuries may not be apparent. The patient presents with abdominal pain, nausea, and fever 2 or 3 days after surgery.[10, 11] Injury to the bladder is uncommon if the bladder is emptied at the beginning of the procedure, but it can occur, particularly with gynecologic procedures. Puncture, laser, or electrocautery can damage the ureters. Complications related to the pneumoperitoneum include pneumothorax and subcutaneous emphysema. In laparoscopic cholecystectomy, the bile duct can be damaged by electrocautery, clips, or cholangiography.

LASERS IN SURGERY

Laser Basics

Laser is an acronym for **l**ight **a**mplification by **s**timulated **e**mission of **r**adiation.[20] The theory on which laser is based, stimulated emission, was formulated by Albert Einstein in 1917. Light is electromagnetic energy released as photons. Visible light is only part of the optical spectrum, which is in turn part of the larger electromagnetic spectrum. The radiation in laser technology is not the ionizing radiation of x-rays. Nonionizing radiation of lasers has no biologic effects or health hazards. Ordinary light travels in waves that have four characteristic properties: (1) wavelength, (2) amplitude, (3) velocity, and (4) frequency. The three characteristics that differentiate laser light from ordinary light are that it is: (1) monochromatic, (2) collimated, and (3) coherent. Monochromatic laser light is all one color; ordinary light is polychromatic. Collimated light waves are parallel to each other and do not diverge as they travel; ordinary light spreads out as it travels. The property of collimation reduces loss of power and allows for focusing with precision. Finally, laser light is coherent, which means that the waves travel in phase and in one direction; ordinary light waves are choppy and travel in many directions.

The general components of a laser are the energy source, the active medium, and a resonant cavity. The active medium may be solid, liquid, or gas. The energy source can be an electrical current, a high-powered lamp, or a chemical reaction. As the light beam passes through the active medium, the photons stimulate other photons, and the energy is continually built up. Collimation could occur because this process occurs in a long tube. For practical purposes, a short cylinder with mirrors at both ends is used to reflect the light back and forth and to create the laser beam. The space between the mirrors is the resonant cavity. One of the mirrors is only partially silvered, allowing the light to leave the cavity as a collimated beam. The beam can be pulsed or continuous. A laser delivery system can use fibers, an articulated arm, or fixed optics. The delivery system can be connected to an operating microscope or used through an endoscope.[20]

Laser-Tissue Interaction

Laser energy has four effects on tissue: (1) reflection, (2) scattering, (3) transmission, and (4) absorption. Reflection can be a positive property in that mirrors can be utilized to get a laser beam into a hard-to-reach area. Reflection can be a hazard if the beam is inadvertently reflected off an instrument. Therefore, special instruments are required for use in laser procedures. Laser beams can be scattered in tissues or back up an endoscope, potentially causing damage to the optics. Some wavelengths are transmitted through tissue with little effect, such as an argon laser going through the eye to the retina and a neodymium:yttrium-aluminum-garnet laser (Nd:YAG) going through fluid to the bladder wall. Absorption of a laser beam is dependent on wavelength and tissue characteristics, such as color, consistency, and water content.

The argon and Nd:YAG beams are absorbed by tissue with high melanin and hemoglobin content. Color is irrelevant to the CO_2 laser absorption because it primarily affects the water molecules in tissue. The cellular water is heated, steams, and bursts the cell membrane. Effects vary with the temperature to which the tissue is heated. Reactions vary from no visible or tissue change at 37°C to 60°C to vaporization, carbonization, and a smoke plume at 100°C. Temperatures between these extremes cause blanching, gray coloration, and puckering, with resultant coagulation, protein denaturization, and drying of tissues.[20]

Laser Types

Lasers are categorized by the active medium utilized. Solid-state lasers use a crystal. Examples include ruby, YAG, yttrium-lithium-fluoride, and yttrium-aluminum-oxide lasers. Gas lasers include helium-neon, CO_2, and argon. Dye lasers have limited applications and require the use of toxic dyes. Semiconductor diode lasers have been used in consumer products and fiberoptic communication systems and are now available for medical use in ophthalmologic and endoscopic applications. Experimental lasers include metal vapor lasers and free-electron lasers.[20]

Ruby Laser. The ruby laser was the first successful medical laser. For most procedures, it has been replaced by newer technology, but it is still used for such applications as removing tattoos.

Nd:YAG Solid-State Laser. The YAG is a garnet crystal of aluminum and yttrium oxides. A minimal portion of the yttrium atoms is replaced with neodymium, creating the Nd:YAG. The resultant crystal can be used in continuous-wave or pulsed laser applications. The wavelength is 1064 nm and creates an invisible beam that penetrates tissue deeply. If the wavelength is halved by combining with certain other crystals to create second harmonic generation, the beam becomes visible and penetration is less deep. The potassium titanyl phosphate YAG produces a green beam. It can be focused to a small diameter for precise procedures, such as those in the middle ear.[21] Other combinations of YAG pulsed lasers include alexandrite, holmium, and erbium.[20]

CO_2 Laser. This laser operates at a 10,500-nm wavelength and utilizes low wattage. It requires an articulating arm system with reflecting mirrors as opposed to fiberoptics because it is absorbed by glass. H_2O molecules absorb the energy superficially, creating a water vapor. It is very effective for cutting.

Excimer Laser. The Excimer laser, used primarily in ophthalmology, is an argon-fluoride laser. It has short-wavelength photons and has photoablative qualities that leave a smooth surface.

Dye Lasers. These lasers have limited applications, such as in photodynamic therapy. The patient is injected with dye 24 to 48 hours before the procedure. Abnormal tissues retain the dye, and the laser selectively destroys that tissue.[21]

Diode Laser. The diode laser for medical use is currently limited mainly to ophthalmic photocoagulation but may have more applications in the future, such as for pain management.

Krypton Laser. This laser is used in ophthalmology as an alternative to the argon laser. Because the retina so readily absorbs this wavelength, this laser is very effective for selective photocoagulation procedures.[21]

Laser Safety

Regulatory Controls

Many regulatory, industry, and professional bodies govern the use of lasers or have recommendations for safe practice. Lasers are considered a class III medical device and are thus subject to the jurisdiction of the United States Food and Drug Administration (FDA). The United States Department of Health and Human Services and the American National Standards Institute (ANSI) subdivide lasers into four classes, with most lasers used in medicine considered class IV.

The Occupational Safety and Health Administration (OSHA) does not have any specific standards related to lasers but has jurisdiction under its general safety clauses. OSHA expects laser users to provide a safe laser program and to follow ANSI general guidelines. If a person were to be injured in the use of a laser, OSHA could inspect the facility in which the laser was operated.

The National Institute for Occupational Safety and Health is a body that conducts research utilized by OSHA in making regulations. The National Institute for Occupational Safety and Health has determined that the plume formed during laser procedures is potentially harmful.

The Center for Devices and Radiological Health is the FDA regulatory agency that is responsible for laser manufacturing standards and the approval of investigational permits for new laser technologies. The Safe Medical Device Act of 1990 mandates the reporting of serious injury or illness related to the use of lasers, as well as any malfunctions that may occur.[22] Not all states regulate lasers, but those that do, including Florida, Texas, Arizona, Alaska, New York, California, Georgia, Illinois, Massachusetts, Oregon, Virginia, and Vermont, have regulations pertaining to the use of lasers. These regulations include such issues as registration of laser devices, training requirements, laser safety officer (LSO) responsibilities, and safety rules.[20]

ANSI is a nongovernmental organization of laser experts that has been establishing standards and recommendations for the safe use of lasers since 1973. Its guidelines define the standard for laser safety and include definition of classes and hazards of lasers, control measures, and medical surveillance.[22]

The Joint Commission on Accreditation of Healthcare Organizations (JCAHO), although not specifically dealing with laser safety, considers lasers as it would any other medical equipment. Staff must be properly trained in the use of equipment, competency must be maintained and documented, equipment must be managed appropriately, and safe practices must be in place.

Laser Safety Program

Laser Safety Committee

The structure of a laser safety program varies from facility to facility. Factors influencing structure include the size of the facility and the number of laser devices and procedures. Laser safety could be under the jurisdiction of an OR committee or a subset of the safety committee. The committee membership varies but might include the LSO, risk management and administration representatives, physician users of laser technology, and the OR director. The committee is charged with guiding and overseeing the use of lasers in the facility, including issues such as education of users, recommendations to the credentialing body on practitioners requesting laser privileges, and monitoring of laser usage.

Laser Safety Officer

Although laser safety is the responsibility of all involved in laser use, the LSO plays an essential role. This role is recommended by ANSI[22] and is required by some states. The LSO must be knowledgeable in the safe use of lasers and must be responsible for imparting that knowledge to all parties involved in the use of the laser. In addition to overseeing the direct use of lasers, the LSO must be educated in all aspects of laser safety and applicable regulations. The LSO monitors and enforces all related safety practices and compliance with regulatory guidelines and institutional policies.

Staff Education

All persons involved in use of lasers must have received education and training before their involvement. A basic laser safety training program includes information about laser biophysics, laser equipment, the laser-tissue interaction, safety procedures, and clinical applications. Knowledge and skills can be verified and updated through staff competency measures developed and facilitated by the LSO.

Physician Credentialing

Physicians who want to perform laser procedures should also demonstrate knowledge and skill before performing such procedures independently. The education of physicians can occur in residency or fellowship programs or in postgraduate courses offered by various sources related to laser usage in medicine. Institutions' bylaws typically specify credentialing requirements. Although there may be variation between settings, proof of both didactic and hands-on training is generally required, and proctoring by a member of the physician staff currently credentialed to perform specific laser procedures is sometimes required. When a physician applies for renewal of laser privileges, scope and currency of experience should be considered. The laser safety committee may serve as a review and recommendation body in matters of physician credentialing and recredentialing.

Protective Measures

Eye Safety

Eye safety measures are essential because the eyes are very susceptible to damage from laser radiation. The CO_2 and the holmium laser can cause scleral and corneal damage because their wavelength is absorbed by these tissues. The argon and the Nd:YAG lasers can cause damage to the retina by passing through the cornea and being focused by the lens. Damage to the retina can be acute or can develop slowly with continual exposure.[20] Early damage may go unnoticed and may be caused by a direct or a reflected beam. In technical terms, the amount of risk to personnel is calculated based on the concepts of maximum permissible exposure and nominal hazard zone.

For practical purposes, anyone entering the OR where a laser is in use is at risk for eye damage. To decrease the risk of eye damage, protective eyewear must be worn by anyone entering the area. The patient's eyes must also be protected, with either eyewear or moist gauze pads. Different lasers require eyewear with optical densities appropriate for filtering the specific wavelength of the laser in use. The applicable wavelength should be clearly marked on the eyewear to prevent confusion. Care must be taken to prevent damage to the protective lenses because scratches compromise the protective filtering capacity. In addition to protective eyewear, filtering devices are available for operative microscopes and endoscopes.[22] Nonreflective instruments must be utilized to prevent reflection of the laser beam, thus causing eye or skin injury.

Eye examinations to establish an ocular history baseline can be performed on personnel routinely involved with laser use, although there is not agreement on the need to do this. Examinations should be performed after any ophthalmic laser exposure incidents. In some states, such exposures must be reported.

Environmental Controls

To alert personnel, the area in which a laser is being used must be easily identified. ANSI standards recommend signs with a specific laser safety symbol. Traffic into areas in which a laser is in use must be limited, and persons in the room must have wavelength-specific eye protection while the laser is in use. Extra goggles should be available outside the room. Glass windows in the room must be covered to prevent nonintentional laser beams from affecting persons outside the room. The laser key must be available only to authorized personnel, not left with the laser.

Fire Safety Measures

When lasers are in use, there is always a risk of fire. Fire prevention measures include education of all those involved in the safe use of the laser. Surgical drapes, anesthesia tubing, and surgical sponges could all be ignited accidentally. Concentration of oxygen, anesthetic gases, or vapors from alcohol-based prep solutions can contribute to flammability. Special drapes and endotracheal tubes can be utilized, sponges should be kept wet, oxygen concentrations should be kept low, and prep solutions should be patted dry to prevent pooling. The foot pedal with which the surgeon activates the laser beam must be placed such that it is not accidentally engaged.[20]

Laser Plume

The smoke produced by the use of the laser is known as *plume*. This plume can contain particles of tissue, toxins, and steam. Many studies about the content of the plume and the risks it poses to caregivers have been performed. At the least, the plume can be irritating, causing burning and watery eyes. At the worst, it may contain viable cells that transmit disease. Of particular concern are viral diseases, such as human papillomavirus, because laser is a common treatment for genital warts. To address concern, smoke evacuators with filters, such as high-efficiency particulate air filters, are used to remove smoke and particles. In addition, persons in the room should wear high-filtration masks to deal with any plume not captured by the smoke evacuator.[20]

OTHER TECHNOLOGIES

Ultrasound

Sound waves are mechanical energy. Waves at frequencies above the audible range are defined as ultrasonic. At lower frequencies, the ultrasonic waves have no tissue effect but are commonly employed for diagnostic purposes. Devices are available that adapt the familiar external modality to laparoscopic applications. At higher frequencies, ultrasound is utilized in two different devices: (1) the cavitational ultrasonic aspirator, and (2) the ultrasonically activated scalpel. The aspirator is utilized in neurosurgical and other procedures to fragment and aspirate tumor cells.

The scalpel, known as the *harmonic scalpel*, is utilized primarily in gynecologic and general surgery. This device can be used in either open or laparoscopic procedures. It employs either multiuse or disposable instruments, such as hooks, coagulators, and shears, and can both cut and coagulate. The harmonic scalpel has some applications in place of lasers or the traditional electrosurgical unit. It can also be used in place of some endoscopic stapling devices used in laparoscopic procedures, such as laparoscopically assisted vaginal hysterectomy. No electric current is transmitted to the patient, as with an electrosurgical unit, thereby eliminating the risk of burns to the patient. There is also little risk of inadvertent damage to adjacent tissues. Because it does not create smoke like the electrosurgical unit or the laser, it eliminates the risk of plume for the surgical team and affords clear visualization during laparoscopic procedures.[23, 24]

Intraoperative Cholangiography

Endoscopic retrograde cholangiopancreatography or intraoperative cholangiography during laparoscopic cholecystectomy can be performed to visualize and remove stones in the biliary tract. Various catheters, baskets, dilators, and balloons are used to manage cholelithiasis. For cholangiography, contrast medium is injected to visualize the biliary tree. Either a flat plate x-ray study or real-time C-arm fluoroscopy can be used. The real time is preferable because the surgeon does not need to wait for films to be developed and read.[25]

Laparoscopic Transcystic Common Duct Exploration. If stones are found via cholangiography, a flexible choledochoscope can be used to explore the common bile duct and to retrieve stones. The duct is first dilated, generally by use of a balloon dilator, although a series of sequential bougie-type dilators can be used. The balloon type is less likely to injure the duct and must be passed over a wire by use of fluoroscopy. The stones themselves are retrieved via a choledochoscope, by use of a basket snare.[26]

Robotics

Although robotics may not be common in the ambulatory setting, this technology was introduced for clinical use in the 1980s. A robot is essentially a combination of mechanical manipulators and a computer. The computer controls the complex movements of the joints and the arms of the manipulators. Robotic applications in minimally invasive procedures have been tested, particularly in the manipulation of the laparoscope. Although this task may seem fairly simple, in reality, maintaining proper alignment of the camera throughout the procedure is difficult. The surgeon relies on stability of the image to maintain orientation to the anatomic structures. Mechanical scope holders are available, but the surgeon must interrupt his or her activities and readjust as needed.[27]

The automated endoscopic system for optimal positioning has been approved by the FDA and has been successfully used for this purpose. This device is anchored to the OR table and is controlled by the surgeon with a foot pedal. The camera does not move unless the surgeon commands it to, so the picture remains stable and upright. This device can actually take over the role of the assistant who is holding the camera, allowing personnel to concentrate on other patient care activities.[28] In a study using the robot for urologic procedures, the device successfully demonstrated this premise.[29]

MANAGEMENT ISSUES

Risk Management

Technology has brought with it many advances in the care of the surgical patient, directly influencing the trend toward more ambulatory procedures. These advances are not without risk and cost. Risk management efforts should include proper training and credentialing of both personnel and physicians. Competence of staff in the performance of procedures and the use of equipment should be assessed at least on an annual basis. Proper maintenance of all equipment and instrumentation is essential.

Staff caring for patients after the procedure must be aware of the signs of complications both in the immediate postoperative period and after the patient goes home. Patients and caregivers must be instructed so that they can recognize complications should they occur. Prompt intervention can make a critical difference in the patient outcome should problems arise.[11, 12] Patients must also be carefully instructed and advised of risks before surgery.

Resource Management

With the revenues from third party payers shrinking as managed care grows and with the competition for contracts being intense, we are challenged to provide high-quality care with the most cost-effective means possible. Surgical services are obvious areas where costs need to be addressed. All parties involved in the care of patients must be cost conscious. Managers are evaluating costs of staffing, changing skill mix, and adding new types of multiskilled workers. The cost of supplies, particularly those used intraoperatively for minimally invasive procedures, has come under intense scrutiny. It is critical for the manager to be fluent in budgeting methods and to maintain a close working relationship with materials management to facilitate purchasing.

Many strategies exist to decrease cost. One of the most obvious is to examine inventory for opportunities to consolidate and streamline inventory and to standardize wherever possible. When using disposables, staff should have available items that the surgeon might need but should not automatically open them when setting up a case. Returning to reusable products rather than disposables is another option. Today's reusables are much improved over their original versions. Disposable trocars, clips, staplers, and instruments account for significant OR costs. These came into vogue because they eliminated the need to reprocess and maintain items and meant that the surgeon always had the assurance of a sharp, sterile item to use. Capital investment, cost of repair and processing, and quality of product must be considered if plans are made to purchase reusables.

Another option, perhaps the most feasible, is to use *resposable* items. A resposable instrument is one that is partially reusable and partially disposable. Several vendors with resposable items are available, including trocars, clip appliers, staplers, and scissors. The sharp part of the instruments is disposable, eliminating the concern of the surgeon and the need to periodically sharpen instruments.[30]

Technology will continue to advance, influencing procedures and activity in the ambulatory surgery setting. Nurses working in ambulatory surgical centers must remain knowledgeable about new procedures and technologies.

References

1. Griffith DP, Wong HY: History of endoscopy. In Janetschek G, Rossweiler J, Griffith DP (eds): Laparoscopic Surgery in Urology. Stuttgart: Thieme, 1996, pp 2–6.
2. Fairchild SS: Perioperative Nursing Principles and Practice, 2nd ed. Boston: Little, Brown & Co, 1996, pp 541–543.
3. Ordica RC, Das S: History of laparoscopy. In Das S, Crawford D (eds): Urological Laparoscopy. Philadelphia: WB Saunders, 1994, pp 3–11.
4. Atkinson LJ, Fortunato NH (eds): Berry & Kohn's Operating Room Technique. St. Louis: CV Mosby, 1996, pp 633–636.
5. Janetschek G, Rassweiler J: Basic laparoscopic technique. In Janetschek G, Rossweiler J, Griffith DP (eds): Laparoscopic Surgery in Urology. Stuttgart: Thieme, 1996, pp 60–77.
6. Janetschek G, Peschel R: Instrumentation and equipment. In Janetschek G, Rossweiler J, Griffith DP (eds): Laparoscopic Surgery in Urology. Stuttgart: Thieme, 1996, pp 8–23.
7. Preminger GM, Potempa DM, Rossweiler J: Video systems in laparoscopic surgery. In Janetschek G, Rossweiler J, Griffith DP (eds): Laparoscopic Surgery in Urology. Stuttgart: Thieme, 1996, pp 24–32.
8. Kavoussi LR, Soper NJ: Establishing the pneumoperitoneum. In Soper NJ, Odem RR, Clayman RV, McDougall EM (eds): Essentials of Laparoscopy. St. Louis: Quality Medical Publishing, 1994, pp 104–147.
9. Eubanks S, Schauer PR: Laparoscopic Surgery. In Sabiston DC Jr, Lyerly HK (eds): Textbook of Surgery: The Biological Basis of Modern Surgical Practice. Philadelphia: WB Saunders, 1997, pp 791–804.
10. The risks of laparoscopic electrosurgery. Health Devices 24:20, 1995.
11. Risk analysis: Laparoscopic electrosurgery. ECRI Hosp Risk Control Bull March 1995, pp 1–15.
12. Rohlf S: Electrosurgical safety considerations for minimally invasive surgery. Minim Invasive Surg Nurs 9:26–29, 1995.
13. McDougall EM, Clayman RV, Soper NJ: Laparoscopic clips and staples. In Soper NJ, Odem RR, Clayman RV, McDougall EM (eds): Essentials of Laparoscopy. St. Louis: Quality Medical Publishing, 1994, pp 184–203.

13a. See WA, Soper NJ: Selection and preparation of the patient for laparoscopic surgery. In Soper NJ, Odem RR, Clayman RV, McDougall EM (eds): Essentials of Laparoscopy. St. Louis: Quality Medical Publishing, 1994, pp 1–10.
14. ACOG educational bulletin: Operative laparoscopy. American College of Obstetricians and Gynecologists. Int J Gynaecol Obstet 59:265–268, 1997.
15. Schmelzer C, Stone N: Laparoscopic cholecystectomy in the cardiac patient: A case study. J Postanesthesia Nurs 10:18–20, 1995.
15a. Quilici PJ: Online Laparoscopic Technical Manual, Interventional Laparoscopy. Available at www.laparoscopy.net. 1997.
16. Monk TG, Weldon BC: Anesthetic considerations for laparoscopic surgery. In Soper NJ, Odem RR, Clayman RV, McDougall EM (eds): Essentials of Laparoscopy. St. Louis: Quality Medical Publishing, 1994, pp 24–33.
17. Fahlenkamp D, Coptcoat MJ: Complications of laparoscopic surgery. In Janetschek G, Rossweiler J, Griffith DP (eds): Laparoscopic Surgery in Urology. Stuttgart: Thieme, 1996, p 81.
18. Wooley DS, Puglisi RN, Bilgrami S, et al: Comparison of the hemodynamic effects of gasless abdominal distention during incremental positive end-expiratory pressure. J Surg Res 58:75–80, 1995.
19. Hunter JC: Laparoscopic pneumoperitoneum: The abdominal compartment syndrome revisited. J Am Coll Surg 181:469–470, 1995.
20. Ball K: Lasers: The Perioperative Challenge. St. Louis: CV Mosby, 1995.
21. Atkinson LJ, Fortunato NH (eds): Berry & Kohn's Operating Room Technique. St. Louis: CV Mosby, 1996, pp 270–279.
22. American National Standards Institute: American National Standards for Safe Use of Lasers in Health Care Facilities. ANSI Z136.3, 1996.
23. Amaral JF: Ultrasonic dissection. Endosc Surg Allied Technol 2:181–184, 1994.
24. Robbins ML, Ferland RJ: Laparoscopic assisted vaginal hysterectomy using the laparoscopic coagulating shears. J Am Assoc Gynecol Laparosc 2:339–343, 1995.
25. Edye M: Cholangiography during laparoscopic cholecystectomy. In Salky B (ed): Laparoscopy for Surgeons. New York/Tokyo: Igoku-Shoin, 1995, pp 113–127.
26. Phillips E: Laparoscopic transcystic common duct exploration. In Salky B (ed): Laparoscopy for Surgeons. New York/Tokyo: Igoku-Shoin, 1995, pp 9–16.
27. Codeddu JA, Stoinovici D, Kavoussi LR: Robotics in urologic surgery. Urology 49:501–506, 1997.
28. Robotic arm returns direct scope control to surgeon. Minim Invasive Surg Nurs 8:87–88, 1994.
29. Partin AW, Adams JB, Moore RG, Kavoussi LR: Complete robot-assisted urological surgery: A preliminary report. J Am Coll Surg 181:552–557, 1995.
30. Abbott P: The best of both worlds: Resposables. Today's Surg Nurse 19:35–38, 1997.

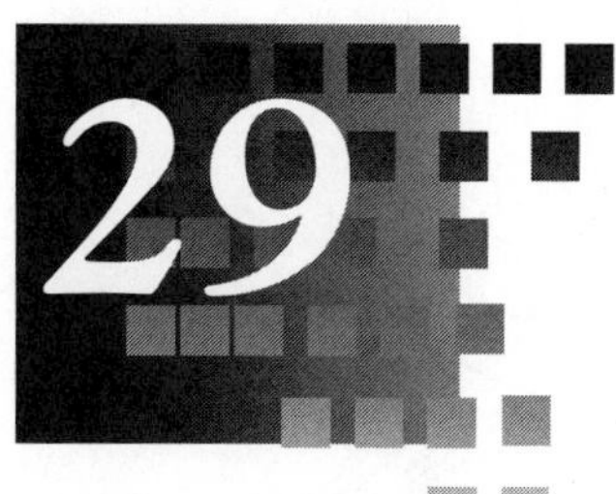

Chapter 29: Ophthalmic Surgery

Linda Anderson Vader

Vision and the appearance of the eyes are essential to an individual's ability to maintain independence, lifestyle, and self-image. Vision loss and facial changes are often threatening on a deeply personal level.[1] Because ophthalmic surgical procedures are frequently performed on an outpatient basis, they are often perceived as a minor inconvenience. Patients undergoing eye surgery are eager to improve their vision or appearance, but they are also anxious about the implications of failure.

Ophthalmic surgery is classified as intraocular or extraocular. Intraocular procedures involve opening the anterior or posterior eyeball and include cataract extraction, corneal transplantation, filtering procedures, retinal procedures, and vitrectomy. Extraocular procedures involve the structures surrounding the eyeball and include lacrimal surgeries, blepharoplasty, ocular muscle repair, scleral buckling, orbital procedures, enucleation, and evisceration.

As illustrated in Figure 29–1, an understanding of normal anatomy and pathologic changes is necessary for the nurse to educate and care for the ophthalmic patient. Table 29–1 defines some of the most commonly used ophthalmic terms and conditions.

PREOPERATIVE CARE

Many people are sensitive about anything in or near their eyes. Some people have a great deal of difficulty allowing the instillation of eyedrops. The nurse should explain the reason for any ophthalmic intervention before touching the patient's face and should use a calm and reassuring approach with patients who involuntarily react with guarding or protective behaviors. Comprehensive preoperative instructions and explanations usually reduce the patient's anxiety level. A three-dimensional model of the eye is helpful, too, for describing the anatomy and for reinforcing the expected outcome. The nurse must also respect the patient who requests not to have the details of the surgery described. Although it is important for the patient to understand the perioperative events, some people are uncomfortable with descriptions of ophthalmic surgery.

It is not uncommon for patients to have exaggerated fears and anxieties about eye surgery. Some of these fears and misconceptions include thinking the eyeball is removed from the socket for the procedure and then replaced or that the patient will see the entire operative procedure being performed. More realistic are the fears of moving during the surgery, the need to go to the bathroom during surgery, and claustrophobia. The nurse should make sure that the patient understands that the eyeball is never removed and that the anesthetized operative eye perceives only light and shadows as opposed to clear images. The nurse should also describe the level of relaxation attained with the type of anesthesia used, the usual draping methods, and the necessity for using the bathroom just before going in to surgery. With some elderly patients, it may be necessary to provide the assurance of padding for urinary incontinence.

Ophthalmic surgery patients may have complicated medical histories, sensory deficits, and complex learning needs. Depending on the surgeon's usual protocol, preoperative and postoperative eye medication schedules can be complicated and confusing. Along with a description of perioperative events, the nurse should dem-

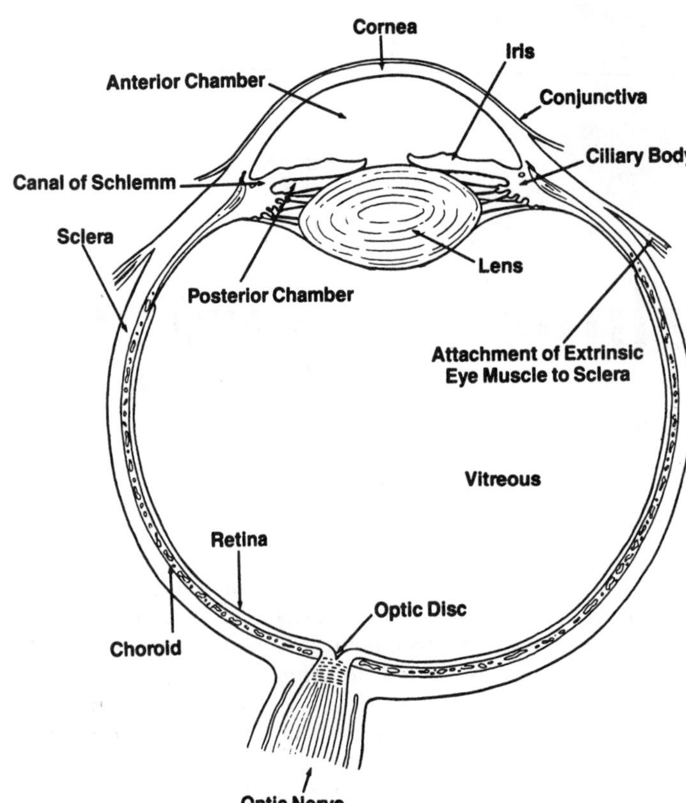

Figure 29–1. Anatomy of the eye. (From Stewart J: Clinical Anatomy and Physiology for the Frustrated and Angry Health Professional. Miami: MedMaster, 1986, p 101.)

onstrate the correct method of eyedrop or ointment instillation (Table 29–2). Patients should be taught to stand in front of a mirror and gently draw down the lower eyelid. The eyedrop or ointment should be instilled in the pocket of the lower eyelid without touching the bottle or tube to the eye (Fig. 29–2). If the patient has shaking hands or is unable to see well enough to stand at the mirror, the patient should be instructed to lie down and draw down the lid. Resting the wrist on the cheek may steady the hand, or the bottle may be placed over the eyebrow to avoid contact with the eye. The patient should also be instructed that more than one drop in the eye is not an overdose and that the extra medication will be blinked away. The eye medication schedule, activity restrictions, diet instructions, and return to previous medications should be written in large print and reviewed by the patient and family before surgery (Box 29–1).

Complications in ophthalmic surgery are rare, but they do occur. The nurse needs to be sensitive to the patient's anxieties. Rather than give the patient false assurances, the nurse should convey a positive, realistic, and competent attitude that encourages confidence in the physicians, staff, and procedure and acknowledges the validity of the patient's concerns.

Before preoperative sedation is given, the correct eye for surgery must be ascertained. The nurse should verify the consent, the scheduled procedure, the medical record, and the patient's understanding before initiating patient care. Discrepancies should be investigated and resolved before the patient is prepared for surgery.

Preoperative preparation for intraocular procedures often includes the instillation of dilating or constricting eyedrops, as well as anti-inflammatory or antibiotic eyedrops. The nurse must check the physician's orders and ensure that the correct medication is given and the correct eye is treated. Dilating a pupil that should be constricted or constricting a pupil that should be dilated could result in delay or cancellation of the procedure.

Most ophthalmic procedures are performed under local anesthesia or conscious sedation (see Chapters 14 and 15). Some ophthalmic surgeons use topical anesthesia in selected patients. General anesthesia may be required for children or for adults who are unable to tolerate or cooperate under local anesthesia.

INTRAOPERATIVE CARE

Before surgery, the perioperative nurse verifies the identification of the patient and checks the operative eye and procedure with the patient, the medical record, the operative consent, the surgery schedule, and the surgeon. The nurse should explain the operating room environment to the patient (bright lights, cool temperature, voices, and noise) and assures the patient that he or she will not be ignored or left alone. During the facial scrub that takes 3 to 5 minutes, the nurse observes the patient for signs of discomfort or anxiety. A pillow or other support may be needed for the patient's back or knees.

The nurse describes the sounds the patient will hear (the beeping of the monitor and other mechanical noises) and instructs the patient that staff in the room will be talking in low voices during the procedure. The nurse should tell the patient not to respond to the conversation and that staff will use the patient's name if they are speaking to them. Patients should also know that the surgeon is most often standing or sitting behind their head and that the anesthesia staff will be at their side. The nurse also explains the draping and that the local block will prevent the patient from blinking or moving the eye.

Before cataract or corneal transplant surgery, a Honan balloon may be applied to reduce intraocular pressure after the local anesthetic has blocked innervation to the eye (see Chapter 14). Some surgeons prefer to manually massage the eyeball. Either method of reducing intraocular pressure may be performed in the holding area or in the operating room. Complications of using a pressure device include reflex bradycardia, tissue damage to the ear from improper placement, or corneal abrasion resulting from improper eyelid closure. Patients undergoing retina or vitreous procedures should know that the lights in the room will be off most of the time. The operating room nurse continues to observe the patient closely during the procedure for signs of discomfort or anxiety.

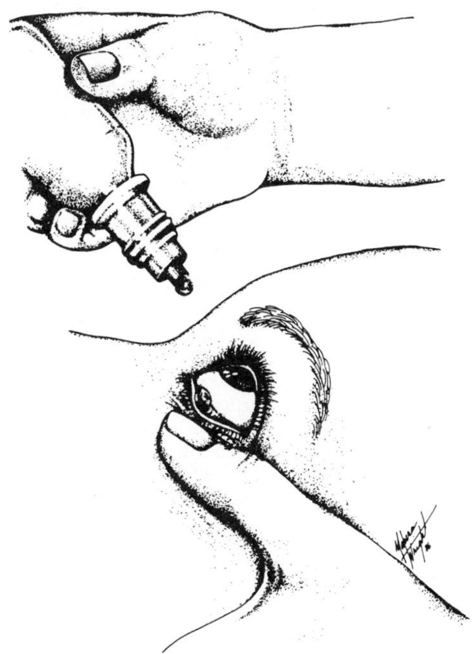

Figure 29–2. Proper technique for instillation of eyedrops. Ask the patient to look upward while gently everting the lower lid. Place the drop in the lower conjunctival sac. Do not touch the tip of the bottle with the fingers or on the eye or lashes. (From Ethicon: Nursing Care of the Patient in the OR, 2nd ed. Somerville, NJ: Ethicon, 1987, p 77.)

Box 29–1. KEY EDUCATION POINTS FOR ADMINISTERING EYE DROPS

1. Wait 5 minutes between administering different types of eyedrops.
2. If more than one drop is instilled in the eye, the excess is not an overdose and will be blinked away.
3. β-Adrenergic blocking eyedrops are absorbed systemically and may affect the heart rate. To decrease systemic absorption of atropine or β-blockers, firmly press on the puncta in the inner corner of the lower eyelid for 5 minutes.
4. Never allow the tip of the eyedrop bottle to touch any part of the eye or lids.
5. Do not rub or press on the eye.
6. Use warm tap water and a clean wash cloth to gently cleanse around the eye. Use a separate washcloth for each eye.
7. Reading and watching television may cause eye fatigue but do not damage the eyes.
8. To apply a metal shield over the eye, use half-inch clear tape on the diagonal from forehead to cheek. Leave the holes in the center open to allow vision. Fold one end of the tape over so that it is easy to grasp.
9. Never use the same tissue on both eyes.
10. Depth perception is decreased when one eye is covered. Carefully approach curbs and steps, and use extra caution when pouring liquids or reaching for objects.
11. If it is difficult to tell whether an eyedrop has gone in the eye, refrigerate the eyedrops to increase sensation.
12. Always wash hands before touching the eye or administering eyedrops.

Table 29–1. Ophthalmic Terms

Term	Definition
Accommodation	Naturally occurring changes in the shape of the lens to allow for far and near vision
Amblyopia	Reduction in visual acuity in an eye that is ophthalmoscopically normal, for instance, due to strabismus or ptosis of the eyelid
Blepharoplasty	Repair of the upper or lower eyelid to remove redundant skin; may be cosmetic or therapeutic when the eyelid interferes with vision
Capsulotomy	Incision (usually laser-induced) into the posterior capsule to improve vision when the posterior capsule tissue has opacified; may occur after extracapsular cataract extraction when debris deposits on the capsular tissue
Cataract	A gradually developing opacity of the lens or lens capsule of the eye most often associated with the normal aging process (senile) but may be congenital, diabetic, traumatic, or toxic as well
Chalazion	A granulomatous inflammation of a meibomian gland (a sebaceous gland) in the upper or lower eyelid
Corneal abrasion	A cut or scratch on the epithelium of the cornea
Cycloplegic	A parasympatholytic drug that dilates the pupil (e.g., homatropine)
Dacryocystorhinostomy	Establishment of a new tear passageway for drainage directly into the nasal cavity
Diplopia	Double vision
ECCE	Extracapsular cataract extraction; removal of the lens of the eye without removal of the posterior capsule; IOL is placed in posterior chamber behind the iris
Ectropion	Outward turning, eversion, of the eyelid
Entropion	Inward turning, inversion, of the eyelid, usually of the lower lid
Enucleation	Removal of the eyeball
Evisceration	Removal of the contents of the eyeball
Fluorescein	A water-soluble dye that stains corneal abrasions; affected areas appear bright green when the stained eye is exposed to an ultraviolet light source; may be a solution or impregnated on a paper strip and released when wet by tears
Glaucoma	Disease in which the reabsorption of aqueous humor into the venous system is blocked; intraocular pressure rises with damage to the retina
Goniotomy	Incision of the trabecular meshwork to relieve congenital glaucoma
Hyperopia	Farsightedness; occurs when the eyeball is shorter than normal and light rays focus behind the retina; corrected by eyeglasses with convex lens
ICCE	Intracapsular cataract extraction; removal of the lens of the eye including the capsule; IOL is placed in anterior chamber, in front of iris
IOL	Intraocular lens; a synthetic lens implanted in either the anterior or posterior chamber to replace the lens removed with cataract extraction
Iridectomy	Removal of a portion of the iris; done in glaucoma to facilitate movement of aqueous humor from posterior to anterior chamber
Iridotomy	Placement of a hole in the iris by means of a laser
Keratoplasty	Removal of an opaque portion of the cornea with replacement by transplantation of a donor cornea
Mydriatic	A sympathomimetic drug that dilates the pupil (e.g., phenylephrine)
Myopia	Nearsightedness; occurs when the eyeball is longer than normal and light rays focus in front of the retina; corrected by eyeglasses with concave lens.
Phacoemulsion	Also called phacoemulsification; removal of the lens of the eye by fragmenting it with ultrasonic vibrations (40,000/sec); simultaneously there is irrigation and aspiration of the fragments without loss of the lens capsule
Proptosis	Downward displacement of the eyeball
Pterygium	A thick, triangular overgrowth of epithelial tissue that extends from the corner of the cornea to the canthus; appearance is pale or white; may grow over the pupillary opening; surgical removal is by excision or curettement of cornea
Ptosis	Drooping of the upper eyelid
Retinal detachment	Separation of a portion of the retina from the pigment layer behind it
Retinopathy	Noninflammatory retinal disorder involving an interference of the eye's blood supply; may be caused by diabetes, hypertension, or occlusion of the central retinal artery or vein
Scleral buckling	A procedure to close retinal holes; after the scleral tissue is "buckled," or indented, a medium is instilled into the vitreous to increase pressure and aid in compressing the retinal hole against the retinal pigment epithelium beneath it until healing occurs
Strabismus	Misalignment of the axes of the eyes in which one or both eyes is turned inward or outward; may require eye muscle surgery
Tarsorrhaphy	Procedure in which the outer edges of the upper and lower lids are united to reduce width, thus permit better closing of the eyelids (e.g., in patients unable to close the eyelid due to facial paralysis)
Trabeculectomy	Excision of a portion of the trabecular meshwork to facilitate drainage of aqueous humor from the posterior chamber to the anterior chamber; for glaucoma treatment
Vitrectomy	Removal of a portion of the vitreous humor; may be done to restore eyesight after hemorrhage into vitreous or because of other causes of opacity; may be necessary if vitreous escapes into anterior chamber during cataract extraction

POSTOPERATIVE CARE

Unless general anesthesia has been administered, the ophthalmic patient is admitted to phase II PACU directly from the operating room. A physical and emotional assessment should occur immediately on arrival. Respiratory management is the priority and should be evaluated by pulse oximetry and breath sounds. While taking the patient's vital signs, the nurse also assesses the patient's level of consciousness and orientation. Patients who are very drowsy or lethargic should be monitored closely until they are recovered from the effects of sedatives and analgesics. Respiratory depression and hypotension may indicate oculocardiac response (decrease in heart rate following manipulation of the eyes or extraocular muscles) similar to a vasovagal reflex, resulting in nausea, vomiting, fainting, or some combination. Raising the head of the bed should always be carried out slowly while the patient's reaction is evaluated.

Retching, vomiting, pain, and hypertension may contribute to increased intraocular pressure that could precipitate intraocular bleeding. Administration of an osmotic diuretic to reduce intraocular pressure may result in hypotension or hypertension as a result of a full bladder.

Bandaging one eye results in a loss of depth perception or may severely reduce the patient's visual acuity if the unoperative eye has poor vision. Patients should be closely evaluated for balance and equilibrium after eye surgery. The operative eye may be patched until the first postoperative visit, which is often the following morning. Patients and family members should be cautioned about depth perception and visual deficits. Reaching for an object such as a cup of hot coffee could result in an accidental burn. Steps and curbs should also be approached with caution. Patients with compromised vision need assistance with meals and help getting to the bathroom until the patch is removed.

Postoperative restrictions vary with the type of procedure and the preferences of the surgeon. Compliance is enhanced with large-print instructions and a verbal review before discharge. The patient should understand the reason for activity restrictions. Reading may cause postoperative discomfort because the operative eye muscles move in tandem with the unoperative eye. Watching television results in less ocular movement and is usually not restricted. Lifting and other activities that increase the heart rate may precipitate bleeding at the operative site. A metal or plastic shield may be placed over the eye patch for protection. Patients are usually advised to wear the shield or their glasses at all times for several weeks after surgery. Patients should ask their surgeon when they may begin activities such as driving and swimming.

All ophthalmic surgical patients must be reminded to not rub the eye. The eye may be gently cleansed at home with tap water and a clean wash cloth. The eye should never be irrigated. Shampooing should be accomplished with the head tilted back instead of forward to avoid getting soap and water in the eye. Above all, patients should be instructed to wash their hands before touching the eye or instilling eyedrops.

Severe postoperative pain is not typical after eye surgery. Corneal transplantation, cataract extraction, and glaucoma filtering procedures usually result in mild-to-moderate discomfort around or in the eye or headache. This discomfort is often relieved with 650 to 1000 mg of acetaminophen. More severe pain, especially if it is accompanied by nausea or vomiting, could indicate increased intraocular pressure and should be reported to the physician. Acute glaucoma may result from blockage of the filtering mechanism by bleeding in the anterior chamber or an inflammatory reaction. Oculoplastic procedures involving the orbit or enucleation often require a stronger opioid analgesic for the first 24 to 48 hours after surgery. Smaller incisions and stronger finer sutures have made postoperative wound leaks and dehiscence extremely rare occurrences. Even more rare is an expulsive hemorrhage. Redness, swelling, and discomfort should all decrease after surgery, and patients should be instructed to call if there is any change in their vision or any increase in redness, swelling, or tenderness.

CATARACT EXTRACTION

Cataract extraction is one of the most frequently performed ambulatory surgical procedures. A cataract is an opacity of the lens that is usually associated with aging changes of the eye. Between the ages of 65 and 74, the prevalence of cataract is about 50%.[2] Opacity of the lens results from chemical changes in the lens (reduced oxygen uptake and an initial increase in water content followed by dehydration, increased sodium and calcium levels, and decreased potassium, ascorbic acid, and protein content), as well as the cumulative effects of ultraviolet light exposure.[2] Other causes of cataracts include systemic disorders such as diabetes, trauma, radiation, exposure to infrared

Table 29–2. Instillation of Eye Drops and Ointments

OVERVIEW

Ophthalmic medications may be used as:
1. Diagnostic agents
2. Treatment agents of ocular conditions
3. Adjuncts to surgical interventions

Ointments are used for their lubricant property and to increase contact time of medication to the ocular surface. Ointments tend to blur the vision when first applied and, therefore, are often used at bedtime.

OBJECTIVE

To deliver medication to the eye by way of ophthalmic drops or ointments

EQUIPMENT

Eye drops or ointment as ordered
Tissue

ACTION	RATIONALE
1. Check the physician's order.	1. Note the correct medication, time, eye, and patient and the expiration date on the label.
2. Wash your hands.	2. Good hygiene
3. Explain the procedure to the patient.	3. Patient cooperation
4. Have the patient in a sitting or supine position.	4. Patient comfort and ease in instilling drops
5. Instruct the patient to tilt the head backward, if in a sitting position, to open the eyes and look up.	5. Reduces blepharospasm
6. Pull down on the lower lid to expose the cul-de-sac.	6.
a. For infants and small children, separate the lids by placing the thumb on the bony prominence below the lid, and index finger on the bony prominence above the lid. Gently pull the lids apart. Do not apply pressure on the eye.	a. For infants and small children, if it is contraindicated or difficult to separate the lids, place the drop of medication in the inner canthus and have the patient remain supine until opening the eye.
7. Gently squeeze the dropper between your thumb and forefinger of the opposite hand to instill the correct amount of medication.	7. If not sure that the drop went in, use another drop. The eye only holds one drop, thus overdosing will not occur.
a. If using ointment, hold the applicator end of the tube close to the eye and squeeze out a 2- to 3-inch ribbon.	
b. Do not touch the lid, lashes, or surface of the eye with the dropper or ointment tip to avoid contamination.	b. If contaminated discard; do not use on multiple patients. Use separate medication bottles perioperatively and for patients with a known infection.

Adapted from Smith S: Standards of Ophthalmic Nursing Practice. ASORN (American Society of Ophthalmic Registered Nurses) in conjunction with AAO (American Academy of Ophthalmologists), 1985, pp 43–44.

light, long-term use of corticosteroids, and infection.

Cataract extraction is usually performed under monitored anesthesia along with a retrobulbar or peribulbar block; however, topical anesthesia may be used in uncomplicated cases.[3] In most cases, an intraocular lens (IOL) is inserted to replace the crystalline lens that is removed. The IOL replaces the need for cataract spectacles or contact lenses to correct the visual defect. The crystalline lens is composed of a nucleus and an outer cortical material encased in a capsule. Removal of the lens can be accomplished by several approaches, including intracapsular, extracapsular, and phacoemulsification.

Intracapsular cataract extraction is the least often performed method and involves the removal of the entire lens and capsule. If an IOL is inserted following intracapsular cataract extraction, it must be placed in the anterior chamber (in front of the iris) because the capsule has been removed from the posterior chamber, leaving no structure to support the position of the lens.

Extracapsular cataract extraction allows the crystalline lens to be removed while leaving the posterior portion of the capsule intact. After removal of the nucleus of the lens, aspiration of any remaining cortical material is accomplished. A viscoelastic agent is usually used to fill and maintain the anterior chamber during surgery to protect the surrounding tissues and prevent corneal collapse that would result in endothelial cell damage. When the procedure is completed, the viscoelastic substance is usually aspirated from the anterior chamber. After the IOL is inserted behind the iris in the posterior capsule, the pupil is constricted with a miotic solution, such as acetylcholine.

Phacoemulsification is a type of extracapsular

Table 29–2. Instillation of Eye Drops and Ointments *Continued*

8. Punctal occlusion:	8.
a. Ask the patient to close both eyes gently without squeezing.	a. Squeezing increases the lacrimal pump shunting the medication away from the eye. In most cases, closing the eyelids provides enough pressure to temporarily occlude the punctal drain.
b. Alternately, place your finger over the patient's lacrimal sac and apply light pressure for one minute or more (or instruct patient to do this if able).	b. Digital punctal occlusion is indicated when: (1) systemic absorption of medication may prove harmful to the patient (i.e., atropine, phospholine iodide, β-blockers such as timolol or betaxolol, or antineoplastic agents such as mitomycin or thiotepa used in treatment of pterygia; (2) prolonged corneal-drug contact is desired; or (3) tasting or feeling of ocular medication in the nasopharyngeal mucosa is distressing to the patient.
9. If using ointment, hold the lower lid down while the ointment melts; then ask the patient to blink gently several times.	9. If the patient blinks immediately, much of the ointment is expressed out of the cul-de-sac. Blinking gently distributes the melted ointment over the cornea.
10. Gently wipe away tears or excess medication with a tissue.	10. Do not apply direct pressure to the eyelid or rub the eye.
11. If adminstering more than one medication to the eye, wait 2 to 5 minutes between medications. Administer drops before ointment.	11. The conjunctival sac cannot hold more than one drop at a time. Allow time for absorption.
12. Date the newly opened bottle or tube of ointment.	12. Policy to establish the length of time to use drops or ointment after being opened should be approved by the local institution Infection Control Committee.
13. Wash your hands.	
14. Document on the medical record.	

STANDARD

All personnel responsible for the instillation of eye drops for the ophthalmic patient will be given proper instruction on the correct method of instilling eye drops and ointments.

OUTCOME

All patients receiving eye drops or ointments will have the procedure performed by trained personnel in a safe and effective manner.

From Smith S: Standards of Ophthalmic Nursing Practice. San Francisco: ASORN (American Society of Ophthalmic Registered Nurses) in conjunction with AAO (American Association of Ophthalmologists), 1985, pp 43–44.

cataract extraction. The cataract is removed through a smaller incision (3 to 4 mm), and the nucleus and cortex of the lens are broken into small pieces by ultrasonic vibrations. Concurrent irrigation and aspiration remove lens material. The posterior lens capsule is left in place to support the IOL.

One intraoperative complication is capsular rupture with leakage of vitreous humor into the anterior chamber. This situation is corrected with removal of the escaped gelatinous material. Anterior vitrectomy during a cataract extraction is accomplished with a battery- or machine-powered handpiece that cuts and suctions away the leaking vitreous. If left in the anterior chamber, vitreous material can cause postoperative opacity with loss of visual acuity. The patient with capsular rupture usually requires an anterior chamber lens.

Potential postoperative complications include secondary glaucoma, macular edema, retinal detachment, wound leakage, corneal opacification, intraocular hemorrhage, infection, and sterile endophthalmitis.[4] As a result of postoperative edema, a certain rise in intraocular pressure is anticipated and expected. It most often resolves without intervention within 24 to 72 hours.[5]

When an IOL is inserted in a cataract extraction, the patient may be given a card that identifies the manufacturer, type, and registration number of the device. The nurse should explain that it should be kept in a safe place for future reference and need not be carried in the person's wallet. The patient should also be told that the same information is attached to the medical record.

LASER POSTERIOR CAPSULOTOMY

After an extracapsular cataract extraction, many people experience reduced vision within the first 2 years. The posterior capsule may become opaque in the same manner as the crystalline lens. This condition is often referred to as a *secondary membrane*, or *aftercataract*. Until recently, an operative capsulotomy was necessary to allow light to pass through the opaque tissue to the retina.

The neodymium:yttrium-aluminum-garnet laser is now routinely used to create the same 2- to 4-mm window in the posterior capsule with topical anesthesia.[5] The procedure requires only a few minutes and is performed in a treatment room or the office rather than in the operating room. The IOL stays in place because the haptics (spring-held feet) maintain the position of the lens at the outer circumference of the posterior capsule. The patient is not required to undress, but it is important to obtain an ophthalmic and allergy history before the treatment. Some physicians order dilating drops before the treatment, and most use apraclonidine (Iopidine) to prevent increased intraocular pressure.[6] Improvement in vision is often immediate. The patient is reminded to wear sunglasses while outdoors because of increased photosensitivity related to pupil dilation. A follow-up appointment is usually scheduled for later that day or the next day to evaluate intraocular pressure and visual acuity.

GLAUCOMA PROCEDURES

Glaucoma includes a group of ocular disorders characterized by increased intraocular pressure, optic nerve atrophy, and visual field loss. The incidence is 1.5% between the ages of 45 and 65. The prevalence is at least five times greater in blacks than in whites.[7] If left untreated, glaucoma results in irreversible blindness.

There are several types of glaucoma. The terms *primary* and *secondary* refer to whether the cause is the disease alone or another condition. *Acute* and *chronic* refer to the onset and the duration of the disorder. *Open (wide)* and *closed (narrow)* refer to the width of the angle between the iris and the cornea (Fig. 29–3). Aqueous humor, the clear fluid that forms the anterior chamber of the eye, is produced by the ciliary body. The fluid flows from behind the iris and exits the anterior chamber through the trabecular meshwork in the anterior chamber angle between the iris and the cornea. After filtering through the trabecular meshwork, the aqueous flows into the canal of Schlemm and is absorbed into the venous network. When the outflow of aqueous is restricted, the intraocular pressure increases, causing atrophy of the optic nerve and resulting in loss of vision. The goal of treatment is to decrease intraocular pressure by intervening pharmacologically or by surgically creating an opening for the aqueous outflow.[8] Generally, medical intervention is attempted before surgical repair.

The most common type of glaucoma is primary open angle. The flow of aqueous humor is hampered by the degeneration and blockage in the trabecular meshwork. The onset is gradual, usually after the age of 45, and there is no associated pain. Loss of peripheral vision, seeing halos around lights, and decreased night vision are symptoms of increased pressure on the optic nerve.

Angle-closure (narrow-angle) glaucoma occurs in people who have an anatomically small anterior chamber angle. The onset is usually acute, resulting from the iris' blocking the outflow of aqueous. The conjunctiva is usually erythematous, the cornea may be cloudy, the pupil may be unresponsive to light, and the patient experiences pain that may be accompanied by nausea and vomiting. Without intervention, this type of glaucoma could result in permanent blindness within several days.[9]

Medical intervention includes pharmacologic agents that may be used alone or in combination. Pilocarpine constricts the pupil, enhancing the outflow of aqueous. β-Adrenergic blockers, such as timolol or betaxolol eyedrops, also lower intraocular pressure by inhibiting the production of aqueous. β-Adrenergic blocking agents should be used with caution in patients with cardiopulmonary conditions because bradycardia and bronchospasm are potential side effects.[10] Acetazolamide (Diamox) and methazolamide (Neptazane) are carbonic anhydrase inhibitors that decrease the production of aqueous. Because these agents are sulfonamides, they should be used with caution in hypersensitive patients. Hyperosmotic agents, such as glycerin, isosorbide, and mannitol, lower intraocular pressure by drawing water into the bloodstream to dilute the high glucose level. When administering mannitol intravenously, the nurse should monitor the patient's vital signs every 15 minutes and assist the patient in managing the diuretic effect.

Surgical intervention is necessary when patients do not respond to medical treatment. Many procedures may be used to improve the flow of aqueous; however, no procedure is uniformly successful. Laser trabeculoplasty employs a laser to create an opening in the trabecular meshwork. The laser produces scars in the trabecular meshwork, causing tightening of the

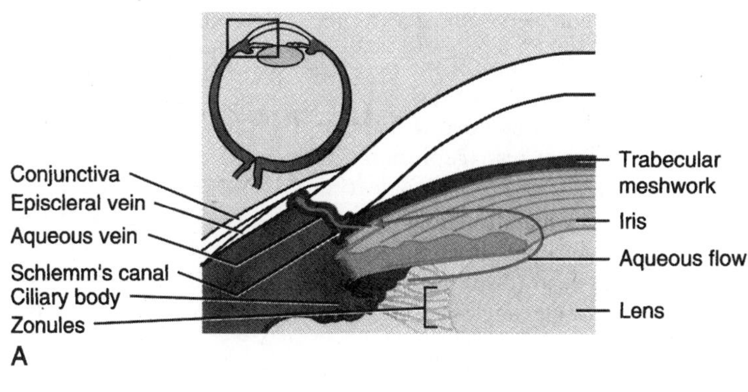

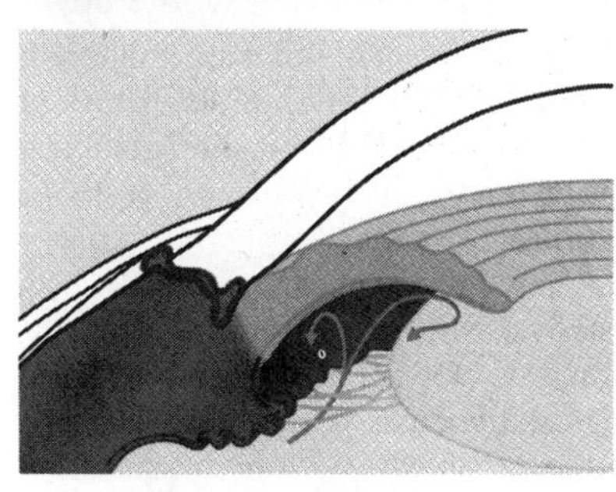

Figure 29–3. *A*, Normal flow of aqueous humor. *B*, Open-angle glaucoma occurs when aqueous humor outflow is impaired by the trabecular meshwork. *C*, Angle-closure glaucoma occurs when the root of the iris occludes the trabecular meshwork. Filtering surgery, *(D)* and iridectomy *(E)* restore flow of aqueous through trabecular meshwork. (From Black JM, Matassarin-Jacobs E: Medical-Surgical Nursing, 5th ed. Philadelphia, WB Saunders, 1997, p 953.)

C

Angle-closure glaucoma occurs when the root of the iris occludes the trabecular meshwork

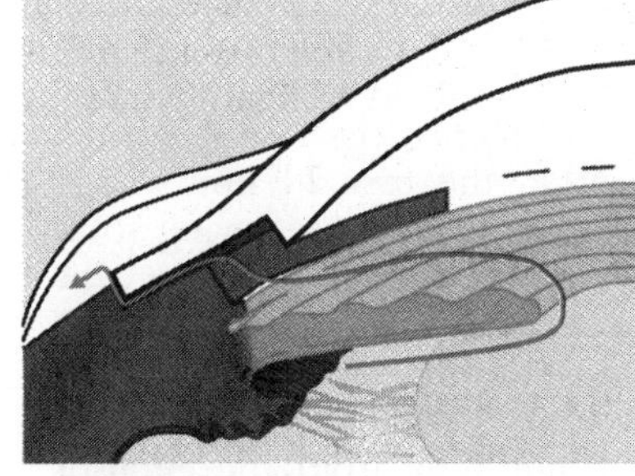

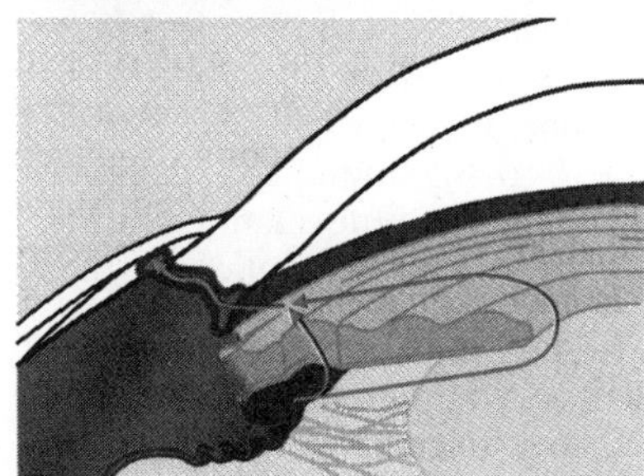

meshwork fibers. The tightened fibers allow for an increase in the outflow of aqueous.[11] The effect of the laser treatment decreases over time, and the procedure may need to be repeated.

Filtering procedures (trephination, thermal sclerostomy, sclerectomy, trabeculotomy) create an outflow channel from the anterior chamber to the subconjunctival space. Aqueous is absorbed through the conjunctival vessels. In about 25% of cases, scar tissue causes the opening to close, and reoperation is necessary. 5-Fluorouracil, mitomycin, and other antimetabolites may be used with filtering procedures to inhibit fibroblast proliferation, thereby decreasing the formation of scar tissue.[12] In patients with complicated types of glaucoma, filtering devices may be used to facilitate the flow of aqueous. The device is sutured to the outer surface of the eyeball on the sclera between the ocular muscles. Iridectomy and iridotomy create a new opening for aqueous flow by removing a section of iris or making a hole in the iris with a laser. Cyclodestructive procedures (cryotherapy, diathermy, high-frequency ultrasound, and the yttrium-aluminum-garnet laser therapy) are used to damage the ciliary body, which decreases the production of aqueous.

CORNEAL TRANSPLANTATION (KERATOPLASTY)

Full (penetrating keratoplasty) or partial-thickness (lamellar keratoplasty) corneal transplantation is indicated in the treatment of corneal opacity owing to corneal dystrophy, keratoconus, or corneal injury or scarring.[13] Keratoplasty is usually performed under intravenous conscious sedation. Donor tissue is obtained from cadavers within the first 24 hours after death and must be stored in a preserving solution. A network of state eye banks around the country provides storage, handling, and coordination of donor tissue with surgeons.

Before surgery, the pupil is constricted to keep the iris flat and away from the anterior chamber angle, which is near the corneal incision. In surgery, the donor cornea is prepared by use of a trephine to cut a corneal button with a radius of 7 to 8.5 mm. The patient's cornea is prepared in the same manner; however, it is usually cut 0.5 mm smaller so that there is an overlap of the donor cornea, which is then sutured into place (Fig. 29–4). An air bubble or sodium hyaluronic acid may be injected to keep the iris from adhering to the cornea. An antibiotic may also be injected or applied topically. The eye is patched, and a metal shield is placed over the patch to protect the eye. There is should be only minimal discomfort after keratoplasty; this is usually relieved by acetaminophen. Some surgeons prescribe one or two doses of acetazolamide after surgery to reduce the transient rise in intraocular pressure that occurs as a result of the inflammation of tissue.

The patch is removed the following morning in the physician's office, and an anti-inflammatory eyedrop is usually prescribed every 1 to 4 hours for a week or more. Postoperative activity restrictions are minimal; however, the patient should wear eyeglasses or the metal shield at all times. Complete corneal healing takes 4 to 6 months. Sutures remain in place for at least 1 year, or indefinitely.

Graft rejection or failure may occur at any time after surgery. The patient should be taught to evaluate the eye on a daily basis for signs of graft rejection by covering the unoperative eye and looking at an object such as a vase or picture in good lighting. The patient should evaluate visual acuity and then look at the operative eye in the mirror. Redness, swelling, visual loss, and pain are the symptoms of graft rejection, and it may be helpful to teach the patient to remember RSVP (the first letter of each symptom) when evaluating the eye.[7]

RETINAL PROCEDURES

Retinal detachment occurs mainly in the adult eye; however, predisposing factors include age, heredity, cataract extraction, degeneration of the retina, trauma, severe myopia, diabetes, and previous retinal detachment.[11] A rhegmatogenous retinal detachment occurs when vitreous traction on the retina creates a hole with subsequent vitreous fluid accumulating between the retina and the blood supply from the choroid layer. Retinal tissue separated from its supply of oxygen results in avascular necrosis.

Before surgery, the eye is widely dilated. General anesthesia is often used because the procedure may take several hours. The use of nitrous oxide is usually avoided because the presence of nitrous oxide gas in the bloodstream may cause the intraocular gas to expand. The goal of surgical repair (scleral buckling) is to place the retina back in contact with the choroid and to seal the accompanying holes or tears.[14] Cryopexy or laser photocoagulation may be used to seal the hole. Scleral buckling involves depressing the sclera externally with a sponge or a band that remains permanently in place. In

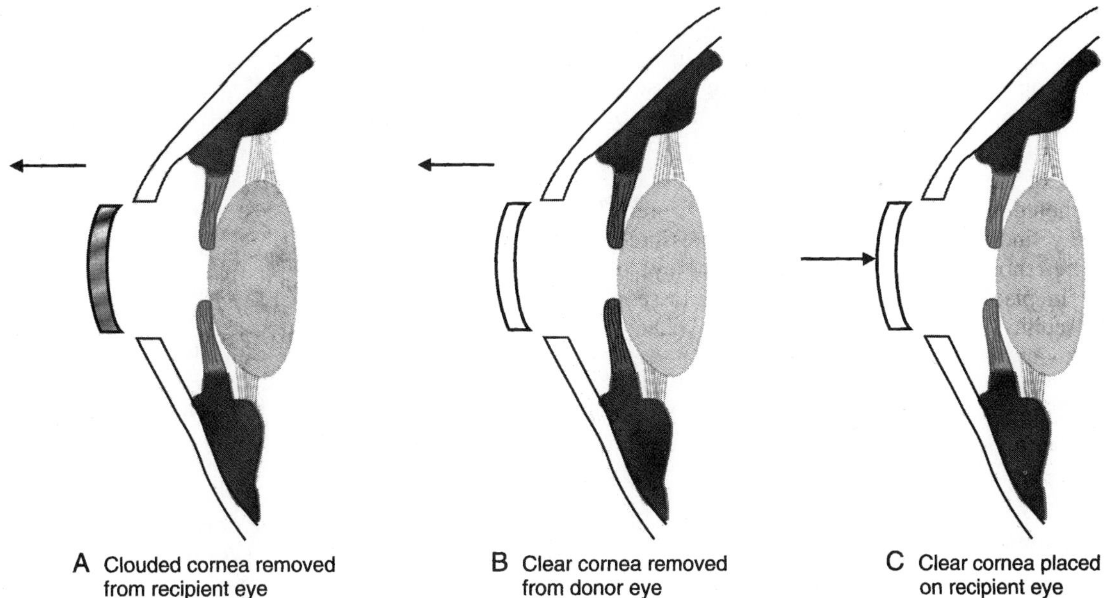

Figure 29–4. Steps involved in corneal transplantation (penetrating keratoplasty). *A*, The diseased cornea is removed with a trephine. *B*, A button of donor cornea is removed with the same trephine so that the cuts are identical. *C*, The donor cornea is placed on the eye and stitched in place with extremely fine suture material. (From Black JM, Matassarin-Jacobs E: Medical-Surgical Nursing, 5th ed. Philadelphia: WB Saunders, 1997, p 967.)

addition to the buckling procedure, an intraocular injection of air, sulfahexafluoride gas, or both, may be used to apply pressure on the retina by gravity during the healing process.[15] Postoperative positioning of the patient's head maximizes the tamponade effect of the air/gas bubble. The bubble is slowly absorbed within days or weeks.

Vitrectomy, removal of vitreous humor, is performed to accomplish extraction of vitreous opacified by blood, to release vitreous traction on the retina, to remove membranes that deform or detach the retina, or to withdraw vitreous in infections (endophthalmitis) to reduce the population of organisms, and inject antibiotics.[16] At the pars plana, the space between the retina and the ciliary body, a small incision is made on each side of the cornea. Tiny plugs hold the incisions open while a fiberoptic light source and a cutting and suction probe are inserted to perform the procedure.

In both scleral buckling and vitrectomy, the extraocular muscles are manipulated, and the eye is rotated frequently during the surgery. The patient may experience moderate-to-severe postoperative pain requiring narcotics. Postoperative inflammation of the tissues in the eye could result in an increase in intraocular pressure requiring intervention with diuretics or, in rare cases, surgery. The surgeon may order the measurement of the intraocular pressure by use of tonometry before discharge from the ambulatory surgery center. It is imperative that the patient and family understand the importance of special positioning (prone, face down, or face to one side). The air/gas bubble can assist in the healing of the retinal tissues only if it is in the correct position. The nurse can offer advice on how to use pillows or cushions to maintain the position. The patient should also be instructed to call if pain is unrelieved by medication or is accompanied by nausea and vomiting, which could indicate a rise in intraocular pressure.

When general anesthesia is used in retina and vitrectomy surgery, the patient is often extubated while still deep under the anesthesia to avoid bucking and coughing. The patient should be observed in phase I PACU for bronchospasm, aspiration, and maintenance of a patent airway. The patient should not be stimulated until some response is observed.

The eye is usually patched, and a metal shield is placed over the eye for protection. A moderate amount of serosanguineous drainage is expected. The tissues around the eye are very edematous and the conjunctiva may be everted for several days after the surgery. The patient and family should be instructed that the swelling and redness will begin to gradually decrease after the first 48 to 72 hours. The patient should be cautioned to avoid rapid eye movements (e.g., those occurring during reading and driving), along with straining, exercise, lifting, or bending over. Rapid eye movements cause discomfort and lifting or straining (including holding back a sneeze) may cause a rise in intraocular pressure.

At home, the eye may be cleaned with warm tap water and a clean washcloth. A combination of antibiotic and anti-inflammatory eyedrops is usually prescribed to be administered several times a day after surgery, as well as a cycloplegic agent, which relaxes the ciliary muscles in order to decrease discomfort and prevent iris adhesions to the cornea (synechiae). Either warm or cold compresses may be applied for comfort several times a day.

LACRIMAL SYSTEM PROCEDURES

Dacryocystitis is an inflammation of the lacrimal gland caused by blockage of the tear duct. The lacrimal drainage system may become obstructed as a result of infection, injury, or lesion. In infants, the tear duct may fail to open. Probing and dilation may be used to open the tear duct, and in chronic conditions, dacryocystorhinoplasty (the formation of an artificial opening between the lacrimal sac and the nasal cavity) may be necessary. A tiny catheter used as a stent to keep the opening patent is secured with absorbable sutures and falls out spontaneously when the sutures absorb.[17] Nasal packing may be inserted for 24 to 48 hours.

After surgery, the patient is cautioned to avoid blowing the nose and to sneeze with the mouth open. Ice packs may be applied to decrease swelling. The patient should also be advised to sleep with the head elevated by three or more pillows to reduce swelling around the eyes. Use of eye makeup should be avoided until approved by the surgeon.

EYELID PROCEDURES

Normal aging changes sometimes result in the relaxation of the orbicularis oculi and the skin around the eyelids. Chronic conjunctivitis or trauma may also result in abnormal eyelid position. Entropion (inversion) and ectropion (eversion) of upper and lower lids may lead to incomplete closure of the lids, which may cause corneal drying or scarring from eyelashes rubbing on the cornea. Sagging or excessive skin around the eyelids may actually interfere with vision. Both ophthalmologists and plastic surgeons perform blepharoplasty and other procedures to provide cosmetic or therapeutic correction.

Ptosis (pronounced toe′ sis), is a drooping of the upper eyelid. Congenital ptosis involves a malfunction of the levator muscle. Ptosis may be acquired from excess skin, eyelid edema, tumors of the lid, third cranial nerve degeneration, Horner's syndrome, goiter, and cervical lymph node enlargement.[17] Unilateral ptosis may be a presenting symptom of myasthenia gravis. Surgical intervention may be necessary to resect or resuspend the levator muscle of the upper eyelid.

Before eyelid surgery, the shape and the symmetry of the patient's eyelids should be documented for later comparison. The patient's baseline visual acuity, as determined by a near-vision card, should also be documented. A near-vision card is held at a comfortable reading distance (around 14 inches). Each line of numbers and letters is smaller and corresponds to the visual acuity lines on the Snellen chart. The nurse should also document whether the patient uses glasses for the evaluation.

Complications in eyelid surgery include hemorrhage, increased intraocular pressure, malposition of the lids, and vision loss. Cool or iced compresses may be used to decrease swelling around the lids. Antibiotic ointment is usually applied to the suture line several times a day. The patient should also be advised to sleep with the head elevated at least 30 degrees to reduce swelling. Sneezing, coughing, and retching should be avoided if possible, and decreased visual acuity (not related to administration of ointment) should be reported immediately. Pain that is unrelieved by analgesics should also be reported because it could indicate increased intraocular pressure.

EYE MUSCLE PROCEDURES

Strabismus, or the misalignment of one or both eyes, is present in about 4% of children. Treatment should begin as soon as a diagnosis is made to ensure the best possible visual acuity and binocular visual function. It is a common misconception that children will "outgrow" crossed eyes. Although primarily a pediatric procedure, both children and adults may require muscle surgery to correct strabismus. Because sets of opposing muscles control the movement of the eye, more than one muscle is generally involved in the operative procedure. Several operative procedures may be necessary to properly strengthen or weaken the muscles to appropriate levels. To strengthen a weak muscle, a portion of the muscle is removed, shortening its length. The opposing muscle usually requires recession, which is the removal of the muscle from its original attachment with reattachment anterior to the original scleral site. This decreases the amount of pull exerted by that muscle and allows the eye to more easily rotate away from that side.

Because it is difficult to judge the exact amount of muscle correction, a reoperation may be necessary. The development of adjustable sutures has provided a great advantage. During the operation, the muscle is reattached to the sclera with a slipknot placed so that it is accessible. After the patient has recovered from the effects of anesthesia and is able to participate in the adjustment process, a topical anesthetic is applied, and the suture is tightened or loosened to position the eye appropriately.

Patients undergoing eye muscle procedures are particularly prone to the oculocardiac response. After surgery, the nurse should observe for signs of bradycardia. If adjustable sutures are used, the adjustment usually takes place several hours after the surgery. Although the eye is anesthetized for the procedure, the manipulation of the ocular muscles may result not only in bradycardia but also in nausea and vomiting. The patient should be encouraged to rest or sleep during the waiting interval. Narcotics should not be used for analgesia, because they interfere with the patient's ability to open the eyes and look straight ahead. It is also advisable to not allow the patient to receive anything by mouth until after the adjustment.

ORBITAL DECOMPRESSION AND REPAIR OF ORBITAL FRACTURES

The most common cause of unilateral or bilateral proptosis (forward protrusion of the eyeball) in adults or children is Graves' ophthalmopathy (eye disease). Although it is usually associated with thyroid disease (both hyperthyroidism and hypothyroidism), it can also occur when there is no thyroid abnormality. Some degree of ophthalmopathy occurs in a high percentage of hyperthyroid patients.[18] Graves' ophthalmopathy is thought to be an autoimmune disorder and is characterized by lymphocytic infiltration and edema of the rectus muscles. The inflamed muscles may become fibrotic and permanently restricted. Proptosis leads to lid retraction, resulting in corneal exposure and drying. Diplopia occurs when the extraocular muscles lose function as a result of enlargement. The extraocular muscles may become so enlarged that there is compression of the optic nerve.

Diplopia, proptosis, and optic nerve compression require intervention. Medical management may include corticosteroids or orbital radiation, but surgical intervention may also be necessary. Orbital decompression may be accomplished by removing the fat pads through the conjunctiva or by fracturing the orbital floor and medial wall to create room for the expanding tissues in the maxillary and ethmoid sinuses. Lid retraction may be corrected by lengthening the lid muscles with donor sclera. Strabismus surgery may be necessary to correct diplopia. Some patients have intractable diplopia despite all attempts.

Before surgery, the nurse should document a baseline visual acuity in both eyes. Beginning in phase I PACU, the visual acuity should be evaluated every 1 to 2 hours and reported to the surgeon if it is below specified parameters. Iced compresses may be applied to reduce swelling. Patients commonly experience nausea and vomiting as a result of blood draining down the throat. Narcotics may be required for pain management. Patients undergoing orbital decompression usually stay in the hospital overnight or in extended observation to monitor the visual acuity and pain control.

ENUCLEATION, EVISCERATION, AND EXENTERATION PROCEDURES

Removal of the eye may be necessary for malignant melanoma, end-stage glaucoma, infection, trauma, or other eye disorders. Enucleation is removal of the complete eyeball, severing nerve, muscle, and vascular attachments. Evisceration is the removal of the contents of the eye, leaving the scleral shell, muscles, innervation, and vascular supply intact. Exenteration is the removal of the entire contents of the orbit, including the eyeball and surrounding tissues.

Although removing the eyeball is performed to prevent the spread of a tumor or infection, to relieve pain, or for cosmetic enhancement, the patient most often experiences anxiety and stress over the loss of a very personal and important part of the body. The patient may be very worried about how he or she will look after the surgery and how his or her appearance will affect others.[19] Adaptation to singular vision may also be a concern. In some cases, the patient and family may have anticipated the surgery and may actually be looking forward to an end to pain or disfigurement. In the case of trauma or malignancy, the urgency of the removal may have given the patient and family little time to adjust. The nurse should carefully explain the perioperative events and should assist the patient and family to identify coping mechanisms.

After surgery, the patient has a pressure dressing over the eye socket, which is usually removed 48 to 72 hours later. The lids are swollen, and a white plastic conformer is visible between the lids. The plastic conformer is placed in the socket so that when the tissues heal, there will be space for the prosthesis. The patient and family members should be instructed to replace the conformer if it accidentally falls out. The conformer should be cleansed with mild soap and tap water and gently replaced between the lids. Fitting for the prosthesis takes place after 6 to 8 weeks. Many patients experience moderate-to-severe discomfort, requiring narcotic analgesics for 48 to 72 hours.

CONCLUSION

Ophthalmic nursing care encompasses a variety of interventions for the physiologic and psychosocial responses to the impact of eye diseases, eye disorders, and loss of vision. The role of the ophthalmic nurse is to assist patients who must find ways to adapt to potential and real problems involving safety, independence, body image, and general health.

References

1. Vader L: The significance of cultural values in vision loss. Assoc Black Nurs Fac J 7:69, 1996.
2. Shock JP, Harper R: The lens. In Vaughan D, Asbury T, Riordan-Eva P (eds): General Ophthalmology, 14th ed. Norwalk, CT: Appleton & Lange, 1995, pp 165–174.
3. Gills J, Loyd T, Chrechio M: Anesthesia, preoperative, and postoperative medications. Curr Opin Ophthalmol 6:32, 1995.
4. Pavan-Langston D: Manual of Ocular Diagnosis and Therapy, 3rd ed. Boston: Little, Brown, 1991.
5. Masket S: Complications of cataract and intraocular lens surgery. Curr Opin Ophthalmol 3:55, 1992.
6. Trobe J: The Physician's Guide to Eye Care. San Francisco: The American Academy of Ophthalmology, 1993.
7. Vader L: Caring for people with visual disorders. In Luckman J (ed): Saunders Manual of Nursing Practice. Philadelpia, WB Saunders, 1997, pp 742–794.
8. Stewart W: The effect of lifestyle on the relative risk to develop open-angle glaucoma. Curr Opin Ophthalmol 6:4, 1995.
9. Gramer E, Tausch M: The risk profile of the glaucomatous patient. Curr Opin Ophthalmol 5:64, 1995.
10. Pavan-Langston D, Dunkel E: Handbook of Ocular Drug Therapy and Ocular Side Effects of Systemic Drugs. Boston: Little, Brown, 1991.
11. Vader L: Eye disorders. In Black J, Matassarin-Jacobs E (eds): Medical-Surgical Nursing, Clinical Management for Continuity of Care, 5th ed. Philadelphia: WB Saunders, 1997, pp 935–979.
12. Khaw P: Antiproliferative agents and the prevention of scarring after surgery: Friend or foe? Br J Ophthalmol 79:627, 1995.
13. Biswell R: Cornea. In Vaughan D, Asbury T, Riordan-Eva P (eds): General Ophthalmology, 14th ed. Norwalk, CT: Appleton & Lange, 1995, pp 123–146.
14. Berrod J: Vitreoretinal separation and fluid-air exchange. Retina 15:445, 1995.
15. Devenyi R: Outpatient postvitrectomy fluid-gas exchange using long-acting gases. Can J Ophthalmol 30:148, 1995
16. O'Malley C: Vitreous. In Vaughan D, Asbury T, Riordan-Eva P (eds): General Ophthalmology, 14th ed. Norwalk, CT: Appleton & Lange, 1995, pp 175–185.
17. Sullivan J: Lids and lacrimal apparatus. In Vaughan D, Asbury T, Riordan-Eva P (eds): General Ophthalmology, 14th ed. Norwalk, CT: Appleton & Lange, 1995, pp 78–94.
18. Sanders M, Graham E: Ocular disorders associated with systemic diseases. In Vaughan D, Asbury T, Riordan-Eva P (eds): General Ophthalmology, 14th ed. Norwalk, CT: Appleton & Lange, 1995, pp 296–329.
19. Allen M, MacDougal F: Origins of beliefs and attitudes toward blindness. J Ophthalmic Nurs Technol 13:279, 1994.

Chapter 30

Otorhinolaryngology and Head and Neck Surgery

Brenda S. Gregory Dawes

Otorhinolaryngologic (ORL) procedures include the skin and soft tissues of the head and neck and upper portions of the respiratory and digestive tracts and the glands. Patients of all ages are scheduled in ambulatory surgery for procedures of the ear, nose, throat, head, and neck. Children are frequently seen for myringotomy with tube insertion, tonsillectomy, adenoidectomy, or foreign body removal. Adults of all ages present for correction, repair, or removal procedures. Table 30–1 lists common terms relating to otorhinolaryngologic surgery.

Laser and endoscopic technologies have increased the number of patients undergoing ORL procedures that can be cared for in the ambulatory surgical center (ASC). The availability of fiberoptic light sources allows physicians to view structures that were previously inaccessible to direct vision, for instance, the sinus cavity. Changes in the surgical approaches and available equipment allow procedures to be completed easier and faster. Patient considerations differ significantly because of the reasons for the procedures or the age group of the patients.

Preoperative Care

Nurses should assess for physical and psychosocial needs specifically and consider age- and procedure-related patient care needs. Potential medical diagnoses for patients with lesions or conditions of the ear, nose, or throat can result in anger, guilt for not seeking medical attention, or denial. For example, the person with polyps on the vocal cord may fear a malignancy, regardless of the support or explanations of the physician. Other patients may deny pathology that they cannot see and delay seeking medical attention until their symptoms are advanced. Patients might also demonstrate a fear of the unknown, such as instrumentation being placed in the airway. Postoperative appearance and cosmetic results might also be a concern, because the head and neck are areas that the patient can see and relate to, in addition to realizing that concealing with clothing might be difficult. Patient teaching and reinforcement of expectations can alleviate anxiety and involve patients in their care. Patients should be aware of potential problems of breathing or swallowing and expected bruising and swelling.

The nursing assessment of physical needs includes obtaining a history of allergies, including latex sensitivity, current medication therapy (e.g., aspirin, hormone therapy, nasal constrictors, preoperative medications); nutritional and systems status; and alcohol and tobacco use. Because of the relative vascularity of the nose, mouth, and pharynx, a detailed history of patient and family bleeding tendencies is obtained. Clotting and bleeding values may be ordered. In addition, the patient should be asked about alternative therapies (e.g., herbal). Patients should have nothing by mouth at least 8 hours before surgery and should discontinue medications that might interfere with clotting. They should sign the operative consent and wash their hair the evening before or morning of the

Table 30–1. Otolaryngologic Definitions

Adenoid	(Pharyngeal tonsil)—lymphoid tissue in the posterior nasopharynx
Auditory tube	(Eustachian tube)—the canal that links the middle ear with the nasopharynx
Cholesteatoma	A cystic mass found in the middle ear that occurs congenitally or as a serious complication of chronic otitis media
Cochlea	Spiral-shaped organ of sound perception in the inner ear
Dysphagia	Difficulty in swallowing
Epiglottis	Cartilaginous structure at the top of the larynx that closes to guard the opening of the airway during swallowing
Leukoplakia	A precancerous change in a mucous membrane Develops slowly and is characterized by firmly attached, thick, white patches that are slightly raised
Lingual tonsil	Lymphatic tissue in the posterior one third of the tongue in the anterior wall of the oropharynx
Mastoid	Air-filled spaces in a portion of the temporal bone
Ossicles	Chain of bones in middle ear that vibrate to transmit sound waves from the tympanic membrane to the inner ear; the bones and their common names are malleus (hammer), incus (anvil), and stapes (stirrup)
Ostium	The opening from a sinus into the nasal cavity
Pinna	(Auricle)—cartilaginous structure of the outer ear
Semicircular ducts	Organ of dynamic equilibrium that responds to changes in position and motion
Sialadenitis	Inflammation of a salivary gland
Sinus	A cavity or large channel within a bone
Tonsil (palatine)	Lymphoid tissue in tonsillar fossa in posterior oropharynx
Turbinate bones	Bones that make up the structure of the lateral walls of the nose
Tympanic membrane	(Eardrum)—separates the outer and middle ear
Vestibular apparatus	Organ of balance and equilibrium in inner ear

procedure. Preoperative audiologic test results, radiographs, or computer-assisted tomography scans should be available. In addition, patients may be asked to complete a "sniff" test. Arthritis, osteoporosis, or other diseases that limit mobility should be identified during the preoperative assessment so that any necessary adjustments in the usual operative position can be planned before the patient's arrival in the operating room (OR). The preoperative nurse should specifically assess for difficulty moving the head and neck. Patients should also have planned to have assistance with care at home after the procedure. The amount (i.e., 24 hours to weeks) and type of assistance vary with the surgical procedure.

The admitting nurse plays a vital role in completing a physical assessment to establish baseline criteria, ensuring that the patient has complied with the physician's preoperative instructions and understands the surgical procedure, the type of anesthesia to be administered, and the risks of both. Patients are informed about the expected plan of care and activities such as transport to the operating room, transfer to the operating room bed, and expectations in the surgical suite. Patients should also be informed about expected postoperative discomfort due to the presence of packing, bloody drainage, and difficulty talking. The nurses should begin discharge planning and teaching before the surgical procedure to reinforce the physician's instructions and to assess the patient for his or her ability to comply with postoperative instructions.

The anesthesia care provider also assesses the patient's airway, presence (or looseness) of teeth, anesthesia and pain tolerance, bleeding tendencies, respiratory status, and other significant information specific to the patient or procedure. Although patients are often positioned supine for the procedures, airway access is often a challenge because of the surgical site. The anesthesia care provider will determine if general anesthesia or monitored anesthesia care is required, the approach for intubation, and anticipated patient care needs.

Intraoperative Care

Although intraoperative considerations vary for each surgical patient, consistent priorities are safety and infection prevention. Positioning safety requires that the patient's bony prominences are protected and that the airway is managed at all times. Although the procedure is near the head and neck, attention to correct body alignment and padding extremities is required. When immobilization of the head is necessary, it must be undertaken with cautious attention to proper anatomic alignment as well as to the patient's particular structural idiosyncrasies. The patient's head should rest in a soft material, such as a foam headrest, to avoid pressure points. If possible, it is beneficial to position the patient for the procedure before administering sedatives to allow the patient to verbalize discomfort with the position.

A primary anesthesia concern is to establish an adequate airway that does not interfere with the surgical field. Suction should be available as soon as the patient arrives in the OR. With otolaryngology procedures performed under general anesthesia, the choice of intubation is almost always nasal or oral. If endotracheal intubation is required, atraumatic tube placement and removal reduce the occurrence of postoperative epistaxis and sore throat. When the procedure involves the mouth or nose, gauze packing of the posterior pharynx helps to prevent aspiration or swallowing of blood, tissue, or other surgical drainage. This area is thoroughly suctioned before removing the packing at the completion of the procedure.

Infiltration of local anesthesia containing epinephrine helps to reduce intraoperative bleeding. However, the practice of injecting epinephrine into the highly vascular areas of the nose, mouth, or throat can lead to systemic uptake, complicating the anesthesiologist's overall management of blood pressure and heart rate. On the other hand, supplemental local anesthesia for surgery helps to reduce the amount of general anesthetic agents required and provides postoperative analgesia.

Toxic reactions to anesthetic agents are possible, particularly because of the vascularity of the head and neck. Because of its potent vasoconstrictive properties, topical cocaine or lidocaine is frequently used, especially for nasal procedures. Because of its high level of toxicity, the anesthesia care provider should be aware of untoward symptoms and should constantly observe each patient.

Prevention of infection requires that intraoperative care is provided using an aseptic technique. Procedures are completed in or near areas of high pathogen counts (i.e., within oral or nasal cavities, hair) that require attention to technique to minimize contamination as much as possible. Hair removal at the surgical site might be necessary and, if this is the case, the hair should be clipped before the patient comes into the operating room if possible. Sterile instruments are used; the patient is draped; and often the skin is prepared as precautionary measures.

Instrumentation for ORL procedures is delicate, and an operative microscope is often used, particularly for ear surgery where the surgical site is very tiny and is bounded by bony structures. Fragile instruments should be handled individually and stored in a protective case. Sponge, needle, and instrument counts are completed.

Medications on the sterile field must be labeled with the patient's name and dosage. Medications might include steroids to minimize edema or airway obstruction. Epinephrine, phenylephrine hydrochloride, or cocaine 4% might be used topically on the vocal cords. Many surgeons use a nasal decongestant for nasal vasoconstriction.

Lasers are frequently used for ORL procedures. Laser safety practices must be followed, including operation of the laser by an individual educated in use and safety precautions. In addition, the patient undergoing an ORL procedure under general anesthesia using laser must be protected from the possibility of endotracheal fire. Specially designed, noncombustible endotracheal (ET) tubes made of copper or stainless steel that reflect the laser energy may be used. If polyvinyl ET tubes are used, they are wrapped with a tape designed from special protective material to shield them from the laser beam. Wet gauze or cottonoids are packed around the cuff of the ET tube, over the patient's eyes, and on other exposed surrounding tissues to protect those areas from stray laser energy. Drapes near the operative site must be covered with wet dressings or towels to avoid combustion and to protect underlying structures.

Postoperative Care

An immediate postoperative concern is airway adequacy, which can be complicated by edema, increased secretions, packing, and bleeding. Although many ORL procedures are accomplished under local anesthesia, those patients who have had general anesthesia are almost always intubated owing to the proximity of the airway to the operative site and because of positioning requirements. Laryngospasm or laryngeal edema may occur secondary to ET intubation or due to irritation from surgical manipulation, instrumentation, or drainage into the airway. Sore throat after intubation is a less serious, but still uncomfortable, symptom for the patient.

The high vascularity of the nose, mouth, and throat make postoperative bleeding another primary concern for the ORL patient. Hemostasis may be difficult to obtain owing to poor visibility in cavities. Postoperative activities such as sneezing, restlessness, coughing, retching, crying, and yelling can encourage bleeding, and nursing care should focus on their avoidance. More subtle symptoms of bleeding such as restlessness, anxiety, tachycardia, frequent swallowing or throat clearing, complaints of postnasal drip, bruising, and swelling or hardness of tissues must be identified and scrutinized so that a large blood loss does not occur without detection. Increased pain can be a symptom of hematoma formation or bleeding within an enclosed cavity such as the ear.

Initial nursing actions to reduce or stop active bleeding depend on the site and source of bleeding. Interventions may include calm reassurance, elevation of and direct pressure to the site, application of ice or cool compresses, protection of the airway by positioning and gentle suctioning, and sometimes sedation to calm a restless patient and to reduce an elevated blood pressure. If active bleeding is identified or suspected, the patient should be allowed nothing by mouth (NPO), and the physician should be notified. To help reduce anxiety in the patient and family, the nurse should keep drainage and blood-stained linens and dressings out of view.

A semi-Fowler position is encouraged for the awake ORL patient unless contraindicated by the surgeon's orders or by excessive vertigo. Head elevation promotes proper drainage of sinuses, helps to decrease edema and pain in the operative area, and facilitates easy respiration. After ear surgery the patient is usually asked to refrain from lying on the side of surgery for at least 24 hours, although some surgeons allow the patient to lie on either side.

The patient might have difficulty talking. Communication may be complicated by the presence of packing or the surgical procedure. Hearing can be diminished owing to occlusive ear dressings or the temporary buildup of fluid in the middle ear. A patient might find it painful to talk. Patients who have undergone procedures involving the larynx or vocal cords may be on enforced voice rest for a period of time and will need an alternate method for communicating, such as a tablet and pencil or a "magic" slate.

After topical or local anesthetic infiltration of the throat or mouth, residual local anesthesia can interfere with talking, chewing, or swallowing. The physician may specify an interval to elapse before allowing oral intake. Once that period has passed and the patient indicates a desire to drink, the nurse should assess the patient's ability to cough and swallow before giving oral fluids. If doubt still exists about the integrity of the patient's protective airway reflexes, a gentle touch on the patient's posterior oral pharynx with a cotton-tipped applicator helps in assessing gag reflex. Water or ice chips should be given before other beverages that would be more damaging if aspirated.

Sensory and motor functions of the structures of the head and neck are dependent upon innervation from the 12 pairs of cranial nerves. Both anesthesia and surgical techniques of the head and neck can temporarily or permanently affect these nerves. The nurse should be aware of their specific functions and the various clinical tests used to determine cranial nerve integrity, as listed in Table 30–2. The following mnemonic may be useful for remembering the names of the cranial nerves, using the first letter of each word to represent the 12 pairs of cranial nerves. "*O*n *o*ld *O*lympus' *t*owering *t*op, *a* *F*inn *a*nd *G*erman *v*iewed *s*ome *h*ops."[1] These first letters relate to *o*lfactory, *o*ptic, *o*culomotor, *t*rochlear, *t*rigeminal, *a*bducens, *f*acial, *a*coustic, *g*lossopharyngeal, *v*agus, *s*pinal accessory, and *h*ypoglossal.

Prevention of infection is extremely important. Many ORL procedures are performed in close proximity to structures of the central nervous system. The sinuses and ears communicate closely with the brain, making the possibility of meningitis a real threat. The high vascularity of the head and neck also increases the possibility of septicemia.

Nutritional status is important to assess because patients need enough nutrients to promote healing. The patient might have had difficulty eating or a lack of desire for food before the procedure, resulting in nutritional compromise. He or she might also experience nausea postoperatively. Encourage patients to eat multiple, small meals and snacks and avoid alcohol intake or tobacco use.

Discharge information about proper home care to avoid infection includes instructions to continue taking all doses of prescribed antibiotics, avoid contact with people with infections, wash the hands before using drops or ointments or handling any dressing, avoid touching the surgical wound, and maintain good nutrition to encourage healing. Symptoms that should be reported to the physician include prolonged or high fever, increased pain or redness of or surrounding the surgical site, stiff neck, severe

Table 30–2. The Cranial Nerves

Nerve	TYPE	FUNCTION	TESTS/ABNORMALITIES
I. Olfactory	S	Smell	Coffee, tobacco
II. Optic	S	Vision	Visual acuity, pupillary reaction, visual fields
III. Oculomotor	M	Eye movement	Ptosis, lateral and downward deviation of the eyeball
IV. Trochlear	M	Eye movement	Medial and upper deviation of eye
V. Trigeminal (3 branches—ophthalmic, maxillary, mandibular)	S	From skin of the face and cornea	Loss of sensation on one side of the face
	M	Masseter and other chewing muscles	Inability to clench teeth on one side or chew symmetrically
VI. Abducens	M	Eye movement	Medial deviation of the eyeball
VII. Facial	S	Taste—anterior tongue	
	M	Muscles of facial expression	Inability to grimace on one side of the face
VIII. Acoustic			
Auditory	S	Hearing	Watch ticking, whispered voice
Vestibulocochlear	S	Equilibrium	Vertigo, nystagmus
IX. Glossopharyngeal	S	Taste on the posterior portion of the tongue	
	M	Pharyngeal muscles	Loss of gag reflex, deviation of the uvula toward the unaffected side
X. Vagus	S	From thoracic and abdominal organs	
	M	Pharyngeal and laryngeal muscles plus thoracic and abdominal organs	Same as IX plus hoarseness
XI. Spinal accessory	M	To sternocleidomastoid and trapezius muscles	Inability to shrug one shoulder or to move chin to one side against pressure from the examiner's hand
XII. Hypoglossal	M	Tongue movement	Deviation of the tongue to the affected side

From Stewart J. Clinical Anatomy and Physiology for the Frustrated and Angry Health Professional. Miami: MedMaster, 1986, p 87.
S, sensory; M, motor.

headache or earache, chills, prolonged nausea and vomiting, or obvious bleeding. Swallowing of blood can result in black or dark stools for a day or more after surgery, and patients should be told that this is a possible, and benign, occurrence.

Patients should be encouraged to use prescribed antiemetics or antimotion sickness drugs as directed and should avoid driving, alcohol, and dangerous activities concurrent with their use. Other suggestions to reduce unpleasant gastrointestinal symptoms at home include darkening the room; limiting noise, lights, and other sensory stimuli; avoiding rapid head movements; walking slowly and only when necessary in the early postoperative period; avoiding rich or spicy foods; and not swallowing postnasal drainage.

The presence of nasal packing increases the patient's general discomfort due to pressure and the resultant mouth breathing. Because nasal packing reduces or obliterates sinus drainage, congestion and headache can occur, and thus antihistamines may be prescribed. Anxiety may accompany real or imagined difficulty in breathing. The patient should be encouraged by the short-term nature of the packing, which is generally removed in the physician's office a few days after surgery. Liquids and soft foods that do not require chewing are best tolerated while the nose is packed. Patients should not swallow through a straw owing to the vacuum that can be created because of the packing. Nose blowing must also be avoided.

Mouthwash or water rinses can be helpful to moisten the mouth and to reduce any bad taste from prolonged mouth breathing or from the presence of drainage-soaked packing or appliances. Peridex, an antibacterial, prescription oral rinse with a chlorhexidine gluconate base, is primarily indicated for the treatment of gingivitis, although some oral surgeons also prescribe this rinse postoperatively. Patients report significantly reduced bad taste and dryness of the mouth after its use.

PROCEDURES OF THE EAR

The ear is divided anatomically into the outer, middle, and inner portions. Outer and middle ear procedures often lend themselves to an ASC. Surgical access to these areas is either through the ear canal or by means of a postauricular incision.

Foreign Body Removal

If sedation is required to remove a foreign body from the ear, the procedure could be scheduled in ASC. If the foreign body is superficial (i.e., has not been in the ear for a long time), it will require an otoscope and forceps to extract the item. If the item has been in the ear for a period of time, it could require an incision to remove the item. The type of item and extent of injury could result in a more extensive procedure.

Myringotomy

Myringotomy is a surgical incision into the tympanic membrane to reduce the pressure in and to allow drainage and ventilation of the middle ear. Most often this procedure is performed bilaterally and is accompanied by the insertion of tympanostomy tubes to maintain patency of the incisions. There are numerous and controversial indications for surgery. The most common application is for the management of recurrent otitis media.

Patients most frequently seen for this procedure are children between the ages of 2 and 7 years. The procedure is accomplished very quickly under general anesthesia and necessitates only a brief separation of the child from the parents. Anesthesia for adults undergoing myringotomy may be local or general depending on the age, physical status, and cooperation of the patient.

Otitis media occurs with chronic or frequent blockage of the eustachian tubes. The air that becomes trapped in the middle ear is absorbed and is replaced by fluid. Small glands appear, which secrete mucus, resulting in hearing loss and infection. Placement of the polyethylene tympanostomy tube, as shown in Figure 30–1, allows drainage of the middle ear, promotes healing of its lining, and provides an alternate path for the entry of air into the middle ear. The procedure is generally done under general anesthesia with anesthetic gases. Approximately 70% of the children experience postoperative pain after these procedures. Suppositories or transnasal injection can be used to improve postoperative pain.[2]

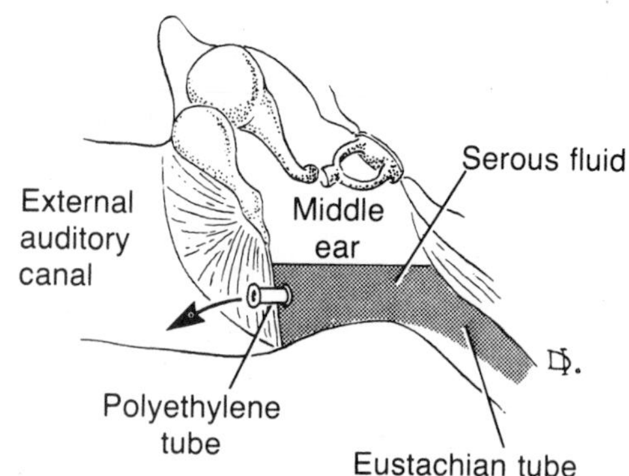

Figure 30–1. Insertion of a myringotomy tube. The flanged tube is inserted through the tympanic membrane. This allows fluid to drain from and air to enter the middle ear. (From Hill G: Outpatient Surgery, 3rd ed. Philadelphia: WB Saunders, 1988, p 182.)

The tubes usually remain for several weeks to several months. The perforations in the tympanic membranes close within 1 week of tube removal. If not removed, tympanostomy tubes fall out spontaneously in about 6 months. Parents or patients should be informed that after several months a small amount of blood may be seen in the ear canal when new tissue forms in an attempt to expel the tube from the tympanic membrane. It is not a dangerous occurrence, and the patient is often given antibiotic eardrops to use if it occurs.

Hearing is usually significantly improved as soon as the fluid has been drained from the middle ear. Postoperatively, the patient may require the temporary, gentle insertion of a small cotton ball or gauze in the outer ear canal to absorb any remaining fluid that drains. The patient may be placed on oral decongestants and should be instructed to keep water out of the ears while the tubes are in place. The obvious reason is to prevent environmental fluids from entering and contaminating the middle ear. Swimming is restricted for a time as directed by the physician. Soft ear plugs that can be molded to the shape of the external ear canal or cotton with petroleum jelly may be used for showering or hairwashing.

Tympanoplasty

Chronic otitis media may result in deafness, persistent ear discharge, and spontaneous perforation of the tympanic membrane. For this or a traumatic perforation, surgical repair may be necessary. Tympanoplasty is ideally performed when there is no current middle ear infection. Small perforations can usually be closed by a transcanal approach. A graft from the temporalis muscle fascia in the postauricular area is used as a patch. Larger perforations or those that have caused loss of continuity between the tympanic membrane and the ossicles (malleus, incus, and stapes) generally require a postauricular approach, again using a graft from the temporalis fascia. The incision is in the postauricular crease. A bulky dressing is applied to protect both the donor and tympanic sites.

After surgery, the physician indicates desired positioning; if not, the patient should be positioned for comfort, usually with the operated ear uppermost. Dizziness, vertigo, and nausea are potential complications. Instructions for home care include keeping the operative ear dressing dry. To help prevent disrupting the graft, the patient is instructed to avoid coughing and nose blowing. Antibiotics are usually prescribed, and the dressing is removed after approximately 1 week.

Mastoidectomy

Chronic otitis media may take a more damaging turn with the formation of a cholesteatoma in the middle ear and mastoid bone. This proliferation of epithelial cells grows and erodes surrounding normal tissues, including portions of the mastoid bone. Infection and deafness eventually follow. As it continues to spread, the cholesteatoma can damage the ossicles and cause facial nerve impairment, brain abscess, or inner ear infringement.

Surgical intervention involves mastoidectomy, which may be simple or radical. The simple removal of portions of the mastoid bone may be undertaken in some ambulatory surgical programs. Radical mastoidectomy involving the removal of large portions of the ear canal along with the ossicles requires hospitalization.

The incision for mastoidectomy is usually postauricular to allow for the best visualization. Owing to the proximity of the surgical site to the facial nerve, the nurse should assess nerve integrity postoperatively by asking the patient to smile, frown, wrinkle the forehead, bare the teeth, close the eyes, and pucker the lips. If the facial nerve is impaired, there can be visible drooping of the mouth or drooling while drinking. The presence of such symptoms or the patient's inability to perform any of the assessment maneuvers should be documented and reported to the physician immediately. Positive symptoms may resolve spontaneously after surgical inflammation and swelling abates or may be permanent if there was direct damage to the nerve.

The patient will have a bulky dressing to protect the surgical site and may have an ear packing in place for several days. The area must be assessed for bleeding, and the patient should be instructed to leave the bandage in place until the physician removes it and to report any bright red bleeding immediately.

As with other ear procedures, nausea and vomiting may complicate the recovery period. Due to the proximity of the mastoid bone to structures of the central nervous system, special care must be taken to avoid infection. The patient should report any symptoms of infection as previously listed to the physician at once.

Stapedectomy

Otosclerosis is the abnormal growth of spongy bone in the labyrinth with adherence to the stapes (stirrup). This fixation prevents transmission of vibrations to the fluids of the inner ear and results in deafness. This condition of unknown cause is more common in women than in men. A hearing aid may provide some relief, but the only definitive treatment is surgical replacement of the affected stapes with one of a variety of prosthetic devices. This transcanal microscopic procedure is called a stapedectomy.

Postoperative care focuses on the prevention or treatment of dizziness, nausea, vomiting, and pain and on the protection and stabilization of the grafted prosthesis. Packing is usually placed in the ear postoperatively and should remain undisturbed. Positioning after a stapedectomy is at the direction of the surgeon, who may prefer that the operated ear remain uppermost to maintain the position of the graft. Some physicians prefer to have the patient lie on the side of surgery to allow for drainage; others allow the patient to choose a comfortable position.

A parenteral analgesic and antiemetic or antimotion sickness medication may be necessary during the first few hours postoperatively. Dizziness can complicate the patient's early recovery after a procedure is done in close proximity to the labyrinth, and thus the patient should avoid rapid head movements and should walk only with assistance. Blowing the nose and coughing can increase pressure in the upper airway and eustachian tube, causing damage to the delicately placed prosthesis.

PROCEDURES OF THE NOSE

The external nose is made up of bone, cartilages, and nasal septum. The internal nose is located between the hard palate, cribriform plate, and nasopharynx. Nasal turbinates project from the lateral walls of the nose. They act as a drainage passage for the sinuses. Nasal disease often presents with nasal discharge or bleedings; a decrease in the sense of smell; or difficulty in breathing from congestion, obstruction, septal deformities, or polyps. A variety of conditions can bring the patient to an ASC for nasal surgery. Nasal polyps, although usually benign, tend to recur, and patients may undergo periodic procedures to have them removed. Correction of nasal deformities that interfere with breathing or that are cosmetically undesirable to the patient constitutes a large portion of the nasal surgeries performed on outpatients.

Septoplasty, Submucous Resection, Rhinoplasty, and Reduction of Nasal Fractures

Septoplasty is to reposition or realign the cartilaginous portions of the septum. The submucous resection is completed to remove osseous or cartilaginous portions of the septum. These procedures are usually completed for septal deviation, nasal polyps, or perforation of the nasal septum. Internal and external nasal procedures can be done in the ASC with local anesthesia supplemented with intravenous sedation. General anesthesia can be used if patients are anxious or apprehensive.

Trauma or congenital deformity may cause the deviated nasal septum. Previous fractures or deformities with deviation of the nasal septum to one side can result in blockage of the nasal passage and sinus openings. Septoplasty or submucous resection of the septum may be undertaken to open those passages and to correct septal deformities that impair nasal drainage or respirations. Polyps occur when the erectile mucosa of the septum becomes engorged because of an inadequate airway on the side of the deviation. Perforation of the nasal septum is a result of ulceration with subsequent perforation of the septal cartilage. This can be caused by trauma, foreign body, previous septal surgery, infection, systemic diseases (e.g., tuberculosis, syphilis), or chemical irritation (e.g., cocaine sniffing, inhalation of chemicals).

In the OR, the surgeon may pack the nose with cottonoids saturated with a hemostatic agent. A local anesthetic can be injected for hemostasis and to increase pain tolerance. A septoplasty requires an intranasal incision in the mucosa. The mucosa is elevated from the cartilage and bony septum, and the septal cartilage is repositioned or straightened. Reduction of a nasal fracture caused by a frontal blow requires a similar procedure. During a submucous resection, the mucoperiosteum is elevated to remove the deviated portion of the septal cartilage. These procedures may be combined with a rhinoplasty, during which the outer structure of the nose is revised, usually for a cosmetic effect.

Internal incisions are not visible on postoperative inspection. Nasal packing is usually placed to provide internal support. The packing helps to keep the septum in the correct position, reduce edema and bleeding, and enhance tissue apposition. This packing is left undisturbed until the physician's office visit several days after surgery, but a small "moustache" dressing (drip pad) is taped over the tip of the nose. It is changed when it becomes wet with surgical drainage. Replacement of the nasal tip dressing should be undertaken with gentleness, because the patient's nose may be extremely tender to touch. The patient and the adult companion should be instructed in and evaluated for the proper technique of changing the dressing at home. A nonallergenic tape is best tolerated by most people and should be repositioned in different areas of the cheeks with periodic dressing changes to decrease skin irritation.

An external splint may be affixed to the bridge of the nose to protect the surgical results. Such devices often are self-adhesive and provide support to the soft tissues of the nose. They also help to decrease postoperative swelling and remind the patient to protect the nose. Internal splints that are designed with ports for breathing are another type of device used by some surgeons.

Further postoperative considerations include maintaining a patent airway by positioning the patient on his or her side if necessary. As soon as feasible after arousal from anesthesia, the patient should be placed in semi-Fowler's position. Excessive secretions may need to be suctioned. The patient may have to be reminded about the nasal packing and the need to take slow, deep breaths through the mouth. Apply ice or cool compresses to the nasal and periorbital areas to help reduce swelling and ecchymosis. Ice should not be applied near the tip of the nose, because circulation could be compromised and the delicate tissues could be damaged. A patient should understand that ecchymosis around the eyes is a common, benign postoperative occurrence. The eyelids may be extensively swollen on the evening of surgery and the next day. Ophthalmic ointment is often applied to the eyes intraoperatively to protect them from blood or surgical drainage, and the patient may have blurred vision in the immediate postoperative period.

Nausea and vomiting can complicate the patient's recovery period, especially if bloody drainage has been swallowed during or after surgery. Antiemetics may be ineffective until blood that has been swallowed is out of the stomach. For a few days postoperatively, soft foods and liquids are easiest for the patient to eat, because chewing and swallowing may be difficult with nasal packing in place. Swallowing is difficult because a vacuum is created in the upper airway when there is complete obliteration of the nasal passages. Use of straws for drinking is prohibited. The patient may also experience bad breath, dry mouth from the need to continuously mouth breathe, sinus congestion, and headache. The physician may prescribe antihistamines, antibiotics, and analgesics.

PROCEDURES OF THE SINUSES

There are four sets of paranasal sinuses on each side of the face. The maxillaries (or antrums) are paired sinuses that lie behind the cheeks. These sinuses are the largest and most often infected. The other sets of sinuses are the frontal sinuses, which are located in the frontal bone; the ethmoid sinus, located in the superior and lateral walls of the nose and medial walls of the orbits; and the sphenoid sinus, located in the sphenoid bone. These sinuses are illustrated in Figure 30–2. Outpatient sinus procedures are generally limited to the maxillary and ethmoid sinuses, because the patient has a greater risk of intracranial complications in procedures of the frontal and sphenoid sinuses because of the potential for contaminating cerebrospinal fluid (CSF).[3]

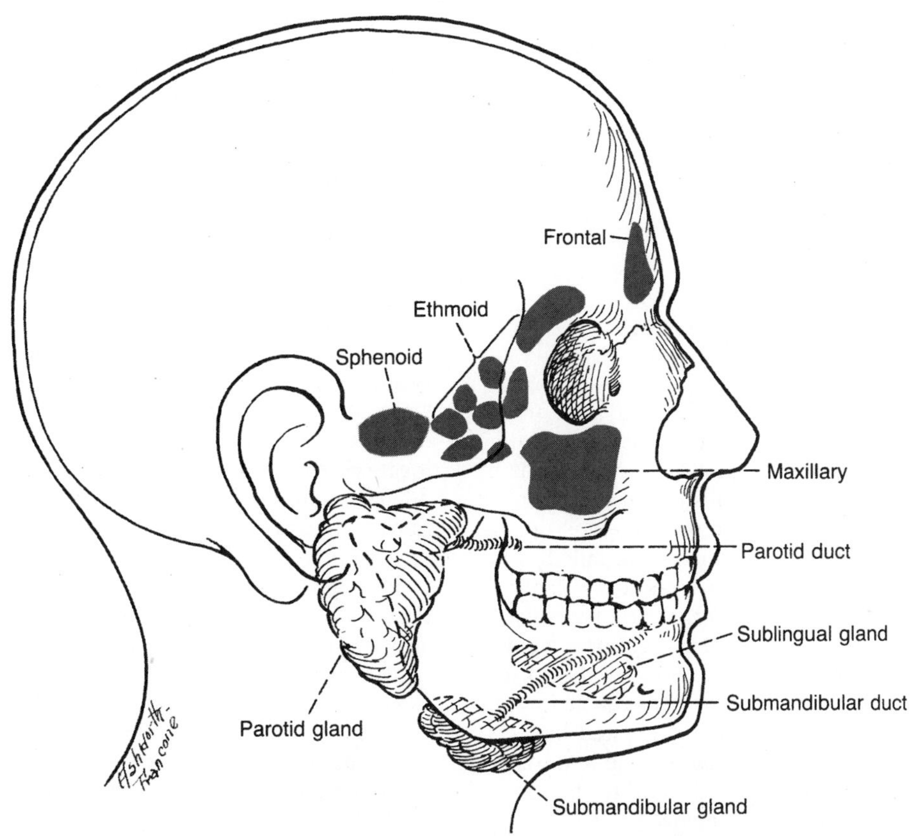

Figure 30–2. Paranasal sinuses. Lateral view of the head showing the paranasal sinuses and salivary glands. (From Jacob S, Francone C: Elements of Anatomy and Physiology, 2nd ed. Philadelphia: WB Saunders, 1989, p 227.)

The sinuses are air-filled mucosa-lined cavities with an unknown function. Fluid accumulates in the sinuses when the ostium (opening) of the sinus into the nose is blocked. The mucosa thickens because of chronic inflammation. The cheeks become tender and painful. When this inflammatory condition becomes chronic, the lining of the sinuses can become thickened and polypoid.[5] Surgical intervention becomes necessary when medical treatment such as antibiotic therapy is ineffective; mucocele or polyps develop in the sinus; or in the event that a tumor is causing the blockage.[4] The ostium is reopened, and an alternate pathway is created for sinus drainage.

Ethmoid sinuses are positioned behind the orbits of the eyes. Surgical entry for removal of diseased tissues can be achieved transantrally or through an incision just below the eyebrow.

Intranasal Antrostomy (Nasal Antral Window)

Intranasal antrostomy (nasal antral window) is one of several surgical procedures that can provide the construction of a permanent, new opening from the maxillary sinus into the nasal cavity. This approach allows for the removal of polyps or diseased mucosa and for irrigation.[4] An opening is created in the medial wall of the maxillary sinus below the inferior turbinate, and purulent secretions are removed by suction. The sinus is packed with antibiotic ointment on gauze or an impregnated gauze, and a moustache dressing is applied.

Radical Antrostomy (Caldwell-Luc Procedure)

The radical antrostomy (Caldwell-Luc procedure) is another approach to treat sinus conditions such as polyps, diseased tissue, or infection. The procedure establishes a large opening in the wall of the inferior meatus. It is undertaken when other procedures have failed. This procedure is becoming less common because of the endoscopic approaches that are available.

In most cases, the patient requires general anesthesia. Through an incision in the canine fossa of the mouth (the area between the upper lip and the gum), a window is created between the antrum and the nasal cavity. The oral mucosal flap is sutured closed at the end of the procedure, but the opening remains permanent between the nasal cavity and the maxillary sinus. Antibiotic on gauze or impregnated packing is placed in the nose and sinus at the end of the procedure with a moustache dressing. The patient will require special attention to mouth care but should avoid gargling and blowing the nose in the early postoperative period. A petroleum-based ointment to the lips to prevent cracking is an appropriate comfort measure.

Complications after a Caldwell-Luc antrostomy are usually self-limiting and transient. The patient may experience temporary numbness of the upper lip, teeth, or cheek. Damage to the maxillary division of the trigeminal nerve (cranial nerve V) will cause permanent loss of sensation to the upper lip. Facial swelling resolves within the first week after the packing is removed. Mild epistaxis can occur after the packing has been removed but it is usually self-limiting.

Further nursing considerations after sinus surgery include the provision of analgesia and positioning of the awake patient in a semi-Fowler position to decrease edema and enhance drainage of the sinuses through the newly established openings. Home instructions include maintaining head elevation and a diet of soft foods and beverages and avoiding sneezing and blowing the nose.

Endoscopic Sinus Surgery

Endoscopic sinus surgery (ESS) has become the state-of-the-art method for gaining access to the sinuses for diagnosis and treatment of inflammatory and chronic infectious processes or anatomic defects such as polyps.[6] Chronic and recurrent sinusitis is the most frequent indication for endoscopic sinus surgery. Improper drainage of the maxillary, frontal, and anterior ethmoid sinuses into the middle meatus often results in chronic or recurrent sinusitis. Inhaled environmental irritants can cause inflammation of the middle turbinate because of its anatomic location in the entrance of the nose (Fig. 30–3). That inflammatory process can spread to the middle meatus and can significantly compromise drainage of the ethmoid and other sinuses. It is believed that most paranasal sinus infections spread from the nose to the sinuses. It has also been demonstrated that in most cases, the spread of inflammation is from the ethmoid sinuses to the frontal and maxillary sinuses. Current treatment, therefore, is primarily directed at removing diseased ethmoid tissue and restoring normal drainage patterns.[7]

Direct visualization of remote sinus areas afforded by transnasal endoscopy prevents tissue trauma and reduces morbidity. This preserva-

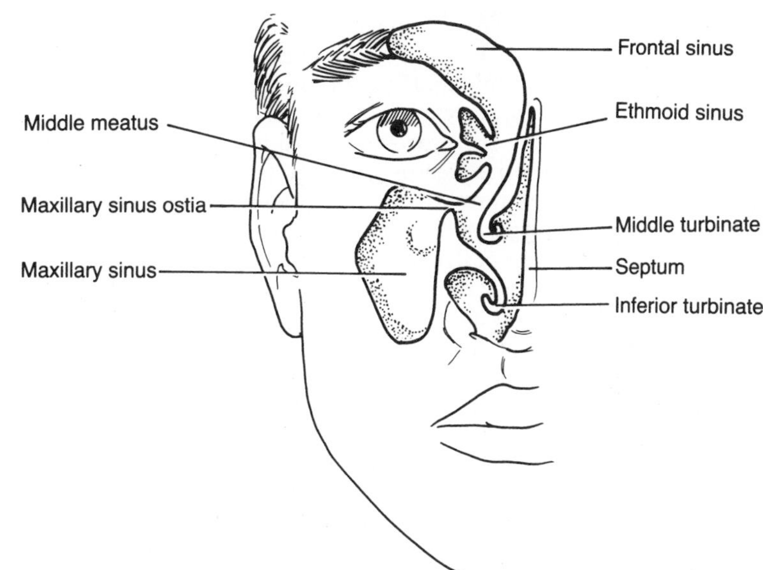

Figure 30–3. Frontal view of the paranasal sinuses.

tion of normal tissue results in an easier postoperative recovery and is considered to be the main advantage of using an endoscopic approach. It is a less invasive procedure; the skin and mucous membrane incisions are avoided; and masses and malformations can be accurately diagnosed by direct visualization. ESS is cost-effective and can be accomplished under local anesthesia with minimal sedation or general anesthesia.

The surgeon inserts a cottonoid soaked with hemostatic agents in the nares. The telescope is inserted into the nares to visualize the nasal cavity. Hand instruments are used to incise the middle turbinate mucosa, excess mucosa, and bone formations or excise polyps or mucocele formations. Sinus lavage can also be accomplished endoscopically. When the procedure is complete, an antibiotic-impregnated nasal splint may be placed in the middle meatus. A moustache dressing is applied.

A nasal decongestant spray may be ordered before surgery. Local anesthesia may be used alone or in conjunction with general anesthesia. Intranasal cocaine provides remarkable vasoconstriction. Methylprednisolone may be injected into the surgical site and into the anterior and inferior turbinates to reduce inflammation and swelling postoperatively.

Potential postoperative complications include bleeding, vision problems, and leakage of CSF (rhinorrhea). In addition, orbital hematoma, orbital subcutaneous emphysema, temporary blindness or diplopia, closure of the natural sinus openings, and tooth pain can follow intranasal endoscopic ethmoidectomy.

As well as observing for such complications, the nurse assesses the patient's general physical status and respiratory effort during the early postoperative period. The surgeon often places an antibiotic/steroid ointment but usually no packing in the nasal cavity. A nasal tip dressing may be needed to collect surgical drainage. If surgical bleeding occurs, the patient may have one or both nares packed with a cocaine-soaked cottonoid that is removed in the postanesthetic care unit (PACU). One practitioner describes the use of a hemostatic balloon that can be taped to the cheek and left in place for several hours or until the next day.

Oral fluids are allowed postoperatively, and the patient is observed for 2 to 4 hours before discharge. At home, the patient should refrain from strenuous activities and from nose blowing. Antibiotics and steroids are not routinely required. Postoperative nasal douching might begin after day 10.[8] Physicians are experiencing positive postoperative results.[9]

PROCEDURES OF THE MOUTH AND THROAT

Laryngoscopy and Microlaryngoscopy

Laryngoscopy is the direct visualization of the larynx to diagnose hoarseness or tumors, to remove foreign bodies, or to determine the cause of an obstructed airway. It can also be done to correct traumatic injury. The preoperative nurse should assess and report neck motion, because positioning and movement of the neck is important to facilitate the procedure. A rigid scope is used. An operative microscope may be connected for close scrutiny of the larynx and related structures. Polyps, nodules, or other lesions of the larynx or vocal cords can be removed with microlaryngoscopy or with a carbon dioxide laser. The carbon dioxide laser is useful to remove webs of the larynx, vocal cord papilloma, or benign endobronchial lesions.

Preoperative NPO restrictions are essential, because aspiration is a serious complication of laryngoscopy. The cooperative adult patient may undergo laryngoscopy under local anesthesia with sedation; children and adults who cannot tolerate that approach are given general anesthesia.

Tonsillectomy and Adenoidectomy

Historically, (palatine) tonsillectomy and adenoidectomy (pharyngeal tonsillectomy) were performed almost exclusively together, in a procedure called adenotonsillectomy. A more recent trend is to selectively remove only those structures that are specifically indicated by the patient's history and clinical symptoms. Tonsillectomy is generally considered an appropriate procedure in an ASC if the patient is an otherwise healthy surgical and anesthesia risk.[10] Contraindications to an ASC for tonsillectomy include unavailability of appropriate home support or poorly controlled systemic diseases, such as sickle cell anemia, kidney or heart disease, sleep apnea disorders, and congenital malformation syndromes.

Certain contraindications exist for these procedures, whether the patient is hospitalized or ambulatory. Patients with immunodeficient states, clotting disorders, active respiratory infections, and symptomatic asthma are treated medically rather than surgically, as are those with severe and poorly controlled systemic diseases. There is controversy regarding the appropriateness of tonsillectomy or adenoidectomy in children younger than 5 or 6 years of age.

For children, eliminating an overnight stay is one way to help reduce psychological sequelae associated with hospitalization and separation from parents. The adult patient may also prefer the home setting after surgery for its comfort and familiarity, depending on the effectiveness of analgesia provided and the availability of an adequate support system. The attending physician knows that the parent is the best judge of the patient's physical and psychological makeup. The parents of small children must be carefully assessed for their ability to provide proper care at home before the child is discharged.

Indications for tonsillectomy vary from one practitioner to another, but those that are generally accepted include recurrent episodes of chronic or acute tonsillitis; airway or swallowing difficulties due to chronic, hypertrophied tonsils; after resolution of a peritonsillar abscess; or complications involving blockage of the eustachian tubes or sinuses. A suspected malignancy is also an indication.

Adenoidectomy is performed when hypertrophy results in nasal obstruction, which can lead to difficulties in breathing or speaking, or when there are recurrent episodes of otitis media with or without hearing loss. Chronic mouth breathing may be an indication as well. Typically, patients who undergo an adenoidectomy are between 4 and 8 years of age. After 8 years of age, the adenoids begin to gradually atrophy. Neither tonsillectomy nor adenoidectomy is done during an acute inflammatory process.

Preoperatively, the patient should be assessed carefully for symptoms that could complicate the postoperative course, for instance, abnormal coagulation studies, loose teeth, inability to open the mouth wide, and pre-existing airway problems or deformities. A nursing history can help identify other potential problem areas, such as easy bruising, petechiae, or poor dietary habits that could predispose to nutritional deficiencies and delayed healing.[11]

Adequate preoperative instructions will help patients and parents deal with later problems such as sore throat, dysphagia, nausea, and the sensation of fullness in the throat. The parents need to understand the essential nature of the NPO requirement, but the patient should be urged to drink fluids up to the beginning of the fasting period to maintain hydration. Parents of young children must closely monitor their child on the day of surgery to prevent the possible ingestion of food, candy, or beverages.

Appropriate beverages and soft foods that do not require much chewing should be available for after surgery. Cool or slightly warm foods are soothing and do not promote bleeding as hot items can. Popsicles and ice chips are soothing and provide fluid intake, particularly for a child who refuses other nourishment.

Tonsils are removed using either sharp or blunt dissection. Adenoids are removed using sharp dissection. A variety of methods are used intraoperatively to maintain hemostasis: direct pressure using dry or chemical-soaked sponges, electrocautery, laser coagulation, and ligation of vessels. Local anesthetics that contain epinephrine are often injected around the operative site after general anesthesia before surgery and prove effective in producing vasoconstriction, which decreases blood loss. Swallowed blood can be vomited and aspirated. A report to the postanesthesia nurse should include the estimated amount of intraoperative bleeding and complications encountered with the procedure.

Local anesthetic injection of the pharynx with a long-acting local anesthetic agent such as bupivacaine is helpful in providing analgesia into the postoperative period. This allows the patient to talk, eat, and drink more comfortably, which bolsters the patient's self-confidence.

The primary postoperative concerns are maintaining airway integrity, protecting against aspiration, and providing adequate analgesia. Postoperative airway management must be meticulous. Once awake, the patient's head is elevated to facilitate venous flow and to prevent aspiration. Sinus drainage is enhanced when the head is elevated, and the patient generally finds this position more comfortable for breathing.

Constant nursing observation should focus on visible bloody drainage or bright red emesis plus the less obvious symptoms of frequent swallowing, apprehension, restlessness, tachycardia, and complaints of postnasal drip. The patient should avoid throat clearing, coughing, and excessive talking in the early recovery period. An ice collar may be applied to the throat for comfort and to deter bleeding.

Adequate analgesia is one method of helping to prevent bleeding due to hyperactivity, straining, or crying, but it should be accompanied by cautious observation because sedation of the patient can mask the more insidious symptoms of bleeding and can promote respiratory depression. In the early recovery period, analgesia may be provided intravenously with titrated doses of fentanyl or morphine. Later, the patient may be given oral liquid acetaminophen with or without codeine.

Intravenous fluid replacement is generally continued until the time of discharge to ensure that the patient is well hydrated. Further observation continues in the Phase II area until discharge criteria are met. Controversy exists about the length of stay required after tonsillectomy. Because it has been determined by some reporters that early bleeding generally occurs within the first hour after surgery, the typical requirement of a 4-, 8-, or 24-hour stay is sometimes questioned. Facility policies and medical directives regarding length of stay must be followed within each institution.

An accompanying responsible adult should be present to receive written and verbal discharge instructions. At home, the patient should be encouraged to avoid: (1) excessive talking; (2) throat clearing; (3) coughing; (4) smoking; (5) spicy or mechanically hard foods; (6) thermal extremes in food and beverages; (7) aspirin, aspirin-containing, or nonsteroidal anti-inflammatory medications; and (8) physical exertion. Bad breath can persist for 7 to 10 days until healing has occurred. The patient may gently rinse the mouth with a commercial mouthwash for oral hygiene, but vigorous gargling should be avoided because it could promote loosening of the tonsillar eschar (scab) and lead to bleeding.

Late bleeding is most likely to occur between the fifth and tenth postoperative days when the operative eschar separates from the underlying tissue. The patient or parent should know the proper response, which is to lie down (side lying is best) and to remain calm and quiet. The patient should be instructed to telephone the physician if the bleeding does not stop within 5 minutes.

Oral fluids are encouraged at home to maintain hydration and to reduce the chance of constipation, which may occur as a result of altered oral intake. One or more bowel movements may be dark or black in the next several days after surgery due to blood that may have been swallowed during and after surgery. The patient usually continues to use an ice collar for the first 24 hours for comfort and to promote hemostasis.

After adenoidectomy the patient may complain of neck stiffness, which should resolve after healing occurs and the adenoidal eschar detaches. A nonprescription antihistamine may be suggested by the physician for rhinitis, which is common postoperatively. A fever of up to 102° F or 103° F is not uncommon. Acetaminophen therapy is usually suggested for any temperature elevation that is over 101° F. A persistently high fever should be reported to the physician.

Other symptoms that should be reported include throat pain that is severe and unrelieved by the analgesics prescribed and prolonged or severe earache. After one day of liquid nourishment, the child who is not nauseated is usually able to eat normal food, because the soft palate closes off the area of the adenoidal site and no food touches that area during swallowing.

Thyroidectomy

Patients having subtotal thyroidectomies in an ASC must be screened carefully to ensure their fitness for early discharge. The physician's technical abilities and prior complication rates for similar surgeries and the expected extent of the procedure are considered. The patient's thyroid status should be as well controlled as possible, and some patients are treated with an oral iodine preparation for 7 to 10 days before surgery to reduce excessive vascularity of the gland.

The patient who expresses anxiety about returning home after thyroidectomy needs special reassurance and specific details about what to expect. Extreme anxiety or fear about early discharge is a contraindication to scheduling the patient in the ASC. Discharge to home is an option if the patient's family can provide appropriate care, but sometimes 23-hour admission or transfer to a recovery care center is appropriate for overnight observation.

Complications are infrequent, but they include incisional bleeding, recurrent laryngeal nerve damage with resultant vocal cord impairment or paralysis, pneumothorax, and tracheal compression due to bleeding or edema. Significant tracheal compression or laryngeal edema can result in partial or complete airway obstruction. Usually, the surgeon dresses the incision loosely, avoiding any circumferential dressing that could become constrictive if swelling occurs.

If injury or inadvertent removal of the parathyroid gland occurs during surgery, signs of hypocalcemia may appear in the postoperative period. These include nervousness, muscle cramps, paresthesias, tingling and numbness of the feet, a positive Chvostek or Trousseau sign, lowered serum calcium levels and, in more severe cases, carpopedal spasms, laryngeal stridor, or convulsions.

Chvostek's sign is the abnormal spasm of facial muscles when the facial nerve is tapped. Trousseau's sign is positive when a sphygmomanometer cuff inflated on the arm higher than the systolic blood pressure for 3 minutes results in carpal spasms. Hospitalization is indicated for such a patient. Treatment is both supportive of presenting symptoms and specific, requiring administration of intravenous calcium gluconate. Symptoms usually reverse within 1 week.

Early postoperative care includes frequent assessment of vital signs and evaluation of the incision, airway, the patient's general comfort level, and signs of complications. Pain can usually be managed with oral analgesics in the home. To make the postoperative course more comfortable, the patient can be told to roll the body to the side, rather than using the upper torso to lift into a sitting position. Some patients find it helpful to use one hand to support the neck when turning or lifting the head.

Airway compromise may present as changes in the rate or depth of respirations, stridor, difficulty in swallowing, complaints of tightness or fullness around the throat, changes in sensorium, or restlessness. Such symptoms require immediate and aggressive intervention to ascertain the extent of compromise and to halt further deterioration. Nursing actions include elevation of the patient's head, oxygen administration, calm reassurance, maintenance of the NPO status until respiratory integrity is ensured, assessment of the incision and surrounding tissues for hematoma formation, evaluation and loosening of any tight dressing, preparations for suture removal and possible subsequent hematoma evacuation, and concurrent notification of the surgeon to assess the patient.

The patient who is having difficulty talking after surgery may be suffering the effects of edema, inflammation, or damage to the recurrent laryngeal nerve and needs reassurance that hoarseness or voice loss usually subsides in a few days. Unilateral recurrent laryngeal nerve damage rarely results in airway problems. Patients are encouraged to rest their voices for the first day or two after surgery to help prevent laryngeal edema. A means of writing should be provided to help the patient communicate.

If bilateral recurrent laryngeal nerve injury occurs intraoperatively, the potential for paralysis of both vocal cords and resultant respiratory problems is significant, and the patient is admitted to a hospital. Subsequent intubation is required if paralysis of both vocal cords occurs. The rare occurrence of direct transection of both recurrent laryngeal nerves requires surgical repair.

Barring early complications, home discharge can occur after a period of observation. The family and patient who have been thoroughly instructed and who have interacted with calm and confident staff members will be better prepared emotionally and physically for the period of home recuperation.

References

1. Rudy E: Advanced Neurological and Neurosurgical Nursing. St. Louis: CV Mosby, 1984.

2. Bennie RE, Boehringer LA, Dierdorf SF, et al: Transnasal butorphanol is effective for postoperative pain relief in children undergoing myringotomy, Anesthesiology 89:385–390, 1998.
3. Kubal WS: Sinonasal anatomy. Neuroimaging Clin N Am 2:14–156, 1998.
4. Piccirillo JF, Thawley SE, Haiduk A, et al: Indications for sinus surgery: How appropriate are the guidelines? Laryngoscope 108:332–338, 1998.
5. Marks SC, Latoni JD, Mathog RH: Mucoceles of the maxillary sinus. Otolaryngol Head Neck Surg 117:18–21, 1997.
6. Krouse HJ, Parker CM, Purcell R, et al: Powered functional endoscopic sinus surgery. AORN J 66:405–414, 1997.
7. Eloy P, Bertrand B, Rombaux P: Medical and surgical management of chronic sinusitis. Acta Otorhinolaryngol (Belg) 51:271–284, 1997.
8. Fernandes SV: Postoperative care in functional endoscopic sinus surgery? Laryngoscope 109:945–948, 1999.
9. Senior BA, Kennedy DW, Tanabodee J, et al: Long-term results of functional endoscopic sinus surgery. Laryngoscope 108:151–157, 1998.
10. Lawson MJ, Lapinski BJ, Velasco EC: Tonsillectomy and adenoidectomy pathway plan of care for the pediatric patient in day surgery. Am Soc Perianesthesia Nurses 12:387–395, 1997.
11. Fina DK: Is it only a tonsillectomy? AORN J 66:1073–1075, 1997.

Chapter 31

Oral and Maxillofacial Surgery

Brenda S. Gregory Dawes

Surgery on the oral and maxillofacial structures should be done by surgeons who specialize in oral/maxillofacial, otorhinolaryngology, or plastic/reconstructive surgery. This is because of the various patient diagnoses and conditions that result in the need for surgery. It is important for the nurse to understand the surgeon's plan of care to anticipate the patient's needs.

The structures involved in oral/maxillofacial procedures are the oral cavity (Fig. 31–1) and skeletal components of the face, including the mandible, maxilla, zygoma, naso-orbital ethmoid complex, and supraorbital structures (Fig. 31–2 *A, B*). The oral cavity includes the lips, teeth, gums, buccal mucosa, tongue, hard and soft palate, tonsils, pharynx, and temporomandibular joint (TMJ). Jaw bones, muscle, and mucosa surround the oral cavity. The cavity forms the beginning of the digestive system and is a major organ of speech and emotional expression.

The trigeminal nerve (cranial nerve V) splits into the maxillary division and the mandibular division (Fig. 31–3 *A, B*). The maxillary division supplies sensation to the upper teeth. There are

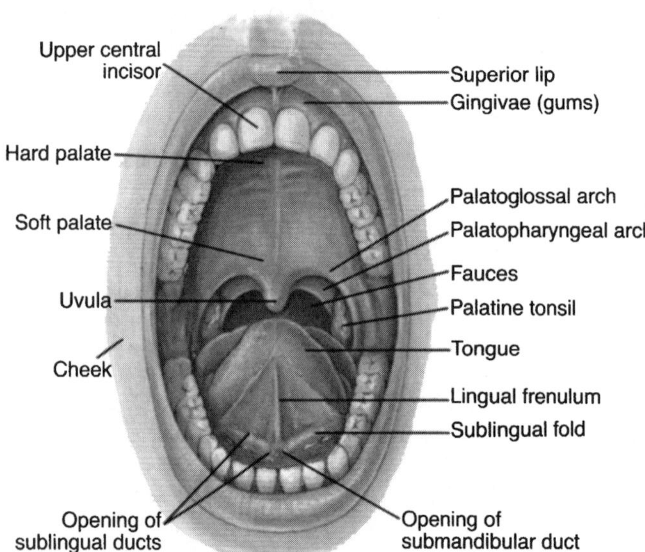

Figure 31–1. Features of the oral cavity. (From Miller-Keane Encyclopedia & Dictionary of Medicine, Nursing & Allied Health, 6th ed. Philadelphia: WB Saunders Co., 1997.)

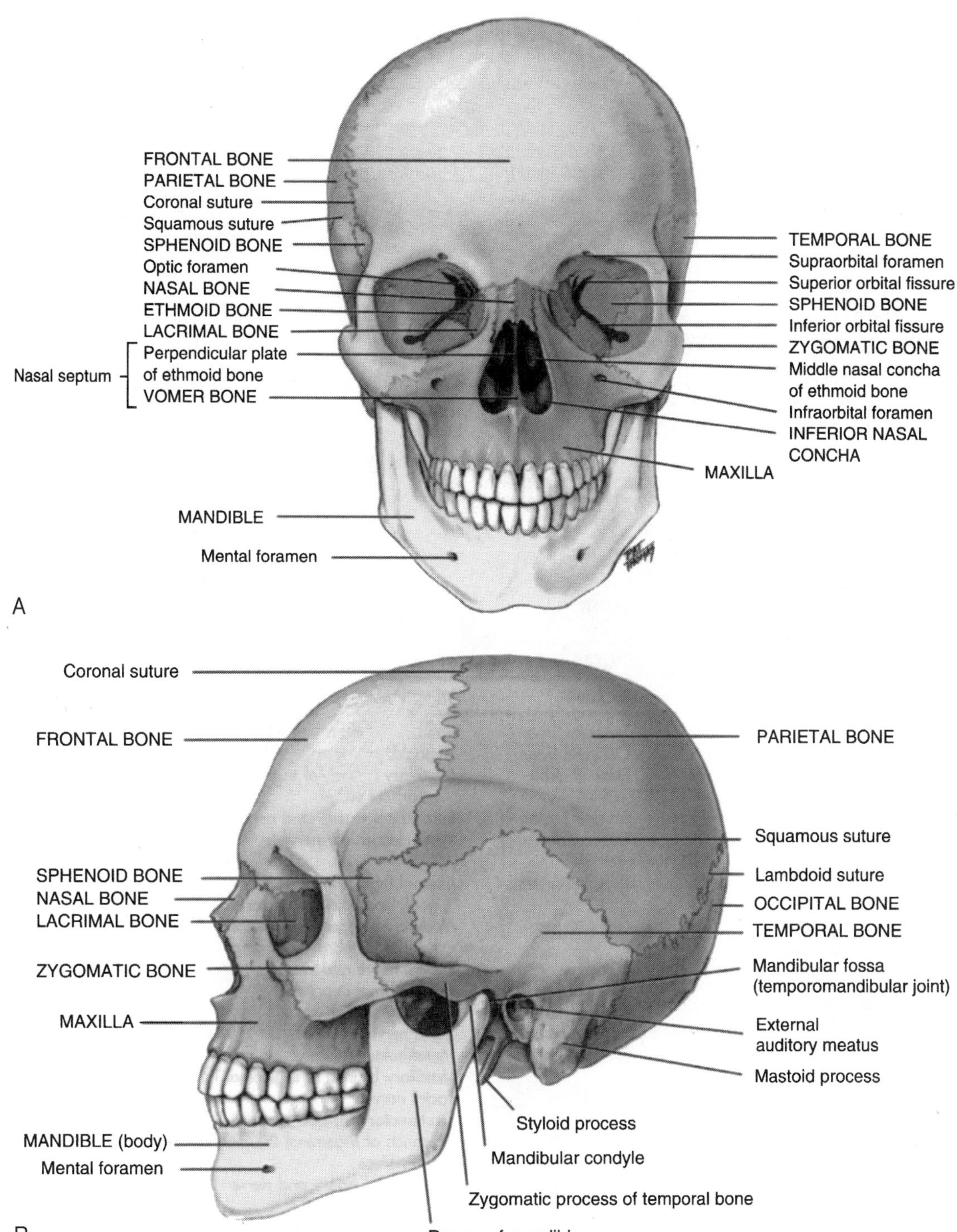

Figure 31–2. *A*, Anterior view of the skull. *B*, Inferior view of the skull. (*A* and *B*, From Applegate EJ: The Anatomy and Physiology Learning System, 2nd ed. Philadelphia: WB Saunders, 1995, p 103.)

three branches that supply sensation to other areas of the mouth and face. The lingual nerve provides sensation to the anterior two thirds of the tongue and the floor of the mouth and gums. The inferior alveolar nerve provides sensation to the premolar and molar teeth of the mandible, and the mental nerve provides sensation to the lower lip and chin.

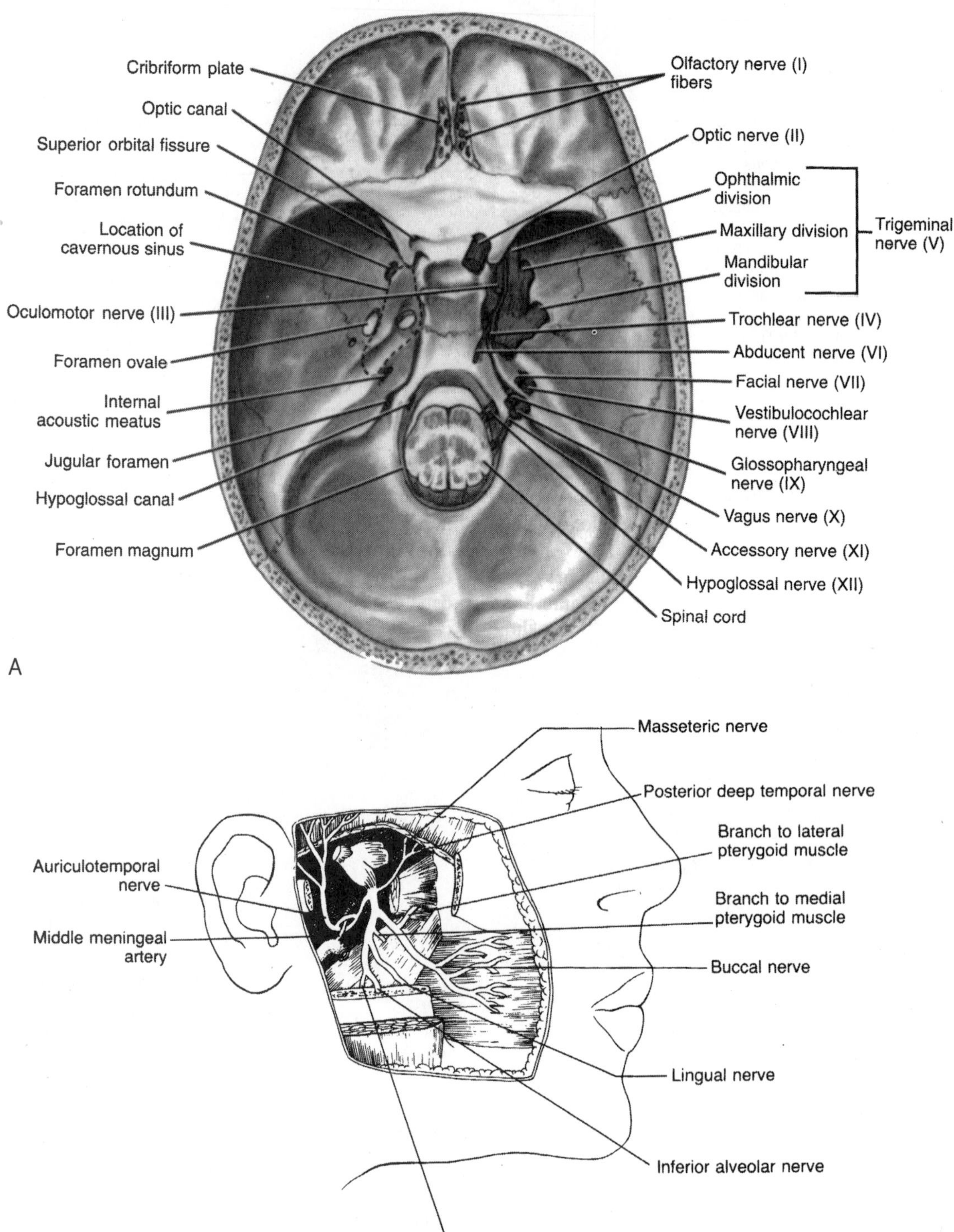

Figure 31–3. *A*, Internal view of the base of the skull showing cranial nerves exiting or entering the skull. (From Fehrenbach MJ, Herring SW: Illustrated Anatomy of the Head and Neck. Philadelphia: WB Saunders, 1996, p 193.) *B*, Mandibular division of the trigeminal nerve. (From Fonseca RJ, et al: Oral and Maxillofacial Trauma, 2nd ed. Philadelphia: WB Saunders, 1997, p 281.)

The mandible and maxilla constitute the bony structure of the jaw. The mandible is a horseshoe-shaped bone that forms the lower jaw. It is the largest and strongest bone in the face. This bone articulates with the TMJ. The maxilla is an irregularly shaped bone that forms the upper jaw. This bone touches every other facial bone except the mandible. It forms the orbit, the nasal cavity, and the palate, and it supports the upper teeth.

Although the TMJ can be compared with other joints in the body, there are distinct differences. The TMJ is a bicondylar joint that is formed by the glenoid fossa of the temporal bone and the mandibular condyle. The meniscus (disk) of connective tissue lies between the bone structures. A capsule of the joint is reinforced laterally by the temporomandibular ligament, which limits the anterior and posterior condylar movements.

Oral and maxillofacial procedures can be restorative or therapeutic or elective or urgent. Examples include dental extractions (odondectomy) or implants, fracture reduction, incision and drainage of abscesses or cysts, and excision of tumors or lesions (Table 31–1). Lasers are used for oral and maxillofacial surgical procedures. Uses include coagulation of angiomatous lesions or TMJ arthroscopy.[1] The nursing care needs of patients undergoing oral and maxillofacial procedures include maintaining the airway and managing nausea and vomiting related to swallowed blood, bad breath, and an unpleasant taste in the mouth. Patients may also experience difficulty chewing and talking after surgery.

Uncooperative patients, small children, and patients who are physically or mentally infirm may be unable to withstand procedures that, under normal circumstances, are performed in an office. These people may be candidates for ambulatory surgical procedures, such as dental extractions or fillings. Procedures that require use of the laser might also be scheduled in the operating room because of equipment availability.

***Table 31–1.* Oral/Maxillofacial Surgery—Terminology**

Alveolectomy	Radical surgical reduction or removal of the alveolar process
Alveoplasty	Bone conserving, surgical contouring, or remodeling of the residual ridge to achieve a denture-bearing surface
Arch bars	Rigid metal bars used to splint and fix the teeth, maxilla, or mandible
Dental implant	A prosthetic implant with an anchoring structure surgically implanted subperiosteally or endosteally
Genioplasty	Correction of chin deformities
Gingivectomy	Removal of all loose, infected, and diseased gingival tissue
Intraoral biopsy	Excisional or incisional removal of abnormal tissue for histiopathologic examination
Marsupialization	Creating an accessory cavity to encourage repair and regeneration; used to eliminate the closed condition of a cyst
Odontectomy	Tooth extraction; can be single or multiple; may be needed because of trauma, recurrent infections, or nonresorbable teeth or to prepare for implants
Vestibuloplasty	Alveolar ridge augmentation for the purpose of making a residual ridge available to use as a denture-bearing surface

PREOPERATIVE CARE

Patients will present with symptoms related to their diagnoses. After a review of systems, the perioperative nurse assesses the facial and oral structures to determine a baseline status. The nurse should observe how far the patient can open his or her mouth and should look for trismus (limited opening), lumps, facial swelling, and skin color and texture. The nurse should assess the intraoral cavity and the tongue for size, mobility, color, and texture. The oral mucosa, alveolar ridges, gingivae, and teeth should also be assessed. The patency of the airway should be verified, and neck mobility should be established. Nutritional status, including that during the preoperative fasting period, should be determined, because pain or injury to the oral and maxillofacial structures might result in decreased desire or inability to eat. Patients should be adequately hydrated before the procedure.

Patient allergies, including possible latex allergy, should be verified. Laboratory values for coagulation or other studies and radiographs or computed tomography scan results should be available. Patients should be asked about previous problems with bleeding and a history of oral surgery procedures to determine reactions to local anesthesia, delayed healing, or alveolalgia ("dry socket"). The patient should sign a consent form and verbally communicate that he or she understands the procedure and risks. One risk that patients must understand is that numbness can occur because of nerve damage. Patients might require preoperative antibiotics if dental implants are planned or if the patient has a history of endocardial damage or valvular surgery.[2] Antibiotics should be systemically infused before the surgery.[3]

Patients should be prepared for the possibility of bloody oral drainage and should secure appropriate supplies for home, including cool and soft foods and beverages, medications prescribed by the physician, and cold therapy (an ice pack), although this may be provided to the patient at the surgery center. Discharge planning should also include general postoperative instructions related to pain management, symptoms to report, and activities.

Patients might be concerned, anxious, or fearful about their resultant body image or might show concern about undergoing a surgical procedure. Many procedures can be done through an incision in the oral cavity; therefore, scarring is not an issue. Patient teaching is important to increase the patient's understanding of the expected outcomes and participation in postoperative care. The perioperative nurses should assess the patient's need for information and the petient's ability to understand instructions.

INTRAOPERATIVE CARE

Patients will be anesthetized using monitored anesthesia care or general anesthesia. Nasal or nasotracheal intubation is commonly used to eliminate interference with the surgical procedure. A moist packing is used to occlude the posterior pharynx. If monitored anesthesia care is required, the choices of agents are

- Midazolam to decrease the emergence of delirium
- Ketamine (glycopyrrolate) to decrease oral secretions and the risk of respiratory depression
- Benzodiazepine with fentanyl
- Propofol or methohexital

Local anesthesia can be used as an adjunct during general anesthesia to minimize bleeding in the operative field, ease dissection, allow for less anesthetic agent, and minimize immediate postoperative pain.

Although every effort is made to maintain aseptic technique, the mouth is an area that harbors pathogens. Prevention of infection is important because a postoperative infection can result in the loss of bone and teeth, endocarditis, loss of implants, or scarring. A steroid medication such as dexamethasone is often given intravenously to reduce edema and inflammation.[4] A sterile field is created, and sterile instruments are used to prevent the introduction of pathogens and also to prevent cross-contamination. A petroleum-based ointment may be used to lubricate the patient's lips to prevent them from cracking. When retracting the mouth to gain operative access, attention must be given to avoid injury to the lips and tongue, because it is easy for them to be pinched owing to the small area of visualization. Hemostatic agents may be requested to manage intraoral bleeding.

At the end of the procedure, the oral cavity is suctioned and pressure packs are placed. The nurse should document the removal of the throat pack and the accuracy of the sponge count, because the patient's airway could be fatally compromised if any foreign object is inadvertently left in place. Sponges may be placed between the patient's teeth or gums and the lip to provide pressure on incisions, but they must be monitored constantly until the patient is alert enough to be aware of their presence and to maintain an adequate airway. An oral or nasal airway may be inserted for transfer to the postanesthesia care unit.

POSTOPERATIVE CARE

The postoperative nurse should receive a report from the anesthesia care provider and intraoperative nurse. Information that should be shared includes the type of procedure, the presence and type of splints, and the location of packing and sutures that were used. If the jaws are wired, wire cutters should be immediately available in the event that the patient vomits or respiratory distress occurs.

Careful postoperative assessment of respiratory status, blood pressure, and pulse, as well as observation of facial and oral structures for changes, is important. Suction should be available in the event that bleeding occurs or secretions collect in the oral cavity. The patient is positioned to facilitate drainage of saliva or bloody secretions. Because of the procedure or local anesthesia that is used, the patient may experience difficulty swallowing. Monitoring vital signs and looking in the oral cavity can help to ensure that there is hemostasis. After some oral and maxillofacial procedures, pressure may be maintained on the surgical sites by having the patient bite gently on folded gauze 4 × 4 pads or 2 × 2-in sponges. Gauze should not be cut for this use, because frayed edges could allow threads to come off in the mouth. Swallowed blood can result in nausea and vomiting. The pressure can increase the chance of bleeding.

Other potential problems after oral and maxillofacial procedures include infection; nerve damage with temporary or permanent paresis of the lips, mouth, or face; inadvertent puncture of the maxillary sinus; damage to other teeth[5]; rarely, fracture of the jaw,[6] and edema. Analgesics should be given to minimize pain. Physicians should be consulted about the use of ice packs on the area of the surgical site for edema owing to the possibility of a rebound effect (increased blood flow) that might occur after the ice pack is removed.

Postoperative edema is expected. At home, the patient should continue intermittent use of ice packs on the jaws for the first 24 to 48 hours or longer to reduce edema and promote healing. Periorbital ecchymosis, swelling of the jaw and cheeks, mouth discomfort, and inability to open the mouth wide are common occurrences. An oral analgesic is usually prescribed for pain, and the patient is warned to avoid taking aspirin in the early postoperative period. Antiemetics, antibiotics, and analgesics (nonsteroidal anti-inflammatory drugs) are usually ordered; medication regimens should be reviewed with the patient.

Swallowing of blood sometimes results in nausea and vomiting. In turn, patients do not want to eat, and their nutritional status and hydration can be compromised. Patients should understand the need to meet nutritional requirements for healing, and they should be encouraged to use antiemetics or other strategies to reduce nausea. Patients will resume a diet appropriate for their procedure. If the procedure is aggressive, the patient can have a clear to full liquid high-calorie diet as tolerated. Some patients might return to a soft (nonchewing) or regular diet. The patient should avoid temperature extremes in food and beverages. Soft foods may or may not be allowed depending on the type of surgery performed. Patients should be taught oral hygiene. For bad breath or taste, the physician may allow the patient to gently rinse with salt water or a commercial mouthwash, but a specific physician's order should be obtained before this instruction. After a tooth extraction, the protective blood clot over the socket may be lost with vigorous gargling or rinsing, resulting in a "dry socket," which exposes the bone and causes severe pain.

The patient may be wearing a prosthetic device in the mouth postoperatively. The nurse should check its proper position and ensure that it does not compromise the airway prior to the patient's discharge. The patient must understand the proper use and care of any device that has been fitted, including whether removal of the device is allowed, necessary cleaning, and the potential problems or restrictions while the prosthesis is in place. If the jaw is stabilized with wires or bands, the patient should be taught how to cut the wires or bands in the event of respiratory distress or vomiting. The patient may also be instructed on how to use dental wax to reduce mucosal irritation (Table 31–2).

***Table 31–2.* Key Education Points**

Report symptoms of infection: increased temperature; pain that cannot be relieved; bleeding from the surgery site.
Keep ice packs on the surgical area for at least 72 hours.
Limit excess movement and lowering the head.
Avoid nose blowing; wipe secretions from the nose.
Do not swallow through straws.
Spit rather than swallow secretions.
Eat small, frequent meals.
Perform oral care and rinse the mouth frequently.
Cut wires or bands if the mouth is secured closed and difficulty in breathing occurs.
Use medications (e.g., analgesics, antibiotics, antihistamines) per the physician's orders.

DENTAL EXTRACTION, INCISION AND DRAINAGE, EXCISION OF NONMALIGNANT TUMORS OR LESIONS

The extraction of teeth involves bony and soft tissues of the oral cavity. Patients might require surgery in an ambulatory surgical center because of their systemic conditions, the extent of the procedure, or anticipated difficulties in removing the teeth that can be managed easier and more comfortably with sedation or anesthesia. Reasons for the extraction might include severe loss of bone structure supporting the teeth, teeth that interfere mechanically with placement of a restorative appliance (i.e., dentures), fractured roots, or nonvital pulps. An alveoplasty or vestibuloplasty might be required, depending on the patient's anatomy.

An abscess or infected area, cyst, tumor, or lesion can form in any area of the oral cavity. Abscesses that will not respond to antibiotics and must be drained or cysts that must be excised are examples of symptoms of patients who might require surgical intervention in the ambulatory surgical center (ASC) for the benefit of having monitored anesthesia care or general anesthesia. Patients might present with symptoms of swelling or pain, depending on the size and location of the abscess or cyst. It is common to culture the drainage to identify the specific bacteria causing the problem. If an abscess is large and there is concern that healing might be difficult, a wound drain might be inserted.

Cysts are a pouch or sac without an opening that contains fluid. Types of cysts include developmental, neoplastic, and retention cysts. Treatment can require complete extraction or the creation of a window in the bone to allow permanent drainage and regrowth of the area (marsupialization).

Nonmalignant tumors or abnormal growths can be found in numerous areas of the oral cavity. These lesions can form in the soft tissue (i.e., gingiva, buccal mucosa, tongue) or bone (i.e., maxilla, mandible, palate). Examples include hyperplasia, fibromas, chondroma, papilloma, or dermoid cysts.[7] An incisional (removing a representative area) or excisional (removing the total lesion) biopsy might require a histiopathologic (frozen section) examination. Exostoses or tori (bone outgrowths) might also occur on the alveolar ridges, palate, or other bone areas requiring excision.

The parotid, submandibular, sublingual, and accessory glands supply saliva through ducts to the oral cavity. The lingual nerves are in close relationship to the submandibular ducts. Tumors, cysts, stones, or trauma may affect salivary glands. Surgery on the ducts is the method of choice to treat lesions of accessory salivary glands, to manage malignant lesions, or to correct traumatic injury.

Postoperative care of these patients varies based on the patient's need for surgery. Airway management is a priority initially and on a long-term basis, because edema could result and requires immediate attention.

DENTAL RESTORATION AND IMPLANTS

The placement of dental implants is a restorative procedure for the permanent anchoring of prosthetic teeth. Implants are placed to improve function, provide comfort, and improve esthetics and emotional and psychological attitude.[8] The procedure provides more natural-appearing and natural-feeling teeth than that provided by traditional dentures. Patients must understand the risks, limitations, cost, and time commitment of implant restorations.[9]

Implant fixtures can be used to anchor single or multiple replacement teeth. The implant fixtures are either buried beneath the mucosal layer or implanted in the periosteal layer (subperiosteal) or in the bone. The dental implant (replacement tooth) fixture is inserted approximately 4 weeks to several months after the insertion of implant fixtures, depending on the time appropriate for the type of implant being used. Implant fixtures are made of titanium, ceramic, or polymer.[10]

Patients undergo the procedure with monitored anesthesia care or a general anesthetic. A local anesthetic is often injected to aid hemostasis and postoperative analgesia. The bone canal is prepared using power equipment. Screws, commonly called implant fixtures, are screwed into the bone of the mandible and maxilla very gently to avoid damage to the bone surrounding the implant.[11] Because the local anesthesia for dental work can spread to nearby structures, the nurse must ensure that the patient is able to swallow properly prior to discharge from the ASC.

The benefits of dental implants over traditional dentures include decreased pain from ill-fitting dentures, improved sense of taste, better dentition and digestion, improved psychological attitude, a more natural look and feel, and sometimes a reduction in problems involving the temporomandibular joint. Oral hygiene is imperative for the success of implants.

TEMPOROMANDIBULAR JOINT ARTHROSCOPY

TMJ disease and dysfunction consists of several conditions. Congenital or developmental deformities of the condylar head, early ankylosis, neoplasia, septic arthritis, or degenerative disease might cause symptoms. It can also be injured by trauma. The TMJ is similar to other joints in that it requires satisfactory function between the disk and bone elements of the joint.

Arthroscopic intervention for TMJ dysfunction has been used in the United States since 1983. Both diagnosis and treatment are possible arthroscopically. It has been reported as an effective technique for treating various stages of internal derangement.[12] Fibrous adhesions in the joint can be lysed, débridements performed, and the disk repositioned through the arthroscope. Often, simple lavage of the joints seems to have a therapeutic effect on decreasing joint symptoms.[13]

Patients who are treated arthroscopically have usually tried more conservative medical treatments without success. Jaw pain, persistent headaches, mechanical restriction, and difficulty in chewing and opening the mouth are typical presenting symptoms. Counseling is important before surgery so that the patient is well informed of the expected outcomes of surgery and the potential risks (e.g., perforation of the external auditory canal and damage to cranial nerve VII with resultant facial paralysis).[14] Insurance reimbursement for TMJ surgery may be restricted; this restriction also creates a financial hardship for the patient.

Before the patient's admission, an occlusive splint is fitted and the patient, surgeon, or the surgeon's staff member usually brings it to the ASC. This appliance is worn in the mouth postoperatively to relieve pressure on the jaw muscles and to maintain proper occlusion.

Intraoperatively, the patient's position is supine. Procedure times vary, depending on the amount of work that is accomplished. Most patients undergo bilateral procedures. Pressure dressings are replaced after 1 to 2 hours with smaller adhesive bandages prior to discharge from the ASC.

Postoperative discomfort may require the use of analgesics. Elevation of the patient's head helps to relieve feelings of pressure, and ice is used to reduce or prevent swelling and reduce pain after the surgery. Physiotherapy to correct trismus may be required after the patient is discharged. At home, the patient often changes to use of moist heat on the following day. The diet is restricted to full liquids for the first 7 to 10 days and is then advanced to foods that require no chewing. It is important for the patient to wear the occlusal splint continuously, to follow instructions regarding diet and activity restrictions, and to take all prescribed medications.[14]

FRACTURE REDUCTION

Closed and open reductions of the mandible can be done in the outpatient setting. A simple fracture can be repaired using general anesthesia and with application of a stabilizing device, such as elastic bands or wires. Arch bars provide maxillomandibular fixation. Numerous interdental eyelet wires (Ivy loop technique) can be placed on the posterior teeth to serve as attachment sites for wires or elastic bands. The wires or splints secure the mandible and maxilla to bring the teeth into normal occlusion.

Open reduction of fractures using plates, screws, or wire might be used to repair a fractured mandible or maxilla or a zygomatic fracture. Frequently, the incision can take place through the oral cavity. The fracture site is exposed, and bone is approximated. The securing devices are applied. Although the patient's tissue is manipulated to implant the securing devices, unless there is concern about the patient's ability to care for himself or herself, airway management, or postoperative bleeding, these patients are candidates for the outpatient setting.

Airway assessment immediately postoperatively is important, because the jaws are wired or elastic bands are applied to secure the jaw in a closed position. Patients are taught about diet and nutrition because they are unable to eat a regular diet or perform oral hygiene or take action in the event of airway difficulties. The use of adequate pain control and cold therapy (ice packs) should be reviewed.

References

1. Bradley PF: A review of the use of the neodymium YAG laser in oral and maxillofacial surgery. Br J Oral Maxillofac Surg 35:26–35, 1997.
2. Archer WH: Oral and Maxillofacial Surgery, 5th ed. Philadelphia: WB Saunders, 1975, p 706.
3. Peterson LJ, Thomas A, Indresano R, et al: Principles of Oral and Maxillofacial Surgery. Philadelphia: JB Lippincott, 1992, pp 35–52. CDC, Guideline for Prevention of Surgical Site Infection, 1999. Am J Infect Control April, 1999, p 108.
4. Steuer K, Addante R, Strong J: Impacted third molars. AORN J 49:1363–1366, 1368–1369, 1989.
5. Ibid.
6. Gustafson N: Wisdom Teeth. Patient Information Library. Daly City, CA: Krames Communications, 1985.
7. Archer WH: Oral and Maxillofacial Surgery, 5th ed. Philadelphia: WB Saunders, 1975, p 423.
8. Pederson GW: Oral Surgery. Philadelphia: WB Saunders, 1988, pp 237–251.
9. Nishimura RD, Beumer J: Implants in the partially edentulous patient: Restorative considerations. Oral Health 10:19–28, 1998.
10. Hobkirk JA, Watson RN: Dental and Maxillofacial Implantology. London: Mosby-Wolfe, 1975.
11. Garg AK: Augmentation grafting of the maxillary sinus for placement of dental implants. Implant Dentistry 8:36–46, 1999.
12. Murakami KI, Tsuboi Y, Bessho K, et al: Outcome of arthroscopic surgery to the temporomandibular joint correlates with stage of internal derangement: Five-year follow-up study. Br J Maxillofac Surg 36:30–34, 1998.
13. Sanders B: Arthroscopic surgery of the temporomandibular joint: Treatment in internal derangement with persistent closed lock. Oral Surgery 62:361, 1986.
14. Bare V: Temporomandibular joint arthroscopy. AORN J 45:1368–1373, 1987.

Suggested Readings

Alpern MC, Wharton MC: The role of arthroscopy in the management of temporomandibular disorders. Oral Surg

Oral Med Oral Pathol Oral Radiol Endod 83:163–166, 1997.

Dolwick, MF: The role of temporomandibular joint surgery in the treatment of patients with internal derangement. Oral Surg Oral Med Oral Pathol Oral Radiol Endod 83:150–155, 1997.

Gerard MW, Laughon MM, Colley JL, et al: Trends in temporomandibular joint surgery. Med Prog Technol 21:171–175, 1996.

Go WS, Teh LY, Peck RH: Clinical experiences in temporomandibular joint arthroscopy. Ann Acad Med Singapore 25:679–682, 1996.

Israel HA: The use of arthroscopic surgery for treatment of temporomandibular joint disorders. Br J Oral Maxillofac Surg 57:579–582, 1999.

Quinn DM: Ambulatory Surgical Nursing Core Curriculum. Philadelphia: WB Saunders, 1999.

Rosenberg I, Goss AN: The outcome of arthroscopic treatment of temporomandibular joint arthropathy. Aust Dent J 44:106–111, 1999.

Chapter 

Plastic and Reconstructive Surgery

Joyce M. Black and Jeanne Prin

The types and extent of procedures available today and in the future are bounded only by the imagination and creativity of plastic and reconstructive surgeons. Modern technologic developments have resulted in the availability of procedures such as laser removal of skin laxity, birthmarks, and tattoos and tissue expansion to provide a suitable amount of skin to cover a defect without the use of a graft from a distant donor site. Patients range in age from infancy to elderly and present with a diversity of backgrounds and clinical needs.

Procedures in an ambulatory surgery center (ASC) range from simple cutaneous excisions to more complex procedures such as face-lifts and breast reductions. Often the patient is able to return directly home postoperatively, but more complicated procedures may be followed by an overnight stay at the surgeon's office with nursing care or at a recovery care center. These approaches are still more cost-effective than hospitalization, although that is another option for postoperative care. Because many plastic surgery procedures are not covered by insurance, cost is an important issue for the patient.

For ASC nurses to provide support and enhance the patient's self-esteem, it is important that they first examine their personal feelings and attitudes about plastic and reconstructive surgery to gain insight about the way that they react to and interact with patients who seek cosmetic changes. It is important to understand that there is often no direct relationship between the extent of the physical characteristic being altered and the level of psychological disturbance that it may create in the patient. Although some people handle extensive problems like burn scars or major facial defects with inner strength and determination, others can be quite affected emotionally by even minor actual or perceived defects.[1]

The specialty of plastic surgery often brings a pleasant climate to an ASC. Generally, patients are enthusiastic and happy because the surgery is the culmination of a personal desire or goal that they have sought for a long time. Most tend to show a high level of cooperation with the care plan and interest in following instructions.

On the other end of the spectrum are those people for whom the procedure is only a first step to wellness, for instance, patients beginning the long course of reconstruction after burns, trauma, or disfiguring surgeries for malignancies. These patients are often struggling with diverse emotions: hope for the future versus fear of disease recurrence; eagerness to see the final cosmetic results versus the despair at the pain and suffering that they must still endure along that path; and weariness of illness versus affirmation of wellness.

PREOPERATIVE CARE

Before scheduling patients for plastic surgery, the surgeon and clinic nurse carefully assess the patients' motivations and expectations. Often, the patient has thought about and debated having the cosmetic procedure for many months or years and may still have reservations about the decision to proceed. Common reasons for seeking cosmetic surgery include uncomfortableness during activities where the body is exposed, embarrassment about developing close relationships, anger over being teased, and inability to buy attractive clothing.[2] Possible reasons for the difficulty in making a decision include fear of pain or the anesthetic, feeling unworthy of the procedure, fear of the reaction of others and what others will think, and financial constraints.

Men requesting cosmetic or reconstructive procedures present some special psychological needs. Although esthetic surgery for men is generally well accepted today, men may be embarrassed when requesting surgery because of traditional cultural restrictions. Pressure to compete with younger and perhaps more attractive peers in the business and social world affects men as well as women. Although there is a scarcity of recent research specific to the male esthetic surgery patient, one study of 1000 men found the factors that most frequently motivated men to seek cosmetic surgery were to look younger and more attractive, to improve body image, to increase self-confidence, and to satisfy the man or his partner.[2a]

Parents of children with congenital deformities often need special support in handling feelings of grief and guilt. They must deal not only with the child's physical defects and special care needs but also with lingering doubts and questions about why their child was afflicted. They may feel totally responsible for acquired defects (e.g., burns or lacerations) even when these defects are the result of an accident. Often parents may feel that they should or could have prevented the accident that injured their child. In addition, the parents may feel guilty or confused about putting the child through the additional pain and stress of surgery. These complex psychological issues illustrate that the parents, as well as the child, are greatly in need of nursing care and support and may also require professional psychological counseling.

The nurse in the ASC should appreciate and use the special relationship that many patients form with the plastic surgical nurse in the surgeon's office. This relationship is often closer than one would see in other types of surgical office nursing specialties as the patient becomes comfortable relating personal goals, fears, and desires to the office nurse. The ASC nurse should encourage and support that relationship in dialogues with the patient and should use the plastic surgical nurse as a resource when planning nursing care. Often the office nurse can provide valuable insight into the patient's social and psychological needs that may otherwise escape the ASC nurse because of the short-term nature of the nurse-patient contact in the ASC.

Privacy is another important perioperative consideration. All patients expect and deserve privacy, but cosmetic surgery patients are often exceptionally concerned that other people in the center will see them or will discuss their surgery with outsiders. The nurse should reassure patients that their need for confidentiality will be strictly honored.

Other preparations for surgery concentrate on the patient's physical needs. Some patients who are extraordinarily concerned with physical appearance may have a long history of extreme eating patterns, including many diets and periods of fasting or starvation. Chemistry studies are important to identify physiologic chemical imbalances that could be harmful perioperatively. The surgeon's office personnel usually secure needed photography and consents. Skin marking by the surgeon is frequently done with the patient sitting or standing. This provides the surgeon with more accurate landmarks and reference points that may be obscured with the patient in a supine position. The ASC must provide both time and privacy protected space for this preoperative marking.

INTRAOPERATIVE CARE

The perioperative nurse addresses all the usual principles of intraoperative nursing care to ensure that the patient's physical and psychological needs are met, including continued sensitivity regarding the patient's need for privacy and confidentiality. Safety measures are employed to ensure that environmental dangers are reduced. The variety of surgical equipment that may be used during surgery includes lasers, electrocautery, extremity tourniquets, and suction lipectomy apparatus. The perioperative nurse must be familiar with the operation and risks associated with each. The use of local anesthesia with epinephrine and associated nursing care has been previously described in Chapter 14.

Because plastic and reconstructive procedures can be lengthy, special attention must be given to the patient's proper anatomic positioning and methods to maintain normal body temperature, skin integrity, and hemodynamic stability. Gel rolls on the operating room (OR) bed can help to alleviate pressure on bony prominences such as the elbows, heels, coccyx, and occiput. Periodic passive range of motion exercises of the legs may be performed during procedures that last for 2 hours. Awake patients may be asked to actively exercise their legs at intervals. Pneumatic compression devices may also be used to prevent the development of deep vein thrombosis during longer procedures and when the patient is asleep.

In procedures involving the scalp, face, or neck, extreme care must be taken to protect the corneas of sedated and anesthetized patients.

POSTOPERATIVE CARE

After many esthetic procedures, bleeding is a threat owing to the high vascularity of the skin, particularly on the face and scalp and also because of the extensive amount of skin that may have been undermined from deeper structures during surgery. At best, the formation of a hematoma can delay healing. At worst, it can lead to significantly altered blood flow to tissue flaps with resultant necrosis and breakdown of the surgical site. Large hematomas and ones that encroach on the airway or optic nerve require that the patient be returned to surgery for immediate evacuation.

The nurse must identify, treat, and, whenever possible, avoid bleeding problems early in their course. The patient requires special observation for edema, ecchymosis, circulatory compromise, hypertensive episodes, or hematoma formation under restrictive bandages that may completely encircle the head, torso, or an extremity. Smoking is particularly detrimental to healing. Use of nicotine leads to peripheral vasoconstriction.[3] Areas along incision lines that are under most tension are known to develop necrosis.

Another potential consequence of plastic or reconstructive surgery is nerve damage. This can occur as a result of direct trauma by instrumentation, inadvertent severing of a nerve, or pressure from edema or hematomas. Nerve damage can be permanent or temporary and can result in sensory or motor loss, or both.

It is important for patients to be aware that a temporary period of depression may follow cosmetic surgery. When this is anticipated and recognized as a normal event in the healing process, the patient is less likely to become alarmed or frightened by it.[4] Preoperative counseling in the physician's office includes a discussion of this possibility. Typically, depression occurs near the second or third postoperative day, but it may occur as late as 2 to 3 weeks after surgery.[5]

One possible reason for postoperative depression is the self-imposed isolation of a patient who remains at home for a lengthy period of recuperation to avoid publicizing the fact that he or she has had cosmetic surgery. This allows a long time for introspection and may contribute to feelings of loneliness. Flaws and postoperative occurrences (e.g., swelling and bruising) may become magnified in the patient's mind. The nurse can suggest to the patient various ways to reduce or eliminate this occurrence, for instance, having worthwhile home projects planned for the period of recuperation, keeping in contact with supportive friends or relatives, using the time for contacting out-of-town friends and family by letters or telephone calls, or taking scenic drives.[5]

TISSUE EXPANSION

Tissue expansion has found application in numerous reconstruction procedures. The pregnant abdomen is the most obvious example of natural tissue expansion and has provided the conceptual basis for current therapy. Although this is a technique rather than a specific procedure, it is discussed here because the concept is used widely in reconstructive procedures. Tissue expansion provides adequate skin coverage for reconstruction of defects without the need to harvest donor tissue from a distant site. The technique is useful in reconstructive breast procedures or when large areas of trauma or lesions result in extensive defects in the skin.

The tissue expander is implanted under the skin next to the area in need of donor tissue. It is filled slowly over a period of time (often several months). The recommended amount of fluid to inject on each subsequent visit for the expansion is 10% to 15% of the total expanded volume. The average interval between injections varies with the site and the amount of skin involved but is approximately every 3 to 9 days. The gradual expansion of the overlying skin is accompanied by an increase in its vascularity. The epidermal thickness remains constant, and thus there is no thinning of the tissues, which is an important feature of the technique.

Some procedures lend themselves to intraoperative tissue expansion. An expander is inserted, inflated to stretch surrounding tissues, and then removed. The expanded tissue is used for reconstruction. This form of tissue expansion does not usually extend beyond 250 ml.

There are both advantages and disadvantages to the use of tissue expanders. The most obvious advantage is the availability of skin that matches in color and texture and has a good blood supply directly adjacent to a defect requiring a graft. This is a simpler approach than the harvesting of donor tissue, which then leaves a defect in another part of the body. There is little risk involved in the procedure, and overall cost efficiency is good because of reduced hospitalization times. Disadvantages include the time element and multiple trips required for the slow expansion of tissue before its use for the intended grafting procedure and the often unappealing esthetic appearance during the expansion period.

Complications are not frequent but include the possibility of infection, hematoma, skin necrosis, expander extrusion, capsular contracture around the expander, deflation, and seroma, which is the accumulation of fluid around the exterior of the expander. Prophylactic antibiotics and wound drains are used to discourage the occurrence of seroma. The most common problem is extrusion of the expander. To reduce the chance of extrusion, tissue expanders should not be implanted in areas with inherently poor blood flow when inflammation or infection is present; furthermore, dressings should not be overly constrictive.

BREAST AUGMENTATION

The first documented breast augmentation was done in 1895 when a surgeon transferred a lipoma from a woman's back to fill in a breast defect. Other physicians followed suit using transplanted fat, paraffin, and other substances, and in the early 1960s, the silicone gel implant was developed. Recent reports of connective tissue diseases linked to leakage of silicone gel have resulted in a shift back to the use of saline-filled prostheses for most women.[6] Although no scientific evidence currently exists to support a linkage of connective tissue disease, silicone gel implants are available only from surgeons involved in randomized clinical trials.[7, 7a, 7b] Perceived problems with breast implants have been aired openly on many daytime talk shows and evening news programs. The intense media "hype" has made many women anxious. The nurse working with women who desire augmentation must keep up-to-date in lay and professional literature on this issue.[8]

Indications for breast augmentation include hypoplasia of breast tissue, asymmetry, trauma, and the patient's desired enhancement of breast size. Augmentation does not adequately correct the ptosis of the breast if the nipple is at or below the inframammary crease, in which case the augmentation procedure may be combined with a mastopexy to lift and reposition the nipple.

Various implantation techniques exist for placement of the incisions and the prostheses. Incisions may be inframammary, axillary, or semicircular around the lower half of the areolar outline. Implants can also be inserted endoscopically through an umbilical incision.[9, 9a] The surgeon's objective is to ensure that postoperative scars are in locations where they will be unnoticed. The inframammary approach is the simplest, and the axillary incision provides the least visible scar postoperatively. However, the axillary approach is associated with web-like scars when patients do not move their arms after surgery.

The breast implant can be placed beneath the mammary tissue or under the muscle layer of the chest. With the latter technique, the pectoralis major and serratus anterior muscles completely cover the implant (Fig. 32–1). Although there is controversy regarding the best site for prosthesis placement, many practitioners believe that positioning beneath the muscle provides the most natural appearance.

Before obtaining consent, the surgeon informs the patient of possible complications. Bleeding, hematoma formation, asymmetry, hypertrophic scarring (mainly in Asian and black patients), implant rupture, temporary or permanent decrease in nipple sensitivity, infection, capsule formation, and extrusion of the implant can occur. Breast cancer is not a complication of breast augmentation; in fact, all statistical studies and in vitro studies have demonstrated a lack of relationship between breast implants and breast cancer.[7b, 10, 10a] Breast-feeding usually remains possible after augmentation.[11]

The scar tissue encapsulation of prostheses (called capsules) that results in firmer-than-desired breasts cannot be adequately explained by any one or two causes; rather, it is believed to be an expected result of healing of a compressed foreign body rather than a true complication. To help prevent encapsulation of the implants by scar tissue contracture, some surgeons inject a long-acting steroid into the pocket or the lumen of the implant during placement to suppress local inflammatory response. Others have used antibiotics, double-lumen implants, varying sized pockets for placement, textured-surface implants, and other approaches to reduce the frequency and degree of encapsulation.

Many surgeons recommend massage of the breasts starting about 2 weeks postoperatively and continuing for up to 1 year after surgery. The theory of the massage technique is that

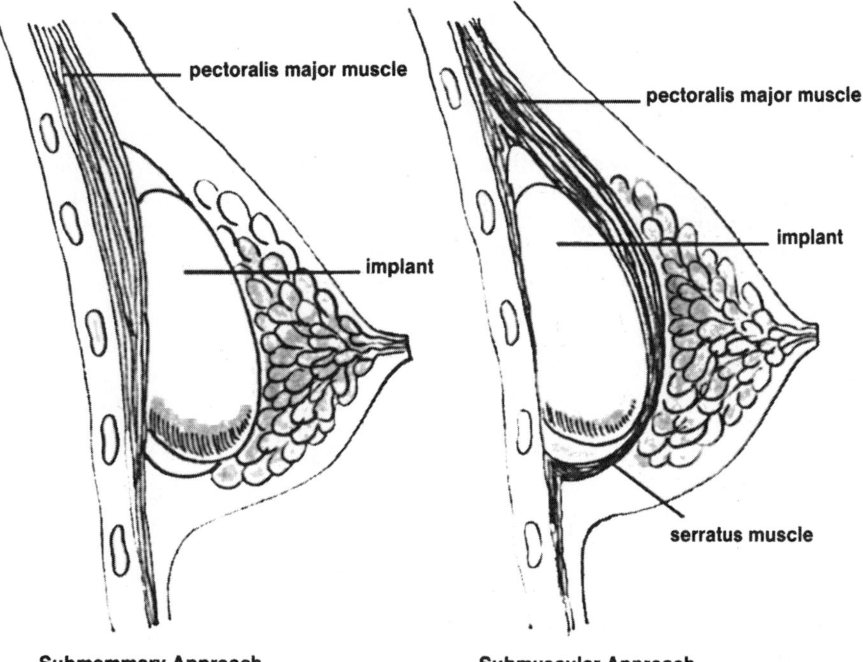

Figure 32–1. Prosthesis placement implants can be placed in a submammary or submuscular position. The most common site is beneath the pectoralis major and serratus anterior muscle. Both muscles are used to cover the implant completely. The other option for placement is submammary with the implant on the anterior surface of the pectoralis muscle. (From Thomas C: Perioperative considerations for the augmentation mammaplasty patient. Plast Surg Nurs 8[3]:93, 1988.)

purposeful movement of the implant helps to maintain the intended size of the pocket into which it was placed. During the early weeks of recuperation, the patient may be instructed by her physician to avoid wearing a brassière to allow free movement of the breast as another tactic to reduce capsule formation. Despite all these theories and attempts to avoid capsule formation, about 10% or more of all patients experience some degree of firmness.

Implant encapsulation can be treated by open capsulotomy. If open surgical correction is necessary, it may be advisable to wait at least 6 months for the fibrous capsule to mature, because some authors have found less recurrence if this waiting period is observed.

Before breast augmentation, the patient should be told to wear a loose-fitting, front-buttoning blouse or shirt, because it is often difficult for the patient to raise her arms above her head to put on a pullover top. During surgery, the patient is most often placed under general anesthesia, although local anesthesia with sedation is a viable alternative. Potential complications during surgery include hemorrhage or rupture of the implant. Inadvertent pneumothorax may occur, particularly with axillary incisions or from the needle used for local anesthesia infiltration. Instruments and equipment for thoracentesis or closed thoracotomy and chest drainage should be quickly available. Documentation in the patient's medical record should include the type, lot, and registration number of the prostheses that are implanted. The manufacturer usually supplies identifying labels that can be affixed to the record. The patient may require aggressive analgesia in the early period of recovery. Intramuscular ketorolac given 45 minutes before the end of surgery or intravenously at the end of surgery has proved to be quite effective in the management of surgical pain. After implantation under the muscle layer, pain is often relieved with an oral muscle relaxant. Some surgeons also advise the intermittent application of ice for the first 24 hours. Because the pain is centered on the chest wall, the need to deep breathe and cough requires emphasis and reinforcement.[10b]

The patient may splint her arms postoperatively, but gentle movement is encouraged to prevent stiffness of the shoulder and elbow joints. When transferring between the bed and chair or to a standing position, the patient should slide to the front edge of a chair before standing, and one should use her legs to lift her body off the chair.

The patient may or may not have compression dressings after surgery. Some practitioners ask the patient to wear a brassière immediately, although others prefer to apply a pressure dressing using elastic tape or a similar wrapping for the first 24 hours. At the next day appointment, bulky dressings are replaced with small incision dressings. Rarely, the patient may have incision drains, in which use the nurse should provide instructions about their care and emptying at home.

The patient and caregiver are instructed to immediately report any symptoms of bleeding or hematoma formation, such as visible blood on the dressing, frequent filling of a drain receptacle, and enlargement, ecchymosis, firmness, or increased pain in one breast. Final breast size will not be achieved until about 6 weeks after surgery when swelling is gone; there may be temporary stimulation of lactation. Women should be encouraged to continue monthly breast self-examinations for cancer screening as before surgery. The physician usually explains that mammography is still necessary postoperatively, but the technician should be informed of the presence of prostheses before performing the mammogram.

The discharging nurse should ensure that the patient's seat belt is fastened snugly for the trip home after surgery. Although all patients should be instructed to wear seat belts, it is especially important after breast procedures to avoid an accidental impact to the chest in case of a sudden stop. Patients are usually not permitted to drive for several days or weeks until arm movement is more normal.[11]

REDUCTION MAMMAPLASTY AND MASTOPEXY

Back pain, postural changes, shoulder grooves, skin rashes, excoriation, and emotional embarrassment are a few of the reasons for reduction and elevation of large or sagging breasts. Breast reduction is performed by excising excess breast tissue and skin and elevating the nipple areolar complex superiorly on the new breast mound (see Fig. 32–1). Breast reduction consists of two parts—excising the extra breast tissue and moving the nipple-areolar complex from its ptotic position back up onto the breast. The nipple is usually moved on an interior pedicle that contains enough blood vessels to maintain its viability and possibly contain the branch of the fourth intercostal nerve, which innervates it. Incisions leave tiny scars typically around the edge of the areola, a vertical scar inferior to the nipple, and a scar in the inframammary fold. Larger breasts have longer pedicles that make nipple transposition more difficult. Viability of the nipple-areolar complex is a major concern after the operation.

This lengthy procedure can result in significant fluid and blood loss and in prolonged anesthesia and surgical time. Some surgeons use a team approach to reduce surgical time. Until recently, breast reduction has been considered an inpatient procedure. Patients are selected for an ASC only after close evaluation of their physical, mental, and emotional status and after determining that the patient has a reliable caregiver at home.

It is recommended that patients be screened preoperatively by physical examination and mammography for underlying malignancies and to establish a baseline for future reference. The woman must be willing to accept the presence of obvious scars, the possibility of permanent loss of nipple sensitivity after surgery, and the probability that breast-feeding will not be possible. Other potential complications include lack of projection of the nipples, asymmetry in the size or shape of the breasts or in nipple location, infection, fat necrosis, and nipple ischemia.

Preoperative instructions are similar to those given to patients undergoing augmentation. Because mild to moderate blood loss may occur, the patient may be instructed to donate one or two units of blood in the few weeks before surgery to be held for autologous transfusion. The nurse should make necessary arrangements for cross-match and availability of autologous blood. For most patients, blood loss is not sufficient to warrant blood replacement; rather, crystalloids are given intravenously. If blood replacement becomes necessary, proper administration procedures must be carried out, as discussed in Chapter 38.

After surgery, important nursing assessments include urinary output, pulse rate, blood pressure, auscultation of lung sounds, skin turgor, and nipple-areolar complex color (if dressing placement allows inspection). The extent of surgical trauma combined with the length of surgery, actual tissue and fluid losses, and third-spacing of a portion of existing body fluids into the extracellular compartment make it imperative that fluid replacement is appropriately and aggressively managed. Large-volume infusions should be warmed to prevent or reduce hypothermia, and the patient should be kept covered to prevent heat loss. The patient's temperature should be monitored, and other methods of rewarming should be instituted when necessary.

After surgery, initial analgesics may be instituted parenterally, but the patient is given oral analgesics for home care. Several hours of observation in an ASC should be provided to manage vital signs and fluid and analgesic needs and to assess for complications, particularly bleeding. An adult who has a calm and confident demeanor and who can be trusted to make sound judgments must be available to provide home care for a patient after breast reduction. Often, antibiotics will be continued in the home.[12]

FACE, BROW, AND NECK LIFTS

Face, brow, and neck lifts are performed to reduce or eliminate age-related sagging of facial skin that has occurred due to loss of elasticity. Rarely, these procedures are undertaken to correct deformities from unilateral facial paralysis. Rhytidectomy, or face-lift, is effective in removing some skin wrinkles from the lower two thirds of the face, except around the eyes and mouth, repositioning soft tissue (jowls) above the mandibular border, and plicating the platysmal band (turkey neck). Submental liposuction may be used to complement the procedure. Incisions are placed along or behind the temporal hairline, in the pre- and postauricular areas, and under the chin when indicated.

A brow lift is performed to correct prominent forehead wrinkles, frown lines, lateral canthal creases (crow's feet), creasing at the bridge of the nose, or ptosis of the eyebrows. This incision line may be along or behind the natural hairline. Many practitioners prefer to use a coronal incision positioned behind the hairline.

It is important for the patient to understand that the final results after facial procedures may be subtle rather than dramatic and that scars will remain after surgery. Expected postoperative occurrences include the presence of ecchymosis, tightness and numbness of skin, elevation of the hairline, and edema.[13] Such symptoms can persist for several weeks or more.

More serious complications after facial procedures include bleeding, hematoma formation, nerve injury with or without loss of motor ability, loss of skin sensation, infection, hypertrophic scar formation, and hair loss. An older estimate of hematoma is at 8.5%. Today, the rate is estimated at less than 5% in normotensive patients. Patients with hypertension have a higher incidence (10%).[14] Other complications are much less frequent—infection (1%), skin slough (1%), and facial nerve injury (0.8%). Hair loss may occur anterior to the incision line because of decreased circulation to the hair follicles. This is usually temporary unless hair follicles are destroyed during the procedure.

Bleeding with or without the formation of a hematoma is the most common postoperative complication. Effective preoperative management of the hypertensive patient is essential, because elevated blood pressure is a major cause of hematoma formation. General anesthesia is advised for the hypertensive patient because of the additional control for maintaining normotension. Hypotensive anesthesia can also be used to reduce risk.

Small hematomas resolve without treatment or with massage and steroid injection, but moderate or large hematomas are surgically evacuated with suction or with open incision to restore proper tissue apposition and healing. Left untreated, large hematomas can inhibit blood flow to the wound edges, contributing significantly to tissue necrosis, which is the most devastating complication of rhytidectomy. Other factors that predispose the patient to skin sloughing and necrosis include excessive surgical trauma, tension on the skin flap or an excessively thin skin flap, dressings that are too tight, inherently impaired circulation from previous surgery or trauma, and, more specifically, delayed identification of hematomas. Gentle handling of tissues and meticulous hemostasis during surgery are the best preventive measures to avoid skin flap necrosis.[15]

Normally, incisions heal with only fine lines that are barely visible, particularly if suture line tension is avoided. Decreased circulation resulting in poor healing or actual tissue necrosis is the main cause of abnormal scar formation, particularly in the postauricular area. The vasoconstrictive effects of smoking (including active smoking and passive inhalation of the smoke from others), wound tension, and inherently poor circulation contribute to poor incision healing. Smoking is discouraged for several weeks before and after surgery. To decrease the visibility of scars that do remain, incisions are placed in the hairline, along existing skin folds, and in hidden areas whenever possible.[16]

Nerve injury is another possible, but rare, complication. Facial nerves can be damaged by forceps, local anesthetic injection, blunt dissection, and use of electrocautery. The great auricular nerve is the one most frequently damaged because of its superficial location. Paresthesia of the earlobe can result. Injury to other nerves can leave the patient with symptoms as diverse as pain and tightness of the neck, unilateral loss of facial expression, or inability to raise the eyebrow or to move a portion of the lip. Permanent paralysis or loss of sensation is rare, and normal function usually returns within a few weeks to a month without intervention. If it is identified that a nerve has been transected during surgery, reattachment is performed under microscopic vision.

Infection is rare after facial procedures (~1%), presumably because of the excellent blood supply to the scalp and face, but prophylactic oral antibiotic therapy is still prescribed. Occasionally, a serious postauricular infection can involve the cartilage if sutures are placed too deeply. The offending sutures are removed, and antibiotic therapy must be instituted to prevent loss of cartilage.[14]

The male patient presents certain technical problems during face-lift surgery because of thicker and larger areas of skin, sparser scalp hair, and shorter hairstyles (making it more difficult to conceal scars). Facial hair complicates the manner in which the facial skin can be manipulated or moved, and increased vascularity leads to increased incidence of hematoma formation.

Preoperatively, the nurse ensures that the patient has on no makeup or skin creams, because their presence in wrinkles, blemishes, and pores can prevent proper skin disinfection and lead to postoperative infection. The physician marks the face and neck just before surgery while the patient is sitting upright. Dentures may remain in the mouth or are replaced after endotracheal intubation to ensure a more natural appearance during surgery.

The choice between using general or local anesthesia with sedation is made jointly by the surgeon, anesthesia care provider, and patient. Local anesthesia with epinephrine is almost universally used for its vasoconstrictive properties. If the patient is awake for the injection, the physician may mix sodium bicarbonate with the local anesthetic to buffer the acidic pH and decrease associated pain. A ratio of 1 ml of sodium bicarbonate to 10 ml of the local agent is usual. This buffered solution may be less effective at pain control, however.

The circulating nurse monitors the cumulative dosage of local anesthesia administered throughout the case and relays that information to the surgeon so that maximal recommended doses are not inadvertently exceeded.

Postoperative nursing care focuses on close attention to the airway, operative sites, and hydration; provision of analgesia; maintenance of normotension; and avoidance of bleeding and nausea. Early head elevation helps to reduce swelling and aids respiration. The compression dressing should not constrict the airway or circulation to the operative sites. Wound drains should be maintained and emptied without occlusion of their tubings.

Pain is not a significant postoperative problem after face-lifts for most patients, but frontal headache is not uncommon after a brow lift, particularly when a snug dressing encircles the forehead. Incisions may have been infiltrated with a long-acting local anesthetic such as bupivacaine, which contributes greatly to the patient's postoperative comfort. Cool compresses or a small ice pack placed at the forehead and periorbital areas may help to reduce both pain and swelling, but an oral or parenteral analgesic may be necessary as well.

Bleeding is the most common postoperative complication, and various methods are used to help reduce its occurrence. Retching, vomiting, coughing, bladder distention, and restlessness should be avoided.[16] A calm environment and adequate analgesia help to prevent or reduce restlessness and hypertension, which can lead to bleeding in the early postoperative period. Ideally, the systolic blood pressure should be kept below 150 mm Hg or within parameters set by the physician. Hypertension that does not respond to analgesics or to sedatives may require definitive pharmacologic intervention. Hydralazine or β-blocking agents are examples of medications that may be given in titrated doses to reduce the blood pressure to acceptable levels. Sublingual nitroglycerin has also proved to be effective.

Although ecchymosis is common after facial procedures, signs of hematoma formation should be reported. Increasing unilateral pain, swelling, tightness, or hardness of the skin, anxiety, trismus (facial muscle spasms), and discoloration of the lips or buccal mucosa can herald significant hematoma formation. Hematomas that infringe on the airway can be life threatening without aggressive intervention to loosen the dressing and evacuate the hematoma. Immediate evacuation by the surgeon and anesthesia care provider is paramount. Supplemental humidified oxygen should be administered, and the patient should not take fluids in expectation of immediate anesthesia and surgery.

After extensive facial procedures, patients often require post-discharge nursing care at home or at the surgeon's office, a recovery care center, or hospital. Discharge instructions may have been reviewed preoperatively, or they may be given on the day of surgery or when the patient is more alert on the following day. Transportation to the secondary recovery site is usually in the company of a nurse or a designated staff member from the receiving facility.[13]

FACIAL RESURFACING

Chronic exposure to the sun causes problems apart from the skin changes caused by aging. Phototrauma is a term used to describe initial insults of exposure to sunlight. Chronic sun exposure leads to skin roughness, mottled areas of hyperpigmentation, sallowness, laxity, and fine and deep wrinkling.[17] The baby-boomers lived through the years when the sun-exposure pendulum promoted the "healthy tan." These people are now seeing the effects of exposure to the sun and may desire facial resurfacing.

Laser

Laser treatment of skin wrinkles is becoming the preferred method of facial resurfacing. The word *laser* is actually an acronym for light amplification by stimulated emission of radiation. It vaporizes intracellular and extracellular water in tissues and releases a plume of tissue fragments and steam.[18] The wound produced is shallow because the energy is absorbed very superficially. An ultrapulse laser is used for facial resurfacing.

The laser can be used with a free-hand technique often under loupe magnification or with the aid of an automated scanning device. Free hand, the area is traced or "painted" with the laser on "pulse" mode. The pulse mode emits laser light for 0.2 second and is then off for 0.2 second. Small dots of white tissue can be seen as the laser treats the area.[19]

Intraoperative care is needed to reduce the risk of inhalation of the plume and fire. Wavelength-specific laser safety glasses or goggles are worn by the patient and all personnel. The door is closed, and "laser in use" warning signs are prominently displayed. Wet drapes are kept nearby. Suction is used to immediately remove the plume.[20]

Laser irradiations are quite painful. Some patients are able to tolerate the procedure with anesthesia provided with local sedation or with topical anesthetics like eutectic mixture of local anesthetic (EMLA). The cream is applied for 1 to 2 hours and covered with an occlusive wrap (cellophane works well). Most patients need nerve blocks and local infiltration. The patient should be told that the laser treatment will feel like multiple pinpricks or like a rubber band snapping against the skin.

At the conclusion, the patient will have skin injury similar to a second-degree burn. There is significant postoperative edema, especially if the periorbital area has been treated. The edema can be reduced somewhat with ice packs and oral corticosteroids for 48 hours. Some patients also experience a burning sensation for 12 to 18 hours after treatment.

In 2 to 4 days, the residual tissue separates and sloughs off. Wound care after that time usually consists of hydrogel dressings. These dressings keep the wound bed moist and occluded, which promotes epithelialization and reduces pain. Hydrogel dressings are used for about 48 hours; after that time thin layers of antibacterial ointments or petrolatum are applied. Both products can create problems—contact dermatitis can develop from antibacterial agents and acne-like lesions can develop from petrolatum.[21]

The skin re-epithelializes in about 5 to 10 days, depending on the depth of the injury. Varying degrees of erythema can remain, but patients can effectively cover the erythema with makeup that has a green color for the foundation. Milia can form and may require tretinoin (Retin-A), or they can be expressed. Sunblocking agents are necessary; hyperpigmentation can develop.[22]

Laser skin resurfacing is a powerful new tool for the treatment of rhytids, scars, and actinic damage and compares favorably with dermabrasion and chemical peel. Whether the results are actually better or not remains to be seen.

Chemical Facial Peeling

There are numerous products in the marketplace today that offer promises of youthful skin. It is important to understand that these products that are available over the counter are working only on the surface of the skin. When a product penetrates the "dead" cells and alters the living cells, it must be prescribed by a physician.

Numerous skin health programs are available by prescription. There are currently three topical products that have been shown to be successful and may even provide results similar to a deep penetrating chemical peel. Those products are hydroquinone, exfoliating acids, and tretinoin. Hydroquinone, in its prescription strength, works as a skin lightener by suppressing the overproduction of melanin. This addresses areas of overpigmentation such as "age" spots, or redness. It also lightens freckles. Exfoliating acids or alpha-hydroxy acids are used to exfoliate the skin. By exfoliating the dead, thick outer layer of skin, the plumper, live tissues are more visible and appear healthier and more youthful. Tretinoin, better known as Retin-A, is the acidic form of vitamin A. Tretinoin stimulates skin to become firmer, tighter, and younger looking.

For deeper, quicker, uniform results of facial chemical peeling, there are phenol, alpha-hydroxy, and trichloroacetic acid peels.

Phenol Peels

The fine lines around the mouth and at the corners of the eyes can be treated with chemical peel. This process employs a caustic solution containing phenol, which produces a controlled chemical burn of the top layers of skin. Chemical peel is best suited for fair-skinned people, because individuals with darker skin tones may experience a change in skin color. Phenol peels are becoming less common, because more people are using alpha-hydroxy acid and tricholoroacetic acid for peels.[23] These solutions cause shallower peels and are usually applied in an office setting.

Before the procedure, the face is washed thoroughly and oil is removed with alcohol or a solvent. For deep peels, intravenous sedation is usually required, because the application of the solution causes a burning sensation until the anesthetic properties of the phenol take effect. Phenol is absorbed systemically and during the procedure; the patient is monitored for dysrhythmias. The peeled area may be covered with several layers of waterproof adhesive tape to enhance penetration of the solution.

Postoperative instructions should address that considerable postoperative edema is common; this can be relieved by keeping the head elevated. If swelling interferes with vision, the patient must have assistance to ensure safety. Limiting talking and drinking a liquid diet through a straw for several days promote comfort. Once the initial dressings are removed, antibiotic ointment may be applied to form a crust, which must be kept dry for several days. With careful washing, the crust will fall away as the tissue beneath it heals. Peeled areas may remain hyperpigmented for some time. These areas should be protected with sunscreen for 1 year. Makeup cannot be worn until all areas have been re-epithelialized. When makeup is worn, it must be easily removable.[24]

Alpha Hydroxy Peels

Alpha-hydroxy acid (AHA) is a natural acid found in many foods. It is used to produce a light peel of the superficial skin and is sometimes called the "minipeel" or "lunchtime peel." The skin is degreased with alcohol or acetone, and the acid is applied to the skin until the skin is thoroughly moist. The acid is left on the skin for up to 5 minutes or until flushing or tingling occurs. The solution is washed off with water or a dilute solution of sodium bicarbonate. The skin is moisturized following the peel. Repeat treatments may be done weekly for 2 to 6 months for full effect. Sun block is critical in preventing skin injury.

Trichloroacetic Acid Peels

Trichloracetic acid peels (TCA) use a stronger solution to peel deeper structures in the skin and can be used to remove subtle lines and large pores, lighten the skin, or improve skin texture. A 20% to 50% solution is used to coagulate the skin, like phenol. The solution is applied until the skin develops a "frost." The solution is removed with water, and the skin is moisturized. Treatment can be combined with other forms of skin peels for improved response. Since evaporation increases concentration of the solution, the body should be immediately covered after use. Sun block is essential in avoiding skin injury.

Dermabrasion

Dermabrasion is a technique for removing the epidermis and portions of the dermis using an abrasive wheel of diamond-tipped brushes driven by a high-speed rotary engine. Dermabrasion can be used to treat acne scars and benign and premalignant facial lesions. Facial skin can heal without scar if the dermabrasion is limited to the dermis above the reticular layer.

The skin is anesthetized with local anesthesia or a cryogenic spray. The OR staff wear extensive barrier protection, because there is a spray from the area being treated. After surgery, biosynthetic dressings are applied for 24 hours. This dressing is covered with nonstick dressings and a precut mask to hold the dressings in place. After removing the dressing and mask, the patient applies topical antibiotic powders. The facial skin will crust and weep for several days. Re-epithelialization takes between 7 and 10 days. Erythema may be present for another 2 to 12 weeks. Makeup can be used to disguise this discoloration. Patients will remain hypersensitive to sun exposure and will need to wear a sunscreen with at least No. 15 sun-protective factor (SPF) for at least 6 months. Milia may develop around 3 to 4 weeks and should be treated with tretinoin (Retin-A) cream or extracted.

EYELID SURGERY

Eyelid surgery is well suited to the ambulatory surgery environment. Entropion (inversion of the upper or lower lid) and ectropion (eversion of the lower lid) are anatomic defects in the position of the eyelids that can often be corrected with plastic surgery techniques. Blepharoplasty is another procedure that is performed strictly for anesthetic results or may be medically corrective when the redundant skin is so extreme that it interferes with vision. Both ophthalmologists and plastic surgeons perform these procedures.

Before eyelid surgery, the shape and symmetry of the patient's face, eyes, and lids should be documented for later comparison. A general assessment of the patient's vision is documented for several reasons. First, visual loss is a potential complication of eyelid surgery, and thus a baseline assessment for comparison is important. In addition, alterations in postoperative vision that were actually pre-existing may be perceived by the patient to be a result of the surgery. If visual changes are noted before surgery, a complete eye examination should be obtained.

Several complications are associated with blepharoplasty. Ptosis of the upper lid and malpositioning of the lower lid can occur. Both conditions usually resolve at least partially without treatment, although subsequent surgical repair may be necessary. Dry eye syndrome is another potential problem. A more devastating complication is loss of vision, which is exceptionally rare and occurs in only 0.04% of all complications.[25]

Various causes for visual loss have been theorized and studied, but it cannot be clearly ascribed to any single cause. Not to be mistaken for blurring caused by eye ointments and drops, loss of vision has been consistently associated with removal of orbital fat. Various other mechanisms that can contribute to vision loss include retrobulbar hemorrhage, which causes pressure that interrupts blood flow to the optic nerve and retina; blood vessel damage secondary to local anesthetic injection; bleeding caused by vasodilatation after epinephrine used in surgery wears off; direct injury to the optic nerve or retinal artery; and increased intraocular pressure, which may be a result of acute narrow-angle glaucoma (Fig. 32–2).

After eyelid procedures, bleeding and hematoma formation are possible. To help avoid such problems postoperatively, patients should be kept calm, comfortable, and normotensive. Appropriate measures should be taken to limit retching, coughing, and sneezing. Antibiotic ointment may be applied to suture lines on the eyelids, which are usually left unbandaged. Cool or iced compresses are often used on the lids for the first 1 or 2 days to reduce swelling, pain, and bleeding. Visual acuity may be diminished

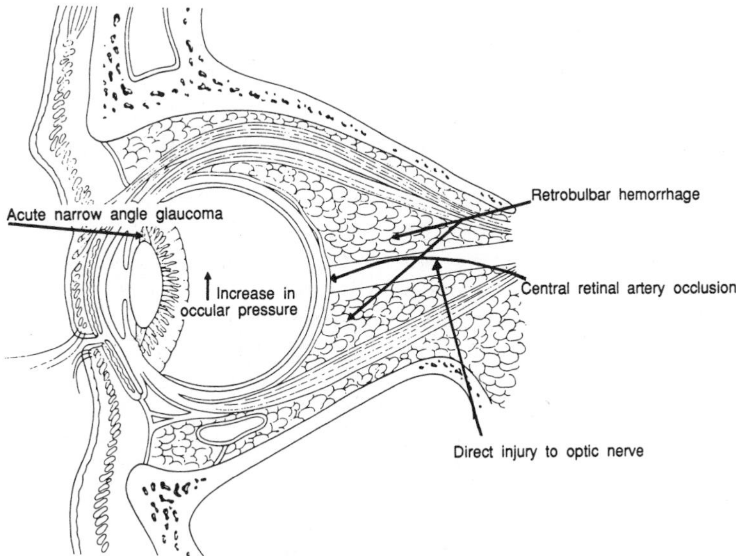

Figure 32–2. Etiologies of visual loss. (From Black J: Complications following blepharoplasty. Plast Surg Nurs 10[4]:155, 1990. Copyright © 1990 Plastic Surgical Nursing. Reprinted with permission of Jannetti Publications, Inc., publisher.)

temporarily if intraocular ointment is used to protect the eye during surgery, and thus the patient may require assistance during early attempts to ambulate and reassurance that visual blurriness is temporary. Patients are treated with eye drops and ointment for use at night. Steroid eye drops should not be used. They can lead to corneal ulceration.[26]

Postoperative instructions are similar to those for other ophthalmic patients. Usual antihypertensive medications should be resumed. Severe pain in and around the eye and persistent nausea should be reported to the physician at once, because they could be signs of acute-angle glaucoma that must be treated immediately.

SUCTION-ASSISTED LIPECTOMY, LIPOPLASTY, OR LIPOLYSIS

Lipoplasty, also called suction-assisted lipectomy (SAL) or lipolysis, is defined as the extraction of subcutaneous fat from local areas using a blunt cannula and high-vacuum suction. Superficial suction lipectomy can be performed with smaller cannulas. This procedure has gained widespread popularity since its beginnings in France in 1978. Refinements in technique have made suction lipectomy suitable for almost every area of the body: neck, face, breasts, abdomen, thighs, buttocks, flank, and extremities, including the knees and ankles. The procedure is major when large amounts of fat are removed because of fluid shifts. Although it is not risk free, it is considered safe for an outpatient setting when the patient is provided with appropriate anesthesia coverage and cardiovascular monitoring and when strict aseptic technique is employed.[27]

Fat distribution is based on gender, heredity, and environmental factors. It is generally accepted that during childhood there is rapid growth of new and expansion of current fat cells, but that new fat cells are not formed in adult life. Diet, exercise, and weight loss are not always successful in eliminating adipose tissue from certain areas of the body, and lipectomy is an alternative for people who desire body contouring in specific areas. The ideal candidate is an adult between 20 and 45 years of age who has good elastic skin tone, is close to an ideal weight, and has relatively isolated areas of fat deposits. As SAL techniques have evolved, it has been used on greater ranges of people outside this "ideal." The nurse may see SAL used in moderately obese patients. It is still contraindicated as a treatment for marked obesity. The patient should be well motivated and emotionally stable and should have realistic expectations about the procedure. Other contraindications to lipectomy include bleeding and clotting disorders, uncontrolled hypertension, and unstable heart disease.

Before scheduling the surgery, the patient is taught that ecchymosis, swelling, and discomfort will follow the procedure. Once the decision is made to proceed, the patient should begin preparing several weeks before surgery. Preparations include limiting or abstaining from alcohol, aspirin, medications containing aspirin (e.g., cold medicine), and vitamin E, all of which can interfere with the clotting mechanism. Multivitamins that include zinc and at least 500 mg of vitamin C are often prescribed for several weeks preoperatively, and the patient is expected to eat a nutritious diet to enhance general healing capacity. If removal of more than 500 ml of fat is anticipated, iron is added to the vitamin preparation. Smoking must be avoided perioperatively. Autologous blood donation during the few weeks before surgery is suggested if removal of a large amount of fat is planned. The patient may bring a lipectomy (compression) garment to the ASC.

Because fatty tissue has a poor blood supply and poor resistance to infection, the patient is asked to shower with an antibacterial soap for several days before surgery. Antibiotics started on the evening before surgery are continued postoperatively.

Because lipectomy is frequently associated with extensive blood and fluid volume losses, the patient's vascular fluid volume should be maintained aggressively on the day of the surgery. Fluid management is an essential element in the patient's overall medical and nursing care. On admission, the patient, who has taken nothing by mouth, is usually considered to already have an approximate 1000 ml fluid deficit, so that amount of lactated Ringer's solution, with or without dextrose, is infused rapidly before surgery.

Differing opinions and formulas for fluid replacement are based on the operative fluid losses and the patient's metabolic needs. One method is to infuse 1500 ml of crystalloid solution plus an amount equal to the volume of fat and fluids removed during the procedure. Replacement is timed so that the total volume is replaced within 30 minutes of the end of surgery. If more than 1500 ml is suctioned, hetastarch, a synthetic colloid, is added to the intravenous regimen. If more than 2000 ml is removed, autologous blood transfusion of one or two units is added. Regardless of the formula for replacement, perioperative nurses should be aware of the patient's fluid and cardiovascular status and should immediately report symptoms of hypovolemia or hypoxia, including hypotension, orthostatic hypotension, tachycardia, thready or weak pulse, pallor, air hunger, faintness or dizziness, and oliguria.

The volume of fat removed is based on the patient's anatomic needs and general medical condition. Most surgeons remove less than 2000 ml; however, removal of larger amounts has been reported without increased morbidity or complications. One authority bases the upper limits of fat to be removed on the preoperative hematocrit. Hematocrit parameters are as follows.

Preoperative Hematocrit	Upper Limit of Fat Removed
45%	2000 ml
40%	1500 ml
35%	750 ml

Intraoperatively, the nurse should keep the surgeon informed of the total volume suctioned. The ratio of blood to fat in the suctioned fluid is usually less than one to four.

Tumescent technique, which was first introduced in 1987 and is frequently used now, involves infusing large volumes (1000 ml) of dilute lidocaine and epinephrine into the operative sites before aspiration. The infusion of such fluids allow greater volumes of fat (and less blood) to be moved.[28] There are several variations of infusing fluids, including Hunstad's formula:

Lactated Ringer's 1000 ml
Lidocaine 1% 50 ml
Epinephrine (1:1000) 1 ml
Warmed to 38°C

It is thought that this large volume infusion of dilute lidocaine/epinephrine promotes vasoconstriction and minimizes bleeding but also provides analgesia intraoperatively and postoperatively. Some clinicians add 10 ml of sodium bicarbonate to the solution too.

Ultrasonic assisted lipoplasty is another refinement in technique. Ultrasonic energy ruptures the fat cell wall and eases aspiration. Areas to be treated are infused with tumescent wetting solution. Accurate assessment of volumes of aspirate in body sites is important in enhancing symmetry.[29, 30]

Postoperative care includes continued management of the fluid status. Because adequacy of urinary output is one indication of adequate cardiovascular volume, the patient should void before discharge from the ASC. In addition to the actual fluid losses observed in surgery, the patient's body fluids shift into extracellular spaces postoperatively owing to surgical trauma. This accumulation of fluid can be up to 6 to 8 ml/kg/hr,[31] and the postoperative fluid replacement should cover this covert loss. Oral intake is usually given as clear liquids after nausea has passed. After extensive liposuctioning, the patient is often anorexic and tolerates only small amounts of liquids orally on the first day. On the following day, a light diet is suggested.

A compression garment designed to provide support to the affected areas and compress the areas suctioned to decrease edema and promote smooth contouring of the body during healing is applied. It is worn for approximately 2 to 3 weeks and is removed only for bathing. After neck and chin procedures, an elastic support strap is worn constantly for the first week postoperatively and then at night for the next 2 weeks.

Despite or because of the compression garments, patients often complain of pain and difficulty in moving. Excessive pain or inability to tolerate oral fluids or pills may require the patient's overnight admission for parenteral fluid and analgesic therapy. Icebags reduce pain in operative sites and reduce ecchymosis.

Other postoperative considerations address the patient's cardiovascular and temperature needs. Hypothermia and shivering are common and are related to intraoperative exposure, general anesthesia, fluid losses, and rapid fluid replacement. Supplemental oxygen addresses increased metabolic demands associated with shivering and any decreased oxygen-carrying capacity secondary to blood loss. External and intravenous fluid warming can help to prevent or reverse hypothermia. Gradual elevation to a reclining position is advised to avoid postural hypotension. Dressings should be checked frequently for bleeding.

Reliability of the responsible adult must be ensured before discharge from an ASC. At home the patient should rest, drink large amounts of fluids, and continue taking oral analgesics as needed. The patient will return to the physician's office on the second or third postoperative day. Vitamins are continued after surgery, and an iron supplement may be added. After several weeks, the patient may begin massage and ultrasound therapy to promote tissue softness and increase circulation to reduce swelling. The effectiveness of this therapy is controversial.

HAND PROCEDURES

An ASC is ideal for a variety of reconstructive and therapeutic hand procedures. A few include repair of traumatic injuries, carpal tunnel release, decompression of de Quervain's disease, tenovaginotomy, release of Dupuytren's contracture, excision of ganglions and neuromas, release of trigger finger or thumb, and separation of webbed fingers (syndactyly). These procedures are performed by plastic surgeons, orthopedic surgeons, and hand surgeons.

Preoperative Care

A number of specific instructions given before the day of surgery help the patient prepare for hand surgery. Handwashing with antibacterial soap for 6 minutes, three times a day, for several days before surgery is undertaken to help reduce the potential for postoperative infection. Jewelry must be removed from the hand before surgery, and the patient should trim long fingernails, remove fingernail polish, and wear sleeveless or large-sleeved clothing to accommodate a bulky dressing or cast after surgery.

The ASC nurse should attempt to identify women who wear prosthetic porcelain or acrylic nails. The cost and emotional importance of prosthetic nails to some women make them reluctant to remove the nails for surgery. Physicians hold varying opinions regarding the need to remove artificial nails on the hand that is to be operated on, and thus the nurse should consult with the surgeon before instructing the patient to do so.

Preoperatively, the patient should understand that he or she may not be able to drive or to perform many usual daily activities for several days or weeks, particularly if surgery involves the dominant hand. The time that a patient must take off from work varies according to the physician's directions and depending on the patient's type of work. The ASC nurse who finds that the patient was unaware that he or she must lose time from work can refer the patient to the physician's office before surgery for further information. With this knowledge, the patient is better able to give informed consent and to plan for the postoperative period.

Intraoperative Care

Regional anesthesia is often chosen for hand surgery. Intravenous regional anesthesia (Bier block) may be used for relatively short procedures. Brachial plexus block is an ideal approach for hand procedures, because it provides excellent motor and sensory anesthesia; it allows the use of an intraoperative tourniquet while the entire arm is anesthetized; and it provides analgesia into the postoperative period.

While positioning the patient's arm for adequate surgical exposure, anatomic factors must be heeded. For instance, the arm should not be extended at the shoulder to an angle greater than 90 degrees to avoid tension and damage to the brachial plexus, and the operative surface should have adequate padding to protect bony prominences. Intraoperative medications may include prophylactic antibiotics and corticosteroids to reduce inflammation. While explaining preparations to the awake patient, the perioperative nurse should include a simple explanation about any grounding pad that is placed on a distant site such as the thigh so the patient does not worry that a wrong area of the body is being prepared for surgery.

Often, a pneumatic tourniquet is used intraoperatively to eliminate bleeding in the operative field. The perioperative nurse who is knowledgeable in the proper operation and application of the tourniquet should document the pressure and length of inflation time on the patient's record. Maximum inflation time is 120 minutes. During particularly lengthy procedures, the surgeon may order the tourniquet to be released temporarily to allow blood flow to the extremity, thus oxygenating peripheral tissues. This practice is especially important for patients with diabetes, alcoholism, and any peripheral vascular deficit. Upper arm tourniquet cuff placement is preferred, because prolonged pressure on the forearm or wrist can result in nerve damage.

Postoperative Care

Special postoperative concerns are controlling pain, monitoring the neurovascular status of the extremity including the effects of constrictive dressings, and ensuring that proper elevation of the hand is maintained in order to prevent injury to the anesthetized arm and hand. The patient is discharged early in the postoperative course, and the responsible adult must be instructed and assessed in his or her ability to accurately evaluate the surgical site and provide appropriate care.

Pain control is probably the most difficult problem following hand surgery. Inadequate analgesia can result in the need for hospitalization or, if the patient is discharged, can be the source of desperate telephone calls from the patient to the physician on the evening of surgery. The physician must anticipate the patient's need for adequate analgesics after the resolution of any regional block based on the type of procedure undertaken and prior knowledge of the patient's personality and tolerance for pain. After the physician writes appropriate prescriptions, the nurse should reinforce the instructions regarding their use and should encourage the patient to begin taking analgesics as soon as the regional anesthesia begins to dissipate. Some surgeons direct the patient to begin oral pain medications immediately after discharge and to take them periodically, regardless of the pain level, for the first day or two after surgery.

Maintaining elevation of the hand helps to reduce postoperative pain and avoid circulatory congestion with resultant edema, which increases pain and throbbing and delays healing of the tissues. Physicians vary in their opinions regarding the postoperative use of arm slings. Some order slings, but others dispute their effectiveness, citing widespread misuse by patients who allow the sling to maintain the elbow at a 90-degree angle or more. These surgeons prefer that the patient consciously and purposefully keep the hand elevated above the level of the heart.

Nursing instructions for the patient who will be wearing a sling include the need to position the hand across the chest and near the opposite shoulder, higher than the elbow and the heart. Unless contraindicated by the type of surgery, the patient should be encouraged to remove the arm from the sling periodically and to gently exercise the elbow and shoulder joints, being careful to maintain hand elevation during this activity. While the patient is resting at home, his or her hand can be propped high on pillows. The sling should fit the patient's arm and be long enough to provide support to the wrist and hand. Padding under the neck strap may be necessary for comfort.

The patient may be discharged after regional block before full motor or sensory return if the hand is supported and protected by a sling. Diminished sensory function can result in inadvertent injury to the hand or arm unless the patient is cautious about positioning and protecting the extremity.

Bandaging that encircles the extremity can result in circulatory compromise owing to tight application or later surgical swelling. Peripheral circulation distal to the bandage is assessed by palpating pulses and by observing skin color and temperature, adequacy of capillary refill, and the presence of edema or bleeding. The use of a pulse oximeter finger probe on the hand of surgery is an excellent adjunct to the assessment of circulatory status. Depending on the type of oximeter device use, it may allow observation of the pulse waveform while all devices measure the oxygen saturation level in affected fingers.

After discharge, the patient and accompanying adult need to know the symptoms of circulatory impairment that should be reported to the physician immediately: blue, black, purple, or flushed discoloration of one or more fingers; return of numbness or tingling in the fingers after anesthesia has worn off; extensive swelling of the fingers; or severe pain that is unrelieved by the prescribed analgesics. Before discharge, staining antiseptics or soaps should be removed from surrounding areas of skin for esthetic reasons, to reduce skin irritation, and to allow easier assessment of the skin tone and nailbed color.

Splints, braces, or elastic wrapping may be used to maintain the hand and wrist in a specific position. The patient must be encouraged to maintain the hand in the intended position and should not remove any splints, braces, or dressings until instructed to do so by the physician.

Hand dressings should be kept dry to reduce the chance of bacterial contamination of the wound. It is particularly tempting for patients to use the affected hand to help squeeze out a washcloth, wipe up a simple spill, or wash the face. It is imperative to keep the dressing completely dry and clean when a drain, joint implant, or hardware is in place, because direct communication of those indwelling devices with subcutaneous tissues and bones increases the threat of infection.

The physician may direct the patient to begin passive and then active exercises of the affected fingers and hand in the early postoperative period or may order complete rest of the affected digits. The ASC nurse should be aware of the individual physician's protocols and reinforce those directives before the patient's discharge. The nurse also encourages the patient to avoid aggressive pushing, pulling, and heavy lifting with the surgical hand for the period specified by the physician.

Surgical Procedures

Various traumatic and pathologic conditions of the hand are amenable to surgical correction. The following discussion explains several types and the corrective procedures. Underlying pathology varies from one disorder to another, but patients' basic perioperative needs and nursing care are similar for most hand procedures.

Traumatic Injuries

Traumatic injuries to the hand may be treated in the ASC primarily as an emergency intervention or later for correction or revision of the original treatment course. The patient who has just sustained an injury presents without the benefit of preoperative instructions or preparation. The patient is often very anxious about the ultimate outcome of the injury and surgery and may be in a state of emotional shock and in pain. If family members are not present because the accident has just occurred, the patient may be frightened about being alone.

If the patient has eaten before the injury, the anesthesia care provider and surgeon will confer to decide the urgency of the surgical intervention. If immediate surgery is necessary to stop bleeding and to re-establish circulation to traumatized or amputated parts of the hand, a regional anesthetic technique that is usually employed for hand procedures affords some protection against aspiration and pulmonary sequelae. A failed or incomplete regional block causes great concern, however, because intraoperative conversion to general anesthesia carries significant risk for the patient with a full stomach.

Other concerns for the patient having unexpected surgery for trauma include: (1) securing an adequate health history and informed consent; (2) assessing and treating extremes of vital signs (i.e., tachycardia, hypotension due to bleeding, or hypertension due to anxiety and pain); (3) providing emotional support to an often frightened patient and family; and (4) providing adequate analgesia preoperatively. The anesthesia care provider may choose to administer the regional anesthetic preoperatively as soon as possible after the patient's admission to provide analgesia. Besides prophylactic parenteral antibiotics, the patient may require a tetanus booster if it was not given in the emergency department. Ongoing assessment of peripheral circulation allows the nurse to quickly report any changes indicative of increasing ischemia.

Dupuytren's Contracture

Dupuytren's contracture is a disease that primarily affects the palmar fascia of the hand and other fascial structures of the body. Its pathology is not clearly understood. The typical flexion contracture associated with Dupuytren's disease is most often noted in the metacarpophalangeal joint (MPJ) in the palm of the hand, but it is also seen in the proximal and distal interphalangeal joints (PIPJ and DIPJ). Although the relationship is unclear, there is an association of the disease with epilepsy, diabetes, and alcoholism.

The usual presenting symptom that prompts the patient to seek medical attention is the presence of nodules in the palm. These nodules may be somewhat painful. Eventually, a tight cord forms proximal to the nodules, resulting in contractures. The condition occurs more often in men. In women, the frequency of the condition increases with advancing age.

The indication for surgery is the occurrence of joint contracture. The goal of surgery is to relieve the contracture while promoting full flexion and extension of the fingers. The procedure performed may be fasciotomy or fasciectomy. Depending on the extent of the contracture, a Z-plasty or W-plasty technique may be necessary to lengthen the thickened contracted palmar fascia. Rarely, a skin graft may be required to provide enough skin to cover the surgical defect.

If a transverse incision is required across the palm, the surgeon may leave a wide incision open to promote drainage and to avoid hematoma formation. These wounds generally heal completely within 3 to 6 weeks and tend to result in less postoperative pain and swelling than incisions that are sutured closed. A hand splint is worn after surgery to maintain extension of the palm and fingers. After about 1 week to 10 days, the patient begins to remove the splint for increasing amounts of time each day to help regain finger flexion.

Complications include loss of finger flexion, bleeding, and sympathetic dystrophy, a condition that can best be prevented by proper elevation of the hand to keep edema to a minimum. Hematomas should be evacuated to reduce the chance of tissue necrosis and sloughing of skin. Intraoperative complications include laceration of the nerve or artery.

Carpal Tunnel Syndrome

Carpal tunnel syndrome (CTS) involves the entrapment of the median nerve by the transverse carpal ligament at the volar surface of the wrist (Fig. 32–3). This entrapment can be caused by thickening of the synovium, trauma, or aberrant muscles. It is one of the most common repetitive motion injuries. CTS is seen in people who work at computer terminals for

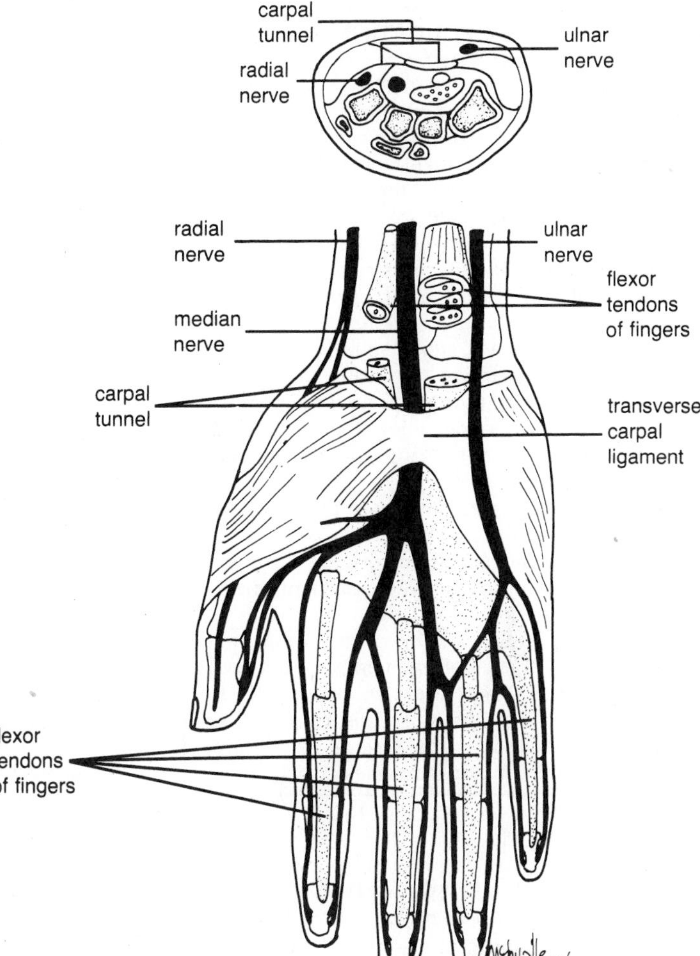

Figure 32–3. A cross-section and palmar view of the carpal tunnel and affected nerves and tendons. (Reprinted with permission from AORN Journal 38:528, 1983. Copyright AORN, Inc., 2170 South Parker Road, #300, Denver, CO 80231-5711.)

long periods or without wrist support. The cause is often unknown, but it may be associated with synovitis or rheumatoid arthritis. Often the condition is seen in people who perform repetitive hand movements. Carpal tunnel syndrome most often affects the dominant hand and frequently occurs bilaterally.

Presenting symptoms include numbness, pain, and tingling of the fingers and weakness of the thumb; symptoms often awaken the patient in the night. Tinel's sign (pain with dorsiflexion and tapping over the canal) and Phalen's sign (pain and flexion of the wrist) are positive. If the condition is long-standing, there may be wasting of the thenar muscle and general weakness of the hand. Symptoms are usually reversible after release of the nerve. Surgical release is by an incision or excision of the carpal ligament, with or without synovectomy. Currently, the endoscope is being used with greater frequency for carpal tunnel release. Conservative medical treatment that may be attempted before surgery includes use of anti-inflammatory agents, splinting to rest the hand, increased consumption of vitamin B_6, or steroid injections.

de Quervain's Disease

de Quervain's disease is stenosing tenosynovitis of the first dorsal compartment of the wrist at the base of the thumb, which results in hand and wrist pain and disability. It commonly occurs in middle-aged women. Symptoms of de Quervain's disease include pain on the radial side of the wrist, especially with attempts to extend the thumb. Diagnosis is made with a positive Finklestein test with pain elicited in the first dorsal compartment when the thumb is purposefully flexed. A second method of diagnosis involves the relief of symptoms when lidocaine is injected into the first dorsal compartment.

Box 32–1 KEY EDUCATION POINTS

- Prepare patients preoperatively, discussing and demonstrating wound or incision, dressing, and drain (when appropriate) care.
- Emphasize to the patient the importance of not smoking, especially for 2 weeks before and 2 weeks after the operative procedure. Smoking can interfere with wound healing.
- Medications that can contribute to bleeding are stopped 2 weeks before surgery. These agents include aspirin, nonsteroidal anti-inflammatory drugs, and vitamin E.[10b]
- Pain may be unexpected or greater than anticipated. Encourage the patient to use prescribed analgesics and other comfort therapies (cold, elevation or position change) to relieve pain and discomfort.
- Reinforce activity restrictions to prevent complications, and encourage wound healing (keeping dressings/incisions dry, elevating extremity, wearing compression garment, maintaining splint).
- Provide the patient and his or her companion with follow-up telephone contact numbers, and encourage the patient or companion to phone if he or she has questions, concerns, or problems related to the surgical procedure, postoperative care, or outcome.

Medical treatment with steroid injections, splinting, heat, hydrotherapy, and anti-inflammatory agents is usually attempted before surgery. If these methods are ineffective at maintaining function and comfort, a simple release of the dorsal compartment is performed. This release allows decompression of the compressed tendons and muscles of the thumb.

Ganglion Excision

Ganglions are soft, mucin-filled cysts that are attached to joint capsules, tendons, retinaculum, or joint pulleys. They account for 50% to 70% of all soft tissue tumors of the hand and are found most often on the dorsal wrist. A ganglion is an outpouching of the synovium that periodically gets larger and smaller. Aspiration may be attempted; however, because the recurrence rate is high, excision is often the only definitive therapy. Pain and limitation of function are the prime indications for surgery, but cosmetic appearance is often a motivation for the patient to seek surgical intervention. Because a portion of the joint capsule is removed during ganglionectomy, instability of the wrist is a possible complication of surgery, and purely cosmetic improvement is not considered by some to be an adequate indication for surgery.

References

1. Maksud D, Congwell-Anderson R: Psychological dimensions of anesthetic surgery: Essentials for nurses. Plast Surg Nurs 15:137–144, 1995.
2. Klassen A: Problems reported by people who request cosmetic surgery. Plast Surg Nurs 20:176–181, 1999.
2a. Banfield R: Preoperative reasons for aesthetic surgery in men. Plast Surg Nurs 9:20–22, 1989.
3. Netscher D, Clamon J: Smoking: Adverse effects on outcomes for plastic surgical patients. Plast Surg Nurs 14:205–210, 1994.
4. Roy D: Caring for the self-esteem of the cosmetic surgery patient. Plast Surg Nurs 6:138–141, 1986.
5. Vinnick M: Self-imposed isolation as a factor in depression following cosmetic surgery. Plast Surg Nurs 6:144–145, 1986.
6. Thomas C: Perioperative considerations for the augmentation mammaplasty patient. Plast Surg Nurs 8:91–95, 1988.
7. Hart D: Women and saline breast implant surgery. Plast Surg Nurs 13:188–200, 1995.
7a. McCain L: A review of autoimmune disorders anecdotally linked to mammary implants. Plast Surg Nurs 15:68–77, 1995.
7b. Stomber RE: Breast implants and the FDA: Past, present and future. Plast Surg Nurs 13:185–187, 200, 1993.
8. Palcheff-Weimer M, Concannon MJ, Conn VS, et al: The impact of the media on women with breast implants. Plast Reconstr Surg 92:775–778, 1993.
9. McCain L, Jones G: Application of endoscopic techniques in aesthetic plastic surgery. Plast Surg Nurs 15:149–160, 1995.
9a. Simler A: Endoscopic augmentation mamoplasty: The umbilical approach. Plast Surg Nurs 14:149–153, 1995.
10. Hart D: Women and saline breast implant surgery. Plast Surg Nurs 13:188–200, 1995.
10a. McCain L: A review of autoimmune disorders anecdotally linked to mammary implants. Plast Surg Nurs 15:68–77, 1995.
10b. Springer RC: Saline augmentation mammaplasty: Nursing implications. Plast Surg Nurs 19:9–14, 1999.
11. Thomas C: Perioperative considerations for the augmentation mammaplasty patient. Plast Surg Nurs 8:91–95, 1988.
12. Fowler M: Body contouring surgery. Nurs Clin North Am 29:753–761, 1994.
13. Springer RC: Rhytidectomy: From consultation to recovery. Plast Surg Nurs 16:27–30, 1996.
14. Salisbury C, Kaye B: Complications following rhytidectomy. Plast Surg Nurs 18:71–77, 89, 1998.
15. Turpin IM: The modern rhytidectomy. Clin Plast Surg 9:383–400, 1992.
16. Hinojosa R: Postoperative nausea and vomiting: How nurses can help. Plast Surg Nurs 15:85–88, 1995.
17. Nicol N, Fenske N: Photodamage: Cause, clinical manifestations and prevention. Plast Surg Nurs 16:9–21, 1996.
18. Vander Kam V, Achauer B: Lasers in plastic surgery: Applications and nursing interventions. Plast Surg Nurs 10:107–111, 125, 1990.
19. Vander Kam V, Achauer B: Laser resurfacing of the face. Plast Surg Nurs 17:134–137, 1997.
20. Pierce L: Laser safety guidelines for plastic surgery nurses. Plast Surg Nurs 17:165–166, 1997.

21. Muiderman K: Postoperative instructions for laser resurfacing of the skin. Plast Surg Nurs 16:254, 1996.
22. Seckel B, Wilson L: Complications of laser resurfacing. Plast Surg Nurs 17:138–143, 1997.
23. Rubin MG: Trichloroacetic acid and other non-phenol peels. Clin Plast Surg 19:525–536, 1992.
24. Ryan F, LaFourcade C: Skin care, chemical face peeling and skin rejuvenation. Plast Surg Nurs 15:51–60, 1995.
25. Black J: Complications following blepharoplasty. Plast Surg Nurs 18:78–83, 1998.
26. Anderson LG, Leroux C: Routine surgery, routine patients? Never. Plast Surg Nurs 16:41–42, 1996.
27. Fowler M: Body contouring surgery. Nurs Clin North Am 29:753–761, 1994.
28. Trolt S, Stool L, Klein K: Anesthetic considerations. In Rohrich R, Beran S, Kenkel J (eds): Ultrasound-Assisted Liposuction. St. Louis: Quality Med Pub, 1998.
29. Ablaza V, Jones M, Gingrass M, et al: Ultrasonic assisted lipoplasty: Overview for nurses. Plast Surg Nurs 18:13–15, 1998.
30. Ablaza V, Jones M, Gingrass M, et al: Ultrasonic Assisted Lipoplasty: Clinical Management. Plast Surg Nurs 18:16–26, 1998.
31. Pettis D, Vogt P: Complications of suction-assisted lipoectomy. Plast Surg Nurs 12:148–154, 1992.

Bibliography

American Society of Plastic and Reconstructive Surgical Nurses: Core Curriculum for Plastic and Reconstructive Surgical Nursing, 2nd ed. Pitman, NJ: Author.

Anderson L: The plastic surgical nurse. Nurs Clin North Am 29:817–825, 1994.

Anderson RC, Larson DL: Patient concerns related to media coverage of silicone implants. Plast Surg Nurs 15:89–91, 1995.

Anderson RC, Maksud D: Psychological adjustments to reconstructive surgery. Nurs Clin North Am 29:711–724, 1994.

Black J: Reconstructive surgery in the elderly. Plast Surg Nurs 11:151–162, 1991.

Black J, Mangan M: Body contouring and weight loss surgery for obesity. Nurs Clin North Am 26:777–788, 1991.

Dillerud E: Abdominoplasty combined with suction lipoplasty: A study of complications, revisions and risk factors in 487 cases. Ann Plast Surg 25:333–343, 1990.

Frioch S, et al: Ambulatory surgery: A study of patient's and helper's experiences. AORN J 52:1000–1009, 1990.

Gellis MB: Preoperative and postoperative instructions for liposuction of the jowl and chin. Plast Surg Nurs 16:57–58, 1996.

Goin M, Burgoyne R, Goin J, et al: A prospective psychological study of 50 female facelift patients. Plast Reconstr Surg 65:436–441, 1998.

Gutek EP, Fowler ME, Heeter C: The forehead lift. Plast Surg Nurs 13:188–200, 1993.

Hinojosa R: Anxiety of elective surgical patients' family members: Relationship between anxiety levels, family characteristics. Plast Surg Nurs 16:43–45, 1996.

Leppa CJ: Cosmetic surgery and the motivation for health and beauty. Nurs Forum 25:25–31, 1990.

Lusis SA: Nursing management of the elderly surgical patient. Plast Surg Nurs 14:139–146, 1994.

McCain L: Making a difference in the breast implant issue. Plast Surg Nurs 12:28–30, 1992.

McCain L, Jones G: Endoscopic techniques in aesthetic plastic surgery. Plast Surg Nurs 15:145–148, 1995.

Napoleon A, Lewis C: Psychological considerations in the elderly cosmetic surgery candidate. Ann Plast Surg 24:165–169, 1990.

Russell B, Russell R: The role of the plastic surgery nurse collagen specialist. Plast Surg Nurs 10:51–60, 1990.

Solomon M, Granick M: Plastic surgery in the elderly. Clin Geriatr Med 6:633–657, 1990.

Spencer KW: Selection and preoperative preparation of plastic surgery patients. Nurs Clin North Am 29:697–710, 1994.

Strzyzewski NM: The cycle of perioperative nursing care for plastic surgery patients. Plast Surg Nurs 15:78–81, 85, 1995.

Tebbetts JB: Blepharoplasty: A refine technique emphasizing accuracy and control. Clin Plast Surg 19:329–350, 1992.

Vander Kam V, Achauer B: Abdominoplasty. Plast Surg Nurs 13:217–220, 222, 1993.

Vander Kam V, Achauer B: Aesthetic rhinoplasty. Plast Surg Nurs 15:182–184, 1995.

Watson D, James D: Intravenous conscious sedation. AORN J 51:1512–1523, 1990.

Wentz MG: Clinical photography simplified: Developing a personal set of uniformed view. Plast Surg Nurs 15:211–215, 1995.

Williams L: Facial rejuvenation. Nurs Clin North Am 29(4):741–752, 1994.

Chapter 33

General Surgery

Linda Pavlak

The broad topic of general surgery encompasses many diverse operations, including hernia repair and breast, abdominal, and rectal procedures. Mastectomy and breast biopsy, partial thyroidectomy, cholecystectomy, pilonidal cystectomy, hemorrhoidectomy, vein ligation, and excision of superficial lesions are just a few of the many procedures performed by the general surgeon in an ambulatory setting. As physician pioneers expand the number and complexity of procedures being done in an ambulatory setting, nurses concurrently ensure that nursing practice changes to safely address patients' ever-changing healthcare needs.

The development and refinement of modern surgical tools and techniques allow more advanced procedures to be accomplished laparoscopically with less trauma to surrounding tissue. Chapter 28 details some recent technical advances. With widespread use of lasers and laparoscopic equipment, the number and types of procedures that can be accomplished with same-day discharge have multiplied dramatically. Modified radical mastectomy is one of the most publicly scrutinized procedures currently performed in ambulatory surgery centers (ASCs).

Another, laparoscopic appendectomy, first was described in 1983 by Semm,[1] the German physician who many consider to be the world's leading expert in operative laparoscopy. Laparoscopic herniorrhaphy is another recent innovation. Robert Moran, MD, along with four other physicians who specialize in hernia repair, founded the National Ambulatory Hernia Institute in California. Moran published results of a study that boasts a recurrence rate of 10% to 12%.[2]

Even more complex procedures, such as bowel resections, thoracic interventions, and splenectomy, are being accomplished via laparoscopy in university and research settings and likely will be embraced by the surgical community within the next few years. A few of the many types of general surgical procedures are addressed in the following discussion.

BREAST PROCEDURES

Breast procedures range from excision of cysts to biopsy to mastectomy. Although many lesions are benign, the incidence of breast cancer is increasing, and it has become the most common cancer in American women. An estimated 180,000 new cases occurred in 1997, with 46,000 attributed deaths.[3]

Most risk factors that are known to increase a women's incidence of cancer cannot be altered: advanced age, white race, family history of breast cancer, late first pregnancy, previous benign or malignant breast disease, and early menarche or late menopause. Although there is conflicting information, excessive weight and high intake of dietary fat are thought to be risk factors that can be altered by changes in the woman's dietary habits.

The value of mammography is well documented as a screening tool for breast cancer. It is estimated that mammography detects carcinoma an average of 2 years before it is palpable.[4] Current recommended standards[3] for mammography and breast self-examination are as follows:

- Age 20–39 years: Monthly breast self-examination, clinical breast examination every 3 years by a healthcare professional.

- Age 40 years and older: Monthly breast self-examination, annual clinical breast examination by a healthcare professional, and annual mammogram.

Once a breast mass has been identified, a fine-needle aspiration or needle biopsy may be performed in the physician's office before a surgical procedure.

Although these techniques often provide valuable information about the mass, results may be inconclusive or false. More definitive therapies include open biopsy, lumpectomy, and partial or superficial mastectomy. In an ambulatory surgery setting, biopsy, excision of benign masses, lumpectomy, and mastectomies are undertaken.

Physicians have begun using a new procedure to identify the "sentinel node" or primary lymph node, located in the axillary area.[5] A small amount of radioisotope is injected, and the sentinel node is identified during a nuclear medicine scan. The node is excised in addition to the malignant breast mass. Researchers are using this procedure, which is much less extensive than an axillary lymph node dissection, in many university settings in the United States.

Patient Education

Patient education plays an important role in the preparation and recovery of the surgical patient. Patients, both male and female, undergoing breast surgery typically have many fears associated with the physiologic effects of breast surgery and the potential diagnosis of carcinoma. These patients need to fully understand the exact procedure that the surgeon is going to perform. Many patients no longer sign consent forms allowing a surgeon to perform additional procedures immediately after a biopsy. The nurse should verify that the patient understands the plan. Any questions or uncertainty should be directed to the physician. Patients should be educated regarding the size and location of the operative site dressing. Dressings are often larger than patients have anticipated.

Postoperative pain management needs to be discussed preoperatively. Facilities are using various pain scales to assist patients in communicating their pain level. By educating patients preoperatively as to how to use a particular scale, the caregivers can further reassure patients that their comfort is extremely important. Facilities should encourage physicians to give patients prescriptions for their postoperative pain medications before the day of the procedure. This allows the patient to have the necessary medications available immediately after discharge.

Female patients need to be instructed to bring a brassiere with them on the day of surgery. Most surgeons recommend that patients wear a brassiere, without underwire, to provide support for several days postoperatively. Patients should also be informed about the potential for swelling and ecchymosis.

Preoperative Care

Regardless of the extent of the surgery intended, the unknown status of the diagnosis plays a significant role in the patient's psychological and behavioral responses. Patients may display a calm demeanor, obvious and extreme emotional distress, or anything in between. Despite what the patient and family may say, it is rare that they are actually calm and confident until benign pathology results are shown.

Patient anxiety may stem from multiple factors. The patient may be confused about appropriate therapy because of the many conflicting opinions held by healthcare providers, the availability of many treatment choices, the tentativeness of providers regarding which definitive treatment is best, the legal ramifications of disclosure of information that is often conflicting and upsetting, and the physician's attitude, which may be less than optimistic.[6] The popular press and Internet represent yet another source of conflicting information. Finally, many patients have had prior personal experiences or may know a friend or family member who has undergone a breast procedure. This historical information cannot help but color the patient's expectations.

Other factors influencing the psychological response include the threat to body image, the value ascribed to the breast in terms of nurturing young, and the associated sexual connotations. Patients have the right to decide on the choice of treatment, but the inherent responsibility creates heightened anxiety related to that choice.

When diagnostic biopsy is performed, the outcome of the biopsy determines further therapy. It has been the practice of some surgeons to obtain the consent of the patient so that, on affirmation of a positive frozen section, definitive intervention can be undertaken during the course of the same anesthesia session. Other practitioners believe that the patient needs more time for consultation and decision-making.

A small lesion may require a preoperative needle localization to identify definitively the mass during surgery. In the radiology department, using radiographic support and local anesthesia, one or more needles are inserted into the area near the mass. A repeat mammogram is done to ensure that the needles accurately identify the mass. The patient goes to surgery with the needles taped in place. This preparation, although not excruciating, is not comfortable for the patient, and the patient may arrive in the admitting area preoperatively in an agitated or frightened state.

The radiographic films from a preoperative needle localization likely will accompany the patient to surgery for the surgeon's reference during the procedure. Postoperatively, the tissue specimen, often with the needles still in place, is reviewed radiologically to ensure that the mass or masses identified preoperatively are, in fact, in the specimen. The surgeon may wait to close the wound until receiving the radiologist's report. This wait can delay the surgical case and cause worry for the family if they have not been informed of the process. Additionally, most patients are sedated, not anesthetized, for this procedure. Any discussions or reports given in the operating room should take into consideration that the patient may be listening to both the words and the tone of voice, searching for a quick answer to the one question that is foremost. What did the pathology show?

Postoperative Care

After most breast procedures, oral analgesics usually are adequate for relieving pain. Concurrent emotional support encourages the patient to voice fears and concerns and seeks to provide the patient with accurate information and a positive, hopeful attitude. The nurse, however, must avoid making unfounded promises or encouraging false or unreasonable hopes.

Discharge instructions depend on the extent of the procedure and the diagnosis. Patients who have undergone a biopsy with negative frozen section report results need instruction about keeping the incision clean and dry. They will return to the physician's office for suture removal and to obtain the full pathology report, which may conflict with that of the initial frozen section.

After mastectomy or other definitive surgery for carcinoma, the patient should be encouraged to continue with all suggested follow-ups for both short- and long-term care. Range-of-motion exercises, as directed by the physician, are encouraged in the affected arm. Exercise promotes circulation and discourages the occurrence of edema.

Literature and contact information can be provided for support groups, such as the American Cancer Society's "Reach for Recovery" program. Providing this information may be a function of the physician's office at a later time. When the patient is cared for in an ambulatory setting rather than in a hospital, the ASC nurse is the only facility nurse involved in the patient's care. Therefore, that nurse should discuss options with the surgeon and ensure that somewhere in the course of aftercare, appropriate information regarding support groups is provided as part of a comprehensive care plan for patients facing recovery from breast cancer. The Internet web site of the American Cancer Society, www.cancer.org, provides a plethora of information in layman's terms.

HERNIORRHAPHY

A hernia is the protrusion of a structure through a weakened area. Various parts of the abdominal wall can be affected from either congenital or acquired weaknesses. Elevation in intra-abdominal pressure related to coughing, sneezing, straining, or intra-abdominal pathology increases the chances of herniation through any weakened area of the abdominal wall. Often the parietal peritoneum is contained within the hernia sac, although a portion of the intestines may be involved as well. If intestinal flow is obstructed, a hernia is said to be incarcerated. When both intestinal and blood flow are obstructed, the hernia is strangulated. Both of these complications require hospitalization of the patient and are not ambulatory surgical procedures.

Hernias are named by their anatomic sites, for example: femoral, umbilical, ventral or incisional, and most commonly, inguinal. Figure 33–1 illustrates these anatomic positions. A poorly healed surgical incision is at risk for herniation, as is the umbilical orifice, particularly in obese people or multiparturient women. Areas above and below the inguinal ligament represent points of weakness because of the course of blood vessels and the lack of muscle mass; thus, hernias often occur there. A hernia below the ligaments is considered femoral, and those above are inguinal.

The terms *direct* and *indirect* refer to two types of inguinal hernias. A direct inguinal hernia exits the abdomen through an area of muscle weakness, whereas an indirect hernia follows the path of a canal, for example, the spermatic cord

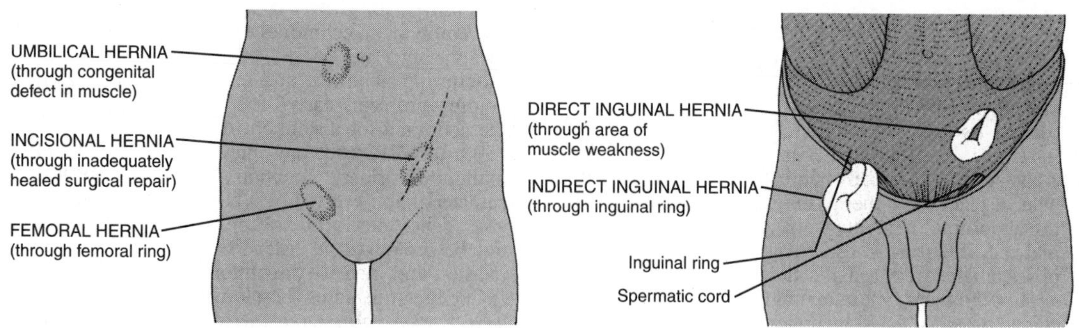

Figure 33–1. Locations of various types of hernias. (From Ignatavicius DD, Workman ML, Mishler MA: Medical Surgical Nursing: A Nursing Process Approach, 2nd ed. Philadelphia: WB Saunders, 1995, p 1599.)

as it exits through the inguinal ring. The indirect hernia is more common in men because of the congenital space that was present to allow for the decent of the testicles. Indirect inguinal hernias in men frequently follow that line where the spermatic cord exits the abdomen and enters the scrotum, eventually involving the scrotum in the hernia. In women, a susceptible area for indirect inguinal hernia surrounds the round ligament.

Femoral hernias are similar in pathophysiology to the indirect inguinal type. They occur at the femoral canal rather than at a point of muscle weakness. They are more common in women and are often associated with strangulation or incarceration. It is not uncommon for the urinary bladder to be involved in a femoral hernia. The most common incision used for a femoral hernia is identical to that for inguinal hernia repair, although a thigh incision can be used.

General, regional, or local anesthesia may be used. Regional blockade of the ilioinguinal and iliohypogastric nerves may be the sole anesthetic or may be used as a supplement to general anesthesia. When administered as an adjunct to general anesthesia, the block is often performed after the patient is asleep but before surgery so that the regional block reduces the amount and depth of general anesthesia required. Bupivacaine (0.5%) is frequently used and provides analgesia for several hours postoperatively.

Complications of this block are rare, although inadvertent block of the femoral nerve can result in temporary weakness of the affected leg. The patient should be monitored closely and assisted with ambulation after surgery until adequate leg strength is ascertained. Before the initial postoperative ambulation, the nurse should explain the possibility of leg weakness to the patient and encourage the patient to bear weight primarily on the unaffected leg.

Specific surgical technique varies, but aspects of the procedure include identification of the hernia; replacement of herniated structures or organs into correct intra-abdominal position; removal of the hernia sac; repair of weakened muscles, ligaments, and other tissues; and closure of the abdominal wall. A synthetic mesh material may be added for strength to prevent recurrence, which can result in a significant economic and medical impact on individual patients and the healthcare system in general. Polypropylene mesh is an inert, nonallergenic, strong fabric that has been used to repair hernia defects. Addition of such a material results in less tension on the sutures because edges of the herniated tissues are not forcibly pulled together.[7]

Patient Education

Patients undergoing surgery for the repair of a hernia may have experienced some degree of pain preoperatively. These patients should be taught to use the facility's accepted pain scale or tool to facilitate their comfort postoperatively. Splinting of incisions should be discussed, and any potential activity, lifting, or bending restrictions should be clarified with the patient. Many physicians or ASCs continue to require postoperative hernia repair patients to void before discharge. This information should be communicated to patients so they can plan transportation based on a realistic length of stay.

Preoperative Care

Patients undergoing all types of hernia repair should be encouraged to empty their urinary bladder immediately before surgery. Bladder distention can impede the reduction of herniated tissue. Patients requiring regional anesthesia should receive nursing support during the administration of those anesthetics. Facility policies differ regarding surgical skin preparation. Facilities requiring clipper preparation or shaving of designated surgical sites should ensure patient privacy during this procedure.

Postoperative Care

Postoperatively, nursing care focuses on anesthesia-related concerns, analgesia, ambulation, assessment for complications, and voiding. Early and aggressive analgesia intervention is important to prevent rather than treat pain. Ambulation, taking and tolerating nourishment, and the patient's general feeling of well-being depend on the patient's comfort level. Local anesthesia infiltration of the skin and subcutaneous tissues surrounding the incision reduces discomfort in the early recovery period. Medications such as narcotics and ketorolac may be necessary, and the patient should be urged to take any oral analgesics that are prescribed for use at home. Local ice application and, in the male patient, support of the scrotum can be palliative.

Adequate analgesia also plays a role in the prevention of nausea and vomiting in the postoperative period. Not only is vomiting unpleasant, but retching can increase incision pain and initiate a circular cause-and-effect pattern. Even with adequate pain relief, gastrointestinal (GI) symptoms may still occur, particularly if there has been a significant manipulation of genitourinary structures. Pharmacologic treatment with antiemetics may be necessary.

The patient's ability to void may be affected after herniorrhaphy. In addition to the physiologic reasons that are discussed in Chapter 35 on urologic procedures, the patient may have discomfort and may be reluctant to attempt voiding because the physical effort is difficult or painful. Further, the emotional climate may be nonconducive to voiding, with staff and family members anxiously awaiting the patient's discharge. The situation can make voiding psychologically stressful, if not impossible, especially for the male patient. Aggressive hydration, analgesia, and positive reinforcement can contribute positively to the patient's voiding.

Instructions for home care stress the return to normal, moderate activity. The patient should be urged to stand erect rather than bent forward. Heavy lifting, strenuous exercise, and driving an automobile are avoided as directed. Some surgeons allow the patient to remove the dressing and to shower on the evening of surgery, whereas others suggest a wait of 48 hours. A diet that is high in fiber with adequate fluid intake contributes to soft stools and reduces strain with bowel movements. A stool softener may be prescribed.

Laparoscopic herniorrhaphy is becoming more popular. Intraoperative times may be longer than with traditional herniorrhaphy; however, as physicians' techniques and experience advance, the time needed for the laparoscopic approach decreases. The reduced discomfort and physical restrictions along with the shorter period of recuperation in the postoperative period make laparoscopic herniorrhaphy an attractive alternative.

ANORECTAL

There are several types of anorectal procedures performed in the ambulatory setting. Hemorrhoidectomy, pilonidal cystectomy, anal fistulectomy, and anal fissurectomy are examples of these procedures.

Hemorrhoidectomy

Internal and external hemorrhoids often present with bleeding, pain, and visible prolapse. Often these varicosities are so painful that their excision leaves the patient with less pain than was present before surgery. Internal hemorrhoids arise from the epithelial lining of the upper two thirds of the anal canal. External hemorrhoids originate in the skin-covered lower one third and can be thrombosed, containing large clots. A number of techniques have been devised for the removal of hemorrhoids, but common to all is the need for adequate postoperative analgesic therapy.

Pilonidal Cystectomy

A pilonidal sinus in the presacral area occurs most often in people younger than 25 years of age and in men. The typical patient is white, has a large amount of body hair, and is subjected to repeated trauma to the area, for example, due to a profession such as truck driving. The word "pilonidal" actually translates for the Latin as *pilus*—"hair" and *nidus*—"nest." In many cases, although not always, hair is contained within the cyst.

A variety of surgical approaches are used, depending largely on the patient's work schedule and personal habits, the size of the cyst, and the patient's ability to care for the wound. The cyst simply may be opened or may be totally excised. In both cases, packing is inserted. Another approach is excision with immediate closure of the wound, allowing quicker return to work. If infection or inflammation is present or if the hygiene is suspect, primary closure is avoided and packing with gradual closure of the open wound by granulation is chosen.

Anal Fistulectomy and Anal Fissurectomy

A fistula in ano occurs as a result of infection. A tract is formed between the anal canal and the skin, often on both sides of the rectum. The tract is opened surgically and most often is packed with the incision left open to heal from the inside by granulation. Sometimes the wound is partially closed with suture.

An anal fissure originates when a tear of the rectal tissue from passing hard stool becomes infected or ulcerated. It may be acute, with associated inflammation, bleeding, burning, and pain on defecation. A fissure also may progress to a chronic state wherein fibrotic tissue forms and results in less acute, but persistent, dull pain. Anal sphincter dilation may be the only surgical treatment necessary, but for chronic conditions, removal of the scarred tissue is recommended.

Patient Education

Preoperatively, patients undergoing anorectal procedures should be instructed to follow the surgeon's desired regimen for cleansing of the GI tract. The patient must understand the need to follow this prescribed method. Satisfactory GI preparation is essential to the procedure and can be accomplished by enemas, cathartic medications, and preoperative dietary restrictions. The nature of anorectal conditions can be embarrassing to patients. The nurse's matter-of-fact manner can help to allay that embarrassment. Patients should be reassured that their dignity and privacy will be respected in all departments of the ASC.

Management of postoperative pain should be discussed with the patient. Allowing the patient to become familiar with whatever scale or method of pain evaluation that the ASC uses promotes patient/nurse communication postoperatively. Surgeons should be encouraged to communicate the need for postoperative medical equipment before surgery. This ensures that the patient can be discharged and the necessary equipment readily available. Sitz baths, rubber rings, and other supportive items are some of the nonpharmacologic comfort measures.

Preoperative Care

On the patient's arrival at the ASC, the nurse should question the patient regarding the adherence to specific orders for diet, medications, and lower GI cleansing. Enemas and shaving of the perirectal area may be necessary. The patient should be provided with privacy for these procedures. Intraoperative positioning can complicate anesthesia management. The prone, jack-knife, lateral, and knee-chest positions are possible options. Patients may have underlying pathologic conditions and may have difficulty assuming some or any of these positions. The admitting nurse should communicate any special positioning issues to the operative team.

Assessment of the patient's functional mobility and documentation and communication of any limitations is needed to ensure patient comfort. All types of anesthesia are used, but regional anesthesia affords long-term postoperative analgesia. It also eliminates the problems associated with airway management of the patient whose position makes continuous hands-on care of the airway impossible.

Postoperative Care

Anorectal pain can be intense because of the extensive innervation of the rectal sphincter and surrounding tissue, and aggressive analgesic therapy is indicated, particularly after the effects of regional anesthesia have passed. Simple comfort measures may help as well. For instance, sitting on a rubber ring may relieve direct rectal pressure. Side-lying and recumbent positions are assumed naturally by the patient to relieve pressure on the surgical site. The surgeon may infiltrate the incision with local anesthetic just before transfer to the postanesthesia care unit.

Another palliative measure that promotes comfort at home is a Sitz bath. Comfortable warm water not only feels soothing but also promotes hygienic cleansing of the rectal area. Sitz baths are usually ordered two or three times a day and after bowel movements. The patient should understand that this bath is not intended for washing, but rather for soaking and relaxing. A rubber ring or padding with a rolled towel can make sitting in the tub more comfortable.

Urinary retention is possible because of rectal spasms or rectal pain.[8]

A packing, often of petroleum jelly gauze, may have been left in the rectum to be removed by the physician or by the postoperative nurse or patient as directed. The plan may be for the packing to remain in place until it falls out naturally with a Sitz bath or a bowel movement. The patient should be told what to expect related to the packing so he or she is not to be surprised or frightened by its presence if it falls out at home. The patient should be instructed about the technique and importance of perianal cleansing after each stool.[9]

Careful attention must be given to the patient's bowel status so that painful constipation and straining are avoided. Adequate hydration, exercise, and fiber intake are coupled with a prescribed stool softener. Strong laxatives are avoided so that potentially irritating diarrhea does not complicate healing of the incision. The physician may order a mild laxative.

LAPAROSCOPIC CHOLECYSTECTOMY

Nonsurgical treatment for gallbladder disease has included low-fat diet, medications to dissolve gallstones, and research into shock wave lithotripsy (SWL). Regardless of the mode used to eliminate gallstones, the chance of recurrence is always present until the gallbladder is actually removed.[10] Until the past decade, traditional open laparotomy was the only surgical choice for removal of the gallbladder. The resultant period of disability and recuperation was approximately 2 to 3 months.

The physical, economic, and psychological advantages of a laparoscopic alternative are significant. It is less invasive than traditional surgery and results in a shorter hospital stay, less postoperative pain, and more rapid ambulation and recuperation. Most people resume full physical activity after approximately 1 week. Nearly 195,000 cholecystectomies were performed in the ambulatory surgical setting in 1994 in the United States.[11] With even more currently being performed, the economic impact of rapid recovery is enormous.

Laparoscopic cholecystectomy (LC) has received tremendous attention both from the public and from the medical community. General surgeons have shown a great interest in learning and applying laparoscopic techniques for a variety of procedures and, in particular, for cholecystectomy.

Care of the cholecystectomy patient takes into account the same general principles of laparoscopic intervention that are described in detail in Chapter 28. Contraindications include patients with severe coagulopathy or peritonitis and pregnant women. Patients who may have intra-abdominal adhesions from previous surgeries are not necessarily eliminated from consideration, although the chance that intraoperative open laparotomy will be needed increases.[12] A massively obese or exceptionally tall patient may pose difficulties because instruments may be too short to reach the gallbladder.[13]

During surgery, the patient is placed in a reverse Trendelenburg position to allow better visualization of the gallbladder and cystic duct. A total of four small abdominal incisions are made, through which a variety of instruments are passed. These small wounds cause minor discomfort compared with a laparotomy incision. Either laser photocoagulation or electrocautery can be used for dissection and control of bleeding. After the gallbladder has been detached from its bed, it is withdrawn from the abdomen with the severed end coming out first. If it is too large to be removed through the small incision because it contains bile and stones, suction and a crushing instrument may be used to empty it before its removal.

The surgeon cannot explore the common duct laparoscopically but can do an intraoperative cholangiogram. If ductal stones are identified by intraoperative cholangiography, the current recommendation is to leave the stones for later treatment by an endoscopist via an intestinal approach. Intraoperative complications include the puncture or rupture of a blood vessel, for example, the aorta or hepatic artery. Perforation of the bladder, bowel, or another viscus is possible and can result in hemorrhage or sepsis.

Patient Education

Some of the key points of preoperative education are pain control, possible referred pain secondary to pneumoperitoneum, and activity restrictions. Many of these patients have experienced episodes of severe pain preoperatively.

Preoperative Care

Preoperatively, the patient's abdomen may be shaved because of the potential need for laparotomy during surgery. The patient should void before surgery to avoid bladder distention that could lead to inadvertent puncture during placement of trocars and instruments into the abdomen.

Postoperative Care

The patient should be assessed periodically for increased abdominal girth, hardness, or tenderness and for other signs that could indicate intra-abdominal bleeding. Less serious complications in the postoperative period include nausea and vomiting, minimal to moderate abdominal discomfort, and referred shoulder pain. After an initial period when parenteral analgesics may be needed, oral pain medications usually suffice for home use.

Discharge is often on the day of surgery, although some patients may require overnight hospitalization for pain or nausea management or urinary problems. At home, the patient is allowed to shower after 48 hours. The patient is encouraged to drink adequate fluids to maintain normal bowel function. Moderate activity is allowed immediately after surgery, and normal exercise and lifting can be resumed after approximately 1 week.

References

1. Semm K: Endoscopic appendectomy. Endoscopy 15:59–64, 1983.
2. Moran R: Inguinal Hernia: Expert Meeting on Hernia Surgery 1995. LaPuente, CA: Karger, 1995, pp 206–211.
3. American Cancer Society, Breast Cancer Statistics, 1998.
4. Bassett L, Manjikian V, Gold R: Mammography and breast cancer screening. Surg Clin North Am 70:775–800, 1990.
5. Veronesi U, Paganelli G, Galimberti V, et al: Sentinel-node biopsy to avoid axillary dissection in breast cancer with clinically negative lymph nodes. Lancet 349:1864–1867, 1997.
6. Schain W: Physician–patient communication about breast cancer. Surg Clin North Am 70:917–936, 1990.
7. Lichtenstein I, Shulman A, Amid P, Willis P: Hernia repair with polypropylene mesh and improved method. AORN J 52:559–565, 1990.
8. Ignatavicius DD, Workman ML, Mishler MA: Medical Surgical Nursing, A Nursing Process Approach, 2nd ed. Philadelphia: WB Saunders 1995, p 1660.
9. Luckman J (ed): Saunders Manual of Nursing Care. Philadelphia: WB Saunders, 1997, p 1286.
10. Nahrwold D, Prystowsky J, Rege R: Biliary lithotripsy. Curr Prob Surg 27:11, 1990.
11. Centers for Disease Control and Prevention, National Center for Health Statistics: Advance Data. Hyattsville, MD: Department of Health and Human Services, 1997, vol 283.
12. Haicken B: Laser laparoscopic cholecystectomy in ambulatory setting. J Anesth Nurs 6:33–39, 1991.
13. Abramowicz M: Laparoscopic cholecystectomy. Med Lett Drugs Ther 32:115–116, 1990.

Chapter 34

Gynecologic and Obstetric Surgery

Brenda S. Gregory Dawes

The female reproductive system is complex. External genital structures differ considerably from one woman to another depending, in large part, on race, age, hereditary factors, and the number of children delivered. Internal organs include the vagina, uterus, and paired fallopian tubes and ovaries. A complex supporting structure of 10 ligaments secures these organs in the bony pelvis, and a rich blood and nerve supply is present (Fig. 34–1).

The usual position of the uterus is anteverted or tipped forward. The uterine position changes with filling and emptying of the urinary bladder and rectum, position changes, age, and during pregnancy. The nonpregnant uterus is approximately 3 × 1½ × ¾ inch. The lining, or endometrium, is a three-layered mucous membrane with rich blood supplies whose two outer layers slough and regenerate with the menstrual cycle. The cervix extends into the vagina and provides

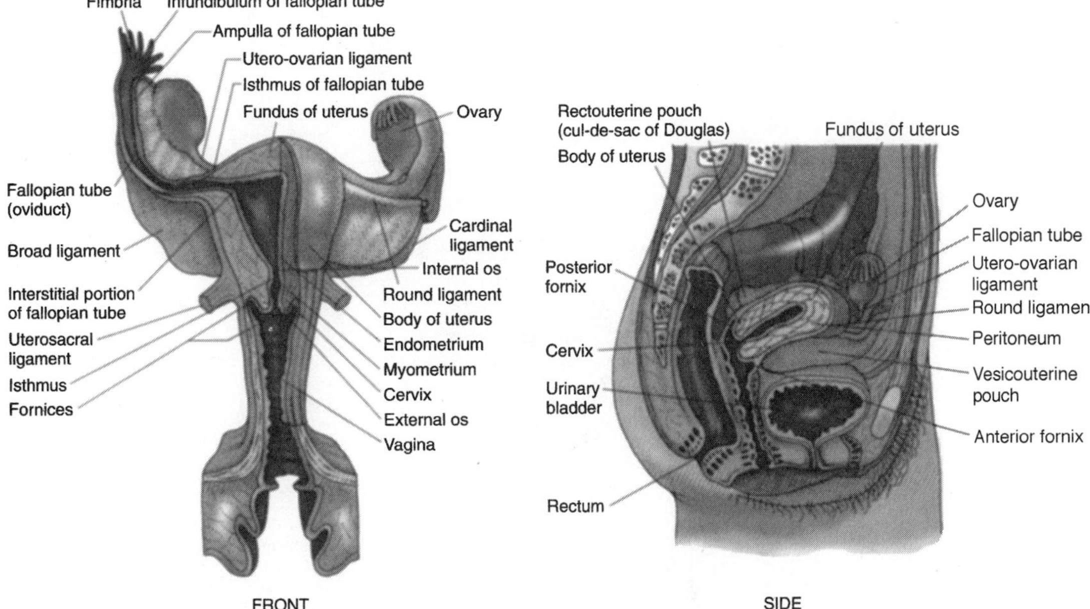

Figure 34–1. Internal female genitalia. (From Ignatavicius DD, Workman ML, Mishler MM: Medical-Surgical Nursing Across the Health Care Continuum, 3rd ed. Philadelphia: WB Saunders, 1999, p 1930.)

external access for menstruation, fertilization, and birth.[1]

Other structures that are not reproductive organs surround the female genitalia (Fig. 34–2). They play a significant role in the pathology and subsequent treatment of gynecologic conditions and must be considered as contributing factors in many cases. Examples include the anus, rectum, urethra, urinary meatus, and bladder. Selected gynecologic definitions appear in Table 34–1.

An ambulatory surgical center (ASC) is ideal for many gynecologic and some obstetric procedures for various reasons. First, many gynecologic procedures lend themselves to early ambulation and do not significantly limit postoperative activity or self-care. Also, the ease and convenience of ambulatory surgery are appealing to many working women. A third reason is the availability and continuous improvement of technologies. Lasers and laparoscopes are devices that decrease the invasiveness of many procedures and reduce the amount of tissue damage. The instrumentation and techniques are constantly being improved.

Gynecology specialists pioneered tremendous advances in the complexity of procedures that are possible and appropriate for ASCs. Laparoscopic tubal sterilization has been a well-accepted procedure for many years, and techniques and equipment now permit outpatient treatment of ectopic pregnancies, infertility, endometriosis, ovarian cysts, and other intraabdominal conditions. Vaginal hysterectomy is being performed in some ASCs. The procedure is done using both laparoscopic and laser applications. Complex procedures may require a 23-hour admission to a hospital or recovery care center.

Women undergoing gynecologic procedures present with a wide variety of conditions, such as abnormal vaginal bleeding or preoperative diagnostic studies, neoplasms, infections, infertility, cysts, lesions, and pelvic pain. Some undergo termination of a pregnancy or sterilization, and others desire artificial fertilization in the hope of becoming pregnant. This diagnostic diversity demands a comprehensive nursing review of each patient's medical history so that counseling and patient teaching can be ethically adapted to each patient's physical and emotional needs.

The elderly gynecologic patient has limitations, such as arthritis or heart disease, that can make preparing and positioning difficult, time consuming, or uncomfortable. Lithotomy positioning, in particular, may require modification of the leg position with less abduction and flexion of the patient's hips. To prevent hypothermia, to which elderly patients are predisposed, warm blankets should be available and the patient should be covered as fully as possible in the cool operating room (OR) environment. This also helps to ensure that the sense of modesty is respected.[2] Other active warming measure may be necessary for longer or more complex procedures where the threat of hypothermia increases.

Other physical problems that are common in an older population have a direct impact on gynecologic conditions. These include decreased vaginal lubrication, constipation or fecal

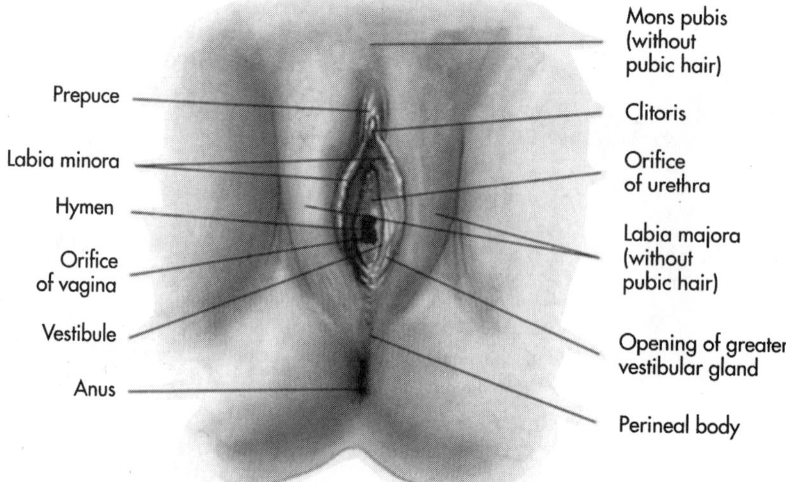

Figure 34–2. External female genitalia. (From Lowdermilk DD, et al: Maternity Nursing, 5th ed. St Louis: Mosby, 1999, p 65.)

***Table 34–1.* Gynecologic Definitions**

Term	Definition
Ablation	Removal or excision of a part of the body or a growth
Abortion	The premature termination of a pregnancy before the fetus is expected to live after birth; may be spontaneous, complete, incomplete, induced, or therapeutic
Adnexa	The structures that are adjacent to another structure; in gynecology, the fallopian tubes and ovaries are adnexa of the uterus
Cerclage	A procedure in which a nonabsorbable suture is placed in the incompetent cervix of a pregnant woman to prevent spontaneous abortion
Colporrhaphy	Repair of the vaginal wall
Condylomata acuminata	Wart-like growths of viral origin commonly seen on the genitals; spread by sexual contact
Cul-de-sac	Cul-de-sac of Douglas; the area between the uterus and the rectum at the top of the posterior vaginal wall
Culdoscopy	Endoscopic examination of the cul-de-sac of Douglas
Cystocele	Prolapse of the urinary bladder into the anterior vaginal wall
Dermoid cyst	Ovarian tumor consisting of embryonic materials such as epithelium, teeth, hair, and bone
Ectopic pregnancy	Implantation of the fertilized ovum in a place other than the upper half of the uterus
Endometriosis	The abnormal growth of endometrial tissue in areas outside of the uterus
Endometrium	The mucous membrane lining the uterus that changes in structure and thickness during the menstrual cycle
Enterocele	Protrusion of the intestine into the cul-de-sac of Douglas—the area between the uterus and the rectum at the top of the posterior vaginal wall
Fibroid	Tumors containing muscle tissue
Fimbrioplasty	Repair of the uterine tube after excision or incision
Hydatid mole	Intrauterine neoplastic mass of chorionic villi of pregnancy; also called molar pregnancy
Hysterectomy	Removal of the uterus
Hysteroscopy	Endoscopic visualization and operation within the uterine cavity
Laparoscopy	Technique of visualization and operation within the abdominal cavity by endoscopic means after inflation of the abdomen to move the abdominal wall away from the viscera
Missed abortion	Condition when a dead fetus is not expelled from the uterus spontaneously
Myoma	A benign, fibroid tumor of the uterine muscle
Myomectomy	Surgical removal of a myoma (fibroid) of the uterus
Oxytocin	A synthetic posterior pituitary hormone used to produce a uterine contraction, induce labor, and promote postpartum or post-abortion contraction of the uterus to control bleeding
Pelviscopy	Procedure for viewing abdominal content using a scope with a wide angle
Perineum	Area of the skin between the vagina and the rectum
Pitressin	Synthetic vasopressin that may be injected into the cervix intraoperatively to reduce bleeding during conization
Pneumoperitoneum	Insufflation of gas into the abdominal peritoneal cavity for the purpose of raising the abdominal wall away from the internal organs; used for laparoscopic procedures
Rectocele	Prolapse of the rectum into the posterior vaginal wall
Salpingotomy	Cutting into the uterine tube
Suction curettage	The suction removal of uterine contents, usually performed after dilatation of the cervix
Urethrocele	Pouch-like protrusion of the urethral wall and thickening of connective tissue around the urethra

impaction, urinary incontinence, and hip and knee joint disease or replacement, which complicates positioning. Prolapsed uterus, rectocele, cystocele, and postmenopausal bleeding are common gynecologic conditions in older women.

The very nature of gynecologic surgery is rife with emotional strain. Not only are physically or pharmacologically induced hormonal changes occurring in many patients, but also the volatile issues of pregnancy, fertility, menstruation, and sexuality are related to gynecologic conditions. Emotions can range from the despondency of a couple over the loss of a baby or discovery of a malignancy to the elation and hope of another woman for obtaining a much-sought pregnancy.

Gynecologic procedures can threaten the patient's body image and sense of sexuality. The nurse can help to alleviate some of the patient's anxieties by exhibiting a confident and calm manner, by answering questions and offering explanations appropriately, and by encouraging the patient's confidence in her physicians.

Each woman places a personal value on these various issues. The nurse in the ASC is challenged to address every patient's emotional needs, but with a gynecologic patient that duty can be complicated by the nurse's (predominantly female) own value system, which may differ considerably from that of the patient. It is important for the nurse to examine personal biases and appropriately separate them from the nursing care given.

Care should be family-centered. Many procedures affect the woman's intimate relationship with a sexual partner, and thus it is helpful to provide both parties with perioperative explanations, instructions, and appropriate emotional support. Inclusion of the patient's partner should not infringe upon the patient's right to privacy. The nurse should provide the patient with opportunities to express her own needs and desires and to ask questions in private.

Patients who have an inadequate home support system need special reassurance and attention from the nurse. The woman may have an emotionally nonsupportive or hostile partner or may have no partner or companion during a time when her need for physical and emotional support may be great. An example is the adolescent undergoing a termination of pregnancy without the support of the child's father or any of her own family members. Such a patient may feel alone, rejected, or frightened and may express her need for reassurance and support verbally or through her actions. Others may cover such feelings with a display of defiance, anger, or casualness. Although nurses attempt to provide nonjudgmental and compassionate care to all patients, this compassion can be difficult to provide to some patients. Often, the very patients who are in the greatest need of the nurse's sincere concern are those whose actions and manner thwart attempts to provide that support.

PREOPERATIVE CARE

Preoperatively, the gynecologic patient may need clarification of instructions or explanations provided by the surgeon. Diagrams and pictures may be helpful in describing anatomic concepts related to the reproductive system. If questions remain that require further clarification by the physician, the nurse should facilitate that dialogue before the patient signs the operative consent.

Providing other specific information before surgery helps the patient to improve the plan for her postoperative needs. Examples include postoperative activity that will be allowed, an estimate of the recovery time, and, if relevant, whether to purchase sanitary napkins rather than tampons for postoperative use. In anticipation of procedures that require a lithotomy position, the nurse might suggest that the patient perform gentle leg stretching exercises during the week before surgery to improve range of motion in the hips. The nurse should stress that only mild exercise is appropriate for women who do not exercise routinely.

The baseline preoperative physical examination includes an abdominal examination to determine any pre-existing distention or discomfort. The patient whose legs will be positioned in stirrups or leg holders should have pedal pulses assessed and documented preoperatively as a valuable baseline for comparison in the rare event of postoperative circulatory complications related to positioning. The patient should also be asked if she experiences back pain and asked to describe the frequency and type to evaluate postoperative complications from the lithotomy position. Patients should void just before surgery to avoid damage to the bladder and to prevent a full bladder from interfering with the surgical procedure.

INTRAOPERATIVE CARE

Because of the personal nature of gynecologic conditions, maintenance of privacy and confidentiality for the patient is a special issue. Provision of warm blankets and demonstration of caring behaviors are simple methods to alleviate patient anxiety. Nursing goals when positioning the patient for surgery are to provide adequate operative exposure while avoiding injury to the patient and maintaining the patient's dignity.

Many procedures require lithotomy procedures. Patients are placed in the lithotomy position after being sedated or anesthetized. Lithotomy positioning requires: (1) elevating and lowering the patient's legs in unison by two people to avoid excess changes in circulatory status; (2) avoiding extreme flexion of the hips; (3) ensuring that the lower back is supported correctly on the operating room (OR) bed, or padding the patient's lumbar region to prevent pressure.

Special care should be taken with patients who have hip prostheses or advanced hip or knee disease that limits movement. Each type of leg holders has specific requirements. Those with straps that encircle the feet and ankles avoid pressure on the popliteal space, but the legs are not supported as when the full leg positioner is used. After placing the patient in the lithotomy position, the nurse should assess the neurovascular status of the patient's legs and feet to ascertain circulatory function.[3]

Other details of positioning are important to prevent injuries. The patient's arms should be placed on her abdomen, chest, or on armboards to avoid injury to her hands when the lower portion of the OR bed is raised at the end of the procedure.[3] During Trendelenburg positioning, the patient may require a padded shoulder brace to prevent discomfort or sliding toward the head of the bed.

POSTOPERATIVE CARE

Immediate postoperative attention is directed to physically assess airway and circulation, but the patient's emotional needs can be significant to her because of the reason for the surgery or the anticipation of an expected outcome. Nurses should immediately determine the outcome of the surgery and collaborate with the surgeon to determine the information that will be shared with the patient.

Postoperative nursing needs relate to vaginal flow, abdominal symptoms, and the effects of intraoperative positioning. Potential complications related to gynecologic surgery will be included in upcoming discussions of specific procedures.

Intraoperative positioning can complicate cardiorespiratory status. Lowering of the legs from the lithotomy position too rapidly, in a well patient or one whose cardiovascular status was previously compromised, can result in hypotension due to the rapid shift of blood volume from the trunk back into the legs. This is particularly true when the sympathetic blockade of a spinal or epidural anesthetic has affected the patient's vasomotor tone. Intravenous (IV) fluid replacement along with gentle postoperative transfer and movement of the patient should be employed until the blood pressure returns to the patient's normal range. After an episode of postoperative hypotension, attempts to ambulate should be gradual with a period of rest and observation between the progressive steps of head elevation, sitting, and walking. Nausea and vomiting related to hypotension are treated with increased IV fluids, maintenance of or return to a horizontal position, and administration of an IV vasopressor such as ephedrine.

Back, leg, hip, or thigh discomfort can be associated with the lithotomy position. To assess for possible nerve or circulatory impairment, the postanesthesia nurse should evaluate and document movement and sensation of the legs and feet as well as bilateral pedal pulses. Because many ASC procedures last for less than 4 hours, neurovascular complications are rare.[4] Other than any obvious neurologic complications, the patient can be reassured that such discomfort is temporary and, most likely, is related to assuming an unusual position.

Another infrequent but potential complication after gynecologic surgery is deep leg vein thrombophlebitis. The patient should be instructed to report any tenderness, swelling, redness, heat, or pain in the calf or other area of the leg. Early ambulation is certainly a favorable deterrent in some patients. This complication is related to three specific predisposing factors: (1) increased coagulation factors, (2) damage to a vessel wall, and (3) venous stasis.

Blood flow in the iliac vein has been reported to decrease during a gynecologic procedure. General risk factors that increase the chance of thrombophlebitis include certain types and lengths of operation, advanced age, obesity, immobility, malignancy or sepsis, severe diabetes, and other conditions that produce venous stasis.

Although most thrombi are either dissolved with treatment or subside spontaneously without treatment, a few result in an embolic incident. When embolism occurs, it is generally in the early postoperative period. Fatal pulmonary embolism is rare after gynecologic procedures;

however, the gynecologic patient should report any chest pain or dyspnea to the physician.

Vaginal flow is related to the type of surgical procedure, the time of surgery related to the woman's menstrual cycle, the underlying pathology, and complications that may have occurred. Nursing assessment includes a count of the number and saturation of perineal pads. Observation and palpation of the abdomen should be performed to identify distention, pain, or tenderness that could indicate perforation of the uterus. It is common for vaginal flow to be somewhat increased after the patient first ambulates. This may be an actual increase in flow, but more often is caused by the movement of pooled blood. Even when the surgical procedure is not intrauterine, vaginal spotting may occur if the surgeon has gripped the cervix with a sharp-toothed tenaculum to assist in movement of the uterus and adnexa. The patient needs reassurance that such spotting is temporary and normal.

The amount of expected vaginal flow or surgical drainage can be difficult to predict because there is a wide variation of normal depending on the type of procedure and the woman's idiosyncrasies. Some procedures such as laser ablation of condylomata may result in a small amount of drainage from operative sites over several weeks or longer. After a dilatation and curettage (D and C), the amount and duration of vaginal flow can range from almost none to flow similar to a menstrual period for a week or more. After a laser vaporization of the cervix, spotting or bleeding may continue for several days.

The important factor is to explain the range of normal and what should be reported to the physician. Explanations should be objective and specific. For instance, passing clots "larger than a lemon" or "saturating an entire pad with bright red blood every hour for several hours" are clear descriptions of what should be reported. They are more precise terms than telling the patient to call if she has "heavy" flow. Foul vaginal odor is also reportable, because it could indicate an infectious process.

Abdominal cramps, similar to menstrual cramps, are common after gynecologic procedures and may require analgesics. An oral medication is usually sufficient, but IV therapy may be required in the postanesthetic care unit (PACU) for rapid pain relief, particularly for the patient receiving oxytocin to promote uterine contraction. General comfort measures such as lateral positioning or knee flexion may be helpful. Anxiety and other psychological responses can alter the patient's perception of pain and cramping, and thus any intervention that helps to calm the patient may be helpful in relieving pain, for instance, reuniting the patient with her family or partner.

Some gynecologic procedures can result in tissue damage or edema in the pelvis, with or without urinary difficulty. Urinary distention, combined with the patient's inability to void, requires catheterization to reduce discomfort and avoid primary urinary bladder damage. The physician's order is followed regarding the requirement of voiding prior to discharge.

Clear written and verbal instructions for aftercare at home should be provided before the patient's discharge from the ASC. These instructions should be discussed in an area that affords the patient privacy. Physicians vary in their approach to postoperative activities, and instructions must meet the particular physician's directives. Discharge information that is important for the gynecologic patient is identified in Table 34–2.

The patient may be embarrassed or may forget to ask her physician about sexual restrictions after the procedure. The nurse should be prepared to answer queries and to provide unsolic-

Table 34–2. Key Education Points

Activity levels (e.g., lifting, swimming, exercise, return to work, driving)
Showering versus bathing
Infection prevention measures (e.g., washing hands before care, changing dressing, keeping the incision site dry, using ointments as ordered)
Symptoms to report (e.g., redness around incision, increased pain, increased temperature)
Expected comfort level (e.g., analgesic therapy, positioning, nausea and vomiting)
Expected norms for vaginal flow (when and what to report to doctor)
Special concerns related to procedure (i.e., potential shoulder pain after pneumoperitoneum, administration of Rh immune globulin)
Menstrual cycle (e.g., interruption or changes)
Medications (e.g., antibiotics, analgesics, instructions for use of vaginal applicators and topical sprays)
Omission of aspirin or other medications that may promote bleeding (according to physician preference)
Douching
Use of tampons versus pads
Prevention of infection (e.g., symptoms to report, washing hands before wound care, reporting fever)
Sexual activity (period of abstinence)
Avoidance of gas-producing food and beverages
Return to the physician's office and follow-up care

ited information as a matter of course prior to discharge. Some patients may mistakenly fear that surgery will cause a permanent loss of sexual interest or performance. Providing the patient and her partner with the reasons to abstain from sexual intercourse for the period of time prescribed by the physician can help to increase their understanding and compliance. Those reasons include limiting the potential for infection, reducing discomfort and bleeding, and avoiding injury to freshly traumatized vaginal and cervical tissues.

The nurse's manner and personal comfort level in discussing sexual issues will be evident. The nurse who comfortably discusses the topic can help the patient to feel at ease. Many older women remain sexually active and should be afforded the same information as younger patients.

BARTHOLIN'S CYST

Bartholin's glands are located at the base of the labia majora, one on either side of the vagina. Each has several ducts for drainage of clear mucus that lubricates the vagina. Bartholin's cyst is actually a cyst of the duct, rather than of the gland. Chronic and acute infections can cause inflammation and result in intense pain.

Initial treatment of an abscessed Bartholin's cyst is usually by simple needle aspiration with subsequent antibiotic therapy. After drainage of an abscess, approximately 80% of women regain patency of the duct. When excision of the cyst is necessary, the procedure can be complicated by a significant amount of bleeding intraoperatively. After surgery, if the skin heals rapidly and obliterates the patency of the duct, fluids secreted by the gland accumulate in surrounding tissues and a chronic abscess can form that requires further treatment.[5]

Subsequent definitive treatment is aimed at preventing further episodes. Two methods are used. The traditional approach is a marsupialization in which the cyst is incised and irrigated, and the lining everted and sutured open with absorbable sutures. In this way, future drainage to the skin is ensured (Fig. 34–3). Packing is not required. The patient is instructed to keep the area clean.

Another treatment is the insertion of a Word catheter. This device resembles a short Foley catheter with a small, inflatable balloon. Unlike a urinary catheter, the Word catheter has no lumen. Some practitioners choose to use a small Foley catheter. The cyst is drained, then the balloon of the catheter is inflated with saline and remains in the cyst for 3 to 4 weeks to ensure the epithelialization of a new tract that will remain patent for drainage of the gland. During the period of time that the catheter remains in place, its distal end can be tucked into the vagina.

Because of the potential for spreading infection and because local anesthetics do not work well in the pH of inflamed tissues, it is difficult for the surgeon to anesthetize the area around Bartholin's abscess. General anesthesia is often indicated. This approach can leave the patient with little or no analgesia into the immediate postoperative period, and IV medication may be needed. Postoperative pain can be intense, although relieving the pressure from the abscess may result in less pain after surgery than before. The patient is usually instructed to take sitz

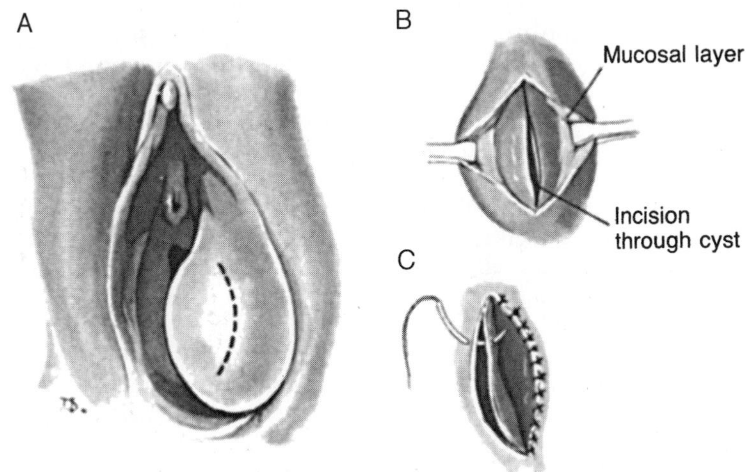

Figure 34–3. Marsupialization of Bartholin's gland cyst. *A*, A longitudinal incision is made along the mucocutaneous junction of the vulva and vagina, overlying the cyst. *B*, The incision is carried down through the cyst wall, and the contents are drained. *C*, The lining of the cyst is everted and sutured to skin with interrupted 3–0 chromic catgut sutures. (From Hill G: Outpatient Surgery, 3rd ed. Philadelphia: WB Saunders, 1988, p 564.)

baths at home, two or three times a day, and after all bowel movements.

HYMENOTOMY

The hymen is a mucosal fold near the introitus (opening) of the vagina. It may require surgical repair if it is very small, rigid, or completely or partially imperforate (closed). A totally imperforate hymen restricts menstrual flow, vaginal instrumentation, and coitus. Technically, the procedure can be accomplished under local anesthesia, but the patient is often tense, frightened, and embarrassed, and general anesthesia is a frequent alternative. Often, the patient is a teenage girl or young adult with little or no previous gynecologic history.

After initial healing after hymenotomy, the patient may be instructed by the physician to digitally stretch the tissues to retain the desired surgical effect. Societal taboos and personal standards or embarrassment can interfere with the patient's compliance. The nurse should encourage the patient to comply with the suggested therapeutic regimen. The patient should also be prepared to review the techniques.

EXTERNAL LESIONS

Vaginal, perineal, perianal, and labial lesions may be removed by a number of methods: sharp dissection, electrocautery, cryotherapy, and laser photocoagulation. The latter is often the treatment modality of choice. Lesions may be neoplastic, precancerous, or infectious.

Venereal disease crosses all borders of age, race, sex, and socioeconomic status. Venereal warts have become a frequent problem in our society. Often, the prognosis for permanent cure is not good, and patients may exhibit signs of fear, anger, and depression. Patients sometimes delay seeking medical treatment, allowing the disease and lesions to become widespread. Several reasons exist for delaying treatment, including no insurance and inability to pay for care, fear or embarrassment, denial or false hope that the lesions will heal spontaneously, self-destructive thoughts, and complicating social lifestyles that are self-abusive.

Condylomata acuminata are venereal lesions caused by the human papilloma virus (HPV). Both external and internal tissues can be affected. Laser vaporization is often the treatment of choice. Postoperative pain is often intense, and thus the surgeon may infiltrate the sites with a long-acting local anesthetic. Other palliative methods employed in the postoperative period include topical creams, sitz baths, and oral analgesics.

When condylomata are present on the cervix, an associated cervical intraepithelial neoplasm is often present as well. Intraoperatively, the surgeon may use a dilute solution of acetic acid on the cervix to make the lesion more visible. Some physicians accompany treatment with the topical application of an antineoplastic cream such as fluorouracil.

DILATATION AND CURETTAGE

D and C is frequently performed in an ASC. Various diagnostic and therapeutic indications exist, for instance, to follow up on abnormal Papanicolaou (Pap) smears, to treat or diagnose the cause of postmenopausal or irregular bleeding, and to remove retained intrauterine devices. Hysteroscopy is considered to be superior for endometrial examination because direct visualization is possible.

During a D and C, uterine perforation is a potential complication, particularly in the older woman whose uterine tissue may be friable. If such a complication occurs, most often no treatment is required and the uterine perforation seals itself closed. It is conceivable, however, that other structures, notably the bowel, can be injured and require surgical repair. Postoperative nursing assessments should focus not only on vaginal bleeding but also on abdominal symptoms. Pain, excessive tenderness, or distention with increased girth could indicate intra-abdominal trauma. Return to normal activity is rapid after uncomplicated surgery, and patients usually resume normal physical and sexual activity immediately.

CERVICAL BIOPSY AND CONIZATION

Abnormal cervical cytology found during a Pap smear is treated by eradication of the abnormal tissue. It is used by some practitioners for chronic intraepithelial neoplasia type III lesions. A punch biopsy and electrocoagulation, cryosurgery, cold-knife cone biopsy, loop electrosurgical excision cone or laser excisional cone are procedures that will provide an adequate histologic specimen. When conization is performed to treat carcinoma in situ, the woman remains at high risk for recurrence and must be closely monitored postoperatively with frequent Pap smears.

Postoperatively, the patient may have a vaginal packing that will be removed at the physician's office. Others may have an absorbable, hemostatic material or none. The patient is at higher risk for bleeding and infection after conization than after a D and C, and postoperative instructions include abstinence from sexual intercourse, douching, and tampon use for up to 6 weeks. The patient should be encouraged to complete all prescribed oral antibiotics.

HYSTEROSCOPY

Hysteroscopy is a procedure that allows direct visualization of the uterine cavity for diagnosis and biopsy of abnormalities and for treatment of uterine pathology. Diagnostic hysteroscopy is planned for the early proliferative phase of the woman's menstrual cycle. Simple procedures may be accomplished with paracervical block with or without supplemental sedation because associated pain is cervical in origin. Some patients prefer or require general or regional anesthesia.

Indications for hysteroscopy include diagnosis and treatment of abnormal bleeding (pre- and postmenopausal), diagnosis and removal of polyps or other intrauterine lesions, diagnosis and division of uterine septa, retrieval of misplaced intrauterine devices or other foreign bodies, and exploration of the uterine cavity in patients with repeated pregnancy losses or infertility. Contraindications include pregnancy, known cervical carcinoma or infection, and profuse uterine bleeding. Concurrent laparoscopy allows the surgeon to monitor the abdominal cavity and to immediately visualize and, if necessary, treat a uterine perforation caused by the hysteroscope.

The uterine cavity is distended during the procedure. This is often accomplished with 32% dextran in dextrose (Hyskon), glycine, carbon dioxide, or a dextrose and water solution.[6] Each has advantages and is chosen by physician preference. Air is not used to dilate the uterine cavity because of its possible entrance into an open blood vessel resulting in an embolism.

Complications are rare, although bleeding, uterine perforation and infection are possible.[7] Reactions to the distending media used in the uterus include anaphylaxis, pulmonary edema due to fluid overload, and bleeding disorders due to excessive infusion of dextran. Carbon dioxide is relatively benign but, if improperly administered, can result in intravasation with hypercarbia and acidosis.

Operative hysteroscopy, for instance for myomectomy or septal division, may require a prolonged period of postoperative nursing observation and care. Twenty-three hour admission is sometimes indicated. The patient should be instructed to report significant vaginal bleeding or a hard, painful abdomen.

ENDOMETRIAL ABLATION

Endometrial ablation involves the destruction of the endometrial uterine lining with either a laser or balloon. The goal is the cessation or reduction of menstrual flow. It is a viable alternative to hysterectomy for the patient with dysfunctional uterine bleeding that is unresponsive to medical treatment.[8]

During neodymium:yttrium-aluminum-garnet (Nd:YAG) laser ablation, the uterine cavity must be bathed continuously with fluids to cool the uterus and remove tissue. Significant absorption of irrigants can occur through tissues and blood vessels. An accurate accounting of the amount of irrigant instilled and retrieved is documented to assess the patient's need for a diuretic to avoid systemic fluid overload. Hyskon is not used during endometrial ablation, because the possible effects of systemic absorption through open blood vessels have not been documented. The use of carbon dioxide or air as a distending medium or the use of gas to cool the fibers of the laser tip increases the possibility of gas embolism, which can be fatal.[9] Sodium chloride (0.9%) or another isotonic solution is the usual medium for uterine distention.

Uterine balloon endometrial ablation offers a fast recovery, is less traumatic and causes less postoperative morbidity. A latex balloon that is attached to a catheter is inserted into the uterus. The balloon is inflated with sterile 5% dextrose in water that allows it to conform to the uterine lining. The solution is heated by a heating element. The combination of pressure and heat result in thermal ablation of the endometrial tissue.[10]

Before surgery, the patient may be given oral or intramuscular medication to cause endometrial atrophy. Usual postoperative instructions include: (1) light activity for several days without any strenuous exercises, (2) avoidance of douching and sexual intercourse, and (3) analgesics and antibiotics as prescribed. Tampons are allowed because no cervical trauma occurs. Watery, bloody, vaginal drainage is common for up to 6 weeks but is generally not copious. Mild abdominal cramping is common on the day of surgery, but subsequent pain is minor.

LAPAROSCOPY OR PELVISCOPY

Laparoscopy, or pelviscopy, is the entry into the abdominal cavity with an endoscope after gas insufflation of the abdomen to lift the abdominal wall away from the viscera. This technique of insufflating the abdomen is called "pneumoperitoneum." A special needle has been developed that reduces or eliminates the risk of visceral injuries. After puncture of the abdominal wall with its sharp point, a self-closing sheath immediate snaps over the point. The appropriate gas is then pumped into the abdomen under pressure.

Several problems can occur during this process. Introduction of the pressurized gas into the vascular system with resultant gas embolism is a rare, but devastating, possibility. Pneumothorax is another rare complication related to increased intra-abdominal pressure. Insufflation of the gas into the abdominal wall or into an organ is also possible.

Once the abdomen has been insufflated, a trocar is positioned. The surgeon must take special care not to puncture the bladder, bowel, stomach, or major vessels when inserting the trocar. One or more sheaths are inserted into the abdomen to contain the laparoscope and instruments. Several puncture sites can be required for additional instrumentation when more complex procedures are undertaken.

Laparoscopy is commonly used for both therapeutic and diagnostic purposes and often negates the need for open laparotomy. Traditional applications for laparoscopy include diagnosis of pathologic conditions, diagnostic infertility workups, and tubal sterilization using coagulation or mechanical banding of the fallopian tubes (Fig. 34–4).

Increasingly complex procedures are now being accomplished by operative laparoscopy, rather than with an open laparotomy, for instance removal of ectopic pregnancies by salpingectomy or salpingotomy, lysis of adhesions, laser-assisted vaginal hysterectomy, ovarian biopsy, and fimbrioplasty, oophorectomy, myomectomy, and appendectomy. Large ovarian cysts may be drained and removed laparoscopically as well. Because of the complexities of procedures now undertaken, some patients require a 23-hour or longer admission program for treatment of associated discomfort and nursing assessment for surgical complications.

When an ectopic pregnancy is suspected, the physician can often confirm the diagnosis and provide treatment laparoscopically. Ectopic pregnancies occur most frequently in the fallopian tubes. Much less frequent sites include the

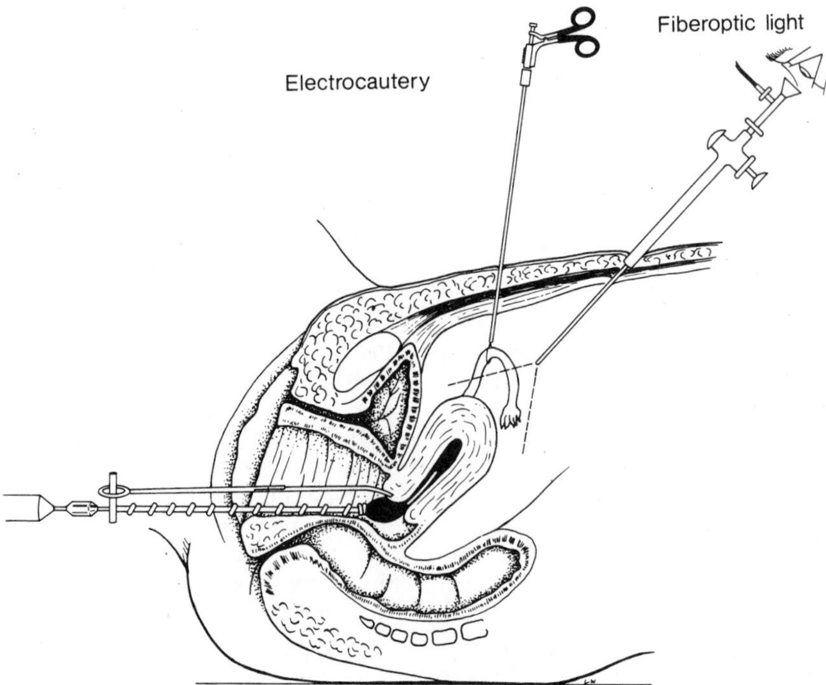

Figure 34–4. Laparoscopy technique for tubal sterilization. The laparoscope has been inserted below the umbilicus with a second probe just above the symphysis pubis. The suprapubic probe can be used for cauterization or for other manipulations. (From Hill G: Outpatient Surgery, 3rd ed. Philadelphia: WB Saunders, 1988, p 574.)

abdominal cavity, ovary, and cervix. Typical symptoms include abdominal pain, amenorrhea, and abnormal vaginal bleeding, which may mask amenorrhea. Nausea, vomiting, and breast enlargement associated with pregnancy do not usually occur owing to the early gestational stage.

Early symptoms are often so innocuous that the woman defers treatment until the pregnancy has advanced to the stage of a tubal rupture. Tubal rupture, which is most common between 8 and 10 weeks after the previous menstrual period, is accompanied by sharp pain on one side of the abdomen. Blood loss can be significant, making open laparotomy necessary.

Laparoscopic treatment of ectopic pregnancy allows a range of treatment alternatives. A salpingectomy may be necessary, although this leaves the woman with only one functioning fallopian tube. Salpingotomy can be done as an alternative to remove the fetus and subsequently repair of the tube. After laparoscopic intervention for ectopic pregnancy, the woman who is Rh negative receives Rh immune globulin to reduce or eliminate Rh sensitization that could affect future pregnancies.

Another application for laparoscopy is treatment of endometriosis, the abnormal occurrence of endometrial tissue in a place other than the lining of the uterus. The etiology of endometriosis is controversial, but theories include: (1) reflux menstruation, (2) spread by lymph and blood, and (3) congenital occurrence. The darkly pigmented patches can be found on pelvic structures, the ovaries, the bowel, and in other locations. Recurrent bleeding from these sites is thought to parallel the menses.

Associated pelvic pain, especially with exercise, intercourse, and pelvic examination, is the most common symptom of endometriosis.[11] Infertility is a less frequent indication for surgery. A patient may be so chronically incapacitated by the associated pain that the patient's physician may begin to consider a psychological cause for the pain. These women need tremendous emotional support and may require larger-than-usual doses of analgesics for postoperative pain due to their histories of preoperative analgesic use. Depending on the extent of the disease, the procedure can last several hours. Although bleeding is not usually a problem during resection of endometriosis from peritoneal tissues, postoperative nausea and discomfort are common and may prolong the postoperative stay.

Patient safety during laparoscopy is decided, in large part, by the skill and the experience of the surgeon, the anesthesia team, and the nursing staff. Although potentially serious and even life-threatening complications are rare, the possibilities include perforated viscus or blood vessels, electrical burns, pulmonary edema, hemorrhage, atelectasis, gas embolism, sciatic nerve damage, and infection. The more common postoperative problems of discomfort, nausea, and vomiting remain less serious but still unpleasant sequelae for the patient. The surgeon can help to reduce complications by thoroughly evacuating gas from the abdomen, instilling local anesthesia at the operative sites, and handling the viscera gently.

Contraindications to laparoscopy have changed with current research, experience, and progressive ideas. Absolute contraindications include the patient's inability to withstand suitable anesthesia, severe bleeding disorders, and acute peritonitis with bowel distention that would complicate or prevent safe entry of sharp instrumentation into the abdomen. Previously, the patient who had undergone numerous laparotomies was not considered a candidate for laparoscopy because of the chance of bowel injury secondary to adhesions, but that philosophy has been challenged.

Endoscopic examination of the intrapelvic and intra-abdominal contents with a pelviscope allows a wide field of vision and depth. Considerations for pelviscopy are similar to those associated with a laparoscopy. A pelviscopy is similar to a laparoscopy, except that there is a difference in the angle of the operative laparoscope. The procedure is beneficial to allow women to have a decreased total cost of the procedure, lower morbidity, and quicker return to full activity.[13]

Preoperative Care

During the preoperative assessment, physical limitations that will complicate intraoperative positioning, usually Trendelenburg and low lithotomy positions, should be noted and discussed with the surgical team. Complicating factors include arthritis, obesity, musculoskeletal deformities, respiratory disease, and pre-existing cardiovascular disease.

Providing the patient with information about the possibility of postoperative shoulder pain may help to allay later fears. Although the surgeon attempts to evacuate the abdomen as thoroughly as possible at the end of the case, some gas can remain. This gas can irritate the diaphragm and the phrenic nerve causing referred pain to one or both shoulders. Sudden onset of severe postoperative shoulder pain can frighten the unsuspecting person who may mistake the symptom for a heart attack or other serious complication. It is important to prepare the patient for the possibility of shoulder pain, but information should be presented in a manner that does not invite the expectation that pain is inevitable.

An empty bladder reduces the risk of bladder perforation upon entry of sharp instrumentation into the abdomen. For lengthy laparoscopic procedures, an indwelling catheter may be inserted to ensure that the bladder does not become distended and, therefore, at higher risk for injury during surgery. Clipping hair on the abdomen is not usually required, except when there is a high probability of conversion to laparotomy, for instance, when treating an ectopic pregnancy or a large ovarian cyst.

Intraoperative Care

During laparoscopy, the role of the registered nurse is complex because of the numerous potential patient-related complications and the sophisticated equipment involved. The circulating nurse must be attentive to many facets of the patient's care and prepared to initiate an immediate open laparotomy if unexpected intraoperative complications require direct abdominal access.

General anesthesia affords certain advantages over other anesthesia approaches, including the ability to control ventilation and prevent hypercarbia, elimination of patient anxiety, excellent control of muscle relaxation, a quiet operative field, and analgesia and amnesia into the postoperative period. Disadvantages are occasional prolonged recovery time and complications of general anesthesia, including increased nausea and vomiting or sore throat after intubation. Other anesthesia-related complications include cardiac arrhythmias, circulatory impairment, pulmonary edema, tracheal irritation or damage, aspiration, hypercarbia, and cardiac arrest. Hypercarbia may occur both from ventilatory insufficiency and secondary to the absorption of carbon dioxide from the peritoneum.

Surgical position and anesthesia complications are interrelated. A combination of Trendelenburg and lithotomy positions is necessary surgically but can lead to complications such as sciatic or perineal nerve damage and cardiorespiratory compromise. Other potential complications from Trendelenburg positioning include pain in the shoulder pads, a sense of facial congestion, tearing of the eyes, and increased jugular pressure. Glaucoma can be aggravated, with the possibility of triggering an acute episode. Retinal detachment may occur.

Respiratory management for the patient in the Trendelenburg position is complex, because lung volume can decrease by 20% and most of the lung is positioned below the level of the left atrium. Left atrial pressure is increased over the alveolar pressure, encouraging transudation into the alveoli. Pulmonary congestion and edema are always possible. The patient with mitral stenosis already has chronically high left atrial pressures and will poorly tolerate this position. Obese patients have increased respiratory difficulty due to the upward shift of abdominal contents as well as the weight of the chest wall, increasing the risk of atelectasis and hypoxemia. Respiratory inadequacy with resultant hypercarbia can predispose the patient to arrhythmias, often benign ventricular premature beats but sometimes requiring treatment.

The risk of aspiration is increased owing to the intra-abdominal pressure related to the pneumoperitoneum. Because of that higher-than-normal risk, preoperative measures to decrease gastric acidity and volume are usually employed. Careful monitoring and positioning are essential while the patient is obtunded.

Circulatory changes begin with increased cardiac output secondary to autotransfusion of 500 to 1000 ml of blood from the lower extremities into the central circulation when the patient is placed in the lithotomy position. Later, the blood pressure and cardiac output drop owing to stimulation of the baroreceptors. Sympathetic blockade from a spinal or epidural anesthetic can promote further hypotension related to vasodilatation. When the legs are lowered at the end of surgery, a further drop in central blood pressure can occur when blood pools in the lower extremities. Hypotension is often prevented or treated with increased IV hydration and a vasopressor such as ephedrine.

Other cardiovascular changes can occur as well. When the abdomen is insufflated with carbon dioxide, pressure on the inferior vena cava can reduce venous return. Bradycardia can develop owing to peritoneal stretching. The cerebral vascular system is also undergoing changes in response to lowering of the patient's head. Intracranial pressure increases along with cerebral vascular resistance.

Potential complications related to surgical technique include gas embolism, pneumothorax, hemorrhage from a ruptured viscus or major vessel, subcutaneous emphysema, electrical injuries, embolism, pulmonary edema, infection, nerve damage, nausea, vomiting, and pain. Long-term complications after a laparoscopic sterilization procedure can include pregnancy from a failed ligation or from recanalization of the tube, tubal pregnancy, and emotional sequelae. Patient anatomy and pre-existing conditions such as obesity and cardiorespiratory disease are also sources of potential complications.

During sterilization procedures, incorrect identification of the fallopian tubes can result in ligation or cautery of ligaments with failure of the sterilization procedure. Many surgeons videotape procedures for documentation that the tube was properly ligated or cauterized. Silastic bands or clips, such as the Falope ring or Yoon ring, have been developed as alternatives to electrocautery of the tubes. They allow tubal occlusion without the dangers associated with use of an electrical current within the abdominal cavity.

Tubal banding is often associated with more postoperative pain than cautery because of resultant ischemia of the fallopian tubes. This ischemic pain is transient but quite severe in some cases.

Postoperative Care

Primary postoperative nursing interventions include cardiorespiratory monitoring and comfort measures to treat or prevent nausea, vomiting, and pain. Supplemental oxygen therapy in the immediate postanesthesia period is not required unless airway difficulty exists. Monitoring the oxygen saturation with pulse oximetry is indicated until the patient is clearly awake, alert, and eupneic. Unpleasant gastrointestinal symptoms can follow intra-abdominal manipulation and gas insufflation. Also, many patients having laparoscopy are young women who are already at higher risk than others for postoperative nausea and vomiting. A lower than normal body temperature should be assessed due to the use of insufflating gases and irrigation fluids. Supplemental IV fluids may be needed to replace deficits and losses owing to the cold, dry instillation gases. Monitor the temperature during the postoperative phase and institute warming measures as appropriate.

Continued postoperative nursing care includes assessment of respirations and circulation, progressive ambulation, and reinforcement of the patient's sense of wellness. The surgical sites are observed for superficial bleeding, and the abdomen is evaluated for distention. Abdominal distention is a sign that most likely indicates retained gas, although internal hemorrhage should be considered in the differential nursing diagnosis. Various surgical techniques employ one, two, or three abdominal puncture sites, and the presence of a number of wounds should be explained to the patient. Complaints of muscle discomfort are not uncommon and general comfort measures such as back rubs, warm blankets, suggestions for relaxation techniques, and repositioning can be very helpful.

Laparoscopy may have been combined with a cervical D and C. Even if a D and C has not been done, vaginal spotting may persist for a few days because a uterine cannula is often placed through the vagina into the uterus to allow manipulation of the uterus and tubes during laparoscopy. Some surgeons use a toothed clamp to grasp the cervix, and thus spotting may occur due to cervical trauma.

Patients who have had a laparoscopy face diverse emotional needs. Outside pressure may have been put on them to undergo a sterilization procedure. Even the woman who freely chooses the procedure is faced with the finality of her decision to end her childbearing capability. Other women may have been informed of an unpleasant diagnosis, and the patient being worked up for infertility or after termination of ectopic pregnancy faces an entirely different set of emotions and may feel relieved, disappointed, guilty, or despondent.

It is helpful for the patient to be allowed to express her feelings in her own manner. Crying may be that outlet in the immediate postoperative period. The nurse can provide a safe, accepting climate and can facilitate an early reunion with the family.

Discharge instructions should include those previously discussed for the gynecologic patient plus specific instructions regarding care of the abdominal puncture wounds. Often the patient is allowed to remove the adhesive bandage strips that cover the incisions and to shower after 1 or 2 days. The surgeon may suggest that the wounds be left uncovered after the first shower or may ask the patient to re-cover them. Some physicians instruct their patients to cleanse the small puncture wounds with hydrogen peroxide or a povidone iodine solution once or twice a day for several days. Swimming and tub bathing are usually restricted for 7 to 10 days. The nurse should reinforce the explanation about potential shoulder pain and should tell the patient to report severe abdominal distention or pain. They should also report increases in temperature up to 72 hours postoperatively that can be indicative of peritonitis. Prior to discharge, the patient's ability to urinate is ascertained.

VAGINAL HYSTERECTOMY

Vaginal hysterectomy in an outpatient setting is a relatively new innovation. Laparoscopic and laser-assisted vaginal hysterectomy are being tried as alternative techniques. Several essential factors combine to make vaginal hysterectomy a safe outpatient procedure. These include careful screening and selection of patients, appropriate anesthesia technique, adequate control of anxiety and pain, and adequate provision for postoperative care at home or in an alternative care setting. The surgeon should be appropriately skilled and should possess a historically low complication record. The physician should also be adaptable and must be willing and able to provide home support for the patient. Physician house calls and the use of recovery care centers are often a part of the overall plan.

The patient must be intellectually able to understand and follow instructions and to identify and report complications appropriately. Home support people must be equally willing and able. The patient's attitude is an especially important factor, because the enthusiastic and positive-thinking woman will certainly approach this innovative procedure with a higher likelihood of successful home discharge as planned.

Hysterectomy has been associated almost universally with hospitalization, and thus it is essential that health care personnel who prepare the patient provide continued positive reinforcement regarding the safety and ease with which the procedure can be adapted to an ASC. There is little serious morbidity associated with vaginal hysterectomy. Symptoms of grave complications such as hemorrhage or intra-abdominal trauma almost always present either during or immediately after surgery.

Although other potential complications are possible, the patient can be honestly assured of a high safety margin for early discharge. Stressing the benefits of early discharge can help to mold a favorable attitude for the patient and family members, for instance, minimal separation from family, quick return to home comforts and routine, minimal interruption of usual activities for other family members, and financial savings. In addition, reduced exposure to the hospital environment decreases the chance of acquiring a nosocomial infection and experiencing personnel-related dangers such as medication errors.

Admission and scheduling times for outpatient vaginal hysterectomy should be early in the day to allow for an adequate length of postoperative observation prior to discharge. An IV antibiotic is given, and a perineal shave is done to reduce the chance of postoperative infection. An indwelling urinary catheter is inserted preoperatively, often in surgery to avoid patient discomfort and embarrassment. Continuous bladder drainage reduces the possibility of surgical injury.

After the initial phase of recovery from anesthesia, the patient is encouraged to ambulate and to take fluids by mouth. Vaginal hysterectomy, uncomplicated by additional vaginal repair such as anterior or posterior colporrhaphy, is not usually associated with a significant amount of postoperative pain, and oral analgesics generally are adequate in the home. The patient can benefit from positive reinforcement preoperatively, suggesting the low level of discomfort that will be experienced after surgery. The effectiveness of this type of counseling has been very specifically illustrated in a study of vaginal hysterectomy patients and can be considered a significant tool for the control of postoperative pain.

Vaginal flow is assessed frequently. The patient should understand that there is a wide range of normal regarding the amount and color of vaginal drainage after hysterectomy. Often only a small amount of bright red to pink spotting is observed. Some women may have almost no flow, whereas others have a larger and longer period of vaginal drainage. Because of the change in position and movement of pooled fluid, it is not uncommon for vaginal flow to increase when the patient ambulates.

Practitioners have varied opinions about the use of a urinary catheter in the postoperative period. Some prefer to remove the catheter in the early recovery period and observe the patient's urinary status throughout the day. Others choose to have the patient discharged with an indwelling catheter that can be removed by a nurse at home or in the alternate care setting on the following day. If the patient is discharged with a catheter, instructions for its care should be provided as discussed in the section on urologic procedures.

Adequate fluid intake must be provided either by mouth or IV to ensure adequate urine production. The patient being discharged without a catheter should void prior to departure. The physician may waive this requirement if the patient will be attended by nursing personnel at home or in an alternate care site. Overdistention of the bladder can cause a temporary paralysis of the detrusor muscle, which can take several days to resolve, making spontaneous urination difficult or impossible. It is essential, therefore, to assess the patient frequently for bladder distention and to intercede appropriately.

The patient's ability to urinate after surgery can be affected by anxiety and pain, administration of narcotics, sympathetic effects of regional anesthesia, and body fluid volume. Also, bladder tone can be affected by local tissue edema or temporary neurologic deficits related to surgery. A rare, but serious, complication is the accidental ligation of a ureter. Unilateral flank pain that increases in intensity could indicate hydronephrosis secondary to ureteral obstruction.

Discharge instructions should be provided to the patient and to the adult who is responsible for her home care. Specific explanations should be provided to identify reportable events, for instance: (1) inability to urinate or very painful urination; (2) unusually heavy vaginal flow or passing of numerous large clots; (3) extreme or painful abdominal distention; (4) flank pain or any unusual pain that is unrelieved by oral analgesics; (5) symptoms of infection such as a high fever or foul-smelling vaginal drainage; and (6) signs of thrombophlebitis such as calf tenderness or redness, chest pain, or dyspnea.[14]

Because the patient often feels very tired and weak after this major surgery, she should be encouraged to rest and to progressively increase activity over the next week to 10 days. Washing is confined to showering until vaginal flow has diminished. Trips outside the home and driving are not advised for several weeks after surgery. Heavy lifting and strenuous activity must be avoided to prevent bleeding and damage to healing tissues. Douching, tampons, and sexual intercourse are avoided until permitted by the physician, usually after 6 weeks.

It should be noted that some women experience depression or other emotional sequelae after a hysterectomy. Postoperative depression is most often self-limiting and temporary and can be related to the woman's self-concept and sexuality. Because the postoperative stay is shortened, the patient is not afforded the benefit of having nurses to assess her emotional status and intercede accordingly. Also, the patient may not realize that such depression is common and is not peculiar to her. Preoperative counseling and instructions can be used to encourage the woman who is so affected to seek advice and counseling from an appropriate source. A family member should be similarly instructed.[15]

TERMINATION OF PREGNANCY

Termination of a pregnancy may be undertaken for therapeutic reasons or at the patient's request. Therapeutic indications include imminent danger to the mother's health or life; a missed, inevitable, or incomplete abortion; or because of a genetically abnormal fetus. The procedure, most often called "suction curettage" or "suction evacuation," may or may not require dilatation of the cervix. Regardless of the reason, emotional and psychological issues always surround abortion for the people involved—the patient, the family, the physician, and the nursing staff.

After therapeutic abortion, the patient and family are often devastated by the loss of their baby. The woman who undergoes a second-trimester abortion because of a fetal deformity often experiences a particularly long and painful period of grieving after the procedure. Not only may the couple have wanted the baby very much, but they also must deal with their conscious decision to terminate the pregnancy. There may be lingering doubts about how severely the baby would have been afflicted and whether they did the right thing. Crying and sadness are frequently observed, and the nurse often experiences a variety of feelings that can range from empathy to a sense of helplessness in providing the patient with support.

Elective abortion is and has been a volatile political, religious, and ethical issue in the United States for many years and is an area in which the individual nurse often has adamant feelings about the procedure and about assisting in the patient's care.[16] Administrators and managers should respect a nurse's reluctance or refusal to participate. On the other hand, those nurses who do provide care to patients should do so without expressing prejudice. Whether the nurse approves of the patient's decision or not, the nurse's duty is to provide care that is nondiscriminatory and respectful.

The woman who has voluntarily chosen to terminate her pregnancy often experiences a wide range of emotions. Sadness, guilt, relief, anger, helplessness, and loneliness are a few of the many possible responses that complicate the patient's psychological state and can heighten her response to pain and cramping. It is a mistake to assume that the woman who is electively terminating her pregnancy experiences no grief or sadness. In fact, it is unlikely that the choice to terminate a pregnancy is ever made without some reservations.

A few of the factors that motivate women

to seek abortions include financial insecurity, ambivalence regarding pregnancy in general, fear of pain or death from pregnancy, having too many children already, lack of emotional closeness or feelings for the father, and being single or a teenager. Some women are uninformed or confused about how and when pregnancy can occur or may not understand how to use or obtain contraceptive devices.

Women and their partners need emotional support during this period surrounding the loss of their baby and should be allowed to grieve in their own manner. The nurse can provide support through kind words, touch, or a silent presence. Facilitating a quick postoperative reunion with the partner or family is a caring gesture that is usually appreciated, as is providing a private place to allow the patient and supporting adult to express their grief.

Most miscarriages and spontaneous abortions occur during the first trimester before many of the physiologic changes of pregnancy have occurred. Physical changes that affect the patient as the term progresses are listed in Table 34–3. In particular, increased acidity of gastric contents and progressive incompetence of the gastroesophageal reflex are associated with advancing pregnancy, thus aspiration poses a real threat to the pregnant patient.

Table 34–3. **Physiologic Changes During Pregnancy**

RESPIRATORY SYSTEM
40% increase in tidal volume
15% increase in respiratory rate
20% increase in oxygen consumption
30% decrease in compliance
35% decrease in resistance

CARDIOVASCULAR SYSTEM
35% increase in blood volume
40% increase in cardiac output
30% increase in stroke volume
15% increase in heart rate
15% decrease in peripheral vascular resistance

CENTRAL NERVOUS SYSTEM
40% decrease in anesthetic requirement (minimum alveolar concentration or MAC)
40% reduction in local anesthetic requirement for spinal anesthesia
Increased neurosensitivity to local anesthetics

GASTROINTESTINAL SYSTEM
Incompetence of gastroesophageal reflux
Delayed gastric emptying
Decreased gastric pH

RENAL SYSTEM
Progressive increase (up to 50%) of glomerular filtration rate (GFR)
Increased renal blood flow

From Litwack Y: Practical points in the care of the obstetric surgical patient. J Past Anesth Nurs 5:3. 1990, p. 183.

If the pregnancy was advanced into the second or third trimester, uterine tone should be assessed postoperatively by palpation of the fundus. Oxytocin (Pitocin or methylergonovine maleate) may be added to the IV infusion intraoperatively to promote uterine contraction. Severe and painful uterine contractions can occur with rapid infusion. Other side effects of oxytocin include nausea and vomiting, anaphylaxis, and cardiac arrhythmias. The possibility of severe hypertension is increased in the presence of local and regional anesthesia. Hypertension related to oxytocic drug administration is treated with vasopressors.

Postoperative bleeding can result from uterine perforation, a cervical tear, a retained placental fragment, or uterine atony. Abdominal palpation should be a part of the postoperative assessment to identify hardness, tenderness, or distention that could indicate intra-abdominal bleeding. Methylergonovine maleate may be given intramuscularly or orally by prescription to treat or prevent uterine atony and associated bleeding. It acts directly on the smooth muscle of the uterus to increase tone and promote contraction. Side effects include hypertension with headache and possibly convulsions, hypotension, nausea, and vomiting. The patient should be instructed to complete taking all doses of any prescribed medication for uterine tone.

Postoperative infection is not a frequent complication, but the chances of infection increase if placental tissue is retained in the uterus. Some practitioners prescribe an oral antibiotic such as prophylaxis against infection. Others think that antibiotic therapy is necessary only in patients with increased risk factors, such as the woman with a history of pelvic inflammatory disease or suspected heart valve disease.

Another issue to consider after termination or loss of a pregnancy is the potential for the Rh-negative mother to become sensitized to the Rh factor of the fetus. The patient's blood type and Rh should be documented on the medical record prior to surgery. In most cases, it is not known if the fetus is Rh negative or positive, and thus administration of the appropriate immune serum generally is advised as a prophylactic measure for all Rh-negative mothers.

The Rh-negative mother does not have a naturally occurring Rh antigen. Her body identifies the blood of an Rh-positive fetus as a foreign antigen, and she produces maternal antibodies to fight that foreign protein. Allowed to proliferate, these antibodies attack and destroy the blood of subsequent Rh-positive fetuses. Rh immune globulin serum is a blood product that will prevent the production of Rh antibodies in the mother. It is administered intramuscularly within 3 days of termination of the pregnancy to prevent sensitization that can affect future pregnancies. This injection is often given in the OR while the patient is still unconscious for patient comfort. An identification card provided by the manufacturer is filled out and given to the patient as a record of her receiving Rh immune globulin.

Discharge instructions should include detailed information about expected vaginal flow that can range from no flow to that equaling a heavy menses. To decrease the occurrence of postoperative infection and bleeding, the patient is instructed to avoid douching, tampons, and sexual intercourse for a period of time specified by the physician. The patient and family should be encouraged to express their emotions honestly and to seek professional counseling if they have prolonged or excessive difficulty in dealing with the emotional impact of the procedure.

IN VITRO FERTILIZATION

The number of in vitro fertilization (IVF) programs in existence continues to increase. Many of these IVF programs utilize an ASC for pre- and postoperative care of patients. In vitro fertilization involves the removal of oocytes from the woman, incubation and fertilization of those oocytes with sperm from the husband or a donor in the laboratory setting, and subsequent implantation of the resultant embryo(s) in the woman's uterus several days later. The entire process is long, and couples who are in the program have committed extensive time, emotional involvement, and money to obtain a desired pregnancy.

Preoperative counseling is extensive and is conducted by a group of multidisciplinary specialists. The nurse in the ASC who provides preoperative instructions, therefore, deals with a patient and spouse who are already knowledgeable about the procedure and the process that will follow. Specific information needs address anesthesia and unit-specific issues such as arrival time, nothing-by-mouth status, and transportation arrangements.

Ovum retrieval can be accomplished in various ways. The laparoscopic approach has been the more traditional manner, but recent technology has spawned the ultrasonographic transvaginal approach to view the ovary. An ultrasound needle is advanced into the follicle to obtain the oocytes under ultrasonic monitoring. Potential complications of this approach include injury to blood vessels or pelvic organs and infection from contamination by normally occurring flora in the vagina. The advantages of this technique over laparoscopic interventions include shorter operative and anesthetic times, sometimes the avoidance of general anesthesia, less surgical trauma to tissues, a usually shorter recovery time, and the ability of the surgeon to view the ovaries on more than one plane.

Postoperatively, the patient's abdomen is observed for distention or extreme tenderness that could indicate an intra-abdominal injury. Recovery is usually rapid, and the patient ambulates and drinks fluids soon after the procedure. Mild cramping usually responds to a nonprescription oral analgesic. An intramuscular injection of progesterone is given prior to discharge to begin preparing the uterine lining to accept and maintain a pregnancy.

Upon and after discharge from the initial retrieval process the couple is often anxious about the question of fertilization, and the nurse should provide encouragement without offering false hope, which indicates assurance of that fertilization. Forty-eight hours after laboratory fertilization has occurred, the woman comes back to the center for implantation of the embryo(s) and begins daily injections of progesterone for 2 weeks. The implantation process is accomplished without anesthesia, and no lengthy recovery period is necessary.

TRANSCERVICAL BALLOON TUBOPLASTY

Tubal occlusion is the primary cause in 25% to 30% of infertile women. Transcervical balloon tuboplasty is an approach that has been developed recently in an attempt to help the woman with blocked fallopian tubes to conceive. The concept is similar to balloon angioplasty. In initial reports at six medical centers where the procedure has been undertaken, 53 women obtained patency of both tubes, 18 had one tube opened, and six women had failure of either tube to recannulate. IV sedation and paracervical block are often the anesthetic approaches of choice, or general anesthesia is given when the procedure is combined with laparoscopy.

After hysterosalpingography using a contrast material to identify areas of blockage in the fallopian tubes, the physician may use this transvaginal procedure in an attempt to open blocked fallopian tubes. Using fluoroscopy, the physician passes small catheters through the cervix and uterus into the tubes. Once in place, a balloon within the catheter is repeatedly inflated, stretching the occluded areas of the tubes to create a patent lumen. A second hysterosalpingography may be performed at the end of the case to verify that patency has been accomplished. Nursing care parallels that for other vaginal procedures.[17]

References

1. Klingman L: Assessing the female reproductive system. AJN 99:37–41, 1999.
2. Leukenotte AG: Gerontologic assessment. In Leukenotte AG (ed): Gerontologic Nursing. St Louis: CV Mosby, 1994, pp 67–100.
3. Meeker M, Rothrock JC: Alexander's Care of the Patient in Surgery, 11th ed. St Louis: CV Mosby, 1999, pp 166–167.
4. Pardanani S, Barbieri RL: Neurovascular complications of the lithotomy position: The four hour rule. J Gynecol Tech 4:143–147, 1998.
5. Cheetham D: Bartholin's cyst, marsupialization or aspiration? Am J Obstet Gynecol 152:569–570, 1985.
6. Bennett KL, Ohrmundt C, Maloni JA: Preventing intravasation in women undergoing hysteroscopic procedures. AORN J 64:792–799, 1996.
7. Issaccson KB: Complications of hysteroscopy. Obstet Gynecol Clin North Am 26:39–51, 1999.
8. Townsend DE, Fields GA, McCausland AM: Operative hysteroscopy: Results in 1000 patients in American Association of Gynecologic Laparoscopists Annual Meeting Proceedings. Santa Fe Springs, CA: American Association of Gynecologic Laparoscopists, 1992.
9. ECRI: Exercise caution during intrauterine laser surgery. Today's OR Nurse 12:35, 1990.
10. Barrow C: Balloon endometrial ablation as a safe alternative to hysterectomy. AORN J 70:79–89, 1999.
11. Petersen N, Rhoe J: Endometriosis. AORN J 48:700–712, 1988.
12. Mirhashemi R, Harlow BL, Ginsburg ES, et al: Predicting risk of complications with gynecologic laparoscopic surgery. Obstet Gynecol 92:327–331, 1998.
13. Levine RL: Pelviscopic surgery in women over 40. J Reprod Med 35:597, 1990.
14. Reiner I: Early discharge after vaginal hysterectomy. Obstet Gynecol 71:416–418, 1988.
15. Mazmanian CM: Hysterectomy: Holistic care is the key. RN 62:32–35, 1999.
16. Ventura MJ: Where nurses stand on abortion. RN 62:44–48, 1999.
17. Confino E, Tur-Kaspa I, DeChurney A, et al: Transcervical balloon tuboplasty: A multi-center study. JAMA 264:2079–2082, 1990.

Chapter 

Genitourinary Surgery

Debra S. Goodwin

Men and women of all ages are treated for a variety of genitourinary (GU) conditions in the ambulatory surgery setting. Endocystoscopic procedures are performed for symptoms ranging from hematuria and dysuria to incontinence or urinary retention. Older men are frequently treated for prostatic obstructive disease and bladder tumors. Procedures are undertaken to diagnose and treat neoplasms, benign growths, infections, strictures, and other anatomic defects. Other therapeutic interventions address male reproductive problems such as infertility, impotence, and the desire for voluntary sterilization.

Figure 35–1 illustrates the paired kidneys and ureters, along with the urinary bladder and urethra that constitute the urinary tract. In the male, a complex reproductive system is integrally connected with the urinary system. The female reproductive tract lies in anatomic proximity to the urinary tract. The male urethra is normally 8 inches long, compared with the 1½-inch-long female urethra.

PREOPERATIVE CARE

Preoperative concerns are similar to many of those of gynecologic patients, such as prevention of infection for both the patient and the caregiver and maintenance of privacy and confidentiality. Any necessary skin shaving and preparation should be carried out quickly and with as little patient exposure as possible. It is a mistake to assume that male patients are any less embarrassed or concerned than their female counterparts about being physically exposed in the perioperative period. The nurse should maintain the modesty of both genders equally.

GU procedures expose the patient to the risk of an acquired urinary tract infection or to a potentially devastating septicemia. Oral and parenteral antibiotics are often prescribed prophylactically before surgery. Postoperative antibiotics are ordered after completion of an invasive procedure during which blood vessels within the urinary tract have been transected.

Many GU procedures expose patients to the possibility of temporary or permanent changes in sexual function. For instance, penile prosthesis implantation is designed to make a substantial and positive change in a man's sexual abilities. Other GU surgeries such as vasectomy, reversal of vasectomy, and varicocelectomy affect reproductive abilities but usually do not, as many patients fear, alter sexual performance in the long term. A patient or partner who expresses fear or appears to have unanswered questions regarding sexual performance should be encouraged to discuss those concerns with the physician before the procedure.

The preoperative nursing history includes a description of the patient's urinary habits: level of continence; color of urine; and presence of dysuria, hematuria, or inability to void. The abdomen is palpated to assess the size, softness, and presence of any painful areas for postoperative comparison. Signs of urinary tract infection that could lead to postponement of the procedure include fever, foul-smelling urine, or dysuria. These must be reported to the surgeon before transfer to the operating room (OR). A patient who is admitted with an indwelling urinary catheter should use a gravity drainage bag system rather than a leg bag while in bed to discourage backflow of urine into the bladder.

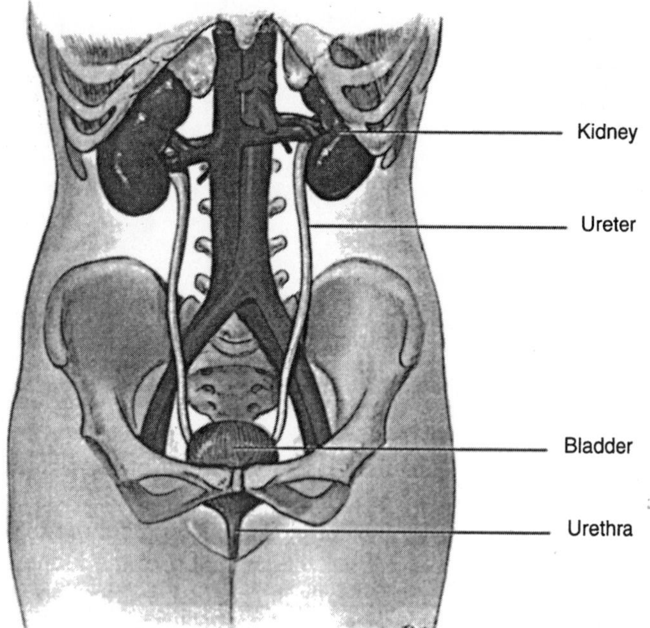

Figure 35–1. The urinary system. (From Applegate EJ: The Anatomy and Physiology Learning System: Textbook. Philadelphia: WB Saunders, 1995, p 372.)

INTRAOPERATIVE CARE

The perioperative nurse ensures a safe and efficient environment within the OR. Care must be employed to ensure that the patient is in an anatomically correct position throughout the procedure and that a safety strap is used to prevent a fall from the OR bed. The use of electrocautery, lasers, or radiographic units demands that appropriate safety practices be observed.

The patient is often placed in a lithotomy position or supine position. Women who are supine may be "frog-legged" for the procedure. These positions, besides being embarrassing, can be uncomfortable and difficult to maintain, particularly for elderly, obese, or awake patients. Simultaneous positioning of both legs helps prevent injury to the patient's back during position changes.

Strict attention to aseptic technique is essential for protecting the patient from nosocomial infection. Preparation of GU instruments entails both sterilization and disinfection methods. Instruments soaked in germicidal solutions between cases should be thoroughly rinsed before reuse. Urinary catheters and irrigation fluids that are used to distend the bladder must be handled aseptically.

POSTOPERATIVE CARE

Postoperatively, patients are assessed for bleeding, comfort level, ability to void, and parameters related to the type of anesthesia used. Oral fluids are encouraged when tolerated, and urinary output is measured. Urine is observed for color and amount, the volume of individual voidings, and the presence of blood and clots. Hematuria is common after cystoscopic procedures. It may persist for the first few voidings or for several days. Also, the patient may experience some burning or pain on urination. Continued bright red urine, passing of large clots, or severe dysuria should be reported to the physician. A careful explanation of normal and abnormal parameters helps the patient avoid under- or over-reporting of hematuria after discharge.

Other symptoms that should be reported to the physician include fever, severe pain on urination, inability to void accompanied by discomfort or bladder fullness, or bladder distention characterized by lower abdominal firmness with or without pain. After ureteroscopy, the presence of a hard, painful abdomen can signal ureteral perforation. Ureteral perforation can result in collection of urine in the retroperitoneum.[1] Occasionally, this complication can lead to a paralytic ileus. Overnight admission is advised when such complications are suspected or confirmed.

After genital surgery, men are instructed to report excessive swelling of the scrotum or penis. Patients will be less anxious if they understand that a small to moderate amount of scrotal swelling and ecchymosis is common and does not affect surgical outcome. Wearing a scrotal support, limiting activity for the first 24 hours, and applying an ice bag to the scrotal area may help reduce these symptoms and provide comfort. Some physicians feel that jockey-style undershorts provide adequate support, at least after the first or second postoperative day. The patient should be provided with this information before the day of surgery so that he can have this style of garment available postoperatively.

Oral analgesics usually are sufficient for pain control. Administration of a local or regional anesthetic blockade of the penis, inguinal region, or spermatic cord is another effective mode of postoperative pain control.[2] Patients should be encouraged preoperatively to report their postoperative comfort level honestly.

Complications after scrotal procedures include bleeding and infection. Hematoma formation, the most common complication, is usually treated conservatively with bedrest and observation. Rarely, drainage of the hematoma may be necessary. The rare person who develops a postoperative infection is treated with antibiotics. On occasion, incision and drainage of an abscess may be necessary.

Discharge instructions should include details of restrictions on sexual intercourse. The physician's advice is often for normal sexual activity as tolerated. Sometimes a specified period of abstinence is required to avoid pain, infection, and bleeding, for instance, after penile procedures such as circumcision or insertion of a penile prosthesis. After male sterilization procedures, specific information must be provided regarding abstinence to avoid undesired pregnancy during the early recovery weeks or months. It is important for the nurse to provide this type of information for all GU patients, because concerns about sexual activity may not be verbalized owing to embarrassment.

Urinary retention is a potential complication after any surgery, but the incidence is highest after procedures of the GU tract, rectum, and pelvis. The urge to void usually occurs when the bladder volume reaches about 150 ml, and urgency is experienced with volumes approaching 400 ml. One or more of the following may cause urinary retention: overdistention of the bladder, prolonged hypotension, incisional pain, perioperative use of narcotics, bladder trauma, benign prostatic hypertrophy, paralysis of the detrusor muscle, spasms of the urinary sphincter, and obstruction of the bladder neck.[3, 4]

In addition, depressed spinal innervation to the bladder associated with spinal or epidural anesthesia can result in an inability to sense bladder fullness and a lack of voluntary muscle coordination to consciously initiate voiding. The anesthetic blocks sympathetic innervation and increases the tone of the urethral sphincter.[4] It was a widely held belief that spinal anesthesia resulted in more urinary retention than general anesthesia, but no difference in incidence was found in a large, classic study of 65,000 patients.[3]

Usually, ambulatory surgical patients do not receive large doses of opioid analgesics that are known to contribute to postoperative urinary retention. Anxiety and pain do occur, and they can cause reflex spasms of the urinary sphincter. Other causes of retention include direct surgical trauma to the detrusor muscle and pelvic nerves and edema at the bladder neck.[5] Additional factors include advanced age, history of retention and urinary tract obstructive disease, dehydration, and administration of drugs such as atropine or glycopyrrolate.

Adequate hydration is essential if the patient is to produce urine. Both oral and intravenous fluids address hydration needs. A patient experiencing bladder discomfort or one who has palpable bladder distention should have reduced fluid intake until the bladder is emptied, either by voiding or by catheterization. Ideally, the patient should void spontaneously, but catheterization may be necessary to prevent overdistention, which can contribute to bladder atony and prolonged disturbances in bladder function.[5] The consequences of contamination of the urethra with catheterization can be devastating, because the membrane that lines the urethra is continuous throughout the urinary tract, and an infection can easily travel to the kidneys.

Voiding usually is a standard requirement for discharge after any GU procedure. However, individual urologists hold varied beliefs about whether every patient should or must void before discharge. If the patient is to be discharged without voiding, a specific written physician's order should be obtained, and the following assessments should be included in the nurse's discharge note:

- The patient's fluid status, including oral and intravenous intake
- An abdominal assessment
- The patient's subjective description regarding pain, bladder fullness, and sense of urinary urge
- Specific instructions provided regarding urinary status and inability to void at home

All patients should have telephone access to the physician to report acute urinary retention. Further, they should be instructed to go to an emergency room in the event of inability to void if they are unable to contact the physician. This information should be provided both verbally and in writing to the patient and family before discharge and should be documented in the patient's record. A patient who experiences any level of urinary distress should not be discharged until the problem is resolved.

Patients may be discharged with an indwelling catheter to be removed by the physician, a home health nurse, or a family member, often on the day following surgery. For a patient and caregiver who have never dealt with an indwelling catheter at home, this can be an intimidating and frightening situation. Instructions for catheter care at home should be given in both written and verbal form before discharge. A brief description of urinary tract anatomy is an excellent way to begin instructions. Providing time for the family member to actually demonstrate proper technique can help enhance learning and reduce anxiety.

Catheter care instructions include proper handwashing before any care or handling of the catheter, observation of the urine for color and amount, and maintenance of a closed system by avoiding separation of the catheter from the drainage tubing. If the tubing becomes separated, the patient should be instructed to avoid touching the ends and to cleanse each with an antiseptic solution or an alcohol swab before rejoining them.[6] Daily cleansing of the urinary meatus with soap and warm water is recommended rather than more frequent or aggressive measures.

The urinary drainage bag should remain lower than the level of the bladder at all times and should be emptied every 8 hours or sooner. The mechanics of the lower drainage clamp for emptying the bag should be explained, but clamping of the tubing between the bladder and the drainage bag is not advised.

Suggestions can be provided for an appropriate receptacle for draining urine from the urinary drainage bag, possibly a disposable plastic canister or a urinal supplied by the surgery center. An ambulatory patient may prefer to empty the bag directly into the toilet. Finally, the drainage tubing should be observed frequently to ensure that it is not looped below the drainage bag, kinked, or otherwise obstructed. Taping the catheter to the thigh prevents pulling on the meatus. Occasionally, there may be specific instructions from the physician regarding irrigation of the catheter at home.

Adequate hydration to encourage urine production should continue during the first few days after surgery. A daily intake of 2 to 3 L of fluid is recommended, except when contraindicated owing to a medical condition such as cardiac insufficiency or renal failure.[7] See Key Patient Education Points (Box 35–1) for a summary of key issues to be included in discharge instructions. Also note Box 35–2 that lists Web sites providing information from the nursing and medical urologic specialty organizations.

Box 35–1. KEY PATIENT EDUCATION POINTS FOR GENITOURINARY SURGERY

Signs and symptoms of urinary tract infection
Sexual function and restrictions
Proper catheter care and drainage
Use of urinary drainage bag versus leg bag
Proper hydration
Addressing urinary retention

CYSTOSCOPIC PROCEDURES

A variety of procedures are undertaken transurethrally, including diagnostic cystoscopy, biopsy and fulguration of bladder tumors, stone removal, dilatation of ureteral strictures, and retrograde radiographic studies. Clinically, a cystoscopic procedure can result in postoperative hematuria, which creates nursing issues regarding catheterization, bladder irrigation, removal of the catheter, and patient discharge. Dysuria and difficulty voiding are also problems that may be encountered. Sound judgment is essential in ensuring that reasoned nursing decisions are made based on the patient's presenting

Box 35–2. INTERNET RESOURCES

http://www.duj.com/suna.html	Society of Urologic Nurses
http://www.auanet.org	American Urologic Association, Inc

urinary symptoms, intellectual abilities, general emotional makeup, and family support.

TRANSURETHRAL RESECTION OF PROSTATE

Transurethral resection of the prostate (TURP) has become the second most common procedure in Medicare-eligible men, second only to cataract removal and lens implantation.[7] Through careful selection of patients and newer surgical techniques, it can now be safely accomplished as an ambulatory procedure, with patients being discharged within 24 hours.

In traditional TURP procedures, the cystoscope is passed through the urethra into the bladder; then a loop or wedge is inserted into the prostate, and excess tissue is excised and removed. Two newer procedures are visual laser ablation prostatectomy (VLAP) and transurethral electrovaporization prostatectomy (TEVP). The tissue is either necrosed (VLAP) or vaporized by electric current (TEVP) and then sloughs into the urine. Coagulation is possible during both procedures; thus postoperative bleeding is significantly decreased compared with standard TURP.[7]

Nursing care of the TURP patient includes assessing the urine for color and consistency. In the VLAP and TEVP procedures, the urine may be cloudy owing to the presence of tissue cells rather than the presence of gross hematuria. The patient may also have continuous bladder irrigation. The flow rate is ordered to keep bleeding and clotting minimal. Accurate intake and output records are maintained. Postoperative bleeding is the most common problem encountered, and if it is severe, treatment with the drug aminocaproic acid may be necessary.[8]

Another rare but serious complication is TURP syndrome. As a result of the absorption of irrigating solution, hyponatremia can occur. Symptoms may include increased blood pressure, decreased heart rate, and confusion. Seizures and fatal arrhythmias may follow. Prompt, aggressive treatment with hypertonic saline and diuretics is necessary.[9]

Discharge teaching includes catheter care (if still present) and the use of a leg bag if ordered. Patients are taught signs and symptoms to report to the physician, including excess bleeding, large clots in the urine, no drainage in the catheter, fever, frequent urges to void, and unrelieved pain. Patients are instructed to drink at least 8 glasses of water a day unless contraindicated. Patients may be instructed to avoid driving, stair climbing, heavy lifting, alcohol, sexual intercourse, and the use of aspirin or warfarin until seeing the urologist for a follow-up visit, usually within 1 week.

There are studies under way regarding radical retropubic prostatectomy in the ambulatory setting.[10] These patients are discharged with a Jackson-Pratt wound drain for 3 days and a urinary catheter for 10 days. Pain management is a major concern but has been successful with the use of epidural anesthesia and pelvic block. Blood loss side effects are offset by the administration of autologous blood infusion. Discharge teaching is clearly vital, including drain and catheter care. A visiting nurse continues to monitor the patient's condition at home.

PROSTATIC BIOPSY

There are two approaches to prostatic needle biopsy, one through the rectal wall and the second through the perineum. In both cases, bleeding is a potential complication. The patient should be observed for frank bleeding and for hematoma formation before discharge and should be instructed to report any excessive swelling or bleeding to the physician. Application of an ice bag to the perineum may promote comfort and reduce bleeding. Understandably, the procedure is often coupled with considerable anxiety regarding pathologic outcome.

PERIURETHRAL-TRANSURETHRAL INJECTION OF COLLAGEN

Contigen is a cross-linked bovine collagen approved by the U.S. Food and Drug Administration in September 1993. Injected with a fine spinal needle, it is used to add bulk around the bladder neck and increase resistance to reduce stress incontinence. The patient must be skin tested within 1 month of the procedure with a test dose of the product. An allergy to eggs may deem the patient an inappropriate candidate. Local or regional anesthesia is most often used. Patients are instructed to notify the physician if urinary retention or signs of urinary tract infection occur.[11] This technique is used with both women and men.

VASECTOMY

Elective male sterilization is accomplished by vasectomy, often in the physician's office, but sometimes in an ambulatory surgery center (ASC) setting. Through small incisions on each side of the scrotum, each vas deferens is identified and separated. Electrocautery is used to occlude the proximal and distal lumina, and the incisions are closed. This is most often accomplished under local anesthesia with or without sedation.

Sterility is not immediate after vasectomy, and unprotected intercourse before semen is found to be free of sperm by laboratory assessment is likely to result in pregnancy. In many instances, two specimens must be determined to be free of sperm before protection is considered adequate. Other discharge instructions include the use of a scrotal support to provide comfort and the application of ice to reduce swelling and pain.

There is much publicity in the popular media regarding successful reversal of this procedure. Thus, some people may believe that vasectomy is always reversible. Although successful reversal is a possibility, a patient who makes the decision to have a vasectomy should first be adequately informed that this method is considered permanent.

VASOVASOSTOMY

Reanastomosis of the previously ligated vas is often successful. Through a scrotal skin incision, the surgeon identifies both the proximal and distal ends of the severed vas deferens. An internal stent may or may not be placed within the vas, and the circumference of the vas is sutured. Postoperative care is similar to that of other scrotal procedures. A semen sample is analyzed in 3 to 4 months. Typically, 95% of patients regain vas patency, and 50% to 60% pregnancy rates have been reported in properly selected patients.[12]

VARICOCELECTOMY

Male fertility may be reduced when a varicocele is present. This engorgement of the venous plexus around the testes results when the gonadal vein places back pressure on the plexus. The engorged veins are ligated, the desired result being increased sperm production and thus increased fertility. This is the most common procedure related to male infertility and has a positive effect on semen quality in 70% of men.[13] The incision is high on the scrotum or low in the inguinal canal, and postoperative care is the same as for other scrotal procedures.

HYDROCELECTOMY

A hydrocele is an accumulation of the fluid within a sac, the tunica vaginalis, in the scrotum. After hydrocelectomy, a drain may be left in the scrotal incision, with a bulky dressing applied and covered with a scrotal support. The patient and caregiver should understand that the presence of a drain in the wound increases the likelihood of surgical drainage. The patient may need to reinforce the dressing in the first 24 hours postoperatively. The drain also increases the patient's risk of acquiring a wound infection. Tub baths or submersion of the wound must be avoided, as should handling of the drain with bare hands.

EXTRACORPOREAL SHOCK WAVE LITHOTRIPSY

Extracorporeal shock wave lithotripsy (SWL) is a noninvasive procedure that became available in the United States in 1984 and is used to manage urinary calculi from the bladder to the kidney.[14] A variety of units are available. Some require partial patient submersion in a tub of water, whereas others use water-filled cushions positioned against the patient's skin through which high-energy shock waves are focused. Third-generation machines include fluoroscopy, ultrasonography, and multifunctioning tables. A portable third-generation machine is available as well.

Before admission, the patient is screened medically. Originally, several conditions were considered contraindications for SWL, including aortic aneurysm, presence of a pacemaker, urosepsis, severe obesity, scoliosis, and difficult fit into the machine. At present, few absolute contraindications exist. One author cites pregnancy, uncorrected bleeding disorders, and obstruction below the stone.[15] Another believes that pregnancy is the only absolute contraindication.[16] Some lithotripters can manage patients up to 450 pounds.

Patients who have pacemakers can be treated successfully when certain criteria are met. These include having had a programmable unit in place for more than 6 months, having a pacemaker representative present to program it, and having cardiologist clearance for the procedure within 1 month.[17] Devices implanted into the abdomen, such as continuous narcotic pumps, might be considered relative contraindications, as the shock waves could damage these units.

Patients may be traveling some distance to have the procedure, because not all locations have a lithotripter. If a preoperative visit is not possible, preoperative assessment can be done by telephone, and preoperative instructions can be sent by mail if necessary. Instructions may include having only clear liquids on the evening before surgery (to facilitate visualization of the stone) and taking nothing by mouth (NPO) after midnight or the time deemed appropriate for the time of the procedure. Patients may be asked to avoid skin powders, oils, and lotions. Showering with a special antibacterial skin cleanser may be part of the instructions.

Laboratory tests may include complete blood count, chemistry panel, prothrombin time, and partial thromboplastin time, and are based on the patient's medical status and needs. Other tests may be included based on patient history.[15] Just before the procedure, a scout KUB (kidney, ureter, and bladder) radiographic film is taken to ascertain the presence and location of the calculi. The patient has an intravenous infusion for fluids and medications. If the patient will be partially submerged in water, it is essential that cardiac electrodes be sealed to maintain contact with the skin. Electrode integrity is essential, because the lithotripter is synchronized to discharge during the refractory period (R wave) of the cardiac cycle.

Shock waves generated by a lithotripter are transmitted to the stone through a liquid medium and are focused on the stones via fluoroscopy or ultrasonography. Repeated shock waves break the calculi into small pieces, sand, or gravel that is passed in the urine when the patient voids. Sometimes ureteral stents are inserted cystoscopically before SWL to ensure a patent pathway for elimination of this gravel. A radiographic examination is repeated after the procedure to ascertain that the stone has been adequately destroyed. The bursts created by the lithotripter are loud, and awake patients are often provided with ear protection.

Anesthesia most often is a combination of analgesia and sedation. Few patients require general anesthesia, and some receive spinal anesthesia. The successful use of patient-controlled analgesia and transcutaneous electrical nerve stimulation has been reported.[15]

After the procedure, the nurse observes and documents the patient's fluid status. Urine is measured and observed for volume, color, and presence of gravel. Some hematuria is normal, but excessive blood in the urine should be reported. Urine straining to assess the amount and composition of gravel passed should continue at home. All fragments should be analyzed to determine the chemical makeup of the stones so that a diet can be prescribed to assist in preventing or reducing the formation of further calculi.

Petechiae and skin bruising are normal over the flank area where the lithotripter was focused, but extensive swelling could indicate hematoma formation. Rarely, the patient may experience temporary or permanent nerve damage to the arms from improper positioning during the procedure. A sudden rise in the patient's temperature can indicate sepsis, which can occur rapidly if infected stones are broken up. Other infrequent complications include renal colic, renal contusion, cardiac arrhythmias, subscapular hematoma, pulmonary edema, and ureteral obstruction.[18, 19]

Cardiovascular status is closely observed, because anesthesia-related hypotension and bradycardia may occur owing to the occasional intraoperative use of cardioactive drugs. A patient who is normally bradycardic may be given atropine to increase the heart rate to expedite the SWL procedure, because shock waves are synchronized with the cardiac cycle.[20] Antidysrhythmic drugs may be necessary in surgery to facilitate the firing process as well.

Postoperatively, the patient is encouraged to drink 2 L or more of fluid daily to ensure adequate flushing of gravel from the urinary tract. Antiemetic medications may be necessary if nausea and vomiting complicate the patient's ability to drink. Patients may complain of discomfort from the urinary catheter or ureteral stent, flank pain, or, rarely, renal colic. Analgesia without sedation is the goal, to facilitate an awake, comfortable patient who is able to ambulate and to drink adequately.

In most instances, any urinary catheter that was placed is removed soon after the procedure. The patient is expected to void before discharge, although exceptions may occur. Postoperative instructions should address access to medical attention in the event of acute urinary retention or obstruction. This access is a particular concern for a patient who lives a long distance from the treatment site and will be traveling home on the same day as the procedure.

PROSTATE BRACHYTHERAPY

Because of the increase in the incidence of prostate cancer in the past 2 decades, treatment with radioactive isotope implantation has become commonplace. More recently it has been accomplished in the ambulatory setting.

Prostate cancer has historically been treated

primarily by radical or simple prostatectomy. If radiotherapy was used, external beam radiation was considered the "gold standard."[21] However, both treatments have significant side effects. Prostatectomy side effects include incontinence and decreased sexual potency. Diarrhea, cystitis, and proctitis in addition to impotence are side effects that often accompany external beam radiation therapy.[21, 22]

Seed implantation offers an alternative that requires less recuperation time and better preservation of continence and potency.[21] Two types of seeds are used today: palladium-103 and iodine-125. Selection of patients is based on the stage of the tumor and whether the physical condition of the patient allows for spinal anesthesia. Excessive TURP defects and very large prostate volumes are relative contraindications.[22]

Preoperative patient preparation before seed implantation includes diagnostic testing based on physical examination and facility protocols, along with the usual nursing assessment and education. Emotional support and direct, honest answers to questions are especially important to help the patient and family prepare for this procedure. The patient may be asked to have only clear liquids for 24 hours before surgery, and a preoperative cleansing enema may be ordered. These preparations are aimed at ensuring a clear ultrasound picture.

During the procedure, the patient is placed in the lithotomy position under spinal anesthesia. An ultrasound-guided transperineal technique is used. Needles carrying the seeds are placed through the perineum directly into the prostate tissue. The needles are removed, and the seeds are left in place permanently. A cystoscopy is performed following seed implantation to assess for and remove any seeds that went into the bladder inadvertently and to remove blood clots.

Immediate care of the patient after the procedure includes monitoring the recession of the spinal blockade, perineal observation, and monitoring of urine flow and for potential hematuria. Hematuria is not uncommon, but clots and gross hematuria may require irrigation. Seeds are sometimes found in the catheter bag. These should be retrieved with forceps and placed in a lead-lined container. The patient may also pass seeds at home. These may be safely flushed with other waste into the sewer system. If the patient retrieves the seed during urine straining, it can be wrapped in foil and returned to the medical facility.[21]

After sensation returns, the patient may experience mild perineal discomfort that can be treated with sitz baths, ice packs, and mild analgesics.

Special isolation of the patient is not required during the recovery phase. However, because the effects of even low-dose radiation are not completely understood, nurses or family members caring for the patient should prevent any unnecessary exposure to the patient's perineum. The catheter bag may be placed toward the patient's head, and limited direct exposure to the perineum when checking dressings or the operative site is prudent. In some facilities, pregnant personnel do not care for these patients.[23, 24] The patient may be discharged once the catheter is removed and the patient has voided. Some patients may be discharged with the catheter in place.

Preoperative teaching should include explanation of the procedure and anesthesia choice. The patient should also be given information regarding expected side effects. These include hematuria, urinary urgency, decreased stream flow, and hesitancy. Other side effects commonly start about 7 to 10 days later. These include urinary obstruction, urethral irritation, frequency, urgency, dysuria, and nocturia. They are usually temporary but should be reported to the physician. Rectal symptoms are rare but could include soft or more frequent stools.

Radiation information is essential. Some patients may consider themselves "radioactive" and isolate themselves. Actually, only minimal restrictions are needed. Close contact with pregnant women or small children (younger than 4 years old) should be limited during the first half-life of the seed. For palladium, this is 17 days, and for iodine, 8 weeks. Activities such as having children sit on the patient's lap should be avoided.[22] Seed implants do not set off metal detectors or interfere with magnetic resonance imaging scans.

Sexual intercourse may be resumed when the physician allows, commonly after 2 weeks. A condom must be worn in case a seed is ejected. This protection is needed for the first month with palladium and for 2 months with iodine seeds.

Patients are given written information regarding the type and amount of radiation implanted. They may wear a bracelet or other identification during the period required for radiation precautions. Postoperative instructions should reinforce preoperative information and include catheter care instructions if the patient is discharged with a catheter in place. Increased fluid intake is encouraged unless contraindicated.

References

1. Luckmann J: Saunders Manual of Nursing Care. Philadelphia: WB Saunders, 1997, p 1236.
2. Cassady J: Regional anesthesia for urologic procedures. Urol Clin North Am 14:43–50, 1987.
3. Badon J, Mazze R: Urinary retention. In Orkin F, Cooperman L (eds): Complications in Anesthesiology. Philadelphia: JB Lippincott, 1983, pp 423–426.
4. Ellis WE: Regional anesthesia. In Nagelhout JJ, Zaglaniczny KL (eds): Nurse Anesthesia. Philadelphia: WB Saunders, 1997, pp 1160–1197.
5. Kemp D, Tabaka N: Postoperative urinary retention. Part I. Overview and implications for the postanesthesia care unit nurse. J Post Anesth Nurs 5:338–341, 1990.
6. D'Angostino J: Sending the patient home with an indwelling Foley catheter. Urol Nurs 10:23, 1990.
7. Churchill JA: Transurethral prostatectomy—new trends. Geriatric Nursing 18:78–80, 1997.
8. Wilson M: Care of the patient undergoing transurethral resection of the prostate. J Perianesth Nurs 12:341–351, 1997.
9. Gillenwater J, Grayhack JT, Howards FS (eds): Adult and Pediatric Urology, 3rd ed. St. Louis: CV Mosby, 1996, p 523.
10. Hajjar JH, Budd HA, Wachtel Z: Ambulatory radical retropubic prostatectomy. Urology 51:443–448, 1998.
11. Stanton SL: Surgical treatment of sphincteric incontinence in women. World J Urol 15:275–279, 1997.
12. Bergant J, Grimes J: Urological surgery of the major ambulatory patient. In Davis J (ed): Major Ambulatory Surgery. Baltimore: Williams & Wilkins, 1986, pp 283–294.
13. Luckmann J: Saunders Manual of Nursing Care. Philadelphia: WB Saunders, 1997, p 1434.
14. O'Reilly M, Mulry K: Postanesthesia care of renal and biliary lithotripsy patients. J Post Anesth Nurs 4:382–389, 1989.
15. Streem SB: Contemporary clinical practice of shock wave lithotripsy: A revolution of contraindications. J Urol 157:1197–1203, 1997.
16. Gillenwater J, Grayhack JT, Howards FS (eds): Adult and Pediatric Urology, 3rd ed. St. Louis: CV Mosby, 1996, pp 913–921.
17. Karlowicz KA: Urologic Nursing: Principles and Practice. Philadelphia: WB Saunders, 1995.
18. Jocham D, Brandl H, Chaussy C, Schmiedt E: Treatment of nephrolithiasis with ESWL. In Gravenstein J, Peter K (eds): Extracorporeal Shock Wave Lithotripsy for Renal Stone Disease. Boston: Butterworth, 1986, pp 35–60.
19. Madler C, Mendl G, Angster R, et al: Anxiety and mood of patients with kidney stones: A comparison between ESWL and invasive therapeutic methods. In Gravenstein J, Peter K (eds): Extracorporeal Shock Wave Lithotripsy for Renal Stone Disease. Boston: Butterworth, 1986, pp 91–98.
20. Odom K: Recovering the ESWL patient. J Post Anesth Nurs 3:14–16, 1988.
21. Cash JC, Dattoli MJ: Management of patients recovering from transperineal palladium-103 prostate implants. Oncol Nurs Forum 24:1361–1367, 1997.
22. Greenburg S, Petersen J, Hansen-Peters I, et al: Interstitially implanted I-125 for prostate cancer using transrectal ultrasound. Oncol Nurs Forum 17:849–854, 1990.
23. Gregory B, Van Valkenburg J: Prostate cancer: Radiation seed implantation without open surgery. J Perianesth Nurs 4:373–376, 1989.
24. Nag S, Petty LR, Parrot S: Comprehensive surgical radiation oncology. AORN J 60:27–37, 1994.

Chapter 36

Orthopedic and Podiatric Surgery

Brenda S. Gregory Dawes

Treatment of orthopedic and podiatric conditions in an ambulatory surgery setting are for diagnostic or therapeutic purposes. Procedures are performed for congenital, traumatic, or acquired conditions that may have resulted in acute or chronic disorders (Table 36–1). These conditions include musculoskeletal disorders caused by abnormality of development, structural disease, degenerative changes, or injury. The disorders might affect any of the bones or supporting structures (Fig. 36–1) of the skeletal system. Procedures on the hand are addressed in the discussion of plastic and reconstructive surgery (see Chapter 32), although they also may be performed by an orthopedic surgeon. Table 36–2 lists common terminology used when caring for the patient undergoing orthopedic procedures.

Caring for patients undergoing procedures on bones or associated structures requires intense assessment and planning to ensure that the procedure is completed in an expedient manner. The ability to decrease the length of stay is a benefit of less invasive procedures but does not preclude the need to spend time preparing for the procedure and teaching the patient. This requires an understanding of the anatomy and associated physiology, specific patient conditions and needs, the plan of care to be provided by other team members (e.g., surgeon, anesthesiologist), the intraoperative interventions, and expected outcomes. In addition to the technique used by the surgeon, the type of anesthetic delivered adds to the benefits recognized when caring for the ambulatory surgery center (ASC) patient. Nursing personnel should become familiar with the options to be provided and readily implement patient care to provide a safe and comfortable environment. The ability to prepare team members and the patient, avoid delays, and ensure safe patient discharge promotes high-quality patient care and physician satisfaction.

The anatomy of the musculoskeletal system includes bony structures, ligaments, tendons, and nerves. The specific patient condition and needs influence the plan of care. Understanding and relating the structures involved and the physiologic condition enables individualized patient and procedure preparation, teaching, and discharge planning. Patients undergoing orthopedic and podiatric procedures are various ages, with varying physical conditions. Their needs provide a challenge to the perioperative and perianesthesia nursing personnel.

Understanding the patient's needs and the plan of care being provided by others complements the preparation for the procedure. Surgeon preferences vary based on level of familiarity with instrumentation and choice of operative technique. This includes implant and repair types. An example includes positioning the patient for a surgical procedure. The position selected is expected to provide exposure without compromising the patients' respiratory, circulatory, or neurovascular status. The nursing intervention is aimed at prevention of patient injury. Understanding the position and equipment specifically used by a physician increases the ability to assess, plan, implement, and evaluate the patient's care.

Table 36–1. Orthopedic Procedures Commonly Performed in the Ambulatory Surgery Center

General Orthopedic Procedures
Arthroscopic procedures (diagnostic and therapeutic)
Arthroplasty—small joints
Bone graft—allograft, autogenous
Cast change
Closed reduction
Cyst removal
Débridement
Epidural steroid injection
Excision of lesion
Fasciectomy
Joint manipulation
Muscle biopsy
Removal of foreign body
Removal of hardware
Tendon exploration, repair, release
Synovectomy
Z-plasty
Foot Procedures
Bone spur excision
Bunionectomy
Hammer toe correction
Osteotomy
Syndactylization of toes
Hand Procedures
Carpal tunnel release
Excision of neuroma
Finger amputation or revision
Flexor tendon sheath release
ORIF fingers
Release of Dupuytren's contracture
Release of trigger finger or trigger thumb
Elbow/Arm
Olecranon bursectomy
Olecranon spur excision
Median nerve decompression
Ulnar nerve transfer
Knee
Prepatellar bursectomy
Anterior cruciate ligament reconstruction
Back
Percutaneous suction lumbar discectomy

ORIF = open reduction internal fixation.

The anesthesia provider's plan of care also influences nursing interventions and can be enhanced if personnel are familiar with the type of anesthetic to be delivered. Regional anesthesia is often chosen for surgeries involving the extremities. It is believed that eliminating general anesthesia agents decreases associated risks.

Studies comparing morbidity of general versus regional anesthesia are inconclusive. Use of regional anesthesia promotes rapid reunion with the family, early ambulation and discharge, and return of mental alertness and encourages self-care, including eating and voiding. Another excellent advantage of regional anesthesia is the postoperative analgesia that it provides.[1–3]

The expected outcome is important to the success of the procedure. A lengthy rehabilitative process may be expected before a patient is recuperated completely. The patient's livelihood or ability to fulfill his or her usual responsibilities within the household may be disturbed temporarily or permanently. Referral for social or financial assistance may be needed, and emotional support becomes even more important for these patients and their families.

PREOPERATIVE CARE

Nursing care provided during the preoperative phase facilitates an uncomplicated procedure. Activities include preparing the patient physically and emotionally, patient teaching, and communicating the assessment data to other team members. Box 36–1 provides educa-

BOX 36–1. KEY EDUCATION POINTS

- Complications of the surgical procedure
  - Nausea, vomiting, or respiratory depression all could be side effects or long-term effects of the anesthetic medications. Dressings should be observed for bleeding or drainage. Questionable outcomes should be reported.
- Ambulation and exercise
  - Passive exercise and ambulation (with crutches as appropriate for the procedure) are started immediately. Active exercises are started in 10 days to 2 weeks. Full range of motion may not return for up to 6 to 8 months. Some procedures may require limited sitting or riding in a vehicle and prohibited lifting, bending, and stooping.
- Prevention of swelling
  - Elevation of the extremity the first 3 to 5 days is beneficial to prevent unnecessary edema. The dependent position should be avoided.
- Healing process
  - Bone healing is slower than the tissue; therefore, activity levels should be increased slowly to previous levels. Bone may not be healed for up to 1 year.
- Pain management
  - Pain medication should be taken according to the physician's instructions. Over-the-counter pain medications may be useful in pain relief.
- Dressing or cast care
  - A dressing can be removed or changed according to the physician's instructions. The cast should remain dry, and objects should never be used to scratch beneath the cast. Protruding pins should be cleaned around the outside daily with alcohol.

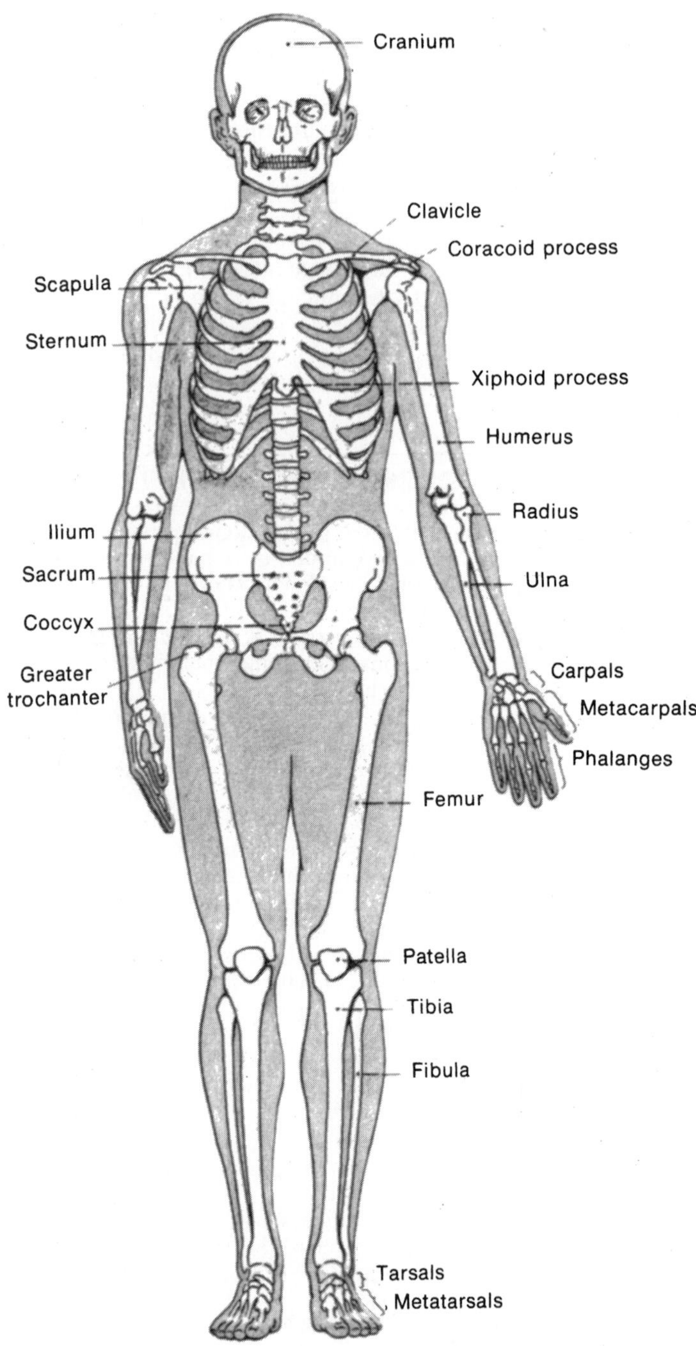

Figure 36–1. Anterior view of the skeleton. (From Jacob S, Francone C: Elements of Anatomy and Physiology, 2nd ed. Philadelphia: WB Saunders, 1989, p 47.)

Table 36–2. Orthopedic Definitions

Term	Definition
Abduction	Drawing away from the midline of the body
Adduction	Bringing toward or nearer the midline of the body
Ankylosis	Immobility and consolidation of a joint
Arthritis	Joint inflammation
Bursa	Synovial bursa; small sac lined with synovial fluid that cushions and prevents friction between two surfaces (for instance, within joints or subcutaneously at the elbow or over the patella)
Chondromalacia patellae	Pain of the patella characterized by roughness of the inner surface of the patella
Dislocation	An abnormal anatomic relationship of bones within a joint; the displacement of a bone from its normal joint position
Epiphysis	The head (end) of a long bone
Extension	Straightening of a joint
Fasciae	Broad bands of fibrous tissue wrapped around muscles to hold the muscles in place
Flexion	Bending of a joint
Ligament	Strong bands of fibrous connective tissue that hold joints together
Meniscus	Curved, fibrous cartilages in the knee
Myositis	Inflammation of voluntary muscles
Neuralgia	Sharp pain that follows the course of a particular nerve
Neuroma	A tumor composed of nerve cells
Osteoporosis	Loss of calcium in the bone
Osteotomy	Cutting of the bone
Paresis	Incomplete or partial paralysis
Paresthesia	A sensation of numbness, prickling, tingling, or heightened sensitivity
Periosteum	Membranous covering of the bones
Phalanges	The bones of the digits
Plication	Folding of tissue
Radicular	Pertaining to a spinal nerve root
Rotation	Movement of a bone around a central axis without undergoing any displacement from the axis (e.g., shoulder joint)
Sprain	Injury to ligaments surrounding a joint, usually from overstress by wrenching or twisting
Subluxation	A partial dislocation of a bone from its normal joint position
Synovectomy	Removal of the synovial membrane
Synovial membrane	The layer of membrane that secretes a thick fluid for lubrication of a freely moving joint

tional points that are applicable. Preoperative care includes patient assessment, identification of the surgical site, implementation of aseptic practices, identifying home care needs, and ensuring that diagnostic results are obtained.

Baseline data are collected to use for postoperative comparison. This includes assessment of the surgical site and distal areas of an associated extremity for skin color, presence of rash, infection, presence and quality of pulses, range of motion, and neurovascular status, including sensation. A pulse oximetry reading obtained on the extremity of surgery provides yet another parameter of assessment.

The site of surgery must be identified carefully and correctly. Because many orthopedic and podiatric procedures involve either the right or left side of the body, this identification may have a greater-than-usual potential for error. One suggestion is to ask the patient to point to the site, or to mark the side of surgery with a skin marker before the patient receives sedation. All staff members who care for the patient should confirm the side and site of surgery with the medical record, the operative consent form, and the patient. It is helpful to tell the patient that, as a safety measure, many staff members will be asking the patient to identify the surgical site even though the information is documented on the chart. This explanation can help to prevent the patient's concern that staff members do not know or remember what has already been told to others.

Implementing and monitoring the principles of aseptic technique promotes infection control.[4, 5] Rigid adherence to aseptic principles is essential in every department of the ASC to prevent nosocomial infection. Infection is a threatening complication because it can be difficult to treat successfully or to confine to one area when bone tissue is involved and may result in a complicated recovery. Methods used to prevent infection include avoidance of skin shaving by using alternate hair removal methods, such as depilatory or clipping. An antimicrobial solution is used for the preoperative skin scrub.

Preoperatively, antibiotics may be administered intravenously and intraoperatively by direct wound irrigation before closure of the incision. If used, the timing of preoperative antibiotics is important to accomplish the expected outcome.[6, 7] The antibiotic must be circulating in the system before inflation of the tourniquet and must have reached the peak systemic effect. The most effective time frame for administration of many antibiotics is within the hour before incision. Oral and topical antibiotics may be prescribed postoperatively. Other measures for infection control are to instruct the patient about careful handwashing before adjusting or changing the dressing and the need to avoid getting the dressing or cast wet after surgery.

Orthopedic or podiatric surgery commonly results in altered mobility after the procedure. Patients face a challenge in performing some of the normal activities of daily living. Plans should be made before the day of surgery to secure necessary home assistance, for example to help with dressing, eating, hygiene, or other activities. Patients should secure necessary ambulatory assistive devices before the day of surgery. The ASC nurse can provide the patient with sources of assistive devices for purchase, rent, or loan. Community services such as fire departments may be one source.

The patient's general mobility and gait should be evaluated, both for comparison after surgery and to identify the potential for related postoperative difficulties. For example, consider the obese 62-year-old woman with rheumatoid arthritis who has joint deformities, advanced loss of function of her hands, and chronic pain in her knees and hips. This patient would likely have difficulty using crutches after surgery, and the nurse might suggest securing a walker or wheelchair for temporary assistance.

Instructions for use of equipment or supplies should begin as soon as it is recognized that the patient will need the assistance. This allows the patient to practice and become comfortable and safe in use of the item. Preoperative crutch-walking instructions may be provided by a physical therapist. When this resource person is not available, the nurse may be called on to provide instructions and to ascertain the proper fit and adjustment of crutches that the patient purchases privately. Specific crutch-walking instructions are illustrated in Table 36–3.

A walker is a more stable device that allows full or partial weight-bearing. When the patient is standing inside the walker, the hand grips should be at the level of the greater trochanter of the hip. The patient's arms should be flexed slightly to approximately 15 to 20 degrees. The patient should be reminded to take small steps and to avoid placing the walker more than 8 to 10 inches in front of the body for each stride.[8]

Other orthopedic devices such as slings, braces, splints, casts, and surgical shoes are dispensed from the surgery center on the day of surgery, and the patient should receive instructions regarding their proper use. A return demonstration or explanation given to the nurse by the patient is helpful in assessing the patient's actual level of understanding. Observation of the patient may also provide hints as to the patient's intended level of cooperation in following postoperative orders.

The nurse can suggest other appropriate preoperative measures to prepare the home before the day of surgery, for example, removal of throw rugs and loose items from the floor. Electric cords and telephone cords should be out of walkways. Household and personal items that will be needed after surgery should be located in easily accessible places. For the patient facing temporary loss of use of the dominant hand or arm, the nurse might suggest (1) assembling clothing that pulls on easily or that buttons up the front; (2) transferring necessary items to containers that can be opened with one hand; and (3) cooking ahead and freezing meals or purchasing easy-to-prepare foods if a companion will not be available after the first day or two. The patient who lives in a two-story house may want to prepare a temporary bed on the first floor.

Because the patient may have a bulky dressing, splint, or cast applied in surgery, loose-fitting clothing should be worn for ease in dressing postoperatively. Blue jeans, one-piece jump suits, and clothes that fit snugly can be particularly difficult to manage. Before the day of surgery, the nurse should provide suggestions for appropriate clothing.

Results of diagnostic imaging tests of the musculoskeletal system, such as those described in Table 36–4, should be on the patient's chart before surgery. Often the surgeon will want the actual diagnostic films to view intraoperatively in addition to the reports. If results of tests are needed intraoperatively, the ASC nurse should ascertain whether these are obtained from the physician's office or from outside sources.

INTRAOPERATIVE CARE

Nursing activities that take place during the intraoperative phase are consistent with those

Table 36–3. **Crutch-Walking Instructions**

FITTING THE CRUTCHES
There should be two to three finger-widths of space between your underarms and the crutches. (Have another person measure when you are standing up straight with the tips of the crutches on the floor just to the outside of your toes.)
Adjust the handpiece to allow your elbow to bend at a 30° angle.
SAFETY PRECAUTIONS
Be sure your crutches have large rubber suction tips.
The arm and handpieces should be fitted with foam rubber pads to relieve pressure on your hands, upper arms, and rib cage.
Wear supportive, sturdy shoes with nonskid soles that fit well. Do not go barefoot or wear "flipflops," sandals, slingbacks, high heels, or slippers while walking with crutches.
Avoid wearing a long bathrobe, skirt, or loose-legged pants that could get tangled in the crutches.
Permanent nerve damage with resulting "crutch paralysis" of the arms can result from leaning your weight on your underarms.
Remove throw rugs and other dangerous objects from your home. Avoid deep-pile carpet and grass when possible. Walk very carefully if you must be on wet or slippery surfaces.
Be sure someone is in attendance to steady you until you feel confident while walking on crutches.
WALKING
Use your hands and arms for weight-bearing, *not* your underarms!
Put both crutches and the weak leg forward at the same time. Then move the strong leg to meet them. Do not take steps that are too large.
Take small, slow steps until you become proficient on the crutches.
For safety, advance your pace only as your physical ability improves.
TO SIT DOWN IN A CHAIR
Hold the crutches by the handpieces to steady your body, bend forward slightly, and sit down. Use the strong leg for bearing weight.
TO STAND UP FROM A CHAIR
Move to the front edge of the chair. Put the strong leg slightly under the seat.
Put both crutches in the hand on the side of the weak leg.
Push down on the handpieces while raising the body to a standing position.
TO GO UP STAIRS OR A CURB
Keep the crutches in place for support.
Step up with the stronger leg first.
Bring the crutches and the weaker leg up to the higher step.
TO GO DOWN STAIRS OR A CURB
Place feet forward as far as possible on the step.
Put the crutches down on the lower step.
Put the weaker leg down while maintaining weight on the crutches and the strong leg.
Lower the strong leg to the lower step.

Data from Smeltzer S, Bare B: Brunner & Suddarth's Textbook of Medical–Surgical Nursing, 7th ed. Philadelphia: JB Lippincott, 1992, pp 232–235; and Luckmann J (ed): Saunders Manual of Nursing Care. Philadelphia: WB Saunders, 1997, pp 1567–1569.

of the hospitalized patient, except the procedures are often less invasive and shorter in length. Two priority goals are that the patient will be free from injury related to positioning or use of equipment and that the patient will be free from infection.

Positioning for orthopedic procedures often is a complex process. The nurse must ensure the patient's proper body alignment, support of all body parts, and padding of bony prominences. Some of the many devices that may be used for positioning include pillows, blanket rolls, sandbags, foam, vacuum beanbag-style cushions, and specialty holding devices.

All appropriate equipment and instrumentation must be available and tested to ensure its proper working condition before admitting the patient to the operating room. Skills must be perfected to properly operate, adjust, and forestall problems with the technical equipment

Table 36–4. Diagnostic Imaging Tests for Musculoskeletal Disorders

NAME OF TEST	INVASIVE OR NONINVASIVE	MODE OF ACTION	ADVANTAGES/ DISADVANTAGES	APPLICATIONS
Computerized transaxial tomography (CT scan, CAT scan)	N or I	Multiple cross-sectional x-rays, give 3-dimensional view Contrast media for some parts of the body	Low radiation exposure Patient must be able to lie still for 30 minutes or more	Some bone and soft tissue tumors (wear no metal jewelry)
Magnetic resonance imaging (MRI)	N	Magnetic field and radio waves	No ionizing radiation exposure More sensitive than CT for diseases associated with ↑ water content Contraindications: obesity > 300 lb or 52-inch girth, pregnancy, presence of ferromagnetic bodies such as implanted metal clips, health status requiring life support Claustrophobic patients may have difficulty tolerating enclosure in the chamber	Ligaments, tendons, muscles, joints, intraspinal contents, spine, intervertebral disks, bones Superior for evaluating in multiple sclerosis (wear no metal jewelry)
Roentgenogram (x-ray, radiography)	N	Simple x-ray	Exposure to ionizing radiation Limited usefulness with soft tissue Positioning/table may cause discomfort Most widely used imaging technique, cost-effective and quick	Fractures of bones, related structures

Arthrogram	I	Air or contrast media injected	Possible allergic reaction Painful joint after exam May require follow-up films after initial film	Joint disorders Soft tissues of joints and related ligaments, capsules (local anesthesia before test)
Bone scan	I	Radioisotope with affinity to bone given IV	Exposure to radioisotope but usually of low dose to be of little or no danger Up to 1 hour on table	Bone tumors and difficult-to-diagnose fractures
Electromyography (EMG)	I	Records electrical activity of skeletal muscles	Discomfort associated with insertion of multiple needles	Assess lower motor neuron function Effects of disk disease
Myelography	I	Radiologic study of spinal cord after injection of radiopaque medium into intrathecal space	Discomfort with positioning or with injection of media Possible allergic reaction Common side effects are headache, nausea, vomiting Seizures/hallucinations very rare After water-soluble dyes—stay in semi-Fowler's for 8–12 hours to prevent dye from traveling up in CSF; force fluids After oil-based dyes—stay supine 4 hours	Diagnosis of spinal stenosis and herniated disk

CSF = cerebrospinal fluid; IV = intravenous.

used in surgery, for example, pneumatic tourniquets, air-powered drills and tools, arthroscopes and associated instrumentation, lasers, light sources, and video equipment.

The principles of electrical safety must be observed conscientiously because a number of electrical devices can be in use simultaneously. At times, the floor might be wet with irrigants and surgical drainage. Personnel safety also becomes a concern in this environment.

Tourniquets are used on the upper or lower extremities to control bleeding. The circulating nurse ensures that the tourniquet is applied properly and monitors pressure settings and the length of inflation time. Inappropriate tourniquet use has been associated with both nerve and muscle damage.[9]

Infection control measures are comparable to other surgical procedures. Some of the considerations for managing the environment include adherence to aseptic technique and sterilization parameters. The implants used must be handled to ensure sterility and that documentation of use is accurate. Skin preparation and draping are more complex because of procedures commonly being performed on the extremity.

POSTOPERATIVE CARE

Nursing care after the procedure initially focuses on stabilization of the patient's condition. Once the patient is stable, their return of alertness and mobility and preparation for discharge should be encouraged. Before discharge, the nurse reinforces teaching and observes the patient by return demonstration and verbalization. The patient and companion must understand the signs and symptoms of complications and the appropriate response.

Potential complications associated with orthopedic and podiatric surgery include neurovascular compromise, bleeding, thrombosis, and embolism. The potential for infection is increased when hardware such as pins, screws, or plates are implanted into the bone, particularly when there is external protrusion, such as with K-wires and external fixation devices. The break in the natural barrier of skin is an easy port of entry for microorganisms.

The operative site and the circulatory and neurologic status of an affected extremity are assessed carefully when the patient is admitted to the postanesthesia care unit and periodically throughout the stay. Whenever possible, the digits should be exposed to allow continuous observation. Assessment of distal pulses, color, and temperature of the skin, range of motion, and sensation should be compared with the opposite extremity and with the preoperative status documented on the medical record. Pulse oximetry on the affected digit may be another helpful assessment parameter.

Bleeding is another potential complication. A compression dressing, elevation of the surgical site, and application of cold to the operative site for the first 24 hours may be ordered to reduce the risk of bleeding and edema. Bleeding at the surgical site may increase the chance of wound infection. Bleeding within a joint (hemarthrosis) usually is self-limiting because of the confines of the space and the tamponade effect. Although self-limiting, hemarthrosis can result in increased pain and may require needle aspiration.

Postoperative elevation of the surgical site above the level of the heart is advantageous for a number of reasons. Because venous return to the heart is enhanced by elevation, the pain and throbbing associated with arterial blood flow are decreased and the chance of bleeding and swelling is reduced. With less effusion into surrounding tissues, incisions heal more quickly. Care must be taken to support adequately all parts of an arm or leg that is being elevated. Pillows should be placed under the elbow or along the full length of the leg for proper support, being careful to avoid popliteal pressure. Active and passive exercises may be ordered by the physician to help increase blood flow and reduce local edema.

Most ambulatory surgical procedures do not require lengthy bedrest or immobilization, therefore the potential for embolism is less than that with more complex orthopedic procedures. However, thrombosis or embolism are still possible because of immobility of an extremity or dislodging of a clot during or after surgery. One preventive measure is active or passive exercise of the extremities as directed by the physician. Careful postoperative physical assessment and patient education are essential to ensure that symptoms suggestive of these grave complications are identified and reported, whether they occur at the surgery center or after discharge.

Signs of thrombosis or embolism depend on the site but can range from painful, red, and swollen tissues in the calf to the sudden onset of chest pain, anxiety, and dyspnea, with or without hemoptysis, when a clot travels to the pulmonary vascular bed. This respiratory complication can quickly lead to shock and severe or fatal cardiovascular sequelae. Initial nursing interventions when pulmonary embolism is suspected include support of respirations through positioning and oxygen administration, oropharyngeal suctioning if needed, monitoring of vital signs, and appropriate fluid therapy to support the blood pressure.

Neurovascular compromise can result from intraoperative trauma or from a constricting dressing, splint, or cast. Intraoperative tourniquet use or regional anesthesia of an extremity can temporarily complicate accurate assessment of both objective and subjective symptoms. Distal extremity coldness, pallor, discoloration, bluishness, decreased pulses, or subjective symptoms such as loss of sensation or prolonged numbness or tingling can herald circulatory or neurologic compromise of an extremity. The patient who has been discharged to home should understand that these symptoms are potentially serious and should be reported to the surgeon without delay.

Neurovascular compromise or the presence of regional anesthetic may decrease the patient's response to cold. An important aspect of patient care and education relates to the safe use of cold therapy. An ice bag is a potentially dangerous treatment, particularly if the patient has not regained full sensory capacity after an anesthetic block. To avoid damage to the tissues caused by cold, the patient is instructed to use intermittent, rather than continuous, cold therapy. Application of ice is avoided directly on the fingers and toes because of the lack of collateral circulation to the digits. Resulting vasoconstriction can cause ischemia and permanent tissue damage.

After upper extremity surgery, the physician may order use of a sling for support and elevation of the surgical site. Without adequate instructions and return demonstration, patients often wear arm slings improperly because they have observed others doing so. A sling should be worn so that the hand is higher than the heart and the elbow. The hand actually rests near the opposite shoulder when the sling is applied properly. Unless contraindicated by the type of surgery, the patient who has had a lower arm or hand procedure should periodically remove the sling each day to exercise the shoulder and elbow joints. Elevation of the lower arm should be maintained during exercise of the joints.

After shoulder, clavicular, or upper arm procedures, the patient may have the affected shoulder and arm immobilized with a commercial immobilizer or an Ace wrap encircling the arm and chest. In this case, the distal pulses should be observed closely because arm flexion can result in reduced blood flow to the hand. Also, opposing skin surfaces between the arm and chest or in the axilla should be protected against possible friction and excoriation by the use of padding.

Prolonged immobilization can be very tiresome and uncomfortable. The patient may be tempted to release the immobilizer prematurely. The nurse should stress the importance of strict compliance with the physician's treatment protocol for immobilization.

A plaster cast or splint requires that the extremity be positioned cautiously until the plaster is dry and hard. Molding of damp plaster cast material can result in undesired pressure to underlying tissues. Leaning the cast on a hard surface should be avoided until the plaster is set. During the 24 to 72 hours it may take for a large plaster cast to completely dry through all layers, the cast should remain uncovered and exposed to the air to enhance drying and subsequent cooling. Patients may require reassurance that it is normal to experience a sensation of heat due to evaporation of water inside the cast while it is drying. Throughout the patient's stay, the nurse should ensure that the cast is not putting pressure on tissues or hindering circulation.[10]

Synthetic cast materials, such as fiberglass, dry very quickly. They are more difficult to mold but are stronger and lighter in weight than plaster, radiolucent, and relatively resistant to water. Weight-bearing, if allowed postoperatively, can begin almost immediately after cast application. A fiberglass cast can be cleaned on the outside with soap and a damp cloth, but water should not be allowed to soak the inside. Moisture held within the cast can lead to tissue maceration, possibly resulting in skin irritation or infection.

Verbal and written instructions for cast care at home include the following points:

1. Avoid getting the cast wet. Report a wet cast to the physician.
2. Avoid putting anything inside the cast to scratch the skin. Also, no powders, lotions, or liquids should be put inside the cast.
3. Do not cut, crush, or otherwise adjust the cast. Report pressure points or areas of skin irritation to the physician.
4. Follow the physician's directions for bearing weight.
5. Keep the affected extremity elevated above heart level as much as possible for the first week.
6. Report any symptoms of circulatory compromise: blue or dusky skin, numbness, or tingling of the toes or fingers.
7. Report a fever, chills, or any foul odors coming from the cast.

8. Report blood stains that increase in size on the cast.
9. Report ongoing or severe pain that is unrelieved by pain medication.

Regardless of the surgical site, orthopedic and podiatric procedures have the potential to complicate mobility. For example, the patient may experience vertigo, weakness of the legs, increased pain on weight-bearing or standing up, inability to feel an anesthetized operative site, or lack of necessary arm and wrist strength to use crutches effectively. During initial attempts to walk, the patient may require both emotional and physical support. Verbal and written discharge instructions should address the physician's directives regarding weight-bearing and the projected number of days or weeks that the patient will be using crutches or a walker.

If the patient received a nerve block, practical and medically appropriate discharge criteria must be established by the ASC. A nerve block may result in prolonged sensory or motor numbness but not prohibit the patient from discharge. The patient should be told what is normal and reminded that normal sensation that would protect the extremity is absent. Extra caution should be taken with ambulation or exposure to hot and cold (such as cooking) or sharp objects.

Discharge by wheelchair may be a requirement of the surgical unit or may be prescribed by the physician or appropriate to the type of procedure performed. Before a wheelchair discharge, it is the nurse's responsibility to ensure that the patient can ambulate effectively and within the bounds of the physician's orders. The patient should demonstrate an adequate gait and, when appropriate, the correct use of crutches or other assistive aids. The accompanying adult should be encouraged to park as close as possible to the entry of the patient's house and to assist the patient into the house.

PROCEDURES

Joint Arthroplasty

Arthroplasty of small joints may be performed in the ambulatory surgical setting. Most common disease processes treated are rheumatoid arthritis and other degenerative processes of the fingers, hand, and wrist. The goals of the procedure are to reestablish or improve function in the joints and reduce pain. The procedure is not recommended solely for cosmetic effect.

Assistance at home is essential for these patients when surgery has been performed on both hands or when the primary degenerative disease has seriously affected function of other joints throughout the body. The nurse should reinforce the importance of following the physician's instructions for pre- and postoperative exercises designed for conditioning and strengthening the hands. The exercise regimen is a key element in the eventual success of the procedure.

After implanting a silicone joint, the normal scarring process encapsulates and provides stability to the new joint. Postoperative management focuses on controlling the scarring process so that an appropriate amount of flexion and extension results. This is accomplished by a progressive splinting program that allows restricted flexion of the fingers with restricted lateral movement of the wrist for at least 6 to 8 weeks. The splinting process is advanced according to the patient's needs, but usually it is not instituted until several days after surgery.

Potential postoperative complications include bleeding, neurovascular compromise of the fingers, infection with or without bone degeneration, dislocation of the new joints, and fracture. Implants may improve joint function, but the disease process plays a part in the amount of return function. The surgeon usually prepares the patient before surgery for a less-than-ideal surgical outcome so that the patient does not have unrealistically high expectations.

Arthroscopy

Arthroscopic technique offers the advantage of less tissue trauma, pain, and patient inconvenience, improved joint visualization, and faster rehabilitation.[11] Arthroscopy, the visual inspection of a joint through a lighted instrument, is one of the most common orthopedic procedures undertaken in the ASC. The technique has decreased tremendously both the length of hospital stay and the overall length of rehabilitation for patients. The patient experiences little external scarring, and the cost of hospitalization is less than with traditional open arthrotomy.

An arthroscopy may be done for diagnostic or therapeutic purposes. Diagnostic procedures may be for patients with pain of unknown origin, limited joint motion, or injuries that result in pain without relief. A variety of therapeutic options are also available during arthroscopy, including joint manipulation and realignment; reconstruction of surrounding structures; repair of tears; excision of loose bodies, synovium, and other tissues; and ligament repair.

Current sophisticated arthroscopic systems with multiple lenses allow extraordinarily clear visualization, television viewing, and videotape recording of the procedure. Cutting, suturing, surface smoothing, coagulation, and laser use are a few of the options possible.

Arthroscopy may be expected to be the only intervention necessary, but the physician usually prepares the patient for the possibility of an open arthrotomy if that approach becomes necessary to correct the pathology identified. The patient often signs a consent form for both alternatives so that treatment can be completed with one anesthetic. If an arthrotomy is necessary, the patient may require hospitalization after surgery for pain management, general nursing care, and physical therapy.

Preoperative preparation for arthroscopy is similar to that for other orthopedic procedures. The uncertainty of the exact surgical approach can be the source of preoperative anxiety for the patient. The patient may have many questions, and further discussion, clarification, or reassurance by the surgeon before surgery may be necessary. Anxiety related to this unknown factor is demonstrated by the many patients who awaken after surgery and immediately ask whether an incision had to be made.

Intraoperative nursing care specific to arthroscopy includes positioning to adequately expose and stabilize the joint, maintenance of the patient's proper body alignment during manipulation and positioning, management of technically complex equipment, and management of irrigation used to maintain distention of the joint.

Usually, joint distention is accomplished with a continuous flow of irrigating solution. Normal saline or lactated Ringer solution is used because it is the closest approximation of physiologic fluid. Sterile water may be needed for joint irrigation in conjunction with the use of an electrocautery unit that will not conduct in saline. Because water is not isotonic, its absorption by cells can result in hemolysis and postoperative burning, and thus, it is not recommended. When the use of sterile water cannot be avoided, it should be for a short duration.

Postoperative nursing care is similar to that provided after other orthopedic procedures. It focuses on pain management, avoidance or early identification and treatment of complications, and support of ambulation and the patient's self-care. The nurse as well as the patient and family must realize that the surgery may have been extensive and that pain experienced after an invasive procedure involving bone may be unexpected in comparison to the appearance of the skin entries. In addition, regional anesthesia often is used to decrease the immediate postoperative pain. Thus, nursing care and patient education require encouraging an appropriate balance between the patient's self-care and the need for rest and recuperation appropriate to the extent of the procedure. Multiple stab wounds and possible retention of irrigating solution within the joint can result in the need for postoperative dressing reinforcement or change.

A multidisciplinary approach to pain management for patients undergoing arthroscopic surgery includes (1) psychological preparation and support; (2) use of local and regional anesthetic techniques; (3) traditional postoperative comfort measures, such as elevation and application of cold; (4) administration of analgesics, including both non-narcotic and narcotic agents and a nonsteroidal anti-inflammatory agent. Occasionally, a transcutaneous electrical nerve stimulator (TENS) unit may be used. Depending on the surgical procedure, the patient may experience mild or no postoperative pain. More extensive procedures such as anterior cruciate ligament repair of the knee and some shoulder procedures may demand more aggressive therapy.

Intra-articular instillation of a long-acting local anesthetic such as bupivacaine is often quite effective in reducing or eliminating postoperative pain. Regional blocks provide a broad and often long-lasting analgesic effect. They may be used alone or as adjuncts to general anesthesia. For example, an interscalene nerve block can provide significant improvement in comfort after shoulder arthroscopy or manipulation. A steroid such as methylprednisolone may be injected to prevent inflammation in the joint. Adequate analgesia should be provided before, rather than after, pain becomes intense.

Complications after arthroscopy are infrequent but include those associated with other orthopedic procedures: infection, neurovascular compromise, bleeding, and phlebitis. Postoperative infections usually require antibiotic therapy and often drainage of the involved joint. Even with treatment, one study showed that more than 19% of patients experiencing postoperative joint infection regained less than 90% of normal motion.[12]

Phlebitis is treated with hospitalization and anticoagulation, followed by up to 6 months of oral anticoagulant therapy. Nerve injury, although rare, can result in permanent deficits.

The surgeon's skill, careful technique, and full understanding of the three-dimensional anatomy of the joint are essential for avoiding injuries that can result from intraoperative overdistention or extensive manipulating of the joint. This is critical in the smaller joints.

Another rare untoward postoperative occurrence is development of reflex sympathetic dystrophy (RSD) that involves excessive sympathetic efferent nerve activity. The resulting pain in affected areas of the body often is described as intense and burning. The pain of RSD remains long past the usual healing period and can lead to muscle atrophy and loss of function. It is treated with intensive physical therapy and sometimes with a series of sympathetic nerve blocks. Even with treatment, RSD can be debilitating and prolonged.

The knee, wrist, shoulder, elbow, and ankle are all amenable to arthroscopic intervention. Table 36–5 lists common disorders of these joints and their arthroscopic treatments. Technologic improvements have allowed arthroscopic access to small joints, such as the wrist, elbow, and ankle, and the completion of more complex procedures, such as anterior cruciate ligament reconstruction of the knee. The following discussion focuses on information regarding specific joints.

Wrist

The wrist consists of eight separate bones that articulate with the radius, the ulna, and the five metacarpal bones. Small arthroscopes and instruments allow entry primarily to address pathology of the ulnar side of the joint. Some procedures undertaken include removal of loose bodies or osteochondral fracture fragments and repair of small tears in the ulnar fibrocartilage.

Often completed under brachial plexus block, wrist arthroscopy has a low incidence of morbidity. Overdistention of the joint by irrigation must be avoided, particularly in the wrist with ligament damage. The ensuing edema can result not only in an obscured view intraoperatively but also in postoperative pressure on the median nerve, causing carpal tunnel–like symptoms.

Elbow

The elbow presents a more difficult problem for the arthroscopist. Diagnostic arthroscopy is fairly common, but several conditions make arthroscopic treatment of elbow pathology difficult. First, the joint is very small. Second, nerves and blood vessels lie in areas in which they can be damaged by instrumentation unless great caution is observed during the procedure. Finally, the articulating surfaces lie in a position that makes visibility and accessibility to areas of the joint difficult. Too much tension placed on the instrumentation by the surgeon in an attempt to reach remote areas around structures in the elbow can result in broken instrumentation within the joint.

An advantage to elbow arthroscopy, however, is the ability to identify pathology that is not readily visible or is difficult to diagnose through other means. Loose bone or cartilage fragments can be removed, and rough areas related to osteochondritis dissecans can be smoothed. Synovectomy, débridement, and lysis of adhesions are other options. Postoperative instillation of bupivacaine into the joint is not advised because of its potential lingering effect on major sensory nerve function. Often, general anesthesia is chosen to ensure patient comfort and to provide ample muscle relaxation for the procedure.

Shoulder

The shoulder's complex structure, illustrated in Figure 36–2, comprises four joints, two of which are amenable to arthroscopic examination. One is the glenohumeral joint, which is the ball-and-socket joint at the end of the humerus. This is the body's most freely mobile joint and allows for the broad range of motion of the normal shoulder. The joint capsule is naturally loose and, under normal conditions, the head of the humerus is able to move away from its usual attachment in the shallow glenoid cavity. Ligaments and the rotator cuff muscle group surround and strengthen this joint. Two other areas of the shoulder that are visualized arthroscopically are the subacromial space and the acromioclavicular joint, which joins the acromion process of the scapula to the clavicle.

Shoulder arthroscopy is performed for a variety of indications, including removal of loose bodies, relief of impingement syndrome, repair of rotator cuff tears or subluxation, lysis of adhesions, diagnosis of persistent shoulder pain, and synovectomy or synovial biopsy. Patients who experience recurrent dislocations, rotator cuff tears, and lesions of the biceps tendon are also candidates for shoulder arthroscopy.[10] Several puncture wounds are used in both the anterior and posterior planes for adequate visualization and access to various areas of the joint.

Neurovascular assessment of the affected arm is indicated because of possible compromise during surgery or positioning. After surgery, the

Table 36–5. **Arthroscopic Treatment of Joint Disorders**

COMMON PATHOLOGY	ARTHROSCOPIC PROCEDURE
Knee	
Torn meniscus	Meniscal resection Meniscal repair
Torn ACL	ACL repair/reconstruction
Patellar dysfunction (compression syndrome; subluxation; dislocation; "chondromalacia")	Lateral release Percutaneous realignment Patellar débridement
Loose body	Removal of loose body
Plica medial synovial shelf (MSS)	Resection of plica/MSS
Osteochondritis dissecans	Drilling, débridement, removal, bone graft, pinning
Osteochondral fracture	Removal, replacement, pinning
Synovial lesions (synovitis, pigmented villonodular synovitis, rheumatoid arthritis, hemophilia)	Synovectomy
Osteoarthritis	Arthroplasty
Shoulder	
Instability (subluxation, dislocation)	Capsular stapling/reefing
Labral tears	Labral resection
Biceps tendon tears (partial)	Débridement
Subacromial impingement	Subacromial bursal resection, coracoacromial ligament resection, acromioplasty
Rotator cuff tear	Débridement/repair
Loose body	Removal of loose body
Synovial lesions	Synovectomy
Ankle	
Impingement (tibial; talus)	Removal of osteophytes, tibia/talus
Osteochondral fracture	Débridement, removal, pinning
Osteochondritis dissecans	Drillings, bone graft, removal, débridement
Post-traumatic arthritis	Débridement
Synovial lesions	Synovectomy
Elbow	
Loose body	Removal of loose body
Impingement (olecranon)	Removal of osteophytes
Osteochondritis dissecans	Removal, drilling, débridement
Synovial lesions	Synovectomy
Hip	
Loose body	Removal of loose body
Synovitis (pigmented villonodular synovitis, nonspecific)	Synovectomy
Wrist	
Torn triangular fibrocartilage complex (TFCC)	Débridement of TFCC
Osteochondral fracture	Débridement

ACL = anterior cruciate ligament.
From Sherman O: The perioperative management of the arthroscopic patient. Clin Sports Med 6:498, 1989.

patient's arm is supported in a sling to relieve tension on the operative shoulder. One or more ice packs are applied to the anterior and posterior aspects of the shoulder for 24 to 48 hours. The dressing may require changing or reinforcing in the early postoperative period because of seepage of irrigant and surgical drainage from multiple puncture wounds.

Some shoulder procedures result in moderate to severe postoperative discomfort, and parenteral analgesics may be necessary in the early recovery phase. Intra-articular instillation of a long-acting local anesthetic and administration of an interscalene nerve block can be very helpful in reducing or eliminating postoperative pain. Depending on the procedure, many patients are encouraged to resume normal activity by that evening or the next day. The physician's specific order regarding movement and exercise versus immobilization of the shoulder must be included in the discharge instructions. A specific exercise routine is prescribed for the home recovery period to aid in strengthening the affected shoulder structures.

Knee

Knee arthroscopy can be accomplished under general, local, or regional anesthesia. Pathology

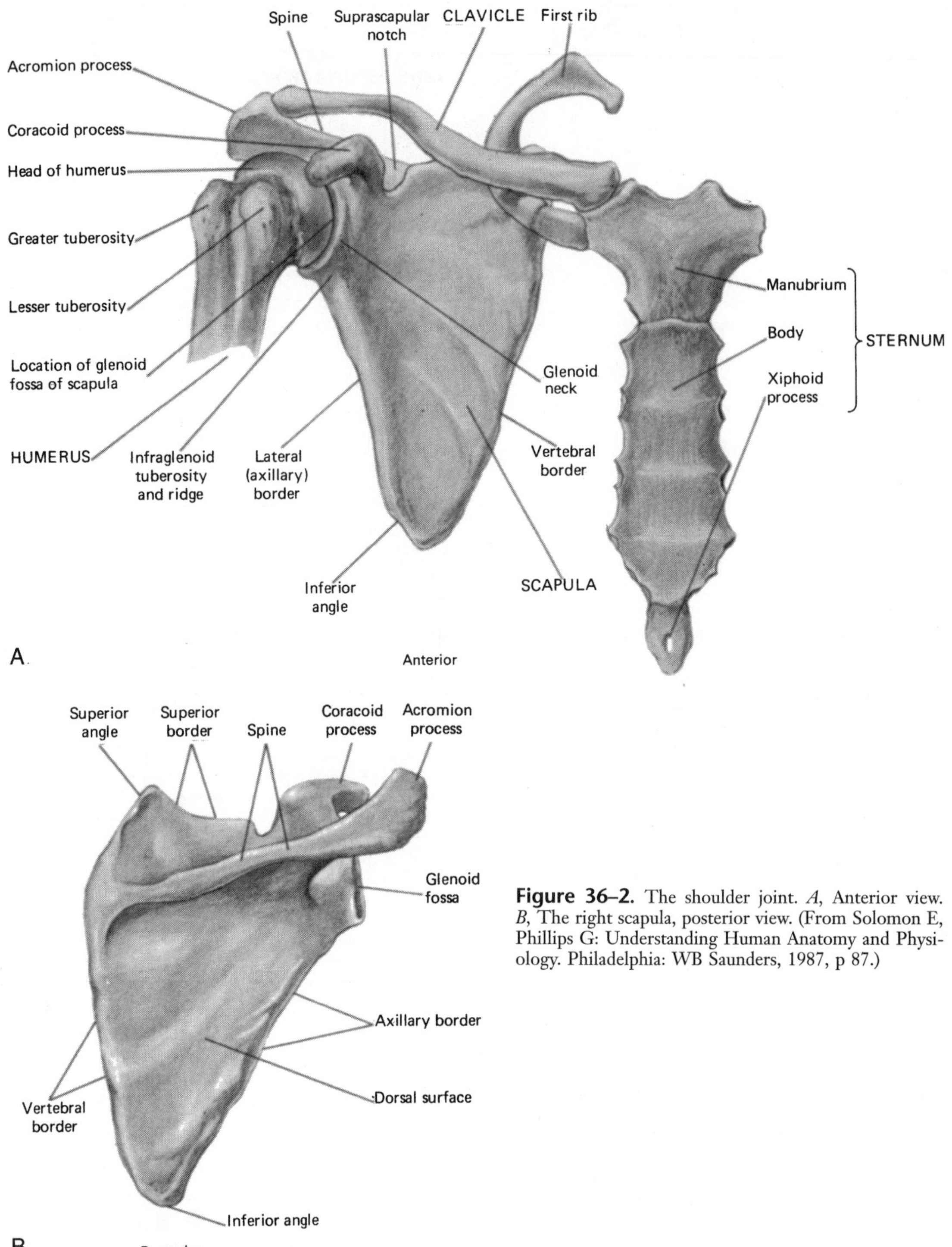

Figure 36–2. The shoulder joint. *A*, Anterior view. *B*, The right scapula, posterior view. (From Solomon E, Phillips G: Understanding Human Anatomy and Physiology. Philadelphia: WB Saunders, 1987, p 87.)

frequently encountered and treated includes chondromalacia patellae, loose bodies within the joint that cause pain and restricted joint movement, meniscal or ligament injuries, fractures, and sports-related injuries.

Two articular disks, or menisci, lie between the femur and tibia of the knee joint (Fig. 36–3). Injuries of the lateral or medial meniscus are the most common knee injuries. Each meniscus is a C-shaped fibrocartilage that acts as a cush-

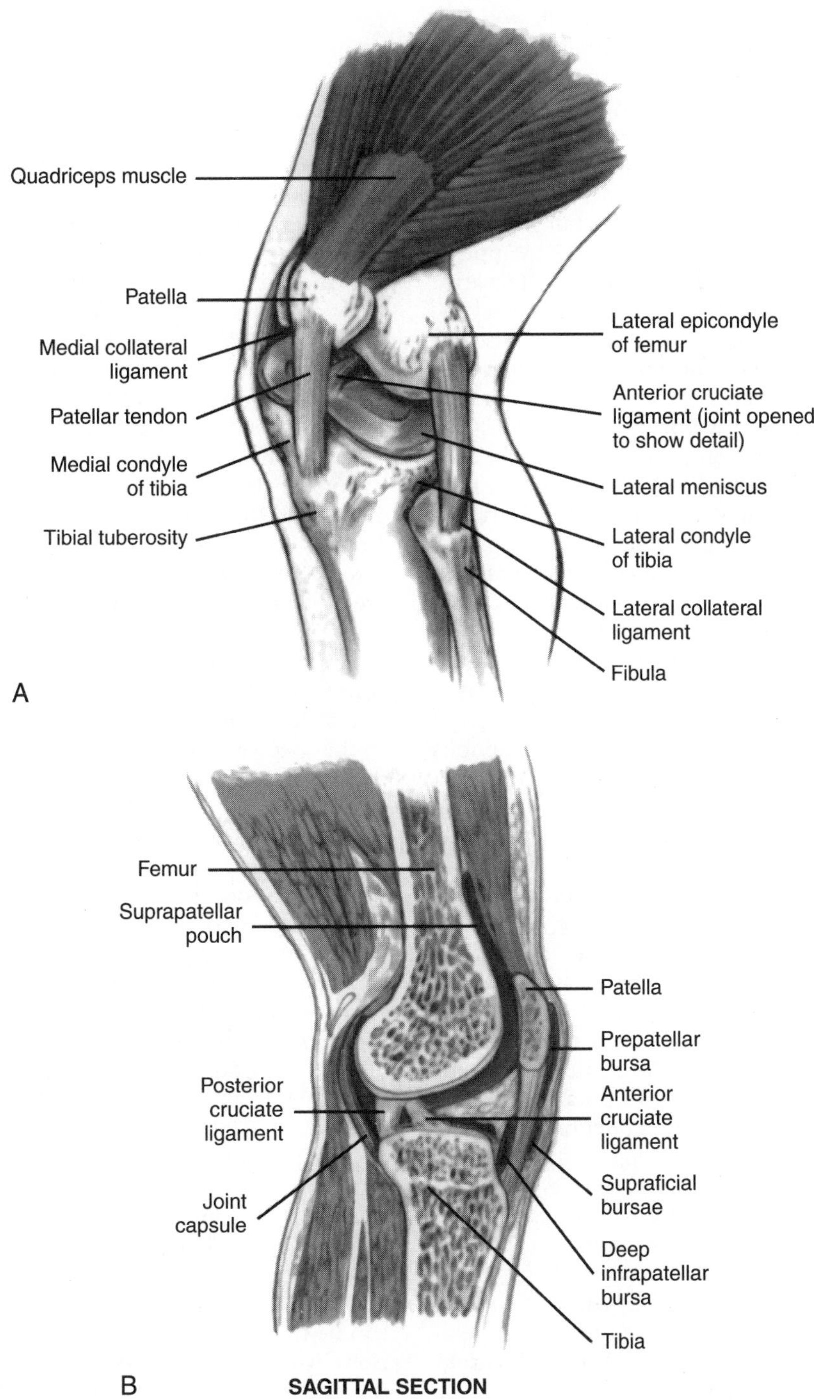

Figure 36–3. Knee ligaments. (From Jarvis C: Physical Examination and Health Assessment. Philadelphia: WB Saunders, 1992, p 669.)

ion between the femur and the tibia, promoting lateral joint support and distributing weight load. Other functions of the meniscus are to lubricate and to limit extremes in flexion and extension. Because of overwhelming evidence indicating the importance of these functions, the present surgical trend is to save as much of the meniscus as possible rather than remove the entire structure, as was common in the past.

Meniscal tears can create significant pain and limitation in joint movement. Partial meniscectomy is the most frequent surgical treatment, although meniscal repair is also an alternative for certain patients. Healing after meniscal repair is enhanced when the tear is in a vascular area of the meniscus and when the site is well supported during the recovery period.

The knee has four major ligaments, including the anterior and posterior cruciate, and the medial and lateral collateral ligament. Tears or ruptures of the ligament also are treated arthroscopically with repair, augmentation, or reconstruction of the ligament. The anterior cruciate ligament (ACL) is probably the most commonly injured ligamentous structure in the knee joint.[12] Techniques used for reconstruction of the ACL vary. A graft may be used as a substitute for the torn ligament. An autogenous graft from the patellar tendon, semitendinous tendon, iliotibial band, gracilis muscle, or fascia lata might be used. An allograft may also be used. The arthroscopic technique is a less invasive procedure than open arthrotomy and can result in less disruption of knee extensor structures.

Care must be taken during knee arthroscopy to maintain the patient's proper body alignment while positioning the operative knee. The thigh is maintained in a foam-lined brace that clamps securely above the knee. This stabilizes the upper leg so that the surgeon can manipulate the knee during the procedure. A pneumatic tourniquet may be placed on the upper thigh to provide a bloodless field. The lingering effects of pressure from both of these devices can be the cause of early postoperative complaints related to localized bruising or tenderness in the thigh. Also, sciatic or femoral nerve palsy can be the result of prolonged tourniquet times. The periodic release of the operative tourniquet during a long procedure does not necessarily ensure adequate circulation to the extremity when the leg brace continues to constrict the leg and act as a second tourniquet. Other rare complications relating to the leg holder are fracture of the femur and ligament sprains.

Neurovascular damage can occur as a result of suturing within the knee. Inadvertent suturing of the peroneal nerve can result in footdrop, diminished sensation, or paresthesia in the foot. Such symptoms should be reported to the surgeon immediately.

Fluids used to distend the joint are often instilled under pressure. This can lead to overdistention or to the escape of fluid from the joint into surrounding tissues. This rare extravasation of fluid can lead to the serious complication of compartment syndrome. Compartment syndrome is described as pressure compromising the circulation and function of tissue. A compartment is any location where bone, blood vessels, nerves, muscle, and soft tissue can collect fluid. A compartment is most commonly at risk in the forearm and leg. Symptoms include decreased or lost sensation in the foot and leg, a sensation of tightness in the calf, and complaints of deep pain unrelated to the operative site and difficult to relieve by ordinary means. Loss of distal pulses is a late sign. Compartment syndrome must be surgically relieved immediately to avoid permanent neurovascular damage to the leg.

Hemarthrosis and thromboembolism are two other possible, but rare, complications. The outcome of an embolic event is related closely to the speed and accuracy of diagnosis and treatment. The nurse must report observed signs, such as pain or tenderness in remote areas, diminished pulses, distal pallor or cyanosis, chest pain, hemoptysis, and dyspnea. Because these events can occur after discharge, the patient should be instructed to report any unusual symptoms to the physician immediately.

Complications with the nonoperative leg can result from intraoperative positioning. When the unaffected leg is allowed to hang over the edge of the operating room bed, pressure to the sciatic nerve and stretching of the femoral nerve can occur. The patient with pre-existing back problems may experience an exacerbation of symptoms. To prevent position-related complications, a leg support or stirrup can be used to elevate the unaffected leg. This allows flexion of the hip joint, relieving pressure on the upper leg and the lumbar area of the patient's back.

The current trend is to have the patient begin isometric exercises postoperatively as soon as the effects of regional anesthesia have resolved. Alternating contraction and relaxation of the leg muscles is most effective at strengthening the knee when each contraction is held for at least 6 seconds. Exercises should be repeated at home 5 to 10 times each day. Straight leg-raising and ankle circles also may be started immediately.

The amount and type of postoperative exercise, weight-bearing, and ambulation allowed after knee arthroscopy depend on the actual procedure undertaken. After partial menisectomy, the patient usually is allowed to bear weight to the tolerance of pain on the day of surgery. Conversely, the patient who has undergone an anterior cruciate ligament graft procedure begins a program of active extension and flexion and passive exercises soon after surgery but avoids weight-bearing or exercising against resistance for up to several months.

Ankle

The ankle can be treated arthroscopically to relieve hemarthrosis; to remove loose bodies; or to repair fractures, ligament instability, or impingement. Some of the complications of maneuvering inside this small joint include broken instruments and damage to structures from the pressure of manipulating instruments within a confined area. The patient with compromised vascularity to the foot or existing infection of surrounding tissues is not an appropriate candidate for ankle arthroscopy.

Entry into the ankle can be made in the anterior or posterior plane. For certain types of surgery, the ankle may require special positioning by means of a distractor. This metal device is affixed with screws into the anterior tibia on one end and into the calcaneus bone of the foot on the other. When the distractor is opened, the ankle joint space is enlarged, allowing better visualization and more room to complete the procedure. Nerve and ligament damage as well as tibial fractures can result from distraction of the joint, and thus, this procedure must be undertaken with great caution.

After ankle arthroscopy, the patient uses crutches but is allowed to bear weight to the tolerance of pain unless the talus was drilled intraoperatively. Elevation of the foot and application of ice are typical protocols, and the patient may require a brace or short leg cast for support. Exercises are instituted immediately to strengthen the ankle, and physical therapy may be started 1 week after surgery.

Procedures of the Foot

The foot is a complex combination of bones, joints, ligaments, and tendons (Fig. 36–4) working in unison. Because the feet are the primary weight-bearing structures of the body, patho-

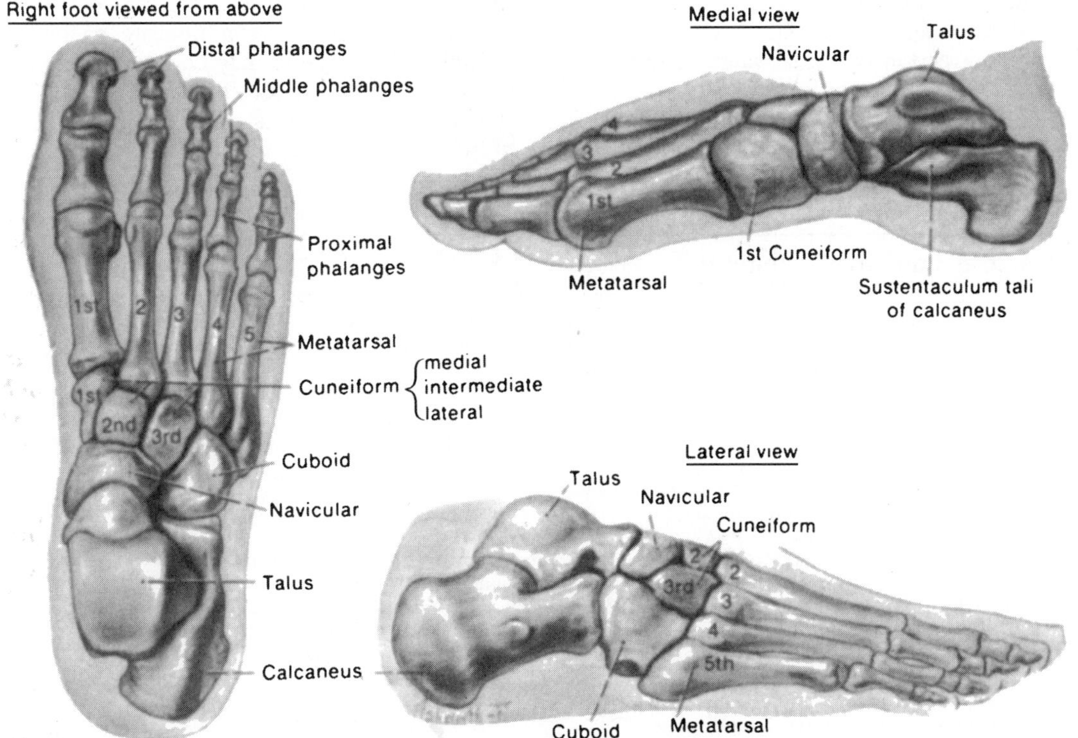

Figure 36–4. Bones of the right foot. (From Jacob S, Francone C: Elements of Anatomy and Physiology, 2nd ed. Philadelphia: WB Saunders, 1989, p 64.)

logic conditions often result in significant pain and difficulty in ambulation, and surgical correction becomes a desirable option for the patient.

Podiatrists and orthopedic surgeons perform a variety of foot procedures in an ambulatory surgery setting. Nursing care is similar to that for other procedures involving the lower extremities, however, there are a few special considerations. The podiatric population is, for the most part, the older generation, bringing with them the varied infirmities and concerns of geriatric care. Typical problems that may be encountered include social isolation, with patients having no family or friends to assist them at home, age-related problems of mobility and ambulation, and a variety of chronic systemic diseases. Foot surgery is rarely an urgent or emergent procedure, but pain, difficulty in mobility, and other problems associated with foot conditions can make the patient eager for a surgical solution.

For each deformity or pathologic process, there may be a variety of corrective surgical approaches, and the ASC nurse is challenged to be familiar with a number of procedures. Some are described anatomically, for example, tenotomy or excision of neuroma. Other procedures may be named after a person who pioneered a specific technique, such as the Silver, Keller, and McBride approaches, all of which are used for the correction of hallux valgus and associated bunion.

A neuroma occurs most frequently between the third and fourth toes, although other interspaces and the medial aspect of the heel are also predisposed to neuroma formation. The etiology of a Morton's neuroma is chronic irritation. This painful mass is caused when the metatarsals entrap, or pinch, the nerve over a period of time. This pressure results in inflammation that can cause pain. If conservative measures do not alleviate the pain, surgical removal is considered. Permanent numbness in the area of the neuroma may occur postoperatively but is generally preferred to the pain the patient experienced before surgery.

Table 36–6 defines a number of podiatric terms. Some abbreviations commonly used in describing procedures include:

DIP—distal interphalangeal, the most distal joint (or "knuckle") in the toe

PIP—proximal interphalangeal, the proximal joint of the toe

MPJ—metatarsal phalangeal joint, the joint between the bones of the foot and those of the toe, at the base of the toe

IS—interspace; this refers to the space on the foot between the toes, most often referred to when describing the location of a neuroma.

The patient undergoing foot surgery should be screened carefully for peripheral vascular insufficiency and for undiagnosed diabetes mellitus because the associated decreased vascular supply to the feet can complicate or prevent healing. The surgeon may choose to defer the procedure if the patient's glucose level is exceptionally high on the morning of surgery. Pedal pulses are assessed before and after surgery, al-

***Table 36–6.* Podiatric Definitions**

Term	Definition
Arthrodesis	Surgical immobilization or fusion of a joint
Arthrolysis	Surgical procedure in which mobility is restored to an ankylosed (fused/immobile) joint
Arthroplasty	Surgical repair or reformation of a joint
Arthrotomy	Incision into a joint
Bunion	Enlargement and inflammation of the joint bursa at the base of the great toe, usually causing the toe to displace laterally; usual etiology is long-term wearing of tight-fitting shoes
Capsulotomy	Incision into the joint capsule
Exostosis	A bony growth on the surface of a bone, also called "osteoma" or "hyperostosis"
Hallux	The great toe
Hallux valgus	Displacement of the great toe laterally toward the other toes; often coexists with a bunion but often the two terms are inaccurately used synonymously
Hammer toe	A deformity in which there is dorsiflexion of the metatarsophalangeal joint (joint between the foot and the toe) or plantar flexion of interphalangeal (IP) joints; when the most distal IP joint is the only one involved, it is called mallet toe
Morton's neuroma	Interdigital nerve entrapment within a metatarsal interspace that causes pain, particularly with weight-bearing
Osteotomy	Incision into a bone
Plantar	Regarding the sole of the foot
Tenotomy	Incision of a tendon, often used to correct hammer toe

though a bulky dressing may make postoperative assessment of pulses difficult or impossible.

Application of cold therapy over the ankle or upper foot may be helpful in reducing swelling, bleeding, and pain. Cold therapy should be avoided directly on or near the toes to prevent ischemia related to vasoconstriction. Depending on the specific procedure, weight-bearing may be restricted, and the patient should be instructed appropriately.

The type of surgical procedure, the presence of a bulky dressing, and the level of discomfort make it impossible for many patients to resume wearing regular shoes immediately. A cast or splint may be applied in surgery, but often a postoperative shoe is ordered. This hard-soled shoe allows the patient to walk without bending the foot. The patient is instructed to wear it whenever bearing weight on the foot to protect the surgical repair, even when walking only a few steps. Ensuring correct fit of the postoperative surgical shoe is important. A shoe that is too short exposes the toes to possible injury from stubbing them against objects while walking. A shoe that is too long increases the potential for a fall.

Percutaneous Lumbar Suction Discectomy

Previously, patients with symptomatic herniated disks of the lumbar spine had the choice among (1) conservative medical therapy, including rest, heat, and anti-inflammatory drugs; (2) epidural steroid injections; or (3) surgical laminectomy to remove the offending disk. Percutaneous lumbar suction discectomy has evolved as a safe and effective alternative for some patients and is performed as an outpatient procedure in many facilities.[13]

For this procedure, a probe is positioned percutaneously into the nucleus pulposus of the bulging disk. The actual herniated portion of the protruding disk is not removed. Rather, aspiration of a portion of the nucleus pulposus material from the center of that disk reduces the overall size of the disk. This technique decreases the amount of herniation of the disk and reduces pressure on the affected spinal nerve.

Minimal tissue damage and scarring occur, although potential complications do exist. These include nerve injury, infection, puncture of the dura, and injury to retroperitoneal structures, which may be in the path of the probe as it is inserted. To avoid the latter complication, radiographic and other diagnostic examinations are done preoperatively to identify the presence and location of retroperitoneal structures.

The procedure generally is performed under local anesthesia with or without sedation. The patient may be prone or in a lateral position with the painful side up. During surgery, the position of the probe used to remove nucleus pulposus material is monitored by fluoroscopy under the C-arm of an image intensifier. This radiographic monitoring is essential to avoid damage to surrounding blood vessels, nerves, and other structures. The probe gently aspirates portions of the nucleus pulposus into a receptacle. If the patient reports radicular pain during the procedure, the surgical trocar and probe must be repositioned. This important subjective evaluation would not be possible if the patient was under general anesthesia.

There are a number of benefits of this procedure compared with those of traditional laminectomy. Foremost is the decreased potential for serious surgical complications. Another benefit is the reduced length of hospital stay and recuperation. Many patients undergoing the percutaneous technique are discharged to home after 8 hours or less compared with 3 days for laminectomy patients. The patient resumes most normal, moderate activities by the end of 1 week and often returns to work after 10 days to a few weeks, depending on the amount of physical exertion associated with the job.

Specific postoperative nursing interventions include assessment for complications, particularly for symptoms of retroperitoneal bleeding. These include flank tenderness or pain; abdominal distention, pain, or masses; or numbness, tingling, or loss of sensation in the lower extremities. The surgical site and the neurovascular status of the lower extremities are monitored. Oral analgesics and anti-inflammatory agents usually provide sufficient pain control.

An important element of postoperative teaching involves educating the patient about proper body mechanics and activities and exercises that are allowed, encouraged, or temporarily contraindicated. There also is emphasis placed on the importance of proper back care as a permanent part of the patient's daily activities.

Before discharge, the patient should receive specific information about lifting, driving, bathing, sexual relations, activities of daily life, exercise, and return to work. Protocols are adjusted by the physician for each patient's particular needs, but a typical plan has patients returning to moderate activity as soon as they feel able. Exercise, lifting, sexual intercourse, and driving are avoided for 1 week. After the initial period of recuperation, many patients are referred to a back school, where various specialists provide detailed instructions about long-term back care.

Nurses in all areas of the ambulatory surgery unit have an essential role in helping the patient to develop a positive attitude about recovery and general well-being after discectomy. Patients who have had chronic or acute back pain may have significant doubts or fears about the success of any treatment. Some may have developed a dependent personality and actually may resist the idea of being cured or relieved of their back pain. Nurses can project a positive attitude and encourage the patient to resume a normal lifestyle within the boundaries of the physician's directives. In particular, patients should be urged to participate actively in the important process of rehabilitation so that they will be better able to avoid recurrence and long-term disability.

References

1. Ramsey D, Thompson G: The case for regional anesthesia for adult outpatient surgery. In Weintraub HD, Levy M (eds): Anesthesia Clinics of North America. Philadelphia: WB Saunders, 1987.
2. Lee TH, Wapner KL, Hecht PJ, et al: Regional anesthesia in foot and ankle surgery. Orthopedics 19:577, 1996.
3. Association of Operating Room Nurses: AORN Standards and Recommended Practices. Denver: AORN, 1997, p 215.
4. Bulls JD, Wolford ET: Timing of perioperative antibiotic administration. AORN J 65:109–114, 1997.
5. Wieck JA, Jackson JK, O'Brien TJ, et al: Efficacy of prophylactic antibiotics in arthroscopic surgery. Orthopedics 2:133–134, 1997.
6. Black J, Matassarin Jacobs E, Luckman J, Sorensen K: Medical Surgical Nursing: A Psychophysiological Approach, 4th ed. Philadelphia: WB Saunders, 1993, p 527.
7. Gregory B: Equipment and supplies. In Gregory B (ed): Orthopaedic Surgery. St. Louis: Mosby–Year Book, 1994.
8. Davids JR, Frick SL, Skewes E, et al: Skin surface pressure beneath an above-the-knee cast: Plaster casts compared with fiberglass casts. J Bone Joint Surg 79:565, 1997.
9. DeLee J: Complications of arthroscopy and arthroscopic surgery: Results of a national survey. Arthroscopy 1:214, 1985.
10. Long JS: Shoulder arthroscopy. Orthop Nurs 15:21, 1996.
11. Brown F: Anterior cruciate ligament reconstruction as an outpatient procedure. Orthop Nurs 15:15, 1996.
12. Jerva MJ: Automated percutaneous lumbar discectomy: A review. Orthop Nur 12:27, 1993.

Chapter 37

Cardiovascular Procedures

Denise O'Brien

The ambulatory surgery arena provides an appropriate setting for a variety of cardiovascular procedures. Varicose vein stripping and ligation, arteriovenous shunts and venous access device placement and removal, temporal artery biopsy, cardiac catheterization, coronary angiography, electrophysiologic studies, and pacemaker and implantable cardioverter-defibrillator generator replacement are among a growing list of procedures. Perfection of new techniques will continue to bring increasingly complex and varied cardiovascular procedures to the outpatient setting.

Maintenance of hemostasis and circulatory adequacy and prevention of infection and thrombosis are important nursing care concerns for the patient undergoing a vascular procedure. Thromboembolism is a potential threat during and after any cannulation of the vasculature. It is important to identify patients who are already at high risk, for instance, those with a history of thrombus formation, older than 40 years, obese, or with malignancy or undergoing prolonged operations (especially operations that interfere with lower extremity blood flow).[1, 2]

Patients should be instructed about measures they can take during the postoperative period to reduce the occurrence and the seriousness of embolic complications. These include avoiding prolonged bedrest, reclining rather than sitting straight upright after vascular procedures involving the pelvis or lower extremities, and resuming activities and exercise to the extent allowed by the surgery and previous ability and health. Isometric exercises of the legs are often suggested for the patient who will be ambulating less in the postoperative period. Patients should know what symptoms must be immediately reported to the physician, for instance, swelling, tenderness, pain, and heat and redness of the calf or other area of the body; fever; generalized chills; and malaise. Patients may be instructed by their physician to take a single aspirin tablet (325 mg) daily to reduce the risk of thrombus formation. However, the physician may instruct other patients to avoid medications that interfere with the clotting mechanism to reduce the risk of bleeding during the perioperative period.

To properly evaluate circulatory adequacy in the postoperative period, the patient's normal baseline status must be assessed and documented before surgery. Appropriate parameters to include are vital signs, heart regularity and rate, skin color and temperature of the extremities, and presence or absence of edema, numbness, tingling, and pain or discomfort in the extremities. A pulse oximetry reading on the affected extremity is another helpful baseline tool. When surgery or intraoperative positioning involves an extremity, preprocedure and postprocedure distal pulses should be taken to determine whether there has been a change in circulation distal to the operative site. A Doppler ultrasound device may be needed to locate the distal pulses in extremities compromised by positioning.

VEIN LIGATION AND STRIPPING

Varicose veins affect more than 20% of the adult population, are more common in women than in men, may develop as a result of pregnancy, and have a familial tendency.[3] Sclerosing agents are used to obliterate some smaller varicosities; vein ligation or stripping remains popular and is the most common treatment for larger or recurrent varicosities. Increased risk of complications is associated with a history of phlebitis, obesity, and extremely enlarged or bilateral extremity involvement. The trend is away from indiscriminate removal (stripping) of the entire saphenous vein system; these veins may be useful for future coronary or peripheral artery bypass procedures, and noninvasive diagnostic methods more accurately identify diseased vessels needing to be stripped.[4]

Before surgery, the physician marks the veins with indelible ink to identify the location of varicosities. The marking is performed while the patient is standing because engorgement is more pronounced and the veins are more visible. Sedative drugs are usually withheld until the surgeon has completed the marking. The patient is screened before surgery for bleeding and for thrombotic tendencies. Incision may be required at various locations along the involved veins: excessive hair growth on the extremity may be clipped at the incision sites before prepping.

Circulation to the legs and feet is not impaired by the procedure. Venous blood that flowed through the now ligated veins is diverted to deeper veins, and adequate superficial collateral circulation develops. The incisions are closed with a single staple or surgical tape strips, covered with gauze pads and bulky dressings, and the leg is wrapped in an elastic compressive bandage, often from the toes to the groin, to reduce bleeding and swelling.

Elevation of the legs is maintained while the patient is observed in the postanesthesia care unit after surgery. The patient may arrive in Trendelenburg's position to enhance venous drainage and reduce swelling of the legs.[4] Flexion at the groin and knees is avoided because related pressure on the pelvic, femoral, and popliteal vasculature can compromise circulation to the legs, causing venous stasis. Depending on the type of operative procedure, minimal movement of the legs may be encouraged to reduce venous stasis. The perioperative nurse's report to the postanesthesia care unit nurse should include the approximate number and locations of multiple incisions.

Postoperative assessment includes observation for bleeding and circulatory compromise. Distal pulses are palpated to the extent allowed by the size and position of the dressings. The color and capillary refill time of the nail beds in the toes are observed. If pulses are not palpable, Doppler ultrasound assessment may be indicated, and the physician should be notified. A tight circumferential bandage may require loosening by, or at the direction of, the physician to improve blood flow to the distal portions of the extremity. The patient should be monitored carefully for bleeding when he or she first ambulates after surgery.

After discharge, the patient should maintain elevation of the legs through the first night. Getting out of bed may be allowed only for trips to the bathroom. With some newer techniques, ambulation is encouraged immediately after surgery.[4] After that first day, the patient is encouraged to either stand, walk, or lie flat and to avoid sitting with prolonged bending at the hips and knees for at least 2 weeks.[4] This positioning helps to prevent venous stasis and ensuing edema of the legs. Although circulatory compromise is uncommon, the patient should be instructed to notify the physician of bleeding or a change in the color, temperature, or sensation of the affected foot or toes. The patient is instructed to lie down, elevate legs, and apply pressure to incision site if bleeding occurs. When adequate hemostasis has been ensured by careful surgical technique, postoperative bleeding rarely occurs, and patient complications are rare.

Complications, if they do occur, include major venous damage, arterial damage, nerve damage, hematoma formation, and venous thromboembolism.[3] Patients should be informed about expected side effects of vein ligation or stripping, including bruising, areas of paresthesia, and scarring, which generally resolve over a few months.[5]

Oral analgesics usually suffice for postoperative pain. Ambulation is encouraged after the first night, and the surgeon may direct the patient to perform isometric leg exercises at home to promote circulation and to discourage thrombus formation in the legs. The patient should be instructed when to remove the bulky dressings and to cover the incisions with individual bandage strips if needed. This change is allowed 1 to 7 days after surgery, depending on the surgeon. After the outer dressings are removed, the patient may shower, using gentle soap to wash over the incisions. The patient is instructed to avoid scrubbing and use of strong soaps, creams, lotions, or alcohol-based solutions near the incisions. Elastic impression bandages or antiembolism stockings are worn for up to 12 weeks to promote venous return and to reduce edema and bleeding.

Long-term goals for avoiding future varicosities should be discussed with the patient. Maintaining a healthy body weight is important, and weight loss may be suggested to reduce the load on the legs. The patient should avoid standing for long periods of time and should elevate the legs whenever possible while resting.

TRANSVASCULAR ENDOMYOCARDIAL BIOPSY

Transvascular heart biopsy was introduced in the 1960s as a diagnostic procedure to replace the more dangerous percutaneous needle biopsy or the complex approach of open thoracotomy. Endomyocardial biopsy is useful in diagnosing myocarditis, cardiomyopathy, etiology of restrictive heart disease, carcinoid heart disease, and cardiac allograft rejection.[6] After initial recovery from the transplant procedure, these biopsies for routine surveillance of rejection status can be performed on an outpatient basis.

As with any invasive cardiac procedure, complications can occur. The most serious complication, although rare, is perforation of the heart wall resulting in hemoperitoneum and cardiac tamponade. Chest pain during the procedure may indicate possible perforation. Immediate pericardiocentesis is required to relieve the tamponade. Other complications of endomyocardial biopsy include arrhythmias, conduction abnormalities, hematoma, infection, pneumothorax, Horner's syndrome, and air embolism.[6, 7]

The endomyocardial biopsy has become the standard for diagnosing cardiac allograft rejection before the appearance of symptoms. Since the introduction of cyclosporine as an immunosuppressant, the common clinical signs of rejection, namely heart failure, an S_3 gallop, arrhythmias, and loss of electrocardiogram (ECG) voltage, are rarely observed.[8] Post-transplant patients initially require weekly biopsies for the first 2 months, then progress to less frequent procedures as time goes on. Although left ventricular biopsy is possible if it is accompanied by systemic heparinization to prevent thromboembolism, the right ventricle of the heart is considered the safer site. It is generally accepted that most pathologic processes can be diagnosed as well from the right ventricle as from any other site in the heart. The two major contraindications to heart biopsies are bleeding disorders and presence of a left ventricular thrombus that could result in release of systemic emboli during or after left ventricular biopsy.

Before surgery, patients need the care of a calm and reassuring staff to promote confidence and to reduce their anxiety concerning this highly invasive procedure. Because these patients are receiving pharmacologic immunosuppressants, caution is employed to prevent infections. These patients may be receiving long-term antibiotic therapy; sulfamethoxazole-trimethoprim is commonly given. Vital signs are assessed to identify abnormalities and to provide a baseline for later reference. The nurse also examines the patient's pedal pulses, observes for ankle edema, and auscultates the lungs.

Biopsy may be performed in an operating room or in a cardiac catheterization laboratory under continuous cardiovascular monitoring. A transvenous approach, usually through the right internal jugular vein, is accomplished by use of local anesthesia. Lidocaine without epinephrine is used to avoid sympathetic stimulation of the heart.[6] Under fluoroscopy, an instrument called a bioptome is threaded through a sheath, and three to five endomyocardial biopsy specimens are obtained from the right ventricle. The taking of multiple specimens increases the accuracy of interpretations. Inadvertent entry into the carotid artery during the procedure requires direct pressure on the site to ensure hemostasis before proceeding. Other possible access sites include the right subclavian vein, either femoral vein, or, for left ventricle biopsy, the femoral or brachial arteries.

At the end of the procedure, pressure is applied to the site for approximately 10 minutes to decrease the chance of postoperative hematoma formation. Topical antibiotics and a single adhesive strip may be used to dress the site.[6] Femoral vein or arterial access sites may require pressure dressings. Complications, although rare, occur without warning; cardiovascular resuscitative drugs, equipment, and supplies required to perform a pericardiocentesis should be immediately available.

Patients return directly to the phase II area of the ambulatory surgery center (ASC) unless complications have occurred that require more intense monitoring in a postanesthesia care unit or a cardiac care unit. The venipuncture site is assessed frequently for bleeding or hematoma formation. After a jugular approach, the head of the bed is elevated, vital signs are assessed, and, barring complications, the patient often can be discharged within 30 minutes.[6] Patients complaining of shortness of breath or, if pneumothorax is suspected, may require a follow-up chest x-ray.

Because the femoral approach is more often associated with bleeding, patients are required to remain supine with the head of the bed elevated no more than 15 to 30 degrees for the first hour. Then, further head elevation is allowed as the patient desires. A No. 5 sandbag may be placed on the femoral site. Pedal pulses are assessed, and vital signs are taken every 15 minutes during the first hour, and then every 30 minutes for another hour. The inguinal puncture site is carefully assessed. If no bleeding or hematoma has occurred after 2 hours of observation, the patient ambulates for 10 or 15 minutes before discharge to ensure that activity is well tolerated without bleeding. After arterial access, a No. 10 sandbag may be used for 4 hours, and the patient is allowed to ambulate after 6 hours.

CARDIAC CATHETERIZATION: DIAGNOSTIC AND THERAPEUTIC INTERVENTIONS

Although cardiac catheterization can be either a diagnostic or a therapeutic procedure, diagnostic applications are more frequently performed in the ambulatory surgery setting (Table 37–1).[9] The most common reason for cardiac catheterization is to diagnose coronary artery disease. Patients may have atypical or progressive angina that does not respond to medical therapy, or they may have an abnormality that has been identified during stress testing. Catheterization may be used to assess cardiac status before heart surgery. Invasive cardiac procedures performed during catheterization include coronary angiography, angioplasty, intravascular ultrasound, and electrophysiologic studies.

One or more catheters are introduced into the heart for many reasons: to obtain blood samples for analysis, to detect shunts, to diagnose congenital abnormalities, to determine various cardiac and pulmonary pressures and blood flow patterns, and to measure cardiac output.[10] Patients considered for ASC care should be hemodynamically stable and free of congestive heart failure, unstable angina, significant arrhythmias, and complicating diseases, such as coagulopathies, uncontrolled systolic hypertension, and renal insufficiency. A pregnancy screening is performed on women of childbearing age because their exposure to radiation is contraindicated.

Specific conditions have been identified by the American College of Cardiology and the American Heart Association that contraindicate same-day discharge after cardiac catheteriza-

***Table 37–1.* Patients Eligible for Outpatient Cardiac Catheterization**

TYPE OF PATIENT	DIAGNOSTIC PROCEDURES	THERAPEUTIC PROCEDURES

Adult	Exclusions
	  High risk for severe CAD
	    Unstable or progressive angina
	    Recent MI (<7 days) with any post-MI symptoms
	    Pulmonary edema as a result of ischemia
	    High risk based on noninvasive testing
	  Congestive heart failure
	    NYHA FC III or IV
	  Advanced age or the very young
	  Certain valvular heart diseases
	    Severe AS or AI
	  Congenital heart disease
	    Any complex congenital heart disease problem
	  High risk for catheterization as a result of other problems
	    Severe peripheral vascular disease
	    Morbid obesity
	    Anticoagulation
	    Uncontrolled systemic hypertension
	    Poorly controlled diabetes mellitus
	    Renal insufficiency (>1.9 creatinine)
	    General debility, mental confusion, cachexia
	    Recent stroke (<1 month)
		None recommended at this time

Pediatric	Stable symptoms whose diagnostic problems are within competence of operator	None recommended at this time
Electrophysiology	Simple diagnostic problems within competence of the operator	Cardioversion

NYHA FC, New York Heart Assoc. functional class; CHF, congestive heart failure; AS, aortic stenosis; AI, aortic insufficiency; CAD, coronary artery disease; MI, myocardial infarction.

Modified from Bashore TM, Wang AG: Cardiac catheterization laboratories. In Pepine CJ (ed): Diagnostic and Therapeutic Cardiac Catheterization, 3rd ed. Baltimore: Williams & Williams, 1998, pp 13–30.

tion.[11] These include recent myocardial infarction, suspected multivessel or main left coronary artery disease, aortic stenosis, various types of cardiomyopathy, significant left ventricular arrhythmias, infective endocarditis, coagulation disorders, constrictive pericarditis, and pulmonary hypertension (Table 37–2).[12]

Complications of cardiac catheterization occur in less than 2% of all cases. These include contrast dye reactions (allergic or toxic), myocardial infarction, stroke, perforation of the heart or vessels, cardiac tamponade, arrhythmias, air embolism, vascular dissection, thromboembolism, bleeding and hematoma, and vasovagal reactions. Thorough preprocedure patient assessment, careful patient selection, appropriately trained and skilled cardiologists and support staff, and properly equipped facilities should limit the patient's risk of complications.[11, 13]

Preoperative care includes taking a thorough nursing history of allergies and medications and a detailed cardiac history. Patients with a history of contrast dye reactions may need premedication to reduce the risk of allergic responses during the procedure. The patient sensitive to contrast dye may be given diphenhydramine, corticosteroids, and histamine$_2$-blocking agents before the procedure.[14] Patients taking metformin should be instructed to discontinue that agent 48 hours before and after their procedure.[15] Patients with a history of renal insufficiency require special monitoring to avoid development of contrast media–associated nephropathy. Other risk factors include dehydration, congestive heart failure, diabetes mellitus, and repeated exposures to contrast agents.[14]

The patient should take nothing by mouth (NPO) except medications with a sip of water for 3 to 6 hours before the procedure. Diagnostic tests that are completed are an ECG, chest x-ray films, and coagulation studies to identify bleeding disorders. An intravenous access is established, and both groins are prepared according to facility policy (antiseptic solution, clipping, shaving) to allow access from either side. Bilateral femoral, posterior tibial, and dorsalis pedis pulses are palpated, marked, and documented to compare with postprocedure status. If access is via the radial artery, an Allen test must be performed before cannulation to ensure satisfactory circulation to the affected hand. Either arm may be used, but the right radial artery is prefered.[16] Other sites include brachial artery or vein, or rarely, subclavian or jugular vein. The procedure room must be fully equipped with appropriate drugs and emergency equipment. Multichannel cardiac monitoring is continued throughout the procedure.

Psychological support to reduce the patient's fear and anxiety includes providing accurate information and allowing the patient to voice specific fears. Explanations should describe the sensory experiences the patient can expect during the procedure (Table 37–3).[17] There is momentary stinging from the injection of local anesthetic that rapidly changes to numbness at the site of catheter entry. During intracardiac manipulation of the catheter, the patient may feel palpitations from extrasystoles. The injection of contrast dye may cause a metallic taste in the mouth, a general feeling of heat, or an urge to

Table 37–2. Exclusion of Patients for Outpatient Cardiac Catheterization; Summary of ACC/AHA Guidelines [33]

Class III

Known or suspected severe cardiac disease (including pulmonary hypertension)
Recent deterioration, e.g., acute ischemic event, active endocarditis
Severe aortic valve disease
Marfan's syndrome with a dilated aortic root
Requirement for continuous anticoagulation
Requirement for left ventricular puncture

Class II

Severely impaired left ventricular function, but clinically in NYHA functional class I or II
Noninvasive investigation suggests a high risk of an adverse outcome
Left ventricular aneurysm
Ejection fraction <35%, or <45% with severe mitral regurgitation
Severe valve disease, but in NYHA functional class I or II
Evaluation of prosthetic valve function
Trans-septal catheterization
Chronic hypoxia
Hypertrophic cardiomyopathy

Class I

Most other conditions not listed under class II or III

Other Characteristics Which Classify Patients Into Class II or III

Severe peripheral vascular disease
Recent stroke
Uncontrolled hypertension
Frequent ventricular arrhythmias
Other coexistent medical problems (e.g., active infection, severe diabetes, renal insufficiency, severe pulmonary disease, morbid obesity or general debility, anemia or electrolyte imbalance)
History of contrast allergy

Modified from Skinner JS, Adams PC: Outpatient cardiac catheterization. Int J Cardiol 53:209–219, 1996.

ACC, American College of Cardiology: AHA, American Heart Association; NYHA, New York Heart Association.

Table 37–3. Explanations to Relieve Anxiety in Patients Undergoing Cardiac Invasive Procedures

- The arterial access may be uncomfortable, but not painful. Although local anesthetic is always used, it stings.
- Back discomfort related to the flat procedure table is a common complaint, but analgesics and positioning with pillows can provide comfort.
- Patients can enhance their comfort by bringing pillows, wearing warm socks, and using their hearing aids and dentures.
- Someone—specifically the "circulator"—will be assigned to meet the patient's needs.
- Feelings of "fluttering" in the chest, caused by dysrhythmias and catheter manipulation, are common and expected.
- Chest pressure or angina from transient coronary ischemia caused by contrast administration into the coronary arteries may occur during angiograms, while a hot flush feeling may be experienced during an angiogram of the left ventricle.
- Angina experienced during interventional procedures may be evaluated on a scale of 1 to 10 for possible treatment with narcotics, nitrates, and oxygen.
- Rotoblator therapy may produce vibrations and burning sensations due to friction from the device spinning in the coronary artery. "Drilling" sounds may be heard during atherectomy, embolectomy, and rotoblator procedures.

From Huddleston E: Cardiac Invasive Procedures: Pre- and Post-procedure Care. Nursing Spectrum Career Fitness Online, Continuing Education. Available at: http://nsweb.nursingspectrum.com/ce/ce178.htm. 1998.

cough.[18] It is helpful for the patient to know that sedation will be administered as necessary and that the nurse will be in constant attendance to support the patient. Also, the patient should be told to report chest pain, headache, lightheadedness, nausea, itching, or dyspnea during the procedure.

The catheterization is performed under aseptic technique by a cardiologist with assistance from registered nurses and technicians experienced in cardiovascular monitoring and radiography. After cannulation of the femoral artery and femoral vein, insertion of a sheath, and introduction of the catheter, heparinized saline is injected to prevent thrombosis of the vessels or clotting within the catheter. Right heart catheterization under fluoroscopy provides valuable information regarding pressures, oxygen saturation, and cardiac output. After cannulation of the left heart, the physician can insert a small catheter tip into the opening of the coronary artery and inject dye to demonstrate the coronary blood supply. Radiographic images are taken throughout the process for later study. Protamine sulfate may be administered to reverse heparinization.[19] Before the patient is transferred to the ASC for observation, manual pressure is applied to the puncture site after removal of the catheter or sheath for no less than 15 minutes and for up to 30 minutes. The site is inspected for hematoma formation before transfer. New hemostatic puncture closure devices (collagen plugs) are undergoing study and may speed initial hemostasis, allow earlier ambulation, and reduce complications. These may eliminate the need for manual pressure after sheath and catheter removal.[17, 20]

Postoperative complications include hypotension, arrhythmias, and bleeding or hematoma formation at the puncture site (Table 37–4).[21] Specific time limitations for positioning vary by facility and access site. Studies have shown that earlier ambulation (3 to 4 hours versus 6 hours) does not appear to increase risk of bleeding and increases patient comfort by decreasing back pain.[22] The patient remains in a supine position at no more than 30-degrees head elevation with the affected leg extended for 2 to 4 hours (for an interventional procedure, it may be 8 hours).[23] If the hemostatic puncture closure device is used, the patient is positioned with affected leg straight and the head flat for 2 hours; then the patient may ambulate and be discharged if no bleeding is noted.

Often, a 5-pound sandbag is placed on the femoral puncture site. New studies are questioning the efficacy of routine use of sandbags and compression dressing for the prevention of vascular complications. Christensen and associates[24] demonstrated that no difference in vascular complications existed between patients with sandbags applied and those who had only a bandage over the access site. Lehmann and colleagues[20] investigated three common dressing techniques (sandbag, pressure dressing, commercially available compression device) that although increasing inconvenience and expense, did not improve patient satisfaction or outcome.

After radial or brachial cannulation, patients may be allowed to sit up after the procedure in the ASC but may have the arm immobilized for a specified time period to limit development of complications.

The site and the vital signs are assessed every 15 minutes for 1 hour, then every 30 minutes for 1 hour, and then hourly. The puncture site is monitored for bleeding, swelling, or hematoma formation. Neurovascular status, including peripheral pulses, color, temperature, and sensation of the affected extremity, is assessed.

Table 37–4. Vascular Complications, Symptoms, and Nursing Interventions

POTENTIAL COMPLICATION	PHYSICAL FINDINGS WITHIN 2–4 HR AFTER PROCEDURE	NURSING INTERVENTIONS
Hematoma	Pain or burning at site Difficulty moving hip or leg Possible tachycardia or hypotension Red or purple discoloration of skin around hematoma	Assess vital signs every 15–30 min until hematoma stabilizes, then every 2–4 hr Measure thigh girth every hour until hematoma stabilizes, then every 4–8 hr Check CBC every 4 hr Measure PTT every 6 hr until it is less than 30 sec
Pseudoaneurysm	Groin pain or burning Back pain Swelling at groin site Ecchymosis, pulsatile mass, bruit	Assess vital signs, groin site, pedal pulses, bruit every 15 min while actively enlarging, then every 2 hr after condition is stable Measure thigh girth every hour Check CBC every 4 hr Measure PTT every 6 hr until it is less than 30 sec
Arteriovenous fistula	Swelling at groin site, pain in leg. May have signs of high output heart failure because of shunting of blood into venous bed. Tachycardia and decreased diastolic BP may occur.	Assess heart and lung sounds every 2–4 hr Assess vital signs and groin site per protocol* but at least every 2 hr Check for decreased pedal pulses and check for bruit every 2 hr
Retroperitoneal hematoma	Moderate to severe back pain Possible groin pain, flank pain, or lower quadrant abdominal pain	Assess vital signs, groin site, pedal pulses every 15 min while patient is actively bleeding Monitor bleeding with abdominal ultrasonography or CT Check CBC every 4 hr Measure PTT every 6 hr until it is less than 30 sec
Arterial occlusion	Pain, pallor, paresthesia, pulselessness of leg	Assess vital signs, leg, pedal pulses, every 15–30 min until circulation is restored Use Doppler ultrasonography for pulse assessment (lesion may require surgical repair)
Neuropathy	Pain, tingling at groin site Numbness at site or down leg Motor difficulty with affected leg Possible decreased patellar tendon reflex Possible weakness or knee extension Symptoms may occur as long as 3 mo after procedure	Check for altered sensation and motor ability Check reflexes and ROM of affected leg and compare with other leg In immediate recovery phase, check vital signs, groin site, and pulses per protocol* and continue checking every 2 hr until symptoms of neuropathy resolve

CBC, complete blood cell count; CT, computed tomography; PTT, partial thromboplastin time; ROM, range of motion; BP, blood pressure.
*Standard assessment protocol: groin check, pulses, vital signs every 15 minutes for an hour, every 30 minutes for 2 hours, every hour for 4 hours, then every 4 hours. (Maintain hourly checks as long as sheaths are in place.) Notify physician of oozing, absence of pulse, hematoma, skin discoloration, or any unusual symptoms or reports from the patient. For arterial bleeding, remove dressing, apply direct pressure just above puncture site for 20 minutes, reapply pressure dressing and retime bedrest period.
Modified from Davis C, Van Riper S, Longstreet J, Moscucci M: Vascular complications of coronary interventions. Heart Lung 26:118–127, 1997.

Coughing, sneezing, or laughing may trigger bleeding from the puncture site.[17] The patient is instructed to apply direct pressure over the site if these situations should occur. The patient may allowed to sit in a chair after 4 hours, walk within 5 hours, and be discharged 6 hours after the end of the procedure.[13] Intravenous hydration may be continued, or oral fluid intake may be encouraged in order to enhance renal clearance of the contrast agent.

Instructions to the patient must address the appropriate actions to take if bleeding occurs after discharge. These include reclining in a supine position, having the responsible adult apply direct pressure to the site without releasing it for at least 15 minutes, and calling the physician immediately. If the physician is not available and the patient is unable to stop the bleeding, the patient should be instructed to call an ambulance or to go to the nearest emergency department as dictated by the amount of bleeding and the patient's general status (Fig. 37–1).

Other discharge instructions include increased oral fluid intake to help eliminate the

UNIVERSITY OF MICHIGAN HOSPITALS
CARDIOLOGY DIVISION

DISCHARGE INSTRUCTIONS FOR OUTPATIENT
CARDIAC CATHETERIZATION FEMORAL ARTERIAL PUNCTURE

A. Activity
- Do not lift or push more than 2–3 pounds the first 2 days after the procedure and then no more than 15 pounds lifting the following 2 days.
- Avoid strenuous activities for next 4 days.
- Do not drive or operate machinery for 24 hours.
- Avoid sitting for more than 1 hour without getting up to stretch and walk around for the next 2 days.
- Support puncture site with your hand when you cough or sneeze over the next 2 days.

B. Bathing
- Do not shower until tomorrow morning.
- Avoid tub bathing for 48 hours.

C. Diet
- Drink 8 glasses of liquids during the first 4 hours following your discharge.
- Resume your normal diet unless otherwise indicated.

D. Puncture Site Care and Observations
- You can expect to have some tenderness in the groin area for up to 1 week.
- You may develop a lump the size of a quarter and/or bruising around the site. The bruising may extend down to your knee as you increase activity. This is normal.
- It is common to have a few drops of blood from site.
- Keep insertion site clean, dry and covered with a Band-Aid for at least 2 days.

E. Call your doctor/seek medical attention if any of the following occur:
- Bleeding: If site suddenly starts to bleed heavily, lay down and apply pressure to the site and go to your nearest Emergency Room.
- Increased tingling and numbness of your affected leg or leg feels cold.
- Sudden onset of chest pain, shortness of breath, dizziness, heart palpitations, nausea and/or itching.
- Sign of infection: Puncture site looks inflamed, drainage from site and/or temperature of greater than 100° F for more than 24 hours.
- Any unusual occurrence that causes you concern.

If you are unable to reach your own Doctor for problems mentioned above, call (313) 936-5625, Monday through Friday, 8:00 am to 5:00 pm, or (313) 936-6267 after 5:00 pm and weekends. (Ask the operator to page the Cardiology Fellow on call).

IP–2054302/DS Rev. 8/95

A

Figure 37–1. *A* and *B*, Discharge Instructions for Outpatient Cardiac Catheterization Femoral Arterial Puncture. (From University of Michigan Hospitals Cardiology Division, Ann Arbor, Michigan.)

UNIVERSITY OF MICHIGAN HOSPITALS
CARDIOLOGY DIVISION

DISCHARGE INSTRUCTIONS FOR OUTPATIENT
CARDIAC CATHETERIZATION FEMORAL VENOUS PUNCTURE

A. Activity During the First 24 Hours After Discharge

- Do not lift or push more than 2–3 pounds.
- Avoid strenuous activities.
- Do not drive or operate machinery for 24 hours.
- Avoid sitting for more than 1 hour without getting up to stretch and walk around.

B. Bathing
- Do not shower until tomorrow morning.
- Avoid tub bathing for 24 hours.

C. Puncture Site Care and Observations

- Examine site daily for swelling or signs of infection.
- You can expect to have some tenderness in the groin area.
- You may develop a lump the size of a quarter and/or bruising around the site. The bruising may extend down to your knee as you increase activity. This is normal.
- It is common to have a few drops of blood from site.
- Keep insertion site clean, dry and covered with a Band-Aid for at least 2 days.

D. Call your doctor/seek medical attention if any of the following occur:

- Bleeding: If site suddenly starts to bleed heavily, lay down and apply pressure to the site and go to your nearest Emergency Room.
- Increased tingling and numbness of your affected leg or leg feels cold.
- Sudden onset of chest pain, shortness of breath, dizziness, heart palpitations, nausea and/or itching.
- Sign of infection: Puncture site looks inflamed, drainage from site and/or temperature of greater than 100° F for more than 24 hours.

If you are unable to reach your own Doctor for problems mentioned above, call (313) 936-5625, Monday through Friday, 8:00 am to 5:00 pm, or (313) 936-6267 after 5:00 pm and weekends. (Ask the operator to page the Cardiology Fellow on call).

IP–2054277/DS Rev. 8/95

B

Figure 37–1 *Continued*

dye from the body. If the catheter insertion site causes discomfort, the physician may order application of an ice bag followed by warm compresses the next day. The patient should avoid heavy lifting or strenuous exercise for several days to lessen the chance of delayed bleeding.

The patient and companion are advised that they will receive a telephone call the following day to answer questions, identify concerns or complications, and discuss any additional follow-up for procedure-related concerns.

ELECTROPHYSIOLOGIC STUDIES

Electrophysiologic (EP) studies, both diagnostic and therapeutic, may be performed on outpatients. The procedure consists of inserting solid electrode catheters under fluoroscopy into a venous access site, similar to a cardiac catheterization (which uses open-lumen catheters to measure pressures), to evaluate rhythm and conduction disturbances. Indications include evaluation of sinus node dysfunction, atrioventricular conduction malfunction, syncope of unknown origin, wide-complex QRS tachycardia, supraventricular tachycardia, and ventricular tachycardia.[25] Therapeutic applications may test responses to pharmacologic agents and arrhythmia induction or select patients for nonpharmacologic control of tachycardias (ablation therapy, pacemakers, or implantable defibrillators).[26]

The patient undergoing EP studies needs a history and physical, 12 lead ECG, blood samples for potassium and other drug levels, and possibly other diagnostic procedures, e.g., neurological evaluation, 24 to 48 hour ambulatory ECG, echocardiogram, stress test and cardiac catheterization.[25] Similar to other cardiovascular procedures, the patient is NPO for at least 3 hours before the procedure.[18] The patient should be prepared for a procedure that may last from 40 minutes to up to several hours. Mild sedation may be given before the procedure. A Foley or condom catheter will be applied or inserted before longer therapeutic procedures.

During the procedure the patient may feel palpitations or a racing heart sensation. If the patient experiences dizziness or lightheadedness, he should notify the nurse or physician.[18] Some patients will undergo therapeutic procedures, such as radiofrequency catheter ablation (RFCA) following diagnostic electrophysiologic studies.

Ablation procedures are used to treat a variety of arrhythmias, those that arise above the atrioventricular node and certain ventricular tachycardias. During the electrophysiologic study, intracardiac stimulation and ECG tracings assist the physician in mapping the arrhythmia amenable to radiofrequency catheter ablation. When the site of an accessory pathway is identified, the catheter tip is positioned to ablate, or burn, that site with a burst of radiofrequency energy. After waiting for 20 to 60 minutes, the physician attempts to elicit the arrhythmia; if the arrhythmia is reproduced, the procedure is repeated.[27]

Complications are uncommon, but therapeutic procedures carry slightly greater risk to the patient.[16] Complications include hemorrhage, venous thromboembolism, phlebitis, pneumothorax, infection, cardiac perforation and tamponade, and refractory ventricular fibrillation.[25]

Postprocedure care is similar to that following other invasive cardiac procedures. Bedrest with no flexion or bending for 4 to 6 hours may be ordered. The puncture site is monitored for bleeding or swelling while vital signs are assessed every 15 minutes for 1 hour, every 30 minutes for 1 hour, and hourly thereafter.[18] A chest x-ray may be ordered to assess for pneumothorax and an ECG to rule out effusion or tamponade.[27] After ablation procedures, the patient may be hospitalized for 1 or 2 days and monitored in a cardiac care or telemetry unit, or the patient may be discharged if recovery is uncomplicated. The outpatient is discharged with instructions to check the puncture site for infection or bleeding and to report any episodes of palpitations, lightheadedness, dizziness, or shortness of breath to the physician.[27]

INTERVENTIONAL PROCEDURES

Interventional cardiology began in the late 1970s with the first percutaneous coronary revascularization procedures. The first procedures were balloon dilation angioplasties. Today, many percutaneous interventions to treat coronary artery disease are used. Table 37–5 describes the more common cardiac interventional procedures.[21, 28] According to Topol and Serruys,[29] interventional cardiology has been revolutionized by stenting procedures. Stents are small metallic mesh tubes, crimped onto angioplasty balloons and inflated.[30] Embedded into the vessel wall, the stents hold the vessels open.

Patients may be admitted for 1 to 2 days for observation and monitoring after the procedures, although some patients may be discharged later on the same day of the procedure.

Table 37–5.* Interventional Procedures

PROCEDURE	DESCRIPTION
Percutaneous transluminal coronary angioplasty (PTCA), also known as balloon angioplasty	Balloon catheter is advanced into coronary artery, inflated to stretch the vessel and flatten the plaque; plaque cracks, scar forms, keeping vessel open. Anticoagulation is given during (heparin) and antiplatelet medications after procedure (aspirin, ticlopidine).
Directional atherectomy	Balloon catheter is used to stabilize cutter in coronary artery; mechanical cutter shaves off layers of plaque, which are removed through the catheter.
Rotational atherectomy	"Roboblator" device is a catheter with a football-shaped tip covered with microscopic diamond crystals; this tip (burr) rotates and cuts through the plaque (best for calcified lesions), creating particles smaller than RBCs.
Transluminal extraction atherectomy	Cutting blades are attached to a hollow catheter with a guide wire inside, guide wire is advanced beyond the lesion to stabilize the device; cutter rotates and cuts off plaque, which is suctioned out through the catheter; intracoronary nitroglycerin is given to prevent vasospasm during the procedure.
Excimer laser angioplasty	Laser beam is used to vaporize the blockade.
Coronary stents	Metal wire meshes or coils surround an angioplasty catheter; catheter is advanced into coronary artery and balloon is inflated, causing mesh or coil stent to expand and compress the lesion; less risk of restenosis; platelet inhibitors required long-term.

*Procedures may be combined; anticoagulation and platelet inhibition similar in all procedures; aftercare similar; facility and physician variations exist.

RBC, red blood cell.

Data from Davis C, VanRiper S, Longstreet J, Moscucci M: Vascular complications of coronary interventions. Heart Lung 26:118–127, 1997.

O'Meara JJ, Dehmer GJ: Care of the patient and management of complications after percutaneous coronary artery interventions. Ann Intern Med 127:458–471, 1997.

The patient is discharged with aspirin and other antiplatelet medications.

PACEMAKER GENERATOR BATTERY CHANGE

Cardiac pacemakers are implanted to regulate the rhythm of the heart. Clinical indications include symptomatic bradydysrhythmias; symptomatic heart block; prophylaxis before or after cardiac surgery or during diagnostic procedures; and tachydysrhythmias.[10] Pacemakers not only pace but can also sense rate changes and are programmed to respond by increasing the heart rate and its duration. After implantation, pacemakers require periodic battery or, more properly, generator replacement to ensure an adequate power supply. A special transmitter allows transtelephonic assessment of pacemaker function. Decreased rate and increased pulse width observed on the transmitted ECG indicate the need for power source replacement.[31] Besides the usual preoperative preparations for surgery, the patient may require special emotional support. The patient may be anxious or frightened about the function of his or her heart, and for those undergoing replacement, may be particularly anxious about the first generator change.

In surgery, ECG electrodes are placed away from the site of the pacemaker, and the chest is prepped. Local anesthesia with or without sedation is usually sufficient for the procedure. The patient's cardiologist may be in attendance with the surgeon. For new pacemaker implants, the incision is generally on the patient's nondominant site, on the anterior chest, just below the clavicle.[31] The generator is placed in this subcutaneous pocket. The leads are placed in either the cephalic or the subclavian veins and attached to the generator. For generator replacement, the incision is made at the site of the original pacemaker insertion. Not only is the generator replaced but the pacemaker leads are also tested and replaced as necessary. Potential intraoperative complications are infrequent but include arrhythmias, bleeding, failure of the new pacemaker generator, inadvertent damage to the pacemaker or leads, and anesthesia-related allergy or toxicity. Lead placement is confirmed by chest x-ray.

Postanesthesia care includes a period of cardiac monitoring to assess pacemaker function. Vital signs are assessed, and the patient is allowed to ambulate soon after surgery. The operative site must be observed for bleeding, and the patient is instructed to call the physician to report excessive bleeding, signs of infection, syncope, palpitations or faintness, or a pulse that is slower than the preset pacemaker rate. The patient should be informed of any change that is made in the preset rate. Pacemaker patients should already be adept at taking their own pulses, but patients with new pacemaker implantation may need instruction and demonstration.

Other instructions for home include avoidance of tight-fitting clothing, extremes of arm movement, and lifting until the wound has healed; resumption of preoperative medications; and attention to all the usual cautions for pacemakers, such as avoiding high voltage, radiation, and magnetic fields and antitheft devices in stores. The patient is instructed to wear appropriate medical identification and to inform all health care providers of their pacemaker.[32]

IMPLANTABLE CARDIOVERTER-DEFIBRILLATOR

Implantable cardioverter-defibrillators monitor cardiac rhythms and deliver shocks to cardiovert or terminate ventricular tachycardia or fibrillation.[33] Implantable cardioverter-defibrillators can provide high energy defibrillation, low-energy cardioversion, and pacing for tachycardia and permanent or postshock bradycardia.[34] Patients who experience ventricular tachycardia or fibrillation episodes are candidates for implantable cardioverter-defibrillator placement. Implantable cardioverter-defibrillator insertion and placement is similar to permanent pacemaker insertion. The patient may require deep sedation or general anesthesia for the procedure. After surgery, the patient may need in hospital observation and monitoring overnight.

Before discharge, the ASC nurse should explain to the patient and companion sensations that the patient may feel if he or she is conscious when the device fires, what to do if the device fires or the patient becomes unconscious and pulseless, and ongoing evaluation of generator function. The patient should wear medical alert identification and should avoid sources of electromagnetic interference.

CARDIOVERSION

Cardioversion is a safe, simple procedure for converting cardiac dysrhythmias to sinus rhythm. Elective cardioversion is most frequently performed for non–life-threatening situations such as atrial flutter, hemodynamically stable sustained fibrillation, and tachyarrhythmias that may be unresponsive to medication or physically exhausting for the patient.[35] Asynchronous cardioversion (defibrillation) is also used to treat ventricular tachycardia and fibrillation in emergency situations.

Patient preparation includes obtaining a nursing history and information regarding the patient's NPO status (4 to 6 hours before procedure), allergy and medication history, potassium and digoxin blood levels, and 12-lead ECG. Patients taking digitalis should not take it on the day of the procedure. After consent is obtained, the patient is positioned supine on the bed or stretcher, and a peripheral intravenous line is started. Supplemental oxygen is supplied, and blood pressure, cardiac rhythm and rate, and O_2 saturation are monitored.

Anesthesia or sedation is induced by an anesthesia care provider with a short-acting drug, such as propofol, midazolam, and etomidate.[36] Emergency airway and resuscitative equipment must be immediately available.

With the defibrillator in the synchronous mode to deliver the shock on the QRS complex, the paddles are placed either from the base of the heart at the sternum to the apex or over the precordium and on the patient's back.[10] Cardioversion usually begins with low-energy current, 20 to 50 J, with successively increasing shocks until the dysrhythmia converts to normal sinus rhythm. As with emergent defibrillation, the operator should ask everyone to stand clear to avoid electrocution.

Complications include atrioventricular nodal dysrhythmias, ventricular dysrhythmias, cardiac arrest, hypotension, pulmonary edema, embolism due to disruption of stagnant clots from the heart chambers, and burn injuries.

After the procedure, the patient is transferred to the recovery area for continued cardiac monitoring and postanesthesia care. A postprocedure 12-lead ECG is obtained. The nurse monitors the patient's vital signs, cardiac rate and rhythm, O_2 saturation, and respiratory status. Supplemental oxygen is given as needed. Intravenous access is maintained. The patient is observed for alterations in level of consciousness, chest pain, shortness of breath, dizziness, heart palpitations or nausea, reddened areas on chest, and changes in vital signs. The physician is notified of changes in cardiac rate and rhythm, respiratory distress, chest pain, and hypotension.

Patients may be monitored up to 24 hours

after the procedure. The patient should receive verbal and written instructions to contact the physician if chest pain, dizziness, or respiratory distress develop. Skin care for abrasions or burns includes cleansing of affected areas with mild soap and application of an ointment or cream if prescribed. A responsible adult companion escorts the patient home from the ASC.

TRANSESOPHAGEAL ECHOCARDIOGRAPHY

An echocardiogram uses sound waves to examine the heart after a probe is placed on the chest wall. Transesophageal echocardiography (TEE) uses the same ultrasound technology but requires insertion of a special probe into the esophagus. If a noninvasive echocardiogram is unsatisfactory or the results do not correlate the patient's clinical status, TEE may be performed. The transesophageal echocardiography may show heart valve diseases, pericardial effusion, congenital heart disease, left ventricular dysfunction, or endocarditis.[18] Transesophageal echocardiography can also be used to monitor heart function intraoperatively.

The patient is NPO for 3 to 6 hours before the procedure. After application of topical anesthetic, the special endoscope is inserted. The transducer tip mounted on the endoscope displays images of the heart for evaluation. After the procedure, the patient is monitored for airway patency; return of swallowing, gag and cough reflexes; and alterations in level of consciousness and vital signs. Discharge instructions include any limitations (activity, driving) that may be necessary if sedation was given for the procedure (see Chapter 15).

INTRAVASCULAR ULTRASOUND

Intravascular ultrasound may be used as an assessment tool and an adjunct to traditional interventions.[37] A flexible catheter with a transducer tip is inserted into a peripheral vessel and advanced into a coronary artery where the transducer is activated. The sound waves generated reflect off the arterial wall or plaque present in the coronary artery. Research demonstrates intravascular ultrasound has greater reliability as an indicator of plaque distribution and composition, arterial dissection, and degree of stenosis than angiography.[37] Intravascular ultrasound can be used for diagnosis of coronary artery disease or as an interventional procedure. Assessment of vessel lesions before and after interventions such as angioplasty, atherectomy, or stenting can be accomplished with intravascular ultrasound.[38]

The most common complication of intravascular ultrasound is vasospasm, which may be treated by catheter withdrawal or intracoronary nitroglycerin.[37] Other complications, which are rare, include occlusion, embolism, myocardial infarction, angina, and coronary dissections.

INSERTION OF VASCULAR ACCESS DEVICES

Vascular access devices are implanted to allow for central venous administration of chemotherapeutic drugs, total parenteral nutrition, and home intravenous therapy of antibiotics and other fluids or drugs. They also provide access for repeated blood samplings and for maintenance hemodialysis. Table 37–6 defines uses for each of the common access devices.[39] Insertion of devices or declotting procedures (thrombectomy) of existing venous catheters and arteriovenous fistulas and shunts may be performed in an ASC. Although same-day discharge is possible, some patients are chronically or acutely ill, and hospitalization may be necessary for associated medical complications.

Nursing care must take into consideration the patient's current state of health and the presence of multiple system diseases. Assessments include preoperative palpation of pulses and observation of the extremity distal to the intended surgical site for comparisons made after surgery. Although a vascular device is heparinized intraoperatively, clotting and subsequent loss of patency or embolic episodes remain potential problems. The patient should be monitored for any signs of embolic activity, including changes in sensorium, speech, and respiratory effort. The patient should be instructed to report such symptoms immediately if they occur after discharge.

After surgery, physical care must be supplemented with psychological support. The patient may express doubts about his or her ability to care for the implanted device and may need reassurance that professional support is available to answer questions. The patient also may experience disturbances of self-image as a result of the need for this access device.

Venous Catheter

Venous catheters may be totally implanted under the skin, for example, the Port-a-Cath

Table 37–6. **Choice of Ambulatory Vascular Access Device**

INDICATION	DEVICE (IN APPROXIMATE ORDER OF PREFERENCE)
Antibiotics 4–6 weeks	Home intravenous therapy (no special device) Peripherally inserted central catheter line Valve-end catheter*
Long-term home total parenteral nutrition	Valve-end catheter* Open-end catheter†
Frequent blood products (Hemophilia, acquired immunodeficiency syndrome)§	Open-end catheter† Port‡
Intermittent ChemoRx	Port‡ Valve-end catheter*
Immediate hemodialysis (also plasma or cell pheresis)	"Surgical" dialysis catheter** "Percutaneous" dialysis catheter††
Permanent hemodialysis	Autologous A-V fistula Prosthetic A-V shunt

A-V, arteriovenous.
*Groshong and others.
†Hickman, Leonard, Broviac, and others.
‡Lifeport, Port-a-Cath, and others.
§Avoiding blood-borne transmission: avoiding the organism (blood) is better with a buried port; avoiding the vector (needle) is better with an external catheter. The best policy is to discuss the specific device with the staff or agency who will actually use it.
**PermaCath and others.
†† Sorensen and others.
Adapted from Schenk WG: Pitfalls in ambulatory vascular access surgery. In Schirmer BD, Rattner DW (eds): Ambulatory Surgery. Philadelphia: WB Saunders, 1998, pp 329–344.

and the Infuse-a-Port, or they may be skin-penetrating devices, such as Broviac and Hickman catheters. Implanted devices reduce the chance of postoperative sepsis but require repeated skin puncture with a needle for accessing the device. They are less cumbersome and allow the patient to maintain a more normal daily lifestyle.

Central venous catheters may be inserted into the superior vena cava through an infraclavicular approach via the subclavian vein, cervically via the internal jugular vein, or an antecubital insertion into the cephalic or basilic vein and threaded into the superior vena cava. The subclavian approach may be complicated by pneumothorax that may or may not require treatment. Tissue injury, hemothorax, air embolism, catheter breakage, and cardiac tamponade are also rare possibilities. This insertion site is well tolerated for long-term management because it does not interfere with neck movement as much as the jugular approach. The internal jugular insertion site is less likely to be associated with pneumothorax but may be difficult to access unless intraoperative ultrasound imaging is used.[39]

The peripherally inserted cental venous catheter allows long-term intravenous therapy with less procedural risk to the patient. With local or topical anesthesia at the site, the catheter is inserted into the cephalic or basilic vein and advanced either at the bedside by the nurse or under fluoroscopy by a physician. Aftercare includes a chest x-ray to verify placement and site care instructions for the patient and companion.

With other venous access devices, the patient's general state of illness is usually best served by avoiding general anesthesia, and the catheter is often placed with the patient under local anesthesia with or without sedation. On completion of the procedure, a chest x-ray is obtained to check device placement and to exclude pneumothorax.[39] After surgery, the insertion site is observed for signs of bleeding or hematoma formation. The patient is instructed to report swelling or frank bleeding after discharge.

Two primary postoperative complications, particularly of devices that penetrate the skin, are infection and thrombosis of the catheter. Careful aseptic technique should be used by nurses caring for the device and should be taught to the patient and to family members. Good handwashing technique and use of universal precautions dictate proper care of the catheter. Before discharge, the patient is instructed to report symptoms that could indicate infection: fever, chills, general malaise, localized redness, and foul-smelling drainage at the catheter site.

A second complication is clotting of the device. Treatment may require: (1) simple aspiration and flushing, (2) a surgical declotting procedure, and (3) administration of streptokinase or another thrombolytic agent. Periodic flushing of the implanted venous catheter with heparinized saline is usually recommended to prevent clot formation. This is especially important after blood sampling.

The patient's discharge instructions include insertion site care, complications to watch for, and how to handle emergency situations, such as breakage, air embolism, and bleeding. Patients with implanted arm ports should not have blood pressures measured on the arm with the port or have blood drawn unless the draw is from the port.

Arteriovenous Fistula

A dependable vascular access site is necessary for the patient who will undergo long-term hemodialysis. The most reliable form is a surgically constructed arteriovenous fistula. Bringing the pressure of arterial blood flow into the vein that will be used for dialysis significantly increases the rate of venous blood flow and allows dialysis can be completed in a reasonable length of time. Initially, the arteriovenous fistula is placed as distal on the arm or hand as possible. This placement allows for future use of more proximal sites. A number of vessels can be used, but the most common site is the radiocephalic fistula on the forearm between the radial artery and the cephalic vein. This has been a standard approach since its development in the 1960s. Benefits include rare infections (less than 3%) and a 65% overall rate of patency at 1 year.[40] Another popular site is the "snuffbox fistula," which is created between the same two vessels but is located more distally on the dorsum of the hand at the origin of the thumb. Preferably vessels of the nondominant arm are used first.

Rather than creating a direct fistula between vessels, some practitioners insert a shunt to provide a communication between the artery and the vein, especially for patients with poor peripheral veins or previously failed arteriovenous fistulas. Autografts from a leg vein, animal grafts, and synthetic materials have all been used. Polytetrafluoroethylene is the most popular material, offering a lower incidence of aneurysm formation than bovine grafts.[40] When this approach is used, the grafted shunt, rather than the patient's vein, is punctured for each use.

The shunt may be totally implanted or externally placed. As with other venous access devices, those grafts that are implanted under the skin are less likely to become infected or thrombosed. While the graft is punctured after surgery, it is important to rotate injection sites to avoid shredding and eventual breakdown of the shunt material.

Because a period of healing is necessary, the arteriovenous fistula should be established before it will be needed for dialysis. Waiting at least 1 to 2 weeks after the shunt placement allows tissue ingrowth, decreasing the risk of hematoma formation from needle punctures.[38] The autologous fistula is allowed to "mature" for at least 6 weeks to ensure adequate blood flow and healing.[39]

Complications include hemorrhage (early) and clotting or thrombosis of the arteriovenous access. Patency may be re-established with surgical thrombectomy under local anesthesia or by interventional radiology, thrombolytic therapy, or thromboemulsification catheter.[39]

Two considerations for discharge are adequate pain control and extremity perfusion with limited edema. Edema of the extremity resolves with elevation and time. Patients should be taught to assess the viability of the fistula or shunt by palpation of a "thrill." Instructions regarding pain management should include encouraging the patient to take the prescribed analgesics until pain diminishes and when to contact the physician—pain is intolerable, no relief is obtained from prescribed analgesic, and the extremity becomes blue, cold, or numb.

TEMPORAL ARTERY BIOPSY

The temporal arteries are normally bilaterally soft and equal in size. They run in front of the ears and supply blood flow to the face. Inflammation and hardening of these arteries can result in bruits and localized tenderness. Temporal arteritis, also defined as giant cell arteritis or vasculitis, may occur acutely or insidiously. Often manifested in headaches, weight loss, fever, and general malaise, sudden blindness can occur as a result of intracranial involvement. Typically, the patient is older than 50 years, white, and female. Women have a three to five times higher incidence than men, and smoking and established atherosclerotic disease are added risk factors.[41]

The patient with such symptoms often is treated with oral corticosteroid therapy. The steroids can prevent but not reverse blindness.[42] Because long-term steroid administration cannot be justified without a definitive diagnosis, biopsy of the temporal artery may be performed to confirm the diagnosis of temporal arteritis by identification of granulomatous cells. This determination is important for establishing or confirming the appropriateness of a therapeutic plan. The biopsy procedure often involves complete ligation and transection of the artery, in which case collateral circulation adequately supplies blood to the affected region.

The biopsy is usually accomplished with local anesthesia that reduces the need for analgesics in the postoperative period. Usually, the patient's postoperative stay is short, although some patients may be already hospitalized for the original symptoms that have become debilitating. Emotional support is important for the patient who has experienced chronic pain or blindness. Surgical complications are few, although the patient should be observed for untoward symptoms at the surgical site. The patient's head is elevated after surgery to decrease the possibility of bleeding. If bleeding or hematoma formation does occur, direct pressure on the site is indicated.

FUTURE OF AMBULATORY CARDIOVASCULAR PROCEDURES

With continuing refinement of techniques; technologic innovations, such as miniaturization; and new therapeutic agents, cardiovascular procedures will most likely become safer and more comfortable for the patient. Capability to continue monitoring via transtelephonic transmissions may revolutionize postprocedure follow-up by allowing the patient to leave the facility sooner without fear that complications may be missed. Interventional procedures will continue to evolve, requiring the nurse working with patients who undergo such procedures to acquire new knowledge continually and to remain aware of ongoing research efforts in this specialty area.

References

1. Polk HC, Cheadle WG: Principles of preoperative preparation of the surgical patient. In Sabiston DC (ed): Textbook of Surgery: The Biological Basis of Modern Surgical Practice, 15th ed. Philadelphia: WB Saunders, 1997, pp 112–117.
2. Hamilton G, Platts A: Deep venous thrombosis. In Beard JD, Gaines PA (eds): Vascular and Endovascular Surgery. Philadelphia: WB Saunders, 1998, pp 351–396.
3. Bradbury AW, Ruckley CV: Varicose veins. In Beard JD, Gaines PA (eds): Vascular and Endovascular Surgery. Philadelphia: WB Saunders, 1998, pp 433–459.
4. Waddell BE, Harkins MB, Lepage PA, et al: The crochet hook method of stab avulsion phlebectomy for varicose veins. Am J Surg 172:278–280, 1996.
5. Minard C, Fellows E: Post-Operative Discharge Instructions for Varicose Vein Stripping and Ligation. Ann Arbor MI: University of Michigan Hospitals and Health System, 1998.
6. Baughman K, Kasper EK: Endomyocardial biopsy. In Uretsky BF (ed): Cardiac Catheterization. Malden MA: Blackwell Science, 1997, pp 306–331.
7. Mills Rm, Young JB: Evaluation for cardiac transplantation and follow-up of the cardiac transplant recipient. In Pepine CJ (ed): Diagnostic and Therapeutic Cardiac Catheterization, 3rd ed. Baltimore: Williams & Wilkins, 1998, pp 960–980.
8. Nanas JN, Anastasiou-Nana MI, Sutton RB, Tsagaris TJ: Effect of acute allograft rejection on exercise hemodynamics in patients who have undergone cardiac transplantation. Chest 107:1517–1521, 1995.
9. Bashore TM, Wang AG: Cardiac catheterization laboratories. In Pepine CJ (ed): Diagnostic and Therapeutic Cardiac Catheterization, 3rd ed. Baltimore: Williams & Wilkins, 1998, pp 13–30.
10. Nettina SM: Lippincott Manual of Nursing Practice, 6th ed. Philadelphia: Lippincott-Raven, 1997 (BiblioMed Textbook Software, Version 2.10, 5/9/97).
11. American College of Cardiology/American Heart Association Ad Hoc Task Force on Cardiac Catheterization: ACC/AHA guidelines for cardiac catheterization and cardiac catheterization laboratories. J Am Coll Cardiol 18:1149–1182, 1991.
12. Skinner JS, Adams PC: Outpatient cardiac catheterization. Int J Cardiol 53:209–219, 1996.
13. Montes P: Managing outpatient cardiac catheterization. Am J Nurs 97:34–37, 1997.
14. Hill JA, Lamber CR, Pepine CJ: Radiographic contrast agents. In Pepine CJ (ed): Diagnostic and Therapeutic Cardiac Catheterization. Baltimore: Williams & Wilkins, 1998, pp 203–216.
15. Mosby GenRx, Mosby: Metformin Hydrochloride product description. Available at: http://www.rxlist.-com/cgi/generic/metformi.htm. 1998.
16. Hill JA, Lambert CR, Vliestra RE, Pepine CJ: Review of techniques. In Pepine CJ (ed): Diagnostic and Therapeutic Cardiac Catheterization. Baltimore: Williams & Wilkins, 1998, pp 106–128.
17. Huddleston E: Cardiac invasive procedures: Pre- and postprocedure care. Nursing Spectrum Career Fitness Online, Continuing Education. Available at: http://nsweb.nursingspectrum.com/ce/ce178.htm. 1998.
18. Fischbach FT: A Manual of Laboratory and Diagnostic Tests, 5th ed. Philadelphia: Lippincott-Raven, 1997 (BiblioMed Textbook Software, Version 2.10, 5/9/97).
19. Deligonul U, Roth R, Flynn M: Arterial and venous access. In Kern MJ (ed): The Cardiac Catheterization Handbook, 2nd ed. St. Louis: CV Mosby, 1995, pp 45–107.
20. Lehmann KG, Ferris ST, Heath-Lange SJ: Maintenance of hemostasis after invasive cardiac procedures: Implications for outpatient catheterization. J Am Coll Cardiol 30:444–451, 1997.
21. Davis C, VanRiper S, Longstreet J, Moscucci M: Vascular complications of coronary interventions. Heart Lung 26:118–127, 1997.
22. Winslow EH: Too much bed rest after cardiac catheterization? Am J Nurs 96:21, 1996.
23. Faxon DP: The cardiac catheterization laboratory: Setup and management. In Uretsky BF (ed): Cardiac Catheterization. Malden MA: Blackwell Science, 1997, pp 63–93.
24. Christensen BV, Manion RV, Iacarella CL, et al: Vascular complications after angiography with and without the use of sandbags. Nurs Res 47:51–53, 1998.
25. Janosik DL, Gamache MC: Electrophysiologic studies

and ablation techniques, In Kern MJ (ed): The Cardiac Catheterization Handbook, 2nd ed. St. Louis: CV Mosby, 1995, pp 208–265.
26. Lexi-Comp: Diagnostic Procedures Handbook. Available at: www.healthgate.com. 1997.
27. Corona GG: Radio waves fight SVT. RN 61:27–31, 1998.
28. O'Meara JJ, Dehmer GJ: Care of the patient and management of complications after percutaneous coronary artery interventions. Ann Intern Med 127:458–471, 1997.
29. Topol EJ, Serruys PW: Frontiers in interventional cardiology. Circulation 98:1802–1820, 1998.
30. Corr LA: The future of interventional cardiology. Lancet Suppl 1:S23–S26, 1996.
31. Lowe JE: Cardiac pacemakers. In Sabiston DC (ed): Textbook of Surgery: The Biological Basis of Modern Surgical Practice, 15th ed. Philadelphia: WB Saunders, 1997, pp 2175–2198.
32. Hasemeier CS: Permanent pacemaker. Am J Nurs 96:30–31, 1996.
33. Portman D, Barden C: Implantable cardioverter defibrillators: Now and in the future. Philadelphia: JB Lippincott Continuing Education Online, AACN/Wyeth-Ayerst Fellows Supplement. Am J Nurs May 1997.
34. Nichols K, Collins J: Update on implantable cardioverter defibrillators: Knowing the difference in devices and their impact on patient care. AACN Clin Issues 6:31–43, 1995.
35. Zuber TJ, Pfenninger JL: Cardioversion. In Pfenninger JL (ed): Procedures for Primary Care Physicians. St. Louis: Mosby-Year-Book, 1994, pp 437–443.
36. Smith I, McCulloch DA: Anesthesia outside the operating room. In White PF (ed): Ambulatory Anesthesia and Surgery. Philadelphia: WB Saunders, 1997, pp 220–232.
37. Strimike C: Understanding intravascular ultrasound. Am J Nurs 96:40–43, 1996.
38. Schlaifer JD, Nissen SE: Intravascular ultrasound. In Pepine CJ (ed): Diagnostic and Therapeutic Cardiac Catheterization. Baltimore: Williams & Wilkins, 1998, pp 301–325.
39. Schenk WG: Pitfalls in ambulatory vascular access surgery. In Schirmer BD, Rattner DW (eds): Ambulatory Surgery. Philadelphia: WB Saunders, 1998, pp 329–344.
40. Haisch CE, Cerilli J: Vascular access procedures for renal dialysis (including peritoneal dialysis). In Sabiston DC (ed): Textbook of Surgery: The Biological Basis of Modern Surgical Practice, 15th ed. Philadelphia: WB Saunders, 1997, pp 429–436.
41. Thompson JM, McFarland GK, Hirsch JE, Tucker SM: Mosby's Clinical Nursing, 4th ed. St. Louis: CV Mosby, 1997.
42. Belch JJF, Ho M: Vasospastic disorders, connective tissue disease and vasculitis. In Beard JD, Gaines PA (eds): Vascular and Endovascular Surgery. Philadelphia: WB Saunders, 1998, pp 201–224.

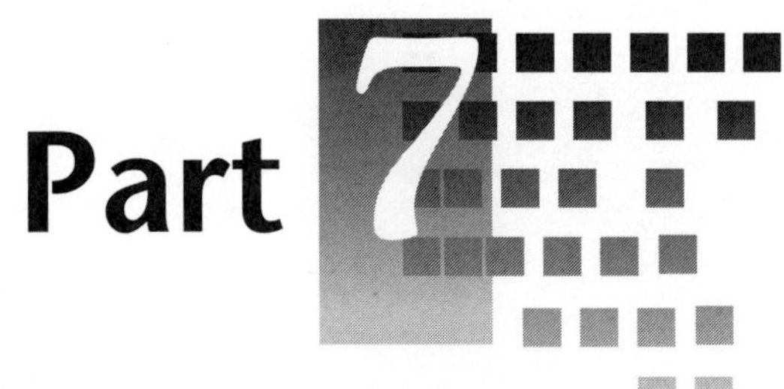

Part 7

The Ambulatory Surgery Center as a Special Procedures Unit

Chapter 38

Special Procedures in the Ambulatory Setting

Denise O'Brien, Virginia A. Walter, and Nancy Burden

CONCEPTS OF CARE RELATED TO SPECIAL PROCEDURES

Many procedures that previously were performed in postanesthesia care units (PACUs), operating rooms, or emergency departments have moved into the ambulatory surgery setting. This change has freed space and nursing time for sicker patients in those critical care areas. It also has moved many nonurgent procedures out of hospital emergency departments. Not only has this change resulted in more efficient hospital resource utilization, but also in most cases, staff trained specifically in the care of this patient population has contributed to more satisfied patients and families.

Facilities differ greatly regarding where and how special procedures are performed. One hospital may consider the ambulatory surgery center (ASC) as an appropriate site for a particular procedure, whereas another does not. The policies of each facility must be based on the physical environment, equipment, nursing personnel, and patient care issues. This chapter should be read with the understanding that the information must be adapted to each facility's policies and available resources.

Developing Special Procedures Programs in the Ambulatory Surgery Center

Use of an ASC for special procedures is related to a number of factors. One is the expedient admission and discharge procedures that have been developed for ease of patient access to the department. The ASC nursing staff is accustomed to accommodating rapid admission and turnover of patients. The versatility and adaptability that the nursing staff typically develops in caring for a broad array of surgical patients is a second reason. Ambulatory surgery (AS) nurses are known to be quickly responsive to unexpected changes in scheduled procedures and caseload.

Some special procedures do not require an operating room but do call for the involvement of anesthesiologists. The close relationship among and frequent presence of anesthesiologists within the ambulatory surgery unit are other positive considerations that make the area an attractive site for performing invasive procedures that do not require overnight stays. Likewise, the nursing staff is knowledgeable about perianesthesia care. Finally, physicians may prefer to work in a "user-friendly and patient-friendly" ASC setting if delays in start times and scheduling conflicts are uncommon.

Before initiating use of an ASC for a particular type of special procedure, carefully developed plans and patient care criteria should be in place. Nurses and other assistive personnel must be adequately trained and should have access to appropriate educational materials. When it is available, hands-on experience in another unit or facility where the procedure is currently being performed is an ideal teaching method.

Each nurse should be knowledgeable not only of the procedures but also of indications for procedures, possible complications, and treatment protocols for those complications. This broad knowledge base prepares the nurse to provide comprehensive patient assessment and education. The physical environment should be properly equipped for the procedure and for potential complications. This preparation includes the availability of an emergency response team.

Nursing policies are developed primarily by unit nurses and nurse managers; however, input and approval should be sought from a multispecialty team. The surgical, medical, anesthesia, nursing, and pharmacy departments all have valuable insights with which to develop safe patient care protocols. The medical director has ultimate responsibility for each patient cared for in an ambulatory surgical center and must be an integral part of the process when planning the addition of new services.

Policies should identify and specify appropriate criteria for patient admission and discharge and for nursing responsibilities before, during, and after the procedure. Pre- and postprocedure patient instructions should be developed, although the physician will customize them for each patient. These policies should be immediately available to personnel for consultation.

Nursing Care Issues

Performing special procedures in an ASC often requires that nurses learn new concepts and perform new skills. Regardless of the type of procedure performed, basic nursing responsibilities and actions are germane to all of them. The patient facing any invasive procedure deserves and requires the same quality of care as the patient undergoing surgery in the traditional sense. Baseline nursing assessments must be obtained: (1) to determine the patient's fitness for the procedure; (2) to identify risk factors and avoid complications; and (3) to use in postprocedure comparisons. This assessment is a responsibility shared by the nurse and the primary physician. Patients with pre-existing illnesses as well as those who are healthy can experience serious complications related to any procedure, and thus, establishing a baseline of information as well as protocols for emergency interventions must be a priority in the ASC.

The fear and anxiety that patients may express or silently endure related to a procedure such as endoscopy or blood transfusion can seem out of proportion to its seemingly minor nature compared to surgery. Fear of the unknown, expectation of discomfort or pain, debilitation or chronicity of a disease, dread of the impending diagnosis, or fear of complications can justifiably unnerve many patients. Whether the patient's fears are valid or unfounded, they are very real. Thus, the AS nurse is challenged to address many emotional, psychological, and social needs in an empathic and effective manner.

Patient education is essential to ensure that the person is properly informed, follows preparatory instructions, and understands what he or she will be experiencing and why. Explanations within the limits of nursing parameters can help to clarify information previously provided by the physician. Unlike surgical patients in many facilities, people having special procedures often do not visit the facility before the day of the procedure. For these patients, instructions may be provided during a telephone call from the ASC nurse or, often, by the physician or the physician's office staff.

When the patient is admitted, the nurse verifies the patient's understanding of the procedure and whether preparations have been completed appropriately. A signed consent must be on the medical record along with documentation that the patient has established adequate home and transportation plans. These issues must be investigated and resolved before beginning or continuing with the procedure.

Unlike surgical patients, many of these people remain in the ASC for their procedures, and the ASC nurses function as procedural assistants and physiologically monitor patients during procedures. One nurse may be sufficient to perform or assist with some procedures; however, for patients who will have sedation or other analgesia, the assistance of a second nurse or another provider may be necessary so as not to compromise the continuous physiologic monitoring of the patient. This is also true for more complicated diagnostic and therapeutic procedures.

Postprocedure care is similar to that for the surgical patient. The intensity of nursing care is dependent upon each patient's clinical needs. Some may require PACU Phase I attention if sedation or analgesia has been given and complications have occurred. Others will be transferred from the procedure area directly to the Phase II PACU or discharge department of the ASC. Discharge instructions should reflect the patient's individual needs for information specific to home aftercare, response to unexpected events, and follow-up by the physician.

During many invasive procedures the nurse administers an intravenous (IV) sedative and analgesics and monitors the patient accordingly. Sedation may be given with or without the addition of local anesthesia by the physician. It is essential that the patient receiving IV sedative and analgesic agents be cared for in a safe environment. Oxygen, suction, and appropriate equipment for monitoring blood pressure, electrocardiogram (ECG), and oxygen saturation must be at the patient's bedside. Emergency equipment, a call-bell system, and knowledgeable emergency assistive personnel should be immediately available. Medications are given under the specific and direct orders of a physician. A more detailed discussion of the nurse's responsibilities during sedation and analgesia is presented in Chapter 15 and should be applied to appropriate areas of care discussed in this chapter.

TYPES OF SPECIAL PROCEDURES PERFORMED IN AMBULATORY SURGICAL CENTERS

Many invasive, nonsurgical procedures are performed in ASCs in both hospital and freestanding facilities. Procedures discussed in this chapter include gastrointestinal endoscopy, bronchoscopy, liver biopsy, paracentesis, thoracentesis, and parenteral therapy. Pain management procedures can be performed in specialized pain clinics or in ASCs. Pain management procedures are discussed in Chapter 39.

Some of these procedures require special environments, yet same-day admission and discharge remain desirable. For those patients, the ASC functions as it does for the surgical patient, providing pre- and postprocedure nursing care. Examples might include cardiac catheterization (see Chapter 37), electroconvulsive shock therapy (ECT), some invasive radiologic studies, and in some facilities, endoscopic procedures.

Nurses who assume the roles of procedure assistant and primary patient monitor require extensive knowledge and training in order to provide comprehensive care during special procedures of a complex nature. It is beyond the scope of this text to provide an inclusive discussion of each procedure. Rather, an overview will be provided to describe the basic concepts and patient needs related to each. The reader is referred to specialty texts to gain a comprehensive insight into the many details related to the various procedures undertaken.

Parenteral Therapy

Parenteral therapy undertaken in the ASC may include the administration of IV fluids, blood and blood products, and IV medications such as antibiotics. Patients requiring such therapies may be debilitated and may require extensive physical and emotional care due to their medical status. The availability of transportation and home care may be a problem. Family members already may have taken considerable time off from work because of the patient's illness, and scheduling should consider the family's needs.

Before beginning parenteral therapy, the facility may or may not require the patient to sign a specific consent and the nurse should ensure compliance to the policy. A specific physician's order must be obtained that includes at least the name of the solution or medication, dose, volume, rate of administration, frequency, if applicable, and route.[1, 2] A designation to keep vein open (KVO) is not considered a specific order for rate and should be further clarified prior to initiating an infusion.

The patient should be provided with a comfortable chair or bed and encouraged to urinate before beginning the therapy. Diversionary items, such as a television, video player, and reading material, may be appropriate when a lengthy stay is projected. A nursing history and physical examination are performed, including specific assessment of potential venipuncture sites and the neurovascular status of areas around and distal to potential venipuncture sites.

In some facilities, a designated IV team is available to perform venipunctures and initiate therapies. In many ASCs, however, this resource is not available and an AS nurse is responsible. Before initiating parenteral therapy, the AS nurse should be knowledgeable and experienced in: (1) basic dosage calculations and drip factors; (2) anatomy and physiology of the circulatory system; (3) signs, symptoms, and treatment of allergic reaction, extravasation, and phlebitis; and (4) the concepts and application of aseptic technique and universal precautions. The nurse must also be familiar with necessary equipment and with the specific medications and products that will be administered, including indications, average dosages, routes and rate of administration, and usual side effects and their treatments. Adequate equipment and supplies must be readily available, including appropriate protective personal apparel and an approved sharps disposal system.

Adequate training should be provided to the staff who perform venipunctures, access ports and other permanent indwelling vascular devices, and initiate and monitor various types of parenteral therapies. Before initiating IV therapy, the nurse should demonstrate an acceptable level of expertise in the technical aspects of the procedure, knowledge of the facility's applicable policies and procedures, and an adequate understanding of the of the principles and practices of IV therapy. Mentoring is appropriate until the individual nurse's skills are ascertained and the nurse feels comfortable undertaking independent practice.

Standards of nursing practice have been established.* The standards address many technical and professional aspects of IV therapy, including physician's orders; use of tourniquets; site preparation and hair removal; cannula selection, placement, and securing; discontinuation of therapy; and others.[3] The standards are applicable to all settings.

The patient's future needs must be considered when choosing a venipuncture site. It is advantageous to select the most distal, yet adequate, vein first so that subsequent venipunctures can be made more proximally on the extremity without interfering with the previous site. Besides the anatomic and physiologic considerations, the patient's wishes and past personal experiences should be taken into account when choosing a site. Patients who have undergone frequent venipunctures can often provide valuable information about past failures or successes. In addition, the patient's comfort is considered in relation to the projected length of time the vein will be in use and the patient's mobility and physical comfort.

It is a rare person who does not dread a venipuncture attempt. Concurrent psychological support and diversion during the procedure can help to alleviate anxiety and discomfort. In addition, facility policy may allow the use of a topical anesthetic cream and/or intradermal lidocaine or saline as a deterrent to pain. Such medications must be used within the policies of the facility. The nurse administering them must be knowledgeable about any untoward effects, including allergic reaction, anaphylaxis, inadvertent vascular injection, and obliteration of the vein.[4]

The nurse provides ongoing monitoring of the site and the component being administered. Volume overload, extravasation with potential for necrosis and sloughing of tissues, allergic or transfusion reactions, embolism, inadvertent intra-arterial injection, bleeding, phlebitis, infection, and septicemia are all complications of parenteral therapy. Peripheral IV infection can be introduced to the patient via many sources, including the healthcare worker's hands, contaminated disinfectants, an improperly prepared venipuncture site, defects in or contamination of equipment, improper techniques of tubing or solution container punctures, and lax use of the principles of universal precautions. Those at highest risk for peripheral infection are the elderly; those who are on immunosuppressors; patients who are malnourished or debilitated; people with pre-existing infections or diseases such as diabetes or heart disease; and those with altered skin flora due to antibiotic therapy.[5]

The transmission of blood-borne pathogens among patients and healthcare workers is a significant danger during parenteral therapy, and all patients should be presumed to be infectious for blood-borne pathogens. The strict implementation of universal precautions described by the Centers for Disease Control and Prevention is a requirement.[6,7] "Recommendations for Prevention of HIV Transmission in Health-Care Settings" applies not only to HIV but to any blood-borne pathogen. These recommendations were published in the *Morbidity and Mortality Weekly Report* (MMWR) of Aug. 21, 1987 (vol 36, 2S) and followed by another document: Update: Universal precautions for prevention of transmission of human immunodeficiency virus, hepatitis B virus, and other blood-borne pathogens in health-care settings. MMWR 37(24):377–388 (6/24/88), which can be obtained from the U.S. Department of Health and Human Services (DHHS), Public Health Service, Centers for Disease Control and Prevention, Atlanta, GA 30333 (www.cdc.gov). Also, the Infection Control Department within each facility should have copies available for reference.

Facility policy should address whether a venipuncture site may be preserved for more than one administration by application of a heparin-flushed resealing device when repeated injections or infusions are ordered for several days. The policy also should identify applicable parameters including the length of time one site may be used before changing to another vein, the frequency of dressing changes and flushing

---

*A comprehensive and authoritative resource for reference is the Revised Intravenous Nursing Standards of Practice formulated by and available through the Intravenous Nurses Society, Fresh Pond Square, 10 Fawcett Street, Cambridge, MA 02138, 617-441-3008, Fax 617-441-3009, www.ins1.org.

of the cannula, and the patient teaching and support that must be provided related to care of the IV port at home. Patient instructions for home care of an IV site should cover the following areas:

- How to tighten connections that become loose or detached
- What to do if the cannula or reseal device falls out
- How to apply pressure to the site for bleeding or dislodgment
- The importance of keeping the site dry
- Symptoms of complications to report to the physician, such as rash or itching, redness, heat, or pain at or above the IV site, fever, or chills.

Antibiotics

Antibiotic therapy may be given in the ASC. Before administration, the nurse should obtain a careful health history from the patient, including tolerance and type of previous antibiotics administered and allergies. The written physician's order should specify the medication and dose, along with the number and frequency of doses to be given. The physician, pharmacist, current drug therapy handbooks, and manufacturer's instructions are all resources for determining the rate of administration, compatibilities, dilution parameters, and untoward effects. Before initiating therapy, the nurse is responsible for questioning and clarifying an incomplete order or an order that the nurse deems to be outside of usual administration parameters.

Blood and Blood Products

The ASC may be chosen for transfusing blood or its components, for instance, packed red blood cells, platelets, coagulation factors, cryoprecipitate, or fresh frozen plasma (FFP), each given for a specific indication. Recipients may be debilitated with systemic illnesses and require comprehensive nursing care that considers pre-existing conditions.

A written physician's order should specify the component, volume, and rate of transfusion, as well as any prophylactic medications to be given before transfusion. An informed consent is obtained. Baseline vital signs should include the patient's temperature, because pre-existing fever could mask the signs or complicate the diagnosis of a later transfusion reaction. The patient should be questioned about any previous transfusions including any untoward reactions. Patient instructions given before the transfusion include advisories on what to expect during the procedure, the expected length of time it will take, and the patient's responsibility to report any unusual symptoms to the nurse immediately, for instance, pain at the venipuncture site, itching, hives, rash, dyspnea, or wheezing respirations.

Further nursing interventions before initiating transfusion therapy should be designed to prevent accidental transfusion of the wrong product. These verification guidelines are provided in Table 38–1. Blood products should be infused through a filter and venous catheter, both of suitable size. A cannula of at least 18 gauge is suggested for adults receiving whole blood or packed red blood cells. The patient should be observed for untoward reactions throughout the treatment and continuously during the first 15 minutes. Further administration guidelines are provided in Table 38–2.

If a warming device is used during blood administration, it should be an approved unit with an upper temperature limit no greater than 42°C.[8] It should have an audible and visual alarm to alert personnel to overheating. Blood should never be warmed under hot tap water, in an unmonitored water bath, or in a microwave oven.[9] The infusion site and vital signs, including temperature, are monitored frequently during administration, according to facility policy. One unit of whole blood should be infused within 4 hours, and no medication or solutions other than 0.9% sodium chloride should be added to blood components.[10]

Even with extensive safety measures implemented, transfusion reactions remain a constant threat to patients. These reactions can be acute or delayed. Acute reactions include: (1) acute hemolytic reaction due to ABO blood type incompatibility; (2) febrile, nonhemolytic reaction, which is the most common; (3) mild allergic reactions; (4) anaphylactic reaction; and (5) circulatory overload or sepsis. Delayed reactions can include a delayed hemolytic response; hepatitis B or C, human immunodeficiency virus (HIV) infection; iron overload; graft-versus-host disease; and other infections. Table 38–3 lists the possible symptoms of a transfusion reaction, and Table 38–4 provides recommended nursing actions when a reaction occurs.

Upon discharge, patients should receive specific instructions regarding signs and symptoms to report in the event a delayed reaction occurs. Symptoms are generally mild but, nonetheless, they must be reported to allow prompt investigation of the reaction.[11]

Gastrointestinal Endoscopy

Endoscopy is defined as "visual inspection of any cavity of the body by means of an endo-

Table 38–1. Verification of Blood Products Before Administration

1. Obtain a blood component from the transfusion service. Inspect it for leaks, abnormal cloudiness, color, clots, excessive air, or bubbles and record in patient chart. If any of these problems are detected, check with the transfusion service before administering the blood component.
2. Record the name of the person issuing blood, person to whom blood is issued, and the date and time of issue. This information is on the chart copy issued by the transfusion service.
3. Read the instructions on the product label and check the expiration date and time. If time is not specified, the product will outdate at 12 midnight on the expiration date.
4. Recheck the physician's order sheet to verify the component ordered.
5. Compare the ABO group and the Rh type on the patient's chart to that on the bag tag and bag label. Verify the consistency and compatibility and the record. Note if the patient should be receiving autologous or designated/ directed unit.
6. Two qualified individuals should verify patient identification and document in the chart:
   a. Compare the name and ID number of the blood bag tag to those on the patient's ID bracelet and transfusion form. They must be the same.
   b. Ask the patient to state his or her full name, if possible; do not state the patient's name in a question that can be answered "yes" or "no." Most transfusion reactions occur as a result of errors in patient or component identification.
7. *Do not* proceed unless all comparisons match *exactly*. Contact the transfusion service immediately if *any* discrepancy exists.
8. Sign the transfusion form immediately before infusion; document identification of individuals and verify the component and the patient.
9. Document the date and time when the transfusion started.
10. Keep all identification attached to blood container until transfusion is completed.

From the National Blood Resource Education Program's Transfusion Therapy Guidelines for Nurses. US Department of Health and Human Services, National Institutes of Health. NIH Publication 90-2668, 1990, p 21.

Table 38–2. Blood Administration Guidelines

1. Start infusion slowly (5 ml/min or less for first 15 min). Observe closely throughout the transfusion. Symptoms of a severe transfusion reaction are usually manifested during the first 50 ml or less of blood infusion. It is advisable to remain with the patient for the first 15 min of the transfusion.
2. Repeat vital signs at 15 min or as patient condition requires and compare to baseline. If there are no signs of transfusion complications, adjust flow to the prescribed rate.
3. Monitor and record vital signs as required by institutional policy.
4. Record on a part of the permanent record the patient name and ID number, component and component number(s), initials of individuals verifying patient ID and starting and ending transfusion times, volume transfused, and immediate response (i.e., no reaction noted, reaction noted).
5. Return empty blood containers to the transfusion service within 24 hours if required by institutional policy.
6. Blood products must be stored only in refrigerators and freezers monitored by the transfusion service. Plasma derivatives (e.g., albumin, and plasma protein fraction) are routinely stored at room temperature and are commonly dispensed through the pharmacy or central stores.

PITFALLS TO AVOID

Do NOT store component in the nursing unit or another unmonitored refrigerator.
Do NOT keep blood out of a monitored refrigerator for more than 30 minutes before beginning the transfusion.
Do NOT warm blood in an unmonitored water bath or sink, or microwave oven.
Do NOT administer any blood component without a blood filter.
Do NOT use the same blood filter for more than 4 hours.
Do NOT transfuse a unit of blood for over 4 hours.
Do NOT add medications, including those intended for IV use, to blood or components or infuse the same administration set as the blood component.
Do NOT allow any solution other than *0.9% normal saline* to come in contact with the blood component or the administration set.

From the National Blood Resource Education Program's Transfusion Therapy Guidelines for Nurses. US Department of Health and Human Services, National Institutes of Health. NIH Publication 90-2668, 1990, p 22.

Table 38–3. Possible Signs and Symptoms of a Transfusion Reaction

GENERAL

Fever (rise of 1°C or 2°F)
Chills
Muscle aches, pain
Back pain
Chest pain
Headache
Heat at site of infusion or along vein

NERVOUS SYSTEM

Apprehension, impending sense of doom
Tingling, numbness

RESPIRATORY SYSTEM

Respiratory rate
- Tachypnea
- Apnea
- Dyspnea
- Cough
- Wheezing
- Rales

GASTROINTESTINAL SYSTEM

Nausea
Vomiting
Pain, abdominal cramping
Diarrhea (may be bloody)

CARDIOVASCULAR SYSTEM

Heart rate
- Bradycardia
- Tachycardia

Blood pressure
- Hypotension, shock
- Hypertension
- Peripheral circulation

Color: cyanosis, facial flushing
Temperature: cool/clammy, hot/flushed/dry
Edema
Bleeding
Generalized (DIC)
Oozing at surgical site

RENAL SYSTEM

Changes in urine volume
- Oliguria, anuria
- Renal failure

Changes in urine color
- Dark, concentrated
- Shades of red, brown, amber may indicate the presence of RBCs (hematuria) or of free hemoglobin (hemoglobinuria)

INTEGUMENTARY SYSTEM

Rashes, hives (urticaria), swelling
Itching
Diaphoresis

SIGNS OF REACTION IN AN UNCONSCIOUS PATIENT

Weak pulse
Fever
Hypotension
Visible hemoglobinuria
Increased operative bleeding (oozing at surgical site)
Vasomotor instability (tachycardia, bradycardia, or hypotension)
Oliguria/anuria

From the National Blood Resource Education Program's Transfusion Therapy Guidelines for Nurses. US Department of Health and Human Services, National Institutes of Health. NIH Publication 90-2668, 1990, p 14.

Reactions from different causes can exhibit similar manifestations; therefore, every symptom should be considered potentially serious and transfusion discontinued until the cause is determined.

scope," which is "an instrument for the examination of the interior of a hollow viscus."[12] An endoscope is a lighted tube-like instrument that can be rigid or flexible. Endoscopy generally refers to gastrointestinal (GI) procedures, but it may include any procedure using a scope to look inside a body cavity.

The GI tract consists of the mouth, pharynx, esophagus, stomach, small intestine (duodenum, jejunum, and ileum) and large intestine (cecum; ascending, transverse, descending colon; and sigmoid colon), rectum, and anus as illustrated in Figure 38–1. Accessory organs of the GI system are the salivary glands, liver, gallbladder, and pancreas, which contribute secretions necessary for the digestive process. The primary function of this organ system is the ingestion, digestion, and absorption of food. Infection, inflammation, and surgery can alter the digestive and absorptive processes, requiring intervention such as endoscopy for diagnosis and treatment.

This discussion will begin with general information about pre-, intra-, and postprocedure care of the GI endoscopy patient and continue with specific information about various GI endoscopy procedures performed in the ASC setting. This discussion is not intended as a review of all procedures, but rather as an overview of the types of patients and procedures that may be seen in the ASC. The reader should refer to texts on GI endoscopy for more information.

Table 38–4. Recommended Nursing Actions During a Transfusion Reaction

When a transfusion reaction occurs:
1. STOP THE TRANSFUSION.
2. Keep the IV open with 0.9% normal saline.
3. Report the reaction to both the transfusion service and the attending physician immediately.
4. Do a clerical check at the bedside of identifying tags and numbers.
5. Treat the symptoms per the physician's order and monitor the patient's vital signs.
6. Send the blood bag with the attached administration set and labels to the transfusion service.
7. Collect blood and urine samples and send them to the lab.*
8. Document thoroughly on the transfusion reaction form and in the patient's chart.

*Check with the transfusion service to determine the specific blood and urine samples needed to evaluate reactions.

From the National Blood Resource Education Program's Transfusion Therapy Guidelines for Nurses. US Department of Health and Human Services, National Institutes of Health. NIH Publication 90-2668, 1990, p 15.

Preprocedure Care

Patients undergoing GI endoscopic procedures require education about the procedure, its preparation, and aftercare. This discussion, staged in the physician's office when the procedure is scheduled, will include information on the procedure; the need for specialized preparation of the GI tract (establishing whether the patient can take anything by mouth, discontinuing or continuing regular medications, and necessary colon preparations); and the need for a responsible adult companion for transportation home after procedures requiring sedation or analgesia. This information is essential to adequately prepare the patient for a procedure. Poor patient preparation can result in delays, cancellations, and frustration for the patient, companion, and ASC staff.

Upon arrival to the ASC on the appointment day, the patient and companion are greeted and proceed to the preparation area, and the patient changes into a gown. A nursing assessment of the patient includes a general health history with specific attention to any GI, cardiac, respiratory, and endocrine system problems; allergies both to medications and other agents; medication history and what medications have been taken on this day; bowel preparation (type and patient compliance with the regimen); NPO status; and adult companion present or available to escort patient home after the procedure. Height, weight, and vital signs, oxygen (O_2) saturation, and temperature are obtained. The physician should be alerted to any deviations from the patient's past history before the procedure. Assuring that the patient has had information related to advance directives (living will, durable power of attorney) may be required under specific state or institutional guidelines. An informed written consent that details the risks of the procedure is also obtained before the procedure. The nurse should be prepared to answer the patient's questions related to the procedure, including the risks and benefits of the procedure. If preprocedure testing (e.g., blood, ECG) has been ordered, these results need to be available and reviewed by the nurse, and report any abnormalities must be reported to the physician performing the procedure. Preprocedure laboratory tests and ECGs are not routinely ordered for GI endoscopy procedures but are based on patient specific needs. Laboratory test results and the ECG report are reviewed; the patient's level of consciousness is assessed, and a physical assessment of the abdomen is completed, focusing on any signs of tenderness, distention, or firmness. Patients are asked to remove all dentures and removable bridgework before an upper endoscopy procedure to prevent aspiration of or obstruction by the appliance. Facility policy may require that dentures be removed before all endoscopy procedures requiring sedation or analgesia. Jewelry, eyeglasses, contact lenses, hearing aids, and prostheses are removed or secured according to ASC policy. Once the patient is positioned on the stretcher or cart, siderails are placed in the up and locked position.

Patient teaching continues at this point. The nurse describes the next phase of the procedure and answers the patient's questions. Description of the sounds, sights, and smells may be helpful in reducing the patient's anxiety and alleviating fears. It is suggested that discharge instructions are reviewed with patients before they are sedated for the procedure.

An IV line using a small-gauge needle (22 to 24 gauge) is usually initiated in the preprocedure area, maintaining venous access with a keep-open line of 5% dextrose in water (D_5W) or normal saline (NS). Location of the IV is determined by the procedure and physician preference. The IV is started using the ASC standard procedure.

The physician should be consulted about orders for antibiotics or any other medications or blood products. Patients with histories of mitral valve prolapse; prosthetic heart valves; or noncardiac prosthetic devices (e.g., artificial joint replacements, arterial grafts, and peritoneal shunts) and patients who are immunosuppressed

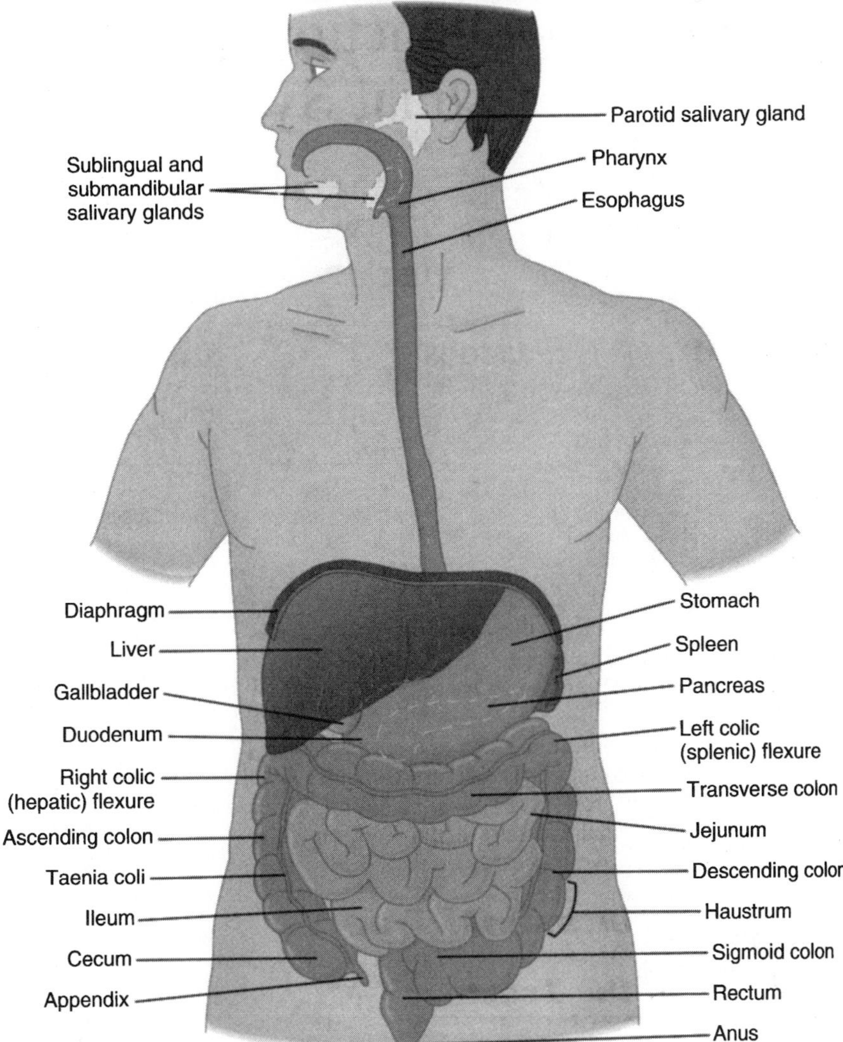

Figure 38–1. The digestive system, showing the path available through the gastrointestinal system for endoscopy. (From Black JM, Matassarin-Jacobs E: Medical-Surgical Nursing: Clinical Management for Continuity of Care, 5th ed. Philadelphia: WB Saunders, 1997, p 1686.)

from drugs or disease may receive prophylactic antibiotic therapy before their procedures. Tables 38–5 to 38–9 delineate current antibiotic prophylaxis recommendations from the American Society of Gastrointestinal Endoscopy[13] and the American Heart Association.[14]

If preparation takes place in the procedure room, the patient may ambulate to the room; otherwise, the patient is transported to the procedure room on a stretcher with appropriate coverings for warmth and dignity and with the siderails up and locked for safety.

Intraprocedure Care

The nurse prepares the appropriate equipment for the scheduled procedure according to ASC policy and procedure and Society of Gastroenterology Nurses and Associates (SGNA) standards.[15] Monitoring equipment including noninvasive blood pressure monitor, cardiac monitor, and pulse oximeter are available. Oxygen, suction and emergency equipment are immediately available.

After the patient is identified, records checked, and consent confirmed, the nurse further explains the procedure and reassures the patient. If the procedure requires topical anesthesia application to the throat to obtund the gag reflex and decrease the discomfort of the passage of the endoscope, the anesthetic is given. Patients who can tolerate a sitting position can have their throat sprayed with topical anesthetic or can gargle and expectorate viscous

Table 38–5. **ASGE Recommendations for Antibiotic Prophylaxis for Endoscopic Procedures**

PATIENT CONDITION	PROCEDURE CONTEMPLATED	ANTIBIOTIC PROPHYLAXIS	COMMENTS
Prosthetic valve, Hx endocarditis, systemic-pulmonary shunt, synthetic vascular graft (less than 1 yr old)	Stricture dilation, varix sclerosis ERCP/ obstructed biliary tree	Recommended	High-risk conditions for development of infectious complication; procedures are associated with relatively high bacteremia rates
	Other endoscopic procedures, including EGD and colonoscopy (with or without biopsy/ polypectomy), variceal ligation	Insufficient data to make firm recommendation; endoscopists may choose on case-by-case basis	While conditions are high-risk, procedures are associated with low rates of bacteremia
Cirrhosis and ascites, immunocompromised patient	Stricture dilation, varix sclerosis ERCP/ obstructed biliary tree	Insufficient data to make firm recommendation; endoscopists may choose on case-by-case basis	Risk for infectious complications related to endoscopic procedures not established
	Other endoscopic procedures, including EGD and colonoscopy (with or without biopsy/ polypectomy), variceal ligation	Not recommended	Procedures are associated with relatively low bacteremia rates
All patients	Endoscopic feeding tube placement	Prophylaxis recommended*	May decrease risk of soft tissue infection
Prosthetic joints	Any endoscopic procedure	Not recommended	No literature to support infectious risk from endoscopic procedures
Rheumatic valvular dysfunction Mitral valve prolapse with insufficiency Hypertrophic cardiomyopathy Most congenital cardiac malformations	Stricture dilation, varix sclerosis ERCP/ obstructed biliary tree	Insufficient data to make firm recommendation; endoscopists may choose on case-by-case basis	Conditions pose lesser risk for infectious complications than prosthetic valve, etc.
	Other endoscopic procedures, including EGD and colonoscopy (with or without biopsy/ polypectomy), variceal ligation	Not recommended	Procedures are associated with relatively low bacteremia rates
Other cardiac conditions (including CABG, pacemakers, implantable defibrillators)	All endoscopic procedures	Not recommended	Conditions are low risk for infectious complications from endoscopic procedures
Obstructed bile duct, pancreatic pseudocyst	ERCP	Recommended	Prudent, but not substitute for definitive drainage

*An acceptable prophylaxis regimen is parenteral ampicillin 2 g and gentamicin 1.5 mg/kg (up to 80 mg) 30 min before the procedure, followed by amoxicillin 1.5 g orally 6 hours after the procedure. Vancomycin 1 g IV is substituted for the penicillin allergic patient.

Note: A summary of the recommendations and comments made in the 1995 guideline on Antibiotic Prophylaxis for Endoscopic Procedures is presented below. There are insufficient data and lack of expert consensus to provide definitive recommendations in certain circumstances. Other factors, including the preferences of patients and referring physicians, must also be considered. It is strongly recommended that each endoscopy unit or center develop a policy appropriate for its specific practice. These recommendations may serve as a template for this process.

From the Standards of Practice Committee of ASGE. Gastrointest Endosc 195:630–635.

lidocaine solution. Simethicone suspension may also be given to the patient at this time to reduce flatus development. The patient is positioned in the left lateral position for most upper and lower GI procedures.

Some degree of sedation is generally necessary to complete the endoscopic procedure. Medications often used for endoscopy include midazolam, diazepam, meperidine, and fentanyl. The medications are given intravenously by the nurse or physician immediately prior to or at the initiation of the procedure. Medication types and doses are documented on the nursing procedure record. When patients receive sedation and analgesia, nurses should follow appropriate guidelines such as those found in the "Practice Guidelines for Sedation and Analgesia by Non-anesthesiologists"[16] and "Guidelines for Nursing Care of the Patient Receiving Sedation and Analgesia in the GI Endoscopy Setting."[17]

***Table 38–6.* Cardiac Conditions Associated With Endocarditis**[2–22]

ENDOCARDITIS PROPHYLAXIS RECOMMENDED

High-risk category
- Prosthetic cardiac valves, including bioprosthetic and homograft valves
- Previous bacterial endocarditis
- Complex cyanotic congenital heart disease (single ventricle states, transposition of the great arteries, tetralogy of Fallot)
- Surgically constructed systemic pulmonary shunts or conduits

Moderate-risk category
- Most other congenital cardiac malformations (other than those listed here)
- Acquired valvar dysfunction (rheumatic heart disease)
- Hypertrophic cardiomyopathy
- Mitral valve prolapse with valvar regurgitation and/or thickened leaflets

ENDOCARDITIS PROPHYLAXIS NOT RECOMMENDED

Negligible-risk category (no greater risk than the general population)
- Isolated secundum atrial septal defect
- Surgical repair of atrial septal defect, ventricular septal defect, or patent ductus arteriosus (without residua beyond 6 mo)
- Previous coronary artery bypass graft surgery
- Mitral valve prolapse without valvar regurgitation
- Physiologic, functional, or innocent heart murmurs
- Previous Kawasaki disease without valvar dysfunction
- Previous rheumatic fever without valvar dysfunction
- Cardiac pacemakers (intravascular and epicardial) and implanted defibrillators

From Dajani AS, Taubert KA, Wilson W, et al: Prevention of bacterial endocarditis: Recommendations by the American Heart Association. JAMA 277:1794–1801, 1997.

Physiologic monitoring of the patient during the procedure includes monitoring blood pressure, heart rate, respiratory rate, oxygen saturation, level of consciousness, pain assessment, and skin color and temperature. ECG monitoring is done according to unit criteria. The criteria should consider age and American Society of Anesthesiologists physical status classification. Depending on ASC policy, patients will either receive supplemental oxygen during the procedure or have it immediately available for use when pulse oximetry indicates a decrease in saturation and stimulation of the patient does not result in an increase in oxygen saturation. O'Connor and Jones studied oxygen desaturation in patients undergoing elective endoscopic procedures.[18] They found that desaturation could not be predicted based on age, medication (sedative and analgesia dose), or the patient's preprocedure oxygen saturation.

Upon completion of the procedure, documentation is completed related to all events and patient status during the procedure, including the following: ECG pattern (if indicated), respiratory status, oxygen saturation, vital signs, discomfort or pain, secretions, signs of obvious distress, shortness of breath, chest pain, abdominal pain, oral or rectal bleeding, hypotension, or dysrhythmias. Although not intended for routine use, naloxone (Narcan) and flumazenil (Romazicon), reversal agents for narcotics and benzodiazepines, respectively, should be immediately available for reversal of sedation as needed, along with resuscitative equipment, oxygen, IV fluids, and emergency drugs.

The procedure, biopsy specimens obtained, type and amount of fluids infused, medications

***Table 38–7.* Other Procedures and Endocarditis Prophylaxis**

ENDOCARDITIS PROPHYLAXIS RECOMMENDED

Respiratory tract
- Tonsillectomy or adenoidectomy
- Surgical operations that involve respiratory mucosa
- Bronchoscopy with a rigid bronchoscope

Gastrointestinal tract*
- Sclerotherapy for esophageal varices
- Esophageal stricture dilatation
- Endoscopic retrograde cholangiography with biliary obstruction
- Biliary tract surgery
- Surgical operations that involve intestinal mucosa

Genitourinary tract
- Prostatic surgery
- Cystoscopy
- Urethral dilatation

ENDOCARDITIS PROPHYLAXIS NOT RECOMMENDED

Respiratory tract
- Endotracheal intubation
- Bronchoscopy with a flexible bronchoscope, with or without biopsy†
- Tympanostomy tube insertion

Gastrointestinal tract
- Transesophageal echocardiography†
- Endoscopy with or without gastrointestinal biopsy†

Genitourinary tract
- Vaginal hysterectomy†
- Vaginal delivery†
- Cesarean section in uninfected tissue:
  - Urethral catheterization
  - Uterine dilatation and curettage
  - Therapeutic abortion
  - Sterilization procedures
  - Insertion or removal of intrauterine devices

Other
- Cardiac catheterization, including balloon angioplasty
- Implanted cardiac pacemakers, implanted defibrillators, and coronary stents
- Incision or biopsy of surgically scrubbed skin
- Circumcision

*Prophylaxis is recommended for high-risk patients; optional for medium-risk patients.

†Prophylaxis is optional for high-risk patients.

From Dajani AS, Taubert KA, Wilson W, et al: Prevention of bacterial endocarditis: Recommendations by the American Heart Association. JAMA 277:1794–1801, 1997.

***Table 38–8.* Prophylactic Regimens for Dental, Oral, Respiratory Tract, or Esophageal Procedures**

SITUATION	AGENT	REGIMEN*
Standard general prophylaxis	Amoxicillin	Adults: 2 g; children: 50 mg/kg orally 1 hr before procedure
Unable to take oral medications	Ampicillin	Adults: 2 g intramuscularly (IM) or intravenously (IV); children: 50 mg/kg IM or IV within 30 min before procedure
Allergic to penicillin	Clindamycin	Adults: 600 mg; children: 20 mg/kg orally 1 hr before procedure
	or Cephalexin† or cefadroxil†	Adults: 2 g; children: 50 mg/kg orally 1 hr before procedure
	or Azithromycin or clarithromycin	Adults: 500 mg; children: 15 mg/kg orally 1 hr before procedure
Allergic to penicillin and unable to take oral medications	Clindamycin	Adults: 600 mg; children: 20 mg/kg IV within 30 min before procedure
	or Cefazolin†	Adults: 1 g; children: 25 mg/kg IM or IV within 30 min before procedure

*The total child's dose should not exceed the adult dose.

†Cephalosporins should not be used for individuals who have an immediate type of hypersensitivity reaction (urticaria, angioedema, or anaphylaxis) to penicillins.

From Dajani AS, Taubert KA, Wilson W, et al: Prevention of bacterial endocarditis: Recommendations by the American Heart Association. JAMA 277:1794–1801, 1997.

given including dosage, patient tolerance to the procedure, and unusual events that occurred during the procedure are documented on the nursing record. Documentation also includes the names of the healthcare personnel in attendance and the types of instruments used for the procedure. Specimens are checked for proper labeling, and laboratory requisitions are completed appropriately. The nurse transports the patient to the appropriate ASC postprocedure recovery area, PACU Phase II, and gives an oral report to the receiving nurse. PACU Phase I is required only if the patient has received anesthesia.

Equipment used for the procedure is cleaned with a high-level disinfectant. High-level disinfection is the recommend standard of care for reprocessing GI endoscopes. Accessory instruments that break the mucosal barrier require sterilization. Those that do not break the mucosal barrier require high-level disinfection. The SGNA "Standards for Infection Control and Reprocessing of Flexible Gastrointestinal Endoscopes" and the SGNA videotape on "Reprocessing Gastrointestinal Endoscopes" offer comprehensive guidelines for reprocessing.[19] Manufacturer's instructions detailing specific features of their instruments and the reprocessing protocol for each instruments should be known and followed.[20]

Meticulous manual cleaning is the first and most important step in the reprocessing of endoscopic equipment. Manual cleaning includes washing the instrument in an enzymatic detergent, brushing all appropriate channels, rinsing, and drying. These steps are required prior to placing the instrument into a liquid chemical germicide to achieve high-level disinfection. Even if an automated reprocessor is used, all the steps of manual cleaning must be done before placing the instrument into the reprocessor.[20]

The most widely used liquid chemical germicide for reprocessing GI endoscopes is a 2% glutaraldehyde 14-day product without surfactants. An exposure time of 20 minutes with 2% glutaraldehyde at room temperature that has tested above its minimum concentration level will achieve high-level disinfection. Peracetic acid used in the STERIS System is another alternative chemical germicide. The only circumstance in which sterilization of the endoscope is required is for use in a sterile operative field. Two additional liquid chemical germicides recently have been cleared by the FDA and are being marketed for reprocessing GI endoscopes. These new products are Sporox, a hydrogen peroxide solution, marketed by Reckitt and Coleman, and Cidex PA, a peracetic acid solution, which is marketed by Advanced Sterilization Systems. There is limited information available concerning use of Sporox and Cidex PA in the GI endoscopy setting. Proper storage of thoroughly cleaned and disinfected scopes is necessary to prevent recontamination or damage. Endoscopes should be hung vertically in a ventilated, enclosed storage cabinet. Accessories

***Table 38–9.* Prophylactic Regimens for Genitourinary Gastrointestinal (Excluding Esophageal) Procedures**

SITUATION	AGENTS*	REGIMEN†
High-risk patients	Ampicillin plus gentamicin	Adults: ampicillin 2 g intramuscularly (IM) or intravenously (IV) plus gentamicin 1.5 mg/kg (not to exceed 120 mg) within 30 min of starting the procedure; 6 hr later, ampicillin 1 g IM/IV or amoxicillin 1 g orally Children: ampicillin 50 mg/kg IM or IV (not to exceed 2 g) plus gentamicin 1.5 mg/kg within 30 min of starting the procedure; 6 hr later, ampicillin 25 mg/kg IM/IV or amoxicillin 25 mg/kg orally
High-risk patients allergic to ampicillin/amoxicillin	Vancomycin plus gentamicin	Adults: vancomycin 1 g IV over 1–2 hr plus gentamicin 1.5 mg/kg IV/IM (not to exceed 120 mg); complete injection/infusion within 30 min of starting the procedure Children: vancomycin 20 mg/kg IV over 1–2 hr plus gentamicin 1.5 mg/kg IV/IM; complete injection/infusion within 30 min of starting the procedure
Moderate-risk patients	Amoxicillin or ampicillin	Adults: amoxicillin 2 g orally 1 hr before procedure, or ampicillin 2 g IM/IV within 30 min of starting the procedure Children: amoxicillin 50 mg/kg orally 1 hr before procedure, or ampicillin 50 mg/kg IM/IV within 30 min of starting the procedure
Moderate-risk patients allergic to ampicillin/amoxicillin	Vancomycin	Adults: vancomycin 1 g IV over 1–2 hr complete infusion within 30 min of starting the procedure Children: vancomycin 20 mg/kg IV over 1–2 hr, complete infusion within 30 min of starting the procedure

*Total child's dose should not exceed the adult dose.

†No second dose of vancomycin or gentamicin is recommended.

From Dajani AS, Taubert KA, Wilson W, et al: Prevention of bacterial endocarditis: Recommendations by the American Heart Association. JAMA 277:1794–1801, 1997.

used, such as biopsy forceps (sterilized), water bottles (sterilization recommended), and mouthpieces should be cleaned and disinfected according to manufacturer's instructions and ASC policy. The procedure room is cleaned prior to use by the next patient according to the ASC policy.

All personnel who are responsible for reprocessing endoscopes and accessories require detailed knowledge of the instruments and specific reprocessing methods required to produce instruments safe for use. This knowledge is obtained through repetition and under the guidance of a preceptor. Competency testing during orientation and annually to assure skill and knowledge is recommended. Each area should limit those responsible for reprocessing to those who have completed their competency testing.[20]

Postprocedure Care

Upon arrival in the postprocedure recovery area, the patient's vital signs, including oxygen saturation and level of consciousness, are obtained and documented. Institutional policy and patient condition dictate the need for further ECG monitoring. Supplemental oxygen by nasal cannula or face mask is initiated as indicated by oxygen saturation and the patient's status and vital signs. Postprocedure scoring, like the postanesthesia recovery score used in a PACU, may also be used to assess the patient and to compare with a preprocedure score for added value in assessment.

Major complications of endoscopy include adverse reactions to analgesics and sedatives, viscous or vessel perforation, and hemorrhage that can occur during, immediately after the procedure, or hours later.[21–23] Vital signs including oxygen saturation are monitored every 15 minutes or more often, as indicated by the patient's condition. Temperature is monitored as indicated. Signs of perforation and hemorrhage include severe or increasing pain, increased temperature, abdominal distention, subcutaneous emphysema, shortness of breath, hypotension, diaphoresis, and obvious bleeding. The patient's level of consciousness and orientation to surroundings should be periodically assessed, and the IV infusion is maintained according to ASC policy and physician preference.

Patients who have received sedation, analgesia, and reversal agents require special attention. Reversal agents may have shorter durations of action than do the sedatives and narcotics they reverse.[24] Patients who have been stimulated during procedures may arrive in the recovery area alert and with stable vital signs. Within a short time and without verbal or tactile stimulation, the patient may "renarcotize" or return to a sedated state. Close monitoring of respiratory status, blood pressure, heart rate, and level of consciousness are necessary to avoid complications. Additional reversal agents may be required, and monitoring and recovery of the patient may be prolonged.

For patients who have had upper GI endoscopies, the gag reflex can be assessed afterward with a tongue blade or swab before giving the patient fluids to drink. Generally, the gag reflex returns within 1 hour of the procedure, depending on the type of topical anesthetic used. It is also important to determine if the patient has any other tests scheduled that require NPO status. Checks with the patient and the patient's record supply this information.

Patient safety continues as a concern for the nurse. Siderails should be up, and the patient should be positioned not only for comfort but, depending on level of consciousness, for safety. The sedated esophagogastroduodenoscopy (EGD) patient is generally positioned flat, in a left lateral position, to facilitate drainage of oral secretions and prevent aspiration. Following esophageal dilation or sclerotherapy, the patient may be placed in a semi-Fowler or high Fowler position for comfort and improved respiratory exchange. The colonoscopy patient may be positioned on either side or on the back, depending on the patient's level of sedation.

After a stay of 30 minutes to 1 hour in the postprocedure recovery area, the patient will usually be ready for discharge, provided the ASC discharge criteria for endoscopy patients are met. The patient should be able to move all extremities as well as before the procedure and should tolerate oral fluids (gag reflex returned) with little or no nausea or vomiting. Pain or discomfort related to the procedure should be minimal, and vital signs and level of consciousness should be stable and consistent with preprocedure levels for the patient to be ready for discharge.

Minor complaints such as throat irritation or hoarseness can be treated with anesthetic throat lozenges or saline gargles. The IV site should be observed and its status documented (i.e., clear, swollen or edematous, reddened or erythematous, complaints of pain at the site by the patient). Bloating and flatus can add to the patient's discomfort. Ambulation and position changes may help relieve distention. Discharge instructions specific for the aftercare of the procedure are reviewed with the patient and companion. Information about diet, medications, activity, emergencies, and follow-up care as determined by the patient's physician are discussed with the patient and companion, both of whom should be able to demonstrate their understanding to the nurse. A copy of the instructions given to the patient is attached to the patient's medical record.

Complications such as bleeding can occur after the patient has left the ASC. Nurses need to explain the potential for postprocedure bleeding, and patients should be instructed to call their physicians or go immediately to a nearby emergency room if complications develop. Bleeding of more than 1 tablespoon, either orally or rectally, or persistent bleeding requires the physician's attention.

The effects of the sedation given for the procedure are explained again, and patients are cautioned not to drive, operate machinery, bathe, swim, drink alcohol, or sign legal documents for a minimum of 12 to 24 hours after the procedure. These times vary by the amount and type of the sedation or analgesia received and by policy of the ASC. Because the findings of the examination and procedure can be potentially life changing, support, reassurance, and appropriate tone and manner are valued by the patients and their companions.

The patient is discharged to the care of a responsible adult companion. A follow-up telephone call on the next day can benefit the patient and ASC staff. The postendoscopic evaluation could include questions related to nausea and vomiting, bleeding, temperature elevation, pain, medication taken and relief afforded, IV site problems, and patient satisfaction with the care received. The follow-up telephone call has numerous benefits, including quality improvement, infection control, good public relations and staff encouragement.[25]

Specific Endoscopy Procedures

Esophagogastroduodenoscopy

Esophagogastroduodenoscopy (EGD) is the examination of the esophagus, stomach, and duodenum with a flexible fiberoptic or video endoscope. For EGD, the endoscope is passed through the oral cavity into the esophagus, stomach, and duodenum.

Indications. Upper endoscopy is often performed on patients with symptoms of dysphagia, recurring indigestion, persistent anemia, regurgitation, substernal pain, and odynophagia (pain upon swallowing). EGD is also used to diagnose esophagitis, hiatal hernia, esophageal varices, esophageal stenosis, achalasia, gastritis, ulcers, neoplasms and obstructive lesions, hemorrhage, diverticula, duodenal ulcers, and foreign bodies.[21, 23, 26]

Preparation. Patients are to have nothing to eat or drink (NPO) for 4 to 8 hours before the procedure. Anesthetic throat spray or gargle and IV sedation are given as ordered by the physician.[27]

Potential Complications. Most patients undergoing EGD receive sedation/analgesia. Patients are at risk for hypotension, cardiac arrhythmias or arrest, respiratory depression or arrest, and drug reactions due to the sedation/analgesia. Other complications include aspiration, infection, hemorrhage, and perforation. Symptoms of perforation include pain, dyspnea, fever, tachycardia, dysphagia, and subcutaneous emphysema in the neck or chest.[23, 28] Crepitus in the neck and pain in the neck or throat can indicate perforation at the cervical level. Substernal or epigastric pain, cyanosis, pleural effusion, and back pain may be signs of a mid-esophageal perforation. A distal esophageal perforation may result in shoulder pain, dyspnea, and symptoms similar to those of a perforated ulcer.[29]

Special Care. The patient should be observed for substernal or epigastric pain, fever, and other signs of perforation and hemorrhage. Vital signs are monitored according to ASC policy. Deeply sedated patients should be positioned and monitored to prevent aspiration of secretions. NPO status is maintained until gag reflex returns. Bloating or gastric distention is common from insufflation during the procedure, and eructation generally relieves this discomfort.

Esophageal Dilatation

Esophageal dilatation is the mechanical stretching or dilating of the esophagus to relieve strictures that prevent or inhibit the passage of food or fluids to the stomach.

Indications. The procedure is intended for relief of esophageal stricture, esophageal web, diffuse esophageal spasm, or scleroderma causing dysphagia or pain. A stricture can have many causes, including peptic esophagitis due to gastroesophageal reflux, nasogastric tubes, Barrett's epithelium and ulcer formation, ingestion of corrosive substances, acute viral or bacterial diseases, sclerotherapy of varices, and rarely, injuries caused by endoscopes.[30, 31] Various types of dilators are used: tungsten-filled (formerly mercury-filled) flexible rubber (Maloney or Hurst), thermoplastic (Savary), hydrostatic balloon, and pneumatic balloon, depending on the etiology and location of the stricture. Postprocedure pain and its severity are variable, depending on the type of dilator used. Maloney or Hurst dilatations do not require endoscopy placement of the dilatation device. Savary, pneumatic dilatation, and hydrostatic balloon dilatation require endoscopy.[27]

Preparation. Preparation is the same as for EGD or gastroscopy plus adjustments to the patient's anticoagulation therapy; nonsteroidal anti-inflammatory drug (NSAID) therapy is indicated. Preprocedure prothombin time should be within normal range.

Potential Complications. Hemorrhage or perforation may be indicated by tachycardia, substernal or epigastric or abdominal pain, fever, and subcutaneous emphysema. Symptoms should be reported to the physician immediately. An esophagogram with contrast dye or a chest x-ray film may be ordered to determine if air in the mediastinum indicates perforation.[28] The patient will require preparation for operative intervention if repair of the perforation or bleeding control is needed. Other potential complications include bacteremia and aspiration.

Special Care. The patient is usually positioned in semi- or high Fowler's position after the procedure to improve respiratory effort and control secretions. Monitoring of respiratory status is essential, and the nurses should reassure the patient that substernal pain or discomfort will decrease. An analgesic or sedative to control pain and anxiety may be necessary after the patient is assessed and the physician determines the course of medical treatment.

Sclerotherapy

Sclerotherapy involves the endoscopic injection of the esophageal varix or the surrounding mucosa with sclerosing agent (e.g., sodium morrhuate, tetradecasulfate, or absolute alcohol). The vein wall is initially inflamed after injection, then fibrosed and thrombosed. Repeated injections over a period of weeks or months may be needed to eradicate or reduce the varices.[21, 29] This procedure is performed both during an acute phase of variceal bleeding to control the bleeding and prophylactically to prevent variceal rebleeding.

Indications. Sclerotherapy is indicated for management of acute hemorrhage from esophageal varices in patients pending "shunt" surgery or for patients who are poor surgical risks. It is also used to eradicate esophageal varices to prevent rebleeding and as a temporary measure to control acute hemorrhage from gastric varices.

Preparation. Preparation is the same for EGD or gastroscopy, including the following: (1) establish a large-bore IV line, and (2) obtain a complete blood cell count (CBC) and type and cross-match if ordered.

Potential Complications. These complications include esophageal perforation, chest pain, mucosal ulcerations, necrosis of the esophagus, sepsis, hemorrhage, esophageal strictures, aspiration, pleural effusions, and portal vein thrombosis.[21, 32]

Special Care. Monitoring includes assessment of the level of comfort, respiratory status, and observation for and management of GI bleeding and perforation.

Endoscopic Variceal Ligation

Endoscopic variceal ligation (EVL) is an additional technique developed in the past 10 years for the treatment of esophageal varices. This technique is as effective as sclerotherapy in controlling active esophageal bleeding. EVL can achieve variceal obliteration in three to four sessions compared with the five or six sessions required for sclerotherapy. The rebleeding rate of EVL is 25% compared with the rebleeding rate of 40% with sclerotherapy. EVL has been used prophylactically to prevent the first variceal bleed.

Indications. The indications are the same as for sclerotherapy.

Preparation. The patient who is not actively bleeding is prepared the same as for an EGD. The actively bleeding patient may be concurrently treated with infusions of vasoconstrictive agents.[48] The nurse will support and monitor these hemodynamically unstable patients as the patient's condition indicates. In addition, the multiband ligator should be prepared for use. A single-band ligator is indicated for patients who would require only one banding. The usual technique for non-bleeding columns is to band just at or below the gastroesophageal junction and proceed cephalad. For small varices, one ligation at the distal esophagus is adequate. Larger varices require a second ligation within a couple of inches above the first ligation site. An average of 5 to 10 ligations are usually performed in the initial session with fewer ligations performed in subsequent sessions. For bleeding varices, the ligations are first performed at or near the bleeding site and then progress to other areas of the bleeding column and to other columns. If the bleeding is not controlled after the first banding session or rebleeding occurs, a second session may be attempted. Balloon tamponade and transjugular portosystemic stent shunt (TIPS) may be required if the previous techniques for controlling bleeding are not effective.[49]

Complications. The overall complication rate of EVL is 5%. Transient substernal pain may last for 24 to 48 hours after the procedure. The more serious complications are bleeding from ligation-induced ulcers, bacteremia, peritonitis, pneumonia, and esophageal laceration due to the passage of an overtube. The overtube is used with the single-band ligator but is not needed with multiple band ligators. Stricture formation in the esophagus is significantly less compared with sclerotherapy.[50–52]

Colonoscopy

Colonoscopy is the examination of the entire colon with a flexible fiberoptic or video endoscope. Biopsy, polypectomy, and electrocautery of bleeding lesions may be performed. Specimens for cytologic, microbiologic, and histologic evaluation may be obtained.

Indications. Colonoscopy can be used for diagnosis of an abnormality found on x-ray examination, unexplained iron deficiency anemia, surveillance for colonic neoplasm, follow-up for prior polypectomy, malignancy, and sometimes treatment of conditions such as inflammatory bowel disease (ulcerative colitis or Crohn's disease), lower GI bleeding, malignancies, strictures, and polyps.[21] Patients may present with a variety of symptoms, including diarrhea, constipation, pain, or bleeding.

Preparation. Various bowel preparations are used, depending on physician preference and patient needs. One requires drinking 4 to 6 L of an isosmolar electrolyte lavage solution such as Colyte or GoLYTELY beginning the day before the procedure. Patients may complain of nausea, vomiting, and hypothermia during and after this type of preparation. Another approach uses sodium biphosphate oral laxative (Fleet's Phospho-Soda) the evening before and again on the morning of the procedure.[21] Magnesium citrate solution by mouth along with a bisacodyl (Dulcolax) suppository may be used as a preparation for selected patients. Generally, a clear liquid diet is allowed with all of these protocols. A clean bowel is essential for a complete colonoscopy examination. A repeat examination may be required if the bowel is not adequately prepared. Incomplete examinations and cancellations of the procedure are frequently due to inadequate bowel preparation.

Blood studies, although not routine, may be indicated for selected patients before the procedure. These studies may include hemoglobin, hematocrit, prothrombin time, partial thromboplastin time, and platelet count, especially for patients expected to undergo biopsy, polypectomy, or electrocautery resection of lesions in which bleeding may be a problem.

Potential Complications. Respiratory depression or arrest, cardiac arrhythmias or arrest, and hypotension are potential complications of colonoscopy.[21] Bleeding and perforation of the colon are also risks.[21] Excessive rectal bleeding or severe cramps should be reported immediately. Perforation is a rare but serious complication. Abdominal distention may be significant. If position changes and the expulsion of flatus do not relieve distention, the physician should be notified.

Special Care. The patient is monitored as above and is observed for rectal bleeding, discomfort, pain, abdominal distention, abnormal breathing, or distress. Positioning is for comfort. If a polypectomy has been performed during which the polyp is not retrieved, the physician may order straining of all stools for polyp retrieval.

Sigmoidoscopy

A sigmoidoscopy is an examination of the sigmoid colon, usually up to 25 cm with a rigid scope or up to 65 cm with a flexible fiberoptic or video endoscope. It is most frequently done with no sedation or analgesia, although an anesthetic lubricant may be used to insert the sigmoidoscope. Rigid proctoscopy or sigmoidoscopy is still performed if disease is suspected in the anorectal region. Rigid instrumentation can be more traumatic for the patient due to awkward positioning and greater risk of bleeding due to larger biopsies.

Indications. Flexible sigmoidoscopy is indicated for screening for colon cancer and for screening in the presence of a strong family history of colorectal cancer or polyps. It is indicated for the evaluation of suspected distal colonic disease, inflammatory bowel disease, chronic diarrhea, pseudomembraneous colitis, sigmoid volvulus, foreign body removal, and lower GI bleeding.[27]

Preparation. A saline or warm tap water or bisacodyl (Fleet) enema may be ordered approximately 2 to 3 hours before the examination. A usual preparation is two bisacodyl (Fleet's) enemas with no dietary restrictions.

Potential Complications. Bowel perforation and bleeding are the most significant complications of sigmoidoscopy, along with complaints of pain, abdominal distention, and shock-like symptoms (increase in blood pressure, decrease in heart rate, pallor, or nausea). Patients may also experience vasovagal stimulation with symptoms of hypotension, bradycardia, diaphoresis, and pallor. The physician should be notified immediately if the patient experiences any of these symptoms after sigmoidoscopy.

Special Care. The patient is observed and monitored according to the ASC standard procedure. Insufflated air during the procedure causes uncontrollable flatus, so the usually alert patient needs supportive reassurance and a private area in which to expel the flatus without embarrassment.

Endoscopic Retrograde Cholangiopancreatography

Endoscopic retrograde cholangiopancreatography (ERCP) is a diagnostic and sometimes therapeutic procedure performed with a side-viewing fiberoptic or video duodenoscope. The pancreatic and biliary ducts are cannulated through the ampulla of Vater and visualized fluoroscopically after retrograde injection of radiopaque contrast medium. Radiographs of the biliary and pancreatic ductal anatomy and direct visualization of the duodenum and periampullary mucosa are possible. Therapeutic ERCP may also be performed, including biliary manometry, sphincterotomy, insertion and removal of biliary stents and drains, dilatation of the pancreatic and biliary ducts, stone lithotripsy, and stone removal.

Indications. ERCP is performed for the evaluation of jaundice, pancreatitis, or persistent abdominal pain; to diagnose cancers of the duodenal papilla, pancreatic or biliary ducts; to identify and treat retained calculi or stenosis of ducts; and to identify extra- and intrahepatic biliary tract disease.[32, 33] It can be employed for evaluation of the biliary system and in an attempt to remove calculi from the common duct before or after a laparoscopic cholecystectomy.

Preparation. Blood studies are patient-specific and may include complete blood cell count, coagulation factors, and liver and enzyme studies. The patient is NPO from midnight. The following medications may be given: (1) topical anesthetic to anesthetize the oral pharynx; (2) antispasmodics (glucagon, atropine) when the hepatopancreatic ampulla is cannulated; (3) IV sedatives and analgesics; (4) an antiflatulant added to the endoscope water bottle or given orally to prevent formation of bile bubbles, which interfere with visualization of intestinal landmarks during the procedure.[33–35]

Potential complications are the same as during other endoscopic procedures with the addition of sepsis, cholangitis (fever, chills, hyperbilirubinemia, hypotension, and gram-negative septicemia), and pancreatitis (upper left quadrant pain, tenderness, elevated serum amylase, and transient hyperbilirubinemia).[27, 32, 34]

Special Care. Nurses monitor and observe vital signs, temperature, and level of comfort and assess gag reflex before giving fluids postprocedure. The patient may complain of colicky abdominal pain for several hours after the procedure and drowsiness from being sedated. The pain should subside after the patient begins eating and drinking.[33] Instructions include telling patients to notify their physicians immediately if they develop prolonged and severe abdominal pain, a temperature greater than 99°F (37.2°C), chills, tachycardia, or nausea and vomiting.[33]

Other Gastrointestinal Procedures

Liver biopsy and paracentesis require sterile technique and local anesthetic. They are often done in the endoscopy suite. These procedures demand careful patient education and preparation to ensure the desired outcome.

Preprocedure preparation is similar to that of the endoscopy patient. After baseline vital signs, including temperature, are obtained, the patient is positioned appropriately for the procedure. Sterile technique is maintained. During the procedure the patient is observed for signs of distress and is supported emotionally.

Following the procedure, the wound site is dressed with a sterile pressure dressing, and the site is observed for bleeding. Specimens are labeled and sent to the laboratory for examination. The liver biopsy patient is transferred to the Phase II PACU for observation. Physical and emotional status including vital signs, temperature, level of consciousness, comfort, and presence of bleeding are assessed. Complications, such as severe pain, fever, and hemorrhage, are reported to the physician immediately.

The liver biopsy patient requires a minimum of 4 hours of recovery time. The patient is discharged with instructions. Discharge should be into the care of a responsible adult who will drive the patient home. The patient should have no complaints of respiratory distress, no bleeding, stable vital signs, and little pain or tenderness at the biopsy or puncture site before discharge.

Liver Biopsy

Liver biopsy is the percutaneous, or closed, retrieval of liver tissue for histologic analysis.

Indications. Liver biopsy is performed to assess acute and chronic jaundice, viral hepatitis and its sequelae, cirrhosis and portal hypertension, drug-related liver disease, unexplained hepatomegaly or abnormalities of liver function, infiltrative neooplastic disease, response to therapy, Wilson's disease, and screening of relatives of patients with familial disease.[27] Post liver transplantation protocols require periodic liver biopsy.

Preparation. The patient is NPO for the procedure. Blood studies often performed before the procedure include hemoglobin and hematocrit, coagulation studies (prothrombin time <3 seconds above control, platelet count <100,000, partial thromboplastin time >20 seconds over control), and blood type and crossmatch, if indicated.[27] An IV line may be started according to ASC policy.

Procedure. The conventional method of biopsy is a blind procedure called the Menghini technique. The patient is in a supine or left lateral position, with the right arm abducted as illustrated in Figure 38–2. The physician will palpate the abdomen, percuss the liver, and mark the desired puncture site. After the skin is cleansed, it is anesthetized with lidocaine.

The nurse instructs the patient to inhale, exhale, and hold the breath for 15 seconds while the physician obtains the specimen. When the needle is removed, the specimen is placed in an appropriately labeled specimen container and sent to the laboratory. A sterile pressure dressing is applied to the site, and the patient is transferred to the recovery area in a right lateral decubitus position to provide continued pressure on the puncture site to promote hemostasis.

Complications. Hemorrhage, liver laceration, perforated gallbladder with or without bile peritonitis, bacteremia, pleurisy and perihepatitis, intrahepatic hepatoma and pneumothorax are potential complications of percutaneous liver biopsy.[27] The nurse observes for pneumothorax, hemorrhage, or tachycardia, and for

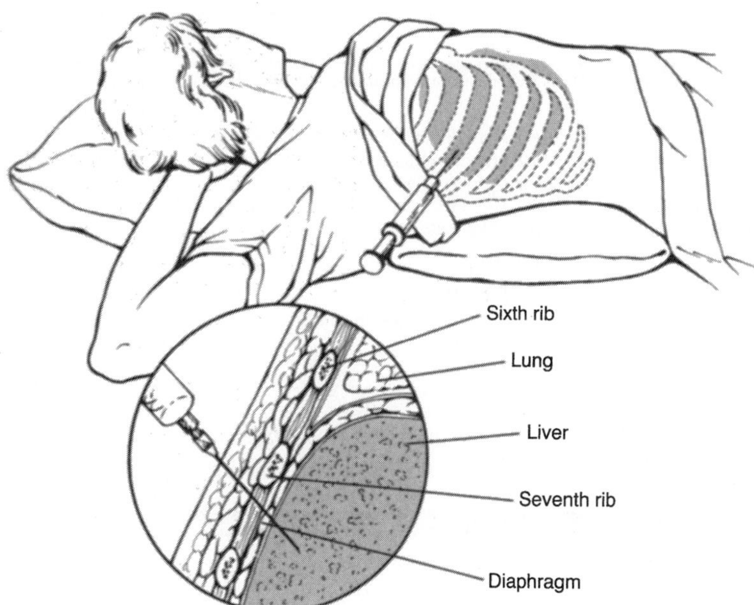

Figure 38–2. The patient is positioned for liver biopsy in a supine or left lateral position with the right arm abducted.

bradycardia and hypotension, which may be transient effects from vagal stimulation during procedure. The latter may be treated with atropine, supplemental C_2 and IV fluids.[21]

Special Care. Observation in the recovery area for 4 to 6 hours after the procedure is recommended. The patient is placed in a right lateral position to put pressure on the puncture site for a period of at least 4 hours after the procedure. Vital signs, temperature, respiratory effort, breath sounds, level of comfort, and bleeding are monitored frequently, for instance, every 15 minutes for 1 hour, then every 30 minutes for 1 hour, then every hour until discharge.

Patients may complain of shoulder pain requiring analgesics. Pain in the right upper quadrant may be due to a subcapsular accumulation of blood or bile, whereas right shoulder pain may result from blood on the undersurface of the diaphragm.[29] The physician should be notified of acute pain, bleeding, fever, or alterations in respiratory status. Discharge instructions specific to the procedure, such as those depicted in Figure 38–3, should be reviewed with the patient and adult companion before discharge from the ASC.

Abdominal Paracentesis

With a large-bore needle, syringe, or gravity drainage, peritoneal fluid for diagnostic and therapeutic purposes can be withdrawn during abdominal paracentesis.

Indications. In the ASC, paracentesis, an invasive treatment, may be used to relieve ascites. Excessive fluid may be causing abdominal pain or respiratory embarrassment such as dyspnea. Paracentesis is also used to evaluate ascites and diagnose perforated viscus following blunt trauma or symptoms of acute abdomen.

Preparation. The patient should void before the procedure.

Procedure. The patient is positioned in Fowler's position or sitting on the edge of the stretcher or cart with feet supported and arms supported on an overbed table. After the skin is cleansed and infiltrated with local anesthetic, a trocar is inserted into the lower abdomen and the ascitic fluid is drained slowly through a catheter into a collection container. Four to 6 L of fluid may be removed over 1 to 3 hours. Colloid replacement with albumin is recommended as an intravascular expander with large volume paracentesis.[21, 27] Culture of bacteria, cytologic testing, cell count, and determination of protein concentration are procedures that are performed on the fluid removed during paracentesis.[23] Upon completion of the procedure, a sterile dressing is applied to the puncture site. Vital signs are monitored and evaluated before discharge. The type and amount of fluid withdrawn are recorded, and fluid specimen are sent to the laboratory when indicated.[27]

Complications. Complications include leakage, fluid and electrolyte imbalances, hemorrhage, bowel perforation, hepatic encephalopathy, hypovolemia, shock, and infection.

Special Care. The patient is observed for leakage from the puncture site, subcutaneous emphysema, scrotal edema, fluid and electrolyte

DATE:

FOLLOW THE INSTRUCTIONS CHECKED BELOW

☐ Minimal physical activity (i.e. cooking and bathroom privileges) for 24 hours following your procedure. Avoid major motor travel and heavy labor for 24 hours following your liver biopsy. No contact sports for 2 weeks.

☐ Remove bandages and replace with fresh gauze or bandaids as needed.

☐ May resume tub bath/shower after 24 hours.

☐ Please call your doctor, Dr. ______________ at ______________ if you develop:

1. severe abdominal pain
2. fever (temperature greater than 100.6° F)
3. lightheadedness
4. vomiting of blood
5. persistent vomiting
6. severe shoulder pain
7. chest pain
8. shortness of breath
9. redness, swelling, redstreaking or pain at your intravenous injection site

If you cannot reach your physician, call (313) 936-6267 and ask for the GI fellow on call.

If you cannot reach a physician and your symptoms persist, go to the Emergency Room.

POST PROCEDURE DIET INSTRUCTIONS

☐ Resume your previous diet as tolerated.

☐ A special diet is recommended as follows: ______________

POST PROCEDURE MEDICATION / INSTRUCTIONS

☐ Resume your daily prescription medication schedule. Exceptions: ______________

Do not take aspirin of any type or non-steroidal anti-inflammatory medication for 48 hours (i.e. all ibuprofen products, Motrin, Advil, Nuprin, etc., Naprosyn, Clinoril, etc.).

☐ New Prescriptions: ______________

POST PROCEDURE BIOPSY FOLLOW UP

☐ A tiny piece of liver tissue (biopsy) has been removed during your procedure.

☐ Please contact Dr. ______________ at ______________ in one week for the pathology results of your liver biopsy.

☐ Follow-up evaluation may be required. Please contact Dr. ______________ at ______________ for a return visit.

☐ Other instructions: ______________

Your procedure has been done by Dr. ______________ **and Dr.** ______________

I hereby acknowledge receipt of the instructions above. I will arrange for follow-up care as instructed.

Physician's Signature/Date	Nurses's Signature/Date	Patient's Signature/Date

PS3538 Rev. 8/97 | PLY 1 – MEDICAL RECORD COPY PLY 2 – DEPARTMENT COPY | University of Michigan Medical Center | **LIVER BIOPSY DISCHARGE INSTRUCTIONS**

Figure 38–3. Liver biopsy discharge instructions. (From the University of Michigan Hospitals Medical Procedures Unit. Ann Arbor, 1997.)

imbalances, and infection. Vital signs and temperature are monitored along with the patient's level of comfort; complaints of abdominal pain are investigated.

Hypovolemic shock with symptoms of tachycardia, hypotension, diaphoresis, pallor, and oliguria may occur. Other complications include peritonitis or infection, which can be typified by fever, abdominal pain, redness, and purulent drainage from the puncture site.[29]

Bronchoscopy and Thoracentesis

The bronchoscopy patient is cared for in a manner similar to that for a GI endoscopy patient, although emphasis is placed on the respiratory tract instead of the GI tract. Preparation for thoracentesis is similar to that for a liver biopsy or paracentesis. This aspiration procedure requires sterile technique and skin preparation.

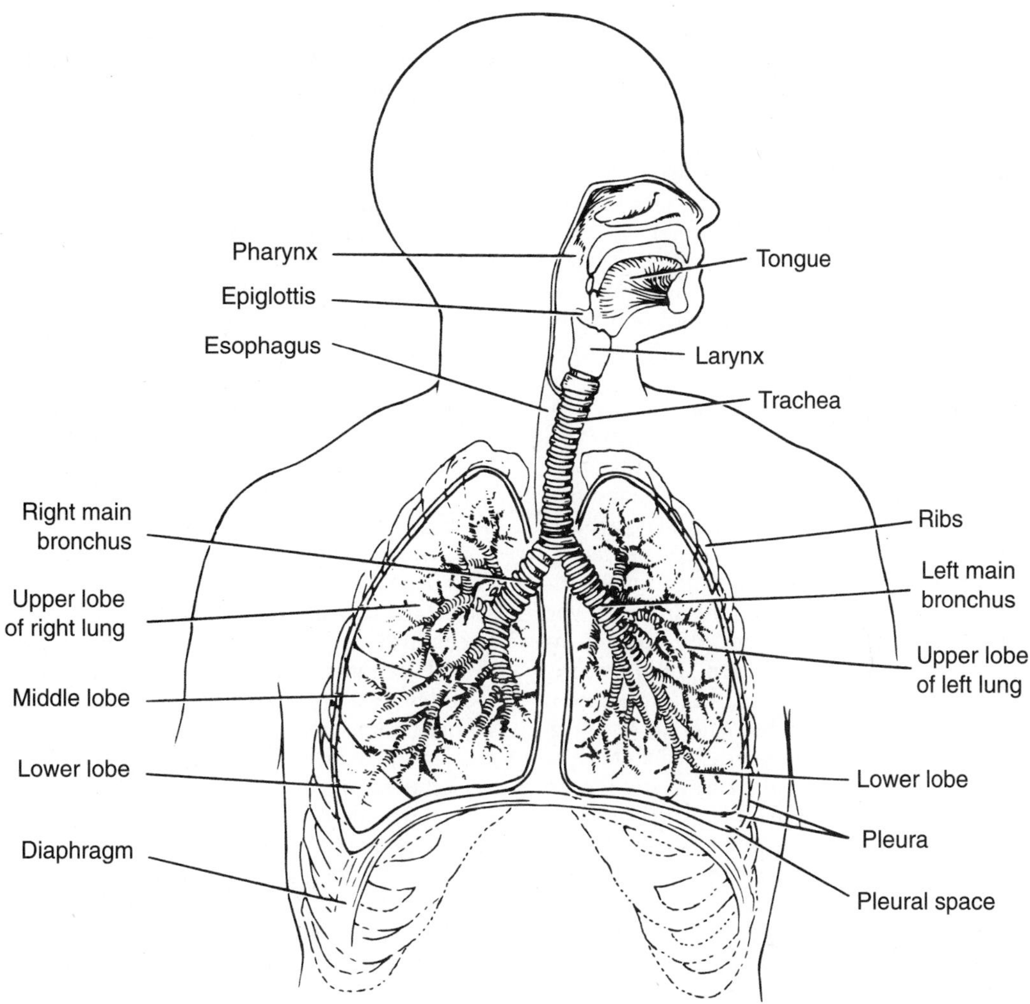

Figure 38–4. The respiratory system, showing the larynx, trachea, and bronchi through which the bronchoscope is passed. (From Phipps WJ, et al: Medical-Surgical Nursing: Concepts and Clinical Practice. St. Louis: CV Mosby, 1995.)

Bronchoscopy

Bronchoscopy is the direct inspection of the larynx, trachea, and bronchi with a thin, fiberoptic or video endoscope using either a transoral or transnasal approach (Fig. 38–4).[23, 32, 36] The procedure is usually done with local anesthesia and sedation and analgesia. It is used to diagnose, treat, and document abnormalities using inspection, biopsy, brush, lavage, and needle aspiration.

Indications. Therapeutic examinations are performed to remove foreign bodies and obstructive secretions such as mucous plugs, for insertion or evaluation of endotracheal tube, and to debride mucosal eschar from burns and other injuries. Diagnostic uses include assessment of airway status, collection of secretions and tissue for cytologic and bacteriologic examination, evaluation of abnormal chest x-ray findings, atelectasis, persistent cough, hemoptysis, and wheezing.[23, 32, 36] Patients who have had a lung transplant require bronchoscopy and biopsy periodically according to protocol.

Preparation. The patient must be NPO for 6 to 8 hours before the procedure. Upon arrival in the procedure area, a nursing assessment is completed including vital signs, O_2 saturation, medication history, allergies, and physical and mental status. Informed consent is necessary for this procedure. Dental prostheses, eyeglasses, and contact lenses are removed.

During the procedure, the patient is monitored by ECG according to unit policy; blood pressure, pulse, respirations, and pulse oximetry are measured; and supplemental O_2 is given. An IV line is in place for medication and fluid during and after the procedure. Analgesics and sedatives are given during the procedure to provide comfort, sedation, and amnesia. Local anesthesia of the nares, pharynx, and tracheobronchial tree is achieved with lidocaine jelly, topical spray or viscous lidocaine, and lidocaine solution, respectively. The patient may be supine, sitting, or in a side-lying position. During the examination, specimens from bronchial washings, brushings, and biopsies are collected and labeled.

Following the procedure, the nurse observes and documents the patient's vital signs, O_2 saturation, respiratory status, level of consciousness, and comfort. A chest x-ray examination may be performed following the bronchoscopy to assess for pneumothorax.[35]

Complications. Bronchospasm, hypoxemia, hemorrhage, pneumothorax, laryngospasm, dysrhythmias, hypoventilation, pulmonary hypertension, fever, infection, aspiration pneumonia, or adverse medication reactions are possible.[36] Sore throat and hoarseness may be observed.[32]

Special Care. The patient should be observed closely after the procedure until full gag and swallowing reflexes return. Monitoring includes vital signs, O_2 saturation, temperature, and auscultation of breath sounds. Assessment should be made for laryngeal edema, dyspnea, shortness of breath, hoarseness, cardiac dysrhythmias, chest pain, bleeding from the biopsy site, and hemoptysis. Supplemental oxygen may be needed. All specimens that are obtained during the procedure should be properly labeled and sent to the laboratory. Return of the gag reflex may be tested by gently touching the posterior pharynx with a tongue blade or swab. Swallowing can be assessed after gag reflex returns by observing the patient drink small sips of water.

When the patient meets the ASC discharge criteria, the patient will be released with verbal and written instructions for aftercare. The patient and the companion are instructed that mild sore throat and small amounts of hemoptysis are not uncommon, but extremes of either should be reported to the physician, as should fever (above 100°F), shortness of breath, and chest pain. Patients receiving sedation should be driven home by a responsible adult.

Thoracentesis

Thoracentesis is the sampling and evacuation of the pleural contents through a needle from the thoracic cavity.[37] Air or fluid may be removed. The drainage relieves lung compression and respiratory distress. Thoracentesis is also used to aid in the diagnosis of inflammatory or neoplastic diseases of the lung or pleura.

Indications. Thoracentesis provides therapeutic relief of dyspnea with large effusions. Smaller amounts of pleural fluid may be removed for diagnostic purposes: suspected malignancy, infection, or inflammation.

Preparation. Preprocedure preparation is similar to that for an endoscopy patient. Occasionally the patient may be sedated for the procedure. The patient is positioned in an upright sitting position, leaning forward over a padded bedside table.[29]

Following skin cleansing and the injection of local anesthesia, the needle is most often placed at the seventh or eighth intercostal space below the angle of the scapula, as illustrated in Figure 38–5.[23, 37] Sterile technique is maintained. During the procedure the patient is observed for signs of distress and is supported emotionally. The pleural fluid is removed slowly, up to 1500 ml at one time.[23, 38]

Following the procedure, the biopsy site is dressed with a sterile pressure dressing and observed for bleeding. Appropriately labeled specimens are sent to the laboratory for examination. Laboratory analysis of the removed fluid includes tests for color and cell count, microscopic and bacteriologic examination, glucose, amylase, protein, pH, and cytologic study.

Complications include vasovagal reflex, hypoxemia, intra-abdominal injury, bacterial contamination of pleural fluid, hemothorax, pneumothorax, air embolism, subcutaneous emphysema, infection, fluid and electrolyte imbalances, hemorrhage, shock, and cardiac distress.[23, 32]

Special Care. The patient is transferred to the PACU for observation. Physical and emotional status including vital signs, temperature, level of consciousness and comfort are assessed. The patient is positioned either recumbent, with the punctured side of the chest up for 1 hour, or in a semi-Fowler position. Assessment for respiratory distress includes auscultation of the entire chest. Untoward occurrences include shock, leakage from the puncture site, pneumothorax, hemoptysis, excessive or persistent coughing, cardiac distress, and pulmonary edema.

Complications, including those noted earlier, and pain, fever, chills, pallor, diaphoresis, nausea, tachycardia, dyspnea, tightness in the chest, and respiratory distress are reported to the physician immediately.[23] A chest x-ray film may be ordered immediately after the procedure or when the patient arrives in the PACU.

Following an appropriate length of stay in the recovery area, the patient is discharged with written and verbal instructions in the care of a responsible adult who will drive if the patient has received sedation. The patient is instructed to contact the physician immediately if respiratory distress, fever, or signs of infection occur.

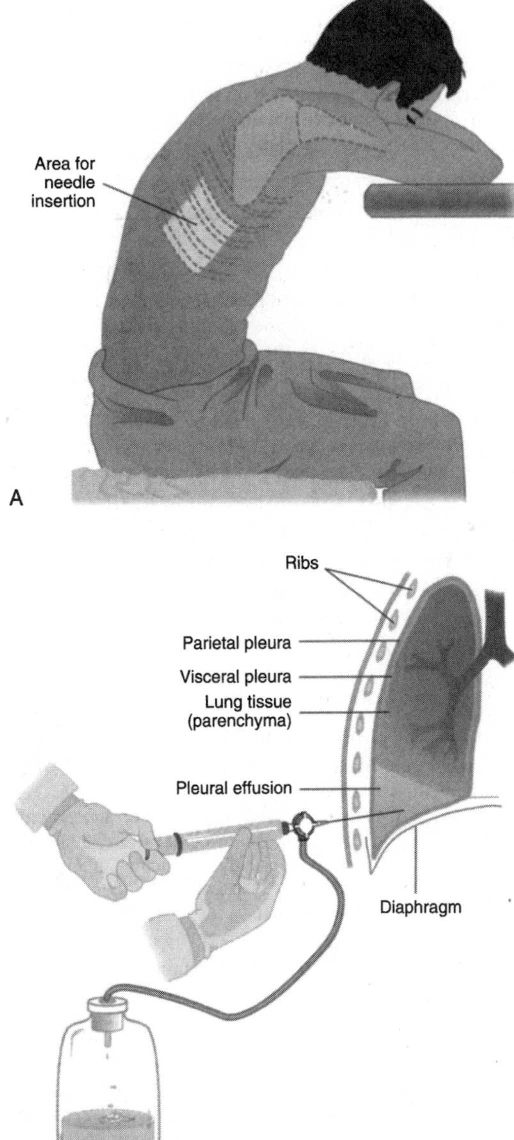

Figure 38–5. Thoracentesis. *A*, Correct position of the client for the procedure. The arms are raised and crossed. The head rests on the folded arms. This position allows the chest wall to be pulled outward in an expanded position. If an institutional overbed table is not available, you may leave the client's arms down, but position them toward the client's hips or cross them in front of the chest. *B*, The usual site for insertion of a thoracentesis needle for a right-sided effusion. The actual site varies, depending on the location and volume of the effusion. The needle is kept as far away from the diaphragm as possible but is inserted close to the base of the effusion so that gravity can help with drainage. (From Black JM, Matassarin-Jacobs E: Medical-Surgical Nursing: Clinical Management for Continuity of Care, 5th ed. Philadelphia: WB Saunders 1997, p 1067.)

Electroconvulsive Therapy

Electroconvulsive therapy (ECT) has been used in the treatment of severe depression since the late 1930s.[39] It is now considered "the safest, least expensive and most effective treatment for depression, having a faster onset than drugs."[40] Scalp electrodes transmit low-voltage alternating current briefly to the brain, causing convulsions and loss of consciousness.

Indications. Electroconvulsive therapy is an effective treatment for depression and, occasionally, other psychiatric illnesses. Patients unresponsive to medication, intolerant of medication side effects, or requiring rapid intervention to treat mental illness are candidates for ECT.[39, 41]

Preparation. Upon the patient's arrival at the ASC, the usual preanesthetic assessment is completed. An informed consent is obtained for the procedure by the physician, and the patient's NPO status of 6 hours or longer is confirmed. Valuables and dental prostheses are removed and secured in accordance with ASC policy, and the patient should void. Baseline vital signs and diagnostic values, which may include a complete blood cell count, serum chemistries, urinalysis, ECG, and chest x-ray films, are checked. Venous access is obtained. Glycopyrrolate or atropine may be administered before ECT to reduce secretions. The administration of anticholinergic agents is controversial and varies by institution and anesthesia care provider.[42, 43]

Procedure. The patient is taken to a private section of the ASC PACU, either walking or on a stretcher. The patient is fully monitored, and emergency resuscitative equipment must be immediately available, including an anesthesia machine or bag-valve-mask device, suction, oxygen, airway and intubation supplies, defibrillator, emergency medications, and IV supplies.[39, 43, 44]

Anesthesia is induced with a short-acting barbiturate, such as methohexital, and a neuromuscular blocking agent, succinylcholine, after preoxygenation and an anticholinergic, such as glycopyrrolate, is given. Ventilation is supported. Because muscle relaxants limit or obliterate motor activity, a blood pressure cuff, applied to an arm or leg, is inflated before induction to monitor seizure movements.[43] Following the application of the electric current and the resultant convulsion, anesthesia is terminated. Transient hypertension and either tachycardia or bradycardia may occur after the treatment.[42] Esmolol may be given as a pretreatment to minimize the hypertension and tachycardia.[42]

Complications. Bradycardia and hypotension can occur owing to parasympathetic stimulation.[42] More commonly, sympathetic effects including hypertension, tachyarrhythmias, increased myocardial oxygen consumption with subsequent myocardial ischemia, and arrhythmias occur.[42, 43]

Special Care. The patient remains in the PACU where close nurse monitoring is essential for patient safety. After the procedure, the patient may awaken confused, agitated, hyperactive, or restless.[44] Memory loss and headache may also be present. Airway, respiratory status, blood pressure, ECG, and O_2 saturation are assessed and monitored while the patient is in the PACU. An oral airway and supplemental oxygen may be required until the patient can support his or her own airway and until O_2 saturation levels return to baseline.[39] The patient exhibiting unstable blood pressure or cardiac arrhythmias must be closely observed, and pharmacologic intervention may be necessary.[45]

When the patient's condition is stable, and when the patient seems oriented and meets Phase I discharge criteria, transfer to the Phase II unit begins the preparation for home discharge. Instructions are reviewed with the patient and companion. Like all patients discharged after general anesthesia, the patient should not drive, drink alcohol, or make important decisions for 24 hours.[44] Adult companionship at home is essential for the first day because of potential lingering confusion or difficulty in cognition.

Rapid Opioid Detoxification

Heroin, a derivative of the opium poppy, is a powder that can be smoked, sniffed, or dissolved in water and injected. Heroin addiction is alarmingly common, with over 8 million users of heroin estimated worldwide. Associated mortality rate and arrest figures continue to rise. Most addicts are concurrently infected with hepatitis C.

The National Household Survey on Drug Abuse,[46] an annual survey conducted by the Substance Abuse and Mental Health Services Administration, estimates the prevalence of illicit drug use in the United States and monitors the trends in use over time. It is based on a representative sample of 25,500 persons from the U.S. population aged 12 and older. The following are some important statistics from this study, published in 1999:

- An estimated 13.6 million Americans were current users of illicit drugs in 1998, meaning they used an illicit drug at least once during the 30 days prior to being interviewed.
- Nearly 1 in 10 (9.9%) youths aged 12 to 17 years were current users of illicit drugs in 1998.
- The survey found that 16.1% of young adults aged 18 to 25 years were current users of illicit drugs in 1998. This rate has been gradually rising, up from 13.3% in 1994.
- In 1998, an estimated 130,000 Americans were current users of heroin, nearly doubling the number in 1993 (68,000). The average age of heroin users is rapidly dropping to 17.6 years old the first time they tried the drug in 1997, from 26.4 years old in 1990.

Other sources estimate a much higher incidence of heroin use.

Given its availability and relatively low cost, heroin is a major threat to youth and adults alike. The toll on lives is enormous, with many users sinking into illegal and other questionable lifestyles to maintain their habits. Family units break down, and economic effects continue to increase.

People may seek treatment for addiction on their own or may be judicially ordered into treatment programs that can be both lengthy and painful. Treatment is actually two-phased. The first phase is detoxification, often thought by the user and others to be the actual end of addiction. This stage is only a beginning; it must be followed by intensive, long-term counseling and other behavior therapies.[47] There is often a high rate of relapse after treatment.

Rapid opioid detoxification (ROD) is a controversial new procedure, often performed in the PACU setting. Called by many names, such as ultrarapid opioid detoxification (UROD), anesthesia-assisted rapid opiate detoxification (AAROD), and others, the process involves the administration of a narcotic antagonist, generally naloxone, after the patient has been given a general anesthetic to eliminate experiencing unpleasant withdrawal symptoms. Infusion of propofol is a common anesthetic method, and promotes rapid awakening upon its discontinuance. Airway management is important because vomiting and aspiration are possible. There is controversy among professionals regarding the need for intubation. Because of the potential for blood pressure fluctuations, vital signs are monitored during and after treatment.

After naloxone has eliminated all the narcotics from receptor sites in the body the patient is slowly awakened and is actually free of opiates, probably for the first time in many months or years. This part of the program must be followed with intensive counseling and other behavioral therapies for any chance of long-term success. Oral medications may supplement the long-term treatment as well; for instance, naltrexone to help prevent relapses by blocking the euphoric effects of heroin and other opiates.

Emotional support and nursing care that is both nonjudgmental and attentive are essential. Current providers consider this type of care to be humane and appropriate for those suffering addictions. Nurses should examine their attitudes and beliefs about addiction prior to caring for these patients. Patients will come from all walks of life and will include professionals who have access to narcotics in their work settings—namely, healthcare providers of all types. Confidentiality is absolutely essential and a right of the patient coming for this type of help.

These patients need encouragement to continue with behavioral therapies and any follow-up medications. Many centers are springing up around the country to provide this type of care and can be found with an easy Internet search. It is important to investigate the credentials and experience of those performing ROD. Whether this procedure becomes common or whether it is a passing fad is yet to be determined. Controlled research is needed along with investigation of the long-term outcomes of people undergoing this approach versus traditional detoxification and rehabilitation.

CONCLUSION

Many patients besides those having surgery take advantage of the benefits of an ASC setting. The efficiency and versatility of the nursing staff play a significant role in the development of these alternative services. Scheduling of the many varied diagnostic and therapeutic procedures in this fast-paced unit requires thorough planning and the implementation of carefully thought-out policies and procedures to ensure the safety and appropriateness of the site for each type of procedure and patient. Information for preprocedural patient preparation and postprocedural instructions regarding home care should be made available to each patient in an appropriate manner. With caution and thoroughness on the part of the nursing staff, the provision of specialized nursing care for the patients described within this chapter is well within the expertise and abilities of the ASC staff.

References

1. Intravenous Nurses Society: Revised Intravenous Nursing Standards of Practice. Cambridge, MA: Intravenous Nurses Society, 1997, p S18.
2. Intravenous Nurses Society: Revised Intravenous Nursing Standards of Practice. Cambridge, MA: Intravenous Nurses Society, 1997, p S19.
3. Intravenous Nurses Society: Revised Intravenous Nursing Standards of Practice. Cambridge, MA: Intravenous Nurses Society, 1997.
4. Intravenous Nurses Society: Revised Intravenous Nursing Standards of Practice. Cambridge, MA: Intravenous Nurses Society, 1997, p S53.
5. Messner R, Pinkerman M: Preventing a peripheral I.V. infection. Nursing 22 (6):34–41, 1992.
6. CDC: Recommendations for prevention of HIV transmission in health care settings. MMWR 36 (suppl 2):1S–18S, 1987.
7. CDC: Update: Universal precautions for prevention of transmission of human immunodeficiency virus, hepatitis B virus, and other bloodborne pathogens in healthcare settings. MMWR 37:377–388, 1988.
8. American Association of Blood Banks, America's Blood Centers and American Red Cross: Circular of Information for the Use of Human Blood and Blood Component. ARC 1751, Rev. Jan. 1999, pp 1–34.
9. US Department of Health and Human Services: Transfusion Therapy Guidelines for Nurses. NIH Publ No 90-2668. Bethesda, MD, US Department of Health and Human Services, 1990.
10. Intravenous Nurses Society: Revised Intravenous Nursing Standards of Practice. Cambridge, MA: Intravenous Nursing Society, 1997, p S28.
11. Butch SH, Oberman HA: Blood Transfusion Policies and Standard Practices. Blood and Transfusion Services, Department of Pathology, University of Michigan Hospitals, Ann Arbor, Michigan, October 1997.

12. Dorland's Illustrated Medical Dictionary, 28th ed. Philadelphia: WB Saunders, 1994.
13. Standards of Practice Committee of the American Society for Gastrointestinal Endoscopy. Antibiotic Prophylaxis for Gastrointestinal Endoscopy. Gastrointestinal Endoscopy 42:630–635, 1995.
14. Dajani AS, Taubert KA, Wilson W, et al: Prevention of bacterial endocarditis: Recommendations by the American Heart Association. JAMA 277:1794–1801, 1997.
15. Society for Gastroenterology Nurses and Associates: Standards of Clinical Nursing Practice and Role Delineation Statements. Publ No 325STP, Chicago, IL, 1998.
16. Task Force on Sedation and Analgesia by Non-anesthesiologists, The American Society of Anesthesiologists: Practice Guidelines for Sedation and Analgesia by Non-anesthesiologists. Anesthesiology 84(2):459–471, 1996.
17. Society for Gastroenterology Nurses and Associates: Guidelines for Nursing Care of the Patient Receiving Sedation and Analgesia in the GI Endoscopy Setting. Publ No 325SED, Chicago, IL, 1997.
18. O'Connor K, Jones S: Oxygen desaturation is common and clinically unappreciated during elective endoscopic procedures. Gastrointest Endosc 36:S2–S4, 1990.
19. Practice Committee of the Society for Gastroenterology Nurses and Associates: Standards for infection control and reprocessing of flexible gastrointestinal endoscopes. Gastroenterol Nurs 20(suppl):1–13s, 1997.
20. ACG, AGA, ASGE, SGNA Position Statement: Reprocessing of flexible gastrointestinal endoscopes. Gastroenterol Nurs 19:109–112, 1996.
21. Society of Gastroenterology Nurses and Associates: Gastroenterology Core Curriculum, 2nd ed. St. Louis: CV Mosby, 1998.
22. Lail L, Cotton P: Risks of retrograde cholangiopancreatography and therapeutic applications. Gastroenterol Nurs 12:239–245, 1990.
23. Melonakos K: Saunders' Pocket Reference for Nurses. Philadelphia: WB Saunders, 1990.
24. Omoigui S: The Anesthesia Drugs Handbook, 2nd ed. St. Louis: Mosby–Year Book, 1995.
25. Burden N: Telephone follow up of ambulatory surgery patients following discharge is a nursing responsibility. J Post Anesth Nurs 7:256–261, 1992.
26. Orringer MB: Esophagoscopy. In Sabiston DC (ed): Textbook of Surgery: The Biological Basis of Modern Surgical Practice, 15th ed. Philadelphia: WB Saunders, 1997, pp 736–744.
27. Schaffner M (ed): SGNA Manual of Gastrointestinal Procedures, 3rd ed. Baltimore: Williams & Wilkins, 1994.
28. Duranceau A: Perforation of the esophagus. In Sabiston DC (ed): Textbook of Surgery: The Biological Basis of Modern Surgical Practice, 15th ed. Philadelphia: WB Saunders, 1997, pp 759–767.
29. Black JM, Matassarin-Jacobs E: Medical-Surgical Nursing: Clinical Management for Continuity of Care, 5th ed. Philadelphia: WB Saunders, 1997.
30. McQuaid KR: Alimentary tract. In Tierney L, McPhee SJ, Papadakis MA (eds): Current Medical Diagnosis and Treatment. Stamford, CT: Appleton & Lange, 1999, pp 538–637.
31. Rothstein RI, Toor A: Dysphagia and esophageal obstruction. In Rakel R (ed): Conn's Current Therapy 1999. Philadelphia: WB Saunders, 1999, pp 472–480.
32. Thompson J, McFarland G, Hirsch J, et al: Mosby's Manual of Clinical Nursing, 4th ed. St. Louis: CV Mosby, 1997.
33. Urban M: Endoscopic retrograde cholangio-pancreatography: A diagnostic outpatient procedure. AORN J, 50:572–581, 1989.
34. McCormick ME: Endoscopic retrograde cholangiopancreatography. Am J Nurs 2:24HH-24JJ, Feb. 1999.
35. Fischbach FT: Manual of Laboratory and Diagnostic Tests, 5th ed. Philadelphia: Lippincott, 1996.
36. Tedder M, Ungerleider RM: Bronchoscopy in Sabiston DC (ed): Textbook of Surgery: The Biological Basis of Modern Surgical Practice, 15th ed. Philadelphia: WB Saunders, 1997, pp 1801–1805.
37. Beart R, Ballantyne G: Fiberoptic endoscopy. In Hill G: Outpatient Surgery, 3rd ed. Philadelphia: WB Saunders, 1988, pp 685–696.
38. Celli BR: Diseases of the diaphragm, chest wall, pleura, and mediastinum. In Bennett JC, Plum F (eds): Cecil Textbook of Medicine, 20th ed. Philadelphia: WB Saunders, 1996.
39. Kradecki D, Tarkinow M: Erasing the stigma of electroconvulsive therapy. J Post Anesth Nurs 7:84–88, 1992.
40. Greenberg C: Consultant's corner. In Hannalah R (ed): Ambulatory Anesthesia. Official Newsletter of the Society for Ambulatory Anesthesia 6:9, 1991.
41. APA Online: Electroconvulsive Therapy (ECT). Public Information, 1/9/96, American Psychiatric Association, www.psych.org.
42. Nimni B: Anesthesia for electroconvulsive therapy. In Atlee JL (ed): Complications in Anesthesia. Philadelphia: WB Saunders, 1999, pp 958–960.
43. Kellner CH, Pritchett JT, Beale MD, Coffey CE: Handbook of ECT. Washington, DC: American Psychiatric Press, 1997.
44. Irvin SM: Treatment of depression with outpatient electroconvulsive therapy. AORN J 65(3):573–582, March 1997.
45. Litwack K, Jones E: Practical points in the care of the post-electroconvulsive therapy patient. J Post Anesth Nurs 3:182–184, 1988.
46. U.S. Department of Justice Drug Enforcement Administration. Accessed at http://www.usdoj.gov/dea/stats/overview.htm on Nov. 28, 1999.
47. Wilson L, DeMaria P, Kane H, et al: Anesthesia-assisted rapid opiate detoxification: A new procedure in the postanesthesia care unit. JOPAN 14(4):207–216, 1999.
48. Sarin SK, Govil A, Jain A, et al: Randomized prospective trial of endoscopic sclerotherapy (EST) vs. endoscopic variceal ligation (EVL) for bleeding esophageal varices: Influence of gastropathy, gastric varices and recurrence. Gastroenterology 108:A1163, 1995.
49. Paptheodoridis GV, Goulis K, Leandro G, et al: Transjugular intrahepatic portosystemic shunt compared with endoscopic treatment for prevention of variceal bleeding: A meta-analysis. Hepatology 30:612–622, 1999.
50. Laine L, Stein C, Sharma V: Randomized comparison of ligation versus ligation plus sclerotherapy in patients with bleeding esophageal varices. Gastroenterology 110:529–533, 1996.
51. Saeed ZA, Stiegmann GV, Ramirez FC, et al: Endoscopic variceal ligation is superior to combined ligation and sclerotherapy for esophageal varices: A multicenter prospective randomized trial. Hepatology 25:71–74, 1997.
52. Dennert B, Ramirez FC, Sanowski RA: A prospective evaluation of the endoscopic spectrum of overtube-related esophageal mucosal injury. Gastrointest Endosc 45:134–137, 1997.

Chapter 39

Chronic Pain Management

Patricia A. Brandon

Pain is a complex part of the human condition that has been present since the beginning of recorded history. As healthcare providers, we are constantly confronted with the challenge of helping people feel more comfortable. The subjective nature of pain makes it difficult for the sufferer to describe its characteristics and the effect it has had on their lives. Treatment that is effective for one patient's pain may have no effect on the pain of another. Frustration is a common emotion felt by both the patient and the healthcare provider when the treatment plan fails to alleviate chronic pain. For pain therapy to be effective, the healthcare provider must show respect for the patient's complaint of pain, assess the pain complaint thoroughly, and offer the patient a pain management plan that the patient believes will relieve the pain. Having a true concern for and interest in the patient's overall needs is an excellent starting point for the healthcare team involved in chronic pain management.

Pain is "an unpleasant sensory and emotional experience arising from actual or potential tissue damage or described in terms of such damage" according to the definition of the International Association for the Study of Pain.[1] The patient scheduled for an appendectomy will be suffering from acute pain postoperatively but may also have chronic back pain. Both complaints are problems that must be managed concomitantly using different strategies.

Acute pain complaints associated with surgery, medical problems, burns, or trauma correlate subjective reports of pain with objective signs of a tissue-injuring process such as swelling, discoloration, abrasion, or crepitus. Acute pain is often treated with various methods, including medications (e.g., analgesics, nonsteroidal anti-inflammatory drugs [NSAIDs], anxiolytics), nerve blocks, heat, massage, rest and comfort measures, transcutaneous electrical nerve stimulation (TENS), distraction, and relaxation techniques. To treat acute pain adequately, it needs to be assessed and reassessed frequently. When treated effectively, the psychological and physiologic risks associated with untreated pain are avoided.

Over time, usually within 6 months, the report of pain and the behavioral response to pain resolves concurrently. However, when pain persists, sensory input from injured tissue reaches the spinal cord neurons and causes subsequent responses to be enhanced. Pain receptors in the periphery also become more sensitive after injury. Recent studies have demonstrated long-lasting changes in cells within spinal cord pain pathways after a brief painful stimulus. Such studies confirm that established pain is more difficult to treat (Table 39–1).[2]

Chronic pain is a persistent seemingly useless burden that inflicts suffering and disability *out of proportion* to any discoverable pathology. Almost one third of Americans have chronic pain and the medical costs of dealing with pain are estimated at over 100 billion dollars annually.[3] It is a condition that lasts beyond its healing period and leads to significant lifestyle alterations, including loss of employment; decreased physical, social, and recreational activities; and psychological changes including depression, drug abuse, and loss of self esteem.[4]

The management of chronic pain is complex and often requires a multidisciplinary approach to pain therapy. Chronic pain complaints range from headaches to sympathetically maintained

Table 39–1. Terms Related to Pain Management

Allodynia—pain resulting from unpleasant simuli that do not normally provoke pain
Anhidrosis—absence of sweat
Causalgia—pain similar to that in reflex sympathetic dystrophy but resulting from a direct nerve injury; terms often used interchangeably
Cephalgia—headache
Epidural—outside of the dura that encases the spinal canal
Ganglion—mass or grouping of nerve tissue outside of the central nervous system
Hyperesthesia—increased sensitivity to stimuli such as touch or pain
Intrathecal—in the spinal canal
Nucleus pulposus—the central portion of an intervertebral disk, which is gelatinous
Paresis—partial paralysis
Paresthesia—tingling, numbness, increased sensitivity or prickling of an area
Radicular—originating from the nerve root; refers to a radiating characteristic
Radiculitis—inflammation of the spinal nerve roots with resultant pain and hyperesthesia
Reflex sympathetic dystrophy—clinical syndrome that can follow a tissue injury; typified by burning pain, hyperesthesia, allodynia, exaggerated sympathetic activity, dystrophy, and eventual atrophy in an affected extremity
Rhizotomy—cutting of the dorsal spinal nerve root to relieve pain
Trigger point—painful areas of tissue that, with direct palpation, cause pain in other areas of the body

pain. Some of the nerve conduction and input changes that can occur in the peripheral and central nervous system are insidious. The problem may not manifest itself for weeks to years after the actual damage has occurred.

The pain specialist must be alert to the possibilities of aberrant pain communications regarding the patient with chronic pain and remain open minded to the complaint of pain. Educating healthcare providers about these problems is part of the responsibility of the pain care specialist, so that patients are referred to them at the earliest possible time.

Chronic pain protocols might include medication management, that is, antidepressants, anticonvulsants, antiarrhythmics, NSAIDs, topical agents (i.e., lidocaine patches or capsaicin), physical therapy (exercise), acupuncture, massage, ultrasound, heat or ice packs, TENS, and invasive neural blockade (nerve blocks). Psychological counseling and therapies such as hypnosis, psychotherapy, biofeedback, distraction, relaxation, guided imagery, and support groups can offer significant help when combined with pharmacologic therapies. The patient suffering from chronic pain should be referred to appropriate resources for information on the financial, legal, and employment/retraining sequelae of the chronic pain syndrome.[5] In addition to reduction of pain, the goals of chronic pain therapy include: (1) eliminating and decreasing nonessential medication use, (2) providing increased coping skills, and (3) increasing physical conditioning and independence.

Multidisciplinary pain management services are found in many communities. Such clinics often offer the services of a physiatrist, physical and occupational therapist, psychologist or psychiatrist, social worker, acupuncturist, and chiropractor. The focus of this chapter is to introduce the nurse to the concept of pain management in the ambulatory care setting under the direction of the anesthesiologist.

Since epidural narcotics were first introduced, we have witnessed the evolution of the anesthesiologist as a pain management provider outside of the operating room, beginning with the obstetric patient and most recently with the management of postoperative pain. Epidural analgesia and patient-controlled analgesia (PCA) are common phrases used in today's population of healthcare professionals.

Surgeons and primary care physicians alike have slowly witnessed the advantage of including the expertise of the anesthesiologist as a consultant in the management of their patients because of their background in neuroanatomy, physiology, and pharmacology. The anesthesiologist assists in identifying the sympathetic or somatic generators of pain via a neural blockade approach, targeting these pain-inciting structures, so that the primary pain management practitioner can design a program that allows the patient to become an active participant in a multidisciplinary program of pain control designed for him or her.

If you practice in a setting that does not have an anesthesiology consultative pain service, you may soon see the development of this service in your institution. Anesthesiologists who are certified in pain management are actively developing practices as pain management consultants. However, this practice is limited because of cost issues and the responsibilities that the anesthesiologist has to the operating room. The anesthesiologist must be skilled in neural blockade techniques and willing to devote the time necessary to manage the immediate effects and side effects of the block, as well as provide follow-up assessment and treatment for the patient. In cases where a formal pain clinic does not exist, the ambulatory care unit or ambulatory surgery center (ASC) provides a setting for the anesthesiologist to schedule nerve blocks for a diagnostic, prognostic, and therapeutic treatment of pain.

The anesthesiology group may not have their own nursing staff working with them. This means that the ASC nurse may be the only professional nurse who the patient meets with for this approach to pain management. Knowledge of basic pain management principles is necessary for the nurse admitting the patient, assisting in the procedure room, or discharging the patient.

The single most important principle of pain management to remember is that the patient's self-report of pain must be accepted and respected. McCaffery and Pasero, authorities in the nursing care of people in pain, explain the importance of the nurse's attitude in communicating with the patient and family.[6] The nurse's role is to express belief in the patient's complaint of pain and the effect that it has had on the patient's life. An individualized care plan should identify the specific pain problem and the expected outcome of the nerve block procedure. It should include support for the emotional and social needs of the patient and the patient's family member(s), or the responsible adult. An expression of belief about the patient's description of his or her pain is necessary for the success of the treatment plan.

Another essential principle to remember is that the patient needs to have time to verbalize his or her feelings. Often the patient has seen several physicians and has had little time to explain his or her symptoms and fears. The patient is rushed from one test to another, never understanding the direction of the treatment plan. Pain has become the patient's lifestyle; the pain controls the patient and everyone who is associated with the patient. The fact that the nurse will listen to the patient describe the pain and the effect that it has had on his or her life may be more therapeutic than the nerve block or medication being offered. Even if the patient leaves the unit with the same amount of pain that he or she entered with, the patient has hope that a solution to the problem may be found, because the pain has been validated by an expression of belief in the patient's pain complaint.

In a busy ambulatory care setting, these patients may be overwhelmed with the activity of the unit. Anxiety and depression are two common emotions associated with chronic pain and may be heightened in the unfamiliar setting of the ambulatory unit. Patients who are admitted before meeting the anesthesiologist may be fearful of the procedure because of the unfamiliar setting and lack of knowledge about the procedure. Notify the anesthesiologist if the patient exhibits severe or panic anxiety. Provide opportunities for the patient and family to express their feelings. Allow them to make decisions such as whether to sit or stand during the interview.[7] It will be important for the nurse to minimize exposure to other patients by assigning a patient to an area away from the busier section of the unit. Closing the curtain around a cubicle, or closing a door to a procedure room may offer the patient the privacy that he or she needs.

Effective pain therapies depend on proper identification of the pain complaint. The patient's assessment of pain should be documented either in the physician's history and physical or as part of the nursing assessment form. Convey that you are assessing the pain complaint because you want to better understand it, not determine if it is present. Assess if the family doubts the pain complaint. It may be necessary to speak privately with the patient, explaining the concept of pain as an individual experience, or explaining the difference between addiction and tolerance to narcotic medication. Listen carefully to the patient's reports of the character of the pain. Your assessment should involve asking the appropriate questions[8]:

- Where is your pain? Use a body figure, noting left and right
- What is the intensity of your pain? Use a visual analog scale or numerical scale (0 to 10; 0 = no pain and 10 = worst pain)
- What is the duration of pain? Is it constant or intermittent?
- What is the character of your pain? Is it sharp, burning, throbbing, dull, or electric?
- What are the factors that precipitate your pain (e.g., walking, sitting)?
- What are the factors that relieve or minimize your pain (e.g., sitting, heat/ice)?
- What medications are you presently taking for pain? List narcotics, NSAIDs, and antidepressants (Fig. 39–1).

Observe the patient's pain behavior. The most important observations include facial expression (e.g., grimacing, movement, posture, and interactions with others). Observing the actions of others is often as important as watching those of the patient. These interactions yield clues to factors that are intensifying or compounding the pain. For example, the patient's pain problem creates a need for a spouse or family mem-

Acute Pain Management
Initial Assessment Tool

Name:______________________________ Date: ______________

I. Place a check by the word(s) that best describes your pain:

A.	Ache, dull	E.	Pulling, stretching
B.	Burning	F.	Numbness
C.	Throbbing	G.	Sharp, knife-like, stabbing
D.	Grabbing, tight		

II. When did your pain start?

III. What causes or increases your pain?

IV. What relieves your pain?

V. Place a check by the word(s) that best describes when you experience your pain:

A.	Constantly	D.	During activity (e.g., walking)
B.	During the day	E.	Standing
C.	At night		

VI. Does your pain affect? (Please circle one answer for each question)

A.	Sleep	Yes	No
B.	Appetite	Yes	No
C.	Physical Activity	Yes	No

VII. What medications are you using for pain control? Please list:

VIII. Is there anything else you do to relieve your pain?

Please circle the appropriate number on the following pain scale that best describes your pain level:

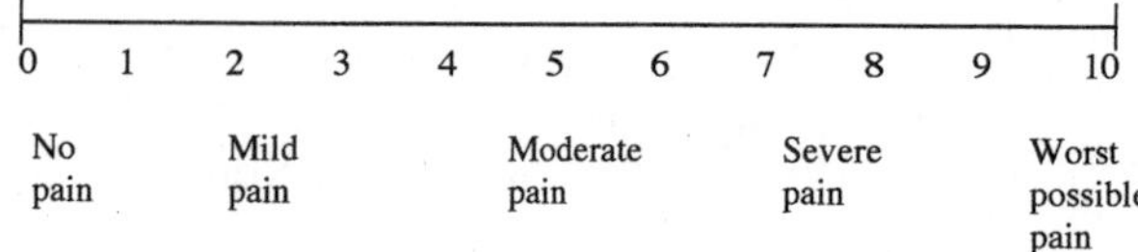

Figure 39–1. Acute Pain Management Initial Assessment Tool. (Courtesy of Ochsner Medical Foundation, New Orleans, LA.)

ber because the patient is dependent and needs help with activities of daily living. However, the pain behavior exhibited by the patient may elicit the attention from the caregiver that the patient seeks. Your observations are important and should be documented on the written assessment. The goals of the clinical assessment process are to characterize the pain experience, to direct the selection of appropriate intervention strategies, and to verify the effectiveness of the pain therapy employed.

Education of the patient about immediate and long-term goals should be completed before proceeding with any intervention for chronic pain management. The physician informs the patient of possible outcomes and risks associated with procedures or protocols and discusses realistic expectations. The nurse clarifies and may expand the information that the patient and his or her caregivers have received from the physician. The ultimate objective is a reduction of pain, not eradication of pain. As stated earlier, pain is such a subjective and personal experience that it is virtually impossible to understand the pain of another person. *Malingerer, hypochondriac*, or *complainer* are terms often used to describe a patient who exhibits chronic pain behavior. Until there is evidence to support that attitude, the healthcare provider must be willing to accept the patient's report of pain and explore all possible explanations for the cause of the pain. Patient education should include an understanding of the chronic pain problem and the role that the patient and the responsible adult are expected to play in the procedure of that day, as well as the role that they will be expected to accept in the long-term plan of therapy.

Questions about sedation and positioning for the procedure, expected reactions during the procedure, and expected outcome of the procedure should be answered by the nurse anesthetist or anesthesiologist performing the block. The patient should sign an informed consent after the physician has discussed the risks associated with the procedure. Sedation for neural blockade is optional and dependent on the patient's intensity of pain and anxiety related to the procedure and by the home support and driver available. The patient and responsible adult must understand that the block approach to pain management is to assist in the diagnosis and treatment of the patient's pain. In addition to the other risks explained, the patient should know that there could be failure of the block(s) to relieve pain or the possibility of worsening pain. The patient must feel comfortable with proceeding and must have a realistic expectation, understanding that if this modality fails to provide effective pain relief, it may not be advisable to continue. The patient must be willing to accept the decision to stop the blocks when the anesthesiologist recommends it and move on to other therapies included in the pain treatment plan. Complementary therapies for pain management are discussed later in this chapter.

NEURAL BLOCKADE (NERVE BLOCKS)

Pain results from the stimulation of nociceptors. These receptors are free nerve endings that are found throughout the body in skin, blood vessels, subcutaneous tissue, muscle, tissue, viscera, joints, and fascia. When they are stimulated, the impulse generated is transmitted to the spinal cord along two types of afferent sensory fibers.

1. A delta fibers are myelinated and conduct painful stimuli quickly. The pain sensation is perceived as sharp, localized pain.
2. C fibers conduct impulses slowly because they are unmyelinated and smaller than A delta fibers. The pain sensation is perceived as dull, diffuse, and persistent pain or burning, aching pain.

Local anesthetic drugs prevent the development of the action potential in a nerve by preventing sodium ions from moving intracellularly through the sodium channels. The anesthesia that results has been referred to as membrane stabilization, in which the resting membrane potential is unaffected by further nerve stimulation. The diameter and myelinization of a nerve fiber determine (to an extent) its sensitivity to local anesthetics as well as its message-carrying function. The drugs from which the anesthesiologist can choose include the esther-derived drugs such as procaine, cocaine, and tetracaine or the amide-derived drugs that include lidocaine, bupivacaine, mepivacaine, and ropivacaine. The risks noted to be associated with neural blockade, include the following:

1. Allergic reactions
2. Seizure
3. Respiratory distress
4. Cardiac toxicity
5. Spinal blockade
6. Vasovagal reaction

When performing a nerve block procedure, proper monitoring and immediate availability of resuscitative equipment must always be ensured (Table 39–2). It should include:

- Monitoring equipment for blood pressure (BP), electrocardiogram (ECG), O_2 saturation
- Intubation equipment, suction, O_2, defibrillator
- Emergency drugs (i.e., thiopental, succinylcholine, ephedrine, epinephrine, atropine)
- Intravenous (IV) fluids

Early signs and symptoms of local anesthetic toxicity include metallic taste, tinnitus, lightheadedness, agitation, and drowsiness. Untoward effects of late central nervous system (CNS) toxicity include hypotension or hypertension, bradycardia or tachycardia, seizures, and unconsciousness. Cardiac and respiratory failure, coma, and death may occur in the late stages of local anesthetic toxicity.[9] See Table 39–3 for a summary of treatment for acute local anesthetic toxicity.

Neural blockade can be used as a diagnostic, prognostic, prophylactic, or therapeutic tool when included as part of a multimodal/interdisciplinary pain management plan. Diagnostic nerve blocks are useful for ascertaining specific pathways, differentiating referred pain from local pain or sympathetic pain from somatic pain, and determining possible mechanisms of chronic pain states. Prognostic nerve blocks may give the patient an opportunity to experience the numbness and other side effects that he or she will experience after a neurolytic or ablative surgical procedure. Prophylactic blocks are most useful in controlling postoperative or post-traumatic pain, preventing complications

Table 39–2. **An Example of Monitoring and Care Parameters for Invasive Pain Management Procedures**

PROCEDURE	IV ACCESS* (PRIOR TO STARTING)	ECG†	NIBP†	PULSE OXIMETER†	MINIMAL RECOVERY OBSERVATION TIME (MIN)	COMMENTS
Epidural steroid injection						
Lumbar	N	N	N	N	30–60 if a local anesthetic used 30 if no local anesthetic is used	Observed for spinal effect
Thoracic	Y	Y	Y	Y	30–60	Perform periodic chest auscultation
Cervical	Y	Y	Y	Y	30–60	Assess level of consciousness
Lumbar sympathetic block	Y	Y	Y	Y	60–90	Monitor temperature of affected extremity
Trigger point injection	N	N	N	N	As needed	
Intercostal nerve block	Y	Y	Y	Y	60–90	Perform periodic chest auscultation
Stellate ganglion block	Y/N	Y	Y	Y	60	Monitor temperature of affected extremity

*The decision to secure intravenous access with a heparin lock or fluids is determined by the physician according to the needs of the patient. This chart represents the usual protocol but is altered on a case-by-case basis according to physician order.
†When monitors are not in use, they should be immediately available at the bedside.
N, no; Y, yes.

that arise from uncontrolled pain. Therapeutic blocks are effective in breaking up the so-called "vicious cycle" that accompanies many chronic pain states, providing temporary relief so that other therapeutic measures may be used (i.e., physical therapy). It is noted that therapeutic injections of a local anesthetic can provide relief that outlasts the pharmacologic action of the local anesthetic.

Preparing the patient for nerve block procedures includes patient assessment, history and physical examination, education, and development of a nursing care plan. Assessment focuses on the patient's pain history and description, previous procedures, analgesic/medication use, and other therapies or comfort measures used by the patient. Education may not only use written booklets or pamphlets but also diagrams, photographs, and anatomic models. A realistic care plan to guide patient care, with achievable goals and measurable outcomes, is established with the patient and caregiver.

When assisting with the nerve block procedure, the nurse's role is to offer support for the patient and to monitor for any signs of adverse reaction or discomfort during the procedure. Instructing patients to make their needs known verbally empowers them. If the patient requests or the nurse observes that the patient needs repositioning, another pillow, or a blanket for support or to halt the procedure, the nurse may advise the anesthesiologist to stop until the patient reports that he or she is ready to proceed. Maintaining an optimistic attitude about the procedure and the outcome expected from the block may facilitate completion of the procedure and a more positive outcome for the patient.

Distraction therapy such as music therapy can help to create an environment that focuses away from the pain. Music therapy may:

1. Provide a positive diversion from negative emotions not compatible with worry
2. Allow the body to relax and act as an effective nonanalgesic sleep aid
3. Increase the positive effects of medications
4. Decrease stress levels (increasing levels of endorphins)
5. Be an effective "helper" during exercise/fitness times by acting as a motivator, positive diversion, time keeper, and pace setter.[10, 11]

Table 39–3. Treatment of Acute Local Anesthetic Toxicity

Establish a clear airway
Breathing
  Oxygen with facemask
  Encourage adequate ventilation
  Artificial ventilation if required
Circulation
  Elevate legs
  IV fluids, increase rate for hypotension
  CVS support drugs (see below)
  Cardioversion if ventricular arrhythmias occur
Drugs
  CNS depressant
    Diazepam 5–10 mg IV
    Thiopental 50 mg IV, incrementally until seizures cease
    Muscle relaxant
      Succinylcholine 1 mg/kg, if inadequate control of ventilation with the aforementioned measures (requires artificial ventilation and may necessitate intubation)
  CVS support
    Atropine 0.6 mg IV if bradycardia occurs
    Ephedrine 12.5–25 mg IV to restore adequate blood pressure
    Epinephrine for profound cardiovascular collapse

CNS, central nervous system; IV, intravenous; CVS, cardiovascular system.

The patient may have been asked to bring a set of relaxation tapes or the pain service may own a set of tapes that can be used by the patient during the procedure and recovery period. Touch is a helpful nursing intervention during the procedure. Handholding or briefly touching or rubbing a shoulder can help to relax the patient, thus allowing the patient to focus away from the pain. Emphasize that the degree to which an individual can be distracted from the pain is unrelated to the existence of or intensity of the pain. Keep the patient informed of the expected serial sensations and progress of the procedure.

Monitor the patient's response to the procedure immediately after the procedure. Has the pain intensity score or character of pain changed? Is there procedural pain? Is medication needed before the patient is discharged? A post block assessment should include:

1. Circulatory and respiratory status (vital signs)
2. Motor and sensory status (e.g., ability to bear weight, ambulate, and pain relief or level)
3. Neurologic status (CNS score)

The nurse should include the family or a responsible adult in education and the discharge plan, reviewing methods the caregiver can assist with such as massage or coaching methods for relaxation therapy. Medication management with NSAIDs, antidepressants, and anticonvulsants is often prescribed by the anesthesiologist as part of the pain management plan for both acute and chronic pain. Educating the patient and family members or the responsible adult about the actions of these medications and known side effects is important if the patient is expected to comply with the prescribed medication plan. A written pain management plan is necessary when starting a new medication regimen. The plan should be communicated to the patient's primary care physician. Most medications on a chronic pain medication plan are not to be taken as needed but on a scheduled dosing regimen. Dose effect is not immediate, but side effects can be and should be reported to the anesthesiologist or primary care physician before discontinuing use of a medication. Side effects reported for common medications are listed in Table 39–4.[12, 13]

Medication instruction, emergency phone numbers, and follow-up appointments should be written on a discharge instruction sheet, which is shared with the person accompanying the patient upon discharge. The nurse will set goals for pain management with the patient and family (Fig. 39–2). The expected outcome of block therapy for pain management includes a reduction in narcotic/analgesic use by the patient, improved flexibility, increased strength, better functioning at home, and a return to employment or educational pursuit.

Table 39–4. Common Side Effects of Selected Medications

Medication	Side Effects
Antidepressants	
Serotonin Selective Reuptake Inhibitors (SSRI)	Anxiety, insomnia (dose in AM), headache, nausea, diarrhea, weight loss, decreased libido
Tricyclic Antidepressants (TCA)	Anticholinergic effects, dry mouth, sedation, urinary retention, constipation
Anticonvulsants	Sedation, dizziness, nausea, fatigue, aplastic anemia, rare
Nonsteroidal anti-inflammatory drugs (NSAID)	Antiplatelet activity, gastrointestinal bleeding, renal insufficiency, hepatotoxicity, headache, vertigo

DISCHARGE ASSESSMENT

TOTAL INTAKE:__________________ OUTPUT:______________

DISCHARGE VITAL SIGNS
B/P_____ P_____ R_____ T_____ TIME__________

MODE OF DISCHARGE
AMBULATORY _____ WHEELCHAIR _____ STRETCHER _____
ACCOMPANIED BY __________________ DESTINATION ______________
DISCHARGE PRESCRIPTIONS AND INSTRUCTIONS GIVEN TO ______________
NAME AND RELATIONSHIP TO PATIENT

DISCHARGE CRITERIA/TRANSFER TO ___ FLOOR FOR ADMIT. ADMITTED FOR __________

☐ YES ☐ NO ☐ N/A SWALLOW, COUGH, GAG REFLEXES PRESENT

☐ YES ☐ NO ☐ N/A ABSENCE OF RESPIRATORY DISTRESS

☐ YES ☐ NO ☐ N/A RESPONSIVE, ORIENTED, __________NEURO SCORE

☐ YES ☐ NO ☐ N/A NAUSEA, VOMITING, DIZZINESS ABSENT

☐ YES ☐ NO ☐ N/A BLEEDING, DRAINAGE MINIMAL

☐ YES ☐ NO ☐ N/A TAKING P.O FLUIDS

☐ YES ☐ NO ☐ N/A VOIDED

☐ YES ☐ NO ☐ N/A DRESSING CHECKED

☐ YES ☐ NO ☐ N/A SENSORY MOTOR FUNCTION RETURNED AFTER REGIONAL

COMMENTS:______________________________________

RN RELEASE (SIGNATURE)______________________________

PHYSICIAN RELEASE (SIGNATURE)______________________________

Figure 39–2. Example of Discharge Assessment. (Courtesy of Ochsner Medical Foundation, New Orleans, LA.)

Acute Pain Treatment to Prevent Chronic Pain

Nerve blocks tend to be effective for relatively acute problems and may actually prevent the development of certain chronic pain syndromes (e.g., reflex sympathetic dystrophy [RSD], phantom limb pain).[14] The diagnoses that most commonly respond to neural blockade are:

Acute herniated nucleus pulposus/radiculopathy
Acute herpes zoster
Sympathetically maintained pain

Each anesthesiologist will follow individualized protocols that should be reviewed with the patient before each procedure and signing of an informed consent (Table 39–5).

Acute Herniated Nucleus Pulposus/Radiculopathy

Low back pain continues to be one of the maladies that few adults escape. In 1994, the Agency for Health Care Policy Research (AHCPR) [1-800-358-9295, *www.ahcpr.gov*] released guidelines for the management of acute low back pain.[15] Pain reported to be related to acute herniated nucleus pulposus requires careful evaluation to discriminate between patients who need aggressive intervention from those who need only time and moderate medical sup-

***Table 39–5.* Common Invasive Pain Management Procedures**

PROCEDURE	TYPICAL INDICATIONS	COMMENTS*
Epidural steroid injection		
Lumbar/thoracic	Low/mid back pain Herniated/leaking intervertebral disk Radiculopathy Degenerative disk disease (DDD) Spinal stenosis/arthritis Herpes zoster and post-herpetic neuralgia (shingles)	May reduce sensory or motor functions May reduce pain immediately if a local anesthetic is used Positioned after block so that gravity keeps the medication in the desired location Observe for "wet tap" with introduction of the needle and medicine into the subarachnoid (spinal) space
Cervical	Neck/arm/upper back pain Headaches Radiculopathy Degenerative disk disease (DDD) Spinal stenosis/arthritis	Cervical epidural space small in circumference, increased potential for spread of medication upward to the ventricles Watch for a spinal effect and cardiovascular, respiratory effects Patient often sitting up for procedure
Epidural sympathetic block	Reflex sympathetic dystrophy/causalgia Phantom limb pain Peripheral vascular disease (PVD)	Full spinal effect possible Monitor for skin temperature changes in affected extremities May be done under fluoroscopy
Trigger point injection	Myofascial pain Low back pain syndrome Reflex sympathetic dystrophy/causalgia Peripheral nerve pain syndromes	Infra-arterial or intravenous injection possible
Intercostal nerve block	Chest wall pain Herpes zoster and post-herpetic neuralgia (shingles) Cancer pain	Pneumothorax always possible Position the arm on the affected side above the head to open up the intercostal spaces Topical anesthetic spray helps reduce pain in an already sensitive area
Stellate ganglion block	RSD† of upper extremity, post-CVA, trauma, surgery Herpes zoster and post-herpetic neuralgia (shingles) Peripheral vascular disease (PVD)	Interrupts sympathetic nerve pathways to the upper extremity Causes vasodilatation, thus increases circulation and improves healing Expect Horner's syndrome (ptosis of the eyelid and pupil constriction on the affected side), possible difficulty swallowing, vasodilatation of scleral and conjunctival blood vessels (bloodshot eyes), stuffy nose, spasm of neck muscles, dizziness, apprehension, lacrimation; hoarseness may occur from recurrent laryngeal and phrenic nerve block Observe for total spinal, bilateral block with bradycardia or cardiac arrest, pneumothorax, hematoma near the trachea

*Complications germane to all invasive nerve blocks include: (1) intra-arterial or intravenous injections with possible toxicity, including respiratory and cardiac arrest; (2) allergic reaction; (3) bleeding; (4) nerve injury; (5) infection.

†RSD—now also known as complex regional pain syndrome, type I.

port. Acute pain of nerve root origin (radiculopathy) may occur due to inflammation of the nerve root through compression of the dorsal root ganglion or by chemical irritation from nucleus pulposus material (Fig. 39–3). Patients with classic radiculopathy describe pain as sharp and stabbing that radiates from the low back through the buttock, down the back of the thigh, and below the knee. The onset is often related to a lifting event but may not be attributable to any one event.

Epidural Steroid Injection

Today, injection of steroid into the epidural space represents one of the most widely used therapeutic modalities in most pain management practices. Epidural steroid injections may be performed at the cervical, thoracic, or lumbar level, or per caudal approach. A thorough evaluation for a complaint of low back pain with radiculopathy should include computed tomography (CT) scanning, magnetic resonance im-

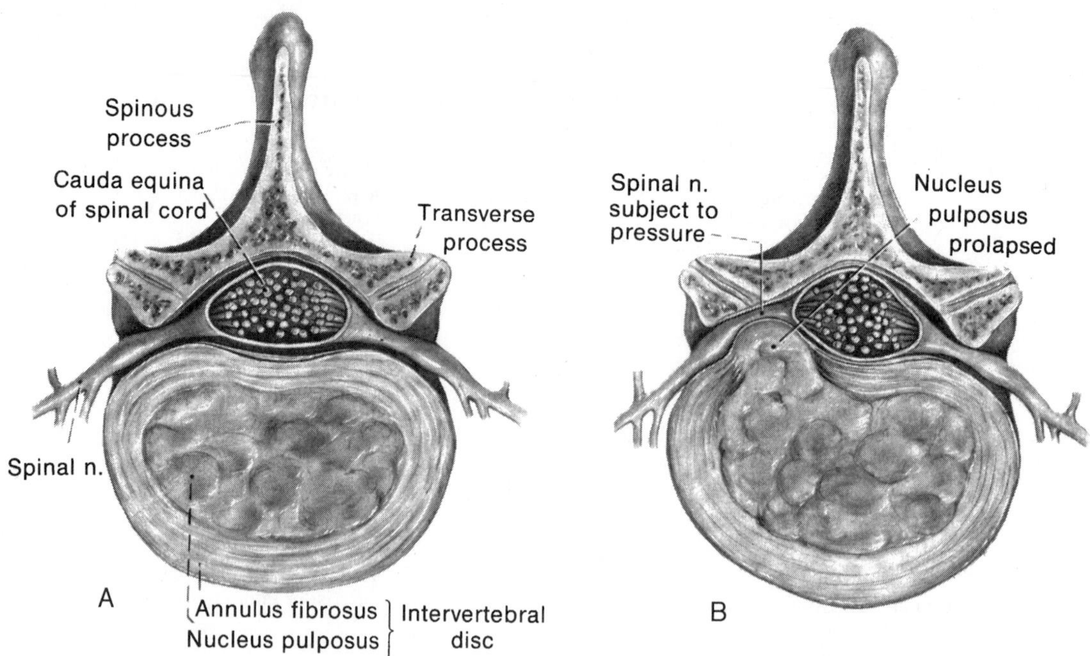

Figure 39–3. A, Normal relationship of the intervertebral disk to the spinal cord and nerve branches. B, Prolapsed nucleus pulposus impinging on the nerve. (From Jacob SW, Francone CA, Lossow WJ: Structure and Function in Man, 5th ed. Philadelphia, WB Saunders, 1982.)

aging (MRI), or electromyelography (EMG). Pain relief may be reported with a single injection or a series of three injections may be necessary. Medical prudence suggests that if the patient has not noticed any improvement after two blocks, other options should be considered.

There are few reports of serious side effects or complications related to epidural steroids. Certainly a review of the literature identifies an element of risk to the procedure, and the patient should be made aware of the possibility of post dural puncture headache, inadvertent injection of a local anesthetic into the spinal fluid or a blood vessel, epidural abscess, reaction to the drugs injected, and epidural hematoma. Probably one of the greatest risks that the patient takes involves a failure of the epidural injection to relieve pain. This risk should not discourage the patient from proceeding with the procedure.

The procedure may be performed in the ambulatory care unit, or the patient may need to be taken to the operating room or radiology department if fluoroscopy is to be used. A minimum suggested recovery period is 30 minutes but the period may be longer pending the use of sedation or narcotic and local anesthetic. Onset of relief may be immediate if a local anesthetic or narcotics are used. However, the steroid effect is not noted for 3 to 5 days after the injection. Patient instruction should include this information so that the patient does not get discouraged if pain returns within hours after the injection. Discharge instructions after an epidural steroid injection should include the following:

1. Driving is not recommended for _____ hours following the procedure.
2. Diabetic patients should be instructed to continue with their routine monitoring of blood sugar and report an increase in blood sugar to their primary care physician for management.
3. Report any signs of emergency or complaint, such as spinal headache, increasing back pain or numbness, weakness of the extremities, or a temperature higher than 101°, to the pain service by calling the following number(s) ______________________________.

Trigger Point Injection

Myofascial pain is often initiated by direct trauma to muscle, chronic muscle strain, arthritis, or nerve root injury. It is characterized by deep regional pain associated with a myofascial trigger point that will differentiate it from fibrositis, a related syndrome. A latent trigger point may restrict movement and cause weakness of the affected muscle. The referred pain, which mimics radicular pain, is dull and aching, occurs at rest or with activity, and is intensified by digital pressure on the trigger point. The trigger point is palpated along the muscle fibers until the maximum point of tenderness is located. The trigger point is fixed between two fingers, and a 25-gauge 1½-inch needle is inserted into it. Local anesthetic with or without steroid is injected. Complications are rare but include inadvertent intravascular or intrathecal injection, pneumothorax (thoracic level injections), or allergic reaction. Pain relief may be immediate or delayed for 1 to 2 days if steroid medication is used for injection. Discharge instructions should include a discussion of the possibility of worsening pain for the first 24-hour period after the injection. Cold or heat packs and massage therapies are often included in the plan following a trigger point injection.

Acute Herpes Zoster

The causative agent of herpes zoster is the small varicella zoster virus (VZV), also responsible for chickenpox in children. Symptoms include unilateral pain or a tingling or a burning sensation limited to a specific part of the body. Erythema is followed within 4 to 5 days by vesicle development. Lymph node swelling may be present. It usually runs a course of 6 to 8 weeks and can be terminated by one or two sympathetic blocks when performed at a level appropriate to the involved area. The block is chosen based on the location of pain and skin eruption and includes a stellate ganglion block, intercostal nerve block (somatic), and epidural blockade. Relief from the severe pain of shingles is greatly appreciated by sufferers.

Possibly even more important is the additional benefit that the incidence of post herpetic neuralgia is reduced when, during the acute phase, pain is aggressively managed.[16] Sympathetic blocks are part of the pain management. However, the success rate of sympathetic blocks decreases with the delay of initiating blocks. Initially, acyclovir for the "specific" treatment of herpes zoster appeared to represent a replacement for the nerve block therapy. However, studies of antiviral treatments, including new agents, remain inconclusive regarding the prevention or reduction of severity of postherpetic neuralgia.[17] Subcutaneous injections of a local anesthetic and a steroid under the areas of eruption have also been shown to provide excellent pain relief. There are no significant complications and the technique is simple and inexpensive.

Reflex Sympathetic Dystrophy or Sympathetically Maintained Pain

Another condition that may respond to nerve blockade is RSD or complex regional pain syndrome, type I. This condition typically follows an injury to bone or tissue in an extremity. The syndrome consists of three stages, which can vary in length and symptoms.[6] During the first stage, or acute stage, the patient experiences diffuse burning pain, edema, and warm or cool skin. This stage may last for about 3 months after the onset of symptoms. Within the first 6 months, stage 2 (or the dystrophic phase), may develop, marked by continued pain, cool skin, decreased hair growth, increased perspiration, and trophic changes. If the syndrome advances to the third stage, known as the atrophic stage, within 2 years of onset, changes may no longer be reversible and may be considered permanent.

Treatment can be successful if initiated during the first stage.[18] Sympathetic blockade with nerve blocks, physical therapy, and oral medications (α-adrenergic tricyclic antidepressants) used in combination may prevent the progression of this syndrome. If the symptoms indicate progression to stage 2, therapy with nerve blocks, physical therapy, and vasodilators may be less successful in restoring function to the affected extremity.[18]

Nerve Blocks Used to Treat Herpes Zoster and Other Painful Conditions

Stellate Ganglion Blockade

A breakout of zoster above the fourth thoracic vertebrae is usually treated with a stellate ganglion block. This block may also be indicated in the treatment of sympathetically mediated pain of the head, neck, or upper extremity. The stellate ganglion is located between the anterior lateral surface of the seventh cervical vertebral (C7) body. Expected effect of stellate ganglion blockade includes Horner's syndrome: ptosis, miosis, conjunctival injection, increased tearing, swelling of the nasal mucosa, temperature increase, and anhidrosis on the arm and half of the face on the side of the blockade. Complications include hematoma, hoarseness, depression of the swallowing reflex, partial block of the brachial plexus, intravascular injection (seizure), high spinal, conduction defects (second-degree atrioventricular block), and spillover to the phrenic nerve, which causes diaphragmatic paralysis and noted difficulty with respiration.

Specific discharge instructions for stellate ganglion blockade should include the following:

- Avoid eating solid food until you swallow without difficulty.
- Avoid driving until your vision is clear.
- Use an arm sling or support if arm weakness is noted.
- Avoid heat or cold application until numbness subsides.
- Report shortness of breath immediately if difficulty is noted.

Intercostal Nerve Blocks

Intercostal nerve blocks are indicated for eruption of vesicles below the fourth thoracic vertebrae. Distal to the spinal ganglia, the thoracic spinal nerves give off the white and gray rami communicantes of the sympathetic system. Distal to this, the nerve trunk divides into the dorsal and ventral branches. The ventral branches each yield a lateral cutaneous branch, first to fifth in the posterior axillary line and sixth to twelfth in the anterior axillary line. Intercostal blockade can be performed at the posterior or anterior axillary line.

The danger of local anesthetic overdose is greater when multiple levels are blocked with higher concentrations or volumes of local anesthetic. High blood levels can occur with accidental IV or arterial injection. At higher blood levels, seizures are more likely to occur with a prodrome of slow speech, jerky movements, tremors, and hallucinations. Raising the seizure threshold by administering midazolam or thiopental may suppress the seizures. The treatment consists primarily of preventing tissue hypoxia, establishing adequate ventilation, and maintaining circulation.

Puncture of the pleura with ensuing pneumothorax is another complication of intercostal blockade. It may be small and asymptomatic. It is important to be suspicious of much more severe outcomes of pneumothorax in persons already compromised with respiratory disease, such as chronic obstructive pulmonary disease. If this patient has a pneumothorax, prolonged observation or admission to a hospital facility may be necessary. A chest radiograph is indicated if the patient displays symptoms of pneumothorax. Oxygen management during the recovery period should continue until the symptoms subside or chest tube placement occurs. Mild analgesics may be indicated.

Numbness along the distribution of the blocks can be noted for several hours, and the patient should be told that he or she may feel a heaviness along the margin area blocked. Specific discharge instructions for intercostal blockade should include:

- Report to the emergency room if severe shortness of breath is noted.
- Avoid heat or cold application until numbness subsides.

Epidural Blockade

Epidural approach to sympathetic blockade may be performed at the cervical, thoracic, or lumbar level. The protocol is the same as that described for herniated nucleus pulposus with radiculopathy, except that the dosage of local anesthetic might be given in a higher volume or concentration. The anesthesiologist is careful to use the lowest concentration and volume of local anesthetic necessary to achieve sympathetic blockade, especially in the elderly or severely debilitated patient. Methylprednisolone or triamcinolone may be added to the local anesthetic injected. Side effects caused by steroids include electrolyte and fluid retention, osteoporosis, hyperglycemia, and infection. Emphasize the potential side effects to the insulin-dependent (type I) diabetic patient. The patient may require additional guidance in monitoring and treating alterations in blood glucose levels following steroid injections. General instructions for epidural blockade are the same as those for epidural steroid injection.

Lumbar Sympathetic Blockade

The lumbar sympathetic block may be used to evaluate and distinguish between sympathetic and somatic components of pain or to increase blood flow to a painful, ischemic limb. The lumbar part of the sympathetic chain and its ganglia lies in the fascial plane close to the anterolateral side of the vertebral bodies, separated from somatic nerve by the psoas muscle and fascia. An injection of a large volume of local anesthetic anywhere in this space will fill the whole space. In most pain clinics today, a single injection of local anesthetic at L2 or L3 is used to achieve sympathetic blockade. In some clinics, injections are performed at two levels. The injections can be performed blindly or with radiologic assistance. The recovery period is 1 hour or longer. Complications include puncture of a major vessel or the renal pelvis, subarachnoid injection, or somatic nerve damage/neuralgia perforation of a disk.

Intravenous Regional Sympathetic Blockade

Intravenous regional sympathetic blockade is based on the "Bier block", a local anesthetic IV regional block. Sympathetic blocking drugs, such as guanethidine (Ismelin) or bretylium tosylate (Bretylol), are added to normal saline or local anesthetic and injected into the vein or artery of the affected extremity, using a double-cuff technique (the cuff is inflated, after the extremity is exsanguinated, for a period of approximately 30 minutes). This technique offers the following advantages: (1) it is less "invasive" and uncomfortable for the patient, (2) it results in significant increased blood flow and decreased pain, and (3) the effects last longer. The patient is monitored until his or her BP has been stabilized. Observe the patient closely for signs of local anesthetic toxicity if the cuff was deflated early (in >30 minutes). For upper extremity blocks, an arm sling may be necessary if a local anesthetic was used in the injection.

Discharge Instructions and Follow-up

General instructions for all of the aforementioned blocks are to:

- Resume the present medication and activity level
- Avoid activities that aggravate the pain, such as lifting, stretching, or long periods of walking or sitting.
- Report the results to the anesthesiology service in ____ days by calling the following number: ______________________

Discharge planning should include a discussion regarding the necessity of continuing with the recommended series of blocks if the anesthesiologist is in favor of doing this. The onset of relief should be immediate, but pain may return within hours to days after the block. A series of blocks is frequently necessary. Patients are often discouraged if the pain returns after the block effect is gone. They see no purpose in continuing with the blocks. More than one injection or block may be needed before the patient experiences long lasting or permanent relief.

Other than keeping his or her appointments with the anesthesiologist, the patient must also be an active participant in other therapies prescribed. It may be necessary to coordinate appointments with other disciplines, such as physiatry or physical medicine and psychology or psychiatry before discharging the patient. Introduction of the idea of complementary therapies is important during the early days of managing the patient with herpes zoster. Expectations are high when therapy starts, and although the blocks may be successful in eliminating severe pain, there is often an element of pain that does not respond to a pharmacologic approach.

The nurse can suggest that the patient plan activities away from home to distract the patient from the pain. Physical activity (e.g., walking) and involvement in activities that are pleasurable and time consuming (e.g., hobbies or arts and crafts) may function as distractions. The patient then needs to understand that stress can contribute to pain, and the combination of stress and pain can alter sleep patterns. The patient feels fatigued and unable to cope with daily routine activities. Encourage the patient to nap in the morning but not in the afternoon, and limit the amount and length of the patient's sleep during the day. At night, a warm bath or warm glass of milk before bedtime may aid in relaxation. A back rub or massage may help to improve sleep. Family members or other support persons can function as coaches for relaxation therapies (e.g., slow, rhythmic breathing) and distraction techniques.

CHRONIC PAIN SYNDROMES

Neuropathic Pain

Neuropathic pain (also called "causalgia" or "deafferentation" pain) results from injury or abnormal functioning of the nerves due to:

1. Disease: painful neuropathy (diabetes, human immunodeficiency virus disease, idiopathic), postherpetic neuralgia, multiple sclerosis, or cancer (direct tumor infiltration and compression of nerves)
2. Injury: minor trauma, thalamic stroke, spinal cord injuries, iatrogenic sources
3. Post surgical syndromes: phantom limb, thoracotomy, nephrectomy
4. Post radiation syndrome
5. Post chemotherapy syndrome

It is characterized by continuous spontaneous pain (burning, aching), paroxysmal lancinating pain (electric shock), or evoked/nonevoked cutaneous sensitivity. Important definitions to remember when discussing neuropathic pain are:

1. Hyperesthesia: increased sensation to evoked non-noxious stimuli, such as cold metal
2. Dysesthesia: unpleasant sensation, evoked or spontaneous

3. Allodynia—painful sensation produced by normally innocuous stimuli such as a cotton wisp or clothes touching, "like a bad sunburn"
4. Paresthesia: abnormal sensation (not necessarily painful) with numbness or tingling
5. Hyperalgesia: increased response to a stimulus that is normally painful, such as a pinprick

Early treatment with sympathetic blockade can often reverse the symptoms. The block can be performed at the cervical, thoracic, or lumbar level as described earlier for acute pain management complaint of herpes zoster. Blocks are often combined with a physical therapy program that follows the block procedure. Treatment usually involves a series of blocks that gradually helps to reverse the cycle of pain. However, if the block fails to give long-term relief, a surgical sympathectomy may be an option for the patient to consider.

For diagnostic and prognostic purposes, short-acting agents (e.g., lidocaine) may be used. However, for therapeutic blocks, sympathetic concentrations of local anesthetic such as bupivacaine or etidocaine are recommended. The epidural technique is preferred by the patient if a series of therapeutic blocks must be scheduled, but when neurolytic blocks are recommended, the lumbar approach is used. A 50% concentration of ethyl alcohol or phenol is the agent used for permanent neurolytic blockade.

Chronic Back Pain

Chronic back pain often originates in the facet or zygapophyseal joints of the cervical or lumbar spine (Fig. 39–4). The only way to know if the pain originates in these joints is to inject them with local anesthetic, with or without steroid. Radiologic assistance is recommended for correct needle placement. Complications of facet injection include neural damage, local anesthetic reaction, systemic steroid effect, spinal headache, and spinal block. Onset of relief is noted in 3 to 5 days after the procedure.

Peripheral Pain Syndromes

Chronic pain, as described earlier, can result from disease, injury, and postsurgical, postradiation, and postchemotherapy syndromes, leading to peripheral pain syndromes. The following nerve blocks may be indicated, in combination with other therapies, for pain alleviation or palliation.

Lumbar Plexus

Included in the branches of the lumbar plexus are the ilioinguinal, genitofemoral, and lateral femoral cutaneous nerves. The purpose of blocking these nerves is for pain related to the groin, scrotum/testicles, and thigh. The agent injected is usually bupivacaine. A steroid preparation (e.g., methylprednisolone) may be added.

Ilioinguinal, Genitofemoral Nerve Blocks

The inguinal region includes the inguinal canal, spermatic cord, and surrounding soft structures. Nerve blocks in this region are used for the management of groin and testicular pain. For the procedure, the patient lies in the dorsal recumbent position with the hands behind the head. The landmarks are identified; the skin is prepared; and the local anesthetic is injected. Pain along the inguinal area is often associated with a previous hernia repair. If there exists a surgical incision that is tender to palpation, the incision can be infiltrated along the margin of the painful area.

Lateral Femoral Cutaneous Block

The lateral femoral cutaneous nerve is a direct branch of the lumbar plexus with contributions from the second and third lumbar nerve roots. It is used in the diagnosis and treatment of meralgia paresthetica, a disease due to the entrapment of the nerve at the inguinal ligament. The patient is positioned in a supine position. Landmarks are identified; the skin is prepared; and 8 to 10 ml of local anesthetic is injected.

Cervical Plexus

The occipital nerves are derived from the branches of the cervical plexus. An occipital block of the greater or lesser occipital nerve is a therapeutic intervention for the complaint of headaches or diagnosis of occipital neuralgia. The procedure is performed with the patient in the seated position with the head and neck slightly flexed. If immediate pain relief is not reported, it may be necessary to repeat the block before discharge, being careful not to exceed the maximum safe dosage of local anesthetic solution for both blocks.

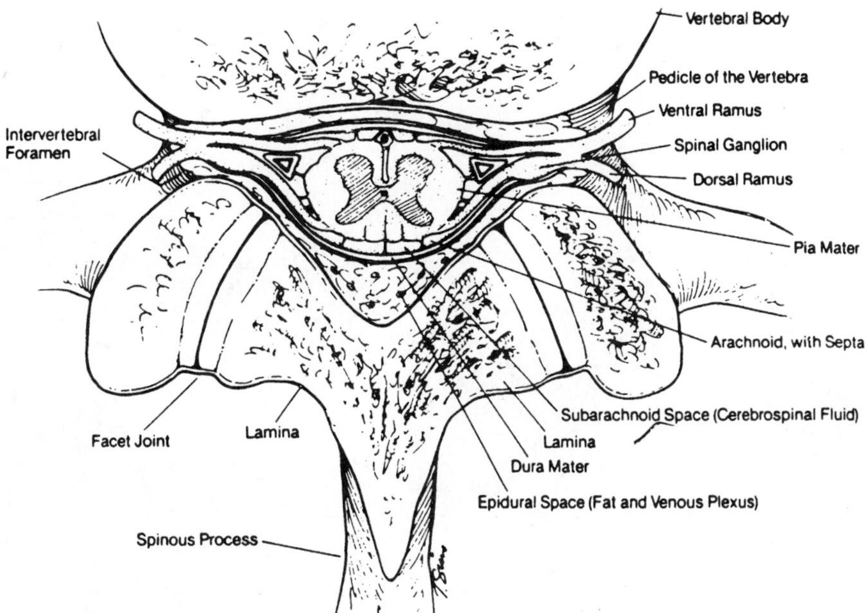

Figure 39–4. Transverse section through the spine. (From RAJ PP: Handbook of Regional Anesthesia. New York: Churchill Livingstone, 1985.)

Discharge Instructions

Patients are instructed to call the pain or anesthesiology service to report the results of procedures in 24 to 48 hours. The onset of relief should be noted within minutes after the injection of local anesthetic. If a steroid medication is injected, the onset of relief from the steroid dose is 24 to 48 hours after the procedure.

Spinal Cord Stimulation

One of the most recent modalities offered for chronic pain is spinal cord stimulation, a nondestructive, reversible method of treating neuropathic pain.[19] Favorable responses have been reported in patients with failed back surgery syndrome, RSD, multiple sclerosis, and peripheral vascular disease.[20] There are two types of systems: (1) a totally internalized system, and (2) an externalized, battery driven system. Introduction of multipolar electrodes, paired with the ability to control the electrical combinations, has increased the flexibility of this procedure. To better forecast the effectiveness of this treatment, a patient undergoes a trial before permanent implant. An electrode is temporarily placed in the epidural space. Patients may be sent home for a day or a week to judge the effectiveness in an environment in which they will be using the spinal cord stimulator. If patients report pain relief, a permanent system is implanted.

Possible mechanisms that may be involved with producing analgesia are:

- Melzack and Wall Gate Control Theory (states that neural mechanisms in the dorsal horn of the spinal cord act like a gate that can enhance or diminish the flow of nerve impulses from peripheral fibers to the spinal cord cells that project to the brain)
- Sympathetic blockade
- Endogenous opiate release

The patient should have a complete psychological evaluation before trial of spinal cord stimulation. Patients with severe psychological disorders or patients who derive significant secondary gain from having persistent pain (i.e., attention from family and friends) do poorly with spinal cord stimulation.

Cancer Pain

Individualizing the regimen for each patient is an essential principle of cancer pain management. Recommendations for pharmacologic therapy begin with the World Health Organization's ladder of analgesic pain management (Fig. 39–5). Strategies that are more complex may be needed for more complicated pain problems. However, the AHCPR guidelines recommend

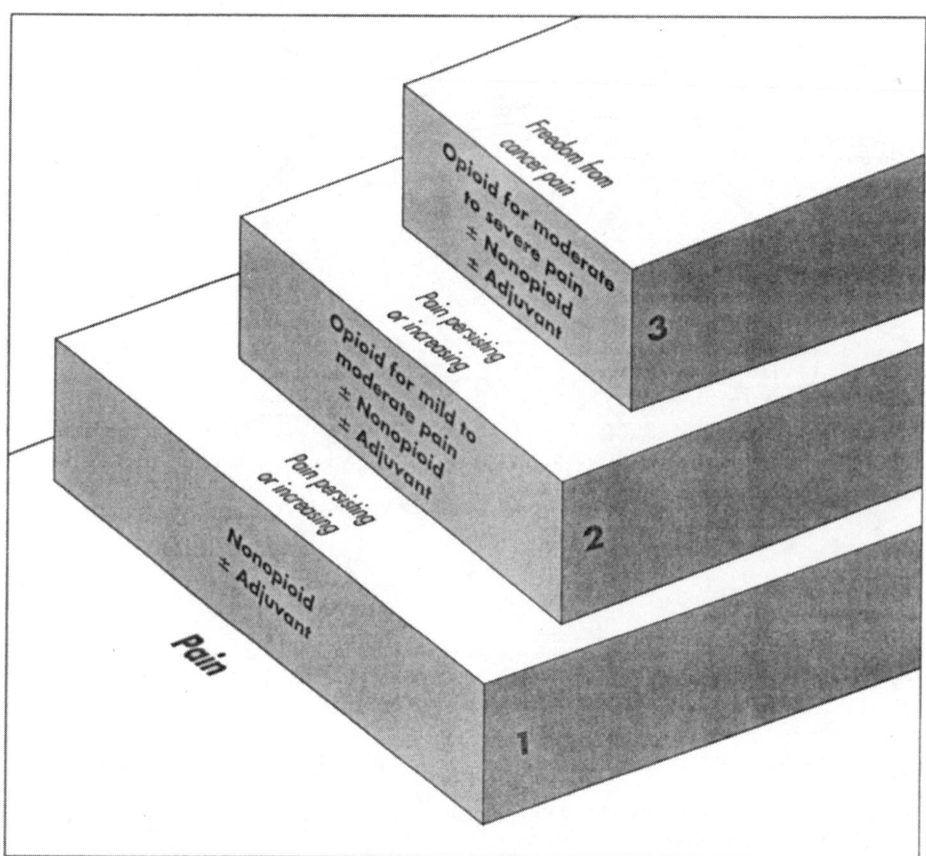

Figure 39–5. The WHO three-step analgesic ladder. (Reproduced by permission of WHO. From Cancer Pain Relief, 2nd ed. Geneva: World Health Organization, 1996.)

interventional strategies such as neuroablative procedures and epidural analgesia to less than 11% of patients with cancer pain and suggest they only be recommended as a final approach to cancer pain.[21, 22] Strict adherence to the World Health Organization's ladder and without consideration of interventional strategies until the systemic analgesic fails may be inappropriate for the patient with increased pain due to cancer.[22]

In selected patients, control of intractable pain due to cancer by a local anesthetic or neurolytic agent is the best choice for pain control. The strategy for controlling intractable cancer pain is targeted at the sympathetic nervous system, which is largely responsible for nociception. There are three essential areas where the plexus of nerve fibers converge. Stellate ganglion blockade has already been discussed. The remaining two nerve plexuses to be discussed are the celiac plexus and the hypogastric plexus.[23]

Celiac Plexus Block

This plexus lies on the anterolateral surface of the aorta from the T12 to L2 vertebral levels. Interruption of autonomic nerve conduction produces sympatholysis and analgesia to most of the upper abdominal organs. A block of this plexus is indicated to control pancreatic pain and chronic visceral cancer pain. This block should also be considered for use in children with cancer pain.[22] Possible complications of celiac blocks include hypotension; intrathecal, epidural, or inter-psoas injection; intravascular injection (aorta, vena cava), and visceral (kidney, intestine, lung) puncture. Pneumothorax has also been reported following celiac plexus blockade.

Hypogastric Plexus Block

This plexus lies over the body of the L5 vertebra and controls sympathetic activity to the pelvis and lower extremities. The block has been used successfully to treat pelvic benign pain and cancer pain and vascular insufficiency in the legs. Complications include urinary/fecal incontinence, visceral (bowel) perforation, and intravascular (iliac) injection.

These blocks are performed initially with local anesthetic (bupivacaine) for two reasons: (1) to allow the patient to experience the effect of a longer lasting neurolytic block before receiving it, and (2) it can itself be therapeutic without producing neurolysis. If a neurolytic substance is injected, the two choices are 3% to 12% phenol or 25% to 100% ethanol. High doses of phenol can produce arrhythmias and convulsions, especially if injected intravascularly. The difference between ethanol and phenol is the pain produced when ethanol is administered. Ethanol is hypobaric, thus the affected nerves should be above the level of the injection. Ethanol produces intense, transient burning when injected. The block produced by phenol tends to be less profound and of shorter duration than that produced by alcohol. Injection of phenol induces warmth followed by numbness.

Discharge instruction should include a discussion about narcotic management following neural blockade. If the patient's pain is relieved, opioids should not be stopped abruptly but should be tapered slowly, lest a withdrawal syndrome be provoked.[21] Activity should increase gradually, noting the potential development of postural lightheadedness that accompanies the intra-abdominal pooling of blood following celiac plexus blockade. Some element of orthostasis accompanies each block. It may be necessary to wrap the legs (toes to thighs) with elastic bandages to allow independence during the adjustment period following neurolytic blockade. Neurologic changes, including leg numbness or weakness, may also be reported with neurolytic blocks. The patient should be instructed to report to the emergency room if increased shortness of breath is noted.

Intraspinal Narcotics

Intraspinal opiates block the transmission of pain at the level of the spinal cord. Catheter placement may be in the epidural or intrathecal space. Epidural and intrathecal introduction of opiates concentrates the drug at the receptors within the dorsal horn of the spinal cord. Injection into the epidural space must diffuse through the dura and arachnoid before entering the cerebrospinal fluid within the intrathecal space. The drug may also be absorbed by the fat within the epidural space, creating a "drug depot," or may be taken up by the venous system in the epidural space, making the intrathecal route a more efficient way to deliver the drug.[6] Therefore, intrathecal injections have a lower dosage and produce fewer side effects.[24]

The systems for intraspinal drug delivery are varied. They include: (1) external access catheters, (2) subcutaneous ports, and (3) implantable pumps (Fig. 39–6). The simplest is the external access catheter. This delivery method is not practical for long-term use because of the risk of infection and catheter dislodgment. It is less costly than an implantable device and may be more economical for a patient whose life expectancy is less than 3 months or for short-term pain management. A family member or support person is taught sterile injection technique and doses the patient with the narcotic dose prescribed by the anesthesiologist.

If a continuous infusion or PCA plus continuous infusion are preferred, a pump delivery system is prescribed and followed by the home health or hospice team. Implantable subcutaneous ports are sometimes preferred over the external catheters because the barrier of the skin protects the entire system. Patients use special needles that penetrate a durable silicone dome and allow the patient to deliver opioids by infusion, bolus injection, or PCA. The cost of these ports is less than that of the implantable pumps, and the port can also be used for intrathecal delivery. One drawback is that the patient or his or her support person must pierce the skin barrier with a needle to initiate therapy.

Implantable pumps for spinal infusion provide a relatively maintenance-free and low infection risk delivery system. The concentration of medication and rate of delivery can be titrated to the analgesic needs of the patient. The cost of inserting these systems is high, and patient selection is very important because the pumps cannot be reused. These systems are used when a patient's pain cannot be controlled with oral, transdermal, subcutaneous, or intravenous routes because side effects such as confusion and nausea limit further dose escalation. Morphine is the most common drug used intraspinally, but fentanyl, hydromorphone, and sufentanil have been used to manage cancer pain. Admixtures may also be used to enhance pain relief. Clonidine, an α_2-adrenergic agonist, has been approved for intrathecal injection in chronic and acute pain states. Patients with a neuropathic pain component appear to gain the most benefit from its addition.[22] Its major side effect is hypotension.

Discharge instructions should include an ex-

External catheter and ambulatory infusion pump

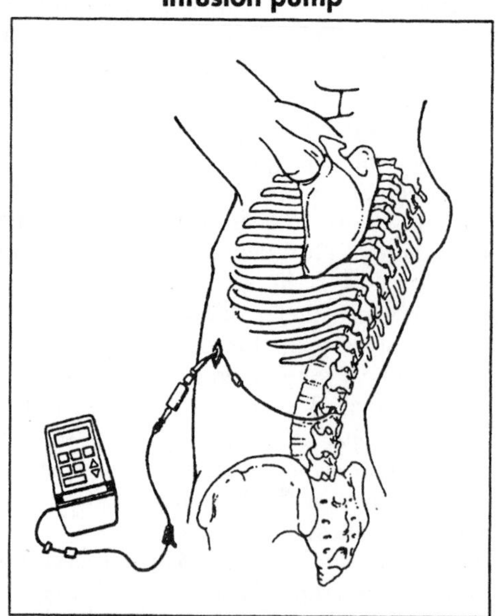

Implantable port and an ambulatory infusion pump

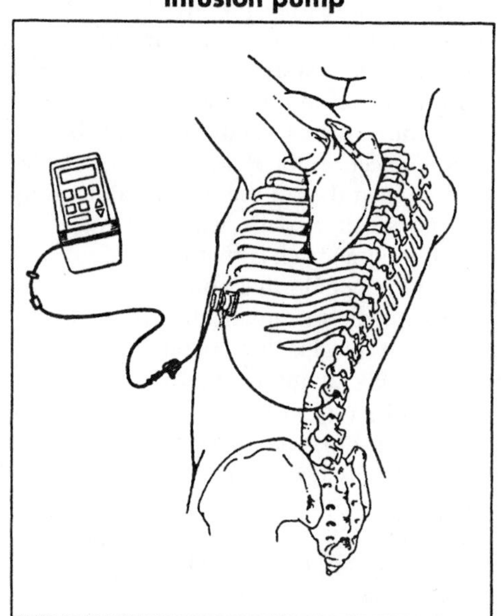

Implantable pump

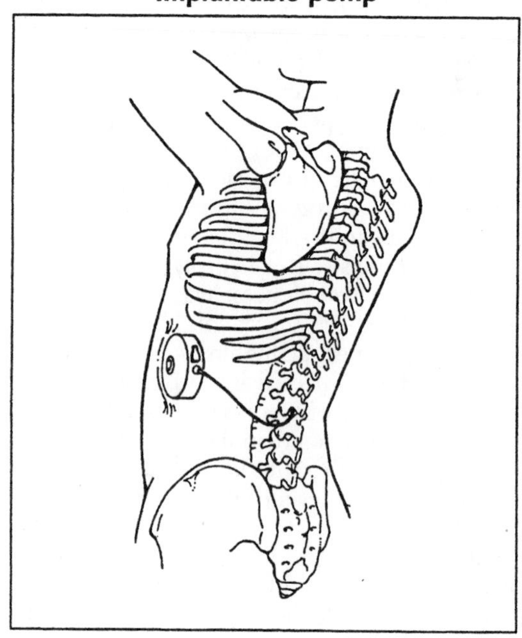

Figure 39–6. Intraspinal delivery systems for chronic pain. (From St. Marie B, Williams A: Management of Cancer Pain with Epidural Morphine [Independent study module]. St. Paul, MN: Sims Deltec, 1994.)

planation of opioids and their side effects. The most common side effects with intrathecal narcotics are urinary retention, pruritus, nausea and vomiting, and respiratory depression. Catheterization of the bladder may be required initially, but tolerance develops rapidly to this effect; thus, patients rarely require repeated catheterization. Pruritus is treated with oral diphenhydramine, nausea with antiemetic therapy, and respiratory depression with naloxone. As with urinary retention, tolerance develops rapidly and these side effects usually disappear if they are seen at all. The risk of respiratory depression appears less in patients who have had previous exposure to systemic opioids.[25] Complications such as infection, catheter failure, and pump malfunction must be discussed, and the support person must understand what to do and who to call in case of any such complication.

Nonpharmacologic Pain Management

Noninvasive pain relief techniques are external measures that influence the person's internal response to pain. They include distraction, cutaneous stimulation, and relaxation. Patients should be told that their reports of pain are believed and these methods are being recommended to increase the effectiveness of the other therapies they are using for pain control. The individual must have the ability and willingness to participate in the method as well as the support of his or her support person(s). Explaining the various types of relief allows the patient to choose one or two methods that he or she would like to try.

Distraction

Distraction is the strategy of focusing one's attention on stimuli other than pain or the accompanying negative emotions.[19] Distraction exercises often include repetitive actions or cognitive activity, such as rhythmic massage or the use of a visual focal point. Examples of distraction methods are:

1. Visual distractions
   - Counting objects
   - Describing objects
2. Auditory distractions (e.g., songs, tapes)
3. Tactile kinesthetic distractions (e.g., stroking, rocking, rhythmic breathing)
4. Guided imagery

Humor is a highly successful distraction strategy that has been proved to improve the release of the body's endorphins. By suggesting pleasant activities on which to focus, the nurse is also intent on giving the patient a sense of personal control over his or her situation. Distraction does not eliminate pain but improves pain tolerance and temporarily makes the pain more acceptable to the patient. It may be used alone to manage mild pain or as an adjunct to analgesic drugs to manage periods of severe pain.

Cutaneous Stimulation

Cutaneous stimulation is stimulation of the skin's surface. Examples of methods are:

1. Massage: Touch and massage are age-old methods of helping others relax.
   - Rub with warm lubricant over the painful part of the body or adjacent part if the actual painful part cannot be massaged. Massage for relaxation is usually done with smooth, long, slow strokes. Try several degrees of pressure along with different types of massage, such as kneading, stroking, and circling. Determine which type is preferred.
2. Application of cold
   - Towel or washcloth soaked in ice water and wrung out
   - Reusable gel pak
   - Ice bags (sealable plastic bag filled with ice water or frozen)

Protect the skin from cold burn. Caution its use on areas of impaired sensation or circulation, or within 48 hours of trauma.

3. Application of heat
   - Warm bath or shower (wrap the feet in a warm, wet towel)
   - Heating pads (moist or dry)
   - Sunbathing

Protect the skin from heat burn. Heat is contraindicated with edema/hemorrhage, vascular insufficiency, and for the first 24 to 48 hours after trauma.

4. Use of external analgesic preparations
   - Products with menthol or methyl salicylate
   - Warm a small bowl of hand lotion in the microwave oven, or place a bottle of lotion in a sink of hot water for about 10 minutes.

Cutaneous stimulation provides an opportunity to include the family member or support person. Setting aside a regular time for the massage or heat or ice treatment gives the patient something to anticipate.

Relaxation

Relaxation is a state of relief from skeletal muscle tension that the person achieves through the practice of deliberate techniques. Examples of relaxation techniques are:

- Biofeedback
- Yoga
- Meditation
- Progressive relaxation exercises

Exercise: Slow rhythmic breathing for relaxation

1. Breathe in slowly and deeply
2. As you breathe out slowly, feel yourself beginning to relax; feel the tension leaving your body.

3. Now breathe in and out slowly and regularly, at whatever rate is comfortable for you. You may wish to try abdominal breathing.
4. To help you focus on your breathing and breathe slowly and rhythmically:
   a. Breathe in as you say silently to yourself, "in, two, three."
   b. Breathe out as you say silently to yourself, "out, two, three." ALTERNATIVELY, each time you breathe out, say silently to yourself a word such as "peace" or "relax."
5. Do steps 1 through 4 only once, or repeat steps 3 and 4 for up to 20 minutes.
6. End with a slow deep breath. As you breathe out say to yourself, "I feel alert and relaxed."

Enlist the aid of a family member or support person as a coach. Praise the family member's participation and concern. These methods do not require a physician's order to implement but instruction of any of these methods should be discussed with the pain management team before initiating the measure.

This chapter describes the numerous pain management options that can be offered in an ASC. Pain management principles and therapies continue to be studied and newer methods of managing pain are being developed. It is a new frontier to explore and research. The nurse's responsibility is to assess the patient before, during, and after procedures and educate, support, and comfort the patient. The nurse must have a working knowledge of the methods used for managing pain and should use this knowledge to decrease suffering and improve the quality of life for the victims of acute and chronic pain. Because each pain experience is individual and the course varies, the clinical approach is to thoroughly assess each situation and then to apply creative intervention, followed by further assessments of pain relief and patient satisfaction. With multimodal therapy, no patient should have to suffer pain.

References

1. International Association for the Study of Pain (IASP) Subcommittee on Taxonomy: Pain terms: A list with definitions and notes on usage. Pain 6 (2):249, 1979.
2. Acute Pain Management Guideline Panel: Acute Pain Management: Operative or Medical Procedures and Trauma. Clinical Practice Guideline. AHCPR Pub. No. 92-0032. Rockville, MD: Agency for Health Care Policy and Research, Public Health Service, U.S. Department of Health and Human Services, February 1992.
3. Sternbach RA: Survey of pain in the United States: The Nuprin pain report. Clin J Pain 2:49–53, 1986.
4. Vasuevan SV: Rehabilitation of the Patient with Chronic Pain. Presentation to the International Pain Symposium, Atlanta, Georgia, April 23, 1992.
5. Schramm DM: The management of chronic pain. Rehab Man 8(4):45–46, 50–53, 1995.
6. McCaffrey M, Pasero C: Pain: Clinical Manual, 2nd ed. St. Louis: CV Mosby, 1999.
7. Carpenito LJ. Nursing Diagnosis, 7th ed. Philadelphia: JB Lippincott, 1997.
8. Carling MA: Pain control: The need for an accurate assessment tool. Analgesia 8 (1):3–8, 1997.
9. Cousins MJ, Bridenbaugh PO (eds): Neural blockade. In Clinical Anesthesia and Management of Pain, 3rd ed. Philadelphia: JB Lippincott, 1988.
10. Putano DB: Music Therapy and Pain Management. Presented to the American Society of Pain Management Nurses, Seattle, WA, March 11, 1997.
11. Kingdon RT, Stanley KJ, Kizior RJ: Cognitive-Behavioral Therapy in Handbook for Pain Management. Philadelphia: WB Saunders, 1998.
12. Davies PS: Treatment of Neuropathic Pain. Presented to the American Society of Pain Management Nurses. Seattle, WA, March 11, 1997.
13. Aronoff GM, Gallagher RM: Pharmacological management of chronic pain: A review. In Aronoff GM (ed): Evaluation and Treatment of Chronic Pain, 3rd ed. Baltimore: Williams & Wilkins, 1998.
14. Jasinski DM, Snyder CJ: Invasive interventions. In Salerno E, Willens JS (eds): Pain Management Handbook. St. Louis: Mosby–Year Book, 1996.
15. Bigos ST, Bowyer OR, Braen GR, et al: Acute low back problems in adults. Clinical Practice Guideline No. 14. AHCPR Pub. No. 95-0642. Rockville, MD, Agency for Health Care Policy and Research, PHS, USDHHS, 1994.
16. Dworkin RH, Portenoy RK: Pain and its persistence in herpes zoster. Pain 67 (2):241–251, 1996.
17. Jackson JL, Gibbons R, Meyer G, et al: The effect of treating herpes zoster with oral acyclovir in preventing postherpetic neuralgia: A meta-analysis. Arch Intern Med 157 (8):909–912, 1997.
18. Veloso KM, Ferrante FM: Chronic pain. In Longnecker DE, Murphy FL (eds): Dripps/Eckenhoff/VanDam Introduction to Anesthesia, 9th ed. Philadelphia: WB Saunders, 1997, pp 466–475.
19. Khan Y, Burgess F, Stamatos J: Spinal Cord Stimulation. Presentation to American Society of Regional Anesthesia, Orlando, FL, April 2, 1995.
20. Kumar K, Toth C, Nath RK, Laing P: Epidural spinal cord stimulation for treatment of chronic pain—some predictors of success: A 15-year experience. Surg Neurol 50:110–121, 1998.
21. Jacox A, Carr DB, Payne R, et al: Management of Cancer Pain: Clinical Practice Guideline No. 9. AHCOR Publication No. 94-0592. Rockville, MD. Agency for Health Care Policy and Research, US Department of Health and Human Services, Public Health Service, March 1994.
22. Staats PS: Cancer pain: Beyond the ladder. J Back Musculoskel Rehab 10:69–80, 1998.
23. Lema Mark J: Cancer Pain. Presentation to American Society of Regional Anesthesia, Orlando, Florida, April 2, 1995.
24. Paice JA, Penn RD: Implanted drug systems for patients with chronic pain. Analgesia 5 (1):7–12, 1994.
25. Paice JA, Winkelmuller W, Burchiel K, et al: Clinical realities and economic considerations: Efficacy of intrathecal pain therapy (Proceedings Supplement). J Pain Symptom Man 14(3):S14–S26, 1997.

Appendix

Legislative Contacts

To Obtain Status of Any National Legislation, Call or Write to the Following:

SENATE
US House Bill Status Office
3669 Office Building, Annex 2
Washington, D.C. 20515
202-225-1772

HOUSE
US Senate Library
The Capitol 5332
Washington, D.C. 20515

To Obtain Copies of Bills and Documents Call or Write to:

SENATE
The Senate Documents Room
The Hart Building
Washington, D.C. 20515
202-224-3121

HOUSE
House Documents Room
The Capitol, B-18 Annex 2
Washington, D.C. 20515
202-224-3121

To Locate Information on Bills, Documents, Executive and Congressional Representatives and Other Legislative Information:

Federal Information Center	800-688-9889 800-326-2996 (Hearing Impaired) *www.gsa.gov/et/fix-firs-fic.html*
Library of Congress	202-707-5000 100 Independence Avenue SE Washington, DC 20540 *www.loc.gov*
House and Senate Bills	*http://thomas.loc.gov*

To contact:

The President of the United States

The Honorable ________________ or
The President
White House
1600 Pennsylvania Avenue
Washington, D.C. 20500
317-226-5555

Dear Mr. President:
Very respectfully yours,

http://www.whitehouse.gov

The Vice President of the United States

The Honorable ______________________ or
The Vice President
Executive Office Building
Washington, D.C. 20500

Dear Mr. Vice President:
Sincerely,

http://www.whitehouse.gov

United States Senator

The Honorable __________________
Senate Office Building
Washington, D.C. 20510

Dear Senator __________________ :
Sincerely,

United States Representative

The Honorable __________________
House of Representatives
Washington, D.C. 20515

Dear Representative ______________ :
Sincerely,

By Telephone
Congressional (Senate & House) Main Switchboard (202) 224-3121

Access for telephone numbers for specific Senators & House Representatives
http://www.cullman.com/government/federal/legislative

To Reach State and Local Government on the Internet

http://www.piperinfo.com/state/states.html

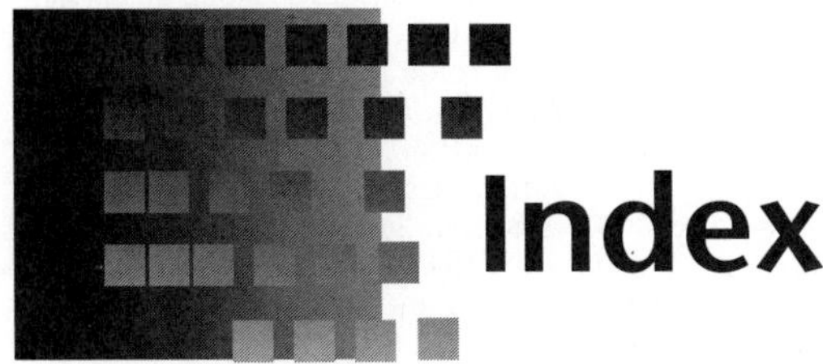

Index

Note: Page numbers in *italics* refer to illustrations; page numbers followed by t refer to tables.